RHEUMATOID ARTHRITIS

RHEUMATOID ARTHRITIS

SECOND EDITION

Edited by

Gary S. Firestein

*Professor of Medicine; Chief, Division of Rheumatology; Allergy and
Immunology Director, UCSD Clinical Investigation Institute,
University of California, San Diego School of Medicine, La Jolla, USA*

Gabriel S. Panayi

Professor of Rheumatology, UMDS Guy's and St Thomas's, London, UK

and

Frank A. Wollheim

Professor of Rheumatology, Lund University Hospital, Lund, Sweden

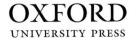

OXFORD
UNIVERSITY PRESS

OXFORD

UNIVERSITY PRESS

Great Clarendon Street, Oxford OX2 6DP

Oxford University Press is a department of the University of Oxford.
It furthers the University's objective of excellence in research, scholarship,
and education by publishing worldwide in

Oxford New York

Auckland Cape Town Dar es Salaam Hong Kong Karachi
Kuala Lumpur Madrid Melbourne Mexico City Nairobi
New Delhi Shanghai Taipei Toronto

With offices in

Argentina Austria Brazil Chile Czech Republic France Greece
Guatemala Hungary Italy Japan Poland Portugal Singapore
South Korea Switzerland Thailand Turkey Ukraine Vietnam

Oxford is a registered trade mark of Oxford University Press
in the UK and in certain other countries

Published in the United States
by Oxford University Press Inc., New York

First published 2000
Second edition 2006

British Library Cataloguing in Publication Data
Data available

Library of Congress Cataloging in Publication Data
Data available

Typeset by Newgen Imaging Systems (P) Ltd., Chennai, India
Printed in Italy
on acid-free paper by Lito Terrazi

ISBN 0–19–856630–1   978–0–19–856630–4

1 3 5 7 9 10 8 6 4 2

Preface to the second edition

Five years have elapsed since the first edition of this book, and we are pleased that the publishers have asked us to collect a second edition. The first edition generated enough interest to be translated into Italian and to sell all available copies. However, much has changed in the last five years. Management of rheumatoid arthritis has undergone more profound changes than during the whole professional career of most rheumatologists. Molecular biology developments have increased insight into the inflammatory and destructive pathways dramatically. Despite these advances, though, the initiation remains as mysterious as ever. Pathogenic similarities between rheumatoid inflammation and atherosclerosis are being established. We have witnessed the successful use of biologics by over half a million patients. Imaging techniques, notably MRI and ultrasonography, have been refined and can now detect pathology earlier than even the most sensitive radiography. Rheumatoid factor is no longer the unchallenged gold standard autoantibody: it now has competition after more than five decades by the anti-citrulline antibodies. Environmental factors influencing both susceptibility and progression rate have been sought, and smoking has emerged as a powerful factor. Steady progress in genetics is finally being made although inheritance is very complex. One day it may be possible to predict rheumatoid arthritis before onset of symptomatic disease. The first 'prophylactic' studies are in progress on a small scale in controlled trials to 'cure' early synovitis.

It is against this background of dynamic developments that a textbook involving a time lag of more than a year between manuscript delivery and printed book faces a real challenge to the foresight and wisdom of the contributors. In some cases, this can present special problems. For instance, the first TNF inhibitors were approved between the time that chapters were written and the first edition was published. This led to frantic attempts to keep the book from becoming out of date before its release! Based on this experience, we have tried to look into the future in the therapeutic chapters and included many agents that are not approved for use at the time that the book is compiled. We have been extremely fortunate in assembling an outstanding team of authors, all experts in their respective fields. Four new chapters have been included in this edition. One-third of the retained topics from the first edition have new authors and are completely new, and all other chapters have been thoroughly revised and updated. We are proud to present the book to a new generation of readers.

La Jolla, London, and Lund   Gary S. Firestein
February 2006   Gabriel S. Panayi
                                                                     Frank A. Wollheim

Preface to the first edition

In the age of information technology proliferation, do we need another textbook on rheumatoid arthritis? The three editors of this book and the publisher that supported us in planning the chapters and selection of contributors clearly think so. Nevertheless, we have asked ourselves if we did the right thing in accepting such a burden: seeing the results now, however, we are very pleased. In the end, it will be the readers who decide if it has been a worthwhile effort. One of the frustrations in this process is the necessary time lag between conceptualization of the project and completion of the finished product. This two year process has seen many changes in the world of rheumatoid arthritis: the approval and rapid acceptance of anti-cytokine therapy, the discovery of new cytokines and signal transduction pathways, new concepts on the pathogenesis of the disease. Although the final editing process allowed us to include some of this information, there is no way to be completely up to date. Despite this limitation, we hope that the book provides a sound basis for scientists and clinicians to understand and appreciate the nuances of rheumatoid arthritis. Several decades ago George Thorn commented after an impressive meeting on rheumatoid arthritis 'We now know all about the disease, except what causes it and how to treat it.' Perhaps this is still true today. However, a new wave of optimism sweeps this field. Advances in cell biology uncover pathways of inflammation and tissue injury, which lead to better understanding of the pathogenesis. The new knowledge opens possibilities for novel attempts to intervene. The marketing of new pharmaceuticals and biologicals for the therapy of rheumatoid arthritis in 2000 is one tangible example, and experienced rheumatologists are speaking of a paradigm shift. We are approaching a situation where the limited availability of motivated and suitable patients for trials of new treatments may hamper new drug development. This stituation calls for the widest possible international co-operation.

TNF inhibition results in impressive symptomatic relief and slowing of structural damage, at least in the short term. One is reminded of the excitement half a century ago, when the early effects of cortisone were presented. It may be good to remember the words of Philip Hench at the famous congress in the Waldorf Astoria: 'this is not the cure for rheumatoid arthritis, but it gives us a new handle to study its nature'. Rheumatoid arthritis is, as all know, a complex disease, and we should not be naïve in hoping for *a* cause or *a* cure. More likely, its pathogenesis will turn out to involve both genetic and environmental factors, and effective control will require a combination of treatments. So, returning to the question on the need for a new textbook, we feel that the explosion of new knowledge has a profound impact on the understanding of rheumatoid arthritis and on the management of our patients, and that this motivates a fresh in-depth text. The 44 chapters cover a wide range of topics and bring together current knowledge from the laboratory to the bedside; drug as well as non-drug therapy; psychological and economic impact. The selection of the team of contributors conveys a truly international state-of-the-art picture at the dawn of the new millennium. We are very grateful for the hard work provided by all the contributors. We also want to thank Oxford University Press for their expert help.

La Jolla, London, and Lund
June 2000

Gary S. Firestein
Gabriel S. Panayi
Frank A. Wollheim

Contents

Contributors

Alarcón, Graciela S.; Division of Clinical Immunology and Rheumatology, The University of Alabama at Birmingham, Birmingham, Alabama, USA.

Aliprantis, Antonios O.; Division of Rheumatology, Immunology and Allergy, Brigham and Women's Hospital, Harvard Medical School, Boston, Massachusetts, USA.

Arend, William P.; Division of Rheumatology, University of Colorado Health Science Center, Denver, Colorado, USA.

Bijlsma, Johannes W. J.; Department of Rheumatology and Clinical Immunology, University Medical Center Utrecht, Utrecht, The Netharlands.

Buckley, Christopher D.; Rheumatology Research Group, MRC Centre for Immune Regulation, University of Birmingham, Birmingham, UK.

Burmester, Gerd-R.; Department of Rheumatology and Clinical Immunology, Charité University Hospital, Humboldt University of Berlin, Germany.

Buttgereit, Frank; Department of Rheumatology and Clinical Immunology, Charité University Hospital, Humboldt University of Berlin, Germany.

Callahan, Leigh F.; Thurston Arthritis Research Center, University of North Carolina, Chapel Hill, North Carolina, USA.

Calvo-Alén, Jaime; Division of Clinical Immunology and Rheumatology, The University of Alabama at Birmingham, Birmingham, Alabama, USA.

Casey, A. T. H.; Department of Surgical Neurology, The National Hospital for Neurology and Neurosurgery and Royal National Orthopaedic Hospital, London, UK.

Cawston, Tim E.; School of Clinical and Medical Sciences, The Medical School, University of Newcastle upon Tyne, Newcastle upon Tyne, UK.

Chatham, W. Winn; Division of Clinical Immunology and Rheumatology, The University of Alabama at Birmingham, Birmingham, Alabama, USA.

Chen, Di; The Center for Musculoskeletal Research, Department of Orthopaedics, University of Rochester Medical Center, Rochester, New York, USA.

Choy, Ernest; Sir Alfred Baring Garrod Clinical Trials Unit, Academic Department of Rheumatology, King's College London, UK.

Chrousos, George P.; First Department of Pediatrics, Athens University Medical School, Athens, Greece, and Pediatric Endocrinology Section, National Institute of Child Health and Human Development, National Institutes of Health, Bethesda, Maryland, USA.

Crockard, H. A.; Department of Surgical Neurology, The National Hospital for Neurology and Neurosurgery, London, UK.

Curtis, Jeffrey R.; Division of Clinical Immunology and Rheumatology, University of Alabama at Birmingham, Birmingham, Alabama, USA.

Day, Richard O.; Department of Clinical Pharmacology, St Vincents Hospital, Victoria St, Darlinghurst, Sydney, Australia.

Emery, Paul; Academic Unit of Musculoskeletal Disease, University of Leeds, Chapel Allerton Hospital, Leeds, UK.

Edberg, Jeffrey C.; Division of Clinical Immunology and Rheumatology, The University of Alabama at Birmingham, Birmingham, Alabama, USA.

Ejbjerg, Bo Jannik; Department of Rheumatology, Department of Radiology and The Danish Research Center of Magnetic Resonance, Copenhagen University Hospital at Hvidovre, Hvidovre, Denmark.

Filer, Andrew; Rheumatology Research Group, MRC Centre for Immune Regulation, University of Birmingham, Birmingham, UK.

Freeston, Jane; Academic Unit of Musculoskeletal Disease, University of Leeds, Chapel Allerton Hospital, Leeds, UK.

Fox, David A.; Division of Rheumatology, University of Michigan, Ann Arbor, Michigan, USA.

Gabay, Cem; Division of Rheumatology, Department of Internal Medicine, University Hospital of Geneva, Geneva, Switzerland.

Gay, Renate; Center for Experimental Rheumatology and WHO Collaborating Center for Molecular Biology and Novel Therapeutic Strategies for Rheumatic Diseases Department of Rheumatology, University Hospital Zurich, Switzerland.

Gay, Steffen; Center for Experimental Rheumatology and WHO Collaborating Center for Molecular Biology and Novel Therapeutic Strategies for Rheumatic Diseases Department of Rheumatology, University Hospital Zurich, Switzerland.

Graham, Garry G.; Department of Clinical Pharmacology, St Vincents Hospital, Victoria St, Darlinghurst, Sydney, Australia.

Gregersen, Peter K.; The Feinstein Institute for Medical Research, North Shore LIJ Health System, Manhasset, New York, USA.

Gulko, Pércio S.; The Feinstein Instiute for Medical Research, North Shore LIJ Health System, Manhasset, New York, USA.

Hamann, Wolfgang; Department of Anaesthetics, King's College, Guy's and Lewisham Hospitals, London, UK.

Heinegård, Dick; Department of Experimental Medical Sciences, Lund University, Lund, Sweden.

Holmdahl, Rikard; Medical Inflammation Research, Lund University, Lund, Sweden.

Jacobs, Johannes W. G.; Department of Rheumatology and Clinical Immunology, University Medical Center Utrecht, Utrecht, The Netherlands.

Kaltsas, Gregory A.; Department of Pathophysiology, University of Athens, Athens, Greece.

Kavanaugh, Arthur; Division of Rheumatology, Allergy and Immunology, University of California, San Diego, USA.

Kidd, Bruce L.; St Bartholomew's and Royal London School of Medicine, London, UK.

Kimberly, Robert P.; Division of Clinical Immunology and Rheumatology, The University of Alabama at Birmingham, Birmingham, Alabama, USA.

Kingsley, Gabrielle; Department of Rheumatology, Lewisham Hospital NHS Trust, London, UK.

Kinne, Raimund W.; Experimental Rheumatology Unit, Department of Orthopedics, Friedrich Schiller University, Jena, Germany.

Kroot, Eric-Jan J. A.; University Hospital, Nijmegen, The Netherlands.

Kvien, Tore Kristian; Department of Rheumatology, Diakonhjemmet Hospital, Oslo, Norway.

Lee, David M.; Division of Rheumatology, Immunology and Allergy, Brigham and Women's Hospital, Harvard Medical School, Boston, Massachusetts, USA.

Leirisalo-Repo, Marjatta; Department of Medicine, Division of Rheumatology, University of Helsinki, Helsinki, Finland.

Lindroth, Ylva; Slottstadens Läkargrupp, Malmö, Sweden.

Luyten, Frank P.; Division of Rheumatology, Department of Musculoskeletal Sciences, University Hospitals KULeuven, Leuven, Belgium.

Månsson, Bengt; Department of Rheumatology, Lund University, Lund, Sweden.

March, Lynette M.; Senior Staff Specialist in Rheumatology and Clinical Epidemiology, Department of Rheumatology, Royal North Shore Hospital, St Leonards, NSW Australia.

Moreland, Larry W.; Division of Clinical Immunology and Rheumatology, University of Alabama at Birmingham, Birmingham, Alabama, USA.

Moritz, Ulrich; Department of Physical Therapy, Lund University, Lund, Sweden.

Müller-Ladner, Ulf; Department of Rheumatology and Clinical Immunology, Justus-Liebig-University Giessen, Bad Nauheim, Germany.

Nigrovic, Peter A.; Division of Rheumatology, Immunology and Allergy, Brigham and Women's Hospital, Harvard Medical School, Boston, Massachusetts, USA.

Nordenskiöld, Ulla; Department of Occupational Therapy, Sahlgrenska University Hospital, Goteborg, Sweden.

Østergaard, Mikkel; Departments of Rheumatology, Copenhagen University Hospitals at Herlev and Hvidovre, Copenhagen, Denmark.

Palombo-Kinne, Ernesta; Experimental Rheumatology Unit, Department of Orthopedics, Friedrich Schiller University, Jena, Germany.

Pap, Thomas; Division of Molecular Medicine of Musculoskeletal Tissue, Department of Orthopaedics, University Hospital Munster, Münster, Germany.

Pitzalis, Costantino; Rheumatology Unit 5th Floor, Thomas Guy House, Guy's St Thomas' and King's College, School of Medicine, London, UK.

Plenge, Robert M.; Broad Institute of MIT and Harvard, Division of Rheumatology, Allergy and Immunology, Brigham and Women's Hospital, Cambridge, Massachusetts, USA.

Pollard, Louise; Department of Rheumatology, King's College Hospital, London, UK.

Rau, Rolf; Department of Rheumatology, Evangelisches Fachkrankenhaus, Ratingen, Germany.

Saxne, Tore; Department of Rheumatology, Lund University, Lund, Sweden.

Rydholm, Urban; Department of Orthopedics, Lund University, Lund, Sweden.

Schwarz, Edward M.; The Center for Musculoskeletal Research, Department of Orthopaedics, University of Rochester Medical Center, Rochester, New York, USA.

Scott, David L.; Department of Rheumatology, King's College Hospital, London, UK.

Scott, Kieran F.; Inflammation Research Laboratory, St Vincent's Hospital Clinical School, The University of New South Wales, L7 Garvan Bldg, 384 Victoria St, Sydney, Australia.

Silverman, Gregg J.; Division of Rheumatology, Allergy and Immunology, Department of Medicine, University of California San Diego, La Jolla, California, USA.

Smedstad, Liv Marit; Hospital for Rehabilitation, Rikshospitalet University Hospital, Norway.

Smolen, Josef S.; Division of Rheumatology, Department of Internal Medicine III, Medical University of Vienna, Vienna, Austria.

Sollerman, Christer; Division E Hand Surgery, Sahlgrenska Hospital, Goteborg, Sweden.

Steiner, Günter; Division of Rheumatology, Department of Internal Medicine III, Medical University of Vienna, Vienna, Austria.

Stuhlmüller, Bruno; Department of Rheumatology and Clinical Immunology, Charité University Hospital, Humboldt University of Berlin, Germany.

Szkudlarek, Marcin; Department of Rheumatology, Copenhagen University Hospital at Hvidovre, Hvidovre, Denmark.

Tak, Paul-Peter; Division of Clinical Immunology and Rheumatology Academic Medical Center, University of Amsterdam, Amsterdam, The Netherlands.

Toivanen, Paavo; The Faculty Office Towers, 510 20th St South Rm 832, Birmingham, AL, USA.

Tutuncu, Zuhre; Division of Rheumatology, Allergy and Immunology, University of California, San Diego, USA.

van Riel, Piet L. C. M.; University Hospital, Nijmegen, The Netherlands.

Weinblatt, Michael; Division of Rheumatology, Immunology and Allergy, Brigham and Women's Hospital, Harvard Medical School, Boston, Massachusetts, USA.

Williams, Kenneth M.; Department of Clinical Pharmacology, St Vincents Hospital, Victoria St, Darlinghurst, Sydney, Australia.

Young, David A.; School of Clinical and Medical Sciences, The Medical School, University of Newcastle upon Tyne, Newcastle upon Tyne, UK.

Zvaifler, Nathan J.; School of Medicine, University of California, San Diego, California, USA.

SECTION 1 | *Etiology*

1 | Genetics of rheumatoid arthritis

Peter K. Gregersen, Robert M. Plenge, and Pércio S. Gulko

Introduction

Over the last five years, it has become apparent that the genetic factors underlying rheumatoid arthritis are more various and more complex than many in the field had originally thought. The major histocompatibility complex (MHC) remains the most important contributor to genetic risk for rheumatoid arthritis (RA), although HLA-DRB1 is clearly not the only locus involved in these MHC associations. The entire field of human genetics, particularly the genetics of complex disease, is currently undergoing dramatic change, driven in part by astounding advances in genotyping technology, accompanied by substantial decreases in costs. This has increasingly permitted a broad-based 'discovery' driven approach to gene identification, as opposed to the more typical 'hypothesis' driven examination of individual candidate genes. The year 2004 may well be viewed as a turning point, since both of these experimental approaches led to the identification of PTPN22, the first major gene that clearly predisposes to multiple autoimmune diseases[1–6], including rheumatoid arthritis[2]; CTLA4 appears to be another example of this[7], although the CTLA4 association with RA is not yet conclusive, as discussed below. These discoveries, together with knowledge of genetic variation in the human genome, have provided support for the view that many of the genes involved in RA are likely to be relatively common genetic variants, each conferring a modest degree of risk. This now sets the stage for an all-out effort to identify all of these risk alleles. As discussed in this chapter, this will require a comprehensive application of high throughput genotyping techniques to large population samples, supplemented by insights from animal models of disease and advances in understanding of cell biology, biochemistry, and immune regulation.

How strong is the genetic component in RA?

The overall strength of the genetic contribution to a complex disorder such as rheumatoid arthritis can be estimated from the extent of familial aggregation combined with information about the epidemiology and population prevalence of the disease[8]. In the case of RA, the sibling recurrence rate (the prevalence of the disease in siblings of affected individuals) is ~2–3%, quite similar to other major autoimmune diseases. In order to establish the relative risk to siblings of affected individuals (commonly referred to as λ_s), one has to also establish an accurate estimate of the prevalence of the disorder in the general population. For a heterogeneous disease like RA, which may vary greatly in severity and accompanying autoimmune phenomena, establishing an accurate estimate of population prevalence is difficult. Prevalence rates of 0.5–1% are generally cited[9], with some estimates even lower[10]. This has led to estimates of λ_s that vary between 3 and 12[11]. It seems likely that for seropositive erosive RA a λ_s between 5 and 10 is a reasonable estimate, a figure that is generally lower than the λ_s for other major autoimmune diseases[8] such as systemic lupus (λ_s ~20), type 1 diabetes (λ_s ~ 15), or multiple sclerosis (λ_s ~20). This lower estimate of λ_s for RA is consistent with the lower monozygotic twin concordance rates in RA, which are in the range of 12–15%, compared with 25–30% for many other autoimmune diseases[12].

These λ_s estimates must be viewed with caution. First, familial aggregation may also be due to shared environment, as well as shared genes. In the case of RA, smoking is now a well established environmental risk factor[13–15]; this probably contributes something to the λ_s calculation. Nevertheless, a formal analysis of heritability has produced estimates of 60% based on twin analysis[16]. so that genes are undoubtedly a major contributor to familial aggregation. It should also be kept in mind that these λ_s estimates relate to the overall clinical syndrome of rheumatoid arthritis. There may be subsets of the disease that exhibit higher heritability. Intermediate phenotypes, for example the presence of anti-citrulline antibodies, will be of interest to examine in this regard. Going forward, the identification of new genes will allow us to refine these estimates, and also will permit identification of additional environmental factors that may interact with these genes. This is one of the important rationales for identifying genes with even moderate risk.

The MHC and RA

Stastny described the first genetic association with rheumatoid arthritis in the late 1970s, using both cellular and serological methods of HLA typing[17]. It is now widely acknowledged that this original DRB1 allele (now known to be DRB1*0401, part of the larger group of DR4-related alleles) confers a higher relative risk (RR ~5) for RA than any other single gene or allele so far identified. The predominance of the MHC in RA genetics has also been confirmed by linkage studies (see below).

Since 1987, the interpretations of the MHC class II associations with RA have been largely centered on the 'shared epitope' hypothesis[18]. As the molecular diversity of HLA-DRB1 alleles was defined in the 1980s, it became apparent that the serologically defined HLA-DR4 allele actually consisted of a family of

Table 1.1 Genotype relative risks of DRB1 genotypes for rheumatoid arthritis[a]

DRB1 genotype	Relative risk	p value
0101/DRX	2.3	10^{-3}
0401/DRX	4.7	10^{-12}
0404/DRX	5.0	10^{-9}
0101/0401	6.4	10^{-4}
0401/0404	31.3	10^{-33}

[a] Data extracted from Ref. 24.

related alleles[19]. Furthermore, the associations with RA also extended to other DR allelic groups, such as DR1[20] and DR10[21]. An examination of the sequence relationships among these disease-associated DRB1 alleles revealed the presence of a shared sequence at positions 70–74 of the DRB1 chain, the so-called shared epitope (^{70}Q K/R R A A^{74}). The DR10 allele (DRB1*1001) is actually an additional variant (^{70}R R R A A^{74}).

Numerous large studies have documented the association of the shared epitope (SE) sequence with susceptibility to RA in white populations[22–25]. Similar associations have been seen in Asian populations[26,27], although the SE is not associated with RA in all ethnic groups[28,29]. In addition, it has become apparent that the shared epitope alone cannot account for the entire genetic signal within the MHC, even in white populations. For example, the strength of the association differs for the different DRB1 alleles. In general, DRB1*0401 and 0404 have a relative risk in the 4–5 range, whereas DRB1*0101 has a relative risk in the range of 1.5–2.5. Certain combinations of alleles, such as the 0401/0404 compound heterozygous genotype, carry very high levels of risk. Some of these relationships are summarized in Table 1.1. In addition, early studies of the tumor necrosis factor (TNF) region suggested that there might be a separate genetic effect in the central MHC[30]. Overall, these data raised the possibility that additional MHC genes, perhaps in linkage disequilibrium with these DRB1 alleles, might also contribute to disease risk.

The A1-B8-DR3 haplotype and RA: importance of the central MHC

A number of recent studies have pointed to the importance of genes in the central MHC for RA susceptibility[30–32], independent of the DRB1-encoded SE alleles. The data further suggest that the relevant genes are derived from an ancestral haplotype that is found commonly in white populations: the A1-B8-DR3 haplotype, also designated the '8.1' haplotype[33]. The entire A1-B8-DR3 haplotype extends to nearly 4 million base pairs, and is fully intact in a substantial fraction of some northern European populations. However, historical meiotic recombination has resulted in the presence of fragments of this haplotype being present in the absence of HLA-DR3 in ~5% of MHC haplotypes. Such fragments of the 8.1 haplotype are associated with RA, independent of DRB1[32]. Currently, the risk haplotype has only been narrowed to around 500 kb[32]. There are at least 50 genes within this fragment that may account for the association with RA, including TNF and IkBL,

both of which have been studied extensively[30,34]. However, because of the strong linkage disequilibrium within this haplotype fragment, it will require dense association mapping in very large populations of cases and controls to narrow the region further and reduce the number of potentially relevant genes.

The A1-B8-DR3 haplotype is of particular interest because it has been associated previously with a wide variety of autoimmune diseases and immunological phenotypes[33]. These include systemic lupus, type 1 diabetes, myasthenia gravis, dermatitis herpetiformis, and common variable immunodeficiency. In addition, the 8.1 haplotype is also implicated in a number of more subtle changes in immune function. Individuals carrying this haplotype exhibit relative unresponsiveness to hepatitis B immunization[35], and carriers of the 8.1 haplotype progress more rapidly to immunodeficiency in the setting of HIV infection[36]. In normal carriers of the 8.1 haplotype, levels of circulating lymphocyte are slightly but significantly lower, and alterations in FcR function have been observed[37–39]. It is likely that different genes on the 8.1 haplotype contribute to these various phenotypes. It has recently been shown that the association with myasthenia gravis is influenced by genes within the central portion of the 8.1 haplotype; paradoxically, the presence of DR3 actually lowers the level of acetylcholine receptor antibodies in this disease[40]. Thus, the A1-B8-DR3 haplotype may carry multiple immunoregulatory alleles that behave differently in the setting of the different diseases. A similar phenomenon may be occurring in RA (see below).

MHC associations with RA: additional complexities

As discussed above, the combination of the DRB1*0401 and *0404 confers very high levels of risk for RA (see Table 1.1), suggesting a genetic interaction between these alleles, or other genes on these haplotypes. It is now apparent that certain 0404 haplotypes are enriched in RA patients compared with controls[32,41]. The differences between the disease-associated 0404 haplotypes have not yet been clearly defined—they may be located in the class I region[32], or within the central MHC[41]. In any case, it appears likely that there is something special about the 0404 haplotypes associated with RA, and this difference is unlikely to be due to the DRB1*0404 alleles themselves, but rather secondary to genetic variation elsewhere in the MHC.

The HLA-DR associations with RA have also been extensively studied with regard to disease phenotypes, particularly the development of bony erosions, as well as the presence of rheumatoid factor[42–44]. The association with rheumatoid factor has been inconstant, while the majority of studies support a positive association between the shared epitope and more rapid progression to erosive disease. More recently, it has become apparent that shared epitope alleles are strongly associated with the development of anti-citrulline antibodies[45]. A recent study of over 1700 RA patients[46] showed that there is a strong association between the SE and anti-CCP antibodies, independent of rheumatoid factor (Table 1.2). In contrast, rheumatoid factor showed only a weak association with SE, independent of anti-CCP (Table 1.3). Interestingly, most of the weak association of the SE with

Table 1.2 The SE is strongly associated with the presence of anti-CCP antibodies, independent of RF status

	RF positive[a]		RF negative[b]	
	SE+	SE−	SE+	SE−
Anti-CCP+	960	128	84	19
Anti-CCP−	95	74	214	149

[a]OR = 5.8, 95% CI: 4.1–8.3, p < 0.0001.
[b]OR = 3.0, 95% CI: 1.8–5.2, p < 0.0001.

Table 1.3 Weak or absent association of SE with RF, independent of anti-CCP status

	Anti-CCP positive[a]		Anti-CCP negative[b]	
	SE+	SE−	SE+	SE−
RF+	960	128	95	74
RF−	84	19	214	149

[a]OR = 1.69, 95% CI: 0.99–2.8, p = 0.07.
[b]OR = 0.89, 95% CI: 0.61–1.3, p = NS.

rheumatoid factor (RF) can be accounted for by the 0401 allele (data not shown). Furthermore, recent data suggests that the rate of progression to an erosive outcome is primarily related to anti-CCP status, with little independent influence of SE[47]. Thus, the previous associations of the SE with RF and with erosive outcome are likely to reflect the primary association of the SE with the production of anti-CCP antibodies.

In addition to the role of SE+DRB1 alleles on anti-CCP production, there is also a highly significant reduction of anti-CCP antibody titers in the presence of HLA-DR3, even when controlling for the presence of a SE on the opposite chromosome[46]. None of the other major HLA-DR alleles exhibit this effect[46]. This result is striking in view of the association of the A1-B8-DR3 haplotype associations with RA discussed above. Indeed it is reminiscent of recent observations in myasthenia gravis, where the 8.1 haplotype is associated with disease, but the DR3 allele itself lowers the titers of acetycholine receptor antibodies[40]. Thus, both positive and negative influences on disease phenotype are found on the same MHC haplotypes. The mechanism by which DR3 lowers anti-CCP titers is not clear, but it is tempting to speculate that this may be related to antigen-specific immune response effects mediated either peripherally or at the level of thymic selection. Of all the SE negative HLA-DRB1 alleles, DR3 is the only one that has a positively charged P4 binding pocket, similar to the shared epitope alleles[48]. Notably, citrullination of arginine residues appears to result in enhanced peptide binding to shared epitope alleles[49], and it has been proposed that the structural features of the P4 pocket explains this result.

Mapping of non-MHC genes: genome-wide approaches based on linkage

There are two basic analytic approaches to mapping disease genes: those based on linkage and those based on association.

Linkage-based approaches have been widely and successfully applied to Mendelian disorders with high penetrance. However, for complex disorders like rheumatoid arthritis, linkage-based methods are severely limited by lack of statistical power[50], in part because the genetic architecture of common diseases is different to Mendelian disorders[51]. The available genetic data suggest that common alleles with low penetrance across many genes contribute to susceptibility of complex diseases such as RA.

In order to perform classical linkage analysis in multiplex families, a disease model is generally required. Thus, one has to specify whether the gene is acting in a dominant or recessive manner, and assign penetrance values to the putative risk genes. Since this is difficult to do for complex disorders such as RA, a 'nonparametric' approach is employed. Most commonly this involves the study of affected sibling pairs, in which there is a search for chromosomal regions that exhibit increased sharing among affected siblings, within families. It should be emphasized that linkage analysis is a family-based approach, so that the particular alleles that are shared among siblings within the entire set of families are not relevant to the analysis. The only relevant parameter is whether sharing among affected individuals in families is present or not. This parameter is compared with the expected degree of sharing, based on the laws of Mendelian segregation. The results can be tabulated as a p value, or a likelihood (LOD) score. Generally, p values of $< 2.2 \times 10^{-5}$ are accepted as evidence of 'significant' linkage for genome-wide linkage studies involving 300–400 markers across the genome[52].

Five genome-wide linkage scans of multiplex families (mainly affected sibling pairs) with RA have been published[53–57]. The largest of these studies combined two separate genome screens for a total of 512 affected sibling pair families[57]. The latter study was carried out by the North American Rheumatoid Arthritis Consortium (NARAC). The data clearly show that no single genetic region has a greater genetic effect than the MHC. Nevertheless, there are a number of chromosomal regions that replicate among the various genome scans, and thus are more likely to actually reflect a true linkage signal, rather than being a false positive result. Among the leading regions are those on chromosome 1p13, 1q41–43, 6q16, 16p and 18q. These regions have shown nominal evidence of linkage on one or more genome-wide scans in Caucasian subjects, and they are the focus of current dense mapping efforts by the NARAC investigators. Notably, none of these regions (including the MHC) was identified in a linkage study in Japanese subjects[54]. This is most likely due to the very small size of this study. However, as reflected in the results of several recent association studies, it is possible that there is some heterogeneity of susceptibility genes among different ethnic populations (see below).

Up until quite recently, whole genome scanning for linkage was carried out using microsatellite markers. These markers contain variable numbers of tandem repeats (VNTRs) of 2, 3 or 4 base pairs in length that are highly polymorphic in the population. Thus, they are very useful for following chromosomal segregation in families. However, it is not widely appreciated outside of the genetics community that there are substantial technical difficulties with using these types of markers. These include the tendency for errors due to allele 'drop out' (failure of polymerase chain reaction (PCR) amplification) and problems with combining data across studies. Genotyping errors are especially difficult to detect when parental DNA is not available for analysis, as is the case for late onset diseases such as RA. The presence of such typing errors is likely to degrade linkage signals in affected sibling pair analysis. Therefore, there is increasing interest in using single nucleotide polymorphisms (SNPs) to repeat these linkage studies, since SNP typing is considerably more robust with reduced typing error. Because SNPs are individually less informative (there are only two alleles), larger numbers of SNPs are required for linkage scans. Currently available platforms generally use between 5000 and 10 000 SNPs across the genome. Genome-wide SNP typing for linkage has recently been reported on a dataset of RA-affected sibling pairs in the UK[58], and a similar approach is being applied to the entire collection of nearly 1000 sibling pairs in the NARAC collection.

Association studies for RA susceptibility genes: assessing the power to find genes of low to moderate risk

Although linkage methods have been widely utilized over the last decade for mapping genes for complex diseases, association methods are likely to be the primary analytic approach for finding new disease genes in the future. These studies may take advantage of

the positional information derived from linkage studies, as discussed above. However, genotyping technologies are now advanced to such a degree that whole genome association studies are fast becoming a reality. This is in stark contrast to the situation just a few years ago, in which association methods were mainly applied to the evaluation of individual candidate genes, usually focused on just a few polymorphisms of interest.

Inasmuch as case control association studies are likely to dominate genetic mapping studies over the next few years, it is useful to review the statistical power of this approach to find genes of low to moderate risk. In the context of RA, a benchmark for a 'high risk' disease susceptibility allele might be DRB1*0401 which confers a relative risk of 4–5. An example of a 'moderate risk' allele might be DRB1*0101, which carries relative risk values in the 1.5–2.5 range. Low risk alleles are those with risks below 1.5. The association of the CTLA4 CT60 polymorphism with type 1 diabetes would be an example of such a low risk allele for autoimmunity.

The sample sizes required to detect associations at this level of risk are highly dependent on the genetic architecture of disease, especially the frequency of the disease allele in the population and the relative risk it confers for the disease or phenotype. Figure 1.1 provides estimates of the sample sizes required to detect associations at various levels of relative risk and allele frequency under a model in which common alleles are responsible for disease risk. The power calculations assume that type 1 error is set at 1% (alpha = 0.01). For allele frequencies in the range of 10% (panel with (p = 0.1 in the figure), there is adequate statistical power to

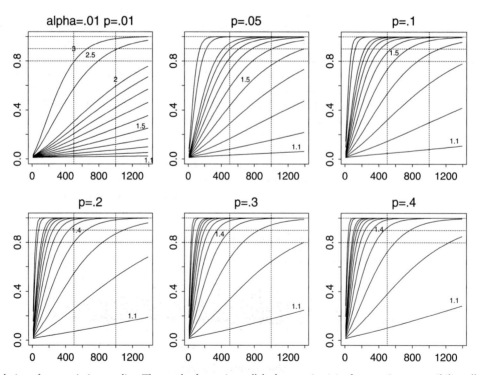

Fig. 1.1 Power calculations for association studies. The results for various allele frequencies (p) of a putative susceptibility allele are shown in each panel. The false positive rate (alpha value) is set at 0.01 for all cases. The curves show the results assuming that the risk allele has an OR of 1.1, increasing to an OR of 2.0, in increments of 0.1. The results for odds ratios of 2.5 and 3.0 are also shown. The odds ratios of certain curves are labeled to facilitate reading the graphs. The abscissa gives the sample size in numbers of cases, assuming an equal number of controls will be studied. The ordinate shows the expected statistical power. (Taken from Ref. 6.)

detect associations with a relative risk of 1.7 or more using ~400 cases and 400 controls. However, for allele frequencies of 5% (p = 0.05), a sample size of 1200 cases and 1200 controls will be required to detect alleles with a RR = 1.5 with 90% power. Thus low frequency, low risk alleles require very substantial sample sizes to detect their effects. These sample size calculations are actually underestimates, since they assume that the allele being tested is identical to, or in complete linkage disequilibrium with, the disease allele. This is unlikely to be the case for an initial screen. Thus, it is probable that many thousands of cases and controls will be required to find alleles of low to moderate risk for rheumatoid arthritis. Until very recently, association studies with these sample sizes were virtually non existent.

Identifying the risk genes in linkage peaks using association

The current linkage data for RA have provided some evidence for the existence of RA susceptibility genes in several regions of the genome. While additional linkage mapping studies may increase confidence in these results, they are unlikely to narrow the candidate regions substantially. In general, these linkage peaks contain 10 million base pairs or more. Narrowing of these intervals will require additional mapping using association methods. The evaluation of each region entails a major commitment of time, money, and effort. The current approach of the NARAC investigators to mapping within the linkage peak on chromosome 18q has been described in some detail in a recent review[6].

When presented with a linkage peak, the first impulse is to examine the region for genes of interest. The linkage region on 18q contains a promising candidate gene, TNFRSF11A, also known as receptor activator of nuclear factor kB (RANK). RANK is known to have a variety of important activities related to osteoclast function and the development of bony erosions in RA[59]. However, a detailed analysis of a large number of SNPs in the RANK gene has failed to show convincing evidence for disease

association (E. Remmers, unpublished data). Therefore, the NARAC investigators have begun to utilize a dense SNP mapping strategy focused on a 10 megabase region surrounding marker D18S858. This marker gives the strongest linkage signal in the region[14], with p < 0.0003 after a combined analysis of 714 affected sibling pair families (C. Amos, unpublished data). A total of 3071 SNPs were selected across the region in consultation with Illumina Inc., a commercial SNP typing firm that is a participant in the worldwide effort to define SNPs across the genome (the International HapMap project—see http://www.hapmap.org/). There were 2303 SNPs with a minor allele frequency of >0.05, and these have been utilized for the initial analyses. These studied 460 independent Caucasian RA cases from the NARAC sibling pair families, along with 460 matched controls.

The result of association for each marker across the region of interest on chromosome 18q is shown in Fig. 1.2. Note that several regions have clusters of markers that approach a significance level of p = 0.001. There are also a number of isolated markers showing significant allele frequency differences between cases and controls at this level of significance. When testing over 2000 markers, it is expected that several markers will achieve a p < 0.001 by chance alone. However, in this case, the number of such 'significant' markers exceeds what is expected. The regions with clusters of associated markers are the least likely to be due to technical artifact of genotyping, so two of these regions have been initially selected for additional study. Interestingly, neither of these associated regions contains obvious candidate genes, and in one case no known functional genes are located in the region. Nevertheless, some of these association results have been replicated in additional datasets, indicating that there are likely to be risk alleles within one or more of these regions. This then presents an analytic challenge which entails extensive resequencing of the region, along with experimental approaches that investigate the effects of these 18q risk haplotypes on intermediate phenotypes and their interactions with the MHC, PTPN22, or other known risk genes. It is likely that similar challenges will be faced in evaluating the other linkage peaks that have been identified for RA.

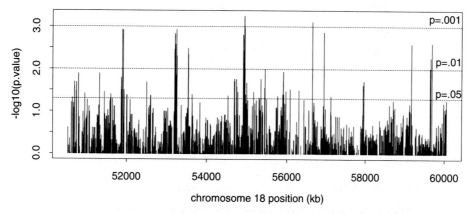

Fig. 1.2 Distribution of p-values (y axis) for SNP associations on chromosome 18q; 460 RA cases from the NARAC sibling pair collection[57] and 460 controls were analyzed. Each bar represents the results for 1 of 2303 SNPs across a 10-million base pairs segment of chromosome 18q. The x axis gives the position on the chromosome in thousands of base pairs. The D18S858 microsatellite marker, which shows maximal evidence of linkage in the NARAC sibling pairs[57], is located roughly in the center of this region.

PTPN22 620W is a risk allele or rheumatoid arthritis: the first fruits of a genome-wide association study of putative functional alleles

The first genome-wide association study of putative functional alleles in RA was carried out in 2003, the result of a collaboration between Celera Diagnostics and the NARAC investigators[2]. The general approach was to focus on a large number of SNPs that appeared to be functional, in the sense that they caused amino acid changes or were located in putative regulatory regions. While this approach does not comprehensively test common variants across the entire genome, it is a cost-effective strategy to test those alleles with a higher prior probability of having phenotypic consequences for association to RA. Broad families of genes in biologically plausible pathways were selected for study, leading to an initial set of ~12 000 SNPs. The study design included examination of both a 'discovery' and a 'replication' dataset[2]. The discovery dataset consisted of 475 cases of seropositive RA. The replication dataset included both seropositive and seronegative cases from 463 NARAC affected sibling pair families. Careful matching of controls to cases was carried out for both datasets. Thus, in view of the statistical power calculations discussed above (Fig. 1.1), this study design had reasonable power to detect causative disease-associated alleles that carry moderate (RR ~ 1.5–2.5) degrees of risk, assuming allele frequencies in at least the 10% range in the general population.

Fortuitously, among the first 100 SNPs tested, a functional SNP (rs24786601, 1858C→T, encoding R620W) in the PTPN22 gene exhibited a strong association in both the discovery (odds ratio (OR) = 1.65, 95% confidence interval (CI): 1.23–2.20) and replication (OR = 1.97, 95% CI: 1.55–2.50) datasets[25]. The risk allele (T) frequency in controls was ~8.5%, whereas the overall allele frequency in the combined cases was 14.7% (OR = 1.80, 95% CI: 1.50–2.17, p < 10^{-12}). The association of the PTPN22 620W allele with rheumatoid arthritis has now been confirmed in several large replication studies around the world[60–63], all in white populations. As of this writing, this finding stands as the only major non-MHC association with RA that has been convincingly replicated in multiple datasets.

PTPN22: a genetic link between RA and other autoimmune disorders

In addition to RA, the PTPN22 620W allele confers a 1.5–2-fold risk for several other autoimmune disorders, including systemic lupus[3], autoimmune thyroid disease, both Hashimoto's thyroiditis[64] and Graves' disease[5] and type 1 diabetes[1,4]. Indeed, the association with type 1 diabetes was the first published report of an association of PTPN22 with an autoimmune disease, discovered through a candidate gene approach[1]. In contrast, it appears that PTPN22 does not confer risk for multiple sclerosis (MS)[65] or

Crohn's disease[62]. This fits the pattern of familial aggregation of these disorders, particularly the fact that type 1 diabetes, autoimmune thyroid disease, and rheumatoid arthritis tend to run together in the same families[66,67]. The data on PTPN22 associations have provided the first direct genetic evidence in humans that common disease mechanisms may underlie some, but not all, of these disorders.

The current data suggest that the PTPN22 association with RA primarily involves the RF+ subset of the disease[2,60], although this has not been universally observed[62,63]. The relationship between PTPN22 and anti-CCP antibodies has not yet been fully examined. However, it is of interest that all of the diseases associated with PTPN22 have a prominent humoral component, and these diseases are frequently preceded by the development of autoantibodies months or years prior to clinical symptoms[68–71]. In contrast, MS and Crohn's disease do not have a prominent humoral component. Interestingly, knockout animals for PTPN22 exhibit alterations in thresholds for T cell signaling, with expansion of T cell populations and the spontaneous development of germinal centers with accompanying increases in immunoglobulin levels[72]. Thus, it is tempting to speculate that the PTPN22 R620 allele acts primarily by predisposing to the development of autoantibodies.

The precise functional consequences of the PTPN22 620W allele have not been determined. The R620W amino acid change is located within one of four SH3 binding sites on the PTPN22 molecule[73,74], and the 620W allele clearly results in reduced binding to Csk, an intracellular protein kinase[1,2]. Both PTPN22 and Csk are involved in regulating phosphorylation of Lck in T cells[75], and loss of PTPN22 expression appears to result in enhanced or prolonged activation of Lck[72]. Nevertheless, the effect of the PTPN22 620W allele on the Lck activation state is unclear. PTPN22 also appears to bind c-Cbl, and may affect the phosphorylation status of Zap70[75–78]. Of note, all of these experimental observations have been made in T cells, whereas PTPN22 is widely expressed in cells of hematopoietic origin[2]. No data are available regarding the function of PTPN22 in these other cell types. Therefore, the mechanism by which the PTPN22 620W allele predisposes to human autoimmune diseases remains to be established.

Candidate gene association studies for complex disease

As discussed above, genetic association studies have been applied to linkage peaks and putative functional genetic variants. However, the vast majority of published genetic association studies on RA and other complex diseases have been focused on candidate genes. Candidate genes have usually been selected based on biological studies of disease pathogenesis. In addition to the lack of statistical power due to inadequate samples sizes (discussed above), another limitation of most published candidate gene studies is that usually only a small fraction of inherited variation within a given gene is examined. It is clear from studies of diverse human populations that the human genome contains ~1 SNP per 1000 base pairs (bp) between any two unrelated chromosomes. The average gene spans over 30 kb of genomic DNA, indicating that at least 30 SNPs with a minor allele frequency > 1% are contained within the average sized gene. A priori, each genetic variant within a gene is a putative causal polymorphism that may explain inherited differences in disease susceptibility, since our knowledge of the function of these variants is still rather limited.

To test all the variants within a candidate gene for an association to RA would quickly become cost prohibitive. However, the problem is mitigated by the extensive linkage disequilibrium (LD), or correlation among neighboring SNPs, so that one SNP often effectively captures the genetic information of several nearby SNPs[79–81]. As a consequence, it is only necessary to test a subset of 'tagging' SNPs to obtain comprehensive coverage of genetic variation within a candidate gene (and eventually the whole genome) in an association study. The intelligent selection of such tagging SNPs depends on knowledge of the patterns of LD within the study population, and this information is still limited. Fortunately, the International HapMap Project is making rapid progress in cataloging the majority of the common human genetic variation across the entire genome. These data are open to the scientific community (www.hapmap.org), and online programs are available to identify the tagging SNPs within a given genetic region (www.broad.mit.edu/mpg/tagger/).

In part due to the lack of statistical power, candidate gene studies in complex diseases frequently fail to replicate. A formal analysis of these studies among complex diseases such as RA has shown that the vast majority of first reports in the literature turn out to be false positive results[82]. In addition, even when replication is achieved, the strength of the association is generally much lower than in the initial report. There are a number of reasons for this state of affairs, the most important of which is probably a bias towards submission and publication of positive studies, especially when they are the first to be performed. This phenomenon has been referred to as the 'winner's curse', where first reports are likely to overestimate the strength of an association. For this reason, it is prudent, and increasingly required by reviewers, that a replication must be included as part of an initial report of a novel candidate gene association. Notably, this approach was taken for the initial studies of PTPN22 and RA[2], as well as type 1 diabetes[1].

Evaluation of reported candidate gene associations with rheumatoid arthritis

With these considerations in mind, it is not surprising that candidate gene association studies applied to RA have led to encouraging, yet inconsistent results. In order to better understand which published genetic association studies represent true positive results, an attempt to replicate previous putative associations in a large collection of RA case-control samples has been recently undertaken[83]. After review of the literature of candidate association studies in RA and other autoimmune diseases, 17 putatively associated alleles were selected from 14 genes to test in over 4000 case-control samples from NARAC and the Epidemiological Investigation of Rheumatoid Arthritis (EIRA) collections[15,84]. The results, summarized in Table 1.4, fail to support most of the

previously reported associations. On the other hand, the data clearly replicate the association of *PTPN22* with the development of seropositive RA using previously untested EIRA samples. Using samples from both the EIRA and NARAC cohorts, there is some support for an association of *CTLA4* (OR 1.13, p-value 0.004) and *PADI4* (OR 1.10, p = 0.02) with the development of RA. The results from *CTLA4* and *PADI4* are less striking than for *PTPN22*, both in terms of the odds ratios and p-values, and will require additional testing in large, independent RA collections to confirm or refute a modest contribution to genetic susceptibility to RA. Importantly, only alleles with evidence of a prior association to RA susceptibility were examined in the above analysis. Consequently, it is still formally possible that genetic variation within the genes that failed to replicate influence the risk (or related phenotype) of RA.

In the last few years, many of the more convincing candidate gene studies have been performed in the Japanese population, leading to the identification of PADI4[85], SLC22A4, and RUNX1[86] as potential susceptibility genes for RA. Of these, only PADI4 gives modest evidence of replication in Caucasians (see above), although published results are conflicting[87]. PADI4 has also been convincingly replicated within the Japanese population[88], but so far large replication studies of the other two genes in Asian populations have not appeared. This at least raises the possibility that different susceptibility genes underlie RA in these racial groups. Clearly, the PTPN22 620W association with RA is unlikely to be replicated in Japan, since this allele is virtually absent in Asian populations (less than 0.1% allele frequency, unpublished data). Alternatively, the same genes may be involved, but the mix of allelic variants may be quite different among different ethnic groups. There is no evidence from other common diseases to support the hypothesis that an allele influences disease susceptibility in one geographic population but not in another[89], although this hypothesis has not been rigorously tested. If observed, this could reflect geographic variation in the environmental factors that contribute to disease. Indeed, historical evidence suggests that RA may be a more ancient disease in populations derived from Asia, compared with the relatively recent appearance of RA phenotypes in Europeans since the Renaissance[90]. Theoretically, a susceptibility allele in one population may be absent from another population (as is the case for PTPN22), although knowledge of genetic variation across the genome suggests that this will be an unusual event. Whether other PTPN22 alleles predispose to RA in an Asian population has not been formally tested. Comparative genetic studies among these various ethnic groups, taking environmental factors into account, will be important to carry out in the future.

Animal models of rheumatoid arthritis: can they lead us to disease susceptibility and severity genes?

Rodent models of arthritis can be induced with pristane, collagen, complete Freund's adjuvant, or squalene. Different strains of animals have dramatically varying degrees of susceptibility to

Table 1.4 Results of testing 11 alleles within 10 genes in over 4000 clinical samples from EIRA and NARAC. Results from the EIRA and NARAC cohorts were combined ('pooled') by Mantel–Haenszel meta-analysis of the odds ratios. Only PTPN22, PADI4, and CTLA4 replicate with a p-value of <0.05

Gene (variant)[a]	dbSNP	Collection	OR (95% CI)	p-value[b]
PTPN22 (R620W)	rs2476601	EIRA	1.30 (1.09–1.54)	0.0015
		NARAC[c]	2.18 (1.76–2.70)	2.15×10^{-13}
		Pooled	*1.59 (1.39–1.82)*	*4.8×10^{-12}*
PADI4 (PADI4_94)	rs2240340	EIRA	1.01 (0.89–1.14)	0.47
		NARAC	1.24 (1.08–1.42)	0.001
		Pooled	*1.10 (1.00–1.21)*	*0.02*
CTLA4 (CT60)	rs3087243	EIRA	1.05 (0.93–1.19)	0.21
		NARAC	1.23 (1.08–1.42)	0.001
		Pooled	*1.13 (1.03–1.24)*	*0.004*
TNFRSF1B (R196M)	rs1061622	EIRA	0.92 (0.80–1.05)	0.90
		NARAC	0.94 (0.79–1.12)	0.77
		Pooled	*0.93 (0.83–1.03)*	*0.92*
RUNX1 (runx1)	rs2268277	EIRA	0.97 (0.86–1.10)	0.68
		NARAC	1.08 (0.94–1.24)	0.16
		Pooled	*1.02 (0.93–1.12)*	*0.36*
MIF (−173 G/C)	rs755622	EIRA	1.03 (0.88–1.19)	0.39
		NARAC	0.98 (0.82–1.18)	0.59
		Pooled	*1.01 (0.90–1.13)*	*0.46*
HAVCR1 (5383_5397del)	rs6149307	EIRA	0.93 (0.79–1.09)	0.83
		NARAC	1.21 (01.00–1.46)	0.03
		Pooled	*1.04 (0.92–1.17)*	*0.28*
HAVCR1 (5509_5511delCAA)	NA	EIRA	0.93 (0.80–1.09)	0.83
		NARAC	0.80 (0.67–0.95)	0.99
		Pooled	*0.87 (0.77–0.98)*	*0.99*
SLC22A4 (slc2F1)	rs2073838	EIRA	1.13 (0.90–1.42)	0.15
		NARAC	1.03 (0.81–1.32)	0.91
		Pooled	*1.09 (0.92–1.28)*	*0.16*
IL3 (rIL3−16)	rs31480	EIRA	0.96 (0.84–1.10)	0.73
		NARAC	1.09 (0.93–1.29)	0.15
		Pooled	*1.01 (0.91–1.12)*	*0.40*
IL4 (−590T)	rs2243250	EIRA	1.12 (0.97–1.30)	0.07
		NARAC	0.88 (0.73–1.05)	0.93
		Pooled	*1.01 (0.90–1.14)*	*0.40*

TNFRSF1B, tumor necrosis factor receptor superfamily, member 1B; alias TNFRII, human tumor necrosis factor receptor II; RUNX1, runt-related transcription factor 1; MIF, macrophage migration inhibitory factor; HAVCR1, hepatitis A virus cellular receptor 1; alias Tim-1, T cell immunoglobulin domain and mucin domain protein 1; SLC22A4, solute carrier family 22.
[a]Unigene identifier with variant ID (alternate gene names listed below).
[b]p-values based on allele frequency, one-tailed using Fisher's Exact Test.
[c]results from PTPN22 previously published by Begovich *et al.* 2004 (Ref. 2).

inflammatory arthritis following these stimuli. Therefore, the development of arthritis can be used for the discovery of genes that regulate this complex trait in these animals. Genetic analyses conducted in intercrosses and backcrosses generated between arthritis-susceptible and resistant inbred strains have already led to the identification of several autoimmune arthritis-regulatory loci[91–96]. This strategy at least partly overcomes some of the difficulties involved in complex trait disease studies in humans, such as genetic and phenotypic heterogeneity, environmental 'noise', and the effects of gene-gene interactions (epistasis). Furthermore, the phenotypic effects accounted for by the identified loci can be confirmed in congenic strains, where a particular genetic region can be investigated in detail, while background genes are kept constant. Using this strategy, it is possible to narrow down particular genetic regions, leading to positional identification of a specific gene. This approach has already led to the identification of *Ncf1* as a susceptibility gene for arthritis in the rat[97].

What is the evidence that studies in rat or mouse models of autoimmune arthritis will actually lead to the identification of RA genes? Clinically and histologically, rodent models of arthritis, particularly those in rats, are very similar to RA, suggesting that similar processes regulate arthritis in both species. In fact, novel drugs or biologic agents used in RA are generally first tested for efficacy in rodent models of arthritis. Additionally, a significant percentage of the arthritis-regulatory loci mentioned above are located in rat chromosomal regions homologous to those containing loci involved in the susceptibility to RA and/or other human autoimmune diseases[98]. One arthritis-regulatory locus, *Cia10*, contains *Ptpn8*, the rat homolog of human PTPN22[99]. Sequencing of the *Ptpn8* gene has so far revealed no differences between the arthritis-susceptible (DA) and resistant (ACI) strains, but these studies are still in progress. In another study, a chromosome 17q22 RA susceptibility locus was identified based on a homology strategy guided by a rat arthritis locus[100]. While the syntenic colocalization of susceptibility genes does not prove that the rat/mouse and human arthritis genes are the same, it is certainly suggestive enough to justify continuing these types of studies.

The fact that rodent models of inflammatory arthritis generally involve an 'induced' form of disease often raises concerns about the relevance of these models to the human phenotype. In addition to the genetic factors, there is also a significant non-genetic component to rheumatoid arthritis; the environmental contributors to RA are only just beginning to be identified[13–15,101]. Certain environmental exposures, such as smoking, in the presence of specific RA-predisposing alleles are likely to be an important factor in disease development. While it remains unclear how these environmental factors operate, it is conceivable that some of them have adjuvant-like properties in humans, stimulating different aspects of immune responses, or interfering with protective or anti-inflammatory pathways. The use of inducible rat models of autoimmune arthritis may well provide a useful parallel with events taking place in human RA. Indeed, this may ultimately facilitate the better understanding of the gene-environment interactions in humans, especially when the disease mechanisms in the animal models become better elucidated.

Another major advantage to animal models is the fact that they permit the study of various phases of disease, as well as particular disease sub-phenotypes. Examples include the identification of loci regulating levels of acute phase reactants[102], rheumatoid factors[103], and autoantibodies against type II collagen[104,105]. Several, but not all, of these loci colocalize with rat arthritis-severity loci, suggesting that some of the arthritis loci operate, for instance, via the regulation of a B cell function or the production of autoantibodies. Furthermore, the effect of some susceptibility genes is likely to be restricted to the early stages in the development of a pathogenic autoimmune response, with a less significant role after arthritis has developed. These genes may provide targets for very early intervention at the time of disease onset. In contrast, genes specifically involved in the regulation of disease severity and joint damage are more likely to generate useful targets for effective treatments of established disease. Genome-wide scans in rodent crosses have identified specific genetic loci regulating disease onset, arthritis severity, chronicity, and joint damage[91–96,106]. The arthritis-regulatory effect of several of these loci has already been confirmed in congenic strains[99,107–109], and in one case the specific gene, *Ncf1*, has been identified[97]. (The role of the *Ncf1* gene in human arthritis remains to be established, in part because the presence of multiple NCF1 pseudogenes in humans has delayed progress.) Studies in congenic strains have also identified loci on rat chromosomes 2 and 10 involved in the regulation of synovial hyperplasia, pannus formation, synovial angiogenesis, and cartilage and bone damage[99] (Brenner *et al.*, unpublished observations). Once identified, these disease severity, or joint damage-regulatory genes can be tested in focused candidate gene or candidate pathway studies using well-characterized and prospectively followed RA cohorts[110].

It is likely that over the next few years the analysis of arthritis models will generate novel and exciting lists of genes involved in the regulation of arthritis susceptibility, severity, and joint damage in rodents. This will lead to an understanding of how these genes regulate arthritis, and this information will be useful for human studies. It is also possible that animal models will facilitate functional studies of risk genes that are first identified in humans; indeed, getting to the bottom of RA genetics and pathogenesis will likely be an iterative process involving both human and animal studies.

Comprehensive whole genome association studies in RA: the beginning of the end?

The field of human genetics is in the midst of a technological 'boom'. Whole genome association studies with hundreds of thousands of SNPs are already a reality, and truly comprehensive genome scans with one million SNPs or more are only a year or two away. There are only two remaining barriers to capturing all the common risk genes for autoimmunity: the availability of very large well-characterized patient populations, and the financial resources to carry out these studies. Both of these barriers are likely to be overcome in the coming years. Once the first comprehensive whole genome association in RA is completed, replication of putative allelic associations will need to be carried out in independent patient collections to confirm the findings. Nevertheless, within the next five years, an extensive list of common risk genes for rheumatoid arthritis will likely become available.

Despite this exciting prospect, it is still unclear whether this will capture the complete catalog of all the genes involved in RA. The power of genetic studies depends upon the genetic architecture of disease, and the exact genetic architecture of common diseases such as RA is still not clear. Most of the current efforts in gene mapping are based on the 'common disease/common variant' hypothesis[111,112]. However, it is still possible that rare genetic variants also have a significant impact on the overall risk of developing disease. Based upon the results from whole genome linkage scans in RA, rare RA susceptibility variants (if they exist) must be distributed among many genes across the genome. On the other hand, it seems likely that common genetic variants with modest effects will contribute substantially to the total genetic burden of RA. This perspective is supported by the examples of the shared epitope alleles and the R620W *PTPN22* allele, as well as other common alleles in other autoimmune diseases. In any case, it is much more difficult to comprehensively test the rare variant hypothesis. This will require further advances in technology, a further expansion of information about the patterns of variation in the human genome, and even larger patient population studies than are now contemplated. Given the extraordinary pace of progress in the last few years, it is probable that this will occur sooner than is now imagined.

References

1. Bottini, N. *et al.* A functional variant of lymphoid tyrosine phosphatase is associated with type I diabetes. *Nat Genet* 2004; **36:** 337–8.
2. Begovich, A. B. *et al.* A missense single-nucleotide polymorphism in a gene encoding a protein tyrosine phosphatase (PTPN22) is associated with rheumatoid arthritis. *Am J Hum Genet* 2004; **75:** 330–7.

3. Kyogoku, C. *et al.* Genetic association of the R620W polymorphism of protein tyrosine phosphatase PTPN22 with human SLE. *Am J Hum Genet* 2004; **75**: 504–7.

4. Smyth, D. *et al.* Replication of an association between the lymphoid tyrosine phosphatase locus (LYP/PTPN22) with type 1 diabetes, and evidence for its role as a general autoimmunity locus. *Diabetes* 2004; **53**: 3020–3.

5. Velaga, M. R. *et al.* The codon 620 tryptophan allele of the lymphoid tyrosine phosphatase (LYP) gene is a major determinant of Graves' disease. *J Clin Endocrinol Metab* 2004; **89**: 5862–5.

6. Gregersen, P. K. Pathways to gene identification in rheumatoid arthritis: PTPN22 and beyond. *Immunol Rev.* 2005; **204**: 74–86.

7. Ueda, H. *et al.* Association of the T-cell regulatory gene CTLA4 with susceptibility to autoimmune disease. *Nature* 2003; **423**: 506–11.

8. Vyse, T. J. and Todd, J. A. Genetic analysis of autoimmune disease. *Cell* 1996; **85**: 311–18.

9. Gabriel, S. The epidemiology of rheumatoid arthritis. *Rheum Dis Clin North Am* 2001; **27**: 269–81.

10. Ward, R. H., Hasstedt, S. J., and Clegg, D. O. Population prevalence of rheumatoid arthritis is lower than formerly supposed. *Arthritis Rheum* 1992; **35** (Suppl. 19): S129.

11. Seldin, M., Amos, C., Ward, R., and Gregersen, P. K. The genetics revolution and the assault on rheumatoid arthritis. *Arthritis Rheum* 1999; **42**: 1071–9.

12. Silman, A. J. *et al.* Twin concordance rates for rheumatoid arthritis: results from a nationwide study. *Br J Rheumatol* 1993; **32**: 903–7.

13. Heliovaara, M., Aho, K., Aromaa, A., Knekt, P., and Reunanen, A. Smoking and risk of rheumatoid arthritis. *J Rheumatol* 1993; **20**: 1830–5.

14. Symmons, D. P. *et al.* Blood transfusion, smoking, and obesity as risk factors for the development of rheumatoid arthritis. *Arthritis Rheum* 1997; **40**: 1955–61.

15. Stolt, P. *et al.* Quantification of the influence of cigarette smoking on rheumatoid arthritis: results from a population based case-control study, using incident cases. *Ann Rheum Dis* 2003; **62**: 835–41.

16. MacGregor, A. J. *et al.* Characterizing the quantitative genetic contribution to rheumatoid arthritis using data from twins. *Arthritis Rheum* 2000; **43**: 30–7.

17. Stastny, P. Association of the B-cell alloantigen DRw4 with rheumatoid arthritis. *N Engl J Med* 1978; **298**: 869–71.

18. Gregersen, P. K., Silver, J., and Winchester, R. J. The shared epitope hypothesis: an approach to understanding the molecular genetics of rheumatoid arthritis susceptibility. *Arthritis Rheum* 1987; **30**: 1205–13.

19. Gregersen, P. K. *et al.* Molecular diversity of HLA-DR4 haplotypes. *Proc Nat Acad Sci* 1986; **83**: 2642–6.

20. Nichol, F. E. and Woodrow, J. C. HLA DR antigens in Indian patients with rheumatoid arthritis. *Lancet* 1981; **1**: 220–1.

21. Sanchez, B. *et al.* HLA-DRw10 confers the highest susceptibility to rheumatoid arthritis in a Spanish population. *Tissue Antigens* 1990; **36**: 174–6.

22. Weyand, C. M., Hicok, K. C., Conn, D. L., and Goronzy, J. J. The influence of HLA-DRB1 genes on disease severity in rheumatoid arthritis. *Ann Intern Med* 1992; **117**: 801–6.

23. Nepom, G. T. Major histocompatibility complex-directed susceptibility to rheumatoid arthritis. *Adv Immunol* 1998; **68**: 315–32.

24. Hall, F. C. *et al.* Influence of the HLA-DRB1 locus on susceptibility and severity in rheumatoid arthritis. *QJM* 1996; **89**: 821–9.

25. Ollier, W. and Winchester, R. The germline and somatic genetic basis for rheumatoid arthritis. *Curr Dir Autoimmun* 1999; **1**: 166–93.

26. Wakitani, S. *et al.* The relationship between HLA-DRB1 alleles and disease subsets of rheumatoid arthritis in Japanese. *Br J Rheumatol* 1997; **36**: 630–6.

27. Lee, H. S. *et al.* Increased susceptibility to rheumatoid arthritis in Koreans heterozygous for HLA-DRB1*0405 and *0901. *Arthritis Rheum* 2004; **50**: 3468–75.

28. Teller, K. *et al.* HLA-DRB1 and DQB typing of Hispanic American patients with rheumatoid arthritis: the 'shared epitope' hypothesis may not apply. *J Rheumatol* 1996; **23**: 1363–8.

29. McDaniel, D. O., Alarcon, G. S., Pratt, P. W., and Reveille, J. D. Most African-American patients with rheumatoid arthritis do not have the rheumatoid antigenic determinant (epitope). *Ann Intern Med* 1995; **123**: 181–7.

30. Mulcahy, B. *et al.* Genetic variability in the tumor necrosis factor-lymphotoxin region influences susceptibility to rheumatoid arthritis. *Am J Hum Genet* 1996; **59**: 676–83.

31. Ota, M. *et al.* A second susceptibility gene for developing rheumatoid arthritis in the human MHC is localized within a 70-kb interval telomeric of the TNF genes in the HLA class III region. *Genomics* 2001; **71**: 263–70.

32. Jawaheer, D. *et al.* Dissecting the genetic complexity of the association between human leukocyte antigens and rheumatoid arthritis. *Am J Hum Genet* 2002; **71**: 585–94.

33. Price, P. *et al.* The genetic basis for the association of the 8.1 ancestral haplotype (A1, B8, DR3) with multiple immunopathological diseases. *Immunol Rev* 1999; **167**: 257–74.

34. Okamoto, K. *et al.* Identification of IkappaBL as the second major histocompatibility complex-linked susceptibility locus for rheumatoid arthritis. *Am J Hum Genet* 2003; **72**: 303–12.

35. Alper, C. A. *et al.* Genetic prediction of nonresponse to hepatitis B vaccine. *N Engl J Med* 1989; **321**: 708–12.

36. Kaslow, R. A. *et al.* A1, Cw7, B8, DR3 HLA antigen combination associated with rapid decline of T-helper lymphocytes in HIV-1 infection: a report from the Multicenter AIDS Cohort Study. *Lancet* 1990; **335**: 927–30.

37. Cryan, E. M. *et al.* Immunoglobulins in healthy controls: HLA-B8 and sex differences. *Tissue Antigens* 1985; **26**: 254–8.

38. Caruso, C. *et al.* HLA-B8, DR3 haplotype affects lymphocyte blood levels. *Immunol Invest* 1997; **26**: 333–40.

39. Lawley, T. J. *et al.* Defective Fc-receptor functions associated with the HLA-B8/DRw3 haplotype: studies in patients with dermatitis herpetiformis and normal subjects. *N Engl J Med* 1981; **304**: 185–92.

40. Vandiedonck, C. *et al.* Pleiotropic effects of the 8.1 HLA haplotype in patients with autoimmune myasthenia gravis and thymus hyperplasia. *Proc Natl Acad Sci U S A* 2004; **101**: 15464–9.

41. Newton, J. L. *et al.* Dissection of class III major histocompatibility complex haplotypes associated with rheumatoid arthritis. *Arthritis Rheum* 2004; **50**: 2122–9.

42. Moxley, G. and Cohen, H. J. Genetic studies, clinical heterogeneity, and disease outcome studies in rheumatoid arthritis. *Rheum Dis Clin North Am* 2002; **28**: 39–58.

43. Mattey, D. *et al.* Independent association of rheumatoid factor and the HLA-DRB-1 shared epitope with radiographic outcome in rheumatoid arthritis. *Arthritis Rheum* 2001; **44**: 1529–33.

44. El-Gabalawy, H. S. *et al.* Association of HLA alleles and clinical features in patients with synovitis of recent onset. *Arthritis Rheum* 1999; **42**: 1696–705.

45. Van Gaalen, F. A. *et al.* Association between HLA class II genes and autoantibodies to cyclic citrullinated peptides (CCPs) influences the severity of rheumatoid arthritis. *Arthritis Rheum* 2004; **50**: 2113–21.

46. Irigoyen, P. *et al.* Regulation of anti-cyclic citrullinated peptide antibodies in rheumatoid arthritis: Contrasting effects of HLA-DR3 and the shared epitope alleles. *Arthritis Rheum* 2005; **52**: 3813–18.

47. Huzinga, T. *et al.* Refining the complex rheumatoid arthritis phenotype based on specificity of the HLA-DRB1 shared epitope for antibodies to citrullinated proteins. *Arthritis Rheum* 2005; **52**: 3433–8.

48. Sturniolo, T. *et al.* Generation of tissue-specific and promiscuous HLA ligand databases using DNA microarrays and virtual HLA class II matrices. *Nat Biotechnol* 1999; **17**: 555–61.

49. Hill, J. A. *et al.* Cutting edge: the conversion of arginine to citrulline allows for a high-affinity peptide interaction with the rheumatoid arthritis-associated HLA-DRB1*0401 MHC class II molecule. *J Immunol* 2003; **171**: 538–41.

50. Risch, N. Linkage strategies for genetically complex traits. II. The power of affected relative pairs. *Am J Hum Genet* 1990; **46**: 229–41.

51. Risch, N. and Merikangas, K. The future of genetic studies of complex human diseases. *Science* 1996; **273**: 1516–17.

52. Lander, E. and Kruglyak, L. Genetic dissection of complex traits: guidelines for interpreting and reporting linkage results. *Nat Genet* 1995; **11**: 241–7.

53. Cornelis, F. *et al*. New susceptibility locus for rheumatoid arthritis suggested by a genome-wide linkage study. *Proc Natl Acad Sci U S A* 1998; **95**: 10746–50.

54. Shiozawa, S. *et al*. Identification of the gene loci that predispose to rheumatoid arthritis. *Int Immunol* 1998; **10**: 1891–5.

55. Jawaheer, D. *et al*. A genome-wide screen in multiplex rheumatoid arthritis families suggests genetic overlap with other autoimmune diseases. *Am J Human Genet* 2001; **68**: 927–36.

56. MacKay, K. *et al*. Whole-genome linkage analysis of rheumatoid arthritis susceptibility loci in 252 affected sibling pairs in the United Kingdom. *Arthritis Rheum* 2002; **46**: 632–9.

57. Jawaheer, D. *et al*. Screening the genome for rheumatoid arthritis susceptibility genes: a replication study and combined analysis of 512 multicase families. *Arthritis Rheum* 2003; **48**: 906–16.

58. John, S. *et al*. Whole-genome scan, in a complex disease, using 11,245 single-nucleotide polymorphisms: comparison with microsatellites. *Am J Hum Genet* 2004; **75**: 54–64.

59. Lubberts, E. *et al*. Increase in expression of receptor activator of nuclear factor kappaB at sites of bone erosion correlates with progression of inflammation in evolving collagen-induced arthritis. *Arthritis Rheum* 2002; **46**: 3055–64.

60. Lee, A. T. *et al*. The PTPN22 R620W polymorphism associates with RF positive rheumatoid arthritis in a dose-dependent manner but not with HLA-SE status. *Genes Immun* 2005; **6**: 129–33.

61. Orozco, G. *et al*. Association of a functional single-nucleotide polymorphism of PTPN22, encoding lymphoid protein phosphatase, with rheumatoid arthritis and systemic lupus erythematosus. *Arthritis Rheum* 2005; **52**: 219–24.

62. van Oene, M. *et al*. Association of the lymphoid tyrosine phosphatase R620W variant with rheumatoid arthritis, but not Crohn's disease, in Canadian Populations. *Arthritis Rheum* 2005; **52**: 1993–8.

63. Simkins, H. *et al*. *Arthritis Rheum* 2005; **52**: 2222–5.

64. Criswell, L. A. *et al*. Analysis of families in the Multiple Autoimmune Disease Genetics Consortium (MADGC) collection: the PTPN22 620W allele associates with multiple autoimmune phenotypes. *Am J Hum Genet* 2005; **76**: 561–71.

65. Begovich, A. B. *et al*. The R620W polymorphism of the protein tyrosine phosphatase PTPN22 is not associated with multiple sclerosis. *Am J Hum Genet* 2005; **76**: 184–7.

66. Torfs, C. P. *et al*. Genetic interrelationship between insulin-dependent diabetes mellitus, the autoimmune thyroid diseases, and rheumatoid arthritis. *Am J Hum Genet* 1986; **38**: 170–87.

67. Lin, J. P. *et al*. Familial clustering of rheumatoid arthritis with other autoimmune diseases. *Hum Genet* 1998; **103**: 475–82.

68. Halldorsdottir, H. D., Jonsson, T., Thorsteinsson, J., and Valdimarsson, H. A prospective study on the incidence of rheumatoid arthritis among people with persistent increase of rheumatoid factor. *Ann Rheum Dis* 2000; **59**: 149–51.

69. Arbuckle, M. R. *et al*. Development of autoantibodies before the clinical onset of systemic lupus erythematosus. *N Engl J Med* 2003; **349**: 1526–33.

70. Hoppu, S. *et al*. Childhood Diabetes in Finland Study Group: GAD65 antibody isotypes and epitope recognition during the pre-diabetic process in siblings of children with type I diabetes. *Clin Exp Immunol* 2004; **136**: 120–8.

71. Strieder, T. G. *et al*. Risk factors for and prevalence of thyroid disorders in a cross-sectional study among healthy female relatives of patients with autoimmune thyroid disease. *Clin Endocrinol (Oxf)* 2003; **59**: 396–401.

72. Hasegawa, K. *et al*. PEST domain-enriched tyrosine phosphatase (PEP) regulation of effector/memory T cells. *Science* 2004; **303**: 685–9.

73. Cloutier J. F. and Veillette A. Cooperative inhibition of T-cell antigen receptor signaling by a complex between a kinase and a phosphatase. *J Exp Med* 1999; **189**: 111–21.

74. Gregorieff, A., Cloutier, J. F., and Veillette, A. Sequence requirements for association of protein-tyrosine phosphatase PEP with the Src

homology 3 domain of inhibitory tyrosine protein kinase p50(csk). *J Biol Chem* 1998; **273**: 13217–22.

75. Mustelin, T., Vang, T., and Bottini, N. Protein tyrosine phosphatases and the immune response. *Nat Rev Immunol* 2005; **5**: 43–57.

76. Hill, R. J. *et al*. The lymphoid protein tyrosine phosphatase Lyp interacts with the adaptor molecule Grb2 and functions as a negative regulator of T-cell activation. *Exp Hematol* 2002; **30**: 237–44.

77. Fournel, M., Davidson, D., Weil, R., and Veillette, A. Association of tyrosine protein kinase Zap-70 with the protooncogene product p120c-cbl in T lymphocytes. *J Exp Med* 1996; **183**: 301–6.

78. Cohen, S. *et al*. Cloning and characterization of a lymphoid-specific, inducible human protein tyrosine phosphatase, Lyp. *Blood* 1999; **93**: 2013–24.

79. Daly, M. J. *et al*. High-resolution haplotype structure in the human genome. *Nat Genet* 2001; **29**: 229–32.

80. Rioux, J. D. *et al*. Genetic variation in the 5q31 cytokine gene cluster confers susceptibility to Crohn disease. *Nat Genet* 2001; **29**: 223–8.

81. Jeffreys, A. J., Kauppi, L., and Neumann, R. Intensely punctate meiotic recombination in the class II region of the major histocompatibility complex. *Nat Genet* 2001; **29**: 217–22.

82. Ioannidis, J. P. *et al*. Replication validity of genetic association studies. *Nat Genet* 2001; **29**: 306–9.

83. Padyukov, L. *et al*. A gene-environment interaction between smoking and shared epitope genes in HLA-DR provides a high risk of seropositive rheumatoid arthritis. *Arthritis Rheum* 2004; **50**: 3085–92.

84. Plenge, R. P. *et al*. Of prior candidate gene association studies to rheumatoid arthritis susceptibility, only *PTPN22*, *CTLA4* and *PADI4* replicate in a collection of over 4,000 samples. *Am J Human Genetics* 2005; **77**: 1044–60.

85. Suzuki, A. *et al*. Functional haplotypes of PADI4, encoding citrullinating enzyme peptidylarginine deiminase 4, are associated with rheumatoid arthritis. *Nat Genet* 2003; **34**: 395–40.

86. Tokuhiro, S. *et al*. An intronic SNP in a RUNX1 binding site of SLC22A4, encoding an organic cation transporter, is associated with rheumatoid arthritis. *Nat Genet* 2003; **35**: 341–8.

87. Barton, A. *et al*. A functional haplotype of the PADI4 gene associated with rheumatoid arthritis in a Japanese population is not associated in a United Kingdom population. *Arthritis Rheum* 2004; **50**: 1117–21.

88. Kuwahara, M. *et al*. Independent confirmation of the association between PADI4 and rheumatoid arthritis. *Arthritis Rheum* 2004; **50**: S353 [abstract].

89. Ioannidis, J. P., Ntzani, E. E., and Trikalinos, T. A. 'Racial' differences in genetic effects for complex diseases. *Nat Genet* 2004; **36**: 1312–18.

90. Firestein, G. S. Evolving concepts of rheumatoid arthritis. *Nature* 2003; **423**: 356–61.

91. Remmers, E. F. *et al*. A genome scan localizes five non-MHC loci controlling collagen-induced arthritis in rats. *Nat Genet* 1996; **14**: 82–5.

92. Vingsbo-Lundberg, C. *et al*. Genetic control of arthritis onset, severity and chronicity in a model for rheumatoid arthritis in rats. *Nat Genet* 1998; **20**: 401–4.

93. Lorentzen, J. C. *et al*. Identification of rat susceptibility loci for adjuvant-oil-induced arthritis. *Proc Natl Acad Sci U S A* 1998; **95**: 6383–7.

94. Gulko, P. S. *et al*. Identification of a new non-major histocompatibility complex genetic locus on chromosome 2 that controls disease severity in collagen-induced arthritis in rats. *Arthritis Rheum* 1998; **41**: 2122–31.

95. Kawahito, Y. *et al*. Localization of quantitative trait loci regulating adjuvant induced arthritis in rats: evidence for genetic factors common to multiple autoimmune diseases. *J Immunol* 1998; **161**: 4411–19.

96. Otto, J. M. *et al*. Identification of multiple loci linked to inflammation and autoantibody production by a genome scan of a murine model of rheumatoid arthritis. *Arthritis Rheum* 1999; **42**: 2524–31.

97. Olofsson, P. *et al.* Positional identification of Ncf1 as a gene that regulates arthritis severity in rats. *Nat Genet* 2003; **33**: 25–32.

98. Griffiths, M. M., and Remmers, E. F. Genetic analysis of collagen-induced arthritis in rats: a polygenic model for rheumatoid arthritis predicts a common framework of cross-species inflammatory/autoimmune disease loci. *Immunol Rev* 2001; **184**: 172–83.

99. Brenner, M. *et al.* The non-MHC quantitative trait locus Cia10 contains a major arthritis gene and regulates disease severity, pannus formation and joint damage. *Arthritis Rheum* 2005; **52**: 322–32.

100. Barton, A. *et al.* High resolution linkage and association mapping identifies a novel rheumatoid arthritis susceptibility locus homologous to one linked to two rat models of inflammatory arthritis. *Hum Mol Genet* 2001; **10**: 1901–6.

101. Mikuls, T. R. *et al.* Coffee, tea, and caffeine consumption and risk of rheumatoid arthritis: results from the Iowa Women's Health Study. *Arthritis Rheum* 2002; **46**: 83–91.

102. Olofsson, P. *et al.* Genetic links between the acute-phase response and arthritis development in rats. *Arthritis Rheum* 2002; **46**: 259–68.

103. Wernhoff, P., Olofsson, P., and Holmdahl, R. The genetic control of rheumatoid factor production in a rat model of rheumatoid arthritis. *Arthritis Rheum* 2003; **48**: 3584–96.

104. Furuya, T. *et al.* Genetic dissection of a rat model for rheumatoid arthritis: significant gender influences on autosomal modifier loci. *Hum Mol Genet* 2000; **9**: 2241–50.

105. Brenner, M. *et al.* The non-mHC quantitative trait locus Cia5 contains three major arthritis genes that differentially regulate disease severity, pennus formation, and joint damage in collagen- and pristane-induced arthritis. *J Immunol* 2005; **174**: 7894–903.

106. Adarichev, V. A. *et al.* Sex effect on clinical and immunologic quantitative trait loci in a murine model of rheumatoid arthritis. *Arthritis Rheum* 2003; **48**: 1708–20.

107. Joe, B. *et al.* Genetic dissection of collagen-induced arthritis in chromosome 10 quantitative trait locus speed congenic rats: evidence for more than one regulatory locus and sex influences. *Immunogenetics* 2000; **51**: 930–44.

108. Remmers, E. F. *et al.* Modulation of multiple experimental arthritis models by collagen-induced arthritis quantitative trait loci isolated in congenic rat lines: different effects of non-major histocompatibility complex quantitative trait loci in males and females. *Arthritis Rheum* 2002; **46**: 2225–34.

109. Ribbhammar, U. *et al.* High resolution mapping of an arthritis susceptibility locus on rat chromosome 4, and characterization of regulated phenotypes. *Hum Mol Genet* 2003; **12**: 2087–96.

110. Sokka, T., Willoughby, J., Yazici, Y., and Pincus, T. Databases of patients with early rheumatoid arthritis in the USA. *Clin Exp Rheumatol* 2003; **21**: S146–53.

111. Smith, D. J. and Lusis, A. J. The allelic structure of common disease. *Hum Mol Genet* 2002; **11**: 2455–61.

112. Pritchard, J. K., and Cox, N. J. The allelic architecture of human disease genes: common disease-common variant . . . or not? *Hum Mol Genet* 2002; **11**: 2417–23.

2 | Epidemiology and determinants of susceptibility

Jaime Calvo-Alén and Graciela S. Alarcón

Introduction

The study of the distribution of rheumatoid arthritis (RA) among distinct human groups, at different times, and its impact on the individual affected with it fall within the scope of Descriptive Epidemiology. Analyses of individuals at risk for developing RA of variable severity (by virtue of a given attribute or risk factor), on the other hand, fall within the realm of Analytical Epidemiology. The knowledge gained from both descriptive and analytical epidemiology may have direct impact in the management of RA patients and it has, therefore, both theoretical and practical implications. We will limit this chapter to adult RA, with a few exceptions.

Descriptive epidemiology

Descriptive studies of diseases still lacking a clear etiology are hampered by the sensitivity, specificity, and positive and negative predictive value of the criteria used to classify cases[1]. In RA, earlier studies (conducted prior to the discovery and widespread utilization of the rheumatoid factor, RF) may have included cases of 'rheumatoid spondylitis'(spondylarthropathies), rheumatic fever, gout, and osteoarthritis. If cases are only diagnosed when typical deformities and/or radiographically demonstrable damage has occurred, there will be relatively little misclassification of cases (with diseases other than RA), but patients with early RA will be totally missed[2]. On the other hand, if RA is defined as the presence of characteristic symmetric synovitis with morning stiffness, early cases will be included but non-RA cases are likely to be included as well. Finally, it should be noted that in the criteria for the classification of RA, adopted by the American College of Rheumatology (ACR) in 1987[3], the categories of probable, definite, and classical disease, as defined in 1958[4], are no longer considered as cases of probable RA are unlikely to meet criteria for RA at later times. Thus, it is hard to merge clinical data obtained using the 1958 classification criteria with more recent studies in which these categories are not used at all. The previous criteria also included a long list of exclusions which were hard to meet in either practice-based or population-based studies and thus they were also dropped. Likewise, since in actual practice tissue from either joint cavities or subcutaneous nodules is not obtained, the histopathological criteria were removed. The

ACR revised criteria were developed using patients from tertiary care facilities but they, too, have been tested in populations (such as the Pima Indian population of Arizona in the USA) and found to perform adequately if present more than at one point in time[5]. Consequently, the revised criteria can be used both in population- and practice-based studies. These and other methodological considerations need to be kept in mind when the epidemiological literature pertaining to RA is examined.

Prevalence

Prevalence studies include all patients with such a condition present in a population at a particular point in time. Although RA is currently described as occurring worldwide in about 1% of the adult population[6], its regional and temporal prevalence has been variable. The disease is about five times more frequent among indigenous populations of the North American subcontinent than in Caucasian populations from either North America or Europe. Asian and African populations, who presumably came in contact with these indigenous populations later than Europeans, have a much lower prevalence of RA than Caucasians[7]. Moreover, evidence for the absence of RA before the seventeenth and twentieth centuries in Europe and in Africa, respectively, have led investigators to hypothesize that RA originated in the American continent and was transported to the Old World by returning Spanish conquistadors[8]. This contrasts with other rheumatic diseases such as ankylosing spondylitis, osteoarthritis, and some infectious arthritis (tuberculosis) for which there is clear pictorial, graphical, and/or physical (skeletal remains) evidence of their existence in the Old World from ancient times[9–11]. RA might thus be a unique disease among chronic rheumatic disorders. It can be argued, however, that RA is much harder to identify both pictorially and in skeletal remains than diseases that primarily affect larger anatomical structures such as the spine or the weight-bearing joints, and thus we may never be able to categorically affirm that the disease was non-existent in Europe prior to the discovery of the Americas. The general impression is that RA has a lower prevalence in developing countries[12]. Although there are not definitive data in which to base this statement, recent epidemiological studies in developing areas seem to support it[13–15]. However, these studies have been hospital-based instead of community-based, which can underestimate the prevalence data. In addition, lack of adequate healthcare for rheumatologic disorders in developing countries can also have some influence in these results, Finally, other factors that can partially account for the lower prevalence of RA in some developing countries such as Indonesia and Pakistan are particular demographic features such as the different age structure of the population, the lower life expectancy, or the relative paucity of older women[16,17], with the consequent decrease in the number of individuals potentially at risk for developing RA. It is intriguing that the risk of developing RA doubles for Pakistanis after living several years in a Western environment such as England[18], although it does not reach the same level as the ethnic English population.

Table 2.1 presents prevalence data for RA in different population groups. These populations have been divided into those with high, intermediate, and low prevalence rates of the disease, which closely agree with the geographic area in which they are located[19–26].

Incidence

Incidence studies include all cases of a given condition arising within a defined population and during a specific period of time. Prevalence data include patients who have moved from other communities after the onset of disease but also exclude patients who die or that have left the area after disease onset, and therefore prevalence data may be difficult to interpret. For this reason incidence data derived from community-based studies are more representative of the real impact a determined condition has in a specific population. The few incidence studies in RA using this methodology performed in indigenous and non-indigenous populations of North America support the data just mentioned, with RA occurring at a higher rate in the Pima Indians and other Native American tribes than in Caucasian populations from Europe and North America[20,27,28]. There are no incidence studies from Latin American or African countries. Nevertheless, the existing data support the hypothesis that RA may have originated in North America. Data from available studies are summarized in Table 2.2[19,22,29,30].

Age and gender influence in the epidemiology of RA

RA occurs more often in women than in men (2:1 to 3:1 ratio in most studies), which suggests the existence of a higher (genetic)

Table 2.1 Prevalence of RA (per 100 population) in different populations[a]

Population	Prevalence[a]
High prevalence	
Yakima Indians, US	6.0
Chippewa Indians, US	5.3
Pima Indians, US	5.3
Intermediate prevalence	
Europe	
Bulgaria	0.9
Denmark	0.9
England	1.1
Greece	0.2
Netherlands	0.9
Sweden	0.9
Spain	0.5
Norway	0.4
Ireland	0.5
France	0.5
North America (Caucasians)	
US	1.0
Sudbury, Massachusetts	0.9
South America and Caribbean	
Brazil	0.6
Colombia	0.1
Jamaica	1.9
Low prevalence	
Asia	
China, a rural island	0.3
China, mainland	0.3
Hong Kong	0.2
Indonesia, rural	0.2
Indonesia, urban	0.3
Japan	0.3
Pakistan	0.1
Philippines	0.2
Taiwan	0.3
Africa	
Lesotho	0.3
Nigeria and Liberia	0
Nigeria	0
South Africa, rural	0
Middle East	
Egypt	0.2
Israel	0.3
Oman	0.4

Figures have been rounded and are shown with only one decimal.
[a] Modified from Abdel-Nasser AM, Rasker JJ, Valkenburg HA. Epidemiological and clinical aspects relating to the variability of rheumatoid arthritis. *Semin Arthritis Rheum* 1997; 27: 123–40.

Table 2.2 Annual incidence rate (per 100 population) of definite RA in different populations[a]

Population	Study period	Incidence
Native Americans		
Alaskan	1970–84	0.09
Pima	1966–73	0.89
Pima	1974–82	0.62
Pima	1983–90	0.38
US (Caucasians)		
Rochester, MI	1950–74	0.04
Rochester, MI	1985–94	0.03
Seattle, WA	1987–89	0.02
Worcester, MA	1987–90	0.03
Europe		
England and Wales	1970–72	0.02
England and Wales	1980–82	0.19
England	1990	0.02
Finland	1974–75	0.04
Finland	1980–90	0.04
France	1980–84	0.01
Greece	1987–95	0.02
The Netherlands	1947–65	0.05
Norway	1969–84	0.02
Norway	1987–96	0.03
Asia		
Japan	1958–64	0.04
Japan	1962–66	0.06
Japan	1965–67	0.09

[a] Modified from Abdel-Nasser AM, Rasker JJ, Valkenburg HA. Epidemiological and clinical aspects relating to the variability of rheumatoid arthritis. *Semin Arthritis Rheum* 1997; 27: 123–40.

threshold requirement for RA in men. Consistent with this model, several studies have shown that the association between genetic markers and RA is stronger in men than in women[31,32]. The role of hormonal factors in triggering or modulating the onset of the disease and its manifestations will be discussed later.

The influence of gender in the clinical expression of the disease continues to be a topic of interest. RA of comparable severity occurs in both men and women, although some clinical forms such as the 'robust' (or 'robustus') is characteristically more common in men who are physical laborers. These patients seem to have only a modest amount of pain and develop little incapacitation over time[33]. An alternative explanation is that the robust type of RA is due to the (stoic) personality of some individuals—preferentially men[34].

Weyand and collaborators, based on data from Olmsted County, Minnesota, have postulated that gender significantly influences the phenotype of the disease, as more women than men experience structural consequences of the disease (measured as the need for surgery) despite the fact that, radiographically, men tend to have more erosive disease. A close examination of these data, however, reveals that the differences in surgical rates are primarily due to foot and hand surgery rather than to large joint arthroplasties, suggesting that reasons other than structural joint damage may be behind the decision to perform these surgical procedures (footwear, appearance, to cite but a few). In any case, the data from Weyand *et al.* substantiate clinical observations made over the years: some extra-articular manifestations, particularly rheumatoid nodules and rheumatoid lung, are more common in men than in women[35]. These phenotypic differences could also result from associated factors such as trauma, smoking, and work-related exposure to toxins rather than to genetic or hormonal differences between the genders[36].

The peak age of onset of RA is in the fifth decade of life[37], although a different pattern has been observed in men vs. women. In men incidence rises steeply with age, whereas in women the incidence reaches a plateau between ages 50 and 75, after which it declines[38]. However, RA may occur as early as in the second decade and in fact the seropositive, polyarticular form of juvenile rheumatoid arthritis (JRA) occurs predominantly in adolescent girls; it is hard to state whether this JRA subtype is one of the tails of the age distribution for RA, as shown in Fig. 2.1[37]. Common clinical, serologic, radiographic, and immunogenetic characteristics of RA and seropositive polyarticular JRA suggest that is the case, as shown in Table 2.3[39,40]. Overall, in

comparison with the experience of a few decades ago, the age of onset of RA appears to be shifting towards later in life, but whether this is a real trend or only an artifact resulting from the aging of the population, and/or an increase in access to specialized care among the elderly, has not been sorted out to date[37,41,42]. In fact, it is not uncommon to see new onset RA in octa- or even nonagenarian individuals, which would have been unheard of a few decades ago[43].

Age at disease onset has been often regarded as a differential marker for a specific type of disease course. Indeed, several reports have described late-onset RA as having special features such as more frequent abrupt onset, weight loss, large joint involvement, and polymyalgia-like symptoms and a lower frequency of IgM-RF[37,44,45]. Late-onset RA has also been said to have a more benign outcome than RA that starts earlier in life [46,47]. However, most of the published studies have been observational, with no direct comparison between patients with late and early disease onset having been made. Moreover, in some of these studies it is unclear whether patients with late-onset RA may have had polymyalgia rheumatica, RS₃PE (the syndrome described by McCarty as seronegative symmetric synovitis with pitting edema, that characteristically occurs in elderly men)[48], or a transient

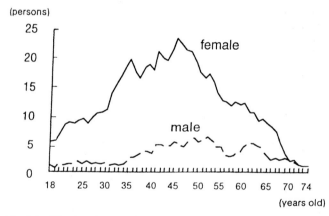

Fig. 2.1 The distribution of age at disease onset for men and women with RA. The polyarticular form of juvenile rheumatoid arthritis (JRA) can be regarded as the left tail of the distribution. (Reproduced with permission from Yukioka M, Wakitani S, Murata N, Toda Y, Ogawa R, Kaneshige T *et al.* Elderly-onset rheumatoid arthritis and its association with HLA-DRB1 alleles in Japanese. *Br J Rheumatol* 1998; 37: 98–101.)

Table 2.3 Comparative features between RA and JRA subtypes

Feature	Rheumatoid arthritis	Polyarticular JRA (positive rheumatoid factor)	Other JRA subtypes
Gender (W:M)	3:1	10% of JRA 3:1	90% of JRA Variable
Clinical	Symmetric polyarthritis	Indistinguishable from RA	Variable
Immunological (autoantibodies other than RF)	Frequent	SSA, SSB may appear during the course of the disease	Infrequent
Radiological	Erosive arthritis	Erosive arthritis	Usually non-erosive
Immunogenetic (HLA-DR4 positivity)	50–83%[a]	≥60%	15%

JRA, juvenile rheumatoid arthritis; SSA; SSB
[a] Frequencies vary from 50% in Caucasians to 83% in some Native American populations.

polyarthritis, rather than RA[49]. More recent studies including both groups of RA patients have not supported the conclusions reached before that late-onset RA may have a more benign course. To the contrary, these studies suggest that late-onset RA may have a similar[50,51], or even a worse, outcome than early-onset RA[52,53].

Secular trends in RA prevalence and incidence

For reasons that are not yet clear, a decline in both the prevalence and incidence of RA, which may have reached an all-time high in the 1960s, has been observed in some Native Americans in the US, Caucasians in North America and Europe, and Japanese in their native country (Fig. 2.2)[28,30,43,54-57]. In contrast, RA appears to be on the rise in African countries, where it appears to have emerged later[58]. The possibility that the decline in the occurrence of RA relates to the introduction of oral contraceptives in the Western world has been considered, based on large epidemiological studies from North America and Europe[59]; the data have not been, however, entirely consistent and thus a final conclusion has not been reached (see below).

The phenotype of the disease also appears to be changing over time. Overall it seems that we are not seeing as many patients with severe articular and extra-articular disease as we saw decades ago[60-62]. In fact, a decrease in the number of hospitalizations for severe manifestations of RA has been recently reported[63]. Thus the number of hospitalizations for RA vasculitis decreased by one-third between the periods 1983–87 and 1998–2001 and those for splenectomy due to Felty's syndrome were 71% lower. This decline in the severity of RA, coupled with a decrease in its incidence and prevalence, as already mentioned, has led some investigators to postulate that RA might eventually disappear from the face of the earth as a human malady[64]. Although we would like to share such optimism and enthusiasm, we think caution is in order, as these observations may result from differences in case ascertainment, case selection, access to healthcare, and other methodological problems rather than from a true decline in the occurrence of the disease or a change in its phenotype.

Impact of RA

According to Fries, the impact of any given disorder should be examined along five defined dimensions: survival, disability, discomfort, iatrogenesis/comorbidities, and economic losses[65]. Some of these dimensions of outcome will be examined in detail in other chapters; thus we will only discuss in this chapter survival and comorbidities directly related to the disease or its treatments.

Survival and causes of death

For the most part, scientific evidence shows that patients with RA die earlier than their peers. Hospital-based studies have shown excess death rates ranging from 30 to 200%[66,67]. In population-based studies excess mortality rates have been less evident, but still significantly higher than in controls[68-70]. Some European investigators have questioned this assertion as they have observed no increased mortality among RA patients seen over the last decade or so[71-73]; an earlier and more aggressive treatment of RA has been suggested as a possible cause of this improvement[72,74]. However, the time of follow-up in these studies has been relatively short, ranging between 8 and 14 years; given that the excess mortality in RA is not evident for 8–10 years after disease onset[75] these data cannot be considered definitive. In fact, recent population-based studies in which patients have been followed up for four decades have confirmed the lower life expectancy RA patients have, which has not changed significantly over the last few decades[75,76]. There is no agreement as to whether gender makes any difference in the increased risk of mortality in RA; in fact some studies have shown a higher risk among men[67,77], whereas others have shown a higher risk among women[75,78]. In general, it can be said that RA appears to decrease the life expectancy of affected individuals by 3–10 years. Survival curves for RA patients from North America are shown in Fig. 2.3[79].

Causes contributing to excess mortality in RA are infectious[77,80,81], renal[77,80,81], respiratory[80], and gastrointestinal diseases[77,82]. Malignancies of the reticuloendothelial system have been reported with increased frequency, but overall, the data on malignancies are controversial[81,83]. The leading cause of death in RA is, however, cardiovascular disease, accounting for almost half of the overall mortality in these patients[69,84]. It is now recognized that patients with RA are at an increased risk of cardiovascular events (some of them silent) and death from cardiovascular causes[85]; this increased risk is not related to traditional risk factors but rather parallels the inflammatory process characteristics of this disease, with patients with evidence of active inflammation (number of swollen joints, serological markers) being at higher risk than those without (or little) evidence of active inflammation[86-89]. The vast majority of patients with RA die from the same causes as the general population, but at a younger age. In populations where other comorbid conditions account for the main causes of death, these are also the causes among patients with RA. That is the case, for example, of the

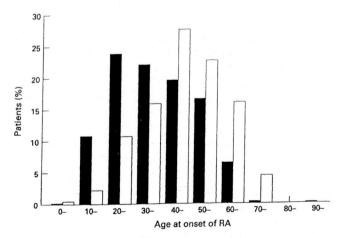

Fig. 2.2   Increase in age at onset of RA in Japan. ■: patients from 1960 to 1965;□: patients from 1985 to 1990. (Reproduced with permission from Imanaka T, Shichikawa K, Inoue K, Shimaoka Y, Takenaka Y, Wakitani S. Increase in age at onset of rheumatoid arthritis in Japan over a 30 year period. *Ann Rheum Dis* 1997; **56**: 313–16.

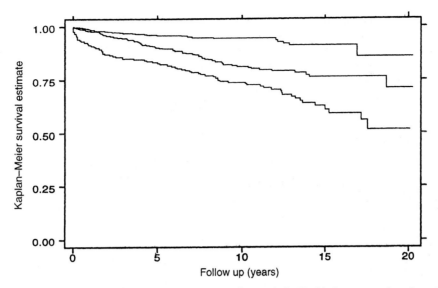

Fig. 2.3 Cumulative probability of survival for a cohort of RA patients according with the Health Assessment Questionnaire (HAQ) Disability index. Scores of 0–1 top, 1–2 intermediate, or 2–3 lower curve. (Reproduced with permission from Wolfe F, Zwillich SH. The long-term outcomes of rheumatoid arthritis: a 23-year prospective, longitudinal study of total joint replacement and its predictors in 1,600 patients with rheumatoid arthritis. *Arthritis Rheum* 1998; **41**: 1072–82.)

Pima Indians of Arizona, where alcohol-related deaths are the leading cause among the general population as well as among RA patients[68].

A greater number of involved joints, older age, fewer (number of) years of education, significant functional losses, and the presence of extra-articular manifestations or comorbid cardiovascular conditions are all significant predictors of mortality in RA[75,90]. In fact, Pincus *et al.* have suggested that, like patients with malignant disorders or coronary artery disease (CAD), patients with RA could simply be 'staged' based on the number of involved joints to correctly predict their probability of survival at 5 or 10 years. Patients with RA and a large number of joints involved (or significant functional impairment) may have a five-year survival probability of only 40–60%, which is comparable to that of patients with stage IV Hodgkin's lymphoma or three-vessel CAD[91]. An increase in the death rate due to cardiovascular and cerebrovascular diseases as a consequence of the utilization of methotrexate (resulting in elevated serum levels of homocysteine) has been proposed but not supported by available data[92,93]. However, more recent and larger studies have shown that methotrexate provides a substantial survival benefit, including a decrease in cardiovascular mortality[94,95]. Finally, a possible increment in the occurrence of lung cancer (and deaths due to it) in methotrexate-treated RA patients was reported in a small study from Canada[96], but such findings have not been corroborated in studies from other centers[97].

Morbidity

RA is capable of inflicting significant structural damage on the affected individual, primarily on the musculoskeletal system. So debilitated may these patients become, that some authors have urged rheumatologists to consider the 'side-effects' of the disease when evaluating the possible 'side-effects' of effective remedies used to treat this condition (and weigh them before making

therapeutic decisions)[98]. Patients with RA may become considerably catabolic, even in the absence of exogenous compounds such as glucocorticoids, probably due to the systemic effects of pro-inflammatory cytokines such as IL-1β, IL-6 or TNF-α. These patients may also experience significant anorexia and their ability to cook may be compromised. Thus, it is possible for RA patients to become markedly malnourished (rheumatoid cachexia)[99]; these malnourished patients tend to have a poorer prognosis than patients who are able to maintain an ideal body weight[100,101]. On the other hand, sedentarism, coupled with extremely poor eating habits, may lead to obesity with detrimental consequences in already damaged weight-bearing joints and other organ systems[102]; this is becoming more common in the US as it is not infrequent for patients to be overweight at disease onset.

As opposed to systemic lupus erythematosus (SLE), a damage index to measure the impact of the disease (or of the drugs used) has yet to be developed in RA. This may relate to the fact that the 'irreversible' damage produced by the disease, at least in the musculoskeletal system, is quite obvious and, in fact, it is measurable; the disease has been staged radiographically for over five decades using the Steinbrocker Staging System, but this system has some deficiencies, including a broad overlap with more detailed scoring methods and its lack of correlation with other outcomes such as disability[103]. More refined radiographic methods have been developed, in Europe and North America (the Larsen[104] and Sharp[105] methods, respectively), and modified subsequently for easier applicability in the clinical setting by Scott[106] and van der Heijde[107]. Only recently investigators from both sides of the Atlantic have developed guidelines for the use of radiographic methods for the assessment of joint destruction (damage) in patients with RA[108].

Glucocorticoids also have a defined and important toxicity profile [109], and although it has been reported that daily oral glucocorticoids, contrary to popular belief, may protect patients from the occurrence of bone and joint destruction[110], this fact has not been borne out in an early RA cohort [111] and it is certainly not the experience of seasoned clinicians. Nevertheless, glucocorticoids are used since they still are the most potent anti-inflammatory drugs available and as such are capable of significantly alleviating the symptoms and signs of inflammation which typify this disease[112].

Felson and collaborators have established a comparative safety (and efficacy) profile for the commonly used disease modifying antirheumatic drugs (DMARDs)[113], and Morgan *et al.* have empirically developed a toxicity index to quantify the side-effects resulting from the administration of methotrexate, an index that proved to be useful in their folic acid supplementation studies[114]. Finally, the long-term toxicity profile of methotrexate is becoming apparent as we are well into the third decade of its widespread utilization in rheumatology. Whereas some clearly folate-deficiency toxicities (abdominal discomfort, alopecia, oral ulcerations) have been curbed with the concomitant administration of folic acid, that is not the case (or it is unclear) with hepatic, pulmonary, and malignant events related to its administration[115–117]. Risk factors for the occurrence of methotrexate-induced clinically significant liver disease include older age and cumulative methotrexate dose (and probably diabetes)[118,119]. For the occurrence of pulmonary toxicity these factors include age older than 60 years, diabetes, hypoalbuminemia, underlying RA pleuropulmonary involvement, and previous use of other DMARD[120,121]. No risk factors have been found, thus far, for Epstein—Barr virus-related (or unrelated) B cell lymphomas occurring in methotrexate-treated RA patients[122,123].

Analytical epidemiology

Although the cause (or causes) of what we currently call RA remains elusive, the general consensus is that factors or attributes contributing to its occurrence and course are probably both genetic and environmental, with RA resulting from their interaction. Genetic factors have been suspected for decades based on the clustering of the disease among families and among individuals from highly inbred populations, as well as by the degree of concordance for the disease among monozygotic twins (15–30%). Nevertheless, the familial risk for RA is certainly small[124,125] and studies of twin concordance have estimated that the shared genetic effect only explains ~50–60% of the occurrence of RA, leaving enough room for the effect of non-genetic factors[126]. Environmental triggers have been also suspected all along, with the number of factors purported to be causal agents of RA rising and falling over the years (see below).

Genetic factors

RA is a complex oligogenic disease in which genetic factors may account for as much as 60% of disease susceptibility[127]. The study of the genetic factors predisposing to the occurrence of RA is relatively recent. It was only two and a half decades ago that the association between RA and some class II human leukocyte antigen (HLA) alleles (*HLA-Dw4*, now *HLA-DRB1*04*) were

reported in Caucasian patients[128]. Since then we have learned that the association is not with *HLA-DRB1*04* per se but with a sequence motif present in the α helical portion (third hypervariable region) of the β chain of the HLA-DRB1 molecule that forms one side of the peptide binding groove. This sequence motif (QKRAA, QRRAA, or RRRAA), also called 'rheumatoid epitope', is encoded by *HLA-DRB1*04* (*0401*, *0404*, and *0405* alleles) and some non-DR4 alleles, such as *HLA-DRB1*01*, *HLA-DRB1*14*, and *HLA-DRB1*10*. The initial studies conducted by Weyand and her collaborators at the Mayo Clinic in 1992 suggested that the rheumatoid epitope (its dose and the alleles carrying it) were important determinants of disease severity as measured by the need for joint surgery, the presence of subcutaneous nodules, and the occurrence of extra-articular manifestations. These studies were, however, conducted in a highly selected sample of Caucasian RA patients with established and advanced disease followed at a tertiary care facility[129]. Based on these data, it was postulated that the course and final outcome of RA could be determined at disease onset based on the genotype of the afflicted person (genotype predicting phenotype) and the patient could be treated accordingly[130]. This initial enthusiasm has been followed by caution as the shared epitope appears less relevant to disease susceptibility in some non-Caucasian ethnic groups, such as North Americans of Hispanic[131] or African descent[132], and Pakistanis[133]. Moreover, in studies of patients with early RA, the frequency of the epitope was comparable among those individuals who evolved to articular destruction and those who completely resolved their articular manifestations, invalidating the value of genotyping to more accurately approach the treatment of patients with early pre-erosive disease. Nevertheless, most studies have shown that there is correlation between disease progression as determined radiographically and the shared epitope[134]. In fact, a recent meta-analysis shows that the presence of the shared epitope doubles the risk for the occurrence of erosions[135] although striking ethnic exceptions were found and, overall, no dose effect was observed. *HLA-DRB1*0404* and, particularly, *HLA-DRB1*0401* appear to be the rheumatoid epitope-carrying alleles most strongly associated with disease severity, being over-represented in those ethnic populations where RA tends to be more severe, whereas the *HLA-DRB1*01* allele is the rheumatoid epitope-carrying allele in population groups, which by and large, tend to have milder forms of the disease. A summary of studies addressing the relationship between the shared epitope with either RA susceptibility or severity across different ethnic groups is shown in Table 2.4[31,31,37,135–152].

The role other major histocompatibility complex (MHC) genes such as HLA-DQB1 may play in susceptibility to RA or its severity remains unclear to date[153,154]. Based on an experimental mouse model of collagen-induced arthritis, it has been proposed that the actual arthritogenic peptide-presenting molecule is HLA-DQ, whereas HLA-DRB1 would play a protective or non-protective role[155]. This theory has been further supported by data from some human studies[156–159]; according to these studies, HLA-DRB1* alleles encoding a DERAA motif instead of the shared epitope are potentially protective. However, other researchers have not confirmed this model; in fact, the associations described may represent only linkage disequilibrium between some HLA-DR and HLA-DQ alleles.

Table 2.4 Association of HLA-DR alleles with RA in various ethnic groups

Allele	Association with susceptibility	Association with severity	Ethnic groups
DRB1*0101	✓		Asian Indians, Jews, Caucasians, Greeks, Japanese, French, Italians, Turkish
DRB1*0102	✓		Israeli Jews
DRB1*0401	✓	✓	Koreans, Caucasians, Greeks, Argentineans, French, Turkish
DRB1*0404	✓	✓	Chinese, Caucasians, Argentineans
DRB1*0405	✓	✓	Koreans, Japanese, Chinese, Spaniard, Greeks, Turkish, Malays
DRB1*0408	✓		Caucasians
DRB1*0410	✓	✓	Japanese, Chinese
DRB1*1001	✓		South Africans, Spaniards, Indians
DRB1*1402	✓		Yakima Indians, Peruvians

Other non-HLA genes located in chromosome 6, and specifically within the MHC region, have been the subject of intense investigation in patients with RA, as their products appear to play a pivotal role in the inflammatory process, which characterizes this condition. One of these is the cytokine tumor necrosis factor (TNF)-α, currently a strong candidate susceptibility gene for RA. Some studies have found associations between certain TNF-α alleles and susceptibility to RA or disease severity[32,160–164], but Gallagher *et al.* could not detect the independent contribution of the TNF genes to the genetic etiology of RA in Caucasians[165]. Finally, other MHC and non-MHC genes have been studied in a large number of affected sib-pairs using either a genome-wide screen strategy or a candidate gene screen approach (Type 2-transporter-associated antigen processing (TAP2), corticotrophin-releasing hormone, estrogen synthase (CYP19), IFN-γ, IL-10 and others)); however, the detailed description of these studies is beyond the scope of this chapter (see Chapter XX for further discussion of the subject).

Environmental factors

Infectious agents

As noted before, the possible infectious etiology of RA has been a theme of interest and discussion within the rheumatology community for decades[166]. Different infectious agents have been implicated in the causation of this disease but, even if they can induce a syndrome clinically indistinguishable from RA, they are relatively infrequent and thus can only explain a fraction of the cases (or of the cause) of RA (attributable risk)[167]. That is the case, for example, for *Borrelia burgdorferi* (Lyme disease), parvovirus B-19 (Fifth disease), or rubella virus, to cite but a few[168,169]. Given the worldwide distribution of RA, more than one microbe must be involved in its causation. It is possible, however, that the infectious agent responsible for RA originated in America and became distributed worldwide after Europeans came into contact with the native populations of the New World[7]. We know that infectious agents may be relatively isolated by geographic barriers, lack of proper ecological requirements to complete their vital cycle, or lack of exposure to humans. In fact syphilis, for example, was unknown to the inhabitants of the Old World prior to Columbus, Lyme disease is limited to ecosystems with the capabilities of sustaining the vital cycle of *Borrelia burgdorferi*, and several viral infections which originated in Africa have only appeared in humans relatively recently (*Ebola* virus, and the human immunodeficiency virus, to cite but two)[170,171].

It is conceivable that, in the genetically predisposed individual, more than one environmental noxa, infectious or not, triggers the development of RA by initiating an immunopathologic reaction leading to a cascade of events initially characterized by inflammation (predominantly at the articular level) and later by joint destruction. If an infectious agent (not necessarily the entire organism, but a microbial product) is involved in RA, it is likely to be through molecular mimicry of specific microbial peptides with autologous molecules such as the rheumatoid epitope or cartilage-derived epitopes rather than by actual conventional seeding of the joint cavity and its structures[172–174].

Hormonal factors

RA, as with many other rheumatic disorders associated with alterations of the immune system/response, occurs more frequently in women (and during their reproductive years) than in men, leading investigators to pursue the role sex hormones may play in disease susceptibility and modulation. In general, estrogens exert a stimulatory effect on the immune system by inhibiting T-cell suppressor function and facilitating T-cell maturation[175].

Pregnancy

The beneficial effect of pregnancy in the clinical manifestations of RA was first reported by Garrod over a century ago and confirmed by Hench during the 1930s[176]. An improvement in the symptoms occurs in about three-quarters of pregnancies, but, with rare exceptions, arthritis returns by the third to fourth month after delivery[177]. This effect was initially linked to the production of steroids by the placenta. Subsequent studies demonstrated that the placenta produces a pregnancy-associated glycoprotein (PAG)[178], an anti-inflammatory/immunomodulatory protein which is present in high concentrations during pregnancy with levels declining in the postpartum period in those women with RA experiencing improvement of their symptoms during pregnancy.

Other non-HLA factors that probably contribute to the amelioration and ultimate reactivation of the disease in pregnancy are IgG galactosylation abnormalities[179]. Healthy individuals, with the exception of the perinatal period and ages older than 40 years, maintain a low proportion of agalactosyl IgG (IgG-G0), a glycosylation pattern also normally found during pregnancy. RA patients exhibit increased IgG-G0, and animal models suggest that these IgGs may be directly involved in the pathogenesis of the disease[180]. The findings of (a) a correlation between changes in disease activity and changes in IgG-G0 during pregnancy and postpartum[181] and (b) an elevation in the IgG-G0 level preceding the first clinical symptoms of RA in Pima Indians, support the hypothesis that IgG galactosylation abnormalities may constitute an independent susceptibility factor in RA[182].

Finally, it has been proposed that remissions occurring during pregnancy relate to the maternal immune response to the paternal HLA antigens, as remissions are more likely to occur when there is maternal—paternal HLA disparity (for HLA-DRB1, -DQA, and -DQB) than when there is none[183]. That there is interplay between the immune system and sex hormones is further supported by the increased occurrence of RA after the first pregnancy in which there was fetal—maternal HLA disparity.

The data reviewed suggest that the remissions observed during pregnancy relate to the transient effect of hormonal and non-hormonal factors. Whatever its cause, the effect reverts or normalizes in the postpartum period, which explains the flares observed at that time in women experiencing remissions of their disease while pregnant. The net effect of pregnancy in the long-term prognosis of women with RA, however, is not known.

The relationship between parity and RA is also being elucidated. Women that have been pregnant are less likely to develop RA than nulliparous women, independent of family history and the use of oral contraceptives. As shown by Dugowson et al. [184], parity has a protective effect, or nulliparity is a risk factor for RA with an odds ratio (OR) of 2.2. In an extension of the prior study, Nelson et al. found that, as compared to nulliparous women, the OR for developing RA 1–2 years after a term pregnancy was 0.40, 0.30 for 2–3 years, and 0.20 from 3–4 years afterwards[177].

Oral contraceptives
The possible protective and modulatory effect of oral contraceptives (OC) in RA has been extensively studied, with data either supporting or denying such effect[59]. Two independently conducted studies in the US and England, published in the late 1970s to early 1980s, supported the possible protective role of the birth control pill in RA[185]. In the US study, a secular declining trend (coinciding with the introduction and utilization of the birth control pill) was observed among women but not men[28], while in the English study RA occurred less frequently among users than among non-users of the pill[185]. A more recent case-control study from Ireland has reinforced this idea[186], although studies that have not supported the protective role of the pill have been interpreted as reflecting differences in the populations studied rather than true differences. So far, one of the most plausible explanations for these discrepancies has come from the meta-analysis conducted by Spector and Hochberg, who divided the studies according to whether they were hospital-based or population-based. The pooled OR from the hospital-based studies was 0.49

whereas it was 0.95 for the population-based studies. These differences suggest that OCs protect against severe disease which requires hospital referral rather than protecting against its occurrence[187]. Overall, however, it has not been possible to reach consensus as to the purported protective effect of OCs in RA[59,188].

Hormonal replacement therapy
The use of hormonal replacement therapy (HRT) during the postmenopausal years has been associated with the occurrence of SLE (relative risk of 2.10 for ever-users and 2.50 for current users) and with lupus flares[189]. In contrast, HRT may have a beneficial effect in RA by ameliorating bone loss without exacerbating the joint disease[190,191]. No evidence has been found about a possible protective effect of HRT for the development of RA[186], although a modest reduction in the risk of developing RA among progestin users has been reported[192].

Androgens
Lower concentrations of androgenic steroids have been found in both men and women with RA[193,194] and it has been proposed that androgens may have a very mild disease-modifying effect in RA[195].

Dietary factors
Several aspects related to the potential role of diets in the development of RA have been studied. For example, inflammatory reactions, which generate free radicals that produce cellular oxidative damage, and free radicals themselves, have been identified in the synovial fluid of RA patients, supporting the role of these compounds in the pathogenesis of RA[196]; antioxidants can ameliorate the effect of free radicals, acting as scavengers of these products and preventing their harmful effects[197]. Based on these facts, it has been hypothesized that a higher intake of antioxidant micronutrients such as vitamin C (ascorbic acid), vitamin E (α-tocoferol), β-carotene, selenium, or β-cryptoxanthin protect from the development of RA. Several case-control studies[198–200] have addressed this issue by examining the serum levels of antioxidants in stored samples of large populations where several incident cases of RA had been observed over time; overall, a negative association between antioxidant levels and RA was found, although for the most part, these associations were weak or not statistically significant. In addition, serum samples that have been stored for a long time may not be reliable as time may affect the stability of the micronutrients; moreover, antioxidant serum levels may not properly reflect their dietary intake other than for β-carotene[201].

Other researchers have focused their attention on the dietary intake of vegetables and fruits (which are rich in antioxidants) and its relationship with the occurrence of RA[202,203]. An inverse association between fruit and vegetable intake and RA has been suggested in these studies, although a negative association between vegetable consumption and RA was found to be significant in only one of them. Only a few studies have specifically investigated the dietary intake of antioxidants; in fact lower levels of vitamin C and β-cryptoxanthin have been found in individuals who developed the disease[203–205]. However, these data have been obtained using questionnaires, which are known to introduce a recall bias; thus firm conclusions about the association of antioxidant intake and RA cannot be reached to date.

The intake of fatty acids have also been investigated in relation to RA. Diverse pro-inflammatory molecules, for example, generic eicosanoids such as prostaglandins and leukotrienes, derive from phospholipids present in cell membranes. The main source of eicosanoids is arachidonic acid, which is synthesized from Ω-6 fatty acids; in contrast, Ω-3 fatty acids are precursors of eicosapentaenoic acid, which is less inflammatory than the eicosanoids. Therefore, a diet rich in Ω-3 fatty acids has been proposed for the treatment of several chronic inflammatory diseases. Supporting this assertion is the fact that Eskimo and some Pacific Islander populations, which adhere to a diet rich in Ω-3 fatty acids, have lower incidence and prevalence rates of RA than other indigenous (and non-indigenous) populations in North America[206]. However, other studies have found a weak association between fish and olive oil consumption (the main dietary sources of 6-3 fatty acids) and lower risk for the occurrence of RA[202,205,207]. Several RA dietary supplementation trials with fish oil, rather than with natural dietary sources, were conducted in the 1980s, with very modest results based on the evidence reviewed[208–210].

Anecdotal reports have associated RA with other dietary components. For example, data from an international study showed a positive correlation between meat and offal intake and the prevalence of RA[211]. Vitamin D has been recently reported to be negatively associated with the occurrence of RA, although the significance was borderline[212]. Finally, in a cross-sectional study a correlation between impaired vitamin B_6 status and disease activity was found[213].

Lifestyle habits

Smoking appears to influence not only the course of the disease in a dose-dependent manner[36,214–216], but also to increase the risk of developing RA[217–219]. Specifically, it has been reported that tobacco use is linearly related to the concentration of RF, and also associates with radiographic damage, pulmonary involvement, and nodule formation[220,221]. Smoking could act as a modulating factor in the genetically predisposed individual, as postulated by Padyukov *et al.*[222]. The effects of smoking affect both genders[223,224], although they appear to be stronger in men than in women[225–227]. Smoking seems to be also more highly associated with the development of seropositive than with seronegative RA[224–226,228] and with the non-familial forms of the disease[220]. Smoking may exert systemic deleterious effects by altering nitric oxide pathways, perturbing local and systemic immune functions, and affecting the vascular endothelium[229]. Tobacco-induced mutations in the p53 tumor suppressor gene have been proposed as another possible mechanism for this etiologic effect in RA. The p53 suppressor gene plays a major role in DNA repair; its mutations are closely related to some types of tumors. Overexpression of this gene has been observed in RA[230] and it has been hypothesized that alterations in its structure and function could play a role in the phenotypic transformations that RA synoviocytes undergo[225].

A relationship between coffee consumption and RA has been suggested but the data have been inconsistent[231,232]. In a recent, well-designed study, such association was not found. Likewise, the possible association between RA and the consumption of alcoholic beverages has been examined by some investigators, with inconclusive results[201].

Others

Some other person-related attributes, particularly years of formal education[233] and marital status[234] (proxies for socioeconomic status), appear to impact the course and ultimate outcome of the disease rather than the susceptibility to its occurrence, although in one study an inverse relation between RA itself and the level of education was found[235]. In the same study, a relationship between RA and a decrease in the occurrence of atopic allergy, being born in households with private wells, and residency in areas with exposure to mold and to farm animals was found[235]. These studies have not considered, however, the possible confounding role of smoking; thus the relationship between markers of low socioeconomic status and outcome in RA deserves to be further examined.

Conclusions

Significant advances have been made over the last few decades in understanding the events leading to joint destruction in patients with RA. As the factors responsible for disease causation and modulation are better understood and new therapies are developed, it is conceivable that patients can be better categorized at disease onset into subsets with divergent expected outcomes, with patients treated accordingly, and the devastating effects of the disease significantly curtailed. Large, multi-center, multinational cohorts of patients with early disease in whom sociodemographic, clinical, radiographic, functional, serologic, cellular, hormonal, genetic, and tissue datasets and repositories are established will certainly be necessary for success to occur. These initiatives are in progress in North America, Continental Europe and the United Kingdom, and have just been initiated in Latin America.

Acknowledgement

To Ella Henderson for her expert assistance in the preparation of this chapter.

References

1. Heyse, S. Design and conduct of collaborative international epidemiological studies of rheumatic diseases. *Rheum Dis Clin North Am* 1990; **16**: 763–72.

2. Allander, E. Conflict between epidemiological and clinical diagnosis of rheumatoid arthritis in a population sample. *Scand J Rheumatol* 1973; **2**: 109–12.

3. Arnett, F. C., Edworthy, S. M., Bloch, D. A., McShane, D. J., Fries, J. F., Cooper, N. S. *et al.* The American Rheumatism Association 1987 revised criteria for the classification of rheumatoid arthritis. *Arthritis Rheum* 1988; **31**: 315–24.

4. Ropes, M. W., Bennett, G. A., Cobb, S., Jacox, R., and Jessar, R. A. 1958 revision of diagnostic criteria for rheumatoid arthritis. *Bull Rheum Dis* 1958; **9**: 175–6.

5. Jacobsson, L. T., Knowler, W. C., Pillemer, S., Hanson, R. L, Pettitt, D. J., McCance, D. R. *et al.* A cross-sectional and longitudinal comparison of the Rome criteria for active rheumatoid arthritis equivalent to the American College of Rheumatology 1958 criteria and the American College of Rheumatology 1987 criteria for rheumatoid arthritis. *Arthritis Rheum* 1994; **37**: 1479–86.

6. Lawrence, R. C., Hochberg, M. C., Kelsey, J. L., McDuffie, F. C., Medsger, T. A., Jr., Felts, W. R. *et al.* Estimates of the prevalence of selected arthritic and musculoskeletal diseases in the United States. *J Rheumatol* 1989; **16**: 427–41.

7. Rothschild, B. M., Woods, R. J., Rothschild, C., and Sebes, J. I. Geographic distribution of rheumatoid arthritis in ancient North America: implications for pathogenesis. *Semin Arthritis Rheum* 1992; **22**: 181–7.

8. Appelboom, T., and Halberg, P. Rheumatoid arthritis and other synovial disorders: history. In *Rheumatology* (Hochberg, M. C., Silman, A. J., Smolen, J. S., Weinblatt, M. E., and Weisman, M. H., eds), pp. 753–56. London: Mosby-Year Book; 2003.

9. Arriaza, B. T., Salo, W., Aufderheide, A. C., and Holcomb, T. A. Pre-Columbian tuberculosis in Northern Chile: molecular and skeletal evidence. *Am J Phys Anthropol* 1995; **98**: 37–45.

10. Martinez-Lavín, M., Mansilla, J., Pineda, C., and Pijoan, C. Ankylosing spondylitis is indigenous to Mesoamerica. *J Rheumatol* 1995; **22**: 2327–30.

11. Rothschild, B. M. Paleopathology, its character and contribution to understanding and distinguishing among rheumatologic disease: perspectives on rheumatoid arthritis and spondyloarthropathy. *Clin Exp Rheumatol* 1995; **13**: 657–62.

12. Kalla, A. A., and Tikly, M. Rheumatoid arthritis in the developing world. *Best Pract Res Clin Rheumatol* 2003; **17**: 863–75.

13. Dai, S. M., Han, X. H., Zhao, D. B., Shi, Y. Q., Liu, Y., and Meng, J. M. Prevalence of rheumatic symptoms, rheumatoid arthritis, ankylosing spondylitis, and gout in Shanghai, China: a COPCORD study. *J Rheumatol* 2003; **30**: 2245–51.

14. Spindler, A., Bellomio, V., Berman, A., Lucero, E., Baigorria, M., Paz, S. *et al.* Prevalence of rheumatoid arthritis in Tucuman, Argentina. *J Rheumatol* 2002; **29**: 1166–70.

15. Anaya, J. M., Correa, P. A., Mantilla, R. D., Jimenez, F., Kuffner T., and McNicholl, J. M. Rheumatoid arthritis in African Colombians from Quibdo. *Semin Arthritis Rheum* 2001; **31**: 191–8.

16. Darmarwan, J., Muirden, K., Vakenburg, H., and Wigley, R. The epidemiology of rheumatoid arthritis in Indonesia. *Br J Rheumatol* 1993; **32**: 357–40.

17. Hameed, K., Gibson, T., Kadir, M., Sultana, S., Fatima, Z., and Syed, A. The prevalence of rheumatoid arthritis in affluent and poor urban communities of Pakistan. *Br J Rheumatol* 1995; **34**: 252–6.

18. Hameed, K., and Gibson, T. A comparison of the prevalence of rheumatoid arthritis and other rheumatic diseases among Pakistanis living in England and Pakistan. *Br J Rheumatol* 1997; **36**: 781–5.

19. Abdel-Nasser, A. M., Rasker, J. J., and Valkenburg, H. A. Epidemiological and clinical aspects relating to the variability of rheumatoid arthritis. *Semin Arthritis Rheum* 1997; **27**: 123–40.

20. Willkens, R. F., Blandau, R. L., Aoyama, D. T., and Beasley, P. Studies of rheumatoid arthritis among a tribe of Northwest Indians. *J Rheumatol* 1976; **3**: 9–14.

21. Harvey, J., Lotze, M., Arnett, F. C., Bias, W. B., Billingsley, L. M., Harvey, E. *et al.* Rheumatoid arthritis in a Chippewa band. II. Field study with clinical, serological, and HLA-D correlations. *J Rheumatol* 1983; **10**: 28–32.

22. Drosos, A. A., Alamanos, I., Voulgari, P. V., Psychos, D. N., Katsaraki, A., Papadopoulos, I. *et al.* Epidemiology of adult rheumatoid arthritis in Northwest Greece 1987–1995. *J Rheumatol* 1997; **24**: 2129–33.

23. Carmona, L., Villaverde, V., Hernandez-Garcia, C., Ballina, J., Gabriel, R., Laffon, A. *et al.* The prevalence of rheumatoid arthritis in the general population of Spain. *Rheumatol* 2002; **41**: 88–95.

24. Riise, T., Jacobsen, B. K., and Gran, J. T. Incidence and prevalence of rheumatoid arthritis in the county of Troms, northern Norway. *J Rheumatol* 2000; **27**: 1386–9.

25. Saraux, A., Guedes, C., Allain, J., Devauchelle, V., Valls, I., Lamour, A. *et al.* Prevalence of rheumatoid arthritis and spondyloarthropathy in Brittany, France. Societe de Rhumatologie de l'Ouest. *J Rheumatol* 1999; **26**: 2622–7.

26. Power, D., Codd, M., Ivers. L., Sant, S., and Barry, M. Prevalence of rheumatoid arthritis in Dublin, Ireland: a population based survey. *Irish J Med Sci* 1999; **168**: 197–200.

27. Jacobsson, L. T., and Pillemer, S. R. What can we learn about rheumatic diseases by studying Pima Indians? *J Rheumatol* 1994; **21**: 1179–82.

28. Linos, A., Worthington, J. W., O'Fallon, W. M., and Kurland, L. T. The epidemiology of rheumatoid arthritis in Rochester, Minnesota: a study of incidence prevalence and mortality. *Am J Epidemiol* 1980; **111**: 87–98.

29. Gabriel, S. E. The epidemiology of rheumatoid arthritis. *Rheum Dis Clin North Am* 2001; **27**: 269–81.

30. Doran, M. F., Pond, G. R., Crowson, C. S., O'Fallon, W. M., and Gabriel, S. E. Trends in incidence and mortality in rheumatoid arthritis in Rochester, Minnesota, over a forty-year period. *Arthritis Rheum* 2002; **46**: 625–31.

31. Wakitani, S., Murata, N., Toda, Y., Ogawa, R., Kaneshige, T., Nishimura, Y. *et al.* The relationship between HLA-DRB1 alleles and disease subsets of rheumatoid arthritis in Japanese. *Br J Rheumatol* 1997; **36**: 630–6.

32. Hajeer, A., John, S., Ollier, W. E., Silman, A. J., Dawes, P., Hassell, A. *et al.* Tumor necrosis factor microsatellite haplotypes are different in male and female patients with RA. *J Rheumatol* 1997; **24**: 217–19.

33. Chopra, A., Raghunath, D., and Singh, A. Chronic inflammatory polyarthritides in a select population of young men: a prospective study. *J Assoc Physicians India* 1989; **37**: 748–51.

34. Barker, J. A., and Sebes, J. I. Rheumatoid arthritis of the robust-reaction type. *Arthritis Rheum* 1998; **41**: 1131–2.

35. Weyand, C. M., Schmidt, D., Wager, U., and Goronzy, J. J. The influence of sex on the phenotype of rheumatoid arthritis. *Arthritis Rheum* 1998; **41**: 817–22.

36. Saag, K. G., Cerhan, J. R., Kolluri, S., Ohashi, K., Hunninghake, G. W., and Schwartz, D. A. Cigarette smoking and rheumatoid arthritis severity. *Ann Rheum Dis* 1997; **56**: 463–69.

37. Yukioka, M., Wakitani, S., Murata, N., Toda, Y., Ogawa, R., Kaneshige, T. *et al.* Elderly-onset rheumatoid arthritis and its association with HLA-DRB1 alleles in Japanese. *Br J Rheumatol* 1998; **37**: 98–101.

38. Symmons, D. P., Barrett, E. M., Bankhead, C. R., Scott, D. G., and Silman, A. J. The incidence of rheumatoid arthritis in the United Kingdom: results from the Norfolk Arthritis Register. *Br J Rheumatol* 1994; **33**: 735–9.

39. Cerna, M., Vavrincova, P., Havelka, S., Ivaskova, E., and Stastny, P. Class II alleles in juvenile arthritis in Czech children. *J Rheumatol* 1994; **21**: 159–64.

40. Thomson, W., Pepper, L., Payton, A., Carthy, D., Scott, D., Ollier, W. *et al.* Absence of an association between HLA-DRB1*04 and rheumatoid arthritis in newly diagnosed cases from the community. *Ann Rheum Dis* 1993; **52**: 539–41.

41. Silman, A. J. Problems complicating the genetic epidemiology of rheumatoid arthritis. *J Rheumatol* 1997; **24**: 194–6.

42. Kaipiainen-Seppanen, O., Aho, K., Isomaki, H., and Laakso, M. Shift in the incidence of rheumatoid arthritis toward elderly patients in Finland during 1975–1990. *Clin Exp Rheumatol* 1996; **14**: 537–42.

43. Imanaka, T., Shichikawa, K., Inoue, K., Shimaoka, Y., Takenaka, Y., and Wakitani, S. Increase in age at onset of rheumatoid arthritis in Japan over a 30 year period. *Ann Rheum Dis* 1997; **56**: 313–16.

44. Shiozawa, K., Tanaka, Y., Imura, S., and Shiozawa, S. Elderly-onset rheumatoid arthritis: ageing as an independent marker for better prognosis. *Arthritis Rheum* 1997; **40**: S151.

45. van Schaardenburg, D., and Breedveld, F. C. Elderly-onset rheumatoid arthritis. *Semin Arthritis Rheum* 1994; **23**: 367–78.

46. Adler, E. Rheumatoid arthritis with the onset in the old age. *Isr J Med Sci* 1966; **2**: 607–13.

47. Corrigan, A. B., Robinson, R. G., Terenty, T. R., Dick-Smith, J. B., and Walters, D. Benign rheumatoid arthritis of the aged. *BMJ* 1974; 1: 444–6.

48. McCarty, D. J., O'Duffy, J. D., Pearson, L., and Hunter, J. B. Remitting seronegative symmetrical synovitis with pitting edema: RS3PE Syndrome. *J Am Med Assoc* 1985; 254: 2763–7.

49. Olivieri, I., Salvarani, C., and Cantini, F. Remitting distal extremity swelling with pitting edema: a distinct syndrome or a clinical feature of different inflammatory rheumatic diseases? *J Rheumatol* 1997; 24: 249–52.

50. van Schaardenburg, D., Hazes, J. M., de Boer, A., Zwinderman, A. H., Meijers, K. A. E., and Breedveld, F. C. Outcome of rheumatoid arthritis in relation to age and rheumatoid factor at diagnosis. *J Rheumatol* 1993; 20: 45–52.

51. Pease, C. T., Bhakta, B. B., Devlin, J., and Emery, P. Does the age of onset of rheumatoid arthritis influence phenotype? A prospective study of outcome and prognostic factors. *Rheumatology* 1999; 38: 228–34.

52. van der Heijde, D. M., van Riel, P. L., van Leeuwen, M. A., van't Hof, M. A., van Rijswijk, M. H., and van de Putte, L. B., Older versus younger onset rheumatoid arthritis: results at onset and after 2 years of a prospective followup study of early rheumatoid arthritis. *J Rheumatol* 1991; 18: 1285–9.

53. Calvo-Alén, J., Corrales, A., Sanchez-Andrada, S., Fernández-Echevarria, M. A., Peña, J. L., and Rodríguez-valverde, V. Outcome of late-onset rheumatoid arthritis. *Clin Rheumatol* 2005; 5 March e-publication ahead of print.

54. Silman, A., Bankhead, C., Rowlingson, B., Brennan, P., Symmons, D., and Gatrell, A. Do new cases of rheumatoid arthritis cluster in time or in space? *Int J Epidemiol* 1997; 26: 628–34.

55. Hochberg, M. C. Changes in the incidence and prevalence of rheumatoid arthritis in England and Wales, 1970–1982. *Semin Arthritis Rheum* 1990; 19: 294–302.

56. Jacobsson, L. T. H., Hanson, R. L., Knowler, W. C., Pillemer, S., Pettitt, D. J., and McCance, D. R. *et al.* Decreasing incidence and prevalence of rheumatoid arthritis in Pima Indians over a twenty-five-year period. *Arthritis Rheum* 1994; 37: 1158–65.

57. Silman, A. J. The changing face of rheumatoid arthritis: why the decline in incidence? *Arthritis Rheum* 2002; 46: 579–81.

58. Adebajo, A. O. Rheumatoid arthritis: a twentieth century disease in Africa? *Arthritis Rheum* 1991; 34: 248–9.

59. Brennan, P., Bankhead, C., Silman, A., and Symmons, D. Oral contraceptives and rheumatoid arthritis: results from a primary care-based incident case-control study. *Semin Arthritis Rheum* 1997; 26: 817–23.

60. Heikkila, S., and Isomaki, H. Long-term outcome of rheumatoid arthritis has improved. *Scand J Rheumatol* 1994; 23: 13–15.

61. Silman, A. J. Trends in the incidence and severity of rheumatoid arthritis. *J Rheumatol* 1992; 32 (Suppl.): 71–3.

62. Laurent, R., Robinson, R. G., Beller, E. M., and Buchanan, W. W. Incidence and severity of rheumatoid arthritis: the view from Australia. *Br J Rheumatol* 1989; 28: 360–1.

63. Ward, M. M. Decreases in rates of hospitalizations for manifestations of severe rheumatoid arthritis, 1983–2001. *Arthritis Rheum* 2004; 50: 1122–31.

64. Buchanan, W. W., and Murdoch, R. M. Hypothesis: that rheumatoid arthritis will disappear. *J Rheumatol* 1979; 6: 324–9.

65. Fries, J. F. Toward an understanding of patient outcome measurement. *Arthritis Rheum* 1983; 26: 697–704.

66. Wolfe, F., Mitchell, D. M., Sibley, J. T., Fries, J. F., Bloch, D. A., and Williams, C. A. *et al.* The mortality of rheumatoid arthritis. *Arthritis Rheum* 1994; 37: 481–94.

67. Martinez, M. S., Garcia-Monforte, A., and Rivera, J. Survival study of rheumatoid arthritis patients in Madrid Spain: a 9-year prospective follow-up. *Scand J Rheumatol* 2001; 30: 195–8.

68. Jacobsson, L. T., Knowler, W. C., Pillemer, S., Hanson, R. L., Pettitt, D. J., and Nelson RG *et al.* Rheumatoid arthritis and mortality: a longitudinal study in Pima Indians. *Arthritis Rheum* 1993; 36: 1045–53.

69. Myllykangas-Luosujarvi, R., Aho, K., Kautiainen, H., and Isomaki, H. Cardiovascular mortality in women with rheumatoid arthritis. *J Rheumatol* 1995; 22: 1065–7.

70. Riise, T., Jacobsen, B. K., Gran, J. T., Haga, H.- J., and Arnesen, E. Total mortality is increased in rheumatoid arthritis: a 17-year prospective study. *Clin Rheumatol* 2001; 20: 123–7.

71. Lindqvist, E., and Eberhardt, K. Mortality in rheumatoid arthritis patients with disease onset in the 1980s. *Ann Rheum Dis* 1999; 58: 11–14.

72. Peltomaa, R., Paimela, L., Kautiainen, H., and Leirisalo-Repo, M. Mortality in patients with rheumatoid arthritis treated actively from the time of diagnosis. *Ann Rheum Dis* 2002; 61: 889–94.

73. Kroot, E. J., van Leeuwen, M. A., van Rijswijk, M. H., Prevoo, M. L., van't Hof, M. A., and van de Putte, L. B. *et al.* No increased mortality in patients with rheumatoid arthritis: up to 10 years of follow up from disease onset. *Ann Rheum Dis* 2000; 59: 954–8.

74. Symmons, D. P., Jones, M. A., Scott, D. L., and Prior, P. Longterm mortality outcome in patients with rheumatoid arthritis: early presenters continue to do well. *J Rheumatol* 1998; 25: 1072–7.

75. Gabriel, S. E., Crowson, C. S., Kremers, H. M., Doran, M. F., Turesson, C., O'Fallon, W. M. *et al.* Survival in rheumatoid arthritis: a population-based analysis of trends over 40 years. *Arthritis Rheum* 2003; 48: 54–8.

76. Gabriel, S. E., Crowson, C. S., and O'Fallon, W. M. Mortality in rheumatoid arthritis: have we made an impact in 4 decades? *J Rheumatol* 1999; 26: 2529–33.

77. Vandenbroucke, J. P., Hazevoet, H. M., and Cats, A. Survival and cause of death in rheumatoid arthritis: a 25-year prospective follow-up. *J Rheumatol* 1984; 11: 158–61.

78. Kvalvik, A. G., Jones, M. A., and Symmons, D. P. Mortality in a cohort of Norwegian patients with rheumatoid arthritis followed from 1977 to 1992. *Scand J Rheumatol* 2000; 29: 29–37.

79. Wolfe, F., and Zwillich, S. H. The long-term outcomes of rheumatoid arthritis: a 23-year prospective, longitudinal study of total joint replacement and its predictors in 1,600 patients with rheumatoid arthritis. *Arthritis Rheum* 1998; 41: 1072–82.

80. Prior, P., Symmons, D. P. M., Scott, D. L., Brown, R., and Hawkins, C. F. Cause of death in rheumatoid arthritis. *Br J Rheumatol* 1984; 23: 92–9.

81. Mutru, O., Laakso, M., Isomaki, H., and Koota, K. Ten year mortality and causes of death in patients with rheumatoid arthritis. *Br Med J Clin Res Ed* 1985; 290: 1811–13.

82. Mitchell, D. M., Spitz, P. W., Young, D. Y., Bloch, D. A., McShane, D. J., and Fries, J. F. Survival, prognosis, and causes of death in rheumatoid arthritis. *Arthritis Rheum* 1986; 29: 706–14.

83. Cibere, J., Sibley, J., and Haga, M. Rheumatoid arthritis and the risk of malignancy. *Arthritis Rheum* 1997; 40: 1580–6.

84. Wallberg-Jonsson, S., Ohman, M. L., and Dahlqvist, S. R. Cardiovascular morbidity and mortality in patients with seropositive rheumatoid arthritis in Northern Sweden. *J Rheumatol* 1997; 24: 445–51.

85. Maradit-Kremers, H., Crowson, C. S., Nicola, P. J., Ballman, K. V., Roger, V. L., and Jacobsen, S. J. *et al.* Increased unrecognized coronary heart disease and sudden death in rheumatoid arthritis: a population-based cohort study. *Arthritis Rheum* 2005; 52: 402–11.

86. Maradit-Kremers, H., Nicola, P. J., Crowson, C. S., Ballman, K. V., and Gabriel, S. E. Cardiovascular death in rheumatoid arthritis: a population-based study. *Arthritis Rheum* 2005; 52: 722–32.

87. Solomon, D. H., Curhan, G. C., Rimm, E. B., Cannuscio, C. C., and Karlson, E. W. Cardiovascular risk factors in women with and without rheumatoid arthritis. *Arthritis Rheum* 2004; 50: 3444–9.

88. Bacon, P. A., Stevens, R. J., Carruthers, D. M., Young, S. P., and Kitas, G. D. Accelerated atherogenesis in autoimmune rheumatic diseases. *Autoimmun Rev* 2002; 1: 338–47.

89. Del Rincon, I., Williams, K., Stern, M. P., Freeman, G. L., O'Leary, D. H., and Escalante, A. Association between carotid atherosclerosis and markers of inflammation in rheumatoid arthritis patients and healthy subjects. *Arthritis Rheum* 2003; 48: 1833–40.

90. Callahan, L. F., Pincus, T., Huston, J. W. I., Brooks, R. H., Nance, E. P., Jr., and Kaye, J. J. Measures of activity and damage in rheumatoid arthritis: depiction of changes and prediction of mortality over five years. *Arthritis Care Res* 1997; 10: 381–94.

91. Pincus, T., Brooks, R. H., and Callahan, L. F. Prediction of long-term mortality in patients with rheumatoid arthritis according to simple

questionnaire and joint count measures. *Ann Intern Med* 1994; **120**: 26–34.

92. Morgan, S. L., Baggott, J. E., Lee J. Y., and Alarcón, G. S. Folic acid supplementation prevents deficient blood folate levels and hyperhomocysteinemia during longterm, low dose methotrexate therapy for rheumatoid arthritis: implications for cardiovascular disease prevention. *J Rheumatol* 1998; **25**: 441–6.

93. Landewe, R. B., van den Borne, B. E., Breedveld, F. C., and Dijkmans, B. A. Methotrexate effects in patients with rheumatoid arthritis with cardiovascular comorbidity. *Lancet* 2000; **355**: 1616–17.

94. Krause, D., Schleusser, B., Herborn, G., and Rau, R. Response to methotrexate treatment is associated with reduced mortality in patients with severe rheumatoid arthritis. *Arthritis Rheum* 2000; **43**: 14–21.

95. Choi, H. K., Hernan, M. A., Seeger, J. D., Robins, J. M., and Wolfe, F. Methotrexate and mortality in patients with rheumatoid arthritis: a prospective study. *Lancet* 2002; **359**: 1173–7.

96. McKendry, R. J. R., and Dale, P. Adverse effects of low dose methotrexate therapy in rheumatoid arthritis. *J Rheumatol* 1993; **20**: 1850–6.

97. Alarcón, G. S., Tracy, I. C., Strand, G. M., Singh, K., and Macaluso, M. Survival and drug discontinuation analyses in a large cohort of methotrexate-treated rheumatoid arthritis patients. *Ann Rheum Dis* 1995; **54**: 708–12.

98. Callahan, L. F., and Pincus, T. Reassessment of twelve traditional paradigms concerning the diagnosis, prevalence, morbidity and mortality of rheumatoid arthritis. *Scand J Rheumatol* 1989; **79** (Suppl.): 67–96.

99. Roubenoff, R., Roubenoff, R. A., Cannon, J. G., Kehayias, J. J., Zhuang, H., and Dawson-Hughes, B. *et al.* Rheumatoid cachexia: cytokine-driven hypermetabolism accompanying reduced body cell mass in chronic inflammation. *J Clin Invest* 1994; **93**: 2379–86.

100. Collins, R., Jr., Dunn, T. L., Walthaw, J., Harrell, P., and Alarcón, G. S. Malnutrition in rheumatoid arthritis. *Clin Rheumatol* 1987; **6**: 391–8.

101. Kremers, H. M., Nicola, P. J., Crowson, C. S., Ballman, K. V., and Gabriel, S. E. Prognostic importance of low body mass index in relation to cardiovascular mortality in rheumatoid arthritis. *Arthritis Rheum* 2004; **50**: 3450–7.

102. Engelhart, M., Kondrup, J., Hoie, L. H., Andersen, V., Kristensen, J. H., and Heitmann, B. L. Weight reduction in obese patients with rheumatoid arthritis, with preservation of body cell mass and improvement of physical fitness. *Clin Exp Rheumatol* 1996; **14**: 289–93.

103. Kaye, J. J., Fuchs, H. A., Moseley, J. W., Nance, E. P., Jr., Callahan, L. F., and Pincus, T. Problems with the Steinbrocker staging system for radiographic assessment of the rheumatoid hand and wrist. *Invest Radiol* 1990; **25**: 536–44.

104. Larsen, A. Radiological grading of rheumatoid arthritis: an interobserver study. *Scand J Rheumatol* 1973; **2**: 136–8.

105. Sharp, J. T., Young, D. Y., Bluhm, G. B., Brook, A., Brower, A. C., and Corbett, M. *et al.* How many joints in the hands and wrists should be included in a score of radiologic abnormalities used to assess rheumatoid arthritis? *Arthritis Rheum* 1985; **28**: 1326–35.

106. Edmonds, J. P., Saudan, A., Lassere, M., and Scott, D. Introduction to reading radiographs by the Scott modification of the Larsen method. *J Rheumatol* 2004; **26**: 740–2.

107. van der Heijde, D. How to read radiographs according to the Sharp/van der Heijde method. *J Rheumatol* 2000; **27**: 261–3.

108. Molenaar, E. T. H., Boers, M., van der Heijde, D. M., Alarcón, G. S., Bresnihan, B., and Cardiel, M. *et al.* Imaging in rheumatoid arthritis: results of a group discussion. *J Rheumatol* 1999; **26**: 749–51.

109. Hansen, M., Florescu, A., Stoltenberg, M., Podenphant, J., Pedersen-Zbinden, B., and Horslev-Petersen, K. *et al.* Bone loss in rheumatoid arthritis: influence of disease activity, duration of the disease, functional capacity, and corticosteroid treatment. *Scand J Rheumatol* 1996; **25**: 367–76.

110. Kirwan, J. R. The effect of glucocorticoids on joint destruction in rheumatoid arthritis. The Arthritis and Rheumatism Council Low-Dose Glucocorticoid Study Group. *N Engl J Med* 1995; **333**: 142–6.

111. Paulus, H. E., DiPrimeo, D., Sanda, M., Lynch, J., Schwartz, B., and Sharp, J. *et al.* Progression of radiographic joint erosion during low dose corticosteroid treatment of rheumatoid arthritis. *J Rheumatol* 2000; **27**: 1632–7.

112. Saag, K. G., Criswell, L. A., Sems, K. M., Nettleman, M. D., and Kolluri, S. Low-dose corticosteroids in rheumatoid arthritis: a meta-analysis of their moderate-term effectiveness. *Arthritis Rheum* 1996; **39**: 1818–25.

113. Felson, D. T., Anderson, J. J., and Meenan, R. F. Use of short-term efficacy/toxicity tradeoffs to select second-line drugs in rheumatoid arthritis: a metaanalysis of published clinical trials. *Arthritis Rheum* 1992; **35**: 1117–25.

114. Morgan, S. L., Baggott, J. E., Vaughn, W. H., Austin, J. S., Veitch, T. A., Lee, J. Y. *et al.* Supplementation with folic acid during methotrexate therapy for rheumatoid arthritis: a double-blind, placebo-controlled trial. *Ann Intern Med* 1994; **121**: 833–41.

115. Ortiz, Z., Shea, B., Súarez-Almazor, M., Moher, D., Wells, G., and Tugwell, P. The efficacy of folic acid and folinic acid in reducing methotrexate gastrointestinal toxicity in rheumatoid arthritis: a metaanalysis of randomized controlled trials. *J Rheumatol* 1998; **25**: 36–43.

116. Bologna, C., Picot, M. C., Jorgensen, C., Viu, P., Verdier, R., and Sany, J. Study of eight cases of cancer in 426 rheumatoid arthritis patients treated with methotrexate. *Ann Rheum Dis* 1997; **56**: 97–102.

117. Kremer, J. M. Safety, efficacy, and mortality in a long-term cohort of patients with rheumatoid arthritis taking methotrexate: followup after a mean of 13.3 years. *Arthritis Rheum* 1997; **40**: 984–5.

118. Walker, A. M., Funch, D., Dreyer, N. A., Tolman, K. G., Kremer, J. M., Alarcón, G. S. *et al.* Determinants of serious liver disease among patients receiving low-dose methotrexate for rheumatoid arthritis. *Arthritis Rheum* 1993; **36**: 329–35.

119. Erickson, A. R., Reddy, V., Vogelgesang, S. A., and West, S. G. Usefulness of the American College of Rheumatology recommendations for liver biopsy in methotrexate-treated rheumatoid arthritis patients. *Arthritis Rheum* 1995; **38**: 1115–19.

120. Alarcón, G. S., Kremer, J. M., Macaluso, M., Weinblatt, M. E., Cannon, G. W., Palmer, W. R. *et al.* Risk factors for methotrexate-induced lung injury in patients with rheumatoid arthritis: a multicenter, case-control study. Methotrexate-Lung Study Group. *Ann Intern Med* 1997; **127**: 356–64.

121. Cannon, G. W. Methotrexate pulmonary toxicity. *Rheum Dis Clin North Am* 1997; **23**: 917–37.

122. Salloum, E., Cooper, D. L., Howe, G., Lacy, J., Tallini, G., Crouch, J. *et al.* Spontaneous regression of lymphoproliferative disorders in patients treated with methotrexate for rheumatoid arthritis and other rheumatic diseases. *J Clin Oncol* 1996; **14**: 1943–9.

123. Thomason, R. W., Craig, F. E., Banks, P. M., Sears, D. L., Myerson, G. E., and Gulley M. L. Epstein-Barr virus and lymphoproliferation in methotrexate-treated rheumatoid arthritis. *Mod Pathol* 1996; **9**: 261–6.

124. Lawrence, J. S., and Ball, J. Genetic studies on rheumatoid arthritis. *Ann Rheum Dis* 1958; **17**: 160–8.

125. Lawrence, J. S., Bremner, J. M., Ball, J., and Burch, T. A. Rheumatoid arthritis in a subtropical population. *Ann Rheum Dis* 1966; **25**: 59–66.

126. MacGregor, A. J., Snieder, H., Rigby, A. S., Koskenvuo, M., Kaprio, J., Aho, K. *et al.* Characterizing the quantitative genetic contribution to rheumatoid arthritis using data from twins. *Arthritis Rheum* 2000; **43**: 30–7.

127. Ollier, W., and MacGregor, A. Genetic epidemiology of rheumatoid arthritis. *BMJ* 1995; **51**: 267–85.

128. Stastny, P. Association of the B-cell alloantigen DRw4 with rheumatoid arthritis. *N Engl J Med* 1978; **298**: 869–71.

129. Weyand, C. M., Hicok, K. C., Conn, D. L., and Goronzy, J. J. The influence of HLA-DRB1 genes on disease severity in rheumatoid arthritis. *Ann Intern Med* 1992; **117**: 801–6.

130. Weyand, C. M., McCarthy, T. G., and Goronzy, J. J. Correlation between disease phenotype and genetic heterogeneity in rheumatoid arthritis. *J Clin Invest* 1995; **95**: 2120–6.

131. Templin, D. W., Boyer, G. S., Lanier, A. P., Nelson, J. L., Barrington, R. A., Hasen J. A. et al. Rheumatoid arthritis in Tlingit Indians: clinical characterization and HLA associations. *J Rheumatol* 1994; 21: 1238–44.

132. McDaniel, D. O., Alarcón, G. S., Pratt, P. W., and Reveille, J. D. Most African-American patients with rheumatoid arthritis do not have the rheumatoid antigenic determinant epitope. *Ann Intern Med* 1995; 123: 181–7.

133. Hameed, K., Bowman, S., Kondeatis, E., Vaughan, R., and Gibson, T. The association of HLA-DRB genes and the shared epitope with rheumatoid arthritis in Pakistan. *Br J Rheumatol* 1997; 36: 1184–8.

134. Toda, Y, Minamikawa, Y, Akagi, S., Sugano, H., Mori, Y, Nishimura, H. et al. Rheumatoid-susceptible alleles of HLA-DRB1 are genetically recessive to non-susceptible alleles in the progression of bone destruction in the wrists and fingers of patients with RA. *Ann Rheum Dis* 1994; 53: 587–92.

135. Toussirot, E., Auge, B., Tiberghien, P., Chabod, J., Cedoz, J. P., and Wendling, D. HLA-DRB1 alleles and shared amino acid sequences in disease susceptibility and severity in patients from eastern France with rheumatoid arthritis. *J Rheumatol* 1999; 26: 1446–51.

136. Nichol, F. E., and Woodrow, J. C. HLA DR antigens in Indian patients with rheumatoid arthritis. *Lancet* 1981; 1: 220–1.

137. Schiff, B., Mizrachi, Y, Orgad, S., Yaron, N., and Gazit, E. Association of HLA-Aw31 and HLA-DR1 with adult rheumatoid arthritis. *Ann Rheum Dis* 1982; 41: 403–4.

138. Christiansen, F. G., Kelly, H., and Dawkins, R. L. Histocompatibility testing. In *Rheumatoid arthritis* (Alber ED, Baur MP, Mayr WR, eds), pp. 378–83. Berlin: Springer-Verlag; 1984.

139. Stavropoulos, C., Spyropoulou, M., Koumantaki, Y, Kappou, I., Kaklamanis, P. V., Linos, A. et al. HLA-DRB1* genotypes in Greek rheumatoid arthritis patients: association with disease characteristics, sex and age at onset. *Br J Rheumatol* 1997; 36: 141–2.

140. Hong, G. H., Park, M. H., Takeuchi, F., Oh, M. D., Song, Y. W., Nabeta, H. et al. Association of specific amino acid sequence of HLA-DR with rheumatoid arthritis in Koreans and its diagnostic value. *J Rheumatol* 1996; 23: 1699–703.

141. MacGregor, A., Ollier, W., Thomson, W., Jawaheer, D., and Silman, A. HLA-DRB1 *0401/0404 genotype and rheumatoid arthritis: increased association in men, young age at onset, and disease severity. *J Rheumatol* 1995; 22: 1032–6.

142. Seglias, J., Li, E. K., Cohen, M. G., Wong, R. W., Potter, P. K., and So, A. K. Linkage between rheumatoid arthritis susceptibility and the presence of HLA-DR4 and DR beta allelic third hypervariable region sequences in Southern Chinese persons. *Arthritis Rheum* 1992; 35: 163–7.

143. Koh, W. H., Chan, S. H., Lin, Y. N., and Boey, M. L. Association of HLA-DRB1*0405 with extraarticular manifestations and erosions in Singaporean Chinese with rheumatoid arthritis. *J Rheumatol* 1997; 24: 629–32.

144. Yelamos, J., García-Lozano, J. R., Moreno, I., Aguilera, I., Gonzales, M. F., García, A. et al. Association of HLA-DR4-Dw15 DRB1*0405 and DR10 with rheumatoid arthritis in Spanish population. *Arthritis Rheum* 1993; 36: 811–14.

145. McDonagh, J. E., Dunn, A., Ollier, W. E., and Walker, D. J. Compound heterozygosity for the shared epitope and the risk and severity of rheumatoid arthritis in extended pedigrees. *Br J Rheumatol* 1997; 36: 322–7.

146. Willkens, R. F., Nepom, G. T., Marks, C. R., Nettles, J. W., and Nepom, B. S. Association of HLA-Dw16 with rheumatoid arthritis in Yakima Indians: further evidence for the 'Shared Epitope' hypothesis. *Arthritis Rheum* 1991; 34: 43–7.

147. Castro, F., Angulo, J., Acevedo, E., Quispe, E., Perich, R., Ciusani, E. et al. [Fenotipo clase II del complejo mayor de histocompatibilidad en artritis reumatoide: Primer reporte en pacientes peruanos]. Type II major histocompatibility complex phenotypes in rheumatoid arthritis: first report in Peruvian patients. *Bol Asoc Peruan Rheum* 1994; 13: 14.

148. Lawrence, J. S. Heberden oration, 1969. Rheumatoid arthritis: nature or nurture? *Ann Rheum Dis* 1970; 29: 357–79.

149. Angelini, G., Morozzi, G., Delfino, L., Pera, C., Dalco, M., Marcolongo, R. et al. Analysis of HLA DP, DQ and DR alleles in adult Italian rheumatoid arthritis patients. *Hum Immunol* 1992; 34: 135–41.

150. Citera, G., Padulo, L. A., Fernandez, G., Lazaro, M. A., Rosemffet, M. G., and Maldonado-Cocco JA. Influence of HLA-DR alleles on rheumatoid arthritis: susceptibility and severity in Argentine patients. *J Rheumatol* 2001; 28: 1486–91.

151. Kong, K. F., Yeap, S. S., Chow, S. K., and Phipps, M. E. HLA-DRB1 genes and susceptibility to rheumatoid arthritis in three ethnic groups from Malaysia. *Autoimmunity* 2002; 35: 235–9.

152. Kinikli, G., Ates, A., Turgay, M., Akay, G., Kinikli, S., and Tokgoz, G. HLA-DRB1 genes and disease severity in rheumatoid arthritis in Turkey. *Scand J Rheumatol* 2003; 32: 277–80.

153. Voskuyl, A. E., Hazes, J. M., Schreuder, G. M., Schipper, R. F., de Vries, R. R., and Breedveld, F. C. HLA-DRB1, DQA1, and DQB1 genotypes and risk of vasculitis in patients with rheumatoid arthritis. *J Rheumatol* 1997; 24: 852–5.

154. Perdriger, A., Chales, G., Semana, G., Guggenbuhl, P., Meyer, O., Quillivic, F. et al. Role of HLA-DR-DR and DR-DQ associations in the expression of extraarticular manifestations and rheumatoid factor in rheumatoid arthritis. *J Rheumatol* 1997; 24: 1272–6.

155. Zanelli, E., González-Gay, M. A., and David, C. S. Could HLA-DRB1 be the protective locus in rheumatoid arthritis? *Immunol Today* 1995; 16: 274–8.

156. Pascual, M., Nieto, A., Lopez-Nevot, M. A., Ramal, L., Mataran, L., Caballero, A. et al. Rheumatoid arthritis in Southern Spain: toward elucidation of unifying role of the HLA class II region in disease predisposition. *Arthritis Rheum* 2001; 44: 307–14.

157. van der Horst-Bruinsma, I. E., Visser, H., Hazes, J. M. et al. HLA-DQ-associated predisposition to and dominant HLA-DR-associated protection against rheumatoid arthritis. *Human Immunol* 1999; 60: 152–8.

158. Vos, K., van der Horst-Bruinsma, I. E., Hazes, J. M. et al. Evidence for a protective role of the human leukocyte antigen class II region in early rheumatoid arthritis. *Rheumatol* 2001; 40: 133–9.

159. Seidl, C., Korbitzer, J., Badenhoop, K., Seifried, E., Hoelzer, D., Zanelli, E. et al. Protection against severe disease is conferred by DERAA-bearing HLA-DRB1 alleles among HLA-DQ3 and HLA-DQ5 positive rheumatoid arthritis patients. *Human Immunol* 2001; 62: 523–9.

160. Moxley, G., Meyer, J., and Han, J. Microsatellite haplotypes of tumor necrosis factor TNFab show linkage disequilibrium with shared-epitope DRB1 alleles TNFa2b1-bearing HLA haplotypes may contribute to rheumatoid arthritis risk. *Arthritis Rheum* 1997; 40: S125. [Abstract.]

161. Mataran, L., Vinasco, J., Beraun, Y, Nieto, A., Fraile, A., Pareja, E. et al. Association of TNF-α polymorphism with outcome of rheumatoid arthritis. *Arthritis Rheum* 1997; 40: S77.

162. Vinasco, J., Beraun, Y, Nieto, A., Fraile, A., Mataran, L., Pareja, E. et al. Polymorphism at the TNF loci in rheumatoid arthritis. *Tissue Antigens* 1997; 49: 74–8.

163. Barton, A., John, S., Ollier, W. E., Silman, A., and Worthington, J. Association between rheumatoid arthritis and polymorphism of tumor necrosis factor receptor II, but not tumor necrosis factor receptor I., in Caucasians. *Arthritis Rheum* 2001; 44: 61–5.

164. Hajeer, A. H., Dababneh, A., Makki, R. F., Thomson, W., Poulton, K., Gonzalez-Gay, M. A. et al. Different gene loci within the HLA-DR and TNF regions are independently associated with susceptibility and severity in Spanish rheumatoid arthritis patients. *Tissue Antigens* 2000; 55: 319–25.

165. Gallagher, G., Eskdale, J., Steven, M., Wordsworth, P., and Field, M. No role for the TNF gene cluster in the genetic predisposition to rheumatoid arthritis or systemic lupus erythematosus. *Arthritis Rheum* 1997; 40: S77.

166. Wilder, R. L. Hypothesis for retroviral causation of rheumatoid arthritis. *Curr Opin Rheumatol* 1994; 6: 295–9.

167. Cole, P., and MacMahon, B. Attributable risk percent in case-control studies. *Brit J Prev Soc Med* 1971; 25: 242–4.

168. Nikkari, S., Roivainen, A., Hannonen, P., Mottonen, T., Luukkainen, R., Yli-Jama, T. et al. Persistence of parvovirus B19 in synovial fluid and bone marrow. *Ann Rheum Dis* 1995; 54: 597–600.

169. Woolf, A. D., and Cohen, B. J. Parvovirus B19 and chronic arthritis: causal or casual association? *Ann Rheum Dis* 1995; **54**: 535–6.

170. Barthold S. W. Globalization of Lyme borreliosis. *Lancet* 1996; **348**: 1603.

171. Le Guenno, B. Haemorrhagic fevers and ecological perturbations. *Arch Virol Suppl* 1997; **13**: 191–9.

172. Albani, S., Keystone, E. C., Nelson, J. L., Ollier, W. E., La Cava, A., Montemayor, A. C. *et al*. Positive selection in autoimmunity: abnormal immune responses to a bacterial dnaJ antigenic determinant in patients with early rheumatoid arthritis. *Nat Med* 1995; **1**: 448–52.

173. Baum, H., and Staines, N. A. MHC-derived peptides and the CD4+ T-cell repertoire: implications for autoimmune disease. *Cytokines Cell Mol Ther* 1997; **3**: 115–25.

174. La Cava, A., Nelson, J. L., Ollier, W. E., MacGregor, A., Keystone, E. C., Thorne JC *et al*. Genetic bias in immune responses to a cassette shared by different microorganisms in patients with rheumatoid arthritis. *J Clin Invest* 1997; **100**: 658–63.

175. Wilder, R. L. Adrenal and gonadal steroid hormone deficiency in the pathogenesis of rheumatoid arthritis. *J Rheumatol* 1996; **44**: 1–2.

176. Hench, P. S. The ameliorating effect of pregnancy on chronic atrophic infectious rheumatoid arthritis, fibrositis and intermittent hydrarthrosis. *Proc Staff Meeting Mayo Clin* 1938; **13**: 161–7.

177. Nelson, J. L., and Ostensen, M. Pregnancy and rheumatoid arthritis. *Rheum Dis Clin North Am* 1997; **23**: 195–212.

178. Roberts, R. M., Xie, S., Nagel, R. J., Low, B., Green, J., and Beckers, J. F. Glycoproteins of the aspartyl proteinase gene family secreted by the developing placenta. *Adv Exp Med Biol* 1995; **362**: 231–40.

179. Perdriger, A., and Chales, G. Influence on non-HLA factors in rheumatoid arthritis: role of enzyme abnormalities in joint destruction. *Rev Rhum Engl Ed* 1997; **64**: 523–6.

180. Rademacher, T. W., Williams, P., and Dwek, R. A. Agalactosyl glycoforms of IgG autoantibodies are pathogenic. *Proc Natl Acad Sci* 1994; **91**: 6123–7.

181. Rook, G. A., Steele, J., Brealey, R., Whyte, A., Isenberg, D., Sumar, N. *et al*. Changes in IgG glycoform levels are associated with remission of arthritis during pregnancy. *J Autoimmun* 1991; **4**: 779–94.

182. Cuchacovich, M., Gatica, H., Grigg, D. M., Pizzo, S. V., and Gonzalez-Gronow, M. Potential pathogenicity of deglycosylated IgG cross reactive with streptokinase and fibronectin in the serum of patients with rheumatoid arthritis. *J Rheumatol* 1996; **23**: 44–51.

183. Nelson, J. L., Hughes, K. A., Smith, A. G., Nisperos, B. B., Branchaud, A. M., and Hansen, J. A. Maternal-fetal disparity in HLA class II alloantigens and the pregnancy: induced amelioration of rheumatoid arthritis. *N Engl J Med* 1993; **329**: 466–71.

184. Nelson, J. L., Koepsell, T. D., Dugowson, C. E., Voigt, L. F., Daling, J. R., and Hansen, J. A. Fecundity before disease onset in women with rheumatoid arthritis. *Arthritis Rheum* 1993; **36**: 7–14.

185. Anonymous. Reduction in incidence of rheumatoid arthritis associated with oral contraceptives. Royal College of General Practitioners' Oral Contraception Study. *Lancet* 1978; **1**: 569–71.

186. Doran, M. F., Crowson, C. S., O'Fallon, W. M., and Gabriel, S. E. The effect or oral contraceptives and estrogen replacement therapy on the risk of rheumatoid arthritis: a population based study. *J Rheumatol* 2004; **31**: 207–13.

187. Spector, T. D., and Hochberg, M. C. The protective effect of the oral contraceptive pill on rheumatoid arthritis: an overview of the analytic epidemiological studies using meta-analysis. *J Clin Epidemiol* 1990; **43**: 1221–30.

188. Pladevall-Vila, M., Delclos, G. L., Varas, C., Guyer, H., Brugues-Tarradellas, J., and Anglada-Arisa, A. Controversy of oral contraceptives and risk of rheumatoid arthritis: meta-analysis of conflicting studies and review of conflicting meta-analyses with special emphasis on analysis of heterogeneity. *Am J Epidemiol* 1996; **144**: 1–14.

189. Bruce, I. N., and Laskin, C. A. Sex hormones in systemic lupus erythematosus: a controversy for modern times. *J Rheumatol* 1997; **24**: 1461–3.

190. Dequeker, J., and Westhovens, R. Low dose corticosteroid associated osteoporosis in rheumatoid arthritis and its prophylaxis and treatment: bones of contention. *J Rheumatol* 1995; **22**: 1013–19.

191. Sanchez-Guerrero, J., Liang, M. H., Karlson, E. W., Hunter, D. J., and Colditz, G. A. Postmenopausal estrogen therapy and the risk for developing systemic lupus erythematosus. *Ann Intern Med* 1995; **122**: 430–3.

192. Koepsell, T. D., Dugowson, C. E., Nelson, J. L., Voigt, L. F., and Daling, J. R. Non-contraceptive hormones and the risk of rheumatoid arthritis in menopausal women. *Int J Epidemiol* 1994; **23**: 1248–55.

193. James, W. H. Further evidence that low androgen values are a cause of rheumatoid arthritis: the response of rheumatoid arthritis to seriously stressful life events. *Ann Rheum Dis* 1997; **56**: 566.

194. Cutolo, M., and Masi, A. T. Do androgens influence the pathophysiology of rheumatoid arthritis? Facts and hypotheses. *J Rheumatol* 1998; **25**: 1041–7.

195. Cutolo, M. Do sex hormones modulate the synovial macrophages in rheumatoid arthritis? *Ann Rheum Dis* 1997; **56**: 281–4.

196. Lunec, J., Halloran, S. P., White, A. C., and Dormandy, T. L. Free radical oxidation peroxidation products in serum and synovial fluid in rheumatoid arthritis. *J Rheumatol* 1981; **8**: 233–45.

197. Silman, A. J., and Pearson, J. E. Epidemiology and genetics of rheumatoid arthritis. *Arthritis Res* 2002; **4**: S265–S272.

198. Heliovaara, M., Knekt, P., Aho, K., Aaran, R. K., Alfthan, G., and Aromaa A. Serum antioxidants and risk of rheumatoid arthritis. *Ann Rheum Dis* 1994; **53**: 51–3.

199. Knekt, P., Heliovaara, M., Aho, K., Alfthan, G., Marniemi, J., and Aromaa, A. Serum selenium, serum alpha-tocopherol, and the risk of rheumatoid arthritis. *Epidemiology* 2000; **11**: 402–5.

200. Comstock, G. W., Burke, A. E., Hoffman, S. C., Helzlsouer, K. J., Bendich, A., Masi, AT *et al*. Serum concentrations of alpha tocopherol, beta carotene, and retinol preceding the diagnosis of rheumatoid arthritis and systemic lupus erythematosus. *Ann Rheum Dis* 1997; **56**: 323–5.

201. Pattison, D. J., Symmons, D. P., and Young, A. Does diet have a role in the aetiology of rheumatoid arthritis? *Proc Nutr Soc* 2004; **63**: 137–43.

202. Linos, A., Kaklamani, V. G., Kaklamani, E., Koumantaki, Y, Giziaki, E., Papazoglou, S. *et al*. Dietary factors in relation to rheumatoid arthritis: a role for olive oil and cooked vegetables? *Am J Clin Nutr* 1999; **70**: 1077–82.

203. Cerhan, J. R., Saag, K. G., Merlino, L. A., Mikuls, T. R., and Criswell, L. A. Antioxidant micronutrients and risk of rheumatoid arthritis in a cohort of older women. *Am J Epidemiol* 2003; **157**: 345–54.

204. Pattison, D. J., Silman, A. J., Goodson, N. J., Lunt, M., Bunn, D., Luben, R. *et al*. Vitamin C and the risk of developing inflammatory polyarthritis: a prospective nested case-control study. *Ann Rheum Dis* 2004; **63**: 843–7.

205. Shapiro, J. A., Koepsell, T. D., Voigt, L. F., Dugowson, C. E., Kestin, M., and Nelson, J. L. Diet and rheumatoid arthritis in women: a possible protective effect of fish consumption. *Epidemiology* 1996; 7: 256–63.

206. Horrobin, D. F. Low prevalences of coronary heart disease, psoriasis, asthma, and rheumatoid arthritis in Eskimos: are they caused by high dietary intake of eicosapentaenoic acid EPA, a genetic variation of essential fatty acid EFA metabolism or a combination of both? *Med Hypotheses* 1987; **22**: 421–8.

207. Linos, A., Kaklamanis, E., Kontomerkos, A., Koumantaki, Y, Gazi, S., Vaiopoulos, G. *et al*. The effect of olive oil and fish consumption on rheumatoid arthritis: a case control study. *Scand J Rheumatol* 1991; **20**: 419–26.

208. Kjeldsen-Kragh, J., Lund, J. A., Riise, T., Finnanger, B., Haaland, K., Finstad, R. *et al*. Dietary omega-3 fatty acid supplementation and naproxen treatment in patients with rheumatoid arthritis. *J Rheumatol* 1992; **19**: 1531–6.

209. Nielsen, G. L., Faarvang, K. L., Thomsen, B. S., Teglbjaerg, K. L., Jensen, L. T., Hansen, T. M. *et al*. The effects of dietary supplementation with n-3 polyunsaturated fatty acids in patients with rheumatoid arthritis: a randomized, double blind trial. *Eur J Clin Invest* 1992; **22**: 687–91.

210. Skoldstam, L., Borjesson, O., Kjallman, A., Seiving, B., and Akesson, B. Effect of six months of fish oil supplementation in stable rheumatoid arthritis: a double-blind, controlled study. *Scand J Rheumatol* 1992; **21**: 178–85.

211. Grant, W. B. The role of meat in the expression of rheumatoid arthritis. *Br J Nutr* 2000; **84**: 589–95.

212. Merlino, L. A., Curtis, J., Mikuls, T. R., Cerhan, J. R., Criswell, L. A., and Saag, K. G. Vitamin D. intake is inversely associated with rheumatoid arthritis: results from the Iowa Women's Health Study. *Arthritis Rheum* 2004; **50**: 72–7.

213. Chiang, E. P., Bagley, P. J., Selhub, J., Nadeau, M., and Roubenoff, R. Abnormal vitamin B6 status is associated with severity of symptoms in patients with rheumatoid arthritis. *Am J Med* 2003; **114**: 283–7.

214. McDonagh, J. E., and Walker, D. J. Smoking and rheumatoid arthritis: observations from a multicase family study. Comment an the article by Silman *et al*. *Arthritis Rheum* 1997; **40**: 594.

215. Masdottir, B., Jonsson, T., Manfredsdottir, V., Vikingsson, A., Brekkan, A., and Valdimarsson, H. Smoking, rheumatoid factor isotypes and severity of rheumatoid arthritis. *Rheumatology* 2000; **39**: 1202–5.

216. Harrison, B. J. Influence of cigarette smoking on disease outcome in rheumatoid arthritis. *Curr Opin Rheumatol* 2002; **14**: 93–7.

217. Masi, A. T., Fecht, T., Aldag, J. C., Malamet, R. L., and Hazes, J. M. Smoking and rheumatoid arthritis: comment on the letter by McDonagh and Walker. *Arthritis Rheum* 1998; **41**: 184.

218. Symmons, D. P., Bankhead, C. R., Harrison, B. J., Brennan, P., Barrett, E. M., Scott, D. G. *et al*. Blood transfusion, smoking, and obesity as risk factors for the development of rheumatoid arthritis: results from a primary care-based incident case-control study in Norfolk, England. *Arthritis Rheum* 1997; **40**: 1955–61.

219. Wolfe, F., and Johnston, D. Smoking is associated with premature development of rheumatoid arthritis and osteoarthritis. *Arthritis Rheum* 1997; **40**: S312.

220. Hutchinson, D., Shepstone, L., Moots, R., Lear, J. T., and Lynch, M. P. Heavy cigarette smoking is strongly associated with rheumatoid arthritis, particularly in patients without a family history of RA. *Ann Rheum Dis* 2001; **60**: 223–7.

221. Wolfe, F. The effect of smoking on clinical, laboratory, and radiographic status in rheumatoid arthritis. *J Rheumatol* 2000; **27**: 630–7.

222. Padyukov, L., Silva, C., Stolt, P., Alfredsson, L., and Klareskog, L. A gene-environment interaction between smoking and shared epitope genes in HLA-DR provides a high risk of seropositive rheumatoid arthritis. *Arthritis Rheum* 2004; **50**: 3085–92.

223. Criswell, L. A., Merlino, L. A., Cerhan, J. R., Mikuls, T. R., Mudano, A. S., Burma, M. *et al*. Cigarette smoking and the risk of rheumatoid arthritis among postmenopausal women: results from the Iowa Women's Health Study. *Am J Med* 2002; **112**: 465–71.

224. Karlson, E. W., Lee, I. M., Cook, N. R., Manson, J. E., Buring, J. E., and Hennekens, C. H. A retrospective cohort study of cigarette smoking and risk of rheumatoid arthritis in female health professionals. *Arthritis Rheum* 1999; **42**: 910–17.

225. Albano, S. A., Santana-Sahagun, E., and Weisman, M. H. Cigarette smoking and rheumatoid arthritis. *Sem Arthritis Rheum* 2001; **31**: 146–59.

226. Uhlig, T., Hagen, K. B., and Kvien, T. K. Current tobacco smoking, formal education, and the risk of rheumatoid arthritis. *J Rheumatol* 1999; **26**: 47–54.

227. Heliovaara, M., Aho, K., Aromaa, A., Knekt, P., and Reunanen, A. Smoking and risk of rheumatoid arthritis. *J Rheumatol* 1993; **20**: 1830–5.

228. Harrison, B. J., Silman, A. J., Wiles, N. J., Scott, D. G., and Symmons, D. P. The association of cigarette smoking with disease outcome in patients with early inflammatory polyarthritis. *Arthritis Rheum* 2001; **44**: 323–30.

229. Farrell, A. J., and Blake, D. R. Nitric oxide. *Ann Rheum Dis* 1996; **55**: 7–20.

230. Firestein, G. S., Echeverri, F., Yeo, M., Zvaifler, N. J., and Green, D. R. Somatic mutations in the p53 tumor suppressor gene in rheumatoid arthritis synovium. *Proc Natl Acad Sci* 1997; **94**: 10895–900.

231. Heliovaara, M., Aho, K., Knekt, P., Impivaara, O., Reunanen, A., and Aromaa, A. Coffee consumption, rheumatoid factor, and the risk of rheumatoid arthritis. *Ann Rheum Dis* 2000; **59**: 631–5.

232. Mikuls, T. R., Cerhan, J. R., Criswell, L. A., Merlino, L., Mudano, A. S., Burma, M. *et al*. Coffee, tea, and caffeine consumption and risk of rheumatoid arthritis: results from the Iowa Women's Health Study. *Arthritis Rheum* 2002; **46**: 83–91.

233. Pincus, T., and Callahan, L. F. Formal education as a marker for increased mortality and morbidity in rheumatoid arthritis. *J Chronic Dis* 1985; **38**: 973–84.

234. Ward, M. M., and Leigh, J. P. Marital status and the progression of functional disability in patients with rheumatoid arthritis. *Arthritis Rheum* 1993; **36**: 581–8.

235. Reckner Olsson, A., Skogh, T., and Wingren, G. Comorbidity and lifestyle, reproductive factors, and environmental exposures associated with rheumatoid arthritis. *Ann Rheum Dis* 2001; **60**: 934–9

3 | Microbes in the pathogenesis of rheumatoid arthritis

Paavo Toivanen

Many diverse concepts and speculations related to the etiopathogenesis of rheumatoid arthritis have been proposed, most of which implicate both genetic and environmental factors. The disease is known to be associated with certain HLA-DRB1 alleles, encoding a common sequence of five amino acids in the hypervariable region of the HLA-DR β chain, the so-called susceptibility epitope. This epitope is found in 80–90% of Caucasoid patients with rheumatoid arthritis and in 40–50% of non-rheumatoid subjects. Disease heritability is estimated to be about 60%, of which HLA accounts for less than a half, and multiple loci outside the HLA region are responsible for the rest[1,2]. Several alternative possibilities have been proposed for the participation of the susceptibility epitope[3], the most common being that it specifies HLA-DR molecules binding arthritogenic peptides. Recently it has become apparent that bacterial colonization of the host could be determined by genetic factors, including HLA, leaving a novel role also for the susceptibility epitope[4].

Among the environmental factors infection and microbes have been one of the most popular alternatives[5–8]. However, despite the extensive and thorough studies carried out during the years only circumstantial evidence supporting the microbial involvement has been obtained, based mostly on the following four types of observations. (a) Certain forms of arthritides are microbially triggered. In addition to septic bacterial and viral arthritis, they include arthritides connected to enterogenic and urogenic infections (reactive arthritis), rheumatic fever, Lyme borreliosis, tuberculosis, leprosy, and Whipple's disease[9–14]. (b) Humoral or cellular immune responses to certain microbes and microbial components have been observed in rheumatoid arthritis[15–17]. (c) The intestinal microbiota of rheumatoid arthritis patients have been found to be different from that in controls[18]. (d) Some antimicrobial agents have been reported to be effective in the treatment of rheumatoid arthritis, though it is not necessarily attributed to the antibacterial effect[19]. (e) Certain bacteria or bacterial components are able to induce experimental chronic arthritis closely resembling rheumatoid arthritis[20–22].

In this chapter, the recent advances in the field will be reviewed, paying attention to infectious agents originating in the outside environment, to the normal or persisting microbiota, and to the information gained from animal experiments. For the previous development in the field, the reader is referred to earlier reviews[5,11,13,23,24].

Viruses

A number of viruses have been implicated in the etiology and pathogenesis of rheumatoid arthritis[25–28] (Table 3.1). Among them, most attention has been given on Epstein-Barr virus (EBV), a widely spread herpesvirus. A possible relationship between EBV and rheumatoid arthritis was suggested by early serologic studies, which showed a high prevalence of antibodies to different EBV-induced antigens in patients with rheumatoid arthritis[29,30]. EBV is a polyclonal activator of B-lymphocytes, resulting in the overproduction of immunoglobulins and rheumatoid factor[31,32]. Patients with rheumatoid arthritis also have increased numbers of circulating EBV-infected B cells and a diminished cytotoxic T cell response to EBV[33,34]. Particularly interesting is the amino acid homology between the EBV gp110 glycoprotein and the third hypervariable region of HLA-DR β chain, the susceptibility epitope[35]. It has been suggested that decreased T cell response to gp110 might lead to poor control of EBV infection especially in individuals with susceptibility epitopes[36,37].

It is difficult to draw conclusions from the presence of herpesviruses in synovial biopsy tissues from rheumatoid arthritis patients, due to limitations and variability of the techniques used. Moreover, there are no suitable animal models available. Epstein-Barr virus (EBV) has been demonstrated, using different methods, in the synovial cells of patients with rheumatoid arthritis[38–42]. Altogether, the conclusions remain controversial, due also to the wide occurrence of the latent EBV in the controls and even in healthy individuals[38,43,44]. The current view about the potential role of EBV in the etiopathogenesis of rheumatoid arthritis can

Table 3.1 Microbes most often discussed as potential etiologic agents in rheumatoid arthritis

Viruses	Bacteria
Adenoviruses	*Mycobacteria*
Cytomegalovirus	*Mycoplasmae*
Epstein–Barr virus	*Proteus mirabilis*
Human T cell leukemia virus type 1	*Clostridium perfringens*
Parvovirus B19	
Rubella virus	

be summarized by stating that considerable evidence for it has accumulated but real causal links do not exist.

In addition to EBV, seven other herpesviruses that affect humans have been identified: herpes simplex virus types 1 and 2 (HSV-1 and HSV-2), cytomegalovirus (CMV), varicella-zoster virus, and the human herpesvirus types 6, 7, and 8 (HHV-6, HHV-7, and HHV-8)[45–47]. With the exception of HSV-2, this family of viruses is ubiquitous, and most people become infected by one or more of them during the first decade of life[48]. They all have a tendency for persistence, with lymphocytes and macrophage-line cells as the favorite sites of latent occurrence[49]. A few reports indicate recovery of HSV-1 from the synovial fluid of patients with monoarticular arthritis after an acute HSV infection, whereas in rheumatoid arthritis the findings have been negative[38,50,51]. The same applies to HSV-2 and HHV-6[38]; for the occurrence of HHV-7 and HHV-8 in joint tissues no information is available.

Similarly to other herpesviruses, CMV has a worldwide distribution with seroprevalence of 50–70% in adult populations, with great tendency for persistence and latency[52]. In addition to these facts, increased antibody response and synovial lymphocyte proliferation against CMV in rheumatoid arthritis have been taken to suggest CMV involvement in the pathogenesis of rheumatoid arthritis[53–56]. Studies using *in situ* hybridization, virus isolation, immunochemistry, or polymerase chain reaction (PCR) have revealed the presence of CMV in the joint tissues of patients with rheumatoid arthritis[42,56–58]. However, in line with studies on EBV, the latent occurrence of CMV in the control populations and healthy individuals casts doubt on the arthritogenic role of CMV.

As a common cause of human infection, parvovirus B19 is also distributed worldwide. Infection may be totally asymptomatic or with mild non-specific symptoms. Of infected adults, 60–80% suffer joint symptoms, usually lasting a few weeks. Several cases of more or less chronic polyarthritis have been described, some of them meeting American College of Rheumatology criteria for rheumatoid arthritis, even with development of rheumatoid factor[59–63]. No clear association with the occurrence of rheumatoid arthritis susceptibility epitope has been observed[64–66]. The virus DNA is often demonstrable in the affected joints[61,62,67–70]. All these findings could be interpreted to indicate that parvovirus B19 might be a real etiological factor in a small proportion of rheumatoid arthritis cases. However, the viral DNA occurs also in joint tissues of trauma patients and in other control samples[69–72], and the virus has a tendency for persistence in a good proportion of the infected patients[73]. Altogether, the general view at present is that parvovirus B19 is not a cause of rheumatoid arthritis[62,70,74–77].

In addition to the viruses mentioned above, a number of other viruses have been discussed and studied as potential participants in the etiopathogenesis of rheumatoid arthritis[13,24,78,79]. They include adenoviruses, rubella, mumps and measles viruses, hepatitis viruses, and exogenous retroviruses. For any of these, real evidence of participation is scanty, or in fact, totally lacking. Therefore, only a brief account of recent studies appears here. A common loophole in several studies searching for viruses in the synovial tissue is concentration on patients with advanced disease. In such cases the initial inflammatory trigger leading to cartilage destruction and autoimmunity has most probably already disappeared. Nevertheless, even when investigating patients with disease duration of less than one year, no evidence has been obtained for the presence of adenoviruses, rubella, or mumps or measles viruses in the synovial tissue of rheumatoid arthritis patients[80,81]. Population studies looking for prevalence of hepatitis C infection in rheumatoid arthritis patients or for occurrence of rheumatoid arthritis in hepatitis patients have found no evidence of a connection[82–85]. A few patients with hepatitis B infection and chronic arthritis fulfilling the American College of Rheumatology criteria for rheumatoid arthritis have been reported[86,87]. Further, it is known that hepatitis B vaccination sometimes causes a complication resembling reactive arthritis[88–90]. Despite these findings, the link between hepatitis B and rheumatoid arthritis remains elusive[91].

Exogenous retroviruses have been considered as potential etiological agents in rheumatoid arthritis because an established animal model with caprine arthritis exists[92]. Likewise, human T-cell leukemia type I (HTLV-I) transgenic mice develop arthritis closely resembling rheumatoid arthritis[93]. Particular interest has been focused on the HTLV-I Tax gene; 25 of 101 HTLV-I/II seronegative rheumatoid arthritis patients carried Tax sequences in the mononuclear cells and had antibodies against its gene product[94]. HTLV-I carriers may present with polyarthritis fulfilling the American College of Rheumatology criteria for rheumatoid arthritis. In an endemic area 111 such patients were observed among 7087 studied[95]. The other exogenous retroviruses considered are human immune deficiency virus (HIV) and human retrovirus-5 (HRV-5). In HIV-infected individuals a number of different articular syndromes have been identified[96], but a real connection to rheumatoid arthritis has not been established. Instead, HRV-5 proviral DNA has been detected in 10–12% of blood samples of rheumatoid arthritis patients[97,98]. However, a similar observation was made in systemic lupus erythematosus, and negative findings have also been reported[99].

Bacterial

A variety of bacteria have attracted attention as possible etiologic agents in rheumatoid arthritis. They include infectious species as well as those belonging to the normal microbiota of the host (Table 3.1). *Mycobacterium tuberculosis* aroused interest after it was demonstrated that synovial T lymphocytes/clones from rheumatoid arthritis patients show increased activity to mycobacterial antigens cross-reactive with the cartilage[16,100]. These findings have given rise to continuing interest in the mycobacterial heat shock proteins potentially preventing development of experimental and human arthritides[101–104]. *Escherichia coli*, the most common cause of urinary tract infections and part of the normal intestinal microbiota, has also been considered an etiologic factor[105,106]. Particular attention has been paid to its heat shock protein DnaJ, which shows molecular mimicry with the HLA-DR sequence. Activation of synovial T cells against DnaJ was observed in patients with early rheumatoid arthritis, but not in controls, indicating that the activated T cells may cross-react with DnaJ *E. coli* heat shock protein, expressed in the joints[107–109].

Mycoplasmas have also been of interest to rheumatologists; altogether 13 different species of mycoplasmas have been implicated in the etiology of arthritides, including rheumatoid arthritis[110–112].

However, mycoplasmas are frequent contaminants of laboratory cultures, and the findings published have not been reproducible[112].

Patients with rheumatoid arthritis have been reported to have an increased prevalence of antibodies against *Proteus mirabilis*[15,113], and to show asymptomatic *P. mirabilis* bacteriuria[114]. This has led to the suggestion that *P. mirabilis* may play an etiologic role in the pathogenesis of rheumatoid arthritis, based on a molecular mimicry between *P. mirabilis* hemolysin and the rheumatoid arthritis susceptibility epitope[115–117]. So far, this suggestion has not received support by other research groups[118,119].

An essential component of the bacterial cell wall is peptidoglycan, which is particularly thick in Gram-positive bacteria (Fig. 3.1). It consists of up to 70 layers of N-acetylmuramic acid and N-acetylglucosamine moieties linked by β-1,4-glycosidic bonds; the layers are bound to each other by peptide bridges. Muramic acid is not found in eukaryotic cells, and its detection indicates that bacteria or bacterial degradation products are present. Using mass spectrometry it has been demonstrated that 60% of young adults have muramic acid within the circulating blood cells, with the frequency of positivity declining with age. Thus, with the present techniques, 2–3% of people at the age of 50–60 years show circulating cells containing muramic acid[120]. In contrast, muramic acid is not observed in the circulation of newborns. Because newborns do not have bacteria within the gastrointestinal tract, it can be concluded that muramic acid in the adult circulation is derived from the intestinal microbiota[121]. Muramic acid has also been observed in the spleen of healthy adult subjects[122]. Therefore, it is no surprise that muramic acid may also end up in the synovial tissue, indicating the presence of bacterially derived peptidoglycan[123–125]. Evidence for bacterial nucleic acids has also been presented in studies on the synovial tissue from a variety of arthritides, including late stage rheumatoid arthritis[126–128]. Such findings indicate the presence of nucleic acids derived from a wide range of bacterial species, and they do not necessarily correlate with the presence of muramic acid in the synovial tissue[125]. Possibly, bacterial nucleic acids, which are quite often present in the blood circulation[129], are trapped in the inflamed joint tissue. It must be noted that the mere presence of bacterial structures within synovial tissues does not necessarily result in inflammation. Both experimental[130,131] and clinical[38,69,132] evidence indicates that microbial components may end up in the synovial tissues without causing inflammation. For synovitis to develop the bacterial components have to be phlogistic. One has also to note that traces of bacterial cell walls present in the synovium could have been derived from a variety of diverse bacterial species.

Arthritogenicity of the Gram-positive bacterial cell wall

The ability of Gram-positive bacterial cell walls to induce chronic, erosive arthritis was first described in the rat by using *Streptococcus pyogenes*[20]. Self perpetuating arthritis, closely resembling human rheumatoid arthritis by histological criteria, develops in susceptible rat strains after a single intraperitoneal injection of the bacterial cell wall. In addition to *S. pyogenes*,

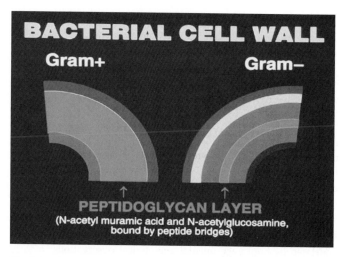

Fig. 3.1 Comparison of Gram-positive and Gram-negative bacterial cell walls. In the Gram-positive cell wall the peptidoglycan consists of up to 70 layers, comprising a continuous net of two alternating amino sugars (N-acetylglucosamine and N-acetylmuramic acid), which are linked to each other by β-1,4-glycosidic bonds. The amino sugar layers are bound to each other by peptides attached to the muramic acid moieties. See also colour plate section.

several bacterial species representing *Lactobacillus*, *Bifidobacterium*, *Eubacterium*, *Collinsella*, and *Clostridium* have been observed to have a similar ability[22,133,134]. Surprisingly, most of these are anaerobic Gram-positive rods belonging to the normal intestinal microbiota in humans.

A typical bacterial cell wall arthritis has also been induced by using an extract from the human intestinal content[135]. In the bacterial cell wall, peptidoglycan has proved to be the decisive component for the induction of arthritis[22,134,136–138]. Peptidoglycan moieties are known as polyclonal stimulators of human and murine lymphocytes, leading to production of potent inflammatory cytokines and monocyte chemoattractant protein 1[139,140], and even of rheumatoid factors[141–143]. However, these properties are not shared by all bacterial peptidoglycans. Certain bacteria have peptidoglycans inducing severe chronic arthritis, whereas others have peptidoglycan that induces only a transient, acute arthritis or no arthritis at all. Most clearly this has been demonstrated by using a pair of strains of *Collinsella aerofaciens*, both isolated from the human intestine[140]. These two bacterial strains are almost identical; 100% identity is observed by polymerase chain reaction of 16S ribosomal genes and only a minor difference in the peptidoglycan structure. Despite their close similarity, only one of these two strains is arthritogenic.

After enzyme digestion, degradation products of the arthritogenic *Collinsella* strain have a five- to eightfold increase in the ability to stimulate production of proinflammatory cytokines in comparison with the intact peptidoglycan. An opposite effect was observed with the degraded fragments of the non-arthritogenic *Collinsella* peptidoglycan—that is, its proinflammatory ability was significantly decreased by enzyme degradation[140]. These findings together with other observations indicate that the chemical composition of the bacterial cell wall peptidoglycan determines whether a particular cell wall can cause chronic arthritis or not[22,134,136–138]. Normal microbiota usually coexist in a peaceful symbiosis with the host[144,145]. On the other hand, cell wall products including peptidoglycan, isolated from intestinal indigenous bacteria, can mount human cytokine responses *in vitro*[146]. The responses are mediated by a group of peptidoglycan recognition molecules present on macrophages and synovial fibroblasts, including CD14 and Toll-like receptor 2[147-151].

Homing of mucosal leukocytes to the joint

Transfer of bacterial products from the intestine to the joint tissue is understandable, since mucosal leukocytes are known to specifically home on the synovium. A putative link between the gut and the joints with regard to leukocyte homing mechanisms has been indicated by both experimental and clinical observations[152,153]. It was first proposed by Jalkanen *et al.*[154] that recirculation routes may be shared between mucosal and synovial tissues. Interestingly, it has been reported that activated gut-derived immunoblasts have dual binding capacity to vessels in mucosa-associated lymphoid tissues and inflamed synovium, but not to peripheral lymph node vessels[155]. *In vivo* animal studies confirmed the ability of lymphocytes originating from mucosal sites to home on the inflamed synovium[156]. Mucosal macrophages are interesting candidates as vehicles transporting exogenous antigens from gut mucosa to joints. In the case of arthritogenic antigens, the final results are endothelial activation and synovitis.

Intestinal microbiota in rheumatoid arthritis

Clostridium perfringens belongs to the normal intestinal microbiota of animals and humans. It was reported by Månsson and Olhagen in 1966 to occur in excess in the fecal flora of patients with rheumatoid arthritis[157,158]. This finding has been discussed and disputed[159-161]. Månsson and coworkers also showed that pigs fed with a barley and oats-based diet supplemented with dry fish developed arthritis with concomitant increase of fecal *C. perfringens*[162,163]. The arthritis had certain clinical and histopathological similarities to rheumatoid arthritis. These experiments were repeated in 1993 by Peltonen *et al.* applying the original protocol as closely as possible[164]. They concluded that a fish diet changed fecal microbiota significantly, but did not induce arthritis. It must be emphasized that even if an increased presence of *C. perfringens* could be documented in patients with advanced rheumatoid arthritis, it may only be secondary to, or accompanying other pathogenic changes.

Analysis of human intestinal microbiota is not an easy task[165]. It has been estimated that, using traditional methods of culture and identification, complete analysis of such a sample comprising 400–500 different bacterial species would take one person-year of laboratory work. To overcome this problem, fatty acids derived from bacterial cell membranes have been analysed in stool samples by gas–liquid chromatography. Each bacterial species has a unique profile of cellular fatty acids. Computerized gas–liquid chromatography of such profiles has successfully been applied to compare intestinal and other complex bacterial samples[166-168]. A study with such a technique showed that patients with early rheumatoid arthritis (disease duration less than six months) have intestinal microbiota significantly different from that in controls. The difference was best seen in patients with erosive or rheumatoid factor positive rheumatoid arthritis. Anaerobic bacteria, which form the overwhelming majority of the gastrointestinal microbiota, were responsible for the difference observed[18]. It is also known that changes in the diet induce changes in the intestinal microbiota. When patients with rheumatoid arthritis underwent a dietary trial with fasting and a vegan/vegetarian diet, the most significant changes in the intestinal microbiota were displayed by those showing clinical improvement[169,170]. Why would the patients with early rheumatoid arthritis have intestinal microbiota different from that in other subjects?

Genetics of intestinal colonization

A few studies have been carried out to clarify whether the composition of gastrointestinal microbiota is influenced by the host genotype. van de Merwe *et al.* analysed stool samples using anaerobic bacterial cultures and concluded that the composition of microbiota in identical twins was considerably more similar than in non-identical twins[171]. Interestingly, a similar conclusion was also reached for bacteria present on the nasal mucosa[172]. Zoetendal *et al.* used electrophoretic analysis of bacterial ribosomal RNA to suggest that the host genotype determines the composition of the bacterial community in the human intestinal tract, without defining the genes involved[173,174]. Studies carried out with congenic mouse strains indicate that the major histocompatibility complex (MHC) may have a prominent effect[168,175,176]. How would such an effect be mediated? It is tempting to speculate that MHC-linked immune responses would lead to elimination of certain bacterial species[168]. However, little is known about the effect of the MHC on antibacterial responses[177,178]. A more probable mechanism is the effect of the MHC on the bacterial adherence to intestinal epithelia, which is a requisite first step in the colonization process. Bacterial surface molecules, adhesins, recognize proteins or glycoproteins on the epithelial cells. Bacteria which cannot adhere are shed. The specificity of the adherence leads to a restricted colonization of the host. As examples, attachment of *Helicobacter pylori* to the human gastric epithelium is selectively mediated by blood group antigen Lewis[b 179], and nasal carriage of *Staphylococcus aureus* is affected by the host genotype[180]. Regarding MHC molecules and bacterial adherence, several immunoglobulin-binding proteins have been demonstrated on the bacterial surfaces. One type of these, fibrous proteins called curli, has been shown to interact with the immunoglobulin-like domains of human class I MHC molecules[181]. The effect of different MHC genotypes was not studied. However, gastric inflammation induced by *Helicobacter felis*, which depends on bacterial attachment and colonization, varies in severity in congenic mice with different MHC[182].

It has been suggested that the normal intestinal microbiota of people developing rheumatoid arthritis harbour bacteria, degradation products of which can induce chronic arthritis[4]. Components

Table 3.2 Four phases in the pathogenesis of rheumatoid arthritis, according to the hypothesis about intestinal microbiota triggering rheumatoid arthritis in genetically susceptible individuals

Phase	Characteristics
Preinduction	Intestinal colonization by arthritogenic bacteria
Induction	Degradation products of arthritogenic bacteria enter joint tissue
Inflammation	Antigen presentation. Production of metalloproteinases, proteases and prostaglandins
Destruction	Pannus formation. Osteoclast activation

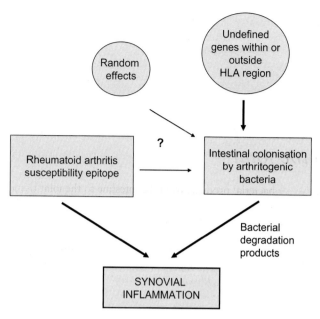

Fig. 3.2 A suggestion about the role of intestinal colonization in the pathogenesis of rheumatoid arthritis; contribution of genetic and environmental factors.

of intestinal bacteria are normally found within circulating blood cells, and they end up in the synovial tissues. The same may occur also with the bacteria which have an arthritogenic ability, resulting in synovial inflammation. Depending on the persistence and other characteristics of the bacterial components, the inflammation is accompanied by production of cytokines, metalloproteinases, proteases, and prostaglandins. All these are known to play a part in the pathogenic process of rheumatoid arthritis, leading to pannus formation and osteoclast activation with cartilage loss, and a self-perpetuating bone erosion (Table 3.2). At the final destruction stage, the inciting bacterial components are not necessarily present any longer in the synovial tissue.

The hypothesis presented does not imply that the genes known as rheumatoid arthritis susceptibility genes are necessarily those favouring the presence of arthritogenic bacteria in the intestinal microbiota[4]. Accordingly, intestinal colonization by arthritogenic bacteria might also be regulated by so-far undefined gene loci, either within the HLA region or outside, or both (Fig. 3.2). Different genes encode for a variety of proteins and glycoproteins present on the intestinal epithelium, allowing adherence of different bacteria. Therefore, the possibility remains that involvement of two or more susceptibility loci is required, some favouring colonization by arthritogenic bacteria and others promoting an inflammatory response to the appropriate bacterial components. In addition, random colonization by arthritogenic bacteria has to be taken into account, owing to the estimated disease heritability of only about 60%[1]. It should be realized that random effects are feasible despite the genetic regulation of the colonization, because the difference between an arthritogenic and non-arthritogenic bacterial strain may be minimal, not affecting the adherence required for the colonization[140].

Peptidoglycans and other persisting components of some bacteria can stimulate production of rheumatoid factor, whereas some other bacteria do not[141,143,183,184], giving a chance of seronegative rheumatoid arthritis to develop. Likewise, the early production of rheumatoid factor, preceding the clinical appearance of the disease[185], is understandable owing to the preinduction period, which may last for years (Table 3.2). Rheumatoid factor in rheumatoid arthritis could be considered a side phenomenon of the host immune response, to some extent similarly to its production in several bacterial and viral infections and as a response to certain vaccinations[184,186,187].

Conclusion

It has become apparent that with the introduction of antimicrobial agents during the past 50 years both the incidence and severity of rheumatoid arthritis have declined in comparison with the pre-antibiotic era[188–190]. Reasons for this may be many, but certainly the effect of the widespread use of antibiotics has to be taken into account, whatever the triggers of rheumatoid arthritis are. Several double blind, placebo-controlled trials with macrolides and tetracyclines have been carried out to treat early and advanced cases of rheumatoid arthritis. It is concluded that the use of antibiotics, in particular of minocycline, results in clinically significant improvement in disease activity. The effect was most marked in patients with disease duration of less than one year[191–196]. However, one should remember that tetracyclines have anti-inflammatory properties, which are independent of their antimicrobial effects[19,197–199].

Monozygotic twins show a concordance rate for the development of rheumatoid arthritis of only 15–30%, which leaves considerable space not only for somatic diversification but also for environmental effects—that is, for participation of diverse microbes, including diverse intestinal colonization. On the other hand, the concordance rate increases with time from the day when the first twin develops rheumatoid arthritis to about 40% during a 30-year follow-up[200], which fits well with the combined effect of genetic and environmental factors. The prevalence of rheumatoid arthritis is remarkably similar worldwide, with estimates varying between 0.5 and 1.0%. However, a prevalence of 5% has been reported in American Indians, and the disease is absent in areas of rural Nigeria. All these findings could be explained by the worldwide occurrence of a variety of arthritogenic microbes, including aberrations in a few isolated areas. Their variable occurrence explains the diversity of the clinical symptoms. In fact, many believe that rheumatoid arthritis is not a single disease. Even monozygotic twins and sibling pairs concordant for rheumatoid arthritis show enormous diversity in the clinical appearance of the disease[201]. Risk factors for rheumatoid arthritis include coffee and smoking[202–204]. It is not difficult to imagine that they both might influence bacterial colonization. Mention of smoking in this context implies that the role of commensal microbiota elsewhere than in the gut, for example in the oral cavity, should not be excluded[196,205,206]. However, the bacterial content in the intestine is overwhelming in comparison with other parts of the body.

References

1. MacGregor, A. J., Snieder, H., Rigby, A. S. *et al.* Characterizing the quantitative genetic contribution to rheumatoid arthritis using data from twins. *Arthritis Rheum* 2000; **43**: 30–7.

2. MacKay, K., Eyre, S., Myerscough, A. *et al.* Whole-genome linkage analysis of rheumatoid arthritis susceptibility loci in 252 affected sibling pairs in the United Kingdom. *Arthritis Rheum* 2002; **46**: 632–9.

3. Firestein, G. S. Evolving concepts of rheumatoid arthritis. *Nature* 2003; **423**: 356–61.

4. Toivanen, P. Normal intestinal microbiota in the aetiopathogenesis of rheumatoid arthritis. *Ann Rheum Dis* 2003; **62**: 807–11.

5. Toivanen, A. Throat streptococci in rheumatoid arthritis. *Acta Med Scand* 1969; **501** (Suppl.): 1–41.

6. Bennett, J. C. The infectious etiology of rheumatoid arthritis. *Arthritis Rheum* 1978; **21**: 531–8.

7. Midtvedt, T. Intestinal bacteria and rheumatic disease. *Scand J Rheumatol* 1987; **64** (Suppl.): 49–54.

8. Hazenberg, M. P., Klasen, I. S., Kool, J., Ruseler-van-Embden, J. G., and Severijnen, A. J. Are intestinal bacteria involved in the etiology of rheumatoid arthritis? *APMIS* 1992; **100**: 1–9.

9. Krause, A., Kamradt, T., and Burmester, G. R. Potential infectious agents in the induction of arthritides. *Curr Opin Rheumatol* 1996; **8**: 203–9.

10. O'Duffy, J. D., Griffing, W. L, Li, C-Y, Abdelmalek, M. F., and Persing, D. H. Whipple's arthritis: direct detection of Tropheryma whippelii in synovial fluid and tissue. *Arthritis Rheum* 1999; **42**: 812–17.

11. Hyrich, K. L., and Inman, R. Infectious agents in chronic rheumatic diseases. *Curr Opin Rheumatol* 2001; **13**: 300–4.

12. Steere, A. C. Lyme disease. *N Engl J Med* 2001; **345**: 115–25.

13. Toivanen, P., and Manninen, R. Microorganisms and the locomotor system. In *Rheumatology*, 3rd edn (Hochberg, M., Silman A., Smolen, J., Weinblatt, M., and Weissman, M., eds), pp. 1039–53. London: Mosby; 2003.

14. Toivanen, A., and Toivanen, P. Reactive arthritis. *Best Pract Res Clin Rheumatol* 2004; **18**: 689–703.

15. Ebringer, A., Ptaszynska, T., Corbett, M. *et al.* Antibodies to Proteus in rheumatoid arthritis. *Lancet* 1985; **2**: 305–7.

16. Holoshitz, J., Koning, F., Coligan, J. E., De Bruyn, J., and Strober, S. Isolation of CD4- CD8- mycobacteria-reactive T lymphocyte clones from rheumatoid arthritis synovial fluid. *Nature* 1989; **339**: 226–9.

17. Klasen, I. S., Melief, M. J., Swaak, T. J. G., Severijnen, A. J., and Hazenberg, M. P. Responses of synovial fluid and peripheral blood mononuclear cells to bacterial antigens and autologous antigen presenting cells. *Ann Rheum Dis* 1993; **52**: 127–32.

18. Eerola, E., Möttönen, T., Hannonen, P. *et al.* Intestinal flora in early rheumatoid arthritis. *Brit J Rheumatol* 1994; **33**: 1030–8.

19. Breedveld, F. C. Minocycline in rheumatoid arthritis. *Arthritis Rheum* 1997; **40**: 794–6.

20. Cromartie, W. J., Craddock, J. G., Schwab, J. H., Anderle, S. K., and Yang C. H. Arthritis in rats after systemic injection of streptococcal cells or cell walls. *J Exp Med* 1977; **146**: 1585–602.

21. Lehman, T. J., Allen, J. B., Plotz, P. H., and Wilder, R. L. Polyarthritis in rats following the systemic injection of Lactobacillus casei cell walls in aqueous suspension. *Arthritis Rheum* 1983; **26**: 1259–65.

22. Simelyte, E., Rimpiläinen, M., Zhang, X., and Toivanen, P. Role of peptidoglycan subtypes in the pathogenesis of bacterial cell wall arthritis. *Ann Rheum Dis* 2003; **62**: 976–82.

23. McKendry, R. J. R. Is rheumatoid arthritis caused by an infection? *Lancet* 1995; **345**: 1319–20.

24. Kingsley, G. Infection in the pathogenesis of rheumatoid arthritis. In *Rheumatoid arthritis: frontiers in pathogenesis and treatment* (Firestein GS, Panayi GS, Wollheim FA, eds), pp. 27–38. Oxford University Press: 2000.

25. Burmester, G. R. Hit and run or permanent hit? Is there evidence for a microbiological cause of rheumatoid arthritis? *J Rheumatol* 1991; **18**: 1443–7.

26. Ford, D. K. The microbiological causes of rheumatoid arthritis [editorial]. *J Rheumatol* 1991; **18**: 1441–2.

27. Fox, R. I., Luppi, M., Pisa, P., and Kang, H. I. Potential role of Epstein-Barr virus in Sjogren's syndrome and rheumatoid arthritis. *J Rheumatol Suppl* 1992; **32**: 18–24.

28. Balandraud, N., Roudier, J., and Roudier, C. Epstein-Barr virus and rheumatoid arthritis. *Autoimmun Rev* 2004; **3**: 362–7.

29. Alspaugh, M. A., Henle, G., Lennette, E. T., Henle, W. Elevated levels of antibodies to Epstein-Barr virus antigens in sera and synovial fluids of patients with rheumatoid arthritis. *J Clin Invest* 1981; **67**: 1134–40.

30. Venables, P. Epstein-Barr virus infection and autoimmunity in rheumatoid arthritis. *Ann Rheum Dis* 1988; **47**: 265–9.

31. Rosen, A., Gergely, P., Jondal, M., Klein, G., and Britton, S. Polyclonal Ig production after Epstein-Barr virus infection of human lymphocytes in vitro. *Nature* 1977; **267**: 52–4.

32. Slaughter, L, Carson, D. A., Jensen, F. C., Holbrook, T. L., Vaughan, J. H. In vitro effects of Epstein-Barr virus on peripheral blood mononuclear cells from patients with rheumatoid arthritis and normal subjects. *J Exp Med* 1978; **148**: 1429–34.

33. Depper, J. M., and Zvaifler, N. J. Epstein-Barr virus: its relationship to the pathogenesis of rheumatoid arthritis. *Arthritis Rheum* 1981; **24**: 755–61.

34. Yao, Q. Y., Rickinson, A. B., Gaston, J. S., and Epstein, M. A. Disturbance of the Epstein-Barr virus-host balance in rheumatoid arthritis patients: a quantitative study. *Clin Exp Immunol* 1986; **64**: 302–10.

35. Roudier, J., Rhodes, G., Petersen, J., Vaughan, J. H., and Carson, D. A. The Epstein-Barr virus glycoprotein gp110, a molecular link between HLA DR4, HLA DR1, and rheumatoid arthritis. *Scand J Immunol* 1988; **27**: 367–71.

36. Saal, J. G., Krimmel, M., Steidle, M. *et al.* Synovial Epstein-Barr virus infection increases the risk of rheumatoid arthritis in individuals with the shared HLA-DR4 epitope. *Arthritis Rheum* 1999; **42**: 1485–96.

37. Toussirot, E., Wendling, D., Tiberghien, P., Luka, J., and Roudier, J. Decreased T cell precursor frequencies to Epstein-Barr virus glycoprotein Gp110 in peripheral blood correlate with disease activity and severity in patients with rheumatoid arthritis. *Ann Rheum Dis* 2000; **59**: 533–8.

38. Zhang, L., Nikkari, S., Skurnik, M. *et al.* Detection of herpesviruses by polymerase chain reaction in lymphocytes from patients with rheumatoid arthritis. *Arthritis Rheum* 1993; **36**: 1080–6.

39. Takei, M., Mitamura, K., Fujiwara, S. *et al.* Detection of Epstein-Barr virus-encoded small RNA 1 and latent membrane protein 1 in synovial lining cells from rheumatoid arthritis patients. *Int Immunol* 1997; **9**: 739–43.

40. Niedobitek, G., Lisner, R., Swoboda, B. *et al.* Lack of evidence for an involvement of Epstein-Barr virus infection of synovial membranes in the pathogenesis of rheumatoid arthritis. *Arthritis Rheum* 2000; **43**: 151–4.

41. Takeda, T., Mizugaki, Y., Matsubara, L. *et al.* Lytic Epstein-Barr virus infection in the synovial tissue of patients with rheumatoid arthritis. *Arthritis Rheum* 2000; **43**: 1218–25.

42. Mehraein, Y., Lennerz, C., Ehlhardt, S. *et al.* Latent Epstein-Barr virus (EBV) infection and cytomegalovirus (CMV) infection in synovial tissue of autoimmune chronic arthritis determined by RNA- and DNA-in situ hybridization. *Mod Pathol* 2004; **17**: 781–9.

43. Ollier, W. Rheumatoid arthritis and Epstein-Barr virus: a case of living with the enemy? *Ann Rheum Dis* 2000; **59**: 497–9.

44. Yang, L., and Hakoda, M., Iwabuchi, K. *et al.* Rheumatoid factors induce signaling from B cells, leading to Epstein-Barr virus and B-cell activation. *J Virol* 2004; **78**: 9918–23.

45. Salahuddin, S. Z., Ablashi, D. V, Markham, P. D. *et al.* Isolation of a new virus, HBLV, in patients with lymphoproliferative disorders. *Science* 1986; **234**: 596–601.

46. Frenkel, N., Schirmer, E. C., Wyatt, L. S. *et al.* Isolation of a new herpesvirus from human CD4+ T cells. *Proc Natl Acad Sci U S A* 1990; **87**: 748–52.

47. Chan, S. R., Bloomer, C., and Chandran, B. Identification and characterization of human herpesvirus-8 lytic cycle-associated ORF 59 protein and the encoding cDNA by monoclonal antibody. *Virology* 1998; **240**: 118–26.

48. Simmons, A., Tscharke, D., and Speck, P. The role of immune mechanisms in control of herpes simplex virus infection of the peripheral nervous system. *Curr Top Microbiol Immunol* 1992; **179**: 31–56.

49. Pellett, P. E., and Tipples, G. Human herpesviruses 6, 7, and 8. In *Manual of clinical microbiology*, 8th edn (Murray, P. R., Baron, E. J., Jorgensen, J. H., Pfaller, M. A., Yolken, R. H., eds), pp. 1341–59. Washington, DC: ASM Press; 2003.

50. Friedman, H. M., Pincus, T., Gibilisco, P. *et al.* Acute monoarticular arthritis caused by herpes simplex virus and cytomegalovirus. *Am J Med* 1980; **69**: 241–7.

51. Shelley, W. B. Herpetic arthritis associated with disseminate herpes simplex in a wrestler. *Brit J Dermatol* 1980; **103**: 209–12.

52. Modrow, S., Falke, D., Truyen, U. Herpesviren. In *Molekulare Virologie*, 2nd edn (Modrow, S., Falke, D., and Truyen, U., eds), pp. 514–613. Heidelberg: Spectrum Akademischer Verlag; 2003.

53. Male, D., Young, A., Pilkington, C., Sutherland, S., and Roitt, I. M. Antibodies to EB virus- and cytomegalovirus-induced antigens in early rheumatoid disease. *Clin Exp Immunol* 1982; **50**: 341–6.

54. Musiani, M., Zerbini, M., Ferri, S. *et al.* Comparison of the immune response to Epstein-Barr virus and cytomegalovirus in sera and synovial fluids of patients with rheumatoid arthritis. *Ann Rheum Dis* 1987; **46**: 837–42.

55. Ford, D. K., da Roza, D. M., Schulzer, M., Reid, G. D., and Denegri, J. F. Persistent synovial lymphocyte responses to cytomegalovirus antigen in some patients with rheumatoid arthritis. *Arthritis Rheum* 1987; **30**: 700–4.

56. Einsele, H., Steidle, M., Müller, C. A. *et al.* Demonstration of cytomegalovirus (CMV) DNA and anti-CMV response in the synovial membrane and serum of patients with rheumatoid arthritis. *J Rheumatol* 1992; **19**: 677–81.

57. Murayama, T., Jisaki, F., Ayata, M. *et al.* Cytomegalovirus genomes demonstrated by polymerase chain reaction in synovial fluid from rheumatoid arthritis patients. *Clin Exp Rheumatol* 1992; **10**: 161–4.

58. Tamm, A., Ziegler, T., Lautenschlager, I. *et al.* Detection of cytomegalovirus DNA in cells from synovial fluid and peripheral blood of patients with early rheumatoid arthritis. *J Rheumatol* 1993; **20**: 1489–93.

59. White, D. G., Woolf, A. D., Mortimer, P. P. *et al.* Human parvovirus arthropathy. *Lancet* 1985; **1**: 419–21.

60. Naides, S. J., Scharosch, L. L., Foto, F., and Howard, E. J. Rheumatologic manifestations of human parvovirus B19 infection in adults: initial two-year clinical experience. *Arthritis Rheum* 1990; **33**: 1297–309.

61. Nikkari, S., Luukkainen, R., Möttönen, T. *et al.* Does parvovirus B19 have a role in rheumatoid arthritis? *Ann Rheum Dis* 1994; **53**: 106–11.

62. Nikkari, S., Roivainen, A., Hannonen, P. *et al.* Persistence of parvovirus B19 in synovial fluid and bone marrow. *Ann Rheum Dis* 1995; **54**: 597–600.

63. Kerr, J. R. Pathogenesis of human parvovirus B19 in rheumatic disease. *Ann Rheum Dis* 2000; **59**: 672–83.

64. Klouda, P. T., Corbin, S. A., Bradley, B. A., Cohen, B. J., and Woolf, A. D. HLA and acute arthritis following human parvovirus infection. *Tissue Antigens* 1986; **28**: 318–19.

65. Jawad, A. S. M. Persistent arthritis after human parvovirus B19 infection [Letter]. *Lancet* 1993; **341**: 494.

66. Gendi, N S., Gibson, K., and Wordsworth, B. P. Effect of HLA type and hypocomplementaemia on the expression of parvovirus arthritis: one year follow up of an outbreak. *Ann Rheum Dis* 1996; **55**: 63–5.

67. Saal, J. G., Steidle, M., Einsele, H. *et al.* Persistence of B19 parvovirus in synovial membranes of patients with rheumatoid arthritis. *Rheumatol Int* 1992; **12**: 147–51.

68. Kerr, J. R., Cartron, J. P., Curran, M. D. *et al.* A study of the role of parvovirus B19 in rheumatoid arthritis. *Brit J Rheumatol* 1995; **34**: 809–13.

69. Söderlund, M., von Essen, R., Haapasaari, J. *et al.* Persistence of parvovirus B19 DNA in synovial membranes of young patients with and without chronic arthropathy. *Lancet* 1997; **349**: 1063–5.

70. Takahashi, Y., Murai, C., Shibata, S. *et al.* Human parvovirus B19 as a causative agent for rheumatoid arthritis. *Proc Natl Acad Sci U S A* 1998; **95**: 8227–32.

71. Mehraein, Y., Lennerz, C., Ehlhardt, S. *et al.* Detection of parvovirus B19 capsid proteins in lymphocytic cells in synovial tissue of autoimmune chronic arthritis. *Mod Pathol* 2003; **16**: 811–17.

72. Peterlana, D., Puccetti, A., Beri, R. *et al.* The presence of parvovirus B19 VP and NS1 genes in the synovium is not correlated with rheumatoid arthritis. *J Rheumatol* 2003; **30**: 1907–10.

73. Kerr, J. R., Curran, M. D., Moore, J. E., and Murphy, P. G. Parvovirus B19 infection: persistence and genetic variation. *Scand J Infect Dis* 1995; **27**: 551–7.

74. Naides, S. J. Rheumatic manifestations of parvovirus B19 infection. *Rheum Dis Clin North Am* 1998; **24**: 375–401.

75. Moore, T L. Parvovirus-associated arthritis. *Curr Opin Rheumatol* 2000; **12**: 289–94.

76. Seishima, M., Oyama, Z., and Yamamura, M. Two-year follow-up study after human parvovirus B19 infection. *Dermatology* 2003; **206**: 192–6.

77. Caliskan, R., Masatlioglu, S., Aslan, M. *et al.* The relationship between arthritis and human parvovirus B19 infection. *Rheumatol Int* 2005; **26**: 7–11.

78. Cooke, S. P., Rigby, S. P., Griffiths, D. J., and Venables, P. J. Viral studies in rheumatic disease. *Ann Med Interne (Paris)* 1998; **149**: 30–3.

79. Carty, S. M., Snowden, N., and Silman, A. J. Should infection still be considered as the most likely triggering factor for rheumatoid arthritis? *J Rheumatol* 2003; **30**: 425–9.

80. Nikkari, S., Luukkainen, R., Nikkari, L., Skurnik, M., and Toivanen, P. No evidence of adenoviral hexon regions in rheumatoid synovial cells and tissue. *J Rheumatol* 1994; **21**: 2179–83.

81. Zhang, D., Nikkari, S., Vainionpää, R. *et al.* Detection of rubella, mumps, and measles virus genomic RNA in cells from synovial fluid and peripheral blood in early rheumatoid arthritis. *J Rheumatol* 1997; **24**: 1260–5.

82. Cacoub, P., Poynard, T., Ghillani, P. *et al.* Extrahepatic manifestations of chronic hepatitis C. MULTIVIRC Group. Multidepartment Virus C. *Arthritis Rheum* 1999; **42**: 2204–12.

83. Maillefert, J. F., Muller, G., Falgarone, G. *et al.* Prevalence of hepatitis C virus infection in patients with rheumatoid arthritis. *Ann Rheum Dis* 2002; **61**: 635–7.

84. Hsu, F. C., Starkebaum, G., Boyko, E. J., and Dominitz, J. A. Prevalence of rheumatoid arthritis and hepatitis C in those age 60 and older in a US population based study. *J Rheumatol* 2003; **30**: 455–8.

85. Rosner, I., Rozenbaum, M., Toubi, E. *et al.* The case for hepatitis C arthritis. *Semin Arthritis Rheum* 2004; **33**: 375–87.

86. Scully, L. J., Karayiannis, P., and Thomas, H. C. Interferon therapy is effective in treatment of hepatitis B-induced polyarthritis. *Dig Dis Sci* 1992; **37**: 1757–60.

87. Csepregi, A., Rojkovich, B., Nemesánszky, E. *et al.* Chronic seropositive polyarthritis associated with hepatitis B virus-induced chronic liver disease: a sequel of virus persistence. *Arthritis Rheum* 2000; **43**: 232–3.

88. Hachulla, E., Houvenagel, E., Mingui, A., Vincent, G., and Laine, A. Reactive arthritis after hepatitis B vaccination. *J Rheumatol* 1990; **17**: 1250–1.

89. Gross, K., Combe, C., Krüger, K., and Schattenkirchner, M. Arthritis after hepatitis B vaccination: report of three cases. *Scand J Rheumatol* 1995; **24**: 50–2.

90. Pope, J. E., Stevens, A., Howson, W., and Bell, D. A. The development of rheumatoid arthritis after recombinant hepatitis B vaccination. *J Rheumatol* 1998; **25**: 1687–93.

91. Csepregi, A., Nemesanszky, E., Rojkovich, B., and Poor, G. Rheumatoid arthritis and hepatitis B virus: evaluating the pathogenic link. *J Rheumatol* 2001; **28**: 474–7.

92. Milhau, N., Renson, P., Dreesen, I. *et al.* Viral expression and leukocyte adhesion after in vitro infection of goat mammary gland cells with caprine arthritis-encephalitis virus. *Vet Immunol Immunopathol* 2005; **103**: 93–9.

93. Iwakura, Y. Roles of IL-1 in the development of rheumatoid arthritis: consideration from mouse models. *Cytokine Growth Factor Rev* 2002; **13**: 341–55.

94. Zucker-Franklin, D., Pancake, B. A, Brown, W. H. Prevalence of HTLV-I Tax in a subset of patients with rheumatoid arthritis. *Clin Exp Rheumatol* 2002; **20**: 161–9.

95. Hasunuma, T., Sumida, T., Nishioka, K. Human T cell leukemia virus type-I and rheumatoid arthritis. *Int Rev Immunol* 1998; **17**: 291–307.

96. Vassilopoulos, D., and Calabrese, L. H. Rheumatic aspects of human immunodeficiency virus infection and other immunodeficient states. In *Rheumatology*, 3rd edn. (Hochberg, M., Silman, A., Smolen, J., Weinblatt, M., Weissman, M., eds), pp. 1115–29. London: Mosby; 2003.

97. Griffiths, D. J., Cooke S. P., Herve C. *et al.* Detection of human retrovirus 5 in patients with arthritis and systemic lupus erythematosus. *Arthritis Rheum* 1999; **42**: 448–54.

98. Brand, A., Griffiths, D. J., Herve, C., Mallon, E., and Venables, P. J. Human retrovirus-5 in rheumatic disease. *J Autoimmun* 1999; **13**: 149–54.

99. Gaudin, P., Moutet, F., Tuke, P. W., and Garson, J. A. Absence of human retrovirus 5 in French patients with rheumatoid arthritis: comment on the article by Griffiths et al. *Arthritis Rheum* 1999; **42**: 2492–4.

100. Holoshitz, J., Klajman, A., Drucker, I. *et al.* T lymphocytes of rheumatoid arthritis patients show augmented reactivity to a fraction of mycobacteria cross-reactive with cartilage. *Lancet* 1986; **2**: 305–9.

101. Gripenberg-Lerche, C., Toivanen, A., and Toivanen, P. *Yersinia*-associated arthritis in rats: effect of 65 kDa heat shock protein, bovine serum albumin and incomplete Freund's adjuvant. *Clin Exp Rheumatol* 1995; **13**: 321–5.

102. Prakken, B. J., Roord, S., Ronaghy, A. *et al.* Heat shock protein 60 and adjuvant arthritis: a model for T cell regulation in human arthritis. *Springer Semin Immunopathol* 2003; **25**: 47–63.

103. Durai, M., Kim, H. R., Moudgil, K. D. The regulatory C-terminal determinants within mycobacterial heat shock protein 65 are cryptic and cross-reactive with the dominant self homologs: implications for the pathogenesis of autoimmune arthritis. *J Immunol* 2004; **173**: 181–8.

104. Quintana, F. J., Carmi, P., Mor, F., and Cohen, I. R. Inhibition of adjuvant-induced arthritis by DNA vaccination with the 70-kd or the 90-kd human heat-shock protein: immune cross-regulation with the 60-kd heat-shock protein. *Arthritis Rheum* 2004; **50**: 3712–20.

105. Aoki, S., Yoshikawa, K., Yokoyama, T. *et al.* Role of enteric bacteria in the pathogenesis of rheumatoid arthritis: evidence for antibodies to enterobacterial common antigens in rheumatoid sera and synovial fluids. *Ann Rheum Dis* 1996; **55**: 363–9.

106. Aoki, S. Rheumatoid arthritis and enteric bacteria. *Jpn J Rheumatol* 1999; **9**: 325–52.

107. Albani, S., Keystone, E. C., Nelson, J. L. *et al.* Positive selection in autoimmunity: abnormal immune responses to a bacterial dnaJ antigenic determinant in patients with early rheumatoid arthritis. *Nat Med* 1995; **1**: 448–52.

108. Hirata, D., Hirai, I., Iwamoto, M. *et al.* Preferential binding with Escherichia coli hsp60 of antibodies prevalent in sera from patients with rheumatoid arthritis. *Clin Immunol Immunopathol* 1997; **82**: 141–8.

109. Puga Yung, G. L., Le, T. D., Roord, S., Prakken, B., and Albani, S. Heat shock proteins (HSP) for immunotherapy of rheumatoid arthritis (RA). *Inflamm Res* 2003; **52**: 443–51.

110. Pönkä, A. The occurrence and clinical picture of serologically verified Mycoplasma pneumoniae infections with emphasis on central nervous system, cardiac and joint manifestations. *Ann Clin Res* 1979; **11** (Suppl. 24): 1–60.

111. Jansson, E., Backman, A, Hakkarainen, K., Miettinen A., and Seniusova, B., Mycoplasmas and arthritis. *Z Rheumatol* 1983; **42**: 315–19.

112. Barile, M. F., Yoshida, H., and Roth, H. Rheumatoid arthritis: new findings on the failure to isolate or detect mycoplasmas by multiple cultivation or serologic procedures and a review of the literature. *Rev Infect Dis* 1991; **13**: 571–82.

113. Ebringer, A., Cox, N. L., Abuljadayel, I. *et al.* Klebsiella antibodies in ankylosing spondylitis and Proteus antibodies in rheumatoid arthritis. *Brit J Rheumatol* 1988; **27** (Suppl. II): 272–85.

114. Senior, B. W., Anderson, G. A., Morley, K. D., and Kerr, M. A. Evidence that patients with rheumatoid arthritis have asymptomatic 'non-significant' Proteus mirabilis bacteriuria more frequently than healthy controls. *J Infection* 1999; **38**: 99–106.

115. Tiwana, H., Wilson, C., Alvarez, A. *et al.* Cross-reactivity between the rheumatoid arthritis-associated motif EQKRAA and structurally related sequences found in Proteus mirabilis. *Infect Immun* 1999; **67**: 2769–75.

116. Wilson, C., Tiwana, H., and Ebringer, A. Molecular mimicry between HLA-DR alleles associated with rheumatoid arthritis and Proteus mirabilis as the aetiological basis for autoimmunity. *Microbes Infect* 2000; **2**: 1489–96.

117. Whiteford, J. R., Wilson, C., Tiwana, H., and Ebringer, A. Genetic diversity in Proteus mirabilis isolates found in the urinary tract of rheumatoid arthritis patients. *J Infection* 2000; **41**: 245–8.

118. Albert, L. J. Infection and rheumatoid arthritis: guilt by association? *J Rheumatol* 2000; **27**: 564–6.

119. Chandrashekara, S., Ramesh, M. N., Shobha, A. *et al.* Proteus mirabilis and rheumatoid arthritis: no association with the disease. *Clin Rheumatol* 2003; **22**: 218–20.

120. Lehtonen, L., Eerola, E., and Toivanen, P. Muramic acid in human peripheral blood leucocytes in different age groups. *Eur J Clin Invest* 1997; **27**: 791–2.

121. Lehtonen, L., Eerola, E., Oksman, P., and Toivanen, P. Muramic acid in peripheral blood leukocytes of healthy human subjects. *J Infect Dis* 1995; **171**: 1060–4.

122. Schrijver, I. A, Melief, M.- J., Markusse, H. M. *et al.* Peptidoglycan from sterile human spleen induces T-cell proliferation and inflammatory mediators in rheumatoid arthritis patients and healthy subjects. *Rheumatology* 2001; **40**: 438–46.

123. Lehtonen, L., Kortekangas, P., Oksman, P. *et al.* Synovial fluid muramic acid in acute inflammatory arthritis. *Brit J Rheumatol* 1994; **33**: 1127–30.

124. van der Heijden, I. M., Wilbrink, B., Tchetverikov, I. *et al.* Presence of bacterial DNA and bacterial peptidoglycans in joints of patients with rheumatoid arthritis and other arthritides. *Arthritis Rheum* 2000; **43**: 593–8.

125. Chen, T., Rimpiläinen, M., Luukkainen, R. *et al.* Bacterial components in the synovial tissue of patients with advanced rheumatoid arthritis or osteoarthritis: analysis with gas chromatography-mass spectrometry and pan-bacterial polymerase chain reaction. *Arthritis Care Res* 2003; **49**: 328–34.

126. Wilbrink, B., van der Heijden, I. M., Schouls, L. M. *et al.* Detection of bacterial DNA in joint samples from patients with undifferentiated arthritis and reactive arthritis, using polymerase chain reaction with universal 16S ribosomal RNA primers. *Arthritis Rheum* 1998; **41**: 535–43.

127. Wilkinson, N. Z., Kingsley, G. H., Jones, H. W. *et al.* The detection of DNA from a range of bacterial species in the joints of patients with a variety of arthritides using a nested, broad-range polymerase chain reaction. *Rheumatology* 1999; **38**: 260–6.

128. Cox, C. J., Kempsell, K. E., and Gaston, J. S. H. Investigation of infectious agents associated with arthritis by reverse transcription PCR of bacterial rRNA. *Arthritis Res Ther* 2003; **5**: R1–R8.

129. Nikkari, S., McLaughlin, I. J., Bi, W., Dodge, D. E., and Relman, D. A. Does blood of healthy subjects contain bacterial ribosomal DNA? *J Clin Microbiol* 2001; **39**: 1956–9.

130. Lehman, T. J. A., Allen, J. B., Plotz, P. H., and Wilder, R. L. Lactobacillus casei cell wall-induced arthritis in rats: cell wall fragment distribution and persistence in chronic arthritis-susceptible LEW/N and -resistant F344/N rats. *Arthritis Rheum* 1984; **27**: 939–42.

131. Gripenberg-Lerche, C., Skurnik, M., and Toivanen, P. Role of YadA-mediated collagen binding in arthritogenicity of *Yersinia enterocolitica* serotype O:8: experimental studies with rats. *Infect Immun* 1995; **63**: 3222–6.

132. Schumacher, H. R., Jr., Arayssi, T., Crane, M. *et al.* Chlamydia trachomatis nucleic acids can be found in the synovium of some asymptomatic subjects. *Arthritis Rheum* 1999; **42**: 1281–4.

133. Severijnen, A. J., van Kleef, R., Hazenberg, M. P., and van de Merwe, J. P. Cell wall fragments from major residents of the human intestinal flora induce chronic arthritis in rats. *J Rheumatol* 1989; **16**: 1061–8.

134. Zhang, X, Rimpiläinen, M., Hoffman, B. *et al.* Experimental chronic arthritis and granulomatous inflammation induced by Bifidobacterium cell walls. *Scand J Immunol* 2001; **54**: 171–9.

135. Kool, J., Ruseler van Embden, J. G., van Lieshout, L. M. *et al.* Induction of arthritis in rats by soluble peptidoglycan-polysaccharide complexes produced by human intestinal flora. *Arthritis Rheum* 1991; **34**: 1611–16.

136. Zhang, X., Rimpiläinen, M., Simelyte, E., and Toivanen, P. What determines arthritogenicity of bacterial cell wall? A study on Eubacterium cell wall-induced arthritis. *Rheumatology* 2000; **39**: 274–82.

137. Simelyte, E., Rimpiläinen, M., Lehtonen, L, Zhang, X, Toivanen, P. Bacterial cell wall-induced arthritis: chemical composition and tissue distribution of four Lactobacillus strains. *Infect Immun* 2000; **68**: 3535–40.

138. Zhang, X., Rimpiläinen, M., Simelyte, E., and Toivanen, P. Characterization of *Eubacterium* cell wall: peptidoglycan structure determines arthritogenicity. *Ann Rheum Dis* 2001; **60**: 269–74.

139. Wang, J. E., Jörgensen, P. F., Almlöf, M. *et al.* Peptidoglycan and lipoteichoic acid from *Staphylococcus aureus* induce tumor necrosis factor alpha, interleukin 6 (IL-6), and IL-10 production in both T cells and monocytes in a human whole blood model. *Infect Immun* 2000; **68**: 3965–70.

140. Zhang, X., Rimpiläinen, M., Simelyte, E., and Toivanen, P. Enzyme degradation and proinflammatory activity in arthritogenic and nonarthritogenic Eubacterium aerofaciens cell walls. *Infect Immun* 2001; **69**: 7277–84.

141. Dziarski, R. Preferential induction of autoantibody secretion in polyclonal activation by peptidoglycan and lipopolysaccharide. II. In vivo studies. *J Immunol* 1982; **128**: 1026–30.

142. Räsänen, L., and Arvilommi, H. Cell walls, peptidoglycans, and teichoic acids of Gram-positive bacteria as polyclonal inducers and immunomodulators of proliferative and lymphokine responses of human B and T lymphocytes. *Infect Immun* 1982; **35**: 523–7.

143. Levinson, A. I., Dziarski, A., Zweiman, B., and Dziarski, R. Staphylococcal peptidoglycan: T-cell-dependent mitogen and relatively T-cell-independent polyclonal B-cell activator of human lymphocytes. *Infect Immun* 1983; **39**: 290–6.

144. Duchmann, R., Neurath, M. F., Meyer, and zum Buschenfelde, K. H. Responses to self and non-self intestinal microflora in health and inflammatory bowel disease. *Res Immunol* 1997; **148**: 589–94.

145. Tlaskalova-Hogenova, H., Stepankova, R., Hudcovic, T *et al.* Commensal bacteria (normal microflora), mucosal immunity and chronic inflammatory and autoimmune diseases. *Immunol Lett* 2004; **93**: 97–108.

146. Chen, T., Isomäki, P., Rimpiläinen, M., and Toivanen, P. Human cytokine responses induced by Gram-positive cell walls of normal intestinal microbiota. *Clin Exp Immunol* 1999; **118**: 261–7.

147. Pierer, M., Rethage, J., Seibl, R. *et al.* Chemokine secretion of rheumatoid arthritis synovial fibroblasts stimulated by Toll-like receptor 2 ligands. *J Immunol* 2004; **172**: 1256–65.

148. Dziarski, R. Peptidoglycan recognition proteins (PGRPs). *Mol Immunol* 2004; **40**: 877–86.

149. Guan, R., Roychowdhury, A., Ember, B. *et al.* Structural basis for peptidoglycan binding by peptidoglycan recognition proteins. *Proc Natl Acad Sci U S A* 2004; **101**: 17168–73.

150. Kielian, T., Esen, N., and Bearden, E. D. Toll-like receptor 2 (TLR2) is pivotal for recognition of S. aureus peptidoglycan but not intact bacteria by microglia. *Glia* 2005; **49**: 567–76.

151. Visser, L., Jan de Heer, H., Boven, L. A. *et al.* Proinflammatory bacterial peptidoglycan as a cofactor for the development of central nervous system autoimmune disease. *J Immunol* 2005; **174**: 808–16.

152. Brandtzaeg, P. Homing of mucosal immune cells: a possible connection between intestinal and articular inflammation. *Aliment Pharm Therap* 1997; **11** (Suppl. 3): 24–39.

153. Salmi, M., and Jalkanen, S. Systemic manifestations of mucosal diseases: trafficking of gut immune cells to joints. In *Mucosal immunology* (Ogra PL, Mestecky J, Lamm ME, Strober W., Bienenstock J, McGhee JR, eds), pp. 1167–74. San Diego; Academic Press: 1999.

154. Jalkanen, S., Steere, A. C., Fox, R. I., and Butcher, E. C. A distinct endothelial cell recognition system that controls lymphocyte traffic into inflamed synovium. *Science* 1986; **233**: 556–8.

155. Salmi, M., Andrew, D. P., Butcher, E. C., and Jalkanen, S. Dual binding capacity of mucosal immunoblasts to mucosal and synovial endothelium in humans: dissection of the molecular mechanisms. *J Exp Med* 1995; **181**: 137–49.

156. Spargo, L. D., Hawkes, J. S., Cleland, L. G., and Mayrhofer, G. Recruitment of lymphoblasts derived from peripheral and intestinal lymph to synovium and other tissues in normal rats and rats with adjuvant arthritis. *J Immunol* 1996; **157**: 5198–207.

157. Månsson, I., and Olhagen, B. Intestinal Clostridium perfringens in rheumatoid arthritis and other connective tissue disorders: studies of fecal flora, serum antitoxin levels and skin hypersensitivity. *Acta Rheum Scand* 1966; **12**: 167–74.

158. Olhagen, B., and Månsson, I. Intestinal Clostridium perfringens in rheumatoid arthritis and other collagen diseases. *Acta Med Scand* 1968; **184**: 395–402.

159. Sapico, F. L., Emori, H., Smith, L. D. S., Bluestone, R., and Finegold, S. M. Absence of relationship of fecal *Clostridium perfringens* to rheumatoid arthritis and rheumatoid variants. *J Infect Dis* 1973; **128**: 559–62.

160. Olhagen, B., and Månsson, I. Fecal *Clostridium perfringens* and rheumatoid arthritis [Letter]. *J Infect Dis* 1974; **130**: 444–7.

161. Shinebaum, R., Neumann, V C., Cooke, E. M., and Wright, V. Comparison of faecal florae in patients with rheumatoid arthritis and controls. *Brit J Rheumatol* 1987; **26**: 329–33.

162. Månsson, I., Norberg, R., Olhagen, B., and Björklund, N.-E. Arthritis in pigs induced by dietary factors: microbiologic, clinical and histologic studies. *Clin Exp Immunol* 1971; **9**: 677–93.

163. Olhagen, B. Arthritis in pigs induced by dietary factors. In *Spondyloarthropathies: involvement of the gut* (Mielants, H., Veys, E. M., eds), pp. 47–60. Amsterdam: Elsevier Science; 1987.

164. Peltonen, R., Eerola, E., Suomi, K. *et al.* Effect of dietary fish powder on intestinal flora and development of arthritis in the pig. *Brit J Rheumatol* 1993; **32**: 1049–54.

165. Guarner, F., Malagelada, J. R. Gut flora in health and disease. *Lancet* 2003; **361**: 512–19.

166. Onderdonk, A. B., Sasser, M. Gas-liquid and high-performance liquid chromatographic methods for the identification of microorganisms. In *Manual of clinical microbiology*, 6th edn (Murray, P. R., Baron, E. J., Pfaller, M. A., Tenover, F. C., Yolken, R. H., eds), pp. 123–9. Washington, DC: ASM Press; 1995.

167. Peltonen, R.-L., Tenovuo, J., Suvanto, O. *et al.* Effect of smoking on oral and faecal microbial flora studied by gas-liquid chromatography of bacterial cellular fatty acids. *Microb Ecol Health Dis* 2001; **13**: 234–9.

168. Toivanen, P., Vaahtovuo, J., and Eerola, E. Influence of major histocompatibility complex on bacterial composition of fecal flora. *Infect Immun* 2001; **69**: 2372–7.

169. Peltonen, R., Kjeldsen-Kragh, J., Haugen, M. *et al.* Changes of faecal flora in rheumatoid arthritis during fasting and one-year vegetarian diet. *Brit J Rheumatol* 1994; **33**: 638–43.

170. Peltonen, R., Nenonen, M., Helve, T *et al.* Faecal microbial flora and disease activity in rheumatoid arthritis during a vegan diet. *Brit J Rheumatol* 1997; **36**: 64–8.

171. van de Merwe, J. P., Stegeman, J. H., and Hazenberg, M. P. The resident faecal flora is determined by genetic characteristics of the host. Implications for Crohn's disease? *Antonie Van Leeuwenhoek* 1983; **49**: 119–24.

172. Hoeksma, A., and Winkler, K. C. The normal flora of the nose in twins. *Acta Leidensia* 1963; **32**: 123–33.

173. Zoetendal, E. G., Akkermans, A. D. L, Akkermans-van Vliet, W. M., and de Visser JAGM, de Vos W. M. The host genotype affects the bacterial community in the human gastrointestinal tract. *Microb Ecol Health Dis* 2001; **13**: 129–34.

174. Zoetendal, E. G., Collier, C. T., Koike, S., Mackie, R. I., and Gaskins, H. R. Molecular ecological analysis of the gastrointestinal microbiota: a review. *J Nutr* 2004; **134**: 465–72.

175. Vaahtovuo, J., Toivanen, P., and Eerola, E. Bacterial composition of murine fecal microflora is indigenous and genetically guided. *FEMS Microbiol Ecol* 2003; **44**: 131–6.

176. Vaahtovuo, J., Eerola, E., and Toivanen, P. Comparison of cellular fatty acid profiles of the microbiota in different gut regions of BALB/c and C57BL/6J mice. *Antonie Van Leeuwenhoek* 2005; **88**: 67–74.

177. Toivanen, P., Koskimies, S., Granfors, K., Eerola, E. Bacterial antibodies in HLA-B27+ healthy individuals. *Arthritis Rheum* 1993; **36**: 1633–5.

178. Mackie, R. I., White, B. A., and Isaacson, R. E. *Gastrointestinal microbiology*. Vol. 2: *Gastrointestinal microbes and host interactions*. New York; Chapman & Hall: 1997.

179. Borén, T., Falk, P., Roth, K A., Larson, G., and Normark, S. Attachment of Helicobacter pylori to human gastric epithelium mediated by blood group antigens. *Science* 1993; **262**: 1892–5.

180. Peacock, S. J., de Silva, I., and Lowy, F. D. What determines nasal carriage of Staphylococcus aureus? *Trends Microbiol* 2001; **9**: 605–10.

181. Olsén, A., Wick, M. J., Mörgelin, M., and Björck, L. Curli, fibrous surface proteins of *Escherichia coli*, interact with major histocompatibility complex class I molecules. *Infect Immun* 1998; **66**: 944–9.

182. Mohammadi, M., Redline, R., Nedrud, J., and Czinn, S. Role of the host in pathogenesis of *Helicobacter*-associated gastritis: *H. felis* infection of inbred and congenic mouse strains. *Infect Immun* 1996; **64**: 238–45.

183. Posnett, D. N., and Edinger, J. When do microbes stimulate rheumatoid factor? *J Exp Med* 1997; **185**: 1721–3.

184. Newkirk, M. M. Rheumatoid factors: host resistance or autoimmunity? *Clin Immunol* 2002; **104**: 1–13.

185. Aho, K., Heliövaara, M., Maatela, J., Tuomi, T., and Palosuo, T. Rheumatoid factors antedating clinical rheumatoid arthritis. *J Rheumatol* 1991; **18**: 1282–4.

186. Nisini, R., Biselli, R., Matricardi, P. M., Fattorossi, A., and D'Amelio, R. Clinical and immunological response to typhoid vaccination with parenteral or oral vaccines in two groups of 30 recruits. *Vaccine* 1993; **11**: 582–6.

187. Kasser, U. R., Seidl, C., Ehrfeld, H., and Schmidt, K. L. Höhe Rheumafaktorentiter durch Vakzination? [A high rheumatoid factor titer caused by vaccination?]. *Z Rheumatol* 2000; **59**: 86–92.

188. Silman, A., Davies, P., Currey, H. L., and Evans, S. J. Is rheumatoid arthritis becoming less severe? *J Chronic Dis* 1983; **36**: 891–7.

189. Silman, A. J. The changing face of rheumatoid arthritis: why the decline in incidence? *Arthritis Rheum* 2002; **46**: 579–81.

190. Doran, M. F., Pond, G. R., Crowson, C. S., O'Fallon, W. M., and Gabriel, S. E. Trends in incidence and mortality in rheumatoid arthritis in Rochester, Minnesota, over a forty-year period. *Arthritis Rheum* 2002; **46**: 625–31.

191. Sigal, L H. Antibiotics for the treatment of rheumatologic syndromes. *Rheum Dis Clin North Am* 1999; **25**: 861–81, viii.

192. O'Dell, J. R., Blakely, K W., Mallek, J. A. *et al*. Treatment of early seropositive rheumatoid arthritis: a two-year, double-blind comparison of minocycline and hydroxychloroquine. *Arthritis Rheum* 2001; **44**: 2235–41.

193. Pillemer, S., Gulko, P., Ligier, S. *et al*. Pilot clinical trial of intravenous doxycycline versus placebo for rheumatoid arthritis. *J Rheumatol* 2003; **30**: 41–3.

194. Stone, M., Fortin, P. R., Pacheco-Tena, C., and Inman, R. D. Should tetracycline treatment be used more extensively for rheumatoid arthritis? Metaanalysis demonstrates clinical benefit with reduction in disease activity. *J Rheumatol* 2003; **30**: 2112–22.

195. Suresh, E., Morris, I. M., and Mattingly, P. C. Use of minocycline in rheumatoid arthritis: a district general hospital experience. *Ann Rheum Dis* 2004; **63**: 1354–5.

196. Voils, S. A., Evans, M. E., Lane, M. T., Schosser, R. H., and Rapp, R. P. Use of macrolides and tetracyclines for chronic inflammatory diseases. *Ann Pharmacother* 2005; **39**: 86–94.

197. Sewell, K. L., Breedveld, F., Furrie, E. *et al*. The effect of minocycline in rat models of inflammatory arthritis: correlation of arthritis suppression with enhanced T cell calcium flux. *Cell Immunol* 1996; **167**: 195–204.

198. Amin, A. R., Attur, M. G., Thakker, G. D. *et al*. A novel mechanism of action of tetracyclines: effects on nitric oxide synthases. *Proc Natl Acad Sci U S A* 1996; **93**: 14014–19.

199. American College of Rheumatology. Guidelines for the management of rheumatoid arthritis: 2002 update. *Arthritis Rheum* 2002; **46**: 328–46.

200. Silman, A. J., MacGregor, A. J., Thomson, W. *et al*. Twin concordance rates for rheumatoid arthritis: results from a nationwide study. *Brit J Rheumatol* 1993; **32**: 903–7.

201. MacGregor, A. J., Bamber, S., Carthy, D. *et al*. Heterogeneity of disease phenotype in monozygotic twins concordant for rheumatoid arthritis. *Brit J Rheumatol* 1995; **34**: 215–20.

202. Heliövaara, M., Aho, K., Knekt, P. *et al*. Coffee consumption, rheumatoid factor, and the risk of rheumatoid arthritis. *Ann Rheum Dis* 2000; **59**: 631–5.

203. Mattey, D. L., Hutchinson, D., Dawes, P. T. *et al*. Smoking and disease severity in rheumatoid arthritis: association with polymorphism at the glutathione S-transferase M1 locus. *Arthritis Rheum* 2002; **46**: 640–6.

204. Olsson, A. R., Skogh, T., and Wingren, G. Aetiological factors of importance for the development of rheumatoid arthritis. *Scand J Rheumatol* 2004; **33**: 300–6.

205. Holmstrup, P., Poulsen, A. H., Andersen, L., Skuldbol, T., and Fiehn, N. E. Oral infections and systemic diseases. *Dent Clin North Am* 2003; **47**: 575–98.

206. Mercado, F. B., Marshall, R. I., and Bartold, P. M. Inter-relationships between rheumatoid arthritis and periodontal disease: a review. *J Clin Periodontol* 2003; **30**: 761–72.

4 | Experimental models for RA

Rikard Holmdahl

Introduction

For a deeper understanding of the complexity of the pathogenesis of rheumatoid arthritis (RA), the use of animal models is a necessity. Obviously a disease identical to RA cannot develop in any experimental animal since they are different species with different genetics and live in a different environment, as compared with humans.

The advantages of using animal models are mainly:

1. The animals can be genetically controlled. Laboratory mouse and rat strains have been inbred, which dramatically facilitates genetic studies.

2. Their environment can be better controlled than for humans.

3. Manipulative experiments can be made. The genome of inbred strains can be changed by mutations, insertions, and deletions. The environment can also be changed in a controlled way; they can be immunized, or infected, which may lead to arthritis.

4. It is more ethical to use animals than humans for experimental research purposes.

To be able to evaluate and select proper animal models for RA it is of value to be able to reproduce some of the basic features of RA. Such hallmarks of RA are;

- *Tissue-specificity*: RA is a characterized by a tissue-specific inflammatory attack affecting diarthrodial, peripheral, and cartilaginous joints. Although systemic manifestations are usually present, the initial inflammatory attack is directed towards peripheral joints.
- *Chronicity*: The disease is chronic and occurs in tissues in which no causative infectious pathogens have so far been demonstrated. Acute joint affections are common manifestations in both physiological responses to infections and in connection with other inflammatory disorders, but in RA chronicity is an essential characteristic. The disease course may proceed with identifiable relapses, but there is usually a steady progression of joint destruction.
- *Autoantibodies*: The development of RA is preceded by, and associated with elevated levels of autoantibodies in serum. Antibodies to citrullinated protein epitopes have the highest specificity and sensitivity, followed by antibodies to immunoglobulin (rheumatoid factors), but antibodies to other antigens do also occur in subsets of patients, like antibodies to type II collagen (CII), RA33 and glucose 6 phosphoisomerase (G6PI).

- *MHC class II association*: The genetic influence is significant but complex. One of the few gene regions so far identified contains the class II genes in the major histocompatibility complex (MHC). In particular certain structures in the peptide-binding pocket of HLA-DR4 molecules are highly associated with RA.

Taken together, these findings suggest that immune-mediated inflammation directed to peripheral joints plays a role in the disease process. One explanation for such a response would be the occurrence of an infectious agent persisting in the joint. However, so far it has not been possible to identify such an agent as an explanation for RA. Alternatively, the immune reaction could be directed to the molecular targets in the joints, in cartilage, or the synovial tissue. Another explanation could relate to a defect in a gene related to peripheral joints, for example leading to cartilage fragility or a gene affecting immune recognition. However, such a genetic defect has not been found. Thus, the cause and driving forces are polygenic and multifactorial, and the understanding of the disease will require a detailed basic analysis of disease mechanisms. Animal models are excellent tools for such an analysis. Recent advances in animal models mimicking different aspects of human diseases, and the improvement in genetic techniques, has dramatically increased their usefulness. The present overview will include not only models for RA, but also models more similar to some related diseases such as psoriasis arthritis, Reiter's disease, ankylosing spondylitis, Lyme disease, and septic arthritis (summarized in Table 4.1).

Arthritis caused by infectious agents, including complete Freund's adjuvant

Several infectious agents may invade joints, persist there, and cause arthritis. As with most persisting infectious agents a balance between the parasite and the host is usually achieved. Thus inflammatory consequences may not only be caused directly by the parasite but also by an aberrant inflammatory response of the host. When microorganisms are present in the target tissue, chronic autoimmunity could be maintained by different mechanisms such as superantigen-mediated T cell activation, a cross-reactive immune response, or the presence of adjuvant material enhancing autoantigen presentation. Several such arthritogenic agents have been described in experimental animals and some of these mimic a corresponding infectious disease in humans.

Table 4.1 Overview of animal arthritis models

Model	Species	Genetics	Disease characteristics
Arthritis caused by infection			
Mycoplasma-induced arthritis	Rats and mice	More pronounced in B cell-deficient mice	Mild chronic arthritis
Borrelia-induced arthritis	Mice	MHC	Severe and erosive arthritis with spirochetes in the joints
Staphylococcus-induced arthritis	Rats and mice	MHC	Severe arthritis
Yersinia-induced arthritis	Rats and mice	LEW and SHR but not DA and BN rats	Severe arthritis with bacteria in the joints
Arthritis caused by bacterial fragments			
Mycobacterium-induced arthritis (MIA)	Rats	MHC, non-MHC genes (LEW > F344)	Acute and generalized inflammatory disease, including erosive arthritis
Streptococcal cell wall-induced arthritis	Mice and rats	Non-MHC genes (LEW > F344) (DBA/1 = Balb/c > B10)	Severe and erosive arthritis
Arthritis induced by adjuvant injection			
Avridine-induced arthritis (AvIA)	Rats	MHC (f)	Very severe, erosive, and chronic arthritis
Oil (mineral oil)-induced arthritis (OIA)	DA rats	non-MHC loci on chr 4, 10	Acute and self-limited inflammation of peripheral joints
Pristane-induced arthritis (PIA)	Rats	MHC, non-MHC loci on chr 1, 4, 6, 12, 14	Chronic and erosive arthritis in peripheral joints
Pristane-induced arthritis (PIA)	Mice	MHC (q, d)? Balb/c, DBA and C3H gene backgrounds	Chronic and generalized inflammatory disease predominately affecting joints
Unmethylated DNA-induced arthritis	Mice	DBA/1	Mild arthritis after intra-articular injection of unmethylated DNA or CpG oligonucleotides
Arthritis induced by cartilage protein immunization			
CII (heterologous or homologous CII in mineral oil)-induced arthritis (CIA)	Rats	MHC (a, l, f and u), non-MHC loci on chr 1, 4, 7, 10	Chronic and erosive arthritis in peripheral joints
CII (heterologous or homologous CII in CFA)-induced arthritis (CIA)	Mice	MHC (q and r), non-MHC loci on chr 1, 2, 3, 6, 7, 8, 10, 15	Erosive arthritis in peripheral joints
CXI (rat CXI in IFA)-induced arthritis	Rats	MHC (f, u)	Severe, chronic arthritis
Human proteoglycan (in CFA)-induced arthritis	BALB/c mice	MHC (d), several non-MHC loci	Chronic arthritis
COMP (in mineral oil)-induced arthritis	Rats	MHC (u)	Acute arthritis
'Spontaneous' arthritis models			
HLA-B27 transgenic animals	Mice and rats	B27 heavy chain transgene	Ankylosing spondylitis, colitis, balanitis, arthritis
The MRL/lpr mouse (mutation in the fas gene controlling apoptosis)	Mice	lpr	Generalized inflammation as a part of lupus disease which also affect joints
Inter-male aggressiveness stress-induced arthritis	DBA/1 mice	Non-MHC genes	Enthesopathic response with no evidence for immune involvement. A model for psoriasis arthritis
TNFα transgenic mice (overproduction of TNFα)	Mice	TNF-α transgene	Erosive arthritis as well as generalized tissue information
ILR antagonist-deficient mouse	Balb/c mice	ILRa deficiency	Erosive arthritis
TCR transgenic mouse (T cell autoreactivity)	Mice	TCR transgene	Severe arthritis mediated by pathogenic antibodies to G6PI
Zap70 mutation	Balb/c mice	Spontaneous mutation in Zap70	Severe arthritis with autoreactivity
HTLV transgenic mouse	Mice	HTLV transgene	Erosive arthritis
HTLV transgenic rat	Rats	HTLV transgene	Generalized tissue inflammation
SCID mouse	Mice	Local injection of fibroblasts into immunodeficient SCID mouse	Sustained destructive arthritis

Mycoplasma arthritides Arthritis associated with mycoplasma infection is endemic among farm animals. It is also possible to induce arthritis in rodents after inoculation with *Mycoplasma arthritidis*. However, Mycoplasma bacteria are not easily found in RA joints, although they may cause arthritis in individuals with severe B cell deficiency[1]. Inoculation of mice induces a mild chronic arthritis in conjunction with the persistence of the microorganism[2]. In accordance with the observations in humans, B cell-deleted mice are more susceptible to Mycoplasma-induced arthritis[3].

Lyme arthritis *Borrelia* is a spirochete that may persist in joints and cause arthritis. The clinical picture is chronic and resembles RA and it is genetically associated with HLA-DR4, as is RA, although the immune response causing the MHC association has not been clarified. Clearly live bacteria persist in the joints but in many patients it has been difficult to identify the spirochete in the arthritic joints. Mice infected with *Borrelia* develop arthritis similar to the human disease[4]. As in humans, MHC controls the susceptibility to arthritis. The persistence of the spirochete seems to be a requirement for the development of the arthritis[5], although some mouse strains do not develop arthritis in spite of high levels of bacteria in the joints.

Staphylococcal arthritis Septic arthritis is most commonly caused by a persistent infection of *Staphylococcus aureus*. The bacteria tend to be encapsulated in tissues, including joint synovia, and persist for years. Inoculation with certain *S. aureus* strains induces septic arthritis in many mouse and rat strains[6,7]. Severe and prolonged arthritis develops in infected joints, mimicking the human situation. Interestingly, protection of the host is critically dependent on the innate defense, such as neutrophils and complement, whereas the adapted immune response is not effective[8]. Instead, the apparently aberrant adapted immune response actually causes the main trouble in the joints[7,9,10].

Arthritis and ankylosing spondylitis induced by intracellular bacteria Some bacteria with the capacity to invade cells upon infection (e.g. *Yersinia*) are known to be related to postinfectious arthritides such as reactive arthritis and ankylosing spondylitis. These diseases are genetically associated with HLA-B27, a MHC class I allele of the B locus. It has been possible to reproduce the human disease to a large extent in HLA-B27 transgenic mice and rats[11]. In B27-transgenic rats, ankylosing spondylitis, balanitis, colitis, dermatitis, and arthritis occur spontaneously. However, if the rats are made germ free the joint manifestations are no longer present, indicating the importance of a so far unknown infectious agent[12]. A similar phenomenon has been shown to occur in B27 transgenic mice[13], in which arthritis occurs only in conventional animal facilities. Inoculation of LEW but not DA rats with *Yersinia* induces arthritis, which persists in the peripheral joints[14].

Arthritis caused by bacterial fragments and complete Freund's adjuvant Post-infectious arthritis may develop after bacterial infections. The occurrence of arthritis can be dependent on several different bacteria-derived compounds, like cell wall fragments, DNA, and heat shock proteins. Bacterial cell wall fragments are difficult to degrade and may cause prolonged activation of macrophages, and synovial macrophages. The first animal model for RA to be described was the so called adjuvant arthritis (= mycobacteria-induced arthritis, MIA) induced in rats after injection of mycobacterium cell walls suspended in mineral oil, that is, complete Freund's adjuvant (CFA)[15]. Surprisingly, only rats (and not mice or primates) have been shown to develop arthritis after mycobacterium challenge[16], although it has been reported that joint-related granuloma formation has occurred in humans treated with mycobacterium-containing vaccine[17]. CFA is a potent adjuvant that stimulates both cellular and humoral immunity. Subcutaneous injection of CFA in rats leads to granulomatous inflammation in many organs, for example the spleen, liver, bone marrow, skin, and eyes, and causes profound inflammation in peripheral joints[18]. MIA is severe but self-limited and the rat recovers within a few months. The mycobacterium cell wall fragments are most likely disseminated throughout the body and engulfed by tissue macrophages, which have difficulties in degrading the bacterial cell wall structures and are therefore transformed into an activated state, which triggers inflammation. MIA can be abrogated by elimination of the classical alpha/beta type of T cells and spleen-derived T cells[19,20] can transfer the disease. The specificity of such T cells has, however, not been reproducibly demonstrated, although some possibilities have been suggested, including bacterial structures and cross-reactive self-components[21,22]. While a role for heat shock proteins in the induction of the disease has not been confirmed, they clearly play an important regulatory role for the development of arthritis[23]. In the search for the minimal arthritogenic structure in mycobacterium it was observed that one of the essential structural elements of the mycobacterium peptidoglycan, muramyl dipeptide, could induce arthritis[24]. Interestingly, T cells do not recognize this structure but it has potent adjuvant capacity indicating that it stimulates innate immune receptors (NOD2) and antigen-presenting cells[25]. The unmethylated DNA of bacteria has also been shown to independently trigger arthritis in mice[26] and contribute to arthritis severity of MIA in rats[27]. The bacterial DNA triggers Toll-like receptors on both antigen-presenting cells and inflammatory macrophages and will therefore interact with both T cell dependent and inflammatory pathways. Another T cell dependent arthritogenic pathway is triggered by the mineral oil in which the mycobacteria are suspended, as will be discussed below in more detail.[19–24] Thus, this classical 'adjuvant-induced arthritis' (MIA) is mediated by different and interacting pathways, dependent on different mycobacterium cell components such as peptidoglycans, DNA, and heat shock proteins but also dependent on adjuvant activity mediated by the oil used to suspend the mycobacteria.

Postinfectious arthritis has also been observed to occur following streptococcal infections. A rapidly developing form of arthritis has been observed after systemic inoculation of streptococcal cell wall fragments in rats[28] and mice[29] but not in primates [16]. Peptidoglycans from the cell wall rapidly disseminate throughout the rat, including the joints[30]. These structures are difficult for the macrophages to degrade and as a consequence synovial macrophages are persistently activated. T cells are necessary for the initiation and perpetuation of the arthritis[31]. Although the precise mechanisms are not known it is possible that there are mechanisms shared with MIA.

Non-bacterial adjuvant-induced arthritis

The induction of arthritis in rats was found to be not only dependent on the mycobacteria but also the oil into which the mycobacterium fragments were suspended. Interestingly, some oils were found to support the induction of arthritis whereas others did not[32]. Many years later it was noted that the mineral oils that supported the induction of arthritis were in fact arthritogenic by themselves[33]. It was also found that subcutaneous administration of adjuvant compounds, such as avridine, pristane, and squalen, which bear no relation to bacteria, were highly effective in inducing arthritis[34–36]. These adjuvant compounds in most cases produce inflammation confined to the joints and offer better experimental models for RA than the earlier commonly used 'adjuvant arthritis' that is, mycobacterium in oil induced arthritis (MIA) model.

Mineral oil-induced arthritis (OIA)[33], avridine-induced arthritis (AvIA)[34], pristane-induced arthritis (PIA)[35], and squalen-induced arthritis[36] in the rat share many common features and differ mainly by the degree of chronic development[37] (Fig. 4.1). They are induced with adjuvant compounds lacking immunogenic capacity, that is, no specific immune responses are elicited. Instead they are rapidly spread throughout the body after a single subcutaneous injection, and penetrate through cell membranes into cells. After a delay of at least one or two weeks arthritis suddenly develops. The arthritis appears in the peripheral joints, with a similar distribution as seen in RA. Occasionally other joints are involved but systemic manifestations in other tissues have so far not been reported[38]. In certain rat strains, especially in the AvIA and PIA models, the arthritis proceeds as a chronic relapsing disease. Surprisingly, no consistent immune response to any specific cartilage component has yet been observed although rheumatoid factors are present in serum[39]. A role for cartilage proteins in regulating disease activity is possible as the disease can be prevented and in fact therapeutically ameliorated by nasal vaccination with various cartilage proteins[40]. Both the initiation and chronic progression of the arthritis is T cell dependent, as shown by *in vivo* administration of antibodies to αβ T cells[35,36,41]. Together with the observation that the chronic disease course is associated with the MHC region[35,36,41], this could implicate the activation of T cells recognizing joint-derived proteins. However, such T cells have not been observed and T cell transfer of the disease has so far failed to identify antigen-specific T cells[42,43]. The inducing agents are all small hydrophobic molecules unable to bind to MHC class II molecules and to be recognized by T cells. A role for environmental infectious agents is not likely since no difference in disease susceptibility could be seen in germ-free rats, although only conventional rats respond to heat shock proteins[44]. There is so far no evidence for recognition by lymphocyte receptors or receptors involved in the innate immune system. Surprisingly, some of the arthritogenic adjuvants are in fact components already present in the body before injection. For example, pristane is a component of chlorophyll and normally ingested by all mammals, including laboratory rats. Pristane is taken up through the intestine and spread throughout the body. However, they all share the capacity to penetrate into cells where they can change membrane fluidity and modulate transcriptional regulation. The injection route and dose is critical, that is, it determines which cell is first activated and to what extent.

As expected the disease is polygenically controlled and a large part of the variance could be explained by less than 20 quantitative trait loci (QTL)[45,46]. These QTLs are often shared between the various forms of adjuvant arthritis and to a lesser degree also with collagen-induced arthritis (CIA)[47]. Interestingly, they seem to control distinct phases of the disease such as arthritis onset, clinical severity, joint erosion, and chronicity[45] (Fig. 4.2). An attractive approach for understanding the complexity of the adjuvant arthritis, and perhaps that of the arthritis process in general, will be to eventually elucidate the underlying genetic polymorphism of these QTLs. One such gene has already been positionally cloned and was found to be Ncf1, controlling the oxidative burst[48]. Surprisingly a higher oxidative burst capacity was associated with more severe arthritis. The effect was found to operate before T cell activation

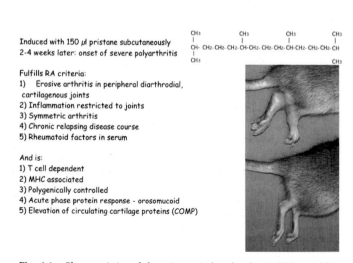

Induced with 150 μl pristane subcutaneously
2-4 weeks later: onset of severe polyarthritis

Fulfills RA criteria:
1) Erosive arthritis in peripheral diarthrodial, cartilagenous joints
2) Inflammation restricted to joints
3) Symmetric arthritis
4) Chronic relapsing disease course
5) Rheumatoid factors in serum

And is:
1) T cell dependent
2) MHC associated
3) Polygenically controlled
4) Acute phase protein response - orosomucoid
5) Elevation of circulating cartilage proteins (COMP)

Fig. 4.1 Characteristics of the pristane induced arthritis (PIA) model in DA rats.

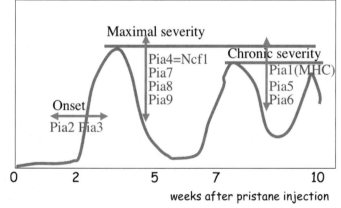

Fig. 4.2 Quantitative trait loci (QTL) identified to control different phases of arthritis induced with pristane.

and therefore also controls the degree of autoimmunity, linking innate and adaptive immunity giving a new perspective on the development of arthritis.

Adjuvant arthritis is not easily inducible in species other than rats. Of the above-mentioned adjuvant-induced arthritis models, only PIA has been described in the mouse[49,50]. The induction of PIA in mouse requires repeated intraperitoneal injections of pristane, which triggers a widespread inflammatory disease with a late and insidious onset. The disease is clearly different from PIA in the rat; the same inducing protocol does not induce disease in the rat and the disease course and characteristics are different. Another adjuvant-related model is the induction of mild arthritis after intra-articular injection of agents activating macrophages like unmethylated DNA[26].

Cartilage protein-induced arthritis

Arthritis is inducible with several different cartilage proteins, such as aggrecan[51], link protein[52], type XI collagen (CXI)[53], cartilage oligomeric matrix protein (COMP)[54], and CII. These various models have different characteristics and genetics. Collagen-induced arthritis (CIA), induced with CII, is today the most commonly used model for RA; it was first demonstrated in the rat[55] and was later reported using other species such as mouse[56] and primates[57], and will be described in more detail.

Collagen (II)-induced arthritis

Immunization with the major collagen in cartilage, CII, leads to an autoimmune response and as a consequence, sudden onset of severe arthritis. Although it is usually necessary to emulsify the CII in adjuvant, such as mineral oil in the rat and complete Freund's adjuvant in the mouse, the disease can be distinguished from the various forms of adjuvant arthritis[58]. However, the CIA model varies considerably depending on the experimental animal species and on whether CII used is of self- or non-self origin.

In both rats and mice immunized with heterologous CII, a severe, erosive polyarthritis suddenly develops 2–3 weeks after immunization (Fig. 4.3). The inflammation usually subsides within 3–4 weeks in the most commonly used DBA/1 strain, whereas in other strains like those with a C57Bl/10 background, the arthritis is milder but eventually later develops into a more chronic relapsing disease course[59–61]. The disease is critically dependent on both a T and a B cell response to CII and pathogenic antibodies play a role in the inflammatory attack on the joints[62]. The collagen antibody-induced arthritis (CAIA) is inducible with certain CII-specific monoclonal antibodies[63]. These CII-specific antibodies bind to the cartilage surface, fix complement, attract neutrophilic granulocytes, and activate macrophages in a process independent of the immune system[64].

The disease induced after immunization with homologous CII in both rats and mice is not as easily inducible, but once started it is severe, and tends to be more chronic than the disease induced with heterologous CII[65]. The pathogenic events in the chronic disease phase are largely unknown but are most likely dependent on both autoreactive B and T cell activity. Nevertheless, the CIA

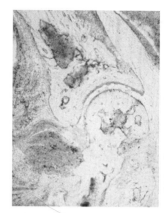
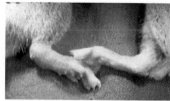

Erosive arthritis in peripheral diarthrodial, cartilagenous joints

Fig. 4.3 Collagen induced arthritis in a DBA/1 mouse. The histology section is from the ankle, showing an inflamed talocrual joint stained with antibodies to MHC class II. The photo demonstrates the clinical occurrence of CIA in the hind pain in the mouse to the left. See also colour plate section.

model is the most extensively investigated model for RA and has given valuable insights into the genetic control of the arthritic process, and of the autoimmune interactions with cartilage. It has also been useful for the development of new therapeutic approaches and for drug screening.

The genetic basis of CIA

Susceptibility to CIA varies dramatically between different inbred strains. The CIA is a complex, polygenic disease, similar to the adjuvant arthritis models described above. In the CIA model the autoimmune process is already determined by the induction through immunization with a defined antigen. Not surprisingly, the MHC class II polymorphism is important for determining susceptibility but there is also a major influence by a large number of other unknown genes. The major gene regions have been identified through genetic segregation experiments in both mice and rats, which have given an overall picture of the genetic inheritance of the susceptibility[66–68]. As in other complex diseases, these genes operate in concert and can only by identified through isolation in a proper genetic and environmental context, that is, as congenic strains used under specified conditions[69,70]. There is an exciting beginning in defining such genes and it is known conclusively that not only MHC class II genes play a role but also genes like Ncf1 and complement C5. The Ncf1 gene was defined through analysis of pristane-induced arthritis[48] but seems to play a similar role in CIA[48]. In fact, when a mutation in the Ncf1 gene is combined with the CIA susceptible MHC class II allele Aq in the C57Bl/10 mice, they developing a chronic relapsing form of CIA[61]. In addition, these mice tend to develop a severe form of chronic arthritis in the postpartum period, with the spontaneous development of autoimmunity to CII. Another genetic polymorphism of importance is the complement C5, which is deficient in many mouse strains. The deficiency leads to a relative resistance to CIA, suggesting a role for complement pathways in arthritis[71], which in fact is opposite to its role in mycoplasma-induced arthritis[72]. Roles for both classical and alternative pathways as well as Fc receptor-mediated pathways have subsequently been demonstrated using both CIA and the CAIA models[73–75].

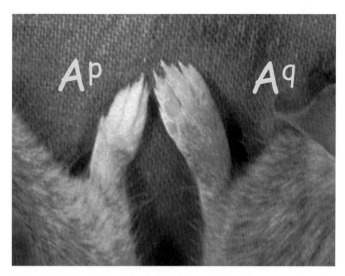

Fig. 4.4 Collagen induced arthritis in mice differing in only one gene, the MHC class II gene Aq. This makes the mouse susceptible to CIA and is the first conclusive evidence that MHC class II is associated with development of arthritis.

The role of the major histocompatibility complex

Early observations using the CIA model in both mice and rats induced with CII indicated a role for the MHC region. In the mouse, CIA induced with either heterologous or homologous CII is most strongly associated with the H2q and H2r haplotypes, whereas most other haplotypes such as b, s, d, and p are relatively resistant but not completely protected from arthritis induced with heterologous CII[76]. The major underlying genes explaining the association with the H2q haplotype has been identified as the Aq beta gene[77] (Fig. 4.4). Moreover, the immunodominant peptide derived from the CII molecule bound to the arthritis-associated q variant of the A (Aq) molecule has been found to be located between positions 260 and 270 of CII[78]. This is a glycopeptide with an oligosaccharide pointing towards the T cell receptor and is recognized by most of the CII-reactive T cells[79]. Interestingly, the peptide-binding pocket of the Aq molecule is very similar to that of the DR4 (DRB1*0401/DRA) and DR1 molecules, that is, the shared epitope, which are associated with RA. Furthermore, mice transgenically expressing DR4 or DR1 are susceptible to CIA and respond to a peptide from the same CII region[80,81] (Table 4.2), and CII reactive T cells from RA patients seem to predominantly recognize the glycopeptide[82]. These findings suggest a model for studies of RA that not only mimic some basic pathogenic events but may also share some critical structural similarities.

Autoimmune recognition of cartilage

It is important to emphasize that the identified structural interaction between MHC class II+peptide complexes and T cells does not give us the answer to the pathogenesis of CIA (or RA), but rather a better tool for further analysis. An important question is how the immune system in fact interacts with the peripheral joints, that is, how autoreactive T and B cells are normally tolerized, and

Table 4.2 MHC class II molecules with the 'shared epitope', associated with CIA in the mouse

MHC class II	CII peptide	MHC binding	T cell activation	CIA	Reference
Aq	259–270	++	++	+	77
Ap	259–270	+	+	−	77
DR4*0401	260–270	++	++	+	81
DR1*0101	260–270	++	++	+	80

what happens in the pathologic situation after their activation by CII immunization. Most of the T cells reactive with the rat CII256–270 peptide do not cross-react with the corresponding peptide from mouse CII. The difference between the heterologous and the homologous peptide is position 266 in which the rat has a glutamic acid (E) and the mouse an aspartic acid (D), which leads to a weaker binding of the mouse peptide to Aq. The importance of this minor difference was demonstrated in transgenic mice expressing CII mutated to express a glutamic acid at this position[83]. When mutated CII was expressed in cartilage the T cell response to CII was partially but not completely tolerized. The mice were susceptible to arthritis but the incidence was low, similar to what is seen in mice immunized with homologous CII. This finding shows that a normal interaction between cartilage and T cells leads to the activation of T cells with less capacity to induce arthritis, or alternatively with regulatory properties. However, the tolerance is not complete since the T cells can still produce effector cytokines such as gamma interferon and give help to B cells. Partially tolerized T cells may under extreme circumstances (such as CII immunization) mediate arthritis. In contrast, B cells reactive with CII are not tolerized and as soon as the T cells are activated, even in a partially tolerized state, they help B cells to produce autoreactive and pathogenic antibodies. It is possible that a similar situation may exist in humans that could explain the difficulties in isolating CII reactive T cells compared with the relative ease in which CII-reactive B cells can be detected in the joints.

Induction of arthritis with other cartilage- and joint-related proteins

Type XI collagen-induced arthritis

The type XI collagen (CXI) is structurally similar to CII and to a large extent colocalized. CXI is a heterotrimer with three different alpha chains, where one is shared with CII (the a3 chain). Both heterologous and homologous CXI have been reported to induce arthritis in rat strains[84,85]. Interestingly, the induction with homologous CXI gives a chronic relapsing disease, which is distinctly different from the heterologous CXI-induced disease and CII-induced CIA.

COMP-induced arthritis

Another cartilage protein is COMP. Homologous COMP induces arthritis in rats. In comparison with CIA, the resulting disease is self-limited, less erosive, and has a different genetic control[54].

Table 4.3 Some environmental effects on mouse CIA

Environmental effect	Effect on arthritis	Reference
Inter-male stress	+	89
Pregnancy	−	114
Postpartum	+	61, 108
Estrogen	−	107
Darkness	+	115

+ = increased arthritis, − = decreased arthritis.

Table 4.4 Some environmental effects on rat arthritis

Environmental effect	Effect on arthritis	Reference
Noise stress	++	116
Predator stress	−	117
Estrogen	−	118
Testosterone	−	118
Infections	−/+	12, 44, 119, 120

+ = increased arthritis, − = decreased arthritis.

Proteoglycan (aggrecan)-induced arthritis

Other major components of joint cartilage are proteoglycans, of which the largest is aggrecan. Repeated immunization of Balb/c mice with fetal human aggrecan induces chronic arthritis[51]. Both B and T cells are involved in the pathogenesis. Autoreactive T cells have been isolated and respond to the G1-domain of aggrecan in which neo-epitopes are created[86]. The disease has been genetically mapped and shown to share many gene regions in common with CIA[87].

Antigen-induced arthritis

Antigen-induced arthritis is a classical model of RA that is induced by immunizing animals with a foreign antigen, usually bovine serum albumin, and subsequently injecting the same antigen into a joint. As a result a pronounced T cell-dependent immune-complex mediated and destructive arthritis develops in the injected joint. The advantage of this model is that a defined part of the pathogenesis leading to arthritis is addressed.

Spontaneous arthritis

Some of the classical inbred mouse strains tend to spontaneously develop arthritis[88,89], in particular under certain environmental influence (see Tables 4.3 and 4.4). In some strains, such as DBA/1, the grouping of males induces inter-male aggressiveness and such stress seems to be associated with development of severe arthritis[89]. This stress-induced arthritis is dependent on a functional immune system and has different histopathology as compared with CIA. Thus, an exaggerated healing process with enthesopathy and new cartilage and bone formation, more similar to psoriasis arthritis than RA[90,91], dominates the joint pathology (Fig. 4.5).

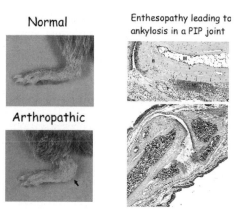

Fig. 4.5 Spontaneous arthropathy in DBA/1 mice. About 50–100% of male DBA/1 mice develop a spontaneous form of arthropathy after challenge with inter-male aggressiveness (i.e. grouping of males from different litters). This is a T cell independent disease; which have both macroscopically and microscopically similarities to psoriasis arthritis.

There are also a number of genetic mutations that strongly enhance arthritis development. One such mutation has been shown to occur in the Fas gene, of critical importance for apoptosis. In the MRL mouse background, arthritis develops together with a severe lupus disease[92]. More recently, a mutation in the T cell receptor-signalling molecule Zap70 was found to be associated with severe arthritis when expressed in the Balb/c mice[93]. The Zap70 mutation led to defective positive selection and the emergence of autoreactive T cells attacking the joints. As a result both rheumatoid factors and CII reactive antibodies were detected in the mice. Just as with the Ncf1 mutation this finding suggests a role of autoreactive T cells in the development of RA-like arthritis in mice.

Spontaneous arthritis has also been observed in a number of different transgenic mouse strains. One such example is a mouse in which TNF-α is overexpressed, leading to inflammation in tissues with elevated TNF-α[94]; another is a mouse deficient for the IL-1 receptor antagonist[95]. Another type of spontaneous arthritis has been shown to develop in T cell receptor transgenic NOD mouse, in which the T cell receptor recognizes a peptide derived from the ubiquitously occurring protein G6PI[96–98]. The pathogenic pathway in this model has been shown to be dependent on antibodies reactive with G6PI. The arthritis can be transferred with such antibodies and bind to the cartilage surface, mimicking the pathogenesis of anti-CII antibodies in the CAIA model. The use of the G6PI antibody-induced arthritis has been instrumental in finding early inflammatory steps in the joint attack, which involves complement activation through the alternative pathway, mast cell activation, and neutrophil infiltration[99,100]. Clearly the joints are specifically targeted in the disease and it remains to be determined how T cells and antibodies recognize this systemically expressed autoantigen in a joint-specific context.

A transgenic model in which spontaneous arthritis has been observed is found in mice and rats transgenic for the envelope protein of human T cell leukemia virus 1[101,102]. In this case there is not only joint inflammation and autoimmunity to CII but also widespread inflammatory infiltrates in skin, salivary glands, and vessels.

Another type of model is the induction of arthritis after transplantation of human synovial fibroblasts into immune-deficient SCID mice[103]. The same type of arthritis develops after transfer of murine fibroblast cell lines[104]. This model is likely to reflect inherent properties of fibroblast-mediated mechanisms showing different features as compared with other arthritis models like CIA and PIA[104].

These models are most likely to represent various aspects of the processes leading to arthritis, which will be determined by the transgene or defective gene, or be due to transplantation of specific cells. They are useful and efficient to work with and will give answers to specific questions, but are not likely to be optimal models for RA, which is not a spontaneous disease with high penetrance and is not believed to be dependent on a dominant genetic defect.

Using animal models

From disease to genes

An ideal model for human RA should mimic the complexity of the human disease in being polygenic and dependent on environmental factors. The animal models have the advantage that both genetics and environment can be better controlled. RA is a syndrome, likely composed of several distinct disease entities, and so are the animal models. The heterogeneity is reflected in the large number of different models with clearly different pathogeneses. It is likely that each of them reflect distinct subsets of RA and provide unique possibilities to study pathogenic pathways in controlled settings. Studies of the animal models need to be performed with the same approach as we investigate RA, starting with the disease to unravel the genetic basis. This provides the proper contextual setting which is critical for understanding the molecular pathogenesis. In this approach the animal models are now genetically dissected to determine the genetic polymorphism that allows the pathogenic development of chronic arthritis. This is a difficult approach, although not as difficult as in humans, but recently progress has been made showing that this will be possible.

From genes to disease

The animal models can also be used to study the role of certain genes in controlling inflammation, that is, from genes to disease. Arthritis models have the advantage that inflammation is easy to follow macroscopically. Consequently, many genes and proteins of potential importance have been targeted and found to play a role in this complex process. With this approach we have gained detailed knowledge on basic physiological mechanisms controlling inflammation, but these are beyond the scope of this present review. This approach is powerful and very informative but the interpretation is sometimes complicated. This is not only because the technology itself may introduce artefacts but also because the genetic setting is difficult to control. Thus, unexpected phenomena are observed that may not be directly relevant for the disease process itself.

Developing new therapeutic strategies

To test new drugs and therapies it will be necessary to select from the different models available. Obviously there is no optimal model for RA and there will never be one. The models described, however, are useful since they represent different aspects of RA pathogenesis. Thus, depending on the questions to be asked or symptoms to be treated, different models may be used. The CIA model, the one most commonly used today for testing new therapeutic approaches, should be included as a reference model. The usefulness of this model has been confirmed with the anti-TNF-α treatment, which was subsequently introduced in RA[105].

It is reasonable that the animal models should display the three hallmark criteria for RA discussed above: tissue specificity, chronicity, and MHC association. A common mistake is to only use acute models and to only use disease prevention and not established chronic disease as a readout. It is also of critical importance to be aware of the specific environmental influences on arthritis development in rodents (see Tables 4.3 and 4.4). Of particular importance are stress effects which are easily produced by mixing mice from different litters in the same cage and which will lead to cage-dependent effects[89]. Other important factors are sex hormones[106–108] and probably also neurohormones[109,110], which play an important role in modulating disease activity—seen as effects by estrous cycling, pregnancy, and light effects. Clearly, not only environmental but also genetic effects need to be controlled. The control of genetics is usually achieved by testing standardized inbred strains. The problem is that these vary considerably between different colonies mainly due to genetic contamination. In spite of these problems, there is no question that both environment and genetics can be better controlled in experimental animal models than can be achieved in studies directly involving the human population.

Ethical considerations

One important drawback of using experimental models for RA is the suffering of animals. However, in the light of various human activities that use animals, the use of them in research seems to be the easiest to defend. In fact, it would be unethical not to use them since it would prohibit further understanding of human diseases, thereby letting humans suffer from something that it will be possible to cure or prevent. It should also be emphasized that the recent development of animal models for RA has refined them to be of more specific use, which has decreased animal suffering. For example, the historically most commonly used model for RA, the mycobacterium-induced adjuvant arthritis, is a systemic and severe inflammatory disease, whereas the collagen-induced arthritis is a much more specific disease of the joints.

Conclusions

Experimental animal models are essential tools not only for investigating the basic mechanisms leading to RA but also for the development of new therapies. Many models have been described and each represents different aspects of the disease, and it is therefore important to use different models. The models for RA described so far can be divided into three principal groups: (a) adjuvant induced, (b) cartilage-protein induced, and (c) spontaneous. It has been emphasized that the models used should reflect essential hallmarks of rheumatoid arthritis such as tissue specificity, chronicity, and MHC class II gene association, and they should reflect the fact that RA is a polygenic disease triggered by unknown and multifactorial environmental factors.

References

1. Franz, A., Webster, A. D., Furr, P. M., and Taylor-Robinson, D. Mycoplasmal arthritis in patients with primary immunoglobulin deficiency: clinical features and outcome in 18 patients. *Br J Rheumatol* 1997; **36**: 661–8.

2. Cole, B. C., Ward, J. R., Jones, R. S., and Cahill J. F. Chronic proliferative arthritis of mice induced by Mycoplasma arthritidis. I. Induction of disease and histopathologic characteristics. *Infection Immunity* 1971; **4**: 344–55.

3. Berglöf, A., Sandstedt, K., Feinstein, R., Bölske, G., and Smith, C. I. B cell-deficient muMT mice as an experimental model for Mycoplasma infections in X-linked agammaglobulinemia. *Eur J Immunol* 1997; **27**: 2118–21.

4. Schaible, U. E., Kramer, M. D., Wallich, R., Tran, T., and Simon, M. M. Experimental Borrelia burgdorferi infection in inbred mouse strains: antibody response and association of H-2 genes with resistance and susceptibility to development of arthritis. *Eur J Immunol* 1991; **21**: 2397–405.

5. Yang, L., Weis, J. H., Eichwald, E., Kolbert, C. P., Persing, D. H., and Weis, J. J. Heritable susceptibility to severe Borrelia burgdorferi-induced arthritis is dominant and is associated with persistence of large numbers of spirochetes in tissues. *Infect Immun* 1994; **62**: 492–500.

6. Bremell, T., Lange, S., Yacoub, A., Ryden, C., and Tarkowski, A. Experimental *Staphylococcus aureus* arthritis in mice. *Infect Immun* 1991; **59**: 2615–23.

7. Bremell, T., Lange, S., Holmdahl, R., Ryden, C., Hansson, G. K., and Tarkowski, A. Immunopathological features of rat Staphylococcus aureus arthritis. *Infect Immun* 1994; **62**: 2334–44.

8. Verdrengh, M., and Tarkowski, A. Role of neutrophils in experimental septicemia and septic arthritis induced by Staphylococcus aureus. *Infect Immun* 1997; **65**: 2517–21.

9. Zhao, Y. X., Abdelnour, A., Holmdahl, R., and Tarkowski, A. Mice with the xid B cell defect are less susceptible to developing Staphylococcus aureus-induced arthritis. *J Immunol* 1995; **155**: 2067–76.

10. Abdelnour, A., Zhao, Y. X., Holmdahl, R., and Tarkowski, A. Major histocompatibility complex class II region confers susceptibility to *Staphylococcus aureus* arthritis. *Scand J Immunol* 1997; **45**: 301–7.

11. Hammer, R. E., Maika, S. D., Richardson, J. A., Tang, J. P., and Taurog, J. D. Spontaneous inflammatory disease in transgenic rats expressing HLA-B27 and human beta2m: an animal model of HLA-B27-associated human disorders. *Cell* 1990; **63**: 1099–112.

12. Taurog, J. D., Richardson, J. A., Croft, J. T., Simmons, W A., Zhou, M., Fernandez-Sueiro, J. L. *et al.* The germfree state prevents development of gut and joint inflammatory disease in HLA-B27 transgenic rats. J Exp Med 1994;180:2359–64.

13. Khare, S. D., Hansen J., Luthra, H. S., and David, C. S. HLA-B27 heavy chains contribute to spontaneous inflammatory disease in B27/human beta2-microglobulin (beta2m) double transgenic mice with disrupted mouse beta2m. *J Clin Invest* 1996; **98**: 2746–55.

14. Hill, J. L., and Yu, D. T. Development of an experimental animal model for reactive arthritis induced by Yersinia enterocolitica infection. *Infect Immun* 1987; **55**: 721–6.

15. Pearson, C. M., and Wood, F. D. Studies of polyarthritis and other lesions induced in rats by injection of mycobacterial adjuvant. I.

General clinical and pathologic characteristics and some modifying factors. *Arthritis Rheum* 1959; **2**: 440–59.

16. Bakker, N. P. M., Van Erck, M. G., Zurcher, C., Faaber, P., Lemmens, A., Hazenberg, M., *et al.* Experimental immune mediated arthritis in rhesus monkeys: a model for human rheumatoid arthritis? *Rheumatol Int* 1990; **10**: 21–9.

17. Torisu, M., Miyahara, T., Shinohara, N., Ohsato, K., and Sonozaki, H. A new side effect of BCG immunotherapy: BCG-induced arthritis in man. *Cancer Immunol Immunother* 1978; **5**: 77–83.

18. Pearson, C. M. Development of arthritis, periarthritis and periostitis in rats given adjuvants. *Proc Soc Exp Biol Med* 1956; **91**: 95–101.

19. Pearson, C. M., and Wood, F. D. Passive transfer of adjuvant arthritis by lymph node or spleen cells. *J Exp Med* 1964; **120**: 547–73.

20. Yoshino, S., Schlipkoter, E., Kinne, R., Hunig, T., and Emmrich, F. Suppression and prevention of adjuvant arthritis in rats by a monoclonal antibody to the alpha/beta T cell receptor. *Eur J Immunol* 1990; **20**: 2805–9.

21. Van Eden, W., Holoshitz, J., Nevo, Z., Frenkel, A., Klajman, A., and Cohen, I. R. Arthritis induced by a T-lymphocyte clone that responds to Mycobacterium tuberculosis and to cartilage proteoglycans. *Proc Natl Acad Sci U S A* 1985; **82**: 5117–20.

22. Van Eden, W., Thole, J. E. R., VanDerZee, R., Noordzij, A., VanEmbden, J. D. A., Hensen, E. J. *et al.* Cloning of the mycobacterial epitope recognized by T lymphocytes in adjuvant arthritis. *Nature* 1988; **334**: 171–3.

23. Anderton, S. M., van der, Zee R., Prakken, B., Noordzij, A., and van Eden, W. Activation of T cells recognizing self 60-kD heat shock protein can protect against experimental arthritis. *J Exp Med* 1995; **181**: 943–52.

24. Kohashi, O., Pearson, C. M., Watanabe, Y., and Kotani, S. Preparation of arthritogenic hydrosoluble peptidoglycans from both arthritogenic and non-arthritogenic bacterial cell walls. *Inf Immun* 1977; **16**: 861–6.

25. Inohara, N., and Nunez, G. NODs: intracellular proteins involved in inflammation and apoptosis. *Nat Rev Immunol* 2003; **3**: 371–82.

26. Deng, G. M., Nilsson, I. M., Verdrengh, M., Collins, L. V., and Tarkowski A. Intra-articularly localized bacterial DNA containing CpG motifs induces arthritis. *Nat Med* 1999; **5**: 702–5.

27. Ronaghy, A., Prakken, B. J., Takabayashi, K., Firestein, G. S., Boyle D., Zvailfler N. J. *et al.* Immunostimulatory DNA sequences influence the course of adjuvant arthritis. *J Immunol* 2002; **168**: 51–6.

28. Cromartie, W. J., Craddock, J. G., Schwab, J. H., Anderle, S. K., and Yang, C. H. Arthritis in rats after systemic injection of streptococcal cells or cell walls. *J Exp Med* 1977; **146**: 1585–602.

29. Koga, T., Kakimoto, K., Hirofuji, T., Kotani, S., Ohkuni, H., Watanabe, K. *et al.* Acute joint inflammation in mice after systemic injection of the cell wall, its peptidoglycan, and chemically defined peptidoglycan subunits from various bacteria. *Infection Immun* 1985; **50**: 27–34.

30. Dalldorf, F. G., Cromartie, W. J., Anderle, S. K., Clark, R. L., and Schwab, J. H. The relation of experimental arthritis to the distribution of streptococcal cell wall fragments. *Am J Pathol* 1980; **100**: 383–402.

31. Yoshino, S., Cleland, L. G., Mayrhofer, G., Brown, R. R., and Schwab, J. H. Prevention of chronic erosive streptococcal cell wall-induced arthritis in rats by treatment with a monoclonal antibody against the T cell antigen receptor alpha beta. *J Immunol* 1991; **146**: 4187–9.

32. Whitehouse, M. W., Orr, K. J., Beck, F. W. J., and Pearson, C. M. Freund¥s adjuvants: relationship to arthritogenicity and adjuvanticity in rats to vehicle composition. *Immunology* 1974; **27**: 311–30.

33. Holmdahl, R., Goldschmidt, T. J., Kleinau, S., Kvick, C., and Jonsson, R. Arthritis induced in rats with adjuvant oil is a genetically restricted, alpha beta T-cell dependent autoimmune disease. *Immunology* 1992; **76**: 197–202.

34. Chang, Y. H., Pearson, C. M., and Abe, C. Adjuvant polyarthritis. IV. Induction by a synthetic adjuvant: immunologic, histopathologic, and other studies. *Arthritis Rheum* 1980; **23**: 62–71.

35. Vingsbo, C., Sahlstrand, P., Brun, J. G., Jonsson, R., Saxne, T., and Holmdahl, R. Pristane-induced arthritis in rats: a new model for rheumatoid arthritis with a chronic disease course influenced by both major histocompatibility complex and non-major histocompatibility complex genes. *Am J Pathol* 1996; **149**: 1675–83.

36. Carlson, B. C., Jansson, A. M., Larsson, A., Bucht, A., and Lorentzen, J. C. The endogenous adjuvant squalene can induce a chronic T-cell-mediated arthritis in rats. *Am J Pathol* 2000; **156**: 2057–65.

37. Holmdahl, R., Lorentzen, J. C., Lu, S., Olofsson, P., Wester, L., Holmberg, J. *et al*. Arthritis induced in rats with non-immunogenic adjuvants as models for rheumatoid arthritis. *Immunol Rev* 2001; **184**: 184–202.

38. Hansson, A. S., Lu, S., and Holmdahl, R. Extra-articular cartilage affected in collagen-induced, but not pristane-induced, arthritis models. *Clin Exp Immunol* 2002; **127**: 37–42.

39. Wernhoff, P., Olofsson, P., and Holmdahl, R. The genetic control of rheumatoid factor production in a rat model for rheumatoid arthritis. *Arthritis Rheum* 2003; **48**: 3584–96.

40. Lu, S., and Holmdahl, R. Different therapeutic and bystander effects by intranasal administration of homologous type II and type IX collagens on the collagen-induced arthritis and pristane-induced arthritis in rats. *Clin Immunol* 1999; **90**: 119–27.

41. Vingsbo, C., Jonsson, R., and Holmdahl, R. Avridine-induced arthritis in rats: a T cell-dependent chronic disease influenced both by MHC genes and by non-MHC genes. *Clin Exp Immunol* 1995; **99**: 359–63.

42. Taurog, J. D., Sandberg, G. P., and Mahowald, M. L. The cellular basis of adjuvant arthritis. I. Enhancement of cellmediated passive transfer by concanavalin A and by immunosuppressive pretreatment of the recipient. *Cell Immunol* 1983; **75**: 271–82.

43. Svelander, L., Mussener, A., Erlandsson-Harris, H., and Kleinau, S. Polyclonal Th1 cells transfer oil-induced arthritis. *Immunology* 1997; **91**: 260–5.

44. Björk, J., Kleinau, S., Midtvedt, T., Klareskog, L., and Smedegård, G. Role of the bowel flora for development of immunity to hsp 65 and arthritis in three experimental models. *Scand J Immunol* 1994; **40**: 648–52.

45. Vingsbo-Lundberg, C., Nordquist, N., Olofsson, P., Sundvall, M., Saxne, T., Pettersson, U. *et al*. Genetic control of arthritis onset, severity and chronicity in a model for rheumatoid arthritis in rats. *Nat Genet* 1998; **20**: 401–4.

46. Lorentzen, J. C., Glaser, A., Jacobsson, L., Galli, J., Fakhrai-Rad, H., Klareskog, L. *et al*. Identification of rat susceptibility loci for adjuvant-oil induced arthritis. *Proc Natl Acad Sci U S A* 1998; **95**: 6383–7.

47. Olofsson, P., Lu, S., Holmberg, J., Song, T., Wernhoff, P., Pettersson, U. *et al*. A comparative genetic analysis between collagen-induced arthritis and pristane-induced arthritis. *Arthritis Rheum* 2003; **48**: 2332–42.

48. Olofsson, P., Holmberg, J., Tordsson, J., Lu, S., Åkerström, B., and Holmdahl, R. Positional identification of Ncf1 as a gene that regulates arthritis severity in rats. *Nat Genet* 2003; **33**: 25–32.

49. Hopkins, S. J., Freemont, A. J., and Jayson, MIV. Pristane-induced arthritis in Balb/c mice. I. Clinical and histological features of the arthropathy. *Int Rheumatol* 1984; **5**: 21–8.

50. Wooley, P. H., Seibold, J. R., Whalen, J. D., and Chapdelaine, J. M. Pristane-induced arthritis: the immunologic and genetic features of an experimental murine model of autoimmune disease. *Arthritis Rheum* 1989; **32**: 1022–30.

51. Glant, T. T., Mikecz, K., Arzoumanian, A., and Poole, A. R. Proteoglycan-induced arthritis in Balb/c mice. *Arthritis Rheum* 1987; **30**: 201–12.

52. Zhang, Y., Guerassimov, A., Leroux, J. Y., Cartman, A., Webber, C., Lalic R *et al*. Induction of arthritis in BALB/c mice by cartilage link protein: involvement of distinct regions recognized by T and B lymphocytes. Am J Pathol 1998; **153**: 1283–91.

53. Cremer, M. A., Ye, X. J., Terato, K., Owens, S. W., Seyer, J. M., and Kang A. H. Type XI collagen-induced arthritis in the Lewis rat: characterization of cellular and humoral immune responses to native types XI, V., and II collagen and constituent alpha-chains. *J Immunol* 1994; **153**: 824–32.

54. Carlsén, S., Hansson, A. S., Olsson, H., Heinegård, D., and Holmdahl, R. Cartilage oligomeric matrix protein (COMP)-induced arthritis in rats. *Clin Exp Immunol* 1998; **114**: 477–84.

55. Trentham, D. E., Townes, A. S., and Kang, A. H. Autoimmunity to type II collagen: an experimental model of arthritis. *J Exp Med* 1977; **146**: 857–68.

56. Courtenay, J. S., Dallman, M. J., Dayan, A. D., Martin, A., and Mosedal, B. Immunization against heterologous type II collagen induces arthritis in mice. *Nature* 1980; **283**: 666–7.

57. Yoo, T. J., Kim, S. Y., Stuart, J. M., Floyd, R. A., Olson, G. A., Cremer, M. A. *et al*. Induction of arthritis in monkeys by immunization with type II collagen. *J Exp Med* 1988; **168**: 777–82.

58. Holmdahl, R., and Kvick, C. Vaccination and genetic experiments demonstrate that adjuvant oil induced arthritis and homologous type II collagen induced arthritis in the same rat strain are different diseases. *Clin Exp Immunol* 1992; **88**: 96–100.

59. Holmdahl, R., Andersson, M., Goldschmidt, T. J., Gustafsson, K., Jansson, L., and Mo, J. A. Type II collagen autoimmunity in animals and provocations leading to arthritis. *Immunol Rev* 1990; **118**: 193–232.

60. Svensson, L., Nandakumar, K. S., Johansson, A., Jansson, L., and Holmdahl, R. IL-4-deficient mice develop less acute but more chronic relapsing collagen-induced arthritis. *Eur J Immunol* 2002; **32**: 2944–53.

61. Hultqvist, M., Olofsson, P., Holmberg, J., Bäckström, B. T., Tordsson, J., and Holmdahl, R. Enhanced autoimmunity, arthritis, and encephalomyelitis in mice with a reduced oxidative burst due to a mutation in the Ncf1 gene. *Proc Natl Acad Sci U S A* 2004; **101**: 12646–51.

62. Stuart, J. M., and Dixon, F. J. Serum transfer of collagen induced arthritis in mice. *J Exp Med* 1983; **158**: 378–92.

63. Holmdahl, R., Rubin, K., Klareskog, L., Larsson, E., and Wigzell, H. Characterization of the antibody response in mice with type II collagen-induced arthritis, using monoclonal anti-type II collagen antibodies. *Arthritis Rheum* 1986; **29**: 400–10.

64. Nandakumar, K. S., Svensson, L., and Holmdahl, R. Collagen type II specific monoclonal antibody induced arthritis (CAIA) in mice: description of the disease and the influence of age, sex, and genes. *Am J Pathol* 2003; **163**: 1827–37.

65. Holmdahl, R., Jansson, L., Larsson, E., Rubin, K., and Klareskog, L. Homologous type II collagen induces chronic and progressive arthritis in mice. *Arthritis Rheum* 1986; **29**: 106–113.

66. Remmers, E. F., Longman, R. E., Du, Y., O'Hare, A., Cannon, G. W., Griffiths, M. M. *et al*. A genome scan localizes five non-MHC loci controlling collagen-induced arthritis in rats. *Nature Genet* 1996; **14**: 82–5.

67. Jirholt, J., Cook, A., Emahazion, T., Sundvall, M., Jansson, L., Nordquist, N. *et al*. Genetic linkage analysis of collagen-induced arthritis in the mouse. *Eur J Immunol* 1998; **28**: 3321–8.

68. Yang, H. T., Jirholt, J., Svensson, L., Sundvall, M., Jansson, L., Pettersson, U. *et al*. Identification of genes controlling collagen-induced arthritis in mice: striking homology with susceptibility loci previously identified in the rat. *J Immunol* 1999; **163**: 2916–21.

69. Johannesson, M., Karlsson, J., Wernhoff, P., Nandakumar, K. S., Lindqvist, A. K., Olsson, L. *et al*. Identification of epistasis through a partial advanced intercross reveals three arthritis loci within the Cia5 QTL in mice. *Genes Immun* 2005; **6**: 175–85.

70. Karlsson, J., Johannesson, M., Lindvall, T., Wernhoff, P., Holmdahl, R., and Andersson A. Genetic interactions in Eae2 control collagen-induced arthritis and the CD4+/CD8+ T cell ratio. *J Immunol* 2005; **174**: 533–41.

71. Watson, W. C., and Townes, A. S. Genetic susceptibility to murine collagen II autoimmune arthritis: proposed relationship to the IgG2 autoantibody subclass response, complement C5, major histocompatibility complex (MHC) and non-MHC loci. *J Exp Med* 1985; **162**: 1878–91.

72. Keystone, E., Taylor-Robinson, D., Pope, C., Taylor, G., and Furr, P. Effect of inherited deficiency of the fifth component of complement

on arthritis induced in mice by Mycoplasma pulmonis. *Arthritis Rheum* 1978; **21**: 792–7.

73. Hietala, M. A., Jonsson, I. M., Tarkowski, A., Kleinau, S., and Pekna, M. Complement deficiency ameliorates collagen-induced arthritis in mice. *J Immunol* 2002; **169**: 454–9.

74. Hietala, M. A., Nandakumar, K. S., Persson, L., Fahlen, S., Holmdahl R., and Pekna, M. Complement activation by both classical and alternative pathways is critical for the effector phase of arthritis. *Eur J Immunol* 2004; **34**: 1208–16.

75. Kleinau, S., Martinsson, P., and Heyman, B. Induction and suppression of collagen-induced arthritis is dependent on distinct fcgamma receptors. *J Exp Med* 2000; **191**: 1611–16.

76. Wooley, P. H., Luthra, H. S., Stuart, J. M., and David, C. S. Type II collagen induced arthritis in mice. I. Major histocompatibility complex (I-region) linkage and antibody correlates. *J Exp Med* 1981; **154**: 688–700.

77. Brunsberg, U., Gustafsson, K., Jansson L., Michaëlsson, E., Åhrlund-Richter, L., Pettersson, S. *et al.* Expression of a transgenic class II Ab gene confers susceptibility to collagen-induced arthritis. *Eur J Immunol* 1994; **24**: 1698–702.

78. Michaëlsson, E., Andersson, M., Engström, A., and Holmdahl, R. Identification of an immunodominant type-II collagen peptide recognized by T cells in H-2q mice: self tolerance at the level of determinant selection. *Eur J Immunol* 1992; **22**: 1819–25.

79. Michaëlsson, E., Malmström, V., Reis, S., Burkhardt, H., Engström, Å., and Holmdahl, R. T cell recognition of carbohydrates on type II collagen. *J Exp Med* 1994; **30**: 745–9.

80. Rosloniec, E. F., Brand, D. D., Myers, L. K., Whittington, K. B., Gumanovskaya, M., Zaller, D. M. *et al.* An HLA-DR1 transgene confers susceptibility to collagen-induced arthritis elicited with human type II collagen. *J Exp Med* 1997; **185**: 1113–22.

81. Andersson, E. C., Hansen, B. E., Jacobsen, H., Madsen, L. S., Andersen C. B., Engberg, J. *et al.* Definition of MHC and T cell receptor contacts in the HLA-DR4 restricted immunodominant epitope in type II collagen and characterization of collagen-induced arthritis in HLA-DR4 and human CD4 transgenic mice. *Proc Natl Acad Sci U S A* 1998; **95**: 7574–9.

82. Bäcklund, J., Carlsen, S., Höger, T., Holm, B., Fugger, L., Kihlberg, J. *et al.* Predominant selection of T cells specific for glycosylated collagen type II peptide (263–270) in humanized transgenic mice and in rheumatoid arthritis. *Proc Natl Acad Sci U S A* 2002; **99**: 9960–5.

83. Malmström, V., Michaëlsson, E., Burkhardt, H., Mattsson, R., Vuorio, E., and Holmdahl, R. Systemic versus cartilage-specific expression of a type II collagen-specific T-cell epitope determines the level of tolerance and susceptibility to arthritis. *Proc Natl Acad Sci U S A* 1996; **93**: 4480–5.

84. Morgan, K., Evans, H. B, Firth, S. A., Smith, M. N., Ayad, S., Weiss, J. B. *et al.* 1α,2α,3α collagen is arthritogenic. *Ann Rheum Dis* 1983; **42**: 680–3.

85. Lu, S., Carlsen, S., Hansson, A-S, and Holmdahl, R. Immunization of rats with homologous type XI collagen leads to chronic and relapsing arthritis with different genetics and joint pathology than arthritis induced with homologous type II collagen. *J Autoimmun* 2002; **18**: 199–211.

86. Zhang, Y., Guerassimov, A., Leroux, J. Y., Cartman, A., Webber, C., Lalic, R. *et al.* Arthritis induced by proteoglycan aggrecan G1 domain in BALB/c mice: evidence for T cell involvement and the immunosuppressive influence of keratan sulfate on recognition of T and B cell epitopes. *J Clin Invest* 1998; **101**: 1678–86.

87. Adarichev, V. A., Valdez, J. C., Bardos, T., Finnegan, A., Mikecz, K., and Glant, T. T. Combined autoimmune models of arthritis reveal shared and independent qualitative (binary) and quantitative trait loci. *J Immunol* 2003; **170**: 2283–92.

88. Bouvet, J. P., Couderc, J., Bouthillier, Y., Franc, B, Ducailar, A., and Mouton D. Spontaneous rheumatoid-like arthritis in a line of mice sensitive to collagen-induced arthritis. *Arthritis Rheum* 1990; **33**: 1716–22.

89. Holmdahl, R., Jansson, L., Andersson, M., and Jonsson, R. Genetic, hormonal and behavioral influence on spontaneously developing arthritis in normal mice. *Clin Exp Immunol* 1992; **88**: 467–72.

90. Corthay, A., Hansson, A. S., and Holmdahl, R. T lymphocytes are not required for the spontaneous development of entheseal ossification leading to marginal ankylosis in the DBA/1 mouse. *Arthritis Rheum* 2000; **43**: 844–51.

91. Lories, R. J., Matthys, P., de Vlam, K., Derese, I., and Luyten, F. P. Ankylosing enthesitis, dactylitis, and onychoperiostitis in male DBA/1 mice: a model of psoriatic arthritis. *Ann Rheum Dis* 2004; **63**: 595–8.

92. Hang, L., Theofilopoulos, A. N., and Dixon, F. J. A spontaneous rheumatoid arthritis-like disease in MRL/l mice. *J Exp Med* 1982; **155**: 1690–701.

93. Sakaguchi, N., Takahashi T., Hata, H., Nomura, T., Tagami, T., Yamazaki, S. *et al.* Altered thymic T-cell selection due to a mutation of the ZAP-70 gene causes autoimmune arthritis in mice. **Nature** 2003; **426**: 454–60.

94. Keffer, J., Probert, L., Cazlaris, H., Georgopoulos, S., Kaslaris, E., Kioussis, D. *et al.* Transgenic mice expressing human tumour necrosis factor: a predictive genetic model of arthritis. *EMBO J* 1991; **10**: 4025–31.

95. Horai, R., Saijo, S., Tanioka, H., Nakae, S., Sudo, K., Okahara, A. *et al.* Development of chronic inflammatory arthropathy resembling rheumatoid arthritis in interleukin 1 receptor antagonist-deficient mice. *J Exp Med* 2000; **191**: 313–20.

96. Kouskoff, V., Korganow, A. S., Duchatelle, V., Degott, C., Benoist, C., and Mathis D. Organ-specific disease provoked by systemic autoimmunity. *Cell* 1996; **87**: 811–22.

97. Matsumoto, I., Staub, A., Benoist, C., and Mathis, D. Arthritis provoked by linked T and B cell recognition of a glycolytic enzyme. *Science* 1999; **286**: 1732–5.

98. Korganow, A. S., Ji, H., Mangialaio, S., Duchatelle, V., Pelanda, R., Martin, T. *et al.* From systemic T cell self reactivity to organ-specific autoimmune disease via immunoglobulins. *Immunity* 1999; **10**: 451–61.

99. Ji, H., Ohmura, K., Mahmood, U., Lee DM, Hofhuis, F. M., Boackle, S. A. *et al.* Arthritis critically dependent on innate immune system players. *Immunity* 2002; **16**: 157–68.

100. Lee, D. M., Friend, D. S., Gurish, M. F., Benoist, C., Mathis, D., and Brenner, M. B. Mast cells: a cellular link between autoantibodies and inflammatory arthritis. *Science* 2002; **297**: 1689–92.

101. Yamazaki, H., Ikeda, H., Ishizu, A., Nakamaru, Y., Sugaya, T., Kikuchi, K. *et al.* A wide spectrum of collagen vascular and autoimmune diseases in transgenic rats carrying the env-pX gene of human T lymphocyte virus type I. *Int Immunol* 1997; **9**: 339–46.

102. Kotani, M., Tagawa, Y., and Iwakura, Y. Involvement of autoimmunity against type II collagen in the development of arthritis in mice transgenic for the human T cell leukemia virus type I tax gene. *Eur J Immunol* 1999; **29**: 54–64.

103. Geiler, T., Kriegsmann, J., Keyszer, G. M., Gay, R E., and Gay, S. A new model for rheumatoid arthritis generated by engraftment of rheumatoid synovial tissue and normal human cartilage into SCID mice. *Arthritis Rheum* 1994; **37**: 1664–71.

104. Lange, F., Bajtner, E., Rintisch, C., Nandakumar, K. S., Sack, U., and Holmdahl, R. Methotrexate ameliorates T cell dependent autoimmune arthritis and encephalomyelitis but not antibody or fibroblast induced arthritis. *Ann Rheum Dis* 2004; **64**: 599–605.

105. Williams, R. O., Feldmann, M., and Maini, R. N. Anti-tumor necrosis factor ameliorates joint disease in murine collagen-induced arthritis. *Proc Natl Acad Sci U S A* 1992; **89**: 9784–8.

106. Holmdahl, R., and Jansson, L., Andersson, M. Female sex hormones suppress development of collagen-induced arthritis in mice. *Arthritis Rheum* 1986; **29**: 1501–9.

107. Jansson, L., Mattsson, A., Mattsson, R., and Holmdahl, R. Estrogen induced suppression of collagen arthritis. V: Physiological level of estrogen in DBA/1 mice is therapeutic on established arthritis, suppresses anti-type II collagen T-cell dependent immunity and stimulates polyclonal B-cell activity. *J Autoimmunity* 1990; **3**: 257–70.

108. Mattsson, R., Mattsson, A., Holmdahl, R., Whyte, A., and Rook, G. A. W. Maintained pregnancy levels of oestrogen afford complete protection from post-partum exacerbation of collagen-induced arthritis. *Clin Exp Immunol* 1991; **85**: 41–7.

109. Mattsson, R., Hansson, I., and Holmdahl, R. Pineal gland in autoimmunity: melatonin-dependent exaggeration of collagen-induced arthritis in mice [Letter]. *Autoimmunity* 1994; **17**: 83–6.

110. Levine, J. D., Clark, R., Devor, M., Helms, C., Moskowitz, M. A., and Basbaum, A. I. Intraneuronal substance P contributes to the severity of experimental arthritis. *Science* 1984; **226**: 547–9.

111. Gripenberg-Lerche, C., Skurnik, M., Zhang, L., Söderström, K O., and Toivanen, P. Role of YadA in arthritogenicity of Yersinia enterocolitica serotype O:8: experimental studies with rats. *Infect Immun* 1994; **62**: 5568–75.

112. Potter, M., and Wax, J. S. Genetics of susceptibility to pristane-induced plasmacytomas in BALB/cAn: reduced susceptibility in BALB/cJ with a brief description of pristane-induced arthritis. *J Immunol* 1981; **127**: 1591–5.

113. Holmdahl, R., Vingsbo, C., Hedrich, H., Karlsson, M., Kvick, C., Goldschmidt, T. J. *et al*. Homologous collagen-induced arthritis in rats and mice are associated with structurally different major histocompatibility complex DQ-like molecules. *Eur J Immunol* 1992; **22**: 419–24.

114. Waites, G. T., and Whyte, A. Effect of pregnancy on collagen-induced arthritis in mice. *Clin Exp Immunol* 1987; **67**: 467–76.

115. Hansson, I., Holmdahl, R., and Mattsson, R. The pineal hormone melatonin exaggerates development of collagen-induced arthritis in mice. *J Neuroimmunol* 1992; **39**: 23–30.

116. Rogers, M. P., Trentham, D. E., Dynesius-Trentham, R., Daffner, K., and Reich, P. Exacerbation of collagen arthritis by noise stress. *J Rheumatol* 1983; **10**: 651–4.

117. Rogers, M. P., Trentham, D. E., McCune, W. J., Ginsberg, B. I., Rennke, H. R., Reich, P. *et al*. Effect of psychological stress on the induction of arthritis in rats. *Arthritis Rheum* 1980; **23**: 1337–41.

118. Holmdahl, R. Female preponderance for development of arthritis in rats is influenced by both sex chromosomes and sex steroids. *Scand J Immunol* 1995; **42**: 104–9.

119. Taurog, J. D., Leary, S. L., Cremer, M., Mahowald, M. L., Sandberg, G. P., and Manning P. J. Infection with mycoplasma pulmonis modulates adjuvant- and collagen-induced arthritis in Lewis rats. *Arthritis Rheum* 1984; **27**: 943–6.

120. Kohashi, O., Kohashi, Y., Takahashi, T., Ozawa, A., and Shigematsu, N. Suppressive effect of Escherichia Coli on adjuvant-induced arthritis in germ-free rats. *Arthritis Rheum* 1986; **29**: 547–53.

SECTION 2 | *Mechanisms of Inflammation*

5 | The role of macrophages in rheumatoid arthritis

Raimund W. Kinne, Bruno Stuhlmüller, Ernesta Palombo-Kinne, and Gerd-R. Burmester

Introduction

Macrophages (Mφs) are of central importance in rheumatoid arthritis (RA), due to their prominent numbers in the inflamed synovial membrane and at the cartilage/pannus junction, their clear activation status[1–4] (see Table 5.1 for details), and their response to successful anti-rheumatic treatment[5]. Although Mφs probably do not occupy a causal pathogenetic position in RA (except for their potential antigen-presenting capacity)[6], they possess broad pro-inflammatory, destructive, and remodeling potential, and contribute considerably to inflammation and joint destruction in acute and chronic RA (see Table 5.2 for details). Also, activation of this lineage extends to circulating monocytes and other cells of the mononuclear phagocyte system (MPS), including bone marrow precursors of the myelomonocytic lineage and osteoclasts[2,7,8] (see Table 5.3).

Thus, before a causal factor for RA is known, monocytes/Mφs remain an attractive research focus for the following reasons: (a) the radiological progression of joint destruction correlates with the degree of synovial Mφ infiltration[1]; (b) the therapeutic efficacy of conventional anti-rheumatic therapy coincides with down-regulation of MPS functions[9–13]; (c) therapies directed at cytokines made predominantly by Mφs are effective in RA[14–16]; (d) conventional or experimental drugs can be selectively targeted to Mφs or their different subcellular compartments[2,17–19]; (e) differential activation of intracellular signal transduction pathways underlie different Mφ effector functions[20]; and (f) more specific inhibitors of key metabolic enzymes and/or particular signal transduction pathways are, or may become available as selective targets of anti-rheumatic therapy[20–22]. In addition, the amplifying role of Mφs in RA has emerged so clearly that the effects of anti-rheumatic therapy (whether specific or conventional) on monocytes/Mφs may become an objective read-out of the effectiveness of treatment[12,13].

Differentiation of the mononuclear phagocyte system in RA

Cells of the myelomonocytic lineage differentiate into several cell types critically involved in disease, that is, monocytes/Mφs, osteoclasts, and dendritic cells (Fig. 5.1A). Due to their marked plas-ticity, these pathways can be influenced by an excess/imbalance of cytokines or growth factors, resulting in altered differentiation/maturation (Fig. 5.1B). In RA, such imbalances clearly occur in inflamed joints, peripheral blood, and bone marrow (Table 5.3 and Fig. 5.1B).

In the RA **synovial membrane**, recently immigrated monocytes differentiate to mature Mφs and differentially colonize the lining and sublining layer (reviewed in Ref. 2). Functional diversity in these areas, indicated by expression of different activation markers and adhesion molecules[23,24] (see Table 5.1 for details), may differentially contribute to disease progression.

Locally, synovial Mφs differentiate into stimulatory or inhibitory subpopulations, known to differentially influence the T-cell reactivity in arthritis[25–27]. In RA, Mφ subpopulations may be responsible for the separate synthesis of pro-inflammatory (e.g., IL-1 and TNF-α) or regulatory cytokines (e.g., IL-10 or TGF-β1), the balance of which is critical to perpetuation of disease[16,28], as well as for the induction of angiogenesis[29,30]. Indeed, the concept of M_1- and M_2-dominant Mφs responses has recently emerged, according to which M_1 or M_2 subsets play a differential role in Th_1 or Th_2 inflammatory responses[26,27].

Also, it has been proposed that the pro-inflammatory Mφs are characterized by the expression of the scavenger receptor CD163[31], a marker of global disease activity in spondyloarthropathy[32]. Interestingly, RA synovial Mφs significantly overexpress oncofetal genes, suggesting embryonal-like de-differentiation; also, their expression is sensitive to starvation/cytokine regulation, possibly reflecting ongoing inflammatory/oxidative stress[33]. Local stress could also underlie the chromosomal aberrations observed in RA synovial Mφs[34].

In the **bone marrow**, patients with active RA display faster generation of CD14+ myelomonocytic cells and faster differentiation into HLA-DR+ cells, which also becomes insensitive to GM-CSF[35]. In addition, CD34+ myeloid precursors appear elevated in the bone marrow adjacent to rheumatoid joints, in correlation with the local levels of IL-1[36]. On the other hand, reduced bone-marrow cellularity has been observed, as well as a defective progenitor-cell reserve and function[37,38]. Common potential triggers for these alterations may be the altered monokine- (e.g., IL-1, IL-6, TNF-α) or growth-factor milieu (e.g., GM-CSF) which builds up in circulation and bone marrow of RA patients[7–9,39] (Fig. 5.1B). The anomalous maturation of CD34+ bone marrow precursor cells extends to endothelial cells (Table 5.3), a finding that correlates with the degree of synovial vascularization[40].

Table 5.1 Activation status of synovial Mφs and/or circulating monocytes in RA

Class of overexpressed molecules	Molecules	(Potential) function
Class-II major histocompatibility (MHC)	HLA-DR	Presentation of antigens relevant to disease initiation or severity (reviewed in Ref. 1)
Cytokines and growth factors	e.g., TNF-α, IL-1, IL-6, IL-10, IL-13, IL-15, IL-18, MIF, GM-CSF, thrombospondin-1	Mediation and regulation of local and systemic inflammation and tissue remodelling (reviewed in Refs 1–4)
Chemokines and chemoattractants	e.g., IL-8, MIP-1, MCP-1, CXCL13	Mediation and regulation of monocyte migration; stimulation of angiogenesis (reviewed in Ref. 5)
Matrix metalloproteinases (MMP)	MMP-9, MMP-12	Tissue degradation, post-injury tissue remodelling[6,7]
Tissue inhibitors of MMP (TIMP)	TIMP-1	Attempt to control excessive tissue destruction[8]
Acute phase reactants	e.g., C-reactive protein (CRP), A-SAA (serum amyloid A)	Integrated, hormone-like activation of hepatocyte by synovial mφs and fibroblasts (mostly via IL-6) (reviewed in Ref. 1, 9)
Other molecules	Neopterin	Produced by IFN-γ-stimulated monocytes/Mφs; induces/enhances cytotoxicity and apoptosis; acts as antioxidant[10,11]
	Cryopyrin	Produced by TNF-α-stimulated Mφs; regulates NF-κB and caspase-1 activation[12]

1. Kinne, R. W., Stuhlmuller, B., Palombo-Kinne, E., and Burmester, G. R. The role of macrophages in the pathogenesis of rheumatoid arthritis. In: *Rheumatoid Arthritis: the new frontiers in pathogenesis and treatment* (ed. F. Wollheim, G. S. Firestein, and G. S. Panayi), pp. 69–87. Oxford University Press: 2000.
2. Feldmann, M., Brennan, F. M., and Maini, R. N. Role of cytokines in rheumatoid arthritis. *Annu Rev Immunol* 1996; **14**: 397–440.
3. Arend, W. P., Malyak, M., Guthridge, C. J., and Gabay, C. Interleukin-1 receptor antagonist: role in biology. *Annu Rev Immunol* 1998; **16**: 27–55.
4. Miossec, P. An update on the cytokine network in rheumatoid arthritis. *Curr Opin Rheumatol* 2004; **16**: 218–22.
5. Koch, A. E. Angiogenesis as a target in rheumatoid arthritis. *Ann Rheum Dis* 2003; **62**: ii60–ii67.
6. Brinckerhoff, C. E. and Matrisian, L. M. Matrix metalloproteinases: a tail of a frog that became a prince. *Nat Rev Mol Cell Biol* 2002; **3**: 207–14.
7. Wang, X., Liang, J., Koike, T., Sun, H., Ichikawa, T., Kitajima, S. *et al.* Overexpression of human matrix metalloproteinase-12 enhances the development of inflammatory arthritis in transgenic rabbits. *Am J Pathol* 2004; **165**: 1375–83.
8. Heller, R. A., Schena, M., Chai, A., Shalon, D., Bedilion, T., Gilmore, J. *et al.* Discovery and analysis of inflammatory disease-related genes using cDNA microarrays. *Proc Natl Acad Sci USA* 1997; **94**: 2150–5.
9. O'Hara, R., Murphy, E. P., Whitehead, A. S., Fitzgerald, O., and Bresnihan, B. Local expression of the serum amyloid A and formyl peptide receptor-like 1 genes in synovial tissue is associated with matrix metalloproteinase production in patients with inflammatory arthritis. *Arthritis Rheum* 2004; **50**: 1788–99.
10. Hahn, G., Stuhlmuller, B., Hain, N., Kalden, J. R., Pfizenmaier, K., and Burmester, G. R. Modulation of monocyte activation in patients with rheumatoid arthritis by leukapheresis therapy. *J Clin Invest* 1993; **91**: 862–70.
11. Hamerlinck, F. F. Neopterin: a review. *Exp Dermatol* 1999; **8**: 167–76.
12. Rosengren, S., Hoffman, H., Bugbee, W., and Boyle, D. L. Expression and regulation of cryopyrin and related proteins in rheumatoid arthritis synovium. *Ann Rheum Dis* 2004; **64**: 708–14.

Table 5.2 Monocyte/Mφ functions and their role in RA

Function	Mechanisms	(Potential) role in RA
Clearance of immune complexes	Binding of immunoglobulins (Ig) to Fc-receptors (Fc-γ-R I, IIA, IIB, IIIA)	Potential clearance of rheumatoid factor (RF), but further activation of monocytes/Mφs; Opsonization of complexes by complement, leading to binding to Mφ complement receptors and further cell activation (reviewed in Refs 1–4); Notably, inhibition of monocyte activation by Fc-γ-R IIB[3]
Complement activation	Binding of complement factors to complement receptors 1(CD35), 3 (CD11b), and 5a (CD88)	Recognition of activated complement (soluble phase or on IgG-immune complexes); Promotion of phagocytosis and activation of monocytes/Mφs[4]
Phagocytosis of particulate antigens	• Conventional (Fc-mediated) →lysosomal degradation and MHC-II antigen processing	Scavenging of debris but potential import of arthritogenic molecules[4]; Antigen presentation and activation of CD4+ and CD8+ T cells, possibly relevant to disease initiation or perpetuation (spreading of autoimmunity) (reviewed in Ref. 1)
	• Coiling phagocytosis → lysosomal degradation and MHC-I antigen processing	Involved in phagocytosis of *Borrelia burgdorferi*, active agent of Lyme arthritis (reviewed in Ref. 1)
Clearance of intracellular pathogens and apoptotic cells	Removal of pathogens and recognition of apoptotic cells via exposed intracellular membrane components	Induction of Mφ-derived cytokines by bacterial toxins or superantigens [4–6]; Modulation of Mφ responses by mycobacterial lipoarabinomannan (LAM)[7,8] or Toll-like receptors (TLR)[9,10]; Persistence of obligate/facultative intracellular pathogens with arthritogenic potential[11,12]
Antigen processing and presentation	**Enzymatic degradation of antigens and binding of antigenic peptides to MHC molecules;** transport to the cell surface	Important cognate functions upon antigen recognition via presentation of antigen on MHC-II molecules[13] and expression of membrane second signal molecules adjacent to T-cells (reviewed in Ref. 1)

Table 5.2 Continued

Chemotaxis and angiogenesis	Attraction of other inflammatory cells; induction of neo-vascularization	Positive feedback between Mφ-derived cytokines and chemotactic factors (e.g., IL-8 and MCP-1); Promotion of angiogenesis by IL-8 and soluble forms of adhesion molecules (e.g., VCAM-1, ELAM-1)[14]
Wound healing	Remodelling of tissue via interaction with fibroblasts	Sustained monocyte recruitment at wound injury sites via monocyte chemoattractant MIP-1α; phagocytosis of matrix debris and endogenous production of IL-1, TNF-a, etc., as well as post-injury tissue remodelling (reviewed in Ref. 1)
Lipid metabolism	Mφ synthesis of prostaglandins (PG)E$_2$ and I$_2$ Expression of scavenger receptor A (uptake of oxidized low-density lipoprotein)	Pro-inflammatory activity of PGE$_2$ and I$_2$ and leukotrienes in RA, but also autocrine negative feedback through peroxisome proliferator-activated receptors α and γ (PPAR-α and -γ) (reviewed in Ref. 1); Fish-based diets are associated with clinical improvement of human and experimental arthritis (reviewed in Ref. 1); Modulation of T cell contact-induced production of IL-1β and TNF-α in Mφs by apolipoprotein A-I[15]

1. Kinne, R. W., Stuhlmuller, B., Palombo-Kinne, E., and Burmester, G. R. The role of macrophages in the pathogenesis of rheumatoid arthritis. In: *Rheumatoid Arthritis: the new frontiers in pathogenesis and treatment* (ed. F. Wollheim, G. S. Firestein, and G. S. Panayi) pp. 69–87. Oxford University Press: 2000.
2. Van Roon, J. A., Bijlsma, J. W., van De Winkel, J. G., and Lafeber, F. P. Depletion of synovial macrophages in rheumatoid arthritis by an anti-Fc{gamma}RI-Calicheamicin immunoconjugate. *Ann Rheum Dis* 2005; **64**: 685–70.
3. Wijngaarden, S., van De Winkel, J. G., Jacobs, K. M., Bijlsma, J. W., Lafeber, F. P., and Van Roon, J. A. A shift in the balance of inhibitory and activating Fcgamma receptors on monocytes toward the inhibitory Fcgamma receptor IIb is associated with prevention of monocyte activation in rheumatoid arthritis. *Arthritis Rheum.* 2004; **50**: 3878–87.
4. Liu, H. and Pope, R. M. Phagocytes: mechanisms of inflammation and tissue destruction. *Rheum Dis Clin North Am* 2004; **30**: 19–39.
5. Giles, J. T. and Bathon, J. M. Serious infections associated with anticytokine therapies in the rheumatic diseases. *J Intensive Care Med* 2004; **19**: 320–34.
6. Hopkins, P. A., Fraser, J. D., Pridmore, A. C., Russell, H. H., Read, R. C., and Sriskandan, S. Superantigen recognition by HLA class II on monocytes up-regulates toll-like receptor 4 and enhances proinflammatory responses to endotoxin. *Blood* 2005; **105**: 3655–62.
7. Dao, D. N., Kremer, L., Guerardel, Y., Molano, A., Jacobs, W. R., Jr., Porcelli, S. A., and Briken, V. Mycobacterium tuberculosis lipomannan induces apoptosis and interleukin-12 production in macrophages. *Infect Immun* 2004; **72**: 2067–74.
8. Briken, V., Porcelli, S. A., Besra, G. S., and Kremer, L. Mycobacterial lipoarabinomannan and related lipoglycans: from biogenesis to modulation of the immune response. *Mol Microbiol* 2004; **53**: 391–403.
9. Seibl, R., Kyburz, D., Lauener, R. P., and Gay, S. Pattern recognition receptors and their involvement in the pathogenesis of arthritis. *Curr Opin Rheumatol* 2004; **16**: 411–18.
10. Mogensen, T. H. and Paludan, S. R. Reading the viral signature by Toll-like receptors and other pattern recognition receptors. *J Mol Med* 2005; **83**: 180–92.
11. Cheevers, W. P., Snekvik, K. R., Trujillo, J. D., Kumpula-McWhirter, N. M., Pretty On Top KJ, and Knowles, D. P. Prime-boost vaccination with plasmid DNA encoding caprine-arthritis encephalitis lentivirus env and viral SU suppresses challenge virus and development of arthritis. *Virology* 2003; **306**: 116–25.
12. Itescu, S. Rheumatic aspects of acquired immunodeficiency syndrome. *Curr Opin Rheumatol* 1996; **8**: 346–53.
13. Iguchi, T., Kurosaka, M., and Ziff, M. Electron microscopic study of HLA-DR and monocyte/macrophage staining cells in the rheumatoid synovial membrane. *Arthritis Rheum* 1986; **29**: 600–13.
14. Koch, A. E. Angiogenesis as a target in rheumatoid arthritis. *Ann Rheum Dis* 2003; **62**: ii60–ii67.
15. Bresnihan, B., Gogarty, M., Fitzgerald, O., Dayer, J. M., and Burger, D. Apolipoprotein A-I infiltration in rheumatoid arthritis synovial tissue: a control mechanism of cytokine production? *Arthritis Res Ther* 2004; **6**: R563–R566.

Table 5.3 Potential sites of myelomonocytic activation in RA and corresponding steps of intermediate or terminal (trans)differentiation

Compartment	Location	Differentiation step
Joint or juxta-articular	Synovial membrane	Recently immigrated monocytes Mφ (M1/M2?) Dendritic cells
	Cartilage–pannus junction	Mφs
	Subchondral bone	Osteoclasts
	Vascular endothelium	–
Extra-articular	Peripheral blood	Circulating monocytes
	Bone marrow	Myelomonocytic precursors Endothelial cells
	Subendothelial space	Mφs/foam cells/pericytes
	Rheumatoid nodules	Epitheloid cells; multinucleated giant cells
	Lung interstitial space	Alveolar Mφs

Bone marrow anomalies may also underlie the presence of highly proliferative potential colony-forming cells in the blood of patients with severe RA and interstitial pulmonary involvement[41]. These facts and the existence of a Mφ activation syndrome in severe systemic juvenile RA[8,42] suggest that arthritis severity is associated with systemic activation of the MPS, as also shown by extra-articular differentiation of Mφ within subcutaneous rheumatoid nodules[43,44] (Table 5.3). The involvement of the MPS system in RA may also explain the mode of action of slow-acting anti-rheumatic drugs (possibly targeting altered precursors)[10] or stem-cell transplantation[45].

(a)

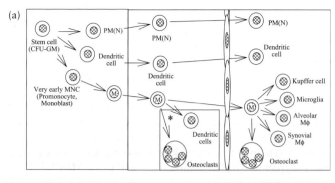

(b)

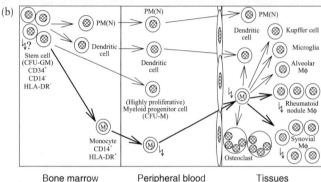

Bone marrow   Peripheral blood   Tissues

Fig. 5.1 (A) Physiological differentiation of the mononuclear phagocyte system (MPS; steady-state cytokine and growth factor milieu). In the human MPS, monocytes (M) differentiate from a CD34+ stem cell via an intermediate step of monoblasts. Monocytes leave the bone marrow and remain in circulation for about three days. Upon entering various tissues, they differentiate into different types of resident macrophages (Mφs), including synovial Mφs. It is believed that these mature cells do not recirculate, surviving for several months in their respective tissues until they senesce and die. Some circulating monocytes retain the potential for differentiating into dendritic cells and osteoclasts (* in the insert). The steady-state myeloid differentiation involves many factors, including GM-CSF, IL-1, IL-6, and TNF-α, which are produced by resident bone marrow Mφs (reviewed in Ref. 2). (B) Increased plasticity of myeloid differentiation and its possible role in RA (augmented cytokine and growth factor milieu). Human bone marrow intermediate cells can differentiate into Mφs or dendritic cells in the presence of c-kit ligand, GM-CSF, and TNF-α. TNF-α, in turn, inhibits the differentiation of monocytes into Mφs *in vitro*, and, together with GM-CSF, directs the differentiation of precursor cells into dendritic cells, another important arm of the accessory cell system. Also, IL-11, or vitamin D3 and dexamethasone, induce the differentiation of bone marrow cells or mature Mφs into osteoclasts, cells involved in the destruction of subchondral bone in RA. Osteoclasts and dendritic cells can also be derived from circulating monocytes upon stimulation with M-CSF or IL-4 plus GM-CSF. This plasticity, and its dependence on growth factors or cytokines that are clearly elevated in peripheral blood and bone marrow of RA patients, may explain some differentiation anomalies in the disease, and also the efficacy of some anti-rheumatic drugs. Non-specific enhancement of monocyte maturation and tissue egression, in turn, are consistent with the known alterations in inflammation (reviewed in Ref. 1). The differentiation paths potentially relevant to RA are indicated by bold arrows. The jagged arrows represent possible sites of cell activation.

Activation of the mononuclear phagocyte system in RA

Synovial and juxta-articular compartments

Synovial membrane

In RA synovial membrane, a surface layer of HLA-DR+, CD14+, and CD68+ Mφ is followed by a layer of fibroblasts[2]. Below these layers, Mφ are distributed in lymphoid aggregates (adjacent to activated CD4+ lymphoid cells) or in diffuse infiltrates near CD8+ T-cells[46], suggesting active participation in (auto)immune processes. In addition, Mφs are located close to synovial fibroblast-like cells with atypical morphology, believed to be centrally involved in tissue destruction[47,48].

Synovial Mφs are clearly activated, as shown by the expression of several markers (see Table 5.1 for details). The degree of Mφ infiltration/activation correlates not only with joint pain and general inflammatory indices[49], but also with the radiological progression of joint damage[1], which ultimately affects the life quality of RA patients. Close correlations are also observed between the density of sublining synovial Mφs and the clinical improvement following effective therapy with several conventional and biological anti-rheumatic treatments, suggesting that synovial Mφ numbers could be used as 'biomarkers' of clinical efficacy[12,13,50].

In chronic RA, certain histological configurations are probably important for the clinical course of disease. High TNF-α and IL-1β production, for example, seems associated to the rare granulomatous synovitis, a condition characterized by a high frequency of subcutaneous rheumatoid nodules[44]. Conversely, these cytokines appear modestly elevated in diffuse synovitis, possibly associated to seronegative RA[44]. This is also consistent with the variable abundance of TNF-α and/or TNF-α receptors in the RA synovial membrane[51,52], and the variable sensitivity to anti-TNF-α therapy[5,15,48]. In addition, differences in joint production of TNF-α may be reflected in differential plasma levels of bioactive TNF-α, compatible with the clinical response of RA patients to anti-TNF-α therapy[53].

Myeloid-derived dendritic cells are also enriched in RA synovial compartments. Their efficacy as antigen-presenting cells and their interdigitating location in perivascular lymphoid aggregates are optimal prerequisites for the presentation of putative arthritogenic antigens to T cells and for the regulation of B cells[54,55]. On the other hand, dendritic cells can also trans-differentiate into osteoclasts under permissive cytokine conditions[56], thus contributing to bone damage.

Cartilage–pannus and bone–pannus junction (subchondral bone)

At the very site of tissue destruction, Mφs express significant amounts of the inflammatory mediators IL-1, TNF-α, and GM-CSF[2] and contribute to the production of matrix metalloproteinases (MMPs) and leukocyte elastase (reviewed in Ref. 57). In general, a number of MMPs have been detected in the RA synovial membrane[58]; also, the synovial tissue remote from the cartilage–pannus junction seems to express a similar spectrum of MMPs compared to the tissue at the cartilage–pannus junction[59].

A particular role in cartilage damage may be played by MMP-9, whose levels positively correlate with RA progression and severity[60], and by the Mφ-specific MMP-12[61]. Nonetheless, the potential of Mφs to directly degrade cartilage matrix components may be modest. Thus, Mφs are conceivably amplifiers (especially via activation of fibroblasts) rather than primary effectors of tissue destruction. Recent studies in RA indicate that the expression of Rel/NF-κB subunits (in particular the p50 NF-κB)[62] is especially high in synovial areas adjacent to the cartilage-pannus junction, suggesting a strong contribution of this site to joint erosion. Likewise, in erosive RA the expression of the MMP inhibitor TIMP-1 at the cartilage-pannus junction is lower than in non-erosive RA[63]. Furthermore, imaging findings show that synovial areas remote from the cartilage-pannus junction respond better to disease-modifying anti-rheumatic drug (DMARD) therapy than areas close to the cartilage-pannus junction[64].

The contribution of Mφ-like cells may be quite different at the bone–pannus junction, where osteoclasts derived from the myelomonocytic lineage (see Fig. 5.1A, B) strongly contribute to bone erosion (reviewed in Ref. 65) (Table 5.3). At this site, the outstanding importance of the osteoprotegerin/RANKL/RANK system for bone destruction has been clearly recognized (reviewed in Ref. 66), so that RANKL blockade or other forms of interference with the balance of this system may become a feasible treatment of RA and other conditions involving bone destruction. Osteoclasts, on the other hand, can be successfully targeted also with novel amino-bisphosphonates, which, through inhibition of osteoclast function, prevent local and systemic bone loss in experimental arthritis and represent means to preserve joint and bone structure in human RA (reviewed in Ref. 65) (see also the section 'Apoptosis-inducing agents').

Extra-articular compartments

Peripheral blood

The active participation of circulating monocytes in RA is documented by: (a) spontaneous production of prostanoids and PGE_2, cytokines and chemokines, soluble CD14, neopterin, and the MMP-inhibitor TIMP (tissue inhibitor of metalloproteinase)-1[9,67-69]; (b) expression of the Mn-superoxide-dismutase, a critical enzyme for the control of oxygen radicals[69]; (c) increased phagocytic activity[70]; (d) increased integrin expression and monocyte adhesiveness[71]; (e) presence of activated suppressor monocytes[25]; (f) more generally, a pattern of gene activation that closely resembles the synovial pattern[7] (see also Table 5.1); and (g) coincidence of the efficacy of conventional anti-rheumatic therapy with down-regulation of monocyte activation[9,10]. Indeed, gold sodium thiomalate and chloroquine reduce the *in vitro* production of pro-inflammatory cytokines (IL-1β, TNF-α)[10]; likewise, steroid treatment down-regulates the expression of Fc-γ-receptor III and ICAM-1[11] and reduces NF-κB activation and TNF-α release in monocytes[13].

Differential analysis of gene patterns in RA monocytes collected upon initial and final therapeutic leukapheresis (which induces clinical remission in severe RA presumably by reducing monocyte activation)[9] shows broad gene-activation patterns in different stages of disease[7]. In addition to the expected cytokines (IL-1α, IL-1β, IL-6, TNF-α), gene activation in the florid stage of disease includes also GRO-α/melanoma growth-stimulatory activity, MIP-2/GRO-β, ferritin, α-1-antitrypsin, lysozyme, transaldolase, EBER-1/EBER-2-associated-protein, thrombospondin-1, an angiotensin receptor-II C-terminal homolog, RNA polymerase-II elongation factor, and other undefined genes[7]. Since a number of these molecules are also (over)expressed in RA joints (see Table 5.1 for details), monocytes appear to be pre-shaped in a 'rheumatoid' phenotype prior to their entry into the inflamed synovial tissue. This is further supported by parallel overexpression of the B cell-attracting chemokine 1 and the late differentiation marker gp39 in circulating monocytes and tissue Mφs[68,72]. Thus, the full extent of systemic monocyte/Mφ activation remains to be explored, both in terms of constitutive activation and response to conventional/experimental anti-rheumatic therapy[71,73,74].

Mφs in the subendothelial space and 'rheumatoid' atherosclerosis

Cardiovascular events are a major cause of mortality in RA patients (reviewed in Ref. 75). Indeed, patients with active RA display not only increased serum levels of lipid peroxidation products, but also a form of dyslipoproteinemia which, due to high lipoprotein lipase activity and fast removal of lipids, leads to low plasma levels of cholesterol and triglycerides (reviewed in Refs 76,77). The paradoxical coexistence of low-risk factors with high mortality for cardiovascular diseases, thus, might be due to a mechanism whereby partially degraded lipoproteins are increasingly cleared by Mφs through scavenger receptors. This excessive removal may lead to formation of foam cells and development of atherosclerotic plaques. The link between disease activity and activation of subendothelial Mφs may be the high TNF-α, IL-1, and IL-6 levels in circulation[77].

Stimulation/regulation of monocyte/Mφ activation in RA

Cell-cell interaction

A significant part of Mφ effector responses is mediated by cell-contact-dependent signaling with different inflammatory or mesenchymal cells.

T cell–Mφ interaction

Accessory, inflammatory, effector, and inhibitory Mφ functions can be stimulated by fixed T cells or their plasma membranes if T cells are pre-activated and express activation surface molecules[78-82]. In response to such interaction, monocytes produce MMP, IL-1α, and IL-1β[78,80,81]. Also, T cells pre-stimulated in an antigen-mimicking fashion stimulate TNF-α and IL-10 production once in contact with monocytes[80,81]. Conversely, fixed T cells stimulated in an antigen-independent fashion (i.e., with IL-15, IL-2, or a combination of IL-6 and TNF-α; so-called Tck cells) induce monocyte production of TNF-α, but not the anti-inflammatory IL-10[80,81,83]. These findings suggest that early RA may reflect antigen-specific T cell-Mφ interactions. Conversely, chronic

RA may be associated with antigen-independent interactions, dominated by an exuberant cytokine milieu and Tck cells. This may also explain the relative paucity of IL-10 in the synovial membrane in chronic RA (see also the section 'Regulatory cytokines').

Several ligand pairs on T cells and monocytes/Mϕs have been implicated in this interaction[80,81], although the individual or combined importance of the ligand pairs remains unclear. This interaction is further modified by several soluble mediators, including the pro-inflammatory cytokines IL-2, IL-15, IL-17, and IL-18, as well as the anti-inflammatory mediators apolipoprotein A-I, IFN-β, GM-CSF, IL-4, and IL-10[81,82]. Finally, the NF-κB pathway, the phosphatidyl-inositol 3-kinase pathway, and the p38 and p42/44 mitogen-activated protein kinase pathways appear central for the induction of TNF-α and IL-10 production in monocytes/Mϕs by contact with T cells[78–82]. Interestingly, T cells isolated from RA synovial tissue show phenotypical and functional features similar to Tck cells and the above-mentioned signal transduction pathways differentially contribute to the induction of TNF-α and IL-10 production in monocytes/Mϕs by co-culture with Tck cells. This creates the hope for selective therapeutic targeting of pro-inflammatory TNF-α and sparing of anti-inflammatory IL-10[80].

Fibroblast-Mϕ interaction

Because of the prominent numbers of Mϕs and fibroblasts and their activated status in RA synovial tissue, the interaction of these cells is critical for the resulting inflammation and tissue damage. Indeed, the mere contact of these cells elicits the production of IL-6, GM-CSF, and IL-8[84]. The cytokine output can be enhanced or down-modulated not only by addition of pro-inflammatory or regulatory cytokines (e.g., IL-4, IL-10, IL-13, or IL-1RA), but also by neutralization of the CD14 molecule[84]. Also, *in vitro* significant cartilage degradation occurs in co-cultures of mouse fibroblasts and Mϕs, a response markedly exceeding that observed with each culture alone[85]. Furthermore, purified human synovial fibroblasts co-cultured with myelomonocytic cells induce cartilage degradation *in vitro*, however, with a strong contribution of soluble IL-1 and TNF-α[86]. Fibroblast-Mϕ interaction can also be demonstrated across species barriers, for example, in the human/murine SCID model induced by transfer of RA synovial fibroblasts into the knee joint of mice, in which both soluble mediators and surface contact contribute to arthritis[87].

Interaction of Mϕ with NK cells and endothelial cells

Upon cell contact, monokine-activated CD56^bright NK cells induce monocytes to the production of TNF-α, thus representing another possible reciprocal loop of activation in RA[88].

The interaction between monocytes and endothelial cells in RA (see Fig. 5.2), critical for the sustained influx of activated monocytes in the synovial membrane, relies on the altered expression of integrin/selectin pairs on the surface of the two cell types (reviewed in Ref. 2). Because the synovial cytokine milieu (including the Mϕ-derived TNF-α) up-regulates the expression of these ligand pairs, a self-perpetuating cycle ensues by which sustained Mϕ-derived mechanisms lead to further influx and activation of

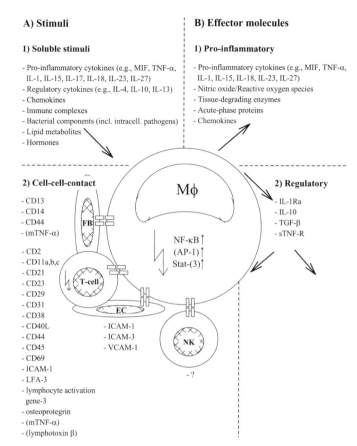

Fig. 5.2 Paracrine, juxtacrine, and autocrine stimuli (*column A*) and effector molecules (*column B*) of Mϕ activation in RA. Most of the regulatory products of activated Mϕs act on Mϕs themselves, creating autocrine regulatory loops whose dysregulation possibly promotes disease severity and chronicity. FB, fibroblasts; EC, endothelial cells; NK, natural killer cells. The jagged arrow in the T cell indicates the necessity of pre-activating T cells for effective juxtacrine stimulation of Mϕs.

circulating monocytes. This may be further aggravated by the release of other pro-inflammatory molecules (e.g., MRP-8 and MRP-14) during monocyte transmigration through the inflamed endothelium[89].

Soluble stimuli

Pro-inflammatory cytokines

An overview of the numerous cytokines with known or potential stimulatory activity on monocytes/Mϕs is provided in Table 5.4. Some cytokines with a particularly relevant role in RA are described in more detail.

Mϕ migration inhibitory factor (MIF) One of the first interleukins discovered, MIF is an early-response cytokine abundantly released by Mϕs. Notably, MIF stimulates a number of Mϕ functions in an autocrine fashion, for example, TNF-α secretion, phagocytosis, and generation of reactive oxygen species (ROS). In addition, MIF confers resistance to apoptosis in Mϕ and synovial fibroblasts, thus prolonging the survival of activated, disease-relevant cells. In RA, MIF is overexpressed in serum and synovial tissue in correlation with disease activity[90]. Also, polymorphisms in the promoter or

Table 5.4 Overview of pro-inflammatory cytokines relevant to Mφ (dys)function in RA

Family	Cytokine	Pro-inflammatory	Dual	Autocrine	Main pathogenetic features
IL-1	IL-1	X	–	X	Predominantly produced by Mφs; critical mediator of tissue damage; autocrine features (see section 'Pro-inflammatory cytokines'
	IL-18	X	–	X	Predominantly produced by Mφs; critical pleiotropic mediator of disease; autocrine features (see section 'Pro-inflammatory cytokines'
IL-18 inducible	IL-32	X	–	–	Unclear[1]
IL-2	IL-7	X	–	–	Elevated in RA, although a relative paucity is also possible[2,3]; induces osteoclastic bone loss in mice[4]
	IL-15	X	–	X	Produced by Mφs; important autocrine mediator of disease processes (see section 'Pro-inflammatory cytokines'
	IL-21	X	–	–	Only IL-21R is expressed by synovial Mφs and fibroblasts[5]
IL-6	IL-6	X	X	–	Predominantly produced by fibroblasts under the influence of Mφs; most strikingly elevated cytokine in acute RA, with phase-dependent differential effects (see section 'Cytokines with a dual role in arthritis')
	IL-31	X	–	–	Induces experimental dermatitis[6]
	LIF	X	–	–	Stimulates proteoglycan resorption in cartilage[7]
	Oncostatin M	X	–	–	Recruits leukocytes to inflammatory sites and stimulates MMP and TIMP production[7]
IFN type I/ IL-10	IL-19	X	–	X	Involved in both Th$_1$ and Th$_2$ inflammatory disorders[8,9]; autocrine features[10,11]
	IL-20	X	–	X	Overexpressed in psoriasis; autocrine features[8]
	IL-22	X	–	–	Relevant to innate immunity and acute-phase response[12]
	IL-24	X	–	–	Possible antagonism with regulatory IL-10[13]
	IL-26	X	–	–	Polymorphism possibly contributes to RA sex-bias susceptibility[14]
	IL-28, IL-29	X	–	X	Involved in microbial recognition by up-regulation of Toll-like receptors; autocrine features[15–17]
IL-12	IL-12	X	–	–	Predominantly produced by synovial Mφs and dendritic cells; promotes Th$_1$ responses[18]
	IL-23	X	–	–	Shares p40 subunit with IL-12 and possibly antagonizes IL-12 (see section 'Pro-inflammatory cytokines')
	IL-27	X	X	X	Produced by Mφs; its neutralization has anti-arthritic effects; autocrine features[19]
IL-17	IL-17	X	–	–	Th$_0$–Th$_1$ lymphokine with pleiotropic, amplifying effects on Mφs (see section 'Pro-inflammatory cytokines')

1. Kim, S. H., Han, S. Y., Azam, T., Yoon, D. Y., and Dinarello, C. A. Interleukin-32: a cytokine and inducer of TNFalpha. *Immunity* 2005; **22**: 131–42.
2. Van Roon, J. A., Glaudemans, K. A., Bijlsma, J. W., and Lafeber, F. P. Interleukin 7 stimulates tumour necrosis factor alpha and Th1 cytokine production in joints of patients with rheumatoid arthritis. *Ann Rheum Dis* 2003; **62**: 113–19.
3. Leonard, W. J. Interleukin-7 deficiency in rheumatoid arthritis. *Arthritis Res Ther* 2005; **7**: 42–43.
4. Toraldo, G., Roggia, C., Qian, W. P., Pacifici, R., and Weitzmann, M. N. IL-7 induces bone loss in vivo by induction of receptor activator of nuclear factor kappa B ligand and tumor necrosis factor alpha from T cells. *Proc Natl Acad Sci USA* 2003; **100**: 125–30.
5. Jungel, A., Distler, J. H., Kurowska-Stolarska, M., Seemayer, C. A., Seibl, R., Forster, A. *et al*. Expression of interleukin-21 receptor, but not interleukin-21, in synovial fibroblasts and synovial macrophages of patients with rheumatoid arthritis. *Arthritis Rheum* 2004; **50**: 1468–76.
6. Dillon, S. R., Sprecher, C., Hammond, A., Bilsborough, J., Rosenfeld-Franklin, M., Presnell, S. R.*et al*. Interleukin 31, a cytokine produced by activated T cells, induces dermatitis in mice. *Nat Immunol* 2004; **5**: 752–60.
7. Wong, P. K., Campbell, I. K., Egan, P. J., Ernst, M., and Wicks, I. P. The role of the interleukin-6 family of cytokines in inflammatory arthritis and bone turnover. *Arthritis Rheum* 2003; **48**: 1177–89.
8. Romer, J., Hasselager, E., Norby, P. L., Steiniche, T., Thorn, C. J., and Kragballe, K. Epidermal overexpression of interleukin-19 and -20 mRNA in psoriatic skin disappears after short-term treatment with cyclosporine a or calcipotriol. *J Invest Dermatol* 2003; **121**: 1306–11.
9. Liao, S. C., Cheng, Y. C., Wang, Y. C., Wang, C. W., Yang, S. M., Yu, C. K.*et al*. IL-19 induced Th2 cytokines and was up-regulated in asthma patients. *J Immunol* 2004; **173**: 6712–18.
10. Parrish-Novak, J., Xu, W., Brender, T., Yao, L., Jones, C., West, J.*et al*. Interleukins 19, 20, and 24 signal through two distinct receptor complexes: differences in receptor-ligand interactions mediate unique biological functions. *J Biol Chem* 2002; **277**: 47517–23.
11. Wolk, K., Kunz, S., Asadullah, K., and Sabat, R. Cutting edge: immune cells as sources and targets of the IL-10 family members? *J Immunol* 2002; **168**: 5397–402.
12. Wolk, K., Kunz, S., Witte, E., Friedrich, M., Asadullah, K., and Sabat, R. IL-22 increases the innate immunity of tissues. *Immunity* 2004; **21**: 241–54.
13. Caudell, E. G., Mumm, J. B., Poindexter, N., Ekmekcioglu, S., Mhashilkar, A. M., Yang, X. H.*et al*. The protein product of the tumor suppressor gene, melanoma differentiation-associated gene 7, exhibits immunostimulatory activity and is designated IL-24. *J Immunol* 2002; **168**: 6041–6.
14. Vandenbroeck, K., Cunningham, S., Goris, A., Alloza, I., Heggarty, S., Graham, C.*et al*. Polymorphisms in the interferon-gamma/interleukin-26 gene region contribute to sex bias in susceptibility to rheumatoid arthritis. *Arthritis Rheum* 2003; **48**: 2773–8.
15. Radstake, T. R., Roelofs, M. F., Jenniskens, Y. M., Oppers-Walgreen, B., van Riel, P. L., Barrera, P.*et al*. Expression of toll-like receptors 2 and 4 in rheumatoid synovial tissue and regulation by proinflammatory cytokines interleukin-12 and interleukin-18 via interferon-gamma. *Arthritis Rheum* 2004; **50**: 3856–65.

16. Pierer, M., Rethage, J., Seibl, R., Lauener, R., Brentano, F., Wagner, U.*et al.* Chemokine secretion of rheumatoid arthritis synovial fibroblasts stimulated by Toll-like receptor 2 ligands. *J Immunol* 2004; **172**: 1256–65.
17. Siren, J., Pirhonen, J., Julkunen, I., and Matikainen, S. IFN-alpha regulates TLR-dependent gene expression of IFN-alpha, IFN-beta, IL-28, and IL-29. *J Immunol* 2005; **174**: 1932–7.
18. Vandenbroeck, K., Alloza, I., Gadina, M., and Matthys, P. Inhibiting cytokines of the interleukin-12 family: recent advances and novel challenges. *J Pharm Pharmacol* 2004; **56**: 145–60.
19. Villarino, A. V. and Hunter, C. A. Biology of recently discovered cytokines: discerning the pro- and anti-inflammatory properties of interleukin-27. *Arthritis Res Ther* 2004; **6**: 225–33.

coding region of the human MIF gene are associated with features of juvenile idiopathic arthritis or adult RA[90,91].

Interestingly, although up-regulated by glucocorticoids, MIF counteracts the anti-inflammatory effects of glucocorticoids on leukocytes, thus neutralization of MIF may achieve a so-called 'steroid-sparing' effect[90]. Indeed, MIF neutralization has clear anti-inflammatory effects in experimental arthritides, and MIF[-/-] mice exhibit reduced arthritis severity compared to wild-type animals[90]. All these effects provide the rationale for the development of anti-MIF treatments in human RA.

Members of the IL-1 family (IL-18)
Interleukin-18 In the RA synovial membrane, this cytokine of the IL-1 family is expressed prominently in CD68[+] Mϕs contained in lymphoid aggregates[92]. CD14[+] Mϕs of the RA synovial fluid also express the IL-18 receptor[92]. IL-18, either alone or in concert with IL-12 and IL-15, strongly enhances the production of IFN-γ, TNF-α, GM-CSF, and nitric oxide by cultured synovial cells. The pro-inflammatory role of IL-18 is indicated by the following findings: (a) IL-18 treatment markedly aggravates experimental arthritis[92,93]; (b) intra-articular overexpression of IL-18 induces experimental arthritis[94]; (c) IL-18 is involved in the development of experimental streptococcal arthritis[95]; (d) IL-18 is selectively overexpressed in the bone marrow in juvenile idiopathic arthritis and Mϕ activation syndrome[8]; and (e) IL-18 can stimulate osteoclast formation through up-regulation of RANKL production by T cells in RA synovitis[96]. Interestingly, IL-18 may mediate its action via several different ways, that is, the classic induction of TNF-α, GM-CSF, and IFN-γ[92]; the induction of functional Toll-like receptors (TLR)-2 and TLR-4 (pattern-recognition receptors for bacterial and endogenous ligands)[97,98]; or the induction of synovial acute phase serum amyloid proteins[99]. The clinical relevance of IL-18 is emphasized by the correlation of its synovial levels with the systemic levels of cyclic AMP receptor protein (CRP), as well as by parallel decreases of IL-18 and CRP in synovial tissue and serum following effective treatment with DMARD[100]. In addition, peripheral blood mononuclear cells of RA patients show low levels of the IL-18 binding protein (a natural inhibitor of IL-18)[101] and reduced sensitivity to stimulation with IL-12/IL-18, indicating profound dysregulation of the IL-18 system[102]. Ongoing clinical studies with IL-18 blockers should answer the question of whether IL-18 is a suitable therapeutic target in human RA[92].

Members of the IL-2 family (IL-15)
Interleukin-15 IL-15, a cytokine with chemoattractant properties for memory T cells, is produced by lining layer cells (including Mϕs) and is increased in RA synovial fluid[103]. Notably, peripheral or synovial T cells stimulated with IL-15 induce Mϕs to produce IL-1β, TNF-α, IL-8, and MCP-1[83,103], but not the regulatory IL-10. Because IL-15 is also produced by Mϕs themselves, this cytokine may (re)stimulate T cells, possibly self-perpetuating a

pro-inflammatory loop[103]. The expression of IL-15 in the RA synovial membrane[103], its biological function[103], and its successful targeting in experimental arthritis have generated large expectations on the use of a fully humanized anti-IL-15 antibody in clinical trials[103,104].

New members of the IL-12 family (IL-23, IL-27)
Interleukin-23 The genuine role of IL-23 is unclear due to the sharing of the p40 subunit with IL-12[105]. IL-23 has prominent pro-inflammatory functions, since transgenic expression in mice leads to multi-organ inflammation and premature death[106]. IL-23 promotes the proliferation of memory T cells, induces IFN-γ production and Th$_1$-mediated immunity, and stimulates the production of the pro-inflammatory cytokine IL-17 in memory T cells[107,108]. Recent studies in experimental arthritis have demonstrated that mice lacking only IL-12 (p35[-/-]) show exacerbated arthritis, whereas mice lacking only IL-23 (p19[-/-]) or lacking both IL-12 and IL-23 (p40[-/-]) are completely protected from arthritis[109]. In addition, activation of Mϕs derived from arthritis-susceptible rats is paradoxically associated with reduced levels of pro-inflammatory mediators (TNF-α, IL-1β, IL-6, IL-10, IL-12 (p35), nitric oxide (NO)) but high expression of IL-23 (p19), whereas non-susceptible rats show the inverse phenotype[108]. If these findings were transferable to human RA, IL-23 would have a pro-inflammatory role and IL-12 a protective one. It is presently unclear whether these findings fit into the recently introduced M$_1$/M$_2$ paradigm of differential Mϕ activation[26,27]. Also, in view of the subunit overlap, the specificity of successful anti-IL-12 therapy (against the shared p40 subunit or against common signal transduction pathways) may have to be re-evaluated[105].

Interleukin-27 IL-27, expressed by monocytes/Mϕs following common inflammatory stimuli, displays a variety of pro- and anti-inflammatory properties[110]. Depending on the immunological environment, IL-27 can either decrease the monocyte expression of IL-6, TNF-α, and IL-12 (as shown in IL-27R[-/-] mice), or else increase the production of IL-1, TNF-α, IL-18, and IL-12[110]. In support of a pro-inflammatory role for IL-27 in arthritis, neutralizing antibodies against IL-27p28 suppresses experimental arthritis[111].

Interleukin-17 This lymphokine, produced in ~90% of RA synovial explant cultures (but only in 16% of osteoarthritis) strongly stimulates Mϕs to produce IL-1 and TNF-α[112]. The TNF-α production can be completely reversed by addition of IL-10[112]. IL-17, present in T cell-rich areas of RA synovial samples, is exclusively produced by Th$_0$ or Th$_1$ clones derived from the synovial membrane or fluid of RA patients[113]. In addition, IL-17 indirectly induces the formation of osteoclasts from progenitor cells[114] and enhances the production of nitric oxide in articular chondrocytes[115], thus potentially contributing to cartilage and bone destruction. As it stands, IL-17 is the only T cell cytokine present in significant amounts in RA joints, thereby potentially representing a major amplifier of the Mϕ-derived cytokines[116], for example by triggering the expression of inducible nitric oxide synthase (iNOS)[117]. Because of its pleiotropic effects on the production of inflammatory mediators and on the degradation of bone and cartilage, IL-17 represents yet another interesting therapeutic target in arthritis[118], possibly in combination with IL-1 or TNF-α blockers[116].

Bacterial/viral components and Toll-like receptors

The ability of bacterial toxins or superantigens to initiate the secretion of Mφ-derived cytokines is relevant in view of a possible microorganism etiology of RA and in view of side-effects of anti-TNF-α therapy, particularly mycobacterial infections[119]. Lipopolysaccharide (LPS), for example, binds to Mφs through the CD14 receptor and, *in vitro*, stimulates the production of IL-1β, TNF-α, and MIP-1α[120]. Staphylococcal enterotoxin-B (SEB), a potent Mφ activator, enhances arthritis in MRL-*lpr/lpr* mice. Anti-TNF-α therapy, in this case, reverses both the severe wasting effects of SEB and the incidence of arthritis, indicating that TNF-α is central in this system[121]. Finally, the staphylococcal enterotoxin A increases the expression of the Toll-like receptor (TLR)-4 in human monocytes by ligation of major histocompatibility complex (MHC)-II, with subsequent enhancement of pro-inflammatory cytokines by known TLR-4 ligands (e.g., LPS[122]).

Lipoarabinomannan (LAM), a mycobacterial lipoglycan involved in attenuating host immune responses and entry of mycobacteria into Mφs, induces monocyte chemotaxis, Th₁-like differentiation, and Mφ production of TNF-α, GM-CSF, IL-1, IL-6, IL-8, and IL-10[123]. Recently, three different families of LAM have been defined, depending on whether the terminal arabinan residues carry mannose caps (ManLAMs), phosphoinositol caps (PILAMs), or do not carry any cap (AraLAMs)[124]. These show strikingly different effects on Mφs, that is, PILAMs induce a potent pro-inflammatory response (apoptosis and IL-12p40 expression), whereas ManLAMs actually inhibit phagosome maturation, apoptosis, and IFN-γ signaling[125]. The pro-inflammatory effects of PILAMs are mediated via TLR-2 (but not TLR-4), indicating selective use of specific elements of the innate immune system.

TLRs are part of the recently discovered cellular pattern-recognition receptors (PPRs), involved in first-line defence of the innate immune system against microbial infections[126,127]. In addition to bacterial or viral components, some PPRs also recognize host-derived molecules, such as the glycoprotein gp96, hyaluronic-acid oligosaccharides, heparan sulfate, fibronectin fragments, and surfactant-protein A (reviewed in Ref. 126). In RA, notably, functional TLR-2 and TLR-4 are expressed in CD16+ synovial Mφs, peripheral blood mononuclear cells, and synovial fibroblasts[97,98,128]. Also, their expression can be up-regulated by cytokines present in the inflamed RA joint (e.g., IL-1β, TNF-α, M-CSF, and IL-10), suggesting that activation of synovial cells via TLRs may contribute to disease processes[126], as supported by findings in experimental arthritis[129].

More generally, the persistence of obligate or facultative intracellular pathogens in Mφs may directly lead to development of arthritis, as in the case of Ross River virus[130] or caprine-arthritis encephalitis lentivirus[131]. The arthritis associated with HIV-1 infection is also due to virus tropism for Mφs[132]. As for the human parvovirus B19[133], the frequency of RA patients with simultaneous positivity for antibodies against B19 (including IgM as indicators of recent infection) and DNA for B19 does not differ from that of other conditions, dampening expectations that B19 infection is relevant to the etiopathogenesis of RA[134].

Hormones

Females are affected by RA at a ratio of ~3:1 compared to males and experience clinical fluctuations during menstrual cycle and pregnancy, indicating a major modulating role for sex hormones[135]. Monocytes/Mφs are strongly involved in hormone modulation of RA, due to their expression of sex-hormone receptors and their cytokine response upon exposure to estrogens[135–137]. Indeed, physiological levels of estrogens stimulate RA Mφs to the production of the pro-inflammatory cytokine IL-1, whereas higher levels inhibit IL-1 production, conceivably mimicking the clinical improvement during pregnancy. Interestingly, selective estrogen-receptor ligands inhibiting NF-κB transcriptional activity (but lacking estrogenic activity) can markedly inhibit joint swelling and destruction in experimental arthritis[138].

Thyroid or other neuroendocrine hormones can also influence RA, at least partially through actions on Mφs[139].

Regulation of monocyte/Mφ activation in RA

Regulatory cytokines

An overview of cytokines that regulate monocyte/Mφ function in RA is provided in Table 5.5.

Interleukin-4 This Th₂-like anti-inflammatory cytokine is believed to play a protective role in arthritis, although its virtual absence from synovial samples indicates a lack of protective mechanisms rather than active regulation[140]. In RA, IL-4 down-modulates monocyte/Mφ cytotoxicity and cytokine/monokine production, including TNF-α and TNF-α receptors[2,141]. Notably, IL-4 decreases IL-1β production while increasing the IL-1RA production, thus providing a 'coordinated' anti-inflammatory approach[142]. IL-4 also decreases the mRNA production of cyclo-oxygenase-2 (COX-2) and cytosolic phospholipase A₂, thereby reducing the levels of PGE₂[143,144]. Importantly, IL-4 reduces bone resorption[140] as well as synovial proliferation *in vitro*[145]. Consistently, treatment with IL-4 clearly suppresses streptococcal cell wall-induced arthritis, a strongly Mφ-dependent model[142]. However, treatment of RA patients with recombinant IL-4 has proven disappointing[146].

Interleukin-10 IL-10, a Th₂- and Mφ-derived cytokine with clear autocrine functions, reduces HLA-DR expression and antigen presentation in monocytes and inhibits the production of pro-inflammatory cytokines, GM-CSF, and Fc-γ-receptors by synovial Mφs[141]. Consistently with cytokine and chemokine down-regulation, IL-10 clearly suppresses experimental arthritis[147]. In spite of IL-10 elevation in serum and synovial compartments of RA patients[141], some studies suggest a relative deficiency of IL-10[148]. A combined IL-4/IL-10 deficiency probably tilts the cytokine balance to a pro-inflammatory predominance. In addition, the *ex vivo* production of IL-10 by RA peripheral blood

Table 5.5 Overview of anti-inflammatory cytokines relevant to Mφ (dys)function in RA

	Anti-inflammatory	Dual	Autocrine	Main pathogenetic features
IL-1RA	X	–	X	Produced by differentiated Mφs and up-regulated by pro-inflammatory mediators, including IL-1 itself or GM-CSF; autocrine contribution to the termination of inflammatory reactions (see section 'Anti-inflammatory/regulatory cytokines')
IL-4	X	–	–	Strong regulator of Mφ functions, but virtually absent in synovial tissue (see section 'Regulatory cytokines')
IL-10	X	–	X	Produced by synovial Mφs strong regulator of Mφ functions, but relatively deficient in RA; autocrine features (see section 'Regulatory cytokines')
IL-11	X	X	–	Regulator of Mφ functions in a paracrine regulatory loop with synovial fibroblasts (see section 'Regulatory cytokines')
IL-13	X	X	–	Selective regulator of Mφ functions; improves experimental arthritis (see section 'Regulatory cytokines')
IL-16	X	X	–	Known as anti-inflammatory[1,2], IL-16 has also pro-inflammatory properties, i.e., correlates with MMP-3 levels, progression of joint destruction, and levels of other pro-inflammatory cytokines[3,4]
IFN-β	X	–	–	Clear anti-inflammatory and anti-destructive effects in experimental arthritides; therapy attempts in human RA are thus far unsuccessful[5]
TGF-β	X	X	X	Produced by Mφs; main regulator of connective tissue remodeling; potent inducer of hyaluronan synthase 1; induces synovial inflammation but also suppresses acute and chronic arthritis; induces inflammation and cartilage degradation in a rabbit model; autocrine features. MMP can affect TGF-β via shedding of latent TGF-β attached to decorin (see section 'Cytokines with a dual role in arthritis')

1. Klimiuk, P. A., Goronzy, J. J., and Weyand, C. M. IL-16 as an anti-inflammatory cytokine in rheumatoid synovitis. *J Immunol* 1999; **162**: 4293–9.
2. Blaschke, S., Schulz, H., Schwarz, G., Blaschke, V., Muller, G. A., and Reuss-Borst, M. Interleukin 16 expression in relation to disease activity in rheumatoid arthritis. *J Rheumatol* 2001; **28**: 12–21.
3. Kaufmann, J., Franke, S., Kientsch-Engel, R., Oelzner, P., Hein, G., and Stein, G. Correlation of circulating interleukin 16 with proinflammatory cytokines in patients with rheumatoid arthritis. *Rheumatology (Oxford)* 2001; **40**: 474–5.
4. Lard, L. R., Roep, B. O., Toes, R. E., and Huizinga, T. W. Enhanced concentrations of interleukin 16 are associated with joint destruction in patients with rheumatoid arthritis. *J Rheumatol* 2004; **31**: 35–9.
5. Tak, P. P. IFN-beta in rheumatoid arthritis. *Front Biosci* 2004; **9**: 3242–7.

mononuclear cells is negatively correlated with radiographic joint damage and progression of joint damage, suggesting that high IL-10 production is protective in RA[149]. Similarly to IL-4, however, treatment with recombinant IL-10 has not produced significant improvement in RA[146]. The inefficacy of IL-10 treatment may be partially explained by up-regulation of Fc-γ-receptors I and IIA on monocytes/Mφs[150].

Interleukin-11 Stromal cell-derived IL-11 is present in synovial membrane, synovial fluid, and sera of RA patients, and blockade of endogenous IL-11 increases endogenous TNF-α production in RA synovium *in vitro*[151], while recombinant human IL-11 reduces the production of TNF-α and IL-12 from activated Mφs[152]. IL-11 may represent another example of paracrine regulatory loops, since IL-1α and TNF-α synergistically stimulate the production of IL-11 in rheumatoid synovial fibroblasts[153]. Treatment with IL-11 decreases clinical severity and prevents joint damage in collagen-induced arthritis[154]. On the other hand, neutralization of IL-11 reduces mBSA/IL-1 arthritis, suggesting that IL-11 can also be pro-inflammatory[155]. Thus far, clinical studies with recombinant human IL-11 have shown very limited therapeutic efficacy in RA[156].

Interleukin-13 Similarly to IL-4 and IL-10, IL-13 exerts suppressive effects in experimental arthritis, likely through a selective effect on monocytes/Mφs[157,158]. Also, exposure of RA synovial tissue explants or synovial fluid mononuclear cells to IL-13 diminishes the production of IL-1 and TNF-α[157]. The potential use of IL-13 as an anti-inflammatory agent in RA, however, is complicated by recent findings showing that overexpression of IL-13 reduces cartilage damage in immune-complex arthritis, but at the same time induces joint inflammation[159].

Monocyte/Mφ effector molecules in RA

Pro-inflammatory cytokines

Tumour necrosis factor-α

TNF-α is a pleiotropic cytokine that increases the expression of cytokines, adhesion molecules, PGE$_2$, collagenase, and collagen by synovial cells. In RA, TNF-α is mostly produced by Mφs in the synovial membrane and at the cartilage-pannus junction, and possibly occupies a proximal position in the RA inflammatory cascade[51]. While an average of ~5% of synovial cells express TNF-α mRNA/protein *in situ*[52,160], the degree of TNF-α expression in the synovial tissue depends upon the prevailing histological configuration, resulting in different clinical variants[44] (see also the section 'Synovial membrane'). Different disease stages and clinical variants are also reflected in serum and synovial fluid levels of TNF-α[9,161].

The critical importance of TNF-α in RA is supported by several experimental observations: (a) TNF-α, in combination with IL-1, is a potent inducer of synovitis[162]; (b) transgenic, deregulated expression of TNF-α causes the development of chronic arthritis[163]; (c) neutralization of TNF-α suppresses experimental arthritides[51,162,164]; (d) TNF-α is produced in synovial membrane and extra-articular/lymphoid organs in experimental arthritides, mimicking the systemic character of RA[165–168].

TNF-α exists in membrane-bound and soluble forms, both acting as pro-inflammatory mediators. Trans-membrane TNF-α is involved in local, cell-contact—mediated processes, and appears the prime stimulator of the R75 receptor[169]. Interestingly, the transgenic expression of this form is alone sufficient to induce chronic arthritis[170]; likewise, a mutant membrane-TNF-α, which utilizes both R55 and R75 receptors, can also cause arthritis[171]. Conversely, the soluble form of TNF-α, shed via MMP cleavage from the membrane-bound form, primarily stimulates the R55 receptor, acting transiently and at a distance[169].

TNF-α receptors

TNF receptors are found in synovial tissue and fluid of RA patients, especially in severe disease[51,52]. There are two known TNF receptors, the R55 (TNF-R1; high-affinity receptor) and the R75 (TNF-R2; low-affinity receptor). The resulting stable or transient character of the ligand/receptor complex, respectively, mediates different cellular responses to soluble and trans-membrane TNF-α[172]. In general, TNF receptors can operate independently of one another, cooperatively, or by 'passing' TNF-α to one another[169]. This complexity may explain the tremendous sensitivity of target cells to minute concentrations of TNF-α, as well as the considerable variety of its effects. TNF receptors can also be shed, binding to soluble TNF-α and hence acting as natural inhibitors in disease. Recent studies have demonstrated that TNF-R1 may be primarily responsible for pro-inflammatory effects of TNF-α, whereas TNF-R2 may predominantly mediate anti-inflammatory effects of TNF-α (reviewed in Ref. 173). Thus, selective blockade of TNF-R1, instead of broad blockade of all effects of TNF-α, may become an attractive therapeutic approach.

Consistent with the pivotal role of TNF-α in arthritis, administration of chimeric/humanized anti-TNF-α monoclonal antibodies or TNF-α receptor constructs has shown remarkable efficacy in acute disease and retardation of radiographic progression[5,15,16] (see also Chapter 27).

Interleukin-1

In RA, IL-1 is found predominantly in CD14+ Mφs[174], and IL-1 levels in the synovial fluid correlate significantly with joint inflammation[28]. This cytokine appears to mediate a large part of the articular damage, as it profoundly influences proteoglycan synthesis and degradation[28,94,162,175]. At the same time, IL-1 induces the production of MMP-1 and MMP-3 and enhances bone

resorption[28], compatible with recent evidence from arthritis models and treatment of RA that the tissue-destruction capacities of IL-1β may outweigh its genuine role in joint inflammation[94,175].

In RA, the balance between IL-1 and its physiological inhibitor IL-1RA is shifted in favour of IL-1, indicating a dysregulation crucial in promoting chronicity[28,175] (see also the section 'Anti-inflammatory/regulatory cytokines').

Chemokines and chemokine receptors

Chemokines, a superfamily subdivided into four subfamilies (CXC, CC, C, and CX3C), are small proteins specialized in differential recruitment of leukocyte populations via a number of transmembrane receptors. Chemokines not only favor monocyte influx in inflamed tissue, but they also play a key role in activation, functional polarization, and homing of patrolling monocytes/Mφs[27]. Notably, monocytes/Mφs express a limited number of the numerous chemokine receptors (e.g., CCR1, 2, 5, 7, and 8, as well as CX3CR1), representing a basis for prominent trafficking of monocyte/Mφs in arthritis. In RA, synovial Mφs produce several chemokines (e.g., CCL3 (or Mφ inflammatory protein 1α), CCL5 (or RANTES), and CX3CL1 (or fractalkine)) and carry at the same time chemokine receptors, indicating the presence of autocrine loops in disease (reviewed in Ref. 176). At the same time, chemokines are up-regulated by the Mφ-derived TNF-α and IL-1[177]. Significantly, some chemokines expressed in synovial Mφs (e.g., IL-8 and fractalkine) are powerful promoters of angiogenesis, thus providing a link between Mφ activation and the prominent neo-vascularization of the RA synovium[29]. In RA, angiogenesis may be further promoted via activation of Mφs by advanced glycation end products[178], whereas thrombospondin 2 seems to down-regulate angiogenesis[24]. Because the enlargement of the vascular bed potentiates the influx of activated monocytes, down-modulation of the chemokine system represents a multi-potential target of anti-rheumatic therapy, as indicated by the promising results of treatment with a CCR1 antagonist in RA[176].

Anti-inflammatory/regulatory cytokines

Mφs also produce anti-inflammatory cytokines, most notably IL-RA and IL-10 (the latter described in the previous section 'Regulatory cytokines'), with both cytokines engaged in autocrine regulatory loops (see also Table 5.5).

Interleukin-1-receptor antagonist (IL-1RA)

Differentiated Mφs constitutively express IL-1RA, which binds to IL-1 receptors without evoking physiological responses[28]. Significantly, this protein is up-regulated by pro-inflammatory mediators, including IL-1 itself or GM-CSF, inducing strong anti-inflammatory effects[28]. By means of this feedback mechanism, Mφs contribute therefore to the termination of inflammatory reactions. The critical relevance of IL-1 in chronic RA, as well as the imbalance between IL-1 and IL-1RA, constitutes the rationale for successful therapy with recombinant IL-1RA[14,28,179].

Cytokines with a dual role in arthritis

Cytokines with a dual role are indicated in Tables 5.4 and 5.5.

Interleukin-6

IL-6 is the most strikingly elevated cytokine in RA, especially in the synovial fluid during acute disease[180]. The acute rise is consistent with the role of IL-6 in acute-phase responses (see also Table 5.1). However, while IL-6 levels in the synovial fluid correlate with the degree of radiological joint damage, and IL-6 and soluble IL-6 receptors promote the generation of osteoclasts[181], this cytokine has phase-dependent effects; for example, it protects cartilage in acute disease but promotes excessive bone formation in chronic disease[182]. While IL-6 is mostly produced by synovial fibroblasts and only partially by Mϕs (reviewed in Ref. 2), two findings suggest that the striking IL-6 rise is a prominent outcome of Mϕ activation: (a) the morphological vicinity of IL-6-expressing fibroblasts with CD14[+] Mϕs in the RA synovial tissue (reviewed in Ref. 2); (b) the co-culture studies showing that IL-1 stimulates IL-6 production[84]. The role of IL-6 in experimental arthritis and the anti-arthritic effects of anti-IL-6 receptor antibodies indicate possible therapeutic applications also in RA (reviewed in Refs 183, 184).

Transforming growth factor-β

TGF-β is a main regulator of connective tissue remodeling, controlling both matrix production and degradation (reviewed in Ref. 2). TGF-β is also a potent inducer of hyaluronan synthase 1, hence promoting the overproduction of hyaluronic acid characteristic of human RA[185]. In animal experiments, TGF-β induces synovial inflammation but also suppresses acute and chronic arthritis (reviewed in Ref. 186). The pro-inflammatory effects of TGF-β are substantiated by induction of Mϕ expression of Fc-γ-receptor III (which elicits the release of tissue-damaging reactive oxygen species); promotion of monocyte adhesion and infiltration during chronic disease (reviewed in Ref. 186); and induction of inflammation and cartilage degradation in a rabbit model[187]. At the same time, TGF-β has anti-inflammatory properties, for example, it counteracts some IL-1 effects, including MMP production and phagocytosis of collagen, although the effects on MMPs are also controversial[188,189]. The effects on TIMPs are also unclear, as the regulation of MMPs and TIMPs may depend on different tissue domains (superficial vs. deep cartilage layers) and may vary for intra- or extracellular digestion of collagen[2,189]. MMPs themselves can also affect TGF-β via shedding of latent TGF-β attached to decorin[190], thereby creating a potential disease-enhancing loop.

In RA, Mϕs express different TGF-β molecules and TGF-β receptors in the lining and sublining layer, at the cartilage–pannus junction, and in the synovial fluid[140,186,191,192]. A protective role of this cytokine in RA has been recently stressed by findings of an association between TGF-β polymorphism and RA severity, that is, alleles associated with low TGF-β expression are correlated with stronger inflammation and poorer outcome[193]. Likewise, experimental arthritis is significantly ameliorated by activation of TGF-β via adenoviral expression of thrombospondin 1[194].

Nitric oxide (NO) and reactive oxygen species (ROS)

In RA, synovial lining Mϕs represent a source of NO[195]. NO levels and inducible NO synthase (iNOS) are elevated in serum and peripheral-blood-derived Mϕs of patients with active RA, respectively[196]. IL-17 seems to play a special role in triggering the expression of iNOS[117]. Synovial cells exposed to NO increase their TNF-α production, possibly adding to the mechanisms that promote synovitis[195]. NO may be relevant to arthritis also for its effects on bone remodeling[197]; however, it can also exert protective effects in experimental autoimmunity[198]. Notably, evidence is growing that not only inducible synthase, but also constitutive forms of NO synthase (NOS; endothelial and neuronal) contribute to the pathogenesis of arthritis, although the evidence points both to pro-inflammatory and anti-inflammatory roles of NO[199].

RA Mϕs also produce ROS, which are involved in distal inflammatory processes[200], including the regulation of MMP production[201]. Enhanced mitochondrial production of ROS in RA blood monocytes correlates with plasma levels of TNF-α, confirming the stimulatory effect of this cytokine on ROS production[200]. ROS cause damage to matrix component by different mechanisms, for example, direct attack on the molecules, reduction of matrix synthesis, induction of apoptosis, or activation of latent MMP[202]. The pathophysiological potential of ROS extends to the activation of pro-inflammatory transcription factors[202]. Interestingly, gene polymorphism for enzymes involved in generation and degradation of ROS or reactive nitrogen species have been identified as risk factors for rheumatic diseases[203].

In general, the link between Mϕ activation and molecules with dual activity (may it be Mϕ products or external stimuli, the latter as soluble, membrane-bound, stimulatory, or suppressive factors), and the number of different receptors involved in such stimulation may result not only in potent pro-inflammatory functions of Mϕs, but also in powerful anti-inflammatory- and tissue repair functions. Finally, Mϕ stimuli and Mϕ responses rely heavily on autocrine regulatory mechanisms, which makes it difficult to discern between the cause and the effect.

Treatment of human RA with conventional anti-Mϕ approaches

The role of Mϕ-derived cytokines in the perpetuation of RA, the pathophysiological dichotomy between joint inflammation and cartilage destruction, and the crucial significance of activated synovial Mϕs in relationship to permanent joint damage[1], have generated a radical re-evaluation of the conventional anti-inflammatory and disease-modifying treatments in relationship to Mϕ parameters, with a focus on potentiation of the therapeutic effects (e.g., via combination approaches[204]) and reduction of the side-effects.

Disease-modifying anti-rheumatic therapy (DMARD) and leflunomide

Empirically introduced DMARDs possess a whole array of anti-Mϕ effects[205].

Methotrexate (MTX)

MTX, a most effective DMARD, impairs chemotaxis of monocytes and production of monokines (including TNF-α), while increasing the production of cytokine inhibitors, including soluble TNF-receptor R75[2,206]. Because MTX shifts the IL-1/IL-1RA balance in favor of IL-RA, this drug may also pharmacologically correct the imbalance between these mediators[206]. This change in the monokine balance may fundamentally decrease the pro-destructive mediators in RA synovial tissue. Thus, the treatment strategy of RA has radically changed in the past few years, and MTX is now recommended in early stages of the disease (mostly in combination with corticosteroids and non-steroidal anti-inflammatory drugs (NSAIDs)) with the aim of preventing joint damage[204]. Despite its clear anti-Mφ effects, MTX therapy can be associated with systemic Mφ activation[207].

Leflunomide

Leflunomide, an anti-proliferative drug known for its effects on T cells, may be effective in RA via its influence on Mφs, with reduction of TNF-α and IL-1β production[208], and on trans-differentiation of monocytes/Mφs into osteoclasts[209,210]. Leflunomide is successfully applied in combination with MTX or the anti-TNF agent infliximab[211,212].

Anti-malarials

Endowed with significant anti-rheumatic effects in early RA, anti-malarials have a tropism for lysosomes. This conceivably causes their slow accumulation in Mφs, in which they inhibit the release of arachidonate and the production of PGE_2 via phospholipase-A_2 inhibition. At high concentrations, anti-malarials also inhibit the production of IL-1 and TNF-α in LPS-stimulated Mφs (reviewed in Ref. 205).

Gold compounds

Gold compounds are conceptually interesting, because they rely on classic Trojan-horse mechanisms (i.e. phagocytosis and lysosomal accumulation) for the therapeutic targeting of Mφs and influence a number of Mφ effector functions (reviewed in Ref. 2).

Corticosteroids

The potent anti-inflammatory effects of corticosteroids in RA can be at least partially explained by their effects on Mφs[12,13]. Indeed, a marked reduction in Mφ infiltration is observed following efficacious oral treatment with prednisolone[12]. Corticosteroids also affect the balance of the functionally distinct membrane-bound and soluble TNF-α[169]. Interestingly, high-dose dexamethasone pulse therapy up-regulates IL-10 production, but down-regulates IFN-γ production, in peripheral blood mononuclear cells, indicating that a relative shift towards Th2 activity may contribute to its therapeutic effects[213]. Corticosteroids also decrease the production of IL-8 and MCP-1[214], therefore limiting the self-perpetuating ingress of monocytes in the inflamed joint.

NSAIDs

Aspirin reduces the production of PGE_2 (in monocytes/Mφs and other cells) through acetylation of the isoforms 1 and 2 of cyclo-oxygenase (COX). While its use in RA is limited by the gastric side-effects (mostly COX-1-dependent), selective inhibitors of the COX-2 isoform have been introduced for RA therapy, which have effects on isolated Mφ, local inflammation, and production of IL-6 (the most prominent cytokine in RA synovial fluid)[215]. More widespread use of COX-2 inhibitors, on the other hand, has recently revealed an increased risk of thrombo-embolic events[216]. A new class of COX inhibitors, combining an NO-donating moiety to conventional NSAIDs, are presently being assessed for their use in the treatment of RA[217]. In general, different NSAIDs clearly down-regulate pro-inflammatory Mφ functions in RA and still belong to the initial *armamentarium* of anti-rheumatic drugs (primarily in combination with MTX and corticosteroids[204]).

Non-conventional and experimental anti-Mφ therapy

Counteraction of monocyte/Mφ activation at a cellular level

Leukapheresis

In RA, repeated leukapheresis removes activated monocytes from the blood, leading to reduced expression of differentiation markers, HLA-DR antigens, cytokines, neopterin, and PGE_2[7,9]. Leukapheresis is a means of treating cases of severe and systemic RA, including cases associated with massive monocyte/Mφ activation[218].

Apoptosis-inducing agents

Physical elimination of disease-relevant cells (e.g., activated Mφs or osteoclasts) by apoptosis is advantageous because it circumvents secondary tissue damage by restraining cellular organelles in apoptotic vesicles. Incorporation of liposome-encapsulated, non-amino-bisphosphonates by activated monocytes, for example, induces apoptosis in these cells[219]. Systemic application of encapsulated bisphosphonates in experimental arthritis not only counteracts joint swelling, but also prevents local joint destruction and subchondral bone damage[220]; in addition, it shows protective effects on remote bone damage[221]. Studies in RA show that a single intra-articular administration of clodronate liposomes leads to Mφ depletion and decreased expression of adhesion molecules in the lining layer of RA synovial tissue[222]. Selective targeting of activated Mφ has also been demonstrated using either apoptosis-inducing immunotoxins coupled to anti-Fc-γ-receptor I (CD64) antibodies or folate receptor-mediated targeting[18,19]. In general, liposome encapsulation can also be exploited for selective delivery of Mφ-modulating drugs[2,3,223] and for gene-therapy constructs[224].

Whereas non-amino-bisphosphonates induce apoptosis in Mφs and osteoclasts, novel amino-bisphosphonates have recently become available that inhibit osteoclast functions. Accordingly, treatment of experimental arthritis with the aminated zolendronic acid is highly effective in reducing local articular damage and systemic bone loss through its effects on osteoclasts (reviewed in Ref. 65).

Control of gene transcription

The transcription of most cytokine genes in monocytes/Mφs depends on the activation of NF-κB and NF-κM transcription factors or that of the AP-1 complex. In RA synovial Mφs, the expression of NF-κB is more pronounced than that of AP-1, a selectivity that may have important therapeutic implications[225]. Accordingly, the anti-arthritic effects of IL-4 may be based on the selective suppression of NF-κB in Mφs. IL-10 also down-regulates the production of pro-inflammatory monokines, inhibiting the nuclear factors NF-κB, AP-1, or NF-IL-6. Unlike IL-4, IL-10 can also enhance degradation of the mRNA for IL-1 and TNF-α (reviewed in Ref. 2). In general, targeted inhibition of 'pro-inflammatory' signal transduction pathways in Mφs represents an attractive therapeutic approach[226].

Gene therapy in arthritis

Gene-therapy approaches have been applied in a number of experimental arthritis models to counteract the monokines IL-1 and TNF-α or to deliver the protective IL-1RA[158,224,227]. The same applies to therapeutic overexpression of the soluble IL-1 type I receptor- and the type I soluble TNF-α receptor-IgG fusion protein, although the latter appears less effective[158,224,227]. Recently, gene-therapy approaches have also been extended to anti-inflammatory cytokines, that is, IL-4, IL-10, IL-13, IFN-β, and TGF-β[158,224,227]. Another goal of gene therapy is to achieve 'molecular synovectomy', either by expression of herpes simplex virus-thymidine kinase (with subsequent administration of ganciclovir) or by overexpression of Fas-ligand/inhibitors of nuclear translocation of NF-κB, resulting in synovial cell apoptosis[158]. Finally, inhibition of synovial cell proliferation is attempted by the expression of cyclin-dependent kinase inhibitors interfering with the cell cycle[158,224,227]. Gene therapy aimed at neutralizing pro-inflammatory Mφ products, overexpressing Mφ-regulating mediators, or simply eliminating overly activated Mφs, is therefore promising for the treatment of arthritis.

Conclusions

The multiplicity and abundance of Mφ-derived mediators in RA and their paracrine and autocrine effects (including those directed to other cells of the myeloid lineage), indicate that Mφs are local and systemic amplifiers of disease severity and perpetuation. The main **local** mechanisms include: (a) self-perpetuating, chemokine-mediated recruitment of inflammatory cells; (b) cytokine-mediated activation of newly immigrated inflammatory cells; (c) cell contact-mediated activation of neighboring inflammatory cells; (d) cytokine- and cell contact-mediated secretion of matrix degrading enzymes; (e) activation of mature dendritic cells and cytokine-mediated differentiation of Mφs (and possibly B cells, T cells, and mesenchymal cells) into antigen-presenting cells, with possible effects on spreading of autoimmunity to cryptic epitopes; (f) neo-vascularization, with potentiation of cellular and exudatory mechanisms; and (g) (trans)differentiation of Mφs into

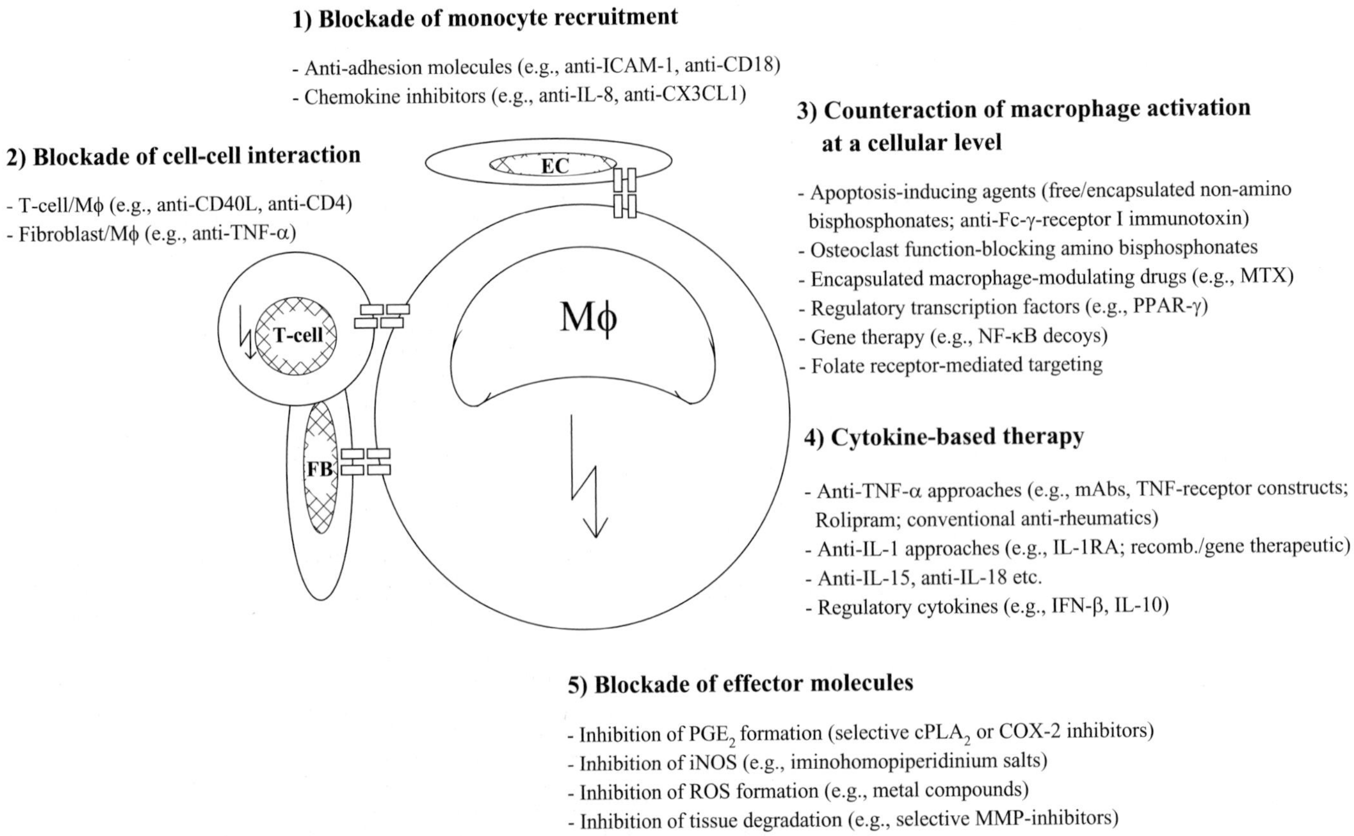

1) Blockade of monocyte recruitment

- Anti-adhesion molecules (e.g., anti-ICAM-1, anti-CD18)
- Chemokine inhibitors (e.g., anti-IL-8, anti-CX3CL1)

2) Blockade of cell-cell interaction

- T-cell/Mφ (e.g., anti-CD40L, anti-CD4)
- Fibroblast/Mφ (e.g., anti-TNF-α)

3) Counteraction of macrophage activation at a cellular level

- Apoptosis-inducing agents (free/encapsulated non-amino bisphosphonates; anti-Fc-γ-receptor I immunotoxin)
- Osteoclast function-blocking amino bisphosphonates
- Encapsulated macrophage-modulating drugs (e.g., MTX)
- Regulatory transcription factors (e.g., PPAR-γ)
- Gene therapy (e.g., NF-κB decoys)
- Folate receptor-mediated targeting

4) Cytokine-based therapy

- Anti-TNF-α approaches (e.g., mAbs, TNF-receptor constructs; Rolipram; conventional anti-rheumatics)
- Anti-IL-1 approaches (e.g., IL-1RA; recomb./gene therapeutic)
- Anti-IL-15, anti-IL-18 etc.
- Regulatory cytokines (e.g., IFN-β, IL-10)

5) Blockade of effector molecules

- Inhibition of PGE_2 formation (selective $cPLA_2$ or COX-2 inhibitors)
- Inhibition of iNOS (e.g., iminohomopiperidinium salts)
- Inhibition of ROS formation (e.g., metal compounds)
- Inhibition of tissue degradation (e.g., selective MMP-inhibitors)

Fig. 5.3 Potential and established approaches for modulation of monocyte/Mφ functions in RA. FB, fibroblasts; EC, endothelial cells.

osteoclasts involved in subchondral bone damage. At a **systemic** level, amplification of disease can proceed at least through the following mechanisms: (a) acute phase response network; (b) systemic production of TNF-α; (c) anomalies in bone marrow differentiation; and (d) chronic activation of circulating monocytes.

Although uncovering the etiology of disease remains the ultimate means of silencing the whole pathogenetic process, the efforts in understanding how activated Mφs influence disease have led to optimization strategies to selectively target Mφs (Fig. 5.3) and to the development of new agents tailored to specific features of Mφ activation in RA. This approach has at least two advantages: (a) it strikes the very cell population that mediates/amplifies most of the irreversible cartilage destruction; and (b) it minimizes adverse effects on other cells that may have no (or marginal) effects on joint damage.

Reducing the numbers of activated Mφs or modulating their functions by means of selective apoptosis-inducing or function-blocking agents, by inhibiting activation signals and/or their specific Mφ receptors, or by selectively counteracting the Mφ products that act as disease amplifiers (Fig. 5.3), are but a few of the possibilities. Nonetheless, future anti-Mφ strategies will have to face the following questions: (a) Do recent findings on the efficacy of anti-B cell treatment[228] provide a rationale for combination approaches? (b) Is systemic targeting of Mφs sufficient or does combined systemic and local treatment provide additional benefit? (c) Is counteration of one (or few) Mφ key mediator(s) sufficient for long-term, efficacious suppression of RA? (d) Can the problem of non-responders be resolved by individual genome-wide scans and/or bioactivity testing for (Mφ) inflammatory mediators in circulation? (e) Does the approach of extreme selectivity bear the inherent risk of sharpening too much the side-effect profile, as indicated by the long-term risks of anti-TNF-α therapy and selective COX-2 inhibitors? (f) Are the increasing healthcare costs and/or the necessity of targeting more than one pro-inflammatory (Mφ) pathway causing a revival of well-established, affordable anti-rheumatics (possibly in connection with better targeting to decrease the required dose and to diminish side-effects)? Research is ongoing to provide answers to these questions, eagerly awaited by rheumatologists and in particular by patients suffering from rheumatic diseases.

Addendum

Recent studies have demonstrated that specific and selective blockade of the TNF-R1 by either pre-ligand assembly domains (173a) or by ligand-induced conformational pertubation (173b) ameliorates murine collagen-induced arthritis, thereby showing that selective blockade of TNF-R1, instead of broad blockade of all effects of TNF-α, may be a therapeutic option also for RA.

References

1. Mulherin, D., Fitzgerald, O., and Bresnihan, B. Synovial tissue macrophage populations and articular damage in rheumatoid arthritis. *Arthritis Rheum* 1996; **39**: 115–24.
2. Kinne, R. W., Stuhlmuller, B., Palombo-Kinne, E., and Burmester, G. R. The role of macrophages in the pathogenesis of rheumatoid arthritis. In *Rheumatoid Arthritis: The New Frontiers in Pathogenesis and Treatment* (Wollheim, F., Firestein, G. S., and Panayi, G. S. eds), pp. 69–87. Oxford University Press; 2000.
3. Kinne, R. W., Brauer, R., Stuhlmuller, B., Palombo-Kinne, E., and Burmester, G. R. Macrophages in rheumatoid arthritis. *Arthritis Res* 2000; **2**: 189–202.
4. Liu, H. and Pope, R. M. Phagocytes: mechanisms of inflammation and tissue destruction. *Rheum Dis Clin North Am* 2004; **30**: 19–39.
5. Smolen, J. S. and Steiner, G. Therapeutic strategies for rheumatoid arthritis. *Nat Rev Drug Discov* 2003; **2**: 473–88.
6. Michaelsson, E., Holmdahl, M., Engstrom, A., Burkhardt, H., Scheynius, A., and Holmdahl, R. Macrophages, but not dendritic cells, present collagen to T cells. *Eur J Immunol* 1995; **25**: 2234–41.
7. Stuhlmuller, B., Ungethüm, U., Scholze, S., Martinez, L., Backhaus, M., Kraetsch, H.-G. *et al.* Identification of known and novel genes in activated monocytes from patients with rheumatoid arthritis. *Arthritis Rheum* 2000; **43**: 775–90.
8. Maeno, N., Takei, S., Imanaka, H., Yamamoto, K., Kuriwaki, K., Kawano, Y., and Oda, H. Increased interleukin-18 expression in bone marrow of a patient with systemic juvenile idiopathic arthritis and unrecognized macrophage-activation syndrome. *Arthritis Rheum* 2004; **50**: 1935–8.
9. Hahn, G., Stuhlmuller, B., Hain, N., Kalden, J. R., Pfizenmaier, K., and Burmester, G. R. Modulation of monocyte activation in patients with rheumatoid arthritis by leukapheresis therapy. *J Clin Invest* 1993; **91**: 862–70.
10. Seitz, M., Valbracht, J., Quach, J., and Lotz, M. Gold sodium thiomalate and chloroquine inhibit cytokine production in monocytic THP-1 cells through distinct transcriptional and posttranslational mechanisms. *J Clin Immunol* 2003; **23**: 477–84.
11. Hepburn, A. L., Mason, J. C., and Davies, K. A. Expression of Fcgamma and complement receptors on peripheral blood monocytes in systemic lupus erythematosus and rheumatoid arthritis. *Rheumatology (Oxford)* 2004; **43**: 547–54.
12. Gerlag, D. M., Haringman, J. J., Smeets, T. J., Zwinderman, A. H., Kraan, M. C., Laud, P. *et al.* Effects of oral prednisolone on biomarkers in synovial tissue and clinical improvement in rheumatoid arthritis. *Arthritis Rheum* 2004; **50**: 3783–91.
13. Lavagno, L., Gunella, G., Bardelli, C., Spina, S., Fresu, L. G., Viano, I., and Brunelleschi, S. Anti-inflammatory drugs and tumor necrosis factor-alpha production from monocytes: role of transcription factor NF-kappaB and implication for rheumatoid arthritis therapy. *Eur J Pharmacol* 2004; **501**: 199–208.
14. Bresnihan, B. Anakinra as a new therapeutic option in rheumatoid arthritis: clinical results and perspectives. *Clin Exp Rheumatol* 2002; **20**: S32–S34.
15. Feldmann, M., Bondeson, J., Brennan, F. M., Foxwell, B. M., and Maini, R. N. The rationale for the current boom in anti-TNFalpha treatment: is there an effective means to define therapeutic targets for drugs that provide all the benefits of anti-TNFalpha and minimise hazards? *Ann Rheum Dis* 1999; **58** (Suppl. 1): I27–I31.
16. Miossec, P. An update on the cytokine network in rheumatoid arthritis. *Curr Opin Rheumatol* 2004; **16**: 218–22.
17. van Rooijen, N. and Kesteren-Hendrikx, E. 'In vivo' depletion of macrophages by liposome-mediated 'suicide'. *Methods Enzymol* 2003; **373**: 3–16.
18. Paulos, C. M., Turk, M. J., Breur, G. J., and Low, P. S. Folate receptor-mediated targeting of therapeutic and imaging agents to activated macrophages in rheumatoid arthritis. *Adv Drug Deliv Rev* 2004; **56**: 1205–17.
19. Van Roon, J. A., Bijlsma, J. W., van De Winkel, J. G., and Lafeber, F. P. Depletion of synovial macrophages in rheumatoid arthritis by an anti-Fc{gamma}RI-Calicheamicin immunoconjugate. *Ann Rheum Dis* 2005; **64**: 865–70.
20. Sweeney, S. E. and Firestein, G. S. Signal transduction in rheumatoid arthritis. *Curr Opin Rheumatol* 2004; **16**: 231–7.
21. Bondeson, J., Browne, K. A., Brennan, F. M., Foxwell, B. M., and Feldmann, M. Selective regulation of cytokine induction by adenoviral gene transfer of IkappaBalpha into human

macrophages: lipopolysaccharide-induced, but not zymosan-induced, proinflammatory cytokines are inhibited, but IL-10 is nuclear factor-kappaB independent. *J Immunol* 1999; **162**: 2939–45.

22. Westra, J., Doornbos-van der Meer, B., de Boer, P., van Leeuwen, M. A., van Rijswijk, M. H., and Limburg, P. C. Strong inhibition of TNF-alpha production and inhibition of IL-8 and COX-2 mRNA expression in monocyte-derived macrophages by RWJ 67657, a p38 mitogen-activated protein kinase (MAPK) inhibitor. *Arthritis Res Ther* 2004; **6**: R384–R392.

23. Pirila, L. and Heino, J. Altered integrin expression in rheumatoid synovial lining type B cells: in vitro cytokine regulation of alpha 1 beta 1, alpha 6 beta 1, and alpha v beta 5 integrins. *J Rheumatol* 1996; **23**: 1691–8.

24. Park, Y. W., Kang, Y. M., Butterfield, J., Detmar, M., Goronzy, J. J., and Weyand, C. M. Thrombospondin 2 functions as an endogenous regulator of angiogenesis and inflammation in rheumatoid arthritis. *Am J Pathol* 2004; **165**: 2087–98.

25. Klareskog, L., Forsum, U., Kabelitz, D., Ploen, L., Sundstrom, C., Nilsson, K. et al. Immune functions of human synovial cells: phenotypic and T cell regulatory properties of macrophage-like cells that express HLA-DR. *Arthritis Rheum* 1982; **25**: 488–501.

26. Mills, C. D., Kincaid, K., Alt, J. M., Heilman, M. J., and Hill, A. M. M-1/M-2 macrophages and the Th1/Th2 paradigm. *J Immunol* 2000; **164**: 6166–73.

27. Mantovani, A., Sica, A., Sozzani, S., Allavena, P., Vecchi, A., and Locati, M. The chemokine system in diverse forms of macrophage activation and polarization. *Trends Immunol* 2004; **25**: 677–86.

28. Arend, W. P., Malyak, M., Guthridge, C. J., and Gabay, C. Interleukin-1 receptor antagonist: role in biology. *Annu Rev Immunol* 1998; **16**: 27–55.

29. Koch, A. E. Angiogenesis as a target in rheumatoid arthritis. *Ann Rheum Dis* 2003; **62**: ii60–ii67.

30. Middleton, J., Americh, L., Gayon, R., Julien, D., Aguilar, L., Amalric, F., and Girard, J. P. Endothelial cell phenotypes in the rheumatoid synovium: activated, angiogenic, apoptotic and leaky. *Arthritis Res Ther* 2004; **6**: 60–72.

31. Fonseca, J. E., Edwards, J. C., Blades, S., and Goulding, N. J. Macrophage subpopulations in rheumatoid synovium: reduced CD163 expression in CD4+ T lymphocyte-rich microenvironments. *Arthritis Rheum* 2002; **46**: 1210–16.

32. Baeten, D., Kruithof, E., De Rycke, L., Boots, A. M., Mielants, H., and Veys, E. M. Infiltration of the synovial membrane with macrophage subsets and polymorphonuclear cells reflects global disease activity in spondyloarthropathy. *Arthritis Res Ther* 2005; **7**: R359–R369.

33. Stuhlmuller, B., Kunisch, E., Franz, J., Martinez-Gamboa, L., Hernandez, M. M., Pruss, A. et al. Detection of oncofetal h19 RNA in rheumatoid arthritis synovial tissue. *Am J Pathol* 2003; **163**: 901–11.

34. Kinne, R. W., Kunisch, E., Beensen, V., Zimmermann, T., Emmrich, F., Petrow, P. et al. Synovial fibroblasts and synovial macrophages from patients with rheumatoid arthritis and other inflammatory joint diseases show chromosomal aberrations. *Genes Chromosomes Cancer* 2003; **38**: 53–67.

35. Hirohata, S., Yanagida, T., Itoh, K., Nakamura, H., Yoshino, S., Tomita, T., and Ochi, T. Accelerated generation of CD14+ monocyte-lineage cells from the bone marrow of rheumatoid arthritis patients. *Arthritis Rheum* 1996; **39**: 836–43.

36. Kotake, S., Higaki, M., Sato, K., Himeno, S., Morita, H., Kim, K. J. et al. Detection of myeloid precursors (granulocyte/macrophage colony forming units) in the bone marrow adjacent to rheumatoid arthritis joints. *J Rheumatol* 1992; **19**: 1511–16.

37. Papadaki, H. A., Kritikos, H. D., Gemetzi, C., Koutala, H., Marsh, J. C., Boumpas, D. T., and Eliopoulos, G. D. Bone marrow progenitor cell reserve and function and stromal cell function are defective in rheumatoid arthritis: evidence for a tumor necrosis factor alpha-mediated effect. *Blood* 2002; **99**: 1610–19.

38. Porta, C., Caporali, R., Epis, O., Ramaioli, I., Invernizzi, R., Rovati, B. et al. Impaired bone marrow hematopoietic progenitor cell function in rheumatoid arthritis patients candidated to autologous hematopoietic stem cell transplantation. *Bone Marrow Transplant* 2004; **33**: 721–8.

39. Jongen-Lavrencic, M., Peeters, H. R., Wognum, A., Vreugdenhil, G., Breedveld, F. C., and Swaak, A. J. Elevated levels of inflammatory cytokines in bone marrow of patients with rheumatoid arthritis and anemia of chronic disease. *J Rheumatol* 1997; **24**: 1504–9.

40. Hirohata, S., Yanagida, T., Nampei, A., Kunugiza, Y., Hashimoto, H., Tomita et al. Enhanced generation of endothelial cells from CD34+ cells of the bone marrow in rheumatoid arthritis: possible role in synovial neovascularization. *Arthritis Rheum* 2004; **50**: 3888–96.

41. Horie, S., Nakada, K., Masuyama, J., Yoshio, T., Minota, S., Wakabayashi, Y. et al. Detection of large macrophage colony forming cells in the peripheral blood of patients with rheumatoid arthritis. *J Rheumatol* 1997; **24**: 1517–21.

42. De Benedetti, F., Pignatti, P., Massa, M., Sartirana, P., Ravelli, A., Cassani, G. et al. Soluble tumour necrosis factor receptor levels reflect coagulation abnormalities in systemic juvenile chronic arthritis. *Br J Rheumatol* 1997; **36**: 581–8.

43. Duke, O. L., Hobbs, S., Panayi, G. S., Poulter, L. W., Rasker, J. J., and Janossy, G. A combined immunohistological and histochemical analysis of lymphocyte and macrophage subpopulations in the rheumatoid nodule. *Clin Exp Immunol* 1984; **56**: 239–46.

44. Klimiuk, P. A., Goronzy, J. J., Bjornsson. J., Beckenbaugh, R. D., and Weyand, C. M. Tissue cytokine patterns distinguish variants of rheumatoid synovitis. *Am J Pathol* 1997; **151**: 1311–19.

45. Verburg, R. J., Sont, J. K., and van Laar, J. M. Reduction of joint damage in severe rheumatoid arthritis by high-dose chemotherapy and autologous stem cell transplantation. *Arthritis Rheum* 2005; **52**: 421–4.

46. Iguchi, T., Kurosaka, M., and Ziff, M. Electron microscopic study of HLA-DR and monocyte/macrophage staining cells in the rheumatoid synovial membrane. *Arthritis Rheum* 1986; **29**: 600–13.

47. Gay, S. Rheumatoid arthritis. *Curr Opin Rheumatol* 2001; **13**: 191–2.

48. Firestein, G. S. Evolving concepts of rheumatoid arthritis. *Nature* 2003; **423**: 356–61.

49. Tak, P. P., Smeets, T. J., Daha, M. R., Kluin, P. M., Meijers, K. A., Brand, R. et al. Analysis of the synovial cell infiltrate in early rheumatoid synovial tissue in relation to local disease activity. *Arthritis Rheum* 1997; **40**: 217–25.

50. Haringman, J. J., Gerlag, D. M., Zwinderman, A. H., Smeets, T. J., Kraan, M. C., Baeten, D. et al. Synovial tissue macrophages: highly sensitive biomarkers for response to treatment in rheumatoid arthritis patients. *Ann Rheum Dis* 2005; **64**: 834–8.

51. Feldmann, M., Brennan, F. M., and Maini, R. N. Role of cytokines in rheumatoid arthritis. *Annu Rev Immunol* 1996; **14**: 397–440.

52. Alsalameh, S., Winter, K., Al-Ward, R., Wendler, J., Kalden, J. R., and Kinne, R. W. Distribution of TNF-alpha, TNF-R55 and TNF-R75 in the rheumatoid synovial membrane: TNF receptors are localized preferentially in the lining layer; TNF-alpha is distributed mainly in the vicinity of TNF receptors in the deeper layers. *Scand J Immunol* 1999; **49**: 278–85.

53. Marotte, H., Maslinski, W., and Miossec, P. Circulating tumour necrosis factor-alpha bioactivity in rheumatoid arthritis patients treated with infliximab: link to clinical response. *Arthritis Res Ther* 2005; **7**: R149–R155.

54. Sibilia, J. Novel concepts and treatments for autoimmune disease: ten focal points. *Joint Bone Spine* 2004; **71**: 511–17.

55. Sakar, S. and Fox, D. A. Dendritic cells in rheumatoid arthritis. *Front Biosci* 2005; **10**: 656–65.

56. Rivollier, A., Mazzorana, M., Tebib, J., Piperno, M., Aitsiselmi, T., Rabourdin-Combe, C. et al. Immature dendritic cell transdifferentiation into osteoclasts: a novel pathway sustained by the rheumatoid arthritis microenvironment. *Blood* 2004; **104**: 4029–37.

57. Brinckerhoff, C. E. and Matrisian, L. M. Matrix metalloproteinases: a tail of a frog that became a prince. *Nat Rev Mol Cell Biol* 2002; **3**: 207–14.

58. Konttinen, Y. T., Ainola, M., Valleala, H., Ma, J., Ida, H., Mandelin, J. et al. Analysis of 16 different matrix metalloproteinases (MMP-1 to MMP-20) in the synovial membrane: different profiles in trauma and rheumatoid arthritis. *Ann Rheum Dis* 1999; **58**: 691–7.

59. Smeets, T. J., Kraan, M. C., Galjaard, S., Youssef, P. P., Smith, M. D., and Tak, P. P. Analysis of the cell infiltrate and expression of matrix metalloproteinases and granzyme B in paired synovial biopsy specimens from the cartilage-pannus junction in patients with RA. *Ann Rheum Dis* 2001; **60**: 561–5.

60. Ahrens, D., Koch, A. E., Pope, R. M., Stein-Picarella, M., and Niedbala, M. J. Expression of matrix metalloproteinase 9 (96-kd gelatinase B) in human rheumatoid arthritis. *Arthritis Rheum* 1996; **39**: 1576–87.

61. Wang, X., Liang, J., Koike, T., Sun, H., Ichikawa, T., Kitajima, S. et al. Overexpression of human matrix metalloproteinase-12 enhances the development of inflammatory arthritis in transgenic rabbits. *Am J Pathol* 2004; **165**: 1375–83.

62. Benito, M. J., Murphy, E., Murphy, E. P., van den Berg, W. B., Fitzgerald, O., and Bresnihan, B. Increased synovial tissue NF-kappa B1 expression at sites adjacent to the cartilage-pannus junction in rheumatoid arthritis. *Arthritis Rheum* 2004; **50**: 1781–7.

63. Kane, D., Jensen, L. E., Grehan, S., Whitehead, A. S., Bresnihan, B., and Fitzgerald, O. Quantitation of metalloproteinase gene expression in rheumatoid and psoriatic arthritis synovial tissue distal and proximal to the cartilage-pannus junction. *J Rheumatol* 2004; **31**: 1274–80.

64. Rhodes, L. A., Tan, A. L., Tanner, S. F., Radjenovic, A., Hensor, E. M., Reece, R. et al. Regional variation and differential response to therapy for knee synovitis adjacent to the cartilage-pannus junction and suprapatellar pouch in inflammatory arthritis: implications for pathogenesis and treatment. *Arthritis Rheum* 2004; **50**: 2428–32.

65. Goldring, S. R. and Gravallese, E. M. Bisphosphonates: environmental protection for the joint? *Arthritis Rheum* 2004; **50**: 2044–7.

66. Hofbauer, L. C. and Schoppet, M. Clinical implications of the osteoprotegerin/RANKL/RANK system for bone and vascular diseases. *JAMA* 2004; **292**: 490–5.

67. Schulze-Koops, H., Davis, L. S., Kavanaugh, A. F., and Lipsky, P. E. Elevated cytokine messenger RNA levels in the peripheral blood of patients with rheumatoid arthritis suggest different degrees of myeloid cell activation. *Arthritis Rheum* 1997; **40**: 639–47.

68. Carlsen, H. S., Baekkevold, E. S., Morton, H. C., Haraldsen, G., and Brandtzaeg, P. Monocyte-like and mature macrophages produce CXCL13 (B cell-attracting chemokine 1) in inflammatory lesions with lymphoid neogenesis. *Blood* 2004; **104**: 3021–7.

69. Heller, R. A., Schena, M., Chai, A., Shalon, D., Bedilion, T., Gilmore, J. et al. Discovery and analysis of inflammatory disease-related genes using cDNA microarrays. *Proc Natl Acad Sci U S A* 1997; **94**: 2150–5.

70. Steven, M. M., Lennie, S. E., Sturrock, R. D., and Gemmell, C. G. Enhanced bacterial phagocytosis by peripheral blood monocytes in rheumatoid arthritis. *Ann Rheum Dis* 1984; **43**: 435–9.

71. Bunescu, A., Seideman, P., Lenkei, R., Levin, K., and Egberg, N. Enhanced Fcgamma receptor I, alphaMbeta2 integrin receptor expression by monocytes and neutrophils in rheumatoid arthritis: interaction with platelets. *J Rheumatol* 2004; **31**: 2347–55.

72. Kirkpatrick, R. B., Emery, J. G., Connor, J. R., Dodds, R., Lysko, P. G., and Rosenberg, M. Induction and expression of human cartilage glycoprotein 39 in rheumatoid inflammatory and peripheral blood monocyte-derived macrophages. *Exp Cell Res* 1997; **237**: 46–54.

73. Van Roon, J. A., van Vuuren, A. J., Wijngaarden, S., Jacobs, K. M., Bijlsma, J. W., Lafeber, F. P. et al. Selective elimination of synovial inflammatory macrophages in rheumatoid arthritis by an Fcgamma receptor I-directed immunotoxin. *Arthritis Rheum* 2003; **48**: 1229–38.

74. Wijngaarden, S., van De Winkel, J. G., Jacobs, K. M., Bijlsma, J. W., Lafeber, F. P., and Van Roon, J. A. A shift in the balance of inhibitory and activating Fcgamma receptors on monocytes toward the inhibitory Fcgamma receptor IIb is associated with prevention of monocyte activation in rheumatoid arthritis. *Arthritis Rheum* 2004; **50**: 3878–87.

75. Sattar, N., McCarey, D. W., Capell, H., and McInnes, I. B. Explaining how 'high-grade' systemic inflammation accelerates vascular risk in rheumatoid arthritis. *Circulation* 2003; **108**: 2957–63.

76. Winyard, P. G., Tatzber, F., Esterbauer, H., Kus, M. L., Blake, D. R., and Morris, C. J. Presence of foam cells containing oxidised low density lipoprotein in the synovial membrane from patients with rheumatoid arthritis. *Ann Rheum Dis* 1993; **52**: 677–80.

77. Monaco, C., Andreakos, E., Kiriakidis, S., Feldmann, M., and Paleolog, E. T-cell-mediated signalling in immune, inflammatory and angiogenic processes: the cascade of events leading to inflammatory diseases. *Curr Drug Targets Inflamm Allergy* 2004; **3**: 35–42.

78. McInnes, I. B., Leung, B. P., and Liew, F. Y. Cell-cell interactions in synovitis: interactions between T lymphocytes and synovial cells. *Arthritis Res* 2000; **2**: 374–8.

79. Brennan, F. M., Hayes, A. L., Ciesielski, C. J., Green, P., Foxwell, B. M., and Feldmann, M. Evidence that rheumatoid arthritis synovial T cells are similar to cytokine-activated T cells: involvement of phosphatidylinositol 3-kinase and nuclear factor kappaB pathways in tumor necrosis factor alpha production in rheumatoid arthritis. *Arthritis Rheum* 2002; **46**: 31–41.

80. Brennan, F. M. and Foey, A. D. Cytokine regulation in RA synovial tissue: role of T cell/macrophage contact-dependent interactions. *Arthritis Res* 2002; **4**: S177–S182.

81. Burger, D. and Dayer, J. M. The role of human T-lymphocyte-monocyte contact in inflammation and tissue destruction. *Arthritis Res* 2002; **4**: S169–S176.

82. Dai, S. M., Matsuno, H., Nakamura, H., Nishioka, K., and Yudoh, K. Interleukin-18 enhances monocyte tumor necrosis factor alpha and interleukin-1beta production induced by direct contact with T lymphocytes: implications in rheumatoid arthritis. *Arthritis Rheum* 2004; **50**: 432–43.

83. Sebbag, M., Parry, S. L., Brennan, F. M., and Feldmann, M. Cytokine stimulation of T lymphocytes regulates their capacity to induce monocyte production of tumor necrosis factor-alpha, but not interleukin-10: possible relevance to pathophysiology of rheumatoid arthritis. *Eur J Immunol* 1997; **27**: 624–32.

84. Chomarat, P., Rissoan, M. C., Pin, J. J., Banchereau, J., and Miossec, P. Contribution of IL-1, CD14, and CD13 in the increased IL-6 production induced by in vitro monocyte-synoviocyte interactions. *J Immunol* 1995; **155**: 3645–52.

85. Janusz, M. J. and Hare, M. Cartilage degradation by cocultures of transformed macrophage and fibroblast cell lines: a model of metalloproteinase-mediated connective tissue degradation. *J Immunol* 1993; **150**: 1922–31.

86. Scott, B. B., Weisbrot, L. M., Greenwood, J. D., Bogoch, E. R., Paige, C. J., and Keystone, E. C. Rheumatoid arthritis synovial fibroblast and U937 macrophage/monocyte cell line interaction in cartilage degradation. *Arthritis Rheum* 1997; **40**: 490–8.

87. Lehmann, J., Jungel, A., Lehmann, I., Busse, F., Biskop, M., Saalbach, A. et al. Grafting of fibroblasts isolated from the synovial membrane of rheumatoid arthritis (RA) patients induces chronic arthritis in SCID mice-A novel model for studying the arthritogenic role of RA fibroblasts in vivo. *J Autoimmun* 2000; **15**: 301–13.

88. Dalbeth, N., Gundle, R., Davies, R. J., Lee, Y. C., McMichael, A. J., and Callan, M. F. CD56bright NK cells are enriched at inflammatory sites and can engage with monocytes in a reciprocal program of activation. *J Immunol* 2004; **173**: 6418–26.

89. Frosch, M., Strey, A., Vogl, T., Wulffraat, N. M., Kuis, W., Sunderkotter, C. et al. Myeloid-related proteins 8 and 14 are specifically secreted during interaction of phagocytes and activated endothelium and are useful markers for monitoring disease activity in pauciarticular-onset juvenile rheumatoid arthritis. *Arthritis Rheum* 2000; **43**: 628–37.

90. Morand, E. F. and Leech, M. Macrophage migration inhibitory factor in rheumatoid arthritis. *Front Biosci* 2005; **10**: 12–22.

91. Gregersen, P. K. and Bucala, R. Macrophage migration inhibitory factor, MIF alleles, and the genetics of inflammatory disorders: incorporating disease outcome into the definition of phenotype. *Arthritis Rheum* 2003; **48**: 1171–6.

92. Gracie, J. A. Interleukin-18 as a potential target in inflammatory arthritis. *Clin Exp Immunol* 2004; **136**: 402–4.

93. Ye, X. J., Tang, B., Ma, Z., Kang, A. H., Myers, L. K., and Cremer, M. A. The roles of interleukin-18 in collagen-induced arthritis in the BB rat. *Clin Exp Immunol* 2004; **136**: 440–7.

94. Joosten, L. A., Smeets, R. L., Koenders, M. I., Van Den Bersselaar, L. A., Helsen, M. M., Oppers-Walgreen, B. *et al.* Interleukin-18 promotes joint inflammation and induces interleukin-1-driven cartilage destruction. *Am J Pathol* 2004; **165**: 959–67.

95. Tissi, L., McRae, B., Ghayur, T., von Hunolstein, C., Orefici, G., Bistoni, F., and Puliti, M. Role of interleukin-18 in experimental group B streptococcal arthritis. *Arthritis Rheum* 2004; **50**: 2005–13.

96. Dai, S. M., Nishioka, K., and Yudoh, K. Interleukin (IL) 18 stimulates osteoclast formation through synovial T cells in rheumatoid arthritis: comparison with IL1 beta and tumour necrosis factor alpha. *Ann Rheum Dis* 2004; **63**: 1379–86.

97. Radstake, T. R., Roelofs, M. F., Jenniskens, Y. M., Oppers-Walgreen, B., van Riel, P. L., Barrera, P. *et al.* Expression of toll-like receptors 2 and 4 in rheumatoid synovial tissue and regulation by proinflammatory cytokines interleukin-12 and interleukin-18 via interferon-gamma. *Arthritis Rheum* 2004; **50**: 3856–65.

98. Pierer, M., Rethage, J., Seibl, R., Lauener, R., Brentano, F., Wagner, U. *et al.* Chemokine secretion of rheumatoid arthritis synovial fibroblasts stimulated by Toll-like receptor 2 ligands. *J Immunol* 2004; **172**: 1256–65.

99. Tanaka, F., Migita, K., Kawabe, Y., Aoyagi, T., Ida, H., Kawakami, A., and Eguchi, K. Interleukin-18 induces serum amyloid A (SAA) protein production from rheumatoid synovial fibroblasts. *Life Sci* 2004; **74**: 1671–9.

100. Rooney, T., Murphy, E., Benito, M., Roux-Lombard, P., Fitzgerald, O., Dayer, J. M., and Bresnihan, B. Synovial tissue interleukin-18 expression and the response to treatment in patients with inflammatory arthritis. *Ann Rheum Dis* 2004; **63**: 1393–8.

101. Kawashima, M., Novick, D., Rubinstein, M., and Miossec, P. Regulation of interleukin-18 binding protein production by blood and synovial cells from patients with rheumatoid arthritis. *Arthritis Rheum* 2004; **50**: 1800–5.

102. Kawashima, M. and Miossec, P. Decreased response to IL-12 and IL-18 of peripheral blood cells in rheumatoid arthritis. *Arthritis Res Ther* 2004; **6**: R39–R45.

103. McInnes, I. B. and Gracie, J. A. Interleukin-15: a new cytokine target for the treatment of inflammatory diseases. *Curr Opin Pharmacol* 2004; **4**: 392–7.

104. Ferrari-Lacraz, S., Zanelli, E., Neuberg, M., Donskoy, E., Kim, Y. S., Zheng, X. X. *et al.* Targeting IL-15 receptor-bearing cells with an antagonist mutant IL-15/Fc protein prevents disease development and progression in murine collagen-induced arthritis. *J Immunol* 2004; **173**: 5818–26.

105. Vandenbroeck, K., Alloza, I., Gadina, M., and Matthys, P. Inhibiting cytokines of the interleukin-12 family: recent advances and novel challenges. *J Pharm Pharmacol* 2004; **56**: 145–60.

106. Wiekowski, M. T., Leach, M. W., Evans, E. W., Sullivan, L., Chen, S. C., Vassileva, G. *et al.* Ubiquitous transgenic expression of the IL-23 subunit p19 induces multiorgan inflammation, runting, infertility, and premature death. *J Immunol* 2001; **166**: 7563–70.

107. Aggarwal, S., Ghilardi, N., Xie, M. H., de Sauvage, F. J., and Gurney, A. L. Interleukin-23 promotes a distinct CD4 T cell activation state characterized by the production of interleukin-17. *J Biol Chem* 2003; **278**: 1910–14.

108. Andersson, A., Kokkola, R., Wefer, J., Erlandsson-Harris, H., and Harris, R. A. Differential macrophage expression of IL-12 and IL-23 upon innate immune activation defines rat autoimmune susceptibility. *J Leukoc Biol* 2004; **76**: 1118–24.

109. Murphy, C. A., Langrish, C. L., Chen, Y., Blumenschein, W., McClanahan, T., Kastelein, R. A., Sedgwick, J. D., and Cua, D. J. Divergent pro- and antiinflammatory roles for IL-23 and IL-12 in joint autoimmune inflammation. *J Exp Med* 2003; **198**: 1951–7.

110. Villarino, A. V. and Hunter, C. A. Biology of recently discovered cytokines: discerning the pro- and anti-inflammatory properties of interleukin-27. *Arthritis Res Ther* 2004; **6**: 225–33.

111. Goldberg, R., Wildbaum, G., Zohar, Y., Maor, G., and Karin, N. Suppression of ongoing adjuvant-induced arthritis by neutralizing the function of the p28 subunit of IL-27. *J Immunol* 2004; **173**: 1171–8.

112. Jovanovic, D. V., DiBattista, J. A., Martel-Pelletier, J., Jolicoeur, F. C., He, Y., Zhang, M., *et al.* IL-17 stimulates the production and expression of proinflammatory cytokines, IL-1beta and TNF-alpha, by human macrophages. *J Immunol* 1998; **160**: 3513–21.

113. Aarvak, T., Chabaud, M., Miossec, P., and Natvig, J. B. IL-17 is produced by some proinflammatory Th1/Th0 cells but not by Th2 cells. *J Immunol* 1999; **162**: 1246–51.

114. Kotake, S., Udagawa, N., Takahashi, N., Matsuzaki, K., Itoh, K., Ishiyama, S., Saito, S. *et al.* IL-17 in synovial fluids from patients with rheumatoid arthritis is a potent stimulator of osteoclastogenesis. *J Clin Invest* 1999; **103**: 1345–52.

115. Shalom-Barak, T., Quach, J., and Lotz, M. Interleukin-17-induced gene expression in articular chondrocytes is associated with activation of mitogen-activated protein kinases and NF- kappaB. *J Biol Chem* 1998; **273**: 27467–73.

116. Stamp, L. K., James, M. J., and Cleland, L. G. Interleukin-17: the missing link between T-cell accumulation and effector cell actions in rheumatoid arthritis? *Immunol Cell Biol* 2004; **82**: 1–9.

117. Miljkovic, D. and Trajkovic, V. Inducible nitric oxide synthase activation by interleukin-17. *Cytokine Growth Factor Rev* 2004; **15**: 21–32.

118. Lubberts, E., Koenders, M. I., Oppers-Walgreen, B., van den Bersselaar, L., Coenen-de Roo, C. J. *et al.* Treatment with a neutralizing anti-murine interleukin-17 antibody after the onset of collagen-induced arthritis reduces joint inflammation, cartilage destruction, and bone erosion. *Arthritis Rheum* 2004; **50**: 650–9.

119. Giles, J. T. and Bathon, J. M. Serious infections associated with anticytokine therapies in the rheumatic diseases. *J Intensive Care Med* 2004; **19**: 320–34.

120. Rodenburg, R. J., Brinkhuis, R. F., Peek, R., Westphal, J. R., Van Den Hoogen, F. H., van Venrooij, W. J., and van de Putte, L. B. Expression of macrophage-derived chemokine (MDC) mRNA in macrophages is enhanced by interleukin-1beta, tumor necrosis factor alpha, and lipopolysaccharide. *J Leukoc Biol* 1998; **63**: 606–11.

121. Edwards, C. K., Zhou, T., Zhang, J., Baker, T. J., De, M., Long, R. E. *et al.* Inhibition of superantigen-induced proinflammatory cytokine production and inflammatory arthritis in MRL-lpr/lpr mice by a transcriptional inhibitor of TNF-alpha. *J Immunol* 1996; **157**: 1758–72.

122. Hopkins, P. A., Fraser, J. D., Pridmore, A. C., Russell, H. H., Read, R. C., and Sriskandan, S. Superantigen recognition by HLA class II on monocytes up-regulates toll-like receptor 4 and enhances proinflammatory responses to endotoxin. *Blood* 2005; **105**: 3655–62.

123. Chatterjee, D. and Khoo, K. H. Mycobacterial lipoarabinomannan: an extraordinary lipoheteroglycan with profound physiological effects. *Glycobiology* 1998; **8**: 113–20.

124. Dao, D. N., Kremer, L., Guerardel, Y., Molano, A., Jacobs, W. R., Jr., Porcelli, S. A., and Briken, V. Mycobacterium tuberculosis lipomannan induces apoptosis and interleukin-12 production in macrophages. *Infect Immun* 2004; **72**: 2067–74.

125. Briken, V., Porcelli, S. A., Besra, G. S., and Kremer, L. Mycobacterial lipoarabinomannan and related lipoglycans: from biogenesis to modulation of the immune response. *Mol Microbiol* 2004; **53**: 391–403.

126. Seibl, R., Kyburz, D., Lauener, R. P., and Gay, S. Pattern recognition receptors and their involvement in the pathogenesis of arthritis. *Curr Opin Rheumatol* 2004; **16**: 411–18.

127. Mogensen, T. H. and Paludan, S. R. Reading the viral signature by Toll-like receptors and other pattern recognition receptors. *J Mol Med* 2005; **83**: 180–92.

128. Iwahashi, M., Yamamura, M., Aita, T., Okamoto, A., Ueno, A., Ogawa, N. *et al.* Expression of Toll-like receptor 2 on CD16+ blood monocytes and synovial tissue macrophages in rheumatoid arthritis. *Arthritis Rheum* 2004; **50**: 1457–67.

129. Frasnelli, M. E., Tarussio, D., Chobaz-Peclat, V., Busso, N., and So, A. TLR2 modulates inflammation in zymosan-induced arthritis in mice. *Arthritis Res Ther* 2005; **7**: R370–R379.

130. Suhrbier, A. and La Linn, M. Clinical and pathologic aspects of arthritis due to Ross River virus and other alphaviruses. *Curr Opin Rheumatol* 2004; **16**: 374–9.

131. Cheevers, W. P., Snekvik, K. R., Trujillo, J. D., Kumpula-McWhirter, N. M., Pretty On Top KJ, and Knowles, D. P. Prime-boost vaccination with plasmid DNA encoding caprine-arthritis encephalitis lentivirus env and viral SU suppresses challenge virus and development of arthritis. *Virology* 2003; **306**: 116–25.

132. Itescu, S. Rheumatic aspects of acquired immunodeficiency syndrome. *Curr Opin Rheumatol* 1996; **8**: 346–53.

133. Takahashi, Y., Murai, C., Shibata, S., Munakata, Y., Ishii, T., Ishii, K. *et al.* Human parvovirus B19 as a causative agent for rheumatoid arthritis. *Proc Natl Acad Sci U S A* 1998; **95**: 8227–32.

134. Caliskan, R., Masatlioglu, S., Aslan, M., Altun, S., Saribas, S., Ergin, S. *et al.* The relationship between arthritis and human parvovirus B19 infection. *Rheumatol Int* 2005; **26**: 7–11.

135. Cutolo, M. and Lahita, R. G. Estrogens and arthritis. *Rheum Dis Clin North Am* 2005; **31**: 19–27.

136. Cutolo, M., Villaggio, B., Seriolo, B., Montagna, P., Capellino, S., Straub, R. H., and Sulli, A. Synovial fluid estrogens in rheumatoid arthritis. *Autoimmun Rev* 2004; **3**: 193–8.

137. Kramer, P. R., Kramer, S. F., and Guan, G. 17 beta-estradiol regulates cytokine release through modulation of CD16 expression in monocytes and monocyte-derived macrophages. *Arthritis Rheum* 2004; **50**: 1967–75.

138. Keith, J. C., Albert, L. M., Leathurby, Y., Follettie, M., Wang, L., Borges-Marcucci, L. *et al.* The utility of pathway selective estrogen receptor ligands that inhibit nuclear factor-kB transcriptional activity in models of rheumatoid arthritis. *Arthritis Res Ther* 2005; **7**: R427–R438.

139. Wilder, R. L. and Elenkov, I. J. Hormonal regulation of tumor necrosis factor-alpha, interleukin-12 and interleukin-10 production by activated macrophages: a disease-modifying mechanism in rheumatoid arthritis and systemic lupus erythematosus? *Ann NY Acad Sci* 1999; **876**: 14–31.

140. Miossec, P., Naviliat, M., Dupuy, d. A., Sany, J., and Bancherau, J. Low levels of interleukin-4 and high levels of transforming growth factor beta in rheumatoid synovitis. *Arthritis Rheum* 1990; **33**: 1180–7.

141. Isomaki, P., Luukkainen, R., Saario, R., Toivanen, P., and Punnonen, J. Interleukin-10 functions as an antiinflammatory cytokine in rheumatoid synovium. *Arthritis Rheum* 1996; **39**: 386–95.

142. Allen, J. B., Wong, H. L., Costa, G. L., Bienkowski, M. J., and Wahl, S. M. Suppression of monocyte function and differential regulation of IL-1 and IL-1ra by IL-4 contribute to resolution of experimental arthritis. *J Immunol* 1993; **151**: 4344–51.

143. Sugiyama, E., Taki, H., Kuroda, A., Mino, T., Yamashita, N., and Kobayashi, M. Interleukin-4 inhibits prostaglandin E2 production by freshly prepared adherent rheumatoid synovial cells via inhibition of biosynthesis and gene expression of cyclo-oxygenase II but not of cyclo-oxygenase I. *Ann Rheum Dis* 1996; **55**: 375–82.

144. Kuroda, A., Sugiyama, E., Taki, H., Mino, T., and Kobayashi, M. Interleukin-4 inhibits the gene expression and biosynthesis of cytosolic phospholipase A2 in lipopolysaccharide stimulated U937 macrophage cell line and freshly prepared adherent rheumatoid synovial cells. *Biochem Biophys Res Commun* 1997; **230**: 40–3.

145. Miossec, P. and van den Berg, W. Th1/Th2 cytokine balance in arthritis. *Arthritis Rheum* 1997; **40**: 2105–15.

146. Van Roon, J. A., Lafeber, F. P., and Bijlsma, J. W. Synergistic activity of interleukin-4 and interleukin-10 in suppression of inflammation and joint destruction in rheumatoid arthritis. *Arthritis Rheum* 2001; **44**: 3–12.

147. Kasama, T., Strieter, R. M., Lukacs, N. W., Lincoln, P. M., Burdick, M. D., and Kunkel, S. L. Interleukin-10 expression and chemokine regulation during the evolution of murine type II collagen-induced arthritis. *J Clin Invest* 1995; **95**: 2868–76.

148. Katsikis, P. D., Chu, C. Q., Brennan, F. M., Maini, R. N., and Feldmann, M. Immunoregulatory role of interleukin 10 in rheumatoid arthritis. *J Exp Med* 1994; **179**: 1517–27.

149. Verhoef, C. M., Van Roon, J. A., Vianen, M. E., Bijlsma, J. W., and Lafeber, F. P. Interleukin 10 (IL-10), not IL-4 or interferon-gamma production, correlates with progression of joint destruction in rheumatoid arthritis. *J Rheumatol* 2001; **28**: 1960–6.

150. van Roon, J., Wijngaarden, S., Lafeber, F. P., Damen, C., van de Winkel, W. J., and Bijlsma, J. W. Interleukin 10 treatment of patients with rheumatoid arthritis enhances Fc gamma receptor expression on monocytes and responsiveness to immune complex stimulation. *J Rheumatol* 2003; **30**: 648–51.

151. Hermann, J. A., Hall, M. A., Maini, R. N., Feldmann, M., and Brennan, F. M. Important immunoregulatory role of interleukin-11 in the inflammatory process in rheumatoid arthritis. *Arthritis Rheum* 1998; **41**: 1388–97.

152. Trepicchio, W. L. and Dorner, A. J. Interleukin-11: a gp130 cytokine. *Ann NY Acad Sci* 1998; **856**: 12–21.

153. Mino, T., Sugiyama, E., Taki, H., Kuroda, A., Yamashita, N., Maruyama, M., and Kobayashi, M. Interleukin-1alpha and tumor necrosis factor alpha synergistically stimulate prostaglandin E2-dependent production of interleukin-11 in rheumatoid synovial fibroblasts. *Arthritis Rheum* 1998; **41**: 2004–13.

154. Walmsley, M., Butler, D. M., Marinova-Mutafchieva, L., and Feldmann, M. An anti-inflammatory role for interleukin-11 in established murine collagen-induced arthritis. *Immunology* 1998; **95**: 31–7.

155. Wong, P. K., Campbell, I. K., Robb, L., and Wicks, I. P. Endogenous IL-11 is pro-inflammatory in acute methylated bovine serum albumin/interleukin-1-induced (mBSA/IL-1)arthritis. *Cytokine* 2005; **29**: 72–6.

156. Moreland, L., Gugliotti, R., King, K., Chase, W., Weisman, M., Greco, T. *et al.* Results of a phase-I/II randomized, masked, placebo-controlled trial of recombinant human interleukin-11 (rhIL-11) in the treatment of subjects with active rheumatoid arthritis. *Arthritis Res* 2001; **3**: 247–52.

157. Woods, J. M., Amin, M. A., Katschke, K. J., Jr., Volin, M. V., Ruth, J. H., Connors, M. A. *et al.* Interleukin-13 gene therapy reduces inflammation, vascularization, and bony destruction in rat adjuvant-induced arthritis. *Hum Gene Ther* 2002; **13**: 381–93.

158. Boissier, M. C. and Bessis, N. Therapeutic gene transfer for rheumatoid arthritis. *Reumatismo* 2004; **56**: 51–61.

159. Nabbe, K. C. A. M., van Lent, P. L. E. M., Holthuysen, A. E. M., Sloetjes, A. W., Koch, A. E., Radstake, T. R. D. J., and van den Berg, W. B. Local IL-13 gene transfer prior to immune-complex arthritis inhibits chondrocyte death and matrix-metalloproteinase-mediated cartilage matrix degradation despite enhanced joint inflammation. *Arthritis Res Ther* 2005; **7**: R392–R401.

160. Firestein, G. S., Alvaro-Gracia, J. M., and Maki, R. Quantitative analysis of cytokine gene expression in rheumatoid arthritis. *J Immunol* 1990; **144**: 3347–53.

161. Klimiuk, P. A., Sierakowski, S., Latosiewicz, R., Cylwik, B., Skowronski, J., and Chwiecko, J. Serum cytokines in different histological variants of rheumatoid arthritis. *J Rheumatol* 2001; **28**: 1211–17.

162. van den Berg, W. B., Joosten, L. A., Kollias, G., and Van De Loo, F. A. Role of tumour necrosis factor alpha in experimental arthritis: separate activity of interleukin 1beta in chronicity and cartilage destruction. *Ann Rheum Dis* 1999; **58**: I40–I44.

163. Kollias, G. Modeling the function of tumor necrosis factor in immune pathophysiology. *Autoimmun Rev* 2004; **3**: S24–S25.

164. Schadlich, H., Ermann, J., Biskop, M., Falk, W., Sperling, F., Jungel, A. *et al.* Anti-inflammatory effects of systemic anti-tumour necrosis factor alpha treatment in human/murine SCID arthritis. *Ann Rheum Dis* 1999; **58**: 428–34.

165. Mussener, A., Klareskog, L., Lorentzen, J. C., and Kleinau, S. TNF-alpha dominates cytokine mRNA expression in lymphoid tissues of rats developing collagen- and oil-induced arthritis. *Scand J Immunol* 1995; **42**: 128–34.

166. Schmidt-Weber, C. B., Pohlers, D., Siegling, A., Schadlich, H., Buchner, E., Volk, H. D. *et al.* Cytokine gene activation in synovial membrane, regional lymph nodes, and spleen during the course of rat adjuvant arthritis. *Cell Immunol* 1999; **195**: 53–65.

167. Simon, J., Surber, R., Kleinstauber, G., Petrow, P. K., Henzgen, S., Kinne, R. W., and Brauer, R. Systemic macrophage activation in locally-induced experimental arthritis. *J Autoimmun* 2001; **17**: 127–36.

168. Nissler, K., Pohlers, D., Huckel, M., Simon, J., Brauer, R., and Kinne, R. W. Anti-CD4 monoclonal antibody treatment in acute and early chronic antigen induced arthritis: influence on macrophage activation. *Ann Rheum Dis* 2004; **63**: 1470–7.

169. Grell, M., Douni, E., Wajant, H., Lohden, M., Clauss, M., Maxeiner, B. *et al.* The transmembrane form of tumor necrosis factor is the prime activating ligand of the 80 kDa tumor necrosis factor receptor. *Cell* 1995; **83**: 793–802.

170. Georgopoulos, S., Plows, D., and Kollias, G. Transmembrane TNF is sufficient to induce localized tissue toxicity and chronic inflammatory arthritis in transgenic mice. *J Inflamm* 1996; **46**: 86–97.

171. Alexopoulou, L., Pasparakis, M., and Kollias, G. A murine transmembrane tumor necrosis factor (TNF) transgene induces arthritis by cooperative p55/p75 TNF receptor signaling. *Eur J Immunol* 1997; **27**: 2588–92.

172. Grell, M., Wajant, H., Zimmermann, G., and Scheurich, P. The type 1 receptor (CD120a) is the high-affinity receptor for soluble tumor necrosis factor. *Proc Natl Acad Sci U S A* 1998; **95**: 570–5.

173. Alsalameh, S., Amin, R. J., Kunisch, E., Jasin, H. E., and Kinne, R. W. Preferential induction of prodestructive matrix metalloproteinase-1 and proinflammatory interleukin 6 and prostaglandin E2 in rheumatoid arthritis synovial fibroblasts via tumor necrosis factor receptor-55. *J Rheumatol* 2003; **30**: 1680–90.

173a. Deng, G. M., Zheng, L., Ka-Ming, C. F., and Lenardo M. Amelioration of inflammatory arthritis by targeting the pre-ligand assembly domain of tumor necrosis factor receptors. *Nat Med* 2005; **11**: 1066–72.

173b. Murali, R., Cheng, X., Berezov, A., Du, X., Schon, A., Freire, E. *et al.* Disabling TNF receptor signaling by induced conformational perturbation of tryptophan-107. *PNAS* 2005; **102**: 10970–5.

174. Wood, N. C., Dickens, E., Symons, J. A., and Duff, G. W. In situ hybridization of interleukin-1 in CD14-positive cells in rheumatoid arthritis. *Clin Immunol Immunopathol* 1992; **62**: 295–300.

175. Dinarello, C. A. The IL-1 family and inflammatory diseases. *Clin Exp Rheumatol* 2002; **20**: S1–S13.

176. Haringman, J. J., Kraan, M. C., Smeets, T. J., Zwinderman, K. H., and Tak, P. P. Chemokine blockade and chronic inflammatory disease: proof of concept in patients with rheumatoid arthritis. *Ann Rheum Dis* 2003; **62**: 715–21.

177. Bedard, P. A. and Golds, E. E. Cytokine-induced expression of mRNAs for chemotactic factors in human synovial cells and fibroblasts. *J Cell Physiol* 1993; **154**: 433–41.

178. Pertynska-Marczewska, M., Kiriakidis, S., Wait, R., Beech, J., Feldmann, M., and Paleolog, E. M. Advanced glycation end products upregulate angiogenic and pro-inflammatory cytokine production in human monocyte/macrophages. *Cytokine* 2004; **28**: 35–47.

179. Dinarello, C. A. Therapeutic strategies to reduce IL-1 activity in treating local and systemic inflammation. *Curr Opin Pharmacol* 2004; **4**: 378–85.

180. Houssiau, F. A., Devogelaer, J. P., Van Damme, J., de Deuxchaisnes, C. N., and Van Snick, J. Interleukin-6 in synovial fluid and serum of patients with rheumatoid arthritis and other inflammatory arthritides. *Arthritis Rheum* 1988; **31**: 784–8.

181. Kotake, S., Sato, K., Kim, K. J., Takahashi, N., Udagawa, N., Nakamura, I. *et al.* Interleukin-6 and soluble interleukin-6 receptors in the synovial fluids from rheumatoid arthritis patients are responsible for osteoclast-like cell formation. *J Bone Miner Res* 1996; **11**: 88–95.

182. Van De Loo, F. A., Kuiper, S., van Enckevort, F. H., Arntz, O. J., and van den Berg, W. B. Interleukin-6 reduces cartilage destruction during experimental arthritis: a study in interleukin-6-deficient mice. *Am J Pathol* 1997; **151**: 177–91.

183. Naka, T., Nishimoto, N., and Kishimoto, T. The paradigm of IL-6: from basic science to medicine. *Arthritis Res* 2002; **4**: S233–S242.

184. Wong, P. K., Campbell, I. K., Egan, P. J., Ernst, M., and Wicks, I. P. The role of the interleukin-6 family of cytokines in inflammatory arthritis and bone turnover. *Arthritis Rheum* 2003; **48**: 1177–89.

185. Stuhlmeier, K. M. and Pollaschek, C. Differential effect of transforming growth factor beta (TGF-beta) on the genes encoding hyaluronan synthases and utilization of the p38 MAPK pathway in TGF-beta-induced hyaluronan synthase 1 activation. *J Biol Chem* 2004; **279**: 8753–60.

186. Chen, W. and Wahl, S. M. TGF-beta: receptors, signaling pathways and autoimmunity. *Curr Dir Autoimmun* 2002; **5**: 62–91.

187. Mi, Z., Ghivizzani, S. C., Lechman, E., Glorioso, J. C., Evans, C. H., and Robbins, P. D. Adverse effects of adenovirus-mediated gene transfer of human transforming growth factor beta 1 into rabbit knees. *Arthritis Res Ther* 2003; **5**: R132–R139.

188. Suto, T. S., Fine, L. G., Shimizu, F., and Kitamura, M. In vivo transfer of engineered macrophages into the glomerulus: endogenous TGF-beta-mediated defense against macrophage-induced glomerular cell activation. *J Immunol* 1997; **159**: 2476–83.

189. Moldovan, F., Pelletier, J. P., Hambor, J., Cloutier, J. M., and Martel-Pelletier, J. Collagenase-3 (matrix metalloprotease 13) is preferentially localized in the deep layer of human arthritic cartilage in situ: in vitro mimicking effect by transforming growth factor beta. *Arthritis Rheum* 1997; **40**: 1653–61.

190. Imai, K., Hiramatsu, A., Fukushima, D., Pierschbacher, M. D., and Okada, Y. Degradation of decorin by matrix metalloproteinases: identification of the cleavage sites, kinetic analyses and transforming growth factor-beta1 release. *Biochem J* 1997; **322**: 809–14.

191. Chu, C. Q., Field, M., Abney, E., Zheng, R. Q., Allard, S., Feldmann, M., and Maini, R. N. Transforming growth factor-beta 1 in rheumatoid synovial membrane and cartilage/pannus junction. *Clin Exp Immunol* 1991; **86**: 380–6.

192. Szekanecz, Z., Haines, G. K., Harlow, L. A., Shah, M. R., Fong, T. W., Fu, R. *et al.* Increased synovial expression of transforming growth factor (TGF)-beta receptor endoglin and TGF-beta 1 in rheumatoid arthritis: possible interactions in the pathogenesis of the disease. *Clin Immunol Immunopathol* 1995; **76**: 187–94.

193. Mattey, D. L., Kerr, J. R., Nixon, N. B., and Dawes, P. T. Association of polymorphism in the transforming growth factor {beta}1 gene with disease outcome and mortality in rheumatoid arthritis. *Ann Rheum Dis* 2005; **64**: 1190–4.

194. Jou, I. M., Shiau, A. L., Chen, S. Y., Wang, C. R., Shieh, D. B., Tsai, C. S., and Wu, C. L. Thrombospondin 1 as an effective gene therapeutic strategy in collagen-induced arthritis. *Arthritis Rheum* 2005; **52**: 339–44.

195. McInnes, I. B., Leung, B. P., Field, M., Wei, X. Q., Huang, F. P., Sturrock, R. D. *et al.* Production of nitric oxide in the synovial membrane of rheumatoid and osteoarthritis patients. *J Exp Med* 1996; **184**: 1519–24.

196. Pham, T. N., Rahman, P., Tobin, Y. M., Khraishi, M. M., Hamilton, S. F., Alderdice, C., and Richardson, V. J. Elevated serum nitric oxide levels in patients with inflammatory arthritis associated with co-expression of inducible nitric oxide synthase and protein kinase C-eta in peripheral blood monocyte-derived macrophages. *J Rheumatol* 2003; **30**: 2529–34.

197. Chae, H. J., Park, R. K., Chung, H. T., Kang, J. S., Kim, M. S., Choi, D. Y., Bang, B. G., and Kim, H. R. Nitric oxide is a regulator of bone remodelling. *J Pharm Pharmacol* 1997; **49**: 897–902.

198. Bogdan, C. The multiplex function of nitric oxide in (auto)immunity. *J Exp Med* 1998; **187**: 1361–5.

199. Wahl, S. M., McCartney-Francis, N., Chan, J., Dionne, R., Ta, L., and Orenstein, J. M. Nitric oxide in experimental joint inflammation: benefit or detriment? *Cells Tissues Organs* 2003; **174**: 26–33.

200. Miesel, R., Murphy, M. P., and Kroger, H. Enhanced mitochondrial radical production in patients which rheumatoid arthritis correlates with elevated levels of tumor necrosis factor alpha in plasma. *Free Radic Res* 1996; **25**: 161–9.

201. Nelson, K. K. and Melendez, J. A. Mitochondrial redox control of matrix metalloproteinases. *Free Radic Biol Med* 2004; **37**: 768–84.

202. Henrotin, Y. E., Bruckner, P., and Pujol, J. P. The role of reactive oxygen species in homeostasis and degradation of cartilage. *Osteoarthritis Cartilage* 2003; **11**: 747–55.

203. Chernajovsky, Y., Winyard, P. G., and Kabouridis, P. S. Advances in understanding the genetic basis of rheumatoid arthritis and osteoarthritis: implications for therapy. *Am J Pharmacogenomics* 2002; **2**: 223–34.

204. Cronstein, B. N. Therapeutic cocktails for rheumatoid arthritis: the mixmaster's guide. *Arthritis Rheum* 2004; **50**: 2041–3.

205. Bondeson, J. The mechanisms of action of disease-modifying antirheumatic drugs: a review with emphasis on macrophage signal transduction and the induction of proinflammatory cytokines. *Gen Pharmacol* 1997; **29**: 127–50.

206. Seitz, M., Loetscher, P., Dewald, B., Towbin, H., Rordorf, C., Gallati, H. *et al.* Methotrexate action in rheumatoid arthritis: stimulation of cytokine inhibitor and inhibition of chemokine production by peripheral blood mononuclear cells. *Br J Rheumatol* 1995; **34**: 602–9.

207. Ravelli, A., Caria, M. C., Buratti, S., Malattia, C., Temporini, F., and Martini, A. Methotrexate as a possible trigger of macrophage activation syndrome in systemic juvenile idiopathic arthritis. *J Rheumatol* 2001; **28**: 865–7.

208. Cutolo, M., Sulli, A., Ghiorzo, P., Pizzorni, C., Craviotto, C., and Villaggio, B. Anti-inflammatory effects of leflunomide on cultured synovial macrophages from patients with rheumatoid arthritis. *Ann Rheum Dis* 2003; **62**: 297–302.

209. Kobayashi, Y., Ueyama, S., Arai, Y., Yoshida, Y., Kaneda, T., Sato, T. *et al.* The active metabolite of leflunomide, A771726, inhibits both the generation and the bone-resorbing activity of osteoclasts by acting directly on cells of the osteoclast lineage. *J Bone Miner Metab* 2004; **22**: 318–28.

210. Urushibara, M., Takayanagi, H., Koga, T., Kim, S., Isobe, M., Morishita, Y. *et al.* The antirheumatic drug leflunomide inhibits osteoclastogenesis by interfering with receptor activator of NF-kappa B ligand-stimulated induction of nuclear factor of activated T cells c1. *Arthritis Rheum* 2004; **50**: 794–804.

211. Hansen, K. E., Cush, J., Singhal, A., Cooley, D. A., Cohen, S., Patel, S. R. *et al.* The safety and efficacy of leflunomide in combination with infliximab in rheumatoid arthritis. *Arthritis Rheum* 2004; **51**: 228–32.

212. Kremer, J., Genovese, M., Cannon, G. W., Caldwell, J., Cush, J., Furst, D. E. *et al.* Combination leflunomide and methotrexate (MTX) therapy for patients with active rheumatoid arthritis failing MTX monotherapy: open-label extension of a randomized, double-blind, placebo controlled trial. *J Rheumatol* 2004; **31**: 1521–31.

213. Verhoef, C. M., Van Roon, J. A., Vianen, M. E., Lafeber, F. P., and Bijlsma, J. W. The immune suppressive effect of dexamethasone in rheumatoid arthritis is accompanied by upregulation of interleukin 10 and by differential changes in interferon gamma and interleukin 4 production. *Ann Rheum Dis* 1999; **58**: 49–54.

214. Seitz, M., Loetscher, P., Dewald, B., Towbin, H., and Baggiolini, M. In vitro modulation of cytokine, cytokine inhibitor, and prostaglandin E release from blood mononuclear cells and synovial fibroblasts by antirheumatic drugs. *J Rheumatol* 1997; **24**: 1471–6.

215. Crofford, L. J., Lipsky, P. E., Brooks, P., Abrahamson, S. B., Simon, L. S., and van de Putte, L. B. A. Current comment: basic biology and clinical application of specific cyclooxygenase-2 inhibitors. *Arthritis Rheum* 2000; **43**: 4–13.

216. Clark, D. W., Layton, D., and Shakir, S. A. Do some inhibitors of COX-2 increase the risk of thromboembolic events? Linking pharmacology with pharmacoepidemiology. *Drug Saf* 2004; **27**: 427–56.

217. Zacharowski, P., Breese, E., Wood, E., Del Soldato, P., Warner, T., and Mitchell, J. NSAIDs increase GM-CSF release by human synoviocytes: comparison with nitric oxide-donating derivatives. *Eur J Pharmacol* 2005; **508**: 7–13.

218. Saniabadi, A. R., Hanai, H., Takeuchi, K., Umemura, K., Nakashima, M., Adachi, T. *et al.* Adacolumn, an adsorptive carrier based granulocyte and monocyte apheresis device for the treatment of inflammatory and refractory diseases associated with leukocytes. *Ther Apher Dial* 2003; **7**: 48–59.

219. Schmidt-Weber, C. B., Rittig, M., Buchner, E., Hauser, I., Schmidt, I., Palombo-Kinne, E. *et al.* Apoptotic cell death in activated monocytes following incorporation of clodronate-liposomes. *J Leukoc Biol* 1996; **60**: 230–44.

220. Kinne, R. W., Schmidt-Weber, C. B., Hoppe, R., Buchner, E., Palombo-Kinne, E., Nurnberg, E., and Emmrich, F. Long-term amelioration of rat adjuvant arthritis following systemic elimination of macrophages by clodronate-containing liposomes. *Arthritis Rheum* 1995; **38**: 1777–90.

221. Oelzner, P., Brauer, R., Henzgen, S., Thoss, K., Wünsche, B., Hersmann, G. *et al.* Periarticular bone alterations in chronic antigen-induced arthritis: free and liposome-encapsulated clodronate prevent loss of bone mass in the secondary spongiosa. *Clin Immunol Immunopathol* 1999; **90**: 79–88.

222. Barrera, P., Blom, A., van Lent, P. L., van Bloois, L., Beijnen, J. H., van Rooijen, N. *et al.* Synovial macrophage depletion with clodronate-containing liposomes in rheumatoid arthritis. *Arthritis Rheum* 2000; **43**: 1951–9.

223. Metselaar, J. M., van den Berg, W. B., Holthuysen, A. E., Wauben, M. H., Storm, G., and van Lent, P. L. Liposomal targeting of glucocorticoids to synovial lining cells strongly increases therapeutic benefit in collagen type II arthritis. *Ann Rheum Dis* 2004; **63**: 348–53.

224. Evans, C. H., Ghivizzani, S. C., and Lechman, E. R. Lessons learned from gene transfer approaches. *Arthritis Res* 1999; **1**: 21–4.

225. Handel, M. L. and Girgis, L. Transcription factors. *Best Pract Res Clin Rheumatol* 2001; **15**: 657–75.

226. Firestein, G. S. NF-kappaB: Holy Grail for rheumatoid arthritis? *Arthritis Rheum* 2004; **50**: 2381–6.

227. Huber, L. C., Pap, T., Muller-Ladner, U., Gay, R. E., and Gay, S. Gene targeting: roadmap to future therapies. *Curr Rheumatol Rep* 2004; **6**: 323–5.

228. Panayi, G. S. B cell-directed therapy in rheumatoid arthritis: clinical experience. *J Rheumatol Suppl* 2005; **73**: 19–24.

6 | *The role of T lymphocytes in rheumatoid arthritis*

David A. Fox

Introduction

The concept that T cells might be important to the pathogenesis of rheumatoid arthritis (RA) is relatively recent. It was little more than 25 years ago that initial evidence was provided that the preponderance of lymphocytes in synovial tissue were in fact T cells, and not antibody-producing cells. A detailed understanding of T cell biology began take shape in the 1980s, in large part due to the development of monoclonal antibodies against a variety of lymphocyte surface structures. In parallel with these advances in basic immunology, the hypothesis for a central role of T lymphocytes in a variety of immune-mediated diseases, such as rheumatoid arthritis, begin to take shape[1]. Data from animal models and from genetic studies were also important factors in the development of a 'T cell hypothesis' for the pathogenesis of RA.

It was not long, however, before elements of this T cell hypothesis came under skeptical scrutiny. At the same time, the importance of other cell types and their secreted products, such as cytokines, became better understood and certain cytokines made primarily by non-T cells proved to be excellent targets for biologic therapeutics. In this context a central role for T cells in RA seemed less well accepted than previously, and strong arguments were made to view RA as either T cell independent[2] or T cell dependent[3].

This chapter will begin with a review of some basic rules that help define our current understanding of T cell development and T cell function. Evidence both for and against the central role of T cells in RA will be presented. Specific aspects of immune mechanisms that are related to the function of T cells in RA will be emphasized, including the role of major histocompatability complex (MHC) determinants, evidence for T cell oligoclonality in RA, the nature of antigen-driven T cell responses in RA, activation pathways for T lymphocytes relevant to joint inflammation, aspects of cytokine biology that control T cell behaviour in RA, and cell—cell interactions involving T lymphocytes in the joint.

In considering the role of T lymphocytes in RA, it is appropriate to bear in mind that definitions of autoimmunity and autoimmune disease are in flux, and that there is no universally agreed, comprehensive model of autoimmunity. Whether or not one regards rheumatoid arthritis as an 'autoimmune disease', with a potential key role for T cells, depends in part on one's definition of autoimmunity. If such a definition requires that a disease be driven by defined lymphocyte responses to a specific autoantigen, the notion that RA is an autoimmune disease remains an unproven hypothesis. If a less narrow definition, such as dysfunction of immune responses resulting in organ-specific tissue damage, were acceptable, one might be able to designate RA as an autoimmune disease. This analysis must occur in the setting of the most updated understanding of the immune system, including the recently developed concepts of innate and adaptive components of the immune response.

Overview of T cell biology

T cell development, activation, and function have become some of the most intensively studied processes in mammalian biology, and space permits only a brief summary of a few key points.

- T lymphocyte development occurs primarily in the thymus, following migration of precursor cells to that organ from the bone marrow. Thymic development is accompanied by (in part mediated through) the sequential appearance and disappearance of critical functional cell membrane glycoproteins, which define stages of thymic selection.
- The T cell receptor (TCR) for antigen is expressed during this developmental process in the thymus, in association with a glycoprotein complex termed CD3, and with a variety of signal transduction molecules.
- Most mature lymphocytes (more than 95% of circulating T cells) express the $\alpha\beta$ TCR, while the remainder express the $\gamma\delta$ TCR.
- The α and γ genes are composed of V, J, and C segments while the β and δ chains are composed of V, D, J, and C segments.
- TCR diversity is achieved by several mechanisms which include: combinatorial rearrangement of germ line gene segments, addition and deletion of nucleotides at junctions of these segments, and variable pairing of α and β chains.
- Most T cells express only one TCR but rare T cells with two distinct TCRs can be found.
- The majority of T cells that develop in the thymus are subject to negative selection and do not form part of the mature T cell repertoire (this is likely to be very important in limiting autoreactivity of the immune system).
- Positive and negative selection both occur in the thymus and are regulated by antigen-presenting MHC molecules expressed in that organ, and by the affinity and abundance of antigens presented to developing T cells by those MHC molecules.
- Unlike B lymphocytes, T lymphocytes do not recognize free antigen, but instead respond to antigenic material displayed by specialized antigen-presenting cells.

- Most T cells recognize processed antigens presented in the peptide binding cleft of MHC molecules; in general CD4[+] T cells recognize antigen on class II MHC due to co-receptor function of CD4 for class II molecules, and CD8[+] T cells recognize antigen on class I MHC due to CD8 co-receptor function for class I molecules.
- Some T cells recognize non-peptide antigens, including lipid- and carbohydrate-containing molecules, which are presented by non-MHC structures such as CD1.
- Superantigens are larger than conventional peptide antigens and do not require the same degree of antigen processing. Superantigens are also presented to the TCR by MHC structures, but through binding sites distinct from the peptide-binding MHC cleft.
- Although a variety of cells can stimulate T cell responses to antigens, the most potent and prototypic initiator of such responses is the dendritic cell. Dendritic cells are phenotypically and functionally heterogeneous, and can inhibit as well as stimulate antigen-specific T cells.
- Activation of T cells requires one or more costimulatory signals in addition to ligation of the TCR; CD28 is the best studied example of a molecule that can deliver such a second signal, but a variety of cell surface glycoproteins may be able to serve a similar function, including cytokine receptors and receptors that recognize cell membrane determinants on antigen-presenting cells.
- T cell activation is accompanied by a complex and rapid sequence of signal transduction events, which leads to changes in gene expression and ultimately proliferation and effector function; a key series of steps involve expression of interleukin 2 (IL-2), the high affinity IL-2 receptor, and delivery of a mitogenic signal by IL-2 binding to the IL-2 receptor. Other cytokines, such as IL-15, can also drive T cell proliferation. At a later stage of T cell activation/differentiation IL-2 mediates activation-induced cell death, and thus IL-2 deficiency can lead to inappropriate T cell survival.
- T lymphocyte trafficking to and from specialized lymphoid organs and inflamed tissues is a regulated process, depending in part on expression of specific adhesion receptors on the T cell surface.
- T cells carry out effector functions through a variety of mechanisms, including direct interactions with other cells (such as lysis of virally infected target cells by cytotoxic T lymphocytes), as well as by secretion of a range of cytokines that regulate the function of other components of the immune response.

- Profiles of cytokine secretion and surface receptor expression have been useful in defining functional subsets of T lymphocytes; Th1 cells have a functional program that includes production of IFNγ while Th2 cells produce IL4 and other cytokines.
- The secretion of IL-12, IL-23, and IL-27 by antigen-presenting cells favors the development of Th1 responses.
- Regulation of mature T cell responses is achieved by a variety of mechanisms. These include production of immunoregulatory cytokines, such as IL-10 and TGFβ, by both regulatory T cell subsets and non-T cells. T cells that are CD4+CD25+ include an important regulatory cell population.
- In parallel with adaptive immune responses, innate immunity is important in host defense, and likely also in immune-mediated diseases. Innate immune responses can occur by activation of certain receptors that typically have less restricted specificity than antibodies or T cell antigen receptors. One example is the family of Toll-like receptors, which recognize molecular patterns of microbial structures. These receptors are expressed by antigen-presenting cells, various tissue cells, and, in some cases, subsets of lymphocytes.
- Innate immune mechanisms are important in initiating and regulating adaptive immune responses.

T cell hypothesis for RA

The foundation for the view that T cells are central to the pathogenesis of RA was first laid in the 1970s, when it was demonstrated that the majority of lymphocytes in the synovial compartment formed rosettes with sheep erythrocytes, at that time the best method for identifying lymphocytes as T cells[4,5] In the early 1980s the hypothesis of RA as a T cell-driven disease was formally articulated[1]. Several impressive lines of evidence support this view of RA (Table 6.1). Use of monoclonal antibodies that identify T lymphocyte-specific lineage differentiation markers has confirmed that the great majority of lymphocytes in RA synovial tissue and synovial fluid are T cells[6–9]. Far smaller numbers of B lymphocytes, plasma cells, and natural killer cells are present. The preponderance of T cells is not unique to RA, but instead is also typical for synovial lesions in other forms of inflammatory arthritis. T cells in synovial tissue form clusters around vascular structures and are most densely distributed in

Table 6.1 Evidence for a central role for T cells in RA

Large numbers of T cells and antigen-presenting cells are present in synovial tissue and fluid
Synovial T cells express activation and memory markers
T cell subsets, and possibly clonal T cell populations, accumulate in RA joints in a non-random manner
RA is associated with specific MHC class II alleles (DR and/or DQ)
T cells and specific clonal T cell populations are central to the induction and regulation of several animal models of RA
T cell-directed therapeutic interventions may be effective in RA, and are clearly effective in animal models
T cell cytokines, such as IFNγ and IL-17, that are present in RA joints, can mediate biological effects highly relevant to the pathogenesis of joint inflammation and damage
Cytokines that favor T cell activation and Th1 differentiation, such as IL-15 and IL-12, are present in RA synovium at functionally relevant concentrations

these regions (Fig. 6.1)[9]. However, T cells are also scattered widely throughout the entire RA synovium, ranging from the sublining layers to the deeper, less cellular regions of RA pannus. Typically, the majority of cells are CD4[+], but the number of CD8[+] cells is more nearly equal to the number of CD4[+] cells than is the case in RA peripheral blood[9,10]. Synovial tissue also contains large numbers of antigen-presenting cells that are required for T cell activation. (Fig. 6.2).

One of the most powerful bodies of evidence for the central role of T cells in RA draws from the extensive investigation of animal models of RA. In many of these models, T cell responses are central to the initiation and maintenance of disease (see

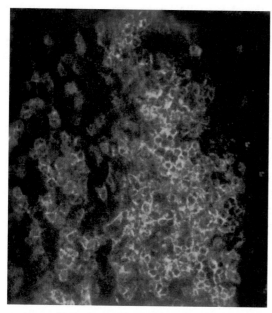

Fig. 6.1 Immunoflourescent micrograph of a frozen section of RA synovial tissue showing a perivascular cluster of T lymphocytes (green fluorescence). The section has been stained with antibody to the CD3 complex, which is associated with the T cell antigen receptor. (Reprinted with permission from Ref. 9). See also Plate 4.

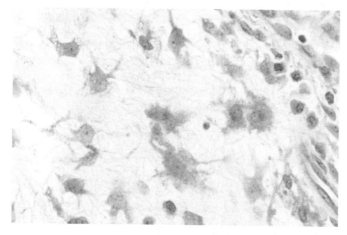

Fig. 6.2 High-power view of a section of fixed, parrafin-embedded synovial tissue, showing T lymphocytes (smaller, rounded cells), in proximity to, and interacting with various antigen-presenting cells, including dendritic cells, macrophages, and fibroblasts. (Reprinted with permission from *Laboratory Investigation* 1995; **73**: 334). See also Plate 5.

Chapter 4). Particularly impressive are studies from the adjuvant arthritis model, in which T cell clones of appropriate specificity can transfer disease to naïve recipients[11]. Moreover, attenuated, arthritogenic T cell clones can be used as vaccines that protect naïve animals. Although the data are quite convincing concerning specific animal models, a major limitation is that no animal model appears to be a perfect replica of human RA. Nonetheless, these models point out the great potential of T cells to initiate immune-mediated mechanisms that lead to joint destruction.

Sakaguchi *et al.* have recently isolated a strain of mice that spontaneously develops an illness similar to RA[12]. Autoimmunity and arthritis in this mouse are due to a subtle mutation in ZAP-70 (zeta chain-associated protein of 70 kilodalton molecular weight), a signaling molecule associated with the T cell antigen receptor complex. This mutation alters ZAP-70 function in a way that leads to inappropriate selection and survival of autoreactive T cells in the thymus. Although there is no evidence at this point that similar mutations are important in RA, this model is an important demonstration that a genetic alteration that has direct effects exclusively on T cell development and function can produce an RA-like disease.

Effects of various therapeutic agents on RA and on animal models also attest to the role of T cells in RA. One example is cyclosporin, which blocks T cell activation by inhibiting transcription of the IL-2 gene through mechanisms that affect activation of essential transcription factors. Other disease-modifying anti-rheumatic drugs also have been postulated to have direct or indirect effects on T cell activation. In the case of anti-malarials and gold salts this may be at the level of antigen-presenting cells. Azathioprine clearly depletes lymphocytes and affects lymphocyte function (reviewed in Ref. 13). Methotrexate has a variety of anti-inflammatory effects, and it is not yet clear that the lymphocyte is the major target for this drug. Therefore, although a variety of the conventional pharmaceutical agents used to treat RA can be shown to affect T cell function, it is not proven that successful treatment of RA requires interference with the action of T lymphocytes. Nevertheless, the recent successful use of CTLA4–Ig in RA[14], an agent that specifically interferes with T cell costimulation, shows that measures that directly impair T cell function can be effective in this disease.

Challenges to the T cell hypothesis for RA

By the mid-1980s, following the elucidation of the structure of the T cell antigen receptor, it seemed that a full understanding of the pathogenesis of RA might be close at hand. The underlying premises were:

1. RA is an autoimmune disease.

2. Autoimmunity arises from a breakdown in normal self/non-self discrimination by the immune system.

3. It would therefore (it was hoped) be possible to identify specific T cell clones targeted to self-antigen that would be principal pathogenic effectors of autoimmunity.

Such concepts derived largely from elegant studies of autoimmune models in inbred rodent strains, in which specific organ-targeted lesions could be induced by autoantigen or by foreign antigen that cross-reacted with autoantigen, in the setting of a defined, homogeneous genetic background.

Unfortunately, none of these three premises has proven to be correct in understanding human autoimmune disease. The difficulties in defining specific pathogenic, or even oligoclonally expanded, populations of lymphocytes in RA are discussed later in this chapter. The ongoing changes in our understanding of autoimmunity have been alluded to earlier. Furthermore, as noted above, it cannot be considered formally proven that RA is indeed an autoimmune disease. With all three premises in doubt, it still would be possible to support a central role for T cells in RA by successful specific targeting of T cells using therapy such as anti-T cell monoclonal antibodies. Earlier, experimental approaches such as lymphocyte depletion by thoracic duct drainage or total lymphoid radiation[15] had supported the concept that RA was a lymphocyte-dependent, and probably T lymphocyte-dependent, disease. On this basis and in light of very favorable effects of anti-T cell monoclonal antibodies in various animal models, numerous studies using cell-depleting monoclonal antibodies specific for T lymphocyte surface markers were conducted in RA patients from the late 1980s through the mid-1990s. In general, the results of such studies were disappointing[16]. Findings that emerge from this body of work that would challenge the T cell hypothesis of RA include:

1. The extent of T cell depletion in peripheral blood by anti-T cell monoclonal antibodies does not differ between 'responders' and non-responders to such treatment[17].

2. In general, controlled studies have not shown consistent benefit of anti-T cell antibody treatment of RA[16].

3. Prolonged T cell lymphopenia does not always lead to remission of RA. In addition, despite prior concepts that RA and HIV infection were absolutely incompatible, sporadic reports of coexistence of AIDS and RA have appeared.

A further challenge to the role of T cells in RA arose from analysis of the cytokine profile within the joint. In general, monocyte-derived cytokines, such as tumor necrosis factor (TNF)-α and IL-1, are very abundant and have readily discernible inflammatory and tissue destructive properties[18]. In contrast, T cell cytokines are either absent or present in low levels compared with other lesions that contain T cells, like tuberculous pleuritis or

chronic tonsillitis[19]. IFNγ can generally be demonstrated in the joint, but at very low levels, while IL-2 is inconsistently detected and IL-4 is generally absent. On the other hand IL-10, which tends to suppress Th1 responses, is abundant[20]. These findings, and others, have led to the hypothesis that RA is largely mediated by activated macrophages and synovial fibroblasts, with a restricted role for T lymphocytes at specific points in the evolution of the disease[2,21]. In contrast to disappointing findings with anti-T cell antibodies, treatment with cytokine blockade, notably neutralization of TNF-α, has been clearly successful in patients with established disease[22]. Although T cells can also make this cytokine, the primary source in RA synovium is the macrophage. The role of membrane-bound T cell cytokines such as TNF-α has been more difficult to assess, although low mRNA levels suggest a minor contribution.

The following sections will explore specific mechanisms of T cell participation in the pathogenesis of RA in order to evaluate further the evidence for and against a central role for T cells in this disease.

Genetics of RA and the role of T cells

The genetic predisposition to RA clearly involves several loci. Several of these could involve T cell function, such as the genes for T cell receptor components, IFNγ, IL-10, TNF, TNF receptors, and the chemokine receptor CCR5—but none of these loci can be considered as definitively proven to have an association with RA. Association of RA with MHC polymorphisms is, in contrast, well established, but extremely complex.

The MHC locus contains genes that encode the antigen-presenting molecules for most T cell responses. Also clustered in the same region are other genes relevant to immune and inflammatory responses, such as the genes for TNF and some complement components.

In the 1970s, Stastny first reported a linkage of RA to the HLADR4 allele[23]. RA, at least in Caucasian patients with seropositive disease, is associated with HLA-DR4 and related DR alleles, which contain a five amino acid sequence from residues 70–74 of the DR β chain termed the 'shared epitope'[24]. This sequence, consisting of amino acids QKRAA or QRRAA, is associated with both susceptibility to RA and severity of RA[25–28]. The effect of the shared epitope on disease severity is present in many, but not all, ethnic groups[29]. In Caucasian patients with RA who have detectable rheumatoid factor, as many as 60–70% of individuals

Table 6.2 Evidence against a central role for T cells in RA

RA has not been proven to be an autoimmune disease
T cell responses to specific antigens have not been shown to trigger or perpetuate RA
Demonstration of oligoclonal T cells in RA synovial tissue and fluid has been difficult, and different oligoclonal populations appear in different patients
T cell-derived cytokines are less abundant in the joint than are cytokines produced by other cell types, especially when compared to other chronic T cell-mediated diseases
Erosion of cartilage and bone does not always correlate with inflammation, and may become independent of regulation by T cells
Depletion of T cells by monoclonal antibodies may not be therapeutic in RA
Association of RA with the HLA-DR 'shared epitope' is not consistently strong in all ethnic or racial groups

carry the DR4 allele, compared to 30% of controls[23,30,31]. The existence of subtypes of HLA-DR4 confers additional complexity to this association, and it is the Dw4 and Dw14 molecules (subtypes of DR4 that are encoded by the DRB1*0401 and DRB1*0404 alleles) which are specifically associated with RA in Caucasians. In Japanese individuals with RA the specific association is with the Dw15 subtype of DR4 encoded by the DRB1*0405 allele[32]. In certain Native American populations and in Israeli Jews non-DR4 alleles (DR6 and DR1, respectively) are associated with risk for RA[33,34]. Clarification of the probable molecular basis for these different genetic associations became clear once the amino acid sequence and three-dimensional structure of MHC molecules were obtained. Each DRB1 susceptibility allele carries the sequence QKRAA or QRRAA from amino acids 69–74 of the DR β chain, while DR alleles not associated with RA have different sequences in this region. (In the amino acid single letter code Q indicates glutamine, K lysine, R arginine, and A alanine.) This stretch of amino acids is positioned along the floor of the antigen-binding groove of the DR molecule, such that it could contribute to the selection of specific peptides presented by DR molecules to CD4 T lymphocytes. While the evidence for linkage of the shared epitope sequence to RA in many populations is strong, the mechanism by which it confers risk remains unknown and several very different alternatives are possible (see below). The shared epitope is more clearly associated with seropositive RA[35] and with male patients who develop RA at a young age[36]. Furthermore, other class II MHC genes have also been proposed to play a role in RA susceptibility[37–40], and in some populations it has been suggested that HLA-DQ is even more important than HLA-DR[39], with homozygosity for DQ3 an especially strong predisposing genotype for RA[41]. Whether DQ alleles confer risk for RA only because of linkage disequilibrium with HLA-DR, or whether they carry independent disease association remains controversial[42–45], and may depend on the specific ethnic group that is analyzed. HLA-DM functions during antigen trafficking and loading on to class II MHC dimers inside antigen-presenting cells. Initial studies suggested that associations of HLA-DM polymorphisms with RA were weak at best[37,46]. A more recent study of a French RA cohort found an altered frequency of alleles at the HLA-DMA locus but not at HLA-DMB[47].

Since the molecules that contain the shared epitope present peptide antigens to CD4+ T cells, it seems straightforward to conclude that the shared epitope is associated with RA because it presents an arthritogenic peptide to specific clones of T cells. However, the situation is likely to be considerably more complicated. There is no certainty yet about the nature of arthritogenic peptide(s) in RA, although some candidate peptides can bind to the shared epitope[48–50], and shared epitope MHC alleles may be selectively overexpressed on the cell surface in RA but not in normal controls[51]. However, even in Caucasian patients with seropositive disease, as many as 27%[35] do not have MHC alleles that contain the shared epitope. Thus far, attempts to isolate unique arthritogenic peptides from RA-associated MHC alleles have not yielded conclusive insights. On the one hand, it has been found that there are distinctions between the peptides that can be externally inserted into molecules bearing the shared epitope compared with other DR molecules, and such distinctions include

some peptides derived from potential autoantigens such as type II collagen, citrullinated peptides, and heat shock proteins[48,49,52–54]. On the other hand, most peptides presented by MHC antigens are loaded on these molecules intracellularly, not inserted externally from the extracellular milieu. Analyses of intracellularly loaded peptides eluted from HLA molecules have not shown unique peptides that are selectively displayed by those MHC structures that bear the shared epitope. However, peptides that are displayed only by non-shared epitope DR molecules have been identified[55].

Some data also suggest that the presence of two copies of the shared epitope confers greater risk of disease and augmented disease severity compared with one copy[25–29]. It would be expected that presentation of an arthritogenic antigen should be a dominant rather than an codominant characteristic. Taken together, these lines of evidence raise the possibility that the shared epitope could augment risk for RA by failing to present an antigen that the immune system must recognize in order to prevent RA, perhaps by clearing a microbial pathogen. In such a model, non-RA-associated DRB1 alleles would be protective, while arthritogenic antigens might be presented by non-DR MHC molecules such as DQ, DP, or class I MHC[56–59]. This possible model has interesting parallels in a transgenic rodent system in which mice that express HLA-DQ8 are susceptible to collagen-induced arthritis, while some alleles of the polymorphic H-2E locus (homologous to HLA-DR) suppress disease[58,60,61]. It has been specifically suggested that MHC alleles containing the sequence DERAA at the same location where the shared epitope sequence is found may be protective against the development of RA[41,56,57,62,63]. The same alleles may also reduce severity of RA[43]. Mechanisms proposed for such protective effects include presentation of HLA-DR-derived peptides by HLA-DQ molecules[58,64], or distinct binding properties between chaperone heat shock proteins and specific HLA-DR molecules[65,66].

The MHC molecules also play an important role in shaping the T cell repertoire during T cell development in the thymus. In this process negative and positive selection are controlled by MHC molecules along with antigenic peptides encountered during thymic development. Analysis of naive CD4+ peripheral blood T cells has led to the hypothesis that the shared epitope molds the expressed TCR repertoire in a unique manner. Furthermore, shared epitope-positive RA patients differ from HLA-matched normal individuals in the repertoire of their resting T cells, which is more restricted in RA patients than in controls[67,68]. Whether such observations truly reflect unique features of intrathymic development, or are linked to T cell responses related to disease, is not yet known. It has been proposed that this contracted T cell repertoire represents premature senescence and distortion of both thymic output and homeostatic T cell proliferation, and leads to over-representation of CD28- and autoreactive T cells[69]. An aberrant pattern of expression of surface markers on circulating memory T cells in RA further supports the concept that T cell differentiation is fundamentally abnormal in this disease[70].

Another possible relationship between the shared epitope and thymic T cell development has been proposed. It is known that MHC sequences can be processed and presented to T cells by other MHC molecules. In view of the finding that synovial fluid T cells from patients with early RA can recognize peptides

Table 6.3 Possible mechanisms for the association of RA with class II MHC polymorphisms

---

Presentation of arthritogenic antigens to CD4+ T cells by RA-associated class II MHC alleles
Specific overexpression of shared epitope alleles favoring presentation of arthritogenic antigens
Linkage to other genes in or near the class II MHC locus
Altered T cell selection in thymic development, leading to expanded populations of potentially arthritogenic T cells
Cross-reactivity between foreign antigen and MHC peptide sequences, particularly the 'shared epitope'
Differences in surface expression and intracellular trafficking of specific MHC alleles
Aberrant signaling through MHC alleles
'Holes' in the T cell repertoire that lead to inability to respond to an antigen that would protect against the development of RA:
 • absence of a particular set of T cell receptors due to negative selection
 • absence of MHC molecules capable of presenting a critical antigen to a particular set of T cell receptors
Lack of protective MHC alleles
Altered affinity of shared epitope peptides for chaperone proteins, causing altered pattern of antigen loading onto MHC molecules
Direct stimulation of T cells by the shared epitope on antigen-presenting cells

---

containing QKRAA (contained in several microbial antigens), it has been suggested that positive selection of T cells reactive with the shared epitope can occur in the thymus, producing lymphocytes that can later create an arthritogenic response after reacting to shared epitope sequences in microbial antigens[71]. A very different potential mechanism for the shared epitope effect springs from the observation that this sequence can alter intracellular trafficking of class II molecules, affecting loading or presentation of antigens as well as the extent of surface expression of MHC proteins[72]. Such differences may reflect variations in stability of the complexes formed between various HLA-DR alleles and intracellular non-antigen class II ligands such as CLIP (class II associated invariant chain peptide)[53]. It has been speculated that low stability of the association of 0404 and 0401 alleles with CLIP could facilitate loading and presentation of autoantigens by these shared epitope alleles. At this time, therefore, it is not possible to reach a conclusion regarding the mechanism by which MHC alleles predispose to RA or affect severity. However, a variety of very distinct and provocative potential mechanisms have been proposed (Table 6.3). The testing of these hypotheses may shed important light on the etiology and pathogenesis of RA. The close relationship of the shared epitope to RA is emphasized by a similar genetic association with a polyarthritis that resembles RA in another species, the dog[73].

T lymphocyte responses to antigen in RA

Activation through the CD3–TCR antigen receptor complex is widely viewed as the primary stimulus that leads to proliferation of mature T cells and acquisition of effector function. It has been reasoned that, within the vast array of diverse T cell clones in the human immune system, detection of oligoclonal expansions would identify antigen- (including autoantigen) stimulated populations that are of primary importance in immune-mediated disease. Therefore, over the past two decades, analysis of the expressed T cell receptor repertoire in RA has attracted enormous attention and effort (reviewed in Ref. 74). Much of this work has been motivated by the hypothesis that it may be possible to identify expanded clones of antigen-specific T cells that are of central importance in the pathogenesis of RA, which could be used to

identify an etiologic antigen, and also serve as a target for specific, biological therapeutics. Initial techniques used to study TCR rearrangements in populations of synovial and peripheral T cells, such as Southern blot analysis, were relatively insensitive. However, more recent approaches have involved precise methods to amplify, measure, clone, and sequence T cell receptor gene segments, using quantitative polymerase chain reaction (PCR) techniques, gel electrophoresis of PCR products, and direct sequencing of TCR gene segments. In patients with RA, there are many problems inherent in attempts to analyze the TCR repertoire. Control subjects should ideally be of similar age, gender, and MHC background. It seems possible that changes in the TCR populations found in blood or joints could either be a part of the cause of RA or be a consequence of inflammation, so that study of patients with early disease might be important. However, identifying such patients and obtaining synovial specimens is often difficult. Additional issues arise in comparison between peripheral blood and synovial tissue or fluid, since the subsets present in the lesional samples are distinct from those in peripheral blood, particularly the expanded proportion with memory markers. Additionally, the effects of medications used in the treatment of RA may be important in altering the pool of lymphocytes available for study.

Nevertheless, more than 50 studies of the expressed T cell repertoire in RA have been published[74]. Most of these examine the αβ TCR, particularly Vβ gene segment usage, while fewer studies examine γδ chain usage. The results of these studies may be summarized as follows:

1. Selective expansion of use of specific TCR V region genes has been frequently observed in the synovial compartment. This is often termed 'skewing' or 'bias' in TCR repertoire expression.

2. The specific V genes overexpressed differ among different studies.

3. There is no evidence yet that TCR expression is distinctive in early versus late RA.

4. There is no evidence yet for functionally significant TCR expression that is unique to RA, compared with other forms of arthritis.

5. Indirect evidence exists to suggest impaired control of expansion and persistence of clonal T cell populations in RA, but

without direct evidence that such clones are selectively autoreactive or arthritogenic, except among CD4+ CD28− cells.

6. Thus far, there is only a tenuous link between the results of TCR usage analysis in RA and antigen-specific responses that might be relevant to joint destruction.

7. Analysis of the γδ TCR shows that the pattern of V gene usage differs between the joint and peripheral blood. However, such tissue specific expression of TCR γδ subtypes is typical for tissue compartments in which γδ cells are found. In some, but not all studies, the proportion of synovial T cells that express TCR γδ is expanded compared to peripheral blood.

8. Clonal populations of T cells are frequently found in peripheral blood in patients with Felty's syndrome and RA, and may be pathogenic in this clinical setting.

At this time, most of the key conceptual issues regarding TCR usage in RA remain unsettled. It has been proposed that some expanded synovial T cell clones are responding to unique antigens in the joint, while other clones are also activated systemically and are detected in peripheral blood. However, it is possible that the representation of T cells found within the joint is no different than T cells that would be present in the peripheral lymphoid organs, such as lymph nodes, of such patients. We do not yet know whether any particular T cell specificity or TCR subset is required for the development of RA. A plausible alternative is that persistent synovial inflammation in RA is maintained by responses to any of a variety of foreign or self-antigens, presented within the joint in the setting of an appropriate cytokine milieu and activation of resident antigen-presenting cells.

A variety of self-antigens and microbial antigens have been studied as potential pathogenic targets for the immune response in RA (Table 6.4). Self antigens include: type II collagen, components of cartilage proteoglycan, a 39 kD cartilage glycoprotein termed gp39, and class II MHC sequences. Microbial antigens of interest have included: Epstein–Barr virus proteins, mycobacterial antigens, microbial peptides with sequences similar to the shared epitope, and bacterial superantigens. The role of microbial agents in RA is considered in detail in Chapter 3.

Despite the frustrating lack of a clear connection between any microbial agent and the etiology of RA, it would be premature to abandon consideration of a central role for an infectious organism or class of organisms in the T cell responses of this disease. The complex interplay between microorganisms and the immune system is by no means fully understood. A variety of potential indirect mechanisms for triggering of RA by microbes remain to be carefully examined. The capacity of RA synovium to retain bacterial products that may be deposited in immune system antigen-presenting cells due to extra-articular infection could be relevant to amplication or even initiation of disease[75]. Since synovial tissue has many of the features of an activated lymphoid organ, it is likely that both primary and secondary immune responses to a variety of microorganisms encountered systemically will be reflected in T cell specificities within synovial tissue. Bacterial antigens that are concentrated in lymphoid organs and that elicit T cell responses in RA[76] can also be detected in RA synovial tissue[77]. Many of these responses have no direct relationship to RA, but instead signify concurrent and essentially unrelated exposure to microbial agents[78]. Enhanced synovial T cell responses to multiple pathogens are consistent with migration to the joint of activated T cells with a variety of specificities[79]. Overall, however, evidence for molecular mimicry between microorganisms and autoantigens as a cause for RA remains distinctly unconvincing[80].

A spectrum of interesting responses to self-antigens that are potentially relevant to disease pathogenesis have been detected in RA[81–100], and one of the earliest to be recognized was the response to type II collagen, the predominant collagen isoform found in articular cartilage[81,97,98]. Although T cell reactivity to collagen is not specific for RA, evidence for a clonally restricted synovial T cell response to specific collagen epitopes has been documented[81,82]. Some T cell epitopes of type II collagen are glycosylated[92]. Type II collagen is arthritogenic in some strains of rodents. Other self-antigens of potential interest in RA include cartilage link protein, a 68 kD glycosylated autoantigen that is also the target of an RA-associated autoantibody, antigens of 25 and 50 kD extracted from RA synovial cells that are absent from control synovial cells, antigens present in RA synovial fluid, and heat shock proteins.

The gp39 antigen is a cartilage glycoprotein that is secreted by cultured chondrocytes and synoviocytes, is found in RA synovium

Table 6.4 Putative antigenic targets for T cells in RA

Microbial antigens	Self-antigens
Superantigens, such as staphylococcal toxins	Collagen (type II and other types)
Epstein–Barr virus antigens	gp39
Heat shock proteins	Cartilage link protein
Mycobacterial antigens	Cartilage proteoglycan
	205 kD synovial fluid antigen
Parvovirus antigens	68 kDa glycoprotein
HTLV-1 proteins	25 kDa/50 kDa synovial cell antigen
	Immunoglobulin-binding protein (BiP)
Peptidoglycan from Gram positive bacteria	Heat shock proteins
	Class II MHC (shared epitope)
	IgG (Fc portion)
	RA33 (heterogeneous nuclear ribonucleoprotein A2)
	Glycosaminoglycans

and cartilage but not in normal joints, and is arthritogenic in mice[83]. T cell-proliferative responses to cartilage gp39 may be more strictly associated with RA than are responses to other autoantigens. Like type II collagen, some peptides of gp39 are presented to T cells by MHC alleles that bear the shared epitope[86]. Immunological techniques have demonstrated the presence in RA synovium of complexes of gp39 peptides bound to HLA-DR4 on the surface of dendritic cells[99]. This was highly specific for RA, and the 60% of RA specimens in which such complexes were detected showed more intense inflammation and more prominent T cell aggregates, compared to the RA subset in which these complexes were absent. When T cell responses to gp39 were analyzed by measuring cytokine production rather than proliferation, a very interesting difference was noted comparing RA and normal peripheral blood lymphocytes[100]. RA patients responded with a Th1 pattern (production of IFNγ) while normal subjects exhibited a regulatory T cell response, with production of IL-10. Responses to gp39 therefore appear to be a useful model for understanding dysregulation of T cell autoreactivity in RA.

T cell subsets in RA

Synovial T cells are distinct in many respects from peripheral blood T cells. Most synovial tissue and synovial fluid T cells bear the CD45 isoforms associated with T cell memory, such as CD45RO, rather than those associated with the 'naïve' T cell subset[101–103]. Moreover, a large proportion of synovial T cells, especially CD8[+] lymphocytes, express class II MHC antigens on the cell surface[6,7], which are only expressed on T cells as a consequence of prior activation. Comparable expression of class II MHC on T cells is only rarely found in RA peripheral blood. Relatively few synovial T cells (generally no more than a few per cent) express high affinity IL-2 receptors on their surface[9], indicating that a relatively small subset of synovial T cells has recently been activated. Paradoxically, many synovial T cells express CD69, also a marker of recent cell activation. Various explanations for this incomplete activation phenotype of synovial T cells have been proposed, but full clarification of this issue is not yet available. It is possible that the surface markers expressed on synovial T cells reflect activation of many of these cells by pro-inflammatory cytokines rather than by antigen recognition[104].

Most T cells express the αβ TCR but a minor subset expresses the γδ TCR. The repertoire of antigens recognized, the mechanisms of antigen presentation, some aspects of receptor stimulation, and intracellular signaling all have unique properties in γδ T cells[105–107]. Some studies have suggested that this subset is expanded in RA synovial fluid and synovial tissue[108–110]. In RA, the role of γδ T cells, which can be either pathogenic or regulatory in animal models of inflammatory arthritis, is not yet clear.

T cells require at least two signals for achieving activation in response to antigen stimulation. The second signal can probably be delivered through a variety of surface receptors or by cytokines. The CD28 molecule is the best-demonstrated example of a surface structure that can deliver such a second signal, upon binding to CD28 of one of its ligands, which are termed B7-1 and B7-2 (CD80 and CD86). Normally, virtually all CD4[+] cells and a substantial subset of CD8[+] cells express CD28.

Synovial T cells generally do express CD28[111], and CD28 ligands are also found in synovial tissues[112]. However, in some RA patients an expanded subset of CD4[+] and CD28[-] cells has been found in peripheral blood and occasionally in the joint[113]. These cells are autoreactive, resistant to apoptosis, and oligoclonal[113–115]. The mechanism by which CD28 might be down-regulated is not established, but it is intriguing that TNF-α can reduce CD28 expression on T cell clones[116]. The means by which a second signal is delivered to such cells is not entirely clear, but it is likely that other T cell surface molecules can perform this function, such as receptors usually found on natural killer cells[117–119], and thrombospondin receptors[120]. These cells do show vigorous proliferation and cytokine production upon CD3–TCR engagement[121], and high circulating numbers of these cells are associated with accelerated atherosclerosis in RA patients[122].

The KIR (killer cell immunoglobulin-like receptor) gene family is expressed on cytotoxic lymphocytes. One study has shown that the KIR2DS2 receptor, which is thought to activate cytotoxic cell function, is found more frequently on the expanded subset of CD4[+] CD28[-] cells in patients with rheumatoid vasculitis, compared to RA or normal controls[123]. This association may reflect a genetic polymorphism in the complex loci that control KIR expression, although direct demonstrations of DNA polymorphisms at such loci in rheumatoid vasculitis are not yet available. Altered allele frequencies of the MHC class I gene HLA-C, a putative ligand for KIR2DS2, were found in the same group of rheumatoid vasculitis patients[123].

Interpretation of the importance of the CD28– T cells in RA is still uncertain, since a fairly small proportion of RA patients has a major expansion of this subset. Moreover, the density of CD28 has been reported to be increased on CD28+ T cells from RA patients with active disease[124].

A variety of structures on the T cell surface other than CD28 could convey costimulatory signals in RA. Some of these other molecules include CD2, CD11a/CD18 (LFA-1), CD6, CD47, and possibly CD60. CD6 is a T cell glycoprotein that has been implicated in autoreactive T cell responses and a ligand for CD6 (ALCAM or CD166) is abundantly expressed in the joint[125]. Recently a second ligand of CD6 has been described, which is expressed on synovial fibroblasts and up-regulated by IFNγ[126]. CD60 is a carbohydrate-bearing determinant found on a minority of peripheral blood T cells, but on a majority of synovial tissue and fluid T cells[9]. Antibody to CD60 is capable of activating T cells[127], including T cell clones derived from RA synovial fluid[9,127]. CD60 is expressed more intensively on memory T cells than on naïve T cells[9,127]. A ligand for CD60 has not yet been determined. The CD40 ligand (CD40L) is a T cell surface molecule induced early in T cell activation, which delivers costimulatory signals to cells with which T cells interact, including B cells, macrophages, and fibroblasts. CD40L expressed on CD8[+] cells has been implicated as having a role in the formation of germinal center-like structures in RA synovium[128]. The importance of costimulatory signals in RA has been further highlighted by the recent demonstration of clinical efficacy of a new biologic agent that inhibits ligand binding to CD28 in the treatment of RA[14,129].

After approximately a decade in which the concept of 'suppressor T cells' fell out of favor, the past several years have seen a prominent re-emergence of what are now termed 'regulatory T cells'. These cells are typically CD4+CD25+, express the transcription factor Foxp3, and often secrete IL-10[130,131]. Such cells seem to be present in RA synovial fluid, but other T cells in patients with RA may be relatively insensitive to these regulatory lymphocytes[132–134]. Regulatory T cells from RA blood were found to be only partly functional, but complete function was restored to such cells from RA patients after systemic administration of TNF-blocking therapy[135]. Although a variety of approaches to induce regulation of arthritis by antigen administration in various animal models of RA have been successful, similar attempts in human RA have yielded an unimpressive level of clinical benefit[136,137]. Nevertheless, restoration of regulatory T cell function by immunomodulatory rather than immunosuppressive approaches would be an attractive goal in RA therapeutics.

T cell survival in RA

Many aspects of the life cycle of synovial T cells remain unknown. It is possible such cells are activated elsewhere, in central or peripheral lymphoid tissue, and then home to synovium. The extent to which synovial T lymphocytes recirculate back through the systemic circulation is also unknown. Studies of mutation frequency in peripheral and lesional T cells in patients with RA (presumably due to oxidative damage) as well as in normal peripheral blood suggest that the synovial compartment is the primary location for activation but that substantial numbers of lymphocytes do recirculate systemically following activation in the joint[138]. The longevity of these cells is also unknown. Despite sensitivity of synovial fluid T cells *ex vivo* to apoptosis induced through the CD95 (Fas) molecule, direct examination of RA tissue sections reveals little evidence of ongoing T cell apoptosis[139].

The complex chemokine family is of great importance in regulating influx of T cells and other leukocytes into RA synovium, through binding of these cytokines (including IL-8, RANTES, MIP-1α, and others) to a family of chemokine receptors that have overlapping expression and function[140]. IL-15 may also play a role in transendothelial migration of T cells in RA[141].

T cells isolated from synovial tissues or synovial fluid are typically hyporesponsive *in vitro* in standard assays of T cell function, such as response to mitogenic lectins or anti-CD3 antibodies[9]. This may be a physiological refractory state due to previous stimulation *in vivo*. Alternatively, it could reflect suppression of T cell activation by immunoregulatory cytokines, such as IL-10, that are present in the synovial compartment. At this point there is no convincing evidence that cells that migrate into the joint have an intrinsic defect in activation pathways or a distinct activation program. However, the environment of oxidative stress found in synovium may perturb redox balance and protein phosphorylations that accompany TCR triggering in synovial T cells[142].

T cell cytokines and effector function in RA

Cytokines that regulate T cell function or that are produced by T cell subsets are often classified as Th1, Th2, or Th3 (also termed type 1, type 2, and type 3). IFNγ is a prototypic Th1 cytokine while IL-4 is a Th2 and TGFβ a Th3 cytokine. Th1 function is associated with delayed type hypersensitivity and cytotoxic T cell responses, while Th2 function is paramount in allergic diseases and some parasitic infections. RA has been viewed as primarily a Th1 disease[143–145]. The myeloid dendritic cell subset that promotes Th1 differentiation is present in RA synovial fluid[146]. Levels of IFNγ detectable in synovial tissue are low but functionally significant[147,148]. T cells taken from synovial tissue or fluid can readily be stimulated to produce IFNγ[149]. Th1 responses dominate whether RA T cells are activated by peptide antigen[149] or by monoclonal antibody to T cell surface structures[150]. The production of IFNγ in RA is partly due to its synthesis by a T cell subset that also bears natural killer cell markers[151]. Biologic effects attributable at least in part to IFNγ (such as strong class II MHC expression on a variety of cell types) are readily demonstrable in RA synovium, and other cytokines associated with activation of Th1 responses, such as IL-12, are also present in synovial tissue[152]. IL-15 and IL-18 probably synergize with IL-12 in supporting Th1 differentiation, and both of these cytokines are readily detectable in RA synovium[153–155]. IL-18 has broad proinflammatory effects that may include chemotactic[156] and angiogenic[157] activities. In contrast, IL-4 is rarely detected[158], and the capacity of synovial T cells to produce IL-4 is lower than their capacity to produce IFNγ[159]. Unexpectedly, individual synovial T cells can sometimes produce both Th1 and Th2 cytokines following *in vitro* stimulation[149]. Rheumatoid nodules consistently show Th1 dominance[160], but more data are needed regarding the T cell cytokine phenotype of other extra-articular RA lesions. Although current concensus views RA as a Th1 disease there are some troubling issues that still require clarification, especially the discrepancy between the levels of IFNγ present in RA synovium and its apparent biologic effects. Whether this discrepancy reflects the short half-life and local action of IFNγ, amplification of IFNγ effects by other cytokines, or independent IFNγ-like actions mediated by other molecules such as GM-CSF (or a combination of these mechanisms) remain open to debate.

IL-2 is barely detectable in RA synovial tissue or fluid[161,162], and a small minority of T cells express the high affinity IL-2 receptor[9]. These findings were viewed at one time as indicating dormancy of T cells in RA synovium, and perhaps only a very limited role for T cells in chronic RA[19]. However, it is now understood that other cytokines, especially IL-15, can have T cell growth factor activity and can substitute for IL-2, even utilizing constitutively expressed subunits of the IL-2 receptor[163]. Thus T cell proliferation can be driven by either paracrine or autocrine mechanisms. The properties of RA synovial T cells can be mimicked by peripheral blood T cells activated by IL-15 or other cytokines more closely than by T cells activated through triggering of the antigen receptor[104]. In addition IL-15 can stimulate oligoclonal T cell expansion[164] and induces expression of CD154, which is critical to T cell interactions with non-T cells[165]. Expression of IL-2 and high affinity IL-2 receptors are transient events in the course of T cell activation and could have occurred in T cells that reside in RA synovium prior to their entry into the joint, in locations such as lymph nodes.

T lymphocytes can also release pro-inflammatory cytokines in RA. In addition to their minor contribution to TNF-α production, T cells in RA synovium make IL-17, which has direct effects on synovial fibroblasts, inducing production of pro-inflammatory mediators such as matrix metalloproteases, prostaglandins, chemikines, nitric oxide, and IL-6[166-169]. IL-17 has multiple isoforms, which can also activate a variety of other cells in the joint[167]. Synthesis of IL-17 can be induced by IL-15[170], thus defining a fibroblast/T cell cytokine axis, relatively independent of the monokines TNF and IL-1, that can also mediate joint destruction both in RA and in animal models[167,169,171]. T cells and other cells in RA also produce macrophage migration inhibitory factor (MIF). MIF activates macrophage cytokine synthesis, antagonizes glucocorticoids, and has multiple other pro-inflammatory effects[172].

The cytokine known as RANK-ligand or RANKL (receptor activator of nuclear factor κB (NF-κB) ligand), or osteoclast differentiation factor (ODF) is critical to osteoclast formation and bone erosion in RA[173]. RANK-ligand can be produced by activated T cells and by osteoblasts, and its osteoclastogenic effects are potentiated by TNF-α[174]. The production of key cytokines by T cells in RA including IFNγ, IL-17, RANK-ligand (and some TNF-α), emphasizes the key role of these cells, together with synovial macrophages and fibroblasts, in the pathogenesis of the destruction of cartilage and bone that is typical of RA.

Immunoregulatory or anti-inflammatory cytokines that are detectable in RA may also become useful as therapeutic agents. IL-10, previously classified as a Th2 cytokine, is now viewed as capable of regulating a variety of T cell responses, and IL-10 is produced within RA synovial tissue[20], but at inadequate levels to control Th1 cells[175]. IL-10 can be produced by a variety of non-T cells as well as by regulatory T cells. Transforming growth factors are a family of cytokines that exist in both latent and active forms. Although TGFβ can have some immunosuppressant and anti-inflammatory effects, its precise role in RA appears to be complex and to some degree pathogenic. Whether members of this cytokine family will be ultimately useful as therapeutic agents is unknown.

T cell interactions with other cells in the RA joint

Entry of T lymphocytes and other inflammatory cells into the synovium requires interactions with specialized vascular endothelium, followed by interactions with a variety of antigen-presenting cells in a milieu rich in pro-inflammatory cytokines. The most potent of these antigen-presenting cells is the dendritic cell (DC).

It was the definition of immune functions mediated by synovial DCs that expressed high levels of Class II MHC molecules that established the importance of DCs in RA. Klareskog and colleagues proposed, in 1982, that RA synovitis resembled a cutaneous delayed type hypersensitivity reaction, with T cell activation mediated by synovial dendritic cells that exhibited similarities to Langerhans cells of the skin[176]. These cells, which were enriched using a gradient centrifugation procedure, were potent stimulators of allogeneic mixed lymphocyte reactions and of antigen responses to peptide antigens, including Type II collagen[176].

Subsequent work by two independent groups, led by Jacob Natvig and Nathan Zvaifler, confirmed and extended these observations[177-179]. These studies showed that (a) DCs could be readily identified and isolated from synovial fluid as well as tissue, and accounted for 5–7% of RA synovial fluid mononuclear cells; (b) T cells formed clusters around individual synovial DCs; (c) synovial DCs stimulated T cell responses more potently than did monocytes, in both allogeneic and autologous mixed lymphocyte reactions; (d) functions of synovial DCs depended on Class II MHC and included induction of T cell responses to a variety of nominal antigens; (e) adhesion of T cells to DCs depended, in part, on interaction of CD2 on the T cell with CD2 ligands on DCs; and (f) DCs could be found in synovial fluids of patients with inflammatory arthritides other than RA.

Table 6.5   Role of cytokines in T cell function in RA synovium. For production of cytokines, quantitative differences between cell types are indicated using arbitrary designations of −, +/−, + and ++. IL-16 is produced by CD8+ and not CD4+ T cells, but acts on CD4+ cells.

Cytokine	Produced by		Target	
	T cells	Synovial macrophages and/or fibroblasts	T cells	Synovial macrophages and/or fibroblasts
IFN-γ	+	−	−	++
IL-1β	+/−	++	+	++
TNF-α	+/−	++	+	++
IL-2	+/−	−	+	−
IL-6	+/−	++	+	+
IL-8	+/−	+	+	−
IL-10	+/−	++	+	+
IL-12	−	+	+	−
IL-15	−	+	+	−
IL-16	+/−	+	+	−
IL-17	+	−	−	+
IL-18	−	+	+	+
RANKL	+	+	−	+
MIF	+	+	+/−	+

Interactions between DCs and lymphocytes are mediated by cell–cell contact through multiple types of receptor-ligand pairs, and also by secretion of cytokines and chemokines. Th1 immune responses are initiated in the context of IL-12 and IL-23 production by DCs. The ability of IL-23 to enhance T cell production of IL-17[180] may be important in RA, since IL-17 can directly activate synovial fibroblasts and augment their response to other signals from T cells[181].

Cells of the monocyte/macrophage lineage (Type A synoviocytes) are abundant in RA synovium, and are competent antigen-presenting cells for T cell responses. In addition, RA T cells may be important activators of the pro-inflammatory potential of synovial monocyte/macrophage cells. Infiltrating T cells and macrophages reside in close proximity in the inflamed RA synovium. This intimate association provides many opportunities for interactions between the cells[182,183]. Evidence supporting T cell participation in TNF-α production by monocytes comes from experiments in which depletion of CD3+ cells from RA synovial cell cultures resulted in decreased TNF-α production, whereas depletion of CD3+ cells from OA cultures did not[104]. These observations suggest that T cells have a direct impact on TNF-α induction in RA joints. To further investigate the role of T cells in TNF-α production, T cells activated by a cytokine cocktail (Tck)[184] were used, as a model for RA T cells, to stimulate monocytes. Tcks were able to induce TNF-α from monocytes via a cell–cell contact-dependent mechanism that mimicked RA T cells, but differed from T cells activated through their TCR and CD28[104]. Another study indicates that Tcks can also induce production of the anti-inflammatory cytokine IL-10 by M-CSF treated monocytes (i.e. macrophages)[185]. These studies imply that RA synovial T cells are similar to bystander activated Tcks in their phenotype, and their effects on monocyte/macrophage cytokine production. The potent effects of Tcks emphasize that a major role for T cells in RA may be independent of recognition of specific antigens or activation of T cells through the TCR.

RANKL has been detected in RA synovial tissue. RANK/RANKL interactions are necessary for the differentiation of osteoclasts from monocytic precursor cells. RANKL was found to localize specifically to CD3+ CD4+ cells, and not other mononuclear cells, in synovial histological sections[186]. In the same study, T cells activated with PHA up-regulated RANKL and effectively induced monocytes to differentiate into osteoclasts.

Antigen presentation by human RA synovial B cells has not been as well characterized as the antigen-presenting cell (APC) role played by synovial dendritic cells. However, it is likely that B cells specific to autoantigens or B cells producing rheumatoid factors are able to bind, internalize, and process antigens for presentation to autoreactive T cells in the ectopic germinal centers of rheumatoid synovium[187,188].

Evidence supporting the dependency of T cell activation on synovial lymphoid architecture, and especially on T cell–B cell interactions, has been obtained through experiments that involve adoptive transfer of T cell clones to SCID mice engrafted with human synovial tissue[189]. To assess the role of B cells in this experimental model, mice engrafted with GC-like synovial tissue were depleted of human B cells with anti-human CD20 antibody prior to adoptive transfer. Pro-inflammatory cytokine production was reduced by B cell depletion in an antibody dose-dependent manner. However, the lack of T cells infiltrating into the engrafted synovial tissue that was depleted of B cells does not allow for determination of whether the essential role of B cells relates to T cell homing or to direct cell–cell interaction between T and B cells in synovium.

T cells in RA synovium can interact not only with a variety of professional antigen-presenting cells (synovial macrophages, dendritic cells, and B lymphocytes), but also with type B fibroblast-like synoviocytes. Early experiments on co-cultures of T cells and fibroblast-like synoviocytes (FLS) demonstrated that phorbol myristate acetate (PMA)-activated T cells triggered IL-1β production in FLSs, dependent on interactions between leukocyte functional antigen-1 (LFA-1/CD11aCD18) and intercellular adhesion molecule 1 (ICAM-1/CD54)[190]. More recent work has documented activation of FLSs and release of pro-inflammatory mediators[181], following co-culture with autologous or allogeneic resting T cells. This effector function of resting T cells is not restricted to a particular T cell subset[181]. Activated FLS showed induction or augmentation of mRNA for stromelysin, IL-6, and IL-8, gene products important in joint inflammation and joint destruction, and IL-17 synergized with T cells to active FLS. Two additional studies have recently provided further support for a role of T cell activation of FLS in antigen-independent systems, and revealed a role for IL-15 production by FLSs in such interactions[191,192]. One study used unstimulated purified T cells[191] and the other used collagen type II (CII)-responsive T cells[192]. Both studies emphasize the importance of IL-15 expression by FLSs and its up-regulation after stimulation by T cells[191,192].

FLS of RA synovium express high levels of MHC II *ex vivo*[193], indicating that the potential for antigen presentation by FLSs in RA. Early studies suggest that FLS can process antigen similarly to professional APCs[194]. In those experiments, FLS were able to take up and present various antigens and present them to T cell clones via an MHC II-restricted mechanism[194]. This gives support to potential antigen specific interaction between T cells and FLS (as APCs). However, antigens relevant to RA were not assayed nor were observed responses robust. IFNγ-treated FLS present superantigens to T cells (Fig 6.3), and induce T cell proliferation which is dependent on MHC II, CD2, LFA-1, and the cytokine IL-2[195].

There is also evidence that FLSs might not activate T cells, but instead induce anergy[196]. These experiments assessed the APC and allostimulatory functions of FLSs. Similar to previous studies, FLSs were able to load antigen onto MHC II. However, allogeneic responses depended upon the addition of accessory cells expressing CD80, and blockade of CD80 abolished the response. When FLSs without accessory cells were cultured with T cells, the T cells adopted a phenotype resembling anergy: upregulation of CD25, reduced proliferation, and reconstitution of proliferation by exogenous IL-2[196]. Interestingly, CD69 on T cells was also up-regulated after T cell culture with FLSs. This study implies that FLSs could cause anergy due to a lack of costimulatory molecules, but that bystander cells expressing costimulatory molecules could overcome this. The potential for accessory costimulation exists abundantly within RA synovium due to the close proximity of FLSs with B cells, macrophages, and dendritic cells.

None of these observations directly address the issue of where critical T cell responses in RA are actually initiated. It is possible that this occurs primarily in lymphoid organs, with the synovium

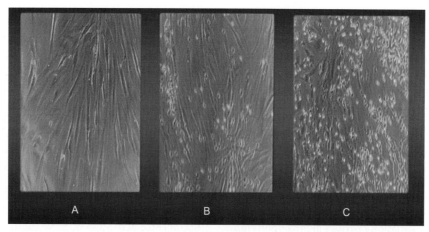

Fig. 6.3   Interaction of T lymphocytes with Type B synoviocytes (synovial fibroblasts) +/− the staphylococcal superantigen SEA (staphylococcal enterotoxin A). A − Synovial fibroblasts, B − Synovial fibroblasts + T cells, C − Synovial fibroblasts + T cells + SEA.

serving as the location for restimulation of T cells and execution of effector functions. It is even possible that APCs such as DCs become loaded with antigens in synovium and then migrate back to regional lymph nodes. Overall, the precise links between the systemic aspects of RA and its local manifestations in joints are poorly understood.

Future directions for analysis of the role of T cells in RA

Current hypotheses regarding the role of T cells in the biology of RA are not necessarily mutually exclusive. Antigen recognition by T cells could be involved either in the initial phases of the disease or in intermittent clinical flares, without the requirement that a unique prototypic antigen is recognized by all patients with RA. Further study of antigen-specific responses in the synovial compartment should not only shed light on the issue of whether RA is truly an autoimmune condition, but should also reveal unique aspects of T cell responses that are shaped by the special cellular and cytokine make-up of the synovial compartment. Future studies will also shed further light on the range of T cell effector mechanisms in the joint. These may extend beyond the traditional roles of immune response regulation and target cell killing, to direct pro-inflammatory effects mediated by cell–cell interactions and secreted cytokines. Useful understanding of the role of T cells in RA will need to place T cell function in context of the incompletely understood cell–cell interactions that are likely to be key to the pathogenesis of this disease[197].

Innate immune responses can be viewed as components of host defense that do not require pre-sensitization to specific antigen. For many years attention was focused primarily on adaptive immune responses—autoantibodies and autoreactive T cells—as central to the pathogenesis and even etiology of RA. Innate immune mechanisms include not only pattern recognition receptors (Toll-like

receptors and others), acute phase reactants, components of the complement cascade, phagocytic cells, and many cytokines, but also natural killer lymphocytes and even some polyreactive antibodies and T cell effector functions. Innate immune responses precede and control the adaptive immune response, and are also engaged by the effector arms of adaptive immunity in ways that blur the boundary between these two systems.

Increasing attention is being focused on the role of innate immunity in RA[198,199]. The functions of T cells described in this chapter that are independent of antigen recognition, such as direct activation of fibroblasts and macrophages, can be viewed as innate immune functions of T lymphocytes. T cells may therefore drive both inflammation and tissue destruction in RA through a variety of immune pathways, which include both innate and adaptive immune responses.

References

1. Janossy, G., Panayi, G., Duke, O., Bofill, M., Poulter, L. W., and Goldstein, G. Rheumatoid arthritis: a disease of T-lymphocyte/macrophage immunoregulation. *Lancet* 1981; **2**: 839–42.
2. Firestein, G. S., and Zvaifler, N. J. How important are T cells in chronic rheumatoid synovitis? II. T cell-independent mechanisms from beginning to end. *Arthritis Rheum* 2002; **46**: 298–308.
3. Smolen, J. S., and Steiner. G. Rheumatoid arthritis is more than cytokines: autoimmunity and rheumatoid arthritis. *Arthritis Rheum* 2001; **44**: 2218–20.
4. Van Boxel, J. A., and Paget, S. A. Predominantly T-cell infiltrate in rheumatoid synovial membranes. *N Engl J Med* 1975; **293**: 517–20.
5. Bankhurst, A. D., Husby, G., and Williams, R. C. Jr. Predominance of T cells in the lymphocytic infiltrates of synovial tissues in rheumatoid arthritis. *Arthritis Rheum* 1976; **19**: 555–62.
6. Burmester, G. R., Yu, D. T., Irani, A. M., Kunkel, H. G., and Winchester, R. J. Ia+ T cells in synovial fluid and tissues of patients with rheumatoid arthritis. *Arthritis Rheum* 1981; **24**: 1370–6.
7. Fox, R. I., Fong, S., Sabharwal, N., Carstens, S. A., Kung, P. C., and Vaughan, J. H. Synovial fluid lymphocytes differ from peripheral blood lymphocytes in patients with rheumatoid arthritis. *J Immunol* 1982; **128**: 351–4.

8. Hemler, M. E., Glass, D., Coblyn, J. S., and Jacobson, J. G. Very late activation antigens on rheumatoid synovial fluid T lymphocytes: association with stages of T cell activation. *J Clin Invest* 1986; 78: 696–702.

9. Fox, D. A., Millard, J. A., Kan, L., Zeldes, W. S., Davis, W. *et al*. Activation pathways of synovial T lymphocytes. Expression and function of the UM4D4/CDw60 antigen. *J Clin Invest* 1990; 86: 1124–36.

10. Veys, E. M., Hermanns, P., Verbruggen, G., Schindler, J., and Goldstein, G. Evaluation of T cell subsets with monoclonal antibodies in synovial fluid in rheumatoid arthritis. *J Rheumatol* 1982; 9: 821–6.

11. Cohen, I. R., Holoshitz, J., van Eden, W., and Frenkel, A. T. lymphocyte clones illuminate pathogenesis and affect therapy of experimental arthritis. *Arthritis Rheum* 1985; 28: 841–5.

12. Sakaguchi, N., Takahashi, T., Hata, H., Nomura, T., Tagami, T., Yamazaki, S. *et al*. Altered thymic T-cell selection due to a mutation of the ZAP-70 gene causes autoimmune arthritis in mice. *Nature* 2003; 426: 454–60.

13. Fox, D. A., and McCune, W. J. Immunologic and clinical effects of cytotoxic drugs used in the treatment of rheumatoid arthritis and systemic lupus erythematosus. *Concepts in Immunopathology* 1989; 7: 20–78.

14. Kremer, J., Westhovens, R., Leon, M., Di Giorgio, E., Alten, R., Steinfeld, S. *et al*. Treatment of rheumatoid arthritis by selective inhibition of T-cell activation with fusion protein CTLA4Ig. *N Engl J Med* 2003; 349: 1907–15.

15. Trentham, D. E., Belli, J. A., Anderson, R. J., Buckley, J. A., Goetzl, E. J., David, J. R. *et al* Clinical and immunologic effects of fractionated total lymphoid irradiation in refractory rheumatoid arthritis. *N Engl J Med* 1981; 305: 976–82.

16. Fox, D. A. Biological therapies: a novel approach to the treatment of autoimmune disease. *Am J Med* 1995; 99: 82–8.

17. Moreland, L. W., Bucy, R. P., Tilden, A., Pratt, P. W., LoBuglio, A. F., Khazaeli, M. *et al*. Use of a chimeric monoclonal anti-CD4 antibody in patients with refractory rheumatoid arthritis. *Arthritis Rheum* 1993; 36: 307–18.

18. Feldmann, M., Brennan, F. M., and Maini, R. N. Role of cytokines in rheumatoid arthritis. *Ann Rev Immunol* 1996; 14: 397–44.

19. Firestein, G. S., and Zvaifler, N. J. How important are T cells in chronic rheumatoid synovitis? *Arthritis Rheum* 1990; 33: 768–73.

20. Katsikis, P., Chu, C. Q., Brennan, F. M., Maini, R. N., and Feldmann, M. Immunoregulatory role of interleukin 10 in rheumatoid arthritis. *J Exp Med* 1994; 179: 1517–27.

21. Nguyen, K. H. Y., and Firestein, G. S. T cells as secondary players in rheumatoid arthritis. In *T cells in arthritis* (Miossec P, van den Berg WB, and Firestein GS, eds), pp. 1–18. Basel: Birkhauser; 1998.

22. Elliott, M. J., Feldmann, M., Kalden, J. R., Antoni, C. Smolen, J. S, Leeb, B. *et al* Randomized double blind comparison of a chimaeric monoclonal antibody to tumor necrosis factor alpha (cA2) versus placebo in rheumatoid arthritis. *Lancet* 1994 344: 1105–10.

23. Stastny, P. Association of the B-cell alloantigen DRw4 with rheumatoid arthritis. *N Engl J Med* 1978; 298: 869–71.

24. Gregersen, P. K., Silver, J., and Winchester, R. J. The shared epitope hypothesis: an approach to understanding the molecular genetics of susceptibility to rheumatoid arthritis. *Arthritis Rheum* 1987; 30: 1205–13.

25. Weyand, C. M., Xie, C., and Goronzy, J. J. Homozygosity for the HLA-DRB1 allele selects for extra-articular manifestations in rheumatoid arthritis. *J Clin Invest* 1992; 89: 2033–9.

26. Weyand, C. M., Hicok, C., Conn, D., and Goronzy, J. J. The influence of HLA-DRB1 genes on disease severity in rheumatoid arthritis. *Ann Intern Med* 1992; 117: 801–6.

27. Evans, T. I., Han, J., Singh, R., and Moxley, G. The genotypic distribution of shared-epitope DRB1 alleles suggests a recessive mode of inheritance of the rheumatoid arthritis disease-susceptibility gene. *Arthritis Rheum* 1995; 38: 1754–61.

28. Moreno, I., Valenzuela, A., Garcia, A., Yelamos, J., Sanchez, B., and Hernanz, W. Association of the shared epitope with radiological severity of rheumatoid arthritis. *J Rheumatol* 1996; 23: 6–9.

29. Gorman, J. D., Lum, R. F., Chen, J. J., Suarez-Almazor, M. E., Thomson, G., and Criswell, L. A. Impact of shared epitope genotype and ethnicity on erosive disease. *Arthritis Rheum* 2004; 50: 400–12.

30. Nepom, G., Byers, P., Seyfried, C., Healey, L. A., Wilske, K. R., Stage, D. *et al*. HLA genes associated with rheumatoid arthritis: identification of susceptibility alleles using specific oligonucleotide probes. *Arthritis Rheum* 1989; 32: 15–21.

31. Wordsworth, B. P., Lanchbury, J. S., Sakkas, L. I., Welsh, K. I., Panayi, G. S., Bell, J. I. *et al*. HLA-DR4 subtype frequencies in rheumatoid arthritis indicate that DRB1 is the major susceptibility locus within the HLA class II region. *Proc Natl Acad Sci U S A* 1989; 86: 10049–53.

32. Takeuchi, F., Matsuta, K., Watanabe, Y., Tokunaga, K., Juji, T., Miyamoto, T. *et al*. Susceptibility epitope on HLA-DR B chain for rheumatoid arthritis and the effect of the positivity on the clinical features. *J Immunogenet* 1989; 16: 475–83.

33. Templin, D., Boyer, G., Lanier, A., Nelson, J., Barrington, R., Jansen, J. *et al*. Rheumatoid arthritis in Tlingit Indians: clinical characterization and HLA associations. *J Rheumatol* 1994; 21: 1238–44.

34. Gao, X., Brautbar, C., Gazit, E., Segal, R., Naparstek, Y., Livneh, A. *et al*. A variant of HLA-DR4 determines susceptibility to rheumatoid arthritis in a subset of Israeli Jews. *Arthritis Rheum* 1991; 34: 547–51.

35. Fries, J., Wolfe, F., Apple, R., Erlich, H., Bugawan, T., Holmes, T. *et al*. HLA-DRB1 genotype associations in 793 white patients from a rheumatoid arthritis inception cohort. *Arthritis Rheum* 2002; 46: 2320–9.

36. del Rincon, I., Battafarano, D., Arroyo, R., Murphy, F., and Escalante, A. Heterogeneity between men and women in the influence of the HLA-DRB1 shared epitope on the clinical expression of rheumatoid arthritis. *Arthritis Rheum* 2002; 46: 1480–8.

37. Reveille J. The genetic contribution to the pathogenesis of rheumatoid arthritis. *Curr Opin Rheumatol* 1998; 10: 187–200.

38. Singal, D., Green, D., Reid, B., Gladman, D., and Buchanan, W. HLA-D region genes and rheumatoid arthritis (RA): importance of DR and DQ genes in conferring susceptibility to rheumatoid arthritis. *Ann Rheum Dis* 1992; 51: 23–8.

39. Zanelli, E., Krco, C., Baisch, J., Cheng, S., and David, C. Immune response of HLA-DQ8 transgenic mice to peptides from the third hypervariable region of HLA-DRB1 correlates with predisposition to rheumatoid arthritis. *Proc Natl Acad Sci U S A* 1996; 93: 1814–19.

40. Pascual, M., Nieto, A., Lopez-Nevot, M., Ramal, L., Mataran, L., Caballero, A. *et al*. Rheumatoid arthritis in southern Spain: toward elucidation of a unifying role of the HLA class II region in disease predisposition. *Arthritis Rheum* 2001; 44: 307–14.

41. Seidl, C., Korbitzer, J., Badenhoop, K., Seifried, E., Hoelzer, D., Zanelli, E. *et al*. Protection against severe disease is conferred by DERRA-bearing HLA-DRB1 alleles among HLA-DQ3 and HLA-DQ5 positive rheumatoid arthritis patients. *Hum Immunol* 2001; 62: 523–9.

42. de Vries, N., van Elderen, C., Tijssen, H., van Riel, P., and van de Putte, L. No support for HLA-DQ encoded susceptibility in rheumatoid arthritis. *Arthritis Rheum* 1999; 42: 1621–7.

43. Wagner, U., Kaltenhauser, S., Pierer, M., Seidel, W., Troltzsch, M., Hantzschel, H. *et al*. Prospective analysis of the impact of HLA-DR and -DQ on joint destruction in recent-onset rheumatoid arthritis. *Rheumatology* 2003; 42: 553–62.

44. Zanelli, E., Breedveld, F., and de Vries R. HLA class II association with rheumatoid arthritis: facts and interpretations. *Hum Immunol* 2000; 61: 1254–61.

45. Fugger, L., and Svejgaard, A. Association of MHC and rheumatoid arthritis: HLA-DR4 and rheumatoid arthritis—studies in mice and men. *Arthritis Res* 2000; 2: 208–11.

46. Pinet, V., Combe, B., Avinens, O., Caillat-Zucman, S., Sany, J., Clot, J. et al. Polymorphism of the HLA-DMA and DMB genes in rheumatoid arthritis. Arthritis Rheum 1997; 40: 854–8.

47. Toussirot, E., Sauvageot, C., Chabod, J., Ferrand, C., Tiberghien, P., and Wendling, D. The association of HLA-DM genes with rheumatoid arthritis in eastern France. Hum Immunol 2000; 61: 303–8.

48. Woulfe, S. L., Bono, C. P., Zacheis, M. L., Kirschmann, D. A., Baudino, T. A., Swearingen, C. et al. Negatively charged residues interacting with the p4 pocket confer binding specificity to DRB1 *0401. Arthritis Rheum 1995; 38: 1744–53.

49. Hammer, J., Gallazzi, F., Bono, E., Karr, R. W., Guenot, J., Valsasnini, P. et al. Peptide binding specificity of HLA-DR4 molecules: correlation with rheumatoid arthritis association. J Exp Med 1995; 181: 1847–55.

50. Szántó, S., Bárdos, T., Szabó, Z., David, C. S., Buzás, E. I., Mikecz, K. et al. Induction of arthritis in HLA-DR4-humanized and HLA-DQ8-humanized mice by human cartilage proteoglycan aggrecan but only in the presence of an appropriate (non-MHC) genetic background. Arthritis Rheum 2004; 50: 1984–95.

51. Kerlan-Candon, S., Louis-Plence, P., Wiedemann, A., Combe, B., Clot, J., Eliaou, J. F. et al. Specific overexpression of rheumatoid arthritis-associated HLA-DR alleles and presentation of low-affinity peptides. Arthritis Rheum 2001; 44: 1281–92.

52. Rosloniec, E., Whittington, K., Zaller, D., and Kang, A. HLA-DR1 (DRB1*0101) and DR4 (DRB1*0401) use the same anchor residues for binding an immunodominant peptide derived from human type II collagen. J Immunol 2002; 168: 253–9.

53. Patil, N., Pashine, A., Belmares, M., Liu, W., Kaneshiro, B., Rabinowitz, J. et al.Rheumatoid arthritis (RA)-associated HLA-DR alleles form less stable complexes with class II-associated invariant chain peptide than non-RA HLA-DR alleles. J Immunol 2001; 167: 7157–68.

54. Hill, J., Southwood, S., Sette, A., Jevnikar, A., Bell, D., and Cairns, E. The conversion of arginine to citrulline allows for a high-affinity peptide interaction with the rheumatoid arthritis-associated HLA-DRB1*0401 MHC class II molecule. J Immunol 2003; 171: 538–41.

55. Kirschmann, D. A., Duffin, K. L., Smith, C. E., Welply, J. K., Howard, S. C., and Schwartz, B. D. Naturally processed peptides from rheumatoid arthritis associated and non-associated HLA-DR alleles. J Immunol 1995; 155: 5655–62.

56. de Vries, N., Tijssen, H., van Riel, P., and van de Putte, L. Reshaping the shared epitope hypothesis: HLA-associated risk for rheumatoid arthritis is encoded by amino acid substitutions at positions 67–74 of the HLA-DRB1 molecule. Arthritis Rheum 2002; 46: 921–8.

57. Vos, K., van der Horst-Bruinsma, I., Hazes, J., Breedveld, F., le Cessie, S., Schreuder, G. et al. Evidence for a protective role of the human leukocyte antigen class II region in early rheumatoid arthritis. Rheumatology 2001; 40: 133–9.

58. Taneja, V., and David, C. Association of MHC and rheumatoid arthritis: regulatory role of HLA class II molecules in animal models of RA—studies on transgenic/knockout mice. Arthritis Res 2000; 2: 205–7.

59. Fox, D. A. Rheumatoid arthritis: heresies and speculations. Perspect Biol Med 1997; 40: 479–91.

60. Zanelli, E., Gonzalez-Gay, M. A., and David, C. Could HLA-DRB1 be the protective locus in rheumatoid arthritis? Immunol Today 1995; 16: 274–8.

61. Nabozny, G. H., Baisch, J. M., Cheng, S., Cosgrove, D., Griffiths, M. M., Luthra, H. S. et al. HLA-DQ8 transgenic mice are highly susceptible to collagen-induced arthritis: a novel model for human polyarthritis. J Exp Med 1996; 183: 27–37.

62. Huizinga, T. Genetics in rheumatoid arthritis. Curr Rheum Reports 2002; 4: 195–200.

63. Tuokko, J., Nejentsev, S., Luukkainen, R., Toivanen, A., and Ilonen, J. HLA haplotype analysis in Finnish patients with rheumatoid arthritis. Arthritis Rheum 2001; 44: 315–22.

64. Snijders, A., Elferink, D., Geluk, A., van Der Zanden, A., Vos, K., Schreuder, G. et al. An HLA-DRB1-derived peptide associated with protection against rheumatoid arthritis is naturally processed by human APCs. J Immunol 2001; 166: 4987–93.

65. Auger, I., Lepecuchel, L., and Roudier, J., Interaction between heat-shock protein 73 and HLA-DRB1 alleles associated or not with rheumatoid arthritis. Arthritis Rheum 2002; 46: 929–33.

66. Maier, J., Haug, M., Foll, J., Beck, H., Kalbacher, H., Rammensee, H. et al Possible association of non-binding of HSP70 to HLA-DRB1 peptide sequences and protection from rheumatoid arthritis. Immunogenetics 2002; 54: 67–73.

67. Walser-Kuntz, D. R., Weyand, C. M., Weaver, A. J., O'Fallon, W. M., and Goronzy, J. J. Mechanisms underlying the formation of the T cell receptor repertoire in rheumatoid arthritis. Immunity 1995; 2: 597–605.

68. Wagner, U., Koetz, K., Weyand, C., and Goronzy, J. Perturbation of the T cell repertoire in rheumatoid arthritis. Proc Natl Acad Sci U S A 1998; 95: 14447–52.

69. Koetz, K., Bryl, E., Spickschen, K., O'Fallon, W., Goronzy, J., Weyand, C. et al. T cell homeostasis in patients with rheumatoid arthritis. Proc Natl Acad Sci U S A 2000; 97: 9203–8.

70. Ponchel, F., Morgan, A., Bingham, S., Quinn, M., Buch, M., Verburg, R. et al. Dysregulated lymphocyte proliferation and differentiation in patients with rheumatoid arthritis. Blood 2002; 100: 4550–6.

71. Albani, S., Keystone, E. C., Nelson, J. L., Ollier, W. E. R., La Cava, A., Montemayor, A. C. et al. Positive selection in autoimmunity: abnormal immune responses to a bacterial dnaJ antigenic determinant in patients with early rheumatoid arthritis. Nat Med 1995; 1: 448–52.

72. Auger, I., Escola, J. M., Gorvel, J. P., and Roudier, J. HLA-DR4 and HLA-DR10 motifs that carry susceptibility to rheumatoid arthritis bind 70–kD heat shock proteins. Nature Med 1996; 2: 306–10.

73. Ollier, W., Kennedy, L., Thomson, W., Barnes, A., Bell, S., Bennett, D. et al. Dog MHC alleles containing the human RA shared epitope confer susceptibility to canine rheumatoid arthritis. Immunogenetics 2001; 53: 669–73.

74. Fox, D. A., and Singer, N. T cell receptor rearrangements in arthritis. In T cells in arthritis (Miossec P, van den Berg WB, and Firestein GS, eds), pp. 19–53. Basel: Birkhauser; 1998.

75. van der Heijden, I., Wilbrink, B., Tchetverikov, I., Schrijver, I., Schouls, L., Hazenberg, M. et al. Presence of bacterial DNA and bacterial peptidoglycans in joints of patients with rheumatoid arthritis and other arthritides. Arthritis Rheum 2000; 43: 593–8.

76. Schrijver, I., Melief, M., Markusse, H., Van Aelst, I., Opdenakker, G., Hazenberg, M. et al. Peptidoglycan from sterile human spleen induces T cell proliferation and inflammatory mediators in rheumatoid arthritis patients and healthy subjects. Rheumatology 2001; 40: 438–46.

77. Schrijver, I., Melief, M., Tak, P., Hazenberg, M., and Laman, J. Antigen-presenting cells containing bacterial peptidoglycan in synovial tissues of rheumatoid arthritis patients coexpress costimulatory molecules and cytokines. Arthritis Rheum 2000; 43: 2160–8.

78. Fazou, C., Yang, H., McMichael, A., and Callan, M. Epitope specificity of clonally expanded populations of CD8+ T cells found within the joints of patients with inflammatory arthritis. Arthritis Rheum 2001; 44: 2038–45.

79. Shadidi, K., Aarvak, T., Jeansson, S., Henriksen, J., Natvig, J., and Thompson, K. T cell responses to viral, bacterial and protozoan antigens in rheumatoid inflammation: selective migration of T cells to synovial tissue. Rheumatology 2001; 40: 1120–5.

80. Albert, L. Infection and rheumatoid arthritis: guilt by association? J Rheumatol 2000; 27: 564–6.

81. Snowden, N., Reynolds, I., Morgan, K., and Holt, L. T cell responses to human type II collagen in patients with rheumatoid arthritis and healthy controls. Arthritis Rheum 1997; 40: 1210–18.

82. Londei, M., Savill, CM., Verhoef, A., Brennan, F., Leech, Z. A., Duance, V. et al. Persistence of collagen type II-specific T-cell clones in the synovial membrane of a patient with rheumatoid arthritis. Proc Natl Acad Sci U S A 1989; 86: 36–40.

83. Verheijden, G. F. M., Rijinders, A. W. M., Bos, E., Coenen-de Roo, C. J., van Staveren, C. J. J., Miltenburg, A. M. M. *et al.* Human cartilage glycoprotein-39 as a candidate autoantigen in rheumatoid arthritis. *Arthritis Rheum* 1997; **40**: 1115–25.

84. Guerassimov, A., Zhang, Y., Banerjee, S., Cartman, A., Leroux, J., Rosenberg, L. *et al.* Cellular immunity to the G1 domain of cartilage proteoglycan aggrecan is enhanced in patients with rheumatoid arthritis but only after removal of keratan sulfate. *Arthritis Rheum* 1998; **41**: 1019–21.

85. Toyosaki, T., Tsuruta, Y., Yoshioka, T., Takemoto, H., Suzuki, R., Tomita, T. *et al.* Recognition of rheumatoid arthritis synovial antigen by CD4+, CD8− T cell clones established from rheumatoid arthritis joints. *Arthritis Rheum* 1998; **41**: 92–100.

86. Cope, A., Patel, S., Hall, F., Coniga, M., Hubers, H., Verheijden, G. *et al.* T cell responses to a human cartilage autoantigen in the context of rheumatoid arthritis-associated and nonassociated HLA-DR4 alleles. *Arthritis Rheum* 1999; **42**: 1497–507.

87. Blass, S., Schumann, F., Hain, N., Engel, J., Stuhlmuller, B., and Burmester, G. p205 is a major target of autoreactive T cells in rheumatoid arthritis. *Arthritis Rheum* 1999; **42**: 971–80.

88. Fritsch, R., Eselbock, D., Skriner, K., Jahn-Schmid, B., Scheinecker, C., Bohle, B. *et al.* Characterization of autoreactive T cells to the autoantigens heterogeneous nuclear ribonucleoprotein A2 (RA33) and filaggrin in patients with rheumatoid arthritis. *J Immunol* 2002; **169**: 1068–76.

89. Wang, J., and Roehrl, M. Glycosaminoglycans are a potential cause of rheumatoid arthritis. *Proc Natl Acad Sci U S A* 2002; **99**: 14362–7.

90. Fang, Q., Sun, Y., Cai, W., Dodge, G., Lotke, P., and Williams, W. Cartilage-reactive T cells in rheumatoid synovium. *Int Immunol* 2002; **12**: 659–69.

91. Kotzin, B., Falta, M., Crawford, F., Rosloniec, E., Bill, J., Marrack, P. *et al.* Use of soluble peptide-DR4 tetramers to detect synovial T cells specific for cartilage antigens in patients with rheumatoid arthritis. *Proc Natl Acad Sci U S A* 2002; **97**: 291–6.

92. Backlund, J., Carlsen, S., Hoger, T., Holm, B., Fugger, L., Kihlberg, J. *et al.* Predominant selection of T cells specific for the glycosylated collagen type II epitope (263–270) in humanized transgenic mice and in rheumatoid arthritis. *Proc Natl Acad Sci U S A* 2002; **99**: 9960–5.

93. Baeten, D., Boots, A., Steenbakkers, P., Elewaut, D., Bos, E., Verheijden, G. *et al.* Human cartilage gp-39+,CD16+ monocytes in peripheral blood and synovium. *Arthritis Rheum* 2000; **43**: 1233–43.

94. Corrigall, V., Bodman-Smith, M., Fife, M., Canas, B., Myers, L., Wooley, P. *et al.* The human endoplasmic reticulum molecular chaperone BiP is an autoantigen for rheumatoid arthritis and prevents the induction of experimental arthritis. *J Immunol* 2001; **166**: 1492–8.

95. Blass, S., Union, A., Raymackers, J., Schumann, F., Ungethum, U., Muller-Steinbach, S. *et al.* The stress protein BiP is overexpressed and is a major B and T cell target in rheumatoid arthritis. *Arthritis Rheum* 2001; **44**: 761–71.

96. Bodman-Smith, M., Corrigall, V., Kemeny, D., and Panayi, G. BiP, a putative autoantigen in rheumatoid arthritis, stimulates IL-10-producing CD8-positive T cells from normal individuals. *Rheumatology* 2003; **42**: 637–44.

97. Rosloniec, E. F., Brand, D. D., Myers, L. K., Whittington, K. B., Gumanovskaya, M., Zaller, D. M. *et al.* An HLA-DR1 transgene confers susceptibility to collagen-induced arthritis elicited with human type II collagen. *J Exp Med* 1997; **185**: 1113–22.

98. Cuesta, I. A., Sud, S., Song, Z., Affholter, J. A., Karvonen, R. L., Fernandez-Madrid, F. *et al.* T cell receptor (Vβ) bias in the response of rheumatoid arthritis synovial fluid T cells to connective tissue antigens. *Scand J Rheumatol* 1997; **26**: 166–73.

99. Baeten, D., Steenbakkers, P. G. A., Rijinders, A. M. W., Boots, A. M., Veys, E. M., and DeKeyser, F. Detection of major histocompatibility complex/human cartilage gp-39 complexes in rheumatoid arthritis synovitis as a specific and independent histologic marker. *Arthritis Rheum* 2004; **50**: 444–51.

100. Van Bilsen, J. H. M., van Dongen, H. V., Lard, L. R., van der Voort, E. I. H., Elferink, D. G., Bakker, A. M. *et al.* Functional regulatory immune responses against human cartilage glycoprotein-39 in health vs. proinflammatory responses in rheumatoid arthritis. *Proc Natl Acad Sci* 2004; **101**: 17180–5.

101. Emery, P., Gentry, K. C., Mackay, I. R., Muirden, K. D., and Rowley, M. Deficiency of the suppressor inducer subset of T lymphocytes in rheumatoid arthritis. *Arthritis Rheum* 1987; **30**: 849–54.

102. Morimoto, C., Romain, P. L., Fox, D. A., Anderson, P., DiMaggio, M., Levine, H. *et al.* Abnormalities in CD4+ T lymphocyte subsets in inflammatory rheumatic diseases. *Am J Med* 1998; **84**: 817–25.

103. Kohem, C. L., Wisbey, H., Tortorella, C., Lipsky, P. E., and Oppenheimer-Marks, N. Enrichment of differentiated CD45RB dim, CD27-memory T cells in the peripheral blood, synovial fluid, and synovial tissue of patients with rheumatoid arthritis. *Arthritis Rheum* 1996; **39**: 844–54.

104. Brennan, F. M., Hayes, A. L., Ciesielski, C. J., Green, P., Foxwell, B. M. J., and Feldmann, M. Evidence that rheumatoid arthritis synovial T cells are similar to cytokine-activated T cells: involvement of phosphatidylinositol 3-kinase and nuclear factor kappaB pathways in tumor necrosis factor alpha production in rheumatoid arthritis. *Arthritis Rheum* 2002; **46**: 31–41.

105. Holoshitz, J., Vila, L. M., Keroack, B. J., McKinley, D. R., and Bayne, N. K. Dual antigenic recognition by cloned γδ T cells. *J Clin Invest* 1992; **89**: 308–14.

106. Tanaka, Y., Morita, C. T., Tanaka, Y., Nieves, E., Brenner, M. B., and Bloom, B. R. Natural and synthetic non-peptide antigens recognized by human gamma delta T cells. *Nature* 1995; **375**: 155–8.

107. Haftel, H. M., Chung, Y., Hinderer, R., Hanash, S., and Holoshitz, J. Induction of the autoantigen proliferating cell nuclear antigen in T lymphocytes by a mycobacterial antigen. *J Clin Invest* 1994; **94**: 1365–72.

108. Lunardi, C., Marguerie, C., Walport, M. J., and So, A. K. T γδ cells and their subsets in blood and synovial fluid from patients with rheumatoid arthritis. *Br J Rheumatol* 1992; **31**: 527–30.

109. Bucht, A., Soderstrom, K., Hultman, T., Uhlen, M., Nilsson, E., Kiessling, R. *et al.* T cell receptor diversity and activation markers in the Vδ1 subset of rheumatoid synovial fluid and peripheral blood T lymphocytes. *Eur J Immunol* 1992; **22**: 567–74.

110. Meliconi, R., Uguccioni, M., D'Errico, A., Cassisa, A., Frizziero, L., and Facchini, A. T-cell receptor γδ positive lymphocytes in synovial membrane. *Br J Rheumatol* 1992; **31**: 59–61.

111. Liu, M., Kohsaka, H., Sakurai, H., Azuma, M., Okumura, K., Saito, I. *et al.* The presence of costimulatory molecules CD86 and CD28 in rheumatoid arthritis synovium. *Arthritis Rheum* 1996; **39**: 110–14.

112. Sfikakis, P., Zografou, A., Viglis, V., Iniotaki-Theodoraki, A., Piskontaki, I., Tsokos, G. *et al.* CD28 expression on T cell subsets in vivo and CD28-mediated T cell response in vitro in patients with rheumatoid arthritis. *Arthritis Rheum* 1995; **38**: 649–51.

113. Schmidt, D., Goronzy, J., and Weyand, C. M. CD4+ CD7− CD28− T cells are expanded in rheumatoid arthritis and are characterized by autoreactivity. *J Clin Invest* 1996; **97**: 2027–37.

114. Vallejo, A., Schirmer, M., Weyand, C., and Goronzy, J. Clonality and longevity of CD4+ CD28null T cells are associated with defects in apoptotic pathways. *J Immunol* 2000; **165**: 6301–7.

115. Wagner, U., Pierer, M., Kaltenhauser, S., Wilke, B., Seidel, W., Arnold, S. *et al.* Clonally expanded CD4+CD28null T cells in rheumatoid arthritis use distinct combinations of T cell receptor BV and BJ elements. *Eur J Immunol* 2003; **33**: 79–84.

116. Bryl, E., Vallejo, A., Weyand, C., and Goronzy, J. Down-regulation of CD28 expression by TNF-a. *J Immunol* 2001; **167**: 3231–8.

117. Warrington, K., Takemura, S., Goronzy, J., and Weyand, C. CD4+,CD28− T cells in rheumatoid arthritis patients combine features of the innate and adaptive immune systems. *Arthritis Rheum* 2001; **44**: 13–20.

118. Namekawa, T., Snyder, M., Yen, J. H., Goehring, B., Leibson, P., Weyand, C. *et al*. Killer cell activating receptors function as costimulatory molecules on CD4+CD28null T cells clonally expanded in rheumatoid arthritis. *J Immunol* 2000; **165**: 1138–45.

119. Groth, V., Bruhl, A., El-Gabalawy, H., Nelson, J., and Spies, T. Stimulation of T cell autoreactivity by anomalous expression of NKG2D and its MIC ligands in rheumatoid arthritis. *Proc Natl Acad Sci* 2003; **100**: 9452–7.

120. Vallego, A. N., Mügge, L. O., Klimiuk, P. A., Weyand, C. M., and Goronzy, J. J. Central role of thrombospondin-1 in the activation and clonal expansion of inflammatory T cells. *J Immunol* 2000; **164**: 2947–54.

121. Fasth, A. E. R., Cao, D., van Vollenhoven, R., Trollmo, C., and Malmström, V. CD28null CD4+ T cells: characterization of an effector memory T-cell population in patients with rheumatoid arthritis. *Scan J Immunol* 2004; **60**: 199–208.

122. Gerli, R., Schillaci, G., Giordano, A., Bocci, E. B., Bistoni, O., Vaudo, G. *et al*. CD4+CD28− T lymphocytes contribute to early atherosclerotic damage in rheumatoid arthritis patients. *Circulation* 2004; **109**: 2744–8.

123. Yen, J., Moore, B., Nakajima, T., Scholl, D., Schaid, D., Weyand, C. *et al*. Major histocompatibility complex class I-recognizing receptors are disease risk genes in rheumatoid arthritis. *J Exp Med* 2001; **193**: 1159–67.

124. Salazar-Fontana, L. I., Sanz, E., Merida, I., Zea, A., Sanchez-Atrio, A., Villa, L. *et al*. Cell surface CD28 levels define four CD4+ T cells subsets: abnormal expression in rheumatoid arthritis. *Clin Immunol* 2001; **99**: 253–65.

125. Bowen, M. A., Patel, D. D., Li, X., Modrell, B., Malacko, A. R., Wang, W. C. *et al*. Cloning, mapping, and characterization of activated leukocyte-cell adhesion molecule [ALCAM], a CD6 ligand. *J Exp Med* 1995; **181**: 2213–20.

126. Saifullah, M. K., Fox, D. A., Sarkar, S., Endres, J., Piktel, J., Haqqi, T. M., and Singer, N. Expression and characterization of a novel CD6 ligand in cells derived from joint and epithelial tissues. *J Immunol* 2004; **173**: 6125–33.

127. Higgs, J. B., Zeldes, W., Kozarsky, K., Schteingart, M., Kan, L., Bohlke, P., Krieger, K. *et al*. A novel pathway of human T lymphocyte activation: identification by a monoclonal antibody generated against a rheumatoid synovial T cell line. *J Immunol* 1998; **140**: 3758–65.

128. Wagner, U. G., Kurtin, P. J., Wahner, A., Brackertz, M., Berry, D. J., Goronzy, J. J. *et al*. The role of CD8+ CD40L+ T cells in the formation of germinal centers in rheumatoid synovitis. *J Immunol* 1998; **161**: 6390–7.

129. Moreland, L. W., Alten, R., Van den Bosch, F., Appelboom, T., Leon, M., Emery, P. *et al*. Costimulatory blockade in patients with rheumatoid arthritis: a pilot dose- finding, double-blind, placebo-controlled clinical trial evaluating CTLA-4Ig and LEA29Y eighty-five days after the first infusion. *Arthritis Rheum* 2002; **46**: 1470–9.

130. Shevach, E. M. Regulatory/suppressor T cells in health and disease. *Arthritis Rheum* 2004; **50**: 2721–4.

131. Baecher-Allan, C., and Hafler, D. A., Suppressor, T. cells in human diseases. *J Exp Med* 2004; **200**: 273–6.

132. Cao, D., Malmström, V., Baecher-Allan, C., Hafler, D., Klareskog, L., and Trollmo, C. Isolation and functional characterization of reg and ulatory CD25bright CD4+ T cells from the target organ of patients with rheumatoid arthritis. *Eur J Immun* 2003; **33**: 215–23.

133. Van Amelsfort, J. M. R., Jacobs, K. M. G., Bijlsma, J. W. J., Lafeber, F. P. J. G., and Taams, L. S. CD4+CD25+ regulatory T cells in rheumatoid arthritis. *Arthritis Rheum* 2004; **50**: 2775–85.

134. Cao, D., van Vollenhoven, R., Klareskog, L., Trollmo, C., and Malmström, V. CD25brightCD4+ regulatory T cells are enriched in inflamed joints of patients with chronic rheumatic disease. *Arthritis Res Ther* 2004; **6**: R335–46.

135. Ehrenstein, M. R., Evans, J. G., Singh, A., Moore, S., Warnes, G., Isenberg, D. A. *et al*. Compromised function of regulatory T cells in rheumatoid arthritis and reversal by anti-TNFα therapy. *J Exp Med* 2004; **200**: 277–85.

136. Choy, E., Scott, D., Kingsley, G., Thomas, S., Murphy, A., Staines, N. *et al*. Control of rheumatoid arthritis by oral tolerance. *Arthritis Rheum* 2001; **44**: 1993–7.

137. Kavanaugh, A., Genovese, M., Baughman, J., Kivitz, A., Bulpitt, K., Olsen, N. *et al*. Allele and antigen-specific treatment of rheumatoid arthritis: a double-blind, placebo controlled phase 1 trial. *J Rheumatol* 2004; **30**: 449–54.

138. Cannons, J. L., Karsh, J., Birnboim, H. C., and Goldstein, R. HRPT-mutant T cells in the peripheral synovial tissue of patients with rheumatoid arthritis. *Arthritis Rheum* 1998; **41**: 1772–82.

139. Firestein, G. S., Yeo, M., and Zvaifler, N. J. Apoptosis in rheumatoid arthritis synovium. *J Clin Invest* 1995; **96**: 1631–8.

140. Koch, A. E., Kunkel, S. L., and Strieter, R. M. Cytokines in rheumatoid arthritis. *J Invest Med* 1995; **43**: 28–38.

141. Oppenheimer-Marks, N., and Lipsky, P. E. Adhesion molecules in arthritis: control of T cell migration into the synovium. In *T cells in arthritis* (Miossec P, van den Berg WB, and Firestein GS, eds), pp. 129–48. Basel: Birkhauser; 1998.

142. Gringhuis, S. I., Leow, A., Papendrecht-van-der, Voort, E. A. M., Remans, P. H. J., Breedveld, F. C., and Verweij, C. L. Displacement of linker for activation of T cells from the plasma membrane due to redox balance alterations results in hyporesponsiveness of synovial fluid T lymphocytes in rheumatoid arthritis. *J Immunol* 2000; **164**: 2170–9.

143. Miossec, P. The Th1/Th2 cytokine balance in arthritis. In *T cells in arthritis* (Miossec P, van den Berg WB, Firestein GS, eds), pp. 93–109. Basel: Birkhauser; 1998.

144. Bakakos, P., Pickard, C., Wong, W., Ayre, K., Madden, J., Frew, A. *et al*. Simultaneous analysis of T cell clonality and cytokine production in rheumatoid arthritis using three-colour flow cytometry. *Clin Exp Immunol* 2002; **129**: 370–8.

145. Gerli, R., Bistoni, O., Russano, A., Fiorucci, S., Borgato, L., Cesarotti, M. *et al*. In vivo activated T cells in rheumatoid synovitis: analysis of Th1- and Th2-type cytokine production at clonal level in different stages of disease. *Clin Exp Immunol* 2002; **129**: 549–55.

146. Santiago-Schwarz, F., Anand, P., Liu, S., and Carsons, S. E. Dendritic cells (DCs) in rheumatoid arthritis (RA): progenitor cells and soluble factors contained in RA synovial fluid yield a subset of myeloid DCs that preferentially activate Th1 inflammatory-type responses. *J Immunol* 2001; **167**: 1758–68.

147. Firestein, G., and Zvaifler, N. Peripheral blood and synovial fluid monocyte activation in inflammatory arthritis. II. Low levels of synovial fluid and synovial tissue interferon suggest that γ-interferon is not the primary macrophage activating factor. *Arthritis Rheum* 1987; **30**: 864–71.

148. Canete, J., Martinez, S., and Farres, J. Differential Th1/Th2 cytokine patterns in chronic arthritis: interferon γ is highly expressed in synovium of rheumatoid arthritis compared with seronegative spondyloarthropathies. *Ann Rheum Dis* 2000; **59**: 263–8.

149. Morita, Y., Yamamura, M., Kawashima, M., Harada, S., Tsuji, K., Shibuya, K. *et al*. Flow cytometric single-cell analysis olf cytokine production by CD4+ T cells in synovial tissue and peripheral blood from patients with rheumatoid arthritis. *Arthritis Rheum* 1998; **41**: 1669–76.

150. Wong, W., Vakis, S., Ayre, K., Ellwood, C., Howell, W., Tutt, A. *et al*. Rheumatoid arthritis T cells produce Th1 cytokines in response to stimulation with a novel trispecific antibody directed against CD2, CD3, and CD28. *Scand J Rheumatol* 2002; **29**: 282–7.

151. Maeda, T., Yamada, H., Nagamine, R., Shuto, T., Nakashima, Y., Hirata, G. *et al*. Involvement of CD4+, CD57+ T cells in the disease activity of rheumatoid arthritis. *Arthritis Rheum* 2002; **46**: 379–84.

152. Morita, Y., Yamamura, M., Nishida, K., Harada, S., Okamoto, H., Inoue, H. *et al*. Expression of interleukin-12 in synovial tissue from patients with rheumatoid arthritis. *Arthritis Rheum* 1998; **41**: 306–14.

153. McInnis, I., Al-Mughales, J., Field, M., Leung, B. P., Huang, F. P., Dixon, R. *et al*. The role of interleukin-15 in T cell migration and activation in rheumatoid arthritis. *Nature Med* 1996; **2**: 175–82.

154. Gracie, J., Forsey, R., Chan, W., Gilmour, A., Leung, B., Greer, M. et al. A pro-inflammatory role for interleukin-18 in rheumatoid arthritis. *J Clin Invest* 1999; **104**: 1393–401.

155. Yamamura, M., Kawashima, M., Taniai, M., Yamauchi, H., Tanimoto, T., Kurimoto, M. et al. Interferon-gamma-inducing activity of interleukin-18 in the joint with rheumatoid arthritis. *Arthritis Rheum* 2001; **44**: 275–85.

156. Komai-Koma, M., Gracie, J., Wei, X., Xu, D., Thomson, N., McInnes, I. et al. Chemoattraction of human T cells by IL-18. *J Immunol* 2003; **170**: 1084–90.

157. Park, C., Morel, J., Amin, M., Connors, M., Harlow, L., and Koch, A. Evidence of IL-18 as a novel angiogenic mediator. *J Immunol* 2001; **167**: 1644–53.

158. Miossec, P., Naviliat M., Dupuy d'Angeac, A., Sany, J., and Banchereau, J. Low levels of interleukin-4 and high levels of transforming growth factor beta in rheumatoid arthritis. *Arthritis Rheum* 1990; **33**: 1180–7.

159. Davis, L., Cush, J., Schulze-Koops, H., and Lipsky, P. Rheumatoid synovial CD4+ T cells exhibit a reduced capacity to differentiate into IL-4 producing T-helper-2 effector cells. *Arthritis Res* 2001; **3**: 54–64.

160. Hessian, P., Highton, J., Kean, A., Sun, C., and Chin, M. Cytokine profile of the rheumatoid nodule suggests that it is a Th1 granuloma. *Arthritis Rheum* 2003; **48**: 334–8.

161. Husby, G., and Williams, R. Immunohistochemical studies of interleukin-2 and interferon-γ in rheumatoid arthritis. *Arthritis Rheum* 1985; **28**: 174–81.

162. Firestein, G., Xu, W., Townsend, K., Broide, D., Alvaro-Gracia, J., Glasebrook, A. et al. Cytokines in chronic inflammatory arthritis. I. Failure to detect T cell lymphokines (interleukin 2 and interleukin 3) and presence of macrophage colony-stimulating factor (CSF-1) and a novel mast cell growth factor in rheumatoid synovitis. *J Exp Med* 1998; **168**: 1573–86.

163. Tagaya, Y., Bamford, R., DeFilippis, A. P., and Waldmann, T. A. IL-15: a pleiotropic cytokine with diverse receptor/signaling pathways whose expression is controlled at multiple levels. *Immunity* 1996; **4**: 329–36.

164. Masuko-Hongo, K., Kurokawa, M., Kobata, T., Nishioka, K., Kato, T. et al. Effect of IL15 on T cell clonality in vitro and in the synovial fluid of patients with rheumatoid arthritis. *Ann Rheum Dis* 2000; **59**: 688–94.

165. Mottonen, M., Isomaki, P., Luukkainen, R., Toivanen, P., Punnonen, J., and Lassila, O. Interleukin-15 up-regulates the expression of CD154 on synovial fluid T cells. *Immunol* 2000; **100**: 238–44.

166. Chabaud, M., Fossiez, F., Taupin, J. L., and Miossec, P. Enhancing effect of IL-17 on IL-1-induced IL-6 and leukemia inhibitory factor production by rheumatoid arthritis synoviocytes and its regulation by Th2 cytokines. *J Immunol* 1998; **161**: 409–14.

167. Miossec, P. Interleukin-17 in rheumatoid arthritis: if T cells were to contribute to inflammation and destruction through synergy. *Arthritis Rheum* 2003; **48**: 594–601.

168. Kehlen, A., Thiele, K., Riemann, D., and Langner, J. Expression, modulation and signalling of IL-17 receptor in fibroblast-like synoviocytes of patients with rheumatoid arthritis. *Clin Exp Immunol* **127**: 539–46.

169. Chabaud, M., Lubberts, E., Joosten, L., van Den Berg, W., and Miossec, P. IL-17 derived from juxta-articular bone and synovium contributes to joint degradation in rheumatoid arthritis. *Arthritis Res* 2001; **3**: 168–77.

170. Ziolkowska, M., Koc, A., Luszczykiewicz, G., Ksiezopolska-Pietrzak, K., Kllimczak, E., Chwalinska-Sadowska, H. et al. High levels of IL-17 in rheumatoid arthritis patients: IL-15 triggers in vitro IL-17 production via cyclosporin A-sensitive mechanism. *J Immunol* 2000; **164**: 2832–8.

171. Bush, K., Farmer, K., Walker, J., and Kirkham, B. Reduction of joint inflammation and bone erosion in rat adjuvant arthritis by treatment with interleukin-17 receptor IgG1 Fc fusion protein. *Arthritis Rheum* 2002; **46**: 802–5.

172. Morand, E., Bucala. R., and Leech, M. Macrophage migration inhibitory factor: an emerging therapeutic target in rheumatoid arthritis. *Arthritis Rheum* 2003; **48**: 291–9.

173. Gravallese, E., and Goldring, S. Cellular mechanisms and the role of cytokines in bone erosions in rheumatoid arthritis. *Arthritis Rheum* 2000; **43**: 2143–51.

174. Lam, J., Takeshita, S., Barker, J., Kanagawa, O., Ross, F., Teitelbaum, S. et al. TNF-α induces osteoclastogenesis by direct stimulation of macrophages exposed to permissive levels of RANK ligand. *J Clin Invest* 2000; **106**: 1481–8.

175. Yudoh, K., Matsuno, H., Nakazawa, F., Yonezaw, T., Kimura, T. et al. Reduced expression of the regulatory CD4+ T cell subset is related to Th1/Th2 balance and disease severity in rheumatoid arthritis. *Arthritis Rheum* 2000; **43**: 617–27.

176. Klareskog, L., Forsum, U., Scheynius, A., Kabelitz, D., and Wigzell, H. Evidence in support of a self-perpetuating HLA-DR-dependent delayed-type cell reaction in rheumatoid arthritis. *Proc Natl Acad Sci U S A* 1982; **70**: 3632–6.

177. Waalen, K., Forre, O., and Natvig, J. B. Dendritic cells in rheumatoid inflammation. *Springer Semin Immunopathol* 1988; **10**: 141–56.

178. Zvaifler, N. J., Steinman, R. M., Kaplan, G., Lau, L. L., and Rivelis, M. Identification of immunostimulatory dendritic cells in the synovial effusions of patients with rheumatoid arthritis. *J Clin Invest* 1985: **76**: 789–800.

179. Tsai, V., and Zvaifler, N. J. Dendritic cell-lymphocyte clusters that form spontaneously in rheumatoid arthritis synovial effusions differ from clusters formed in human mixed leukocyte reactions. *J Clin Invest* 1988; **82**: 1731–45.

180. Aggarwal, S., Ghilardi, N., Xie, M. H., de Sauvage, F. J., and Gurney, A. L. Interleukin-23 promotes a distinct CD4 T cell activation state characterized by the production of interleukin-17. *J Biol Chem* 2003; **278**: 1910–14.

181. Yamamura, Y., Gupta, R., Morita, Y., He, X., Chung, K., Freiberg, A. et al. Effector function of resting T cells: activation of synovial fibroblasts. *J Immunol* 2001; **166**: 2270–5.

182. Burger, D., and Dayer, J. M. The role of human T lymphocyte-monocyte contact in inflammation and tissue destruction. *Arthritis Res* 2002; **4**: S169–S176.

183. McInnes, I. B., Leung, B. P., and Liew, F. Y. Cell-cell interactions in synovitis: interactions between T lymphocytes and synovial cells. *Arthritis Res* 2000; **2**: 374–8.

184. Unutmaz, D., Pileri, P., and Abrignani, S. Antigen-independent activation of naïve memory resting T cells by a cytokine combination. *J Exp Med* 1994; **180**: 1159–64.

185. Foey, A., Green, P., Foxwell, B., Feldmann, M., and Brennan, F. Cytokine-stimulated T cells induce macrophage IL-10 production dependent on phosphatidylinositol 3-kinase and p70S6K: implications for rheumatoid arthritis. *Arthritis Res* 2002; **4**: 64–70.

186. Kotake, S., Udagawa, N., Hakoda, M., Mogi, M., Yano, K., Tsuda, E. et al. Activated human T cells directly induce osteoclastogenesis from human monocytes: possible role of T cells in bone destruction in rheumatoid arthritis patients. *Arthritis Rheum* 2001; **44**: 1003–12.

187. Roosnek, E., and Lanzavecchia, A. Efficient and selective presentation of antigen-antibody complexes by rheumatoid factor B cells. *J Exp Med* 1997; **173**: 487–9.

188. Patil, N. S., Hall F. C., Drover, S., Spurrell, D. R., Bos, E., Cope, A. P. et al. Autoantigenic HCgp39 epitopes are presented by the HLA-DM-dependent presentation pathway in human B cells. *J Immunol* 2001; **166**: 33–41.

189. Takemura, S., Klimiuk, P. A., Braun, A., Goronzy, J. J., and Weyand, C. M. T cell activation in rheumatoid synovium is B cell dependent. *J Immunol* 2001; **167**: 4710–18.

190. Nakatsuka, K., Tanaka, Y., Shubscher, S., Abe, M., Wake, A., Saito, K. et al. Rheumatoid synovial fibroblasts are stimulated by the cellular adhesion to T cells through lymphocyte function associated antigen-1/intercellular adhesion molecule-1. *J Rheumatol* 1997; **24**: 458–64.

191. Miranda-Carus, M. E., Balsa, A., Benito-Miguel, M., Pérex de Ayala, C., and Martíin-Mola, E. IL-15 and the initiation of cell contact-dependent synovial fibroblast-T lymphocyte cross-talk in

rheumatoid arthritis: effect of methotrexate. *J Immunol* 2004; **173**: 1463–76.

192. Cho, M. L., Yoon, C. H., Hwang, S. Y., Park, M. K., Min, S. Y., Lee, S. H. *et al.* Effector function of type II collagen-stimulated T cells from rheumatoid arthritis patients: cross-talk between T cells and synovial fibroblasts. *Arthritis Rheum* 2004; **50**: 776–84.

193. Zimmermann, T., Kunischm, E., Pfeiffer, R., Hirth, A., Stahl, H. D., Sack, U. *et al.* Isolation and characterization of rheumatoid arthritis synovial fibroblasts from primary culture: primary culture cells markedly differ from fourth-passage cells. *Arthritis Res* 2001; **3**: 72–6.

194. Boots, A. M., Wimmers-Bertens, A. J. and Rijnders, A. W. Antigen-presenting capacity of rheumatoid synovial fibroblasts. *Immunology* 1994; **82**: 268–74.

195. Tsai, C., Diaz, L. A., Jr, Singer, N. G., Li, LL, Kirsch, A.H., Mitra R. *et al.* Responsiveness of human T lymphocytes to bacterial superantigens presented by cultured rheumatoid arthritis synoviocytes. *Arthritis Rheum* 1669; **39**: 125–36.

196. Corrigall, V. M., Solau-Gervais, E., and Panayi, G. S. Lack of CD80 expression by fibroblast-like synoviocytes leading to anergy in T lymphocytes. *Arthritis Rheum* 2000; **43**: 1606–15.

197. Fox, D. A. The role of T cells in the immunopathogenesis of rheumatoid arthritis. *Arthritis Rheum* 2000; **4**: 598–609.

198. Arend, W. The innate immune system in rheumatoid arthritis. *Arthritis Rheum* 2001; **44**: 2224–34.

199. Klinman, D. Does activation of the innate immune system contribute to the development of rheumatoid arthritis? *Arthritis Rheum* 2003; **48**: 590–3.

7 | *The role of neutrophils in the pathogenesis of rheumatoid arthritis*

W. Winn Chatham, Jeffrey C. Edberg, and Robert P. Kimberly

Introduction

The classical paradigm of the loss of tolerance as a breakdown in the discrimination between self and non-self and as central to the development of autoimmune disease has been challenged by more recent insights into the innate immune system[1,2]. Rather than positing recognition of non-self as opposed to self as the pivotal event in an acquired immune response, the distinctions between infectious/non-infectious and between dangerous/not dangerous may be the critical elements[3–6]. These distinctions, often made by components of the innate immune system[7–10], regulate the delivery of a 'second signal' to T cells that is required for development of an acquired immune response. Given the central role of innate immunity in this perspective, a re-consideration of the contributions of the neutrophil, as well as those of macrophages and natural killer cells, to autoimmunity and chronic inflammatory diseases such as rheumatoid arthritis is timely.

Classically, studies of the role of the neutrophil have focused on its role in effector mechanisms of inflammation and in the enzymatic degradation of cartilage with the development of cartilage erosions (reviewed in Refs 11, 12). Neutrophils elaborate LTB4, IL-8, TGF-β, and GRO-α, powerful chemoattractants that recruit other neutrophils and mononuclear cells to the rheumatoid joint. Neutrophils synthesize IL-1, and in the context of the rheumatoid joint, corresponding synthesis of IL-1ra may be down-regulated, thereby producing a net balance favoring IL-1. Neutrophils have the capacity for a potent oxidative burst with the production of superoxide, hydrogen peroxide, and, in the presence of myeloperoxidase, hypochlorous acid. Among their many effects, these reactive oxygen intermediates, working in conjunction with granule enzymes, can depolymerize hyaluronic acid, decrease the viscosity of synovial fluid, and generate free hyaluronic acid capable of altering cartilage proteoglycan synthesis. More recently, nitric oxide synthase has been demonstrated in the primary granules of neutrophils[13–14], and an important role for neutrophils in the generation of the potent oxidant peroxynitrite (ONOO-) and in the nitration and chlorination of tyrosine residues has been identified[15–18]. Indeed, elevated nitrite levels have been identified in synovial fluid and other body fluids of rheumatoid arthritis patients[19–25] and rheumatoid arthritis (RA) synovial tissues are substantially nitrosylated.

The intracellular granules of neutrophils contain a variety of potent degradative enzymes, which in the context of oxidant-mediated enhancement of protease activity[26] are capable of cartilage destruction. Neutrophils are found at the pannus–cartilage junction, where they secrete procollagenase, elastase, and other degradative enzymes[27–29]. Cartilage from rheumatoid arthritis patients contains immunoglobulin embedded in the superficial layers[30–32], and partially degraded cartilage can bind anticollagen antibodies. Such surface-bound immunoglobulin effectively displays ligand for specific immunoglobulin receptors expressed on the neutrophil plasma membrane. Engagement of surface-bound Ig promotes cell adhesion to cartilage and may create a restricted subjacent space inaccessible to antiproteinases at the same time that it amplifies both the production of oxidants and the exocytosis of granules into that space. This milieu, with elastase, cathepsin G, and oxidants to activate collagenase, facilitates further cartilage degradation and destruction.

Each of these activities provides an important role for neutrophils in the pathogenesis of rheumatoid arthritis, but they do not address the potential for neutrophils to help shape the nature of the acquired immune response[33–38], or to provide targets for the acquired immune response through delivery of granule proteins[39–43], or through chemical modification of other endogenous proteins rendering them antigenic. Furthermore, the classical framework for the roles of neutrophils has not considered the role of oxidants as modulators of the intracellular redox state and of signal transduction capacity[44], nor has it considered the potential for oxidants to induce somatic mutations in key regulatory genes which might facilitate a transformed phenotype for synoviocytes[45]. When one adds the recent recognition that neutrophil Fcγ receptors bind ligands of both the innate (C reactive protein)[46,47] and acquired (IgG) immune systems, that complement receptors recognizing C3b selectively regulate the degranulation of primary azurophilic granules[48,49], and that genetic polymorphisms in these receptors substantially alter function[50–52], a much more complex role for neutrophils in rheumatoid arthritis becomes evident. Indeed the presence of a 'neutrophil signature' in the transcriptome of leukocytes in some inflammatory diseases, the identification of the important role for neutrophils in the KRN model of rheumatoid arthritis and the recognition of IL-17, the T cell-derived cytokine associated with autoimmune disease, as a potent chemoattractant for neutrophils each underscore an exciting frontier in neutrophil biology for the pathogenesis and treatment of rheumatoid arthritis and other inflammatory diseases[53–55].

Neutrophil structure and function

Neutrophils, basophils, and eosinophils have distinct developmental lineages, with neutrophils sharing a progenitor with the monocytic lineage distinct from basophils and eosinophils. All granulocytic cells are rich in cytoplasmic granules but are distinguished from each other by, among other things, the composition of these granules[56]. Neutrophil granules contain a variety of catalytic and degradative enzymes (see below) and show no preference for acidic or basic stains. In contrast, basophil granules are rich in histamine and react with basic dyes while eosinophil granules contain cationic granule proteins with high affinity for eosin and other acidic stains. Neutrophils, the predominant granulocyte in blood and synovial fluid, are important sources of inflammatory mediators. As they participate in inflammatory reactions, they respond to microbial products as well as to mediators of both the innate and acquired immune systems[57]. These mediators include myeloid and lymphoid-derived cytokines, lipid-based mediators, immunoglobulin aggregates, and complement split-products (especially C3 and C5 derived products).

Degranulation

The neutrophil has four distinct intracellular granular organelles: the primary (azurophilic), secondary (specific), and tertiary (gelatinase) granules, and the secretory vesicle[58–60]. The primary granules appear first during neutrophil maturation and comprise approximately one-third of the granule content in mature neutrophils. Primary granules contain hydrolases, proteases, peroxidases, and a diverse group of cationic antimicrobial proteins. In addition to secretion of contents through exocytosis, these granules fuse with the intracellular phagolysosomal vacuole formed during phagocytosis and facilitate the killing and degradation of internalized microorganisms. Myeloperoxidase, a major constituent of primary granules and the enzyme responsible for the characteristic yellow-green color of pus, is critical for the conversion of hydrogen peroxide to microbiocidal hypochlorous acid. Primary granules also include elastase, cathepsins D and G, and proteinase 3, each of which has been implicated in inflammatory tissue damage: elastase can cleave collagen cross-linkages, proteoglycans, and the elastin components of vessels and supporting tissues; cathepsin G is a broad spectrum protease that activates latent collagenase; and proteinase 3 is a potent serine protease.

Secondary granules appear later in neutrophil maturation at the metamyelocyte stage and contain leukocyte-specific proteins, lactoferrin, and vitamin B_{12}-binding protein. These granules are more easily mobilized for exocytosis than primary granules and their contents have an important role in regulating the inflammatory response[58–60]. In this regard, specific granules contain numerous cell surface-associated proteins including the β2 integrin CD11b/CD18, which is also a receptor of the C3 split product iC3b, and receptors for laminin, vitronectin, thrombospondin, tumor necrosis factor, and formyl peptides. An important component of the NADPH oxidase complex, cytochrome b558, is also contained within specific granule membranes. Specific granules also contain procollagenase, heparanase, plasminogen activator, and the chitinase YKL-40 (HC gp-39) that is also expressed in articular cartilage[42,43]. Procollagenase, when activated by oxidants or cathepsins, can degrade type I and type II collagen and, to a lesser degree, type III collagen[11,61]. Collagen breakdown products have chemotactic activity towards neutrophils, monocytes, and fibroblasts[11].

At times, constituents of granules may be the target of an acquired immune response[39–41,62]. The occurrence of antineutrophil cytoplasmic antibodies (ANCA) with specificity for granule proteins provides an additional novel mechanism for neutrophil activation[63,64]. In patients with RA, the most common ANCA target is the secondary (specific) granule component lactoferrin. Given the recent insight that the HC gp-39 (YKL-40) chitinase is also expressed in neutrophil secondary granules and in human cartilage[42,43], acquired immune responses to this protein may result in a specific anticartilage reaction leading to cartilage destruction as well as an antineutrophil reaction promoting neutrophil activation[63,64].

Some constituents are found in several different types of granules. For example CD11b/CD18 is found in secondary granules, tertiary granules, and secretory vesicles. Nonetheless, differential regulation of the granule organelles in the degranulation response is an important determinant of the neutrophil response at sites of inflammation. This regulation is determined by the nature and intensity of the activation signal and can be modified by counterbalancing receptor-specific negative signals[65]. Variations in the intensity of both the activating and de-activating signals may reflect genetic polymorphisms in membrane-associated receptors[51,52].

The oxidative burst

The neutrophil respiratory burst is characterized by increased consumption of oxygen and the generation of multiple pro-inflammatory and cytotoxic products (reviewed in Refs 66, 67). Activated through cell surface receptors for Fc region of immunoglobulin, complement activation (C5a, C1q), lipid mediators (PAF, LTB_4), or bacterial products (lipopolysaccharide (LPS), fMLP), the respiratory burst starts with the assembly of the NADPH oxidase complex. This complex is composed of the membrane-associated cytochrome b558 which contains an α-chain ($gp91^{phox}$) and a β-chain ($p22^{phox}$). This flavin (FAD)-binding complex also binds NADPH and contains two heme groups. Upon proper activation, three cytosolic proteins ($p67^{phox}$, $p47^{phox}$, and $p21^{rac}$) associate with flavocytochrome b558 to form the complete oxidase. Once assembled, NADPH is the electron donor for the oxidase that converts O_2 to superoxide (O_2^-) with the generation of $NADP + H^+$. Superoxide can be transported across membranes via anion channels, and while it probably does not have direct toxic effects, it is a precursor or substrate for formation of other toxic products, including singlet oxygen, hydroxyl radical, $OH^•$, and hydrogen peroxide and peroxynitrite[16]. Hydrogen peroxide can also be produced directly from divalent oxygen through the action of glucose oxidase or from dismutation of superoxide generated by xanthine oxidase. In a reaction catalyzed by myeloperoxidase, hydrogen peroxide may be used as a substrate for the generation of hypochlorous acid (HOCl), a regulator of protease activity. The most toxic of all of these compounds may be the hydroxyl radical, a powerful one-electron oxidant capable of reacting with a wide range of compounds to form new radicals that can then oxidize other substrates.

Soluble mediators of inflammation

Lipid-derived inflammatory mediators produced by neutrophils include eicosanoids and leukotrienes (reviewed in Ref. 68). Activation of neutrophils by cell surface receptors can induce phospholipase activity. Phospholipase A_2 releases arachidonic acid from the sn-2 position of membrane phospholipids which then can be metabolized by the cyclo-oxygenase and lipoxygenase pathways. Prostaglandins and thromboxanes (particularly PGE_2 and PGI_2), products of the cyclo-oxygenases, enhance vascular permeability, can potentiate the effects of agents such as histamine and bradykinin, and enhance pain perception. In some models, however, PGE_2 can have an anti-inflammatory effect, probably through increased cAMP production. Metabolism of arachidonic acid by the lipoxygenase pathway can lead to the production of mono-, di-, and trihydroxyeicosatetraenoic acids (HETEs)—precursors of leukotrienes. These lipid-derived mediators can also have potent pro-inflammatory effects. 5,12-HETE is pro-inflammatory through its leukocyte chemoattractant activity, and LTB4, in addition to being chemoattractant, stimulates cell adhesion, superoxide anion generation, and degranulation. Generation of these lipid mediators, by both the cyclo-oxygenase and lipoxygenase pathways, are important mechanisms for perpetuation of the chronic inflammatory reaction typically observed in the affected joints of patients with RA.

Cytokines

While the release of degradative enzymes and the generation of reactive oxygen intermediates by neutrophils are widely appreciated, the role of neutrophils in modulating the inflammatory reaction through production of cytokines has been less clear. Careful analysis of the biosynthetic capacity of neutrophils, however, has shown that these cells can activate transcription in response to stimulation. The synthesis and secretion of cytokines[35–37], T cell chemoattractants including α-defensins[69], and B cell stimulatory factors such as BLyS[70,71] can play an important role in shaping both the inflammatory response and the corresponding adaptive immune response (reviewed in Ref. 72). Indeed, constituents of rheumatoid synovial fluid can delay neutrophil apoptosis, thereby extending the opportunity for cytokine synthesis[73]. Of the cytokines typically found in rheumatoid synovial fluid, IL-1β, IL-6, IL-8, TNF (tumor necrosis factor)-α, TGF-β, and IL-1ra can all be released by neutrophils. The ability of neutrophils to be transcriptionally active should not come as a great surprise given the ample evidence of receptor-mediated activation of intracellular signaling cascades known to lead to the activation of transcription factors in other cell types. For example both the ras pathway and the MAP kinase pathways are active in neutrophils[11,74] and probably play a key regulatory role in the ability of neutrophils to modulate inflammation through the secretion of cytokines.

Neutrophil surface receptors

Neutrophils respond to inflammatory mediators through cell surface receptors, and our knowledge of the mechanisms by which these receptors regulate neutrophil function has increased substantially. For instance the complexity in the signaling cascades initiated by neutrophil surface receptors extends beyond G protein-mediated signals to networks of phosphorylation/dephosphorylation reactions and formation of lipid-based signaling intermediates. Furthermore, there is increased recognition of the role of antigen non-specific pattern recognition systems in regulating inflammatory reactions[2–6].

The range of stimuli that a neutrophil encounters includes chemotactic factors and chemokines, adhesion receptors/counter-receptors, immunoglobulin and complement breakdown products in the context of immune complexes, cytokines and lymphokines, lipid-based mediators such as prostaglandins and leukotrienes, and reactive oxygen/nitrogen-based compounds. While a detailed consideration of all of the receptors for these agonists and the mechanisms by which they activate neutrophils is well beyond the scope of this chapter, there are a number of general principles important for consideration.

Chemokine receptors

The ability of neutrophils to migrate to sites of inflammation is regulated by a variety of chemotactic factors that include bacterially derived peptides such as fMLP, complement fragments (especially C5a), and chemokines. These agonists can also initiate degranulation and the oxidative burst. Neutrophils express three chemokine receptors, CXCR1, CXCR2, and CXCR4, which bind to CXC chemokines such as IL-8, melanoma growth stimulatory activity (GROα/β/γ), neutrophil activating peptide 2 (NAP-2), epithelial activating peptide 78 (ENA78), granulocyte chemotactic protein 2 (GCP-2), and stromal-derived factor (SDF-1)[75,76]. RA synovial fluid neutrophils also express CCRL2, an orphan receptor with homology to CC chemokine receptors. Expression of this receptor mediates neutrophil responses to CCL2, CCL5, CCL7, and CCL8[77,78].

Intense investigation of chemokines and chemokine receptors has identified structural polymorphisms both in chemokines and their receptors[79–81]. The 32 bp deletion in CCR5, which has an allele frequency approaching 0.10, blocks the uptake of human immunodeficiency virus (HIV), and is associated with delay in HIV disease progression, provides a compelling example of an association between a polymorphism and clinical phenotype[79,81]. Such findings open up the possibility that polymorphisms in the chemokine receptor family or in chemokines themselves may also play a role in chronic inflammatory diseases such as RA. Indeed, preliminary data suggest that homozygosity of the CCR5⁻ allele might protect against RA[82]. Insight into mechanisms of functional blockade of receptor binding or inhibition of receptor function may also be fruitful areas of future investigation.

Perhaps not surprisingly given the common functional responses elicited by chemotactic agents, the receptors for each of these factors share many common structural and functional features[11,82–84]. All members of the superfamily of seven-transmembrane-domain family of receptors signal through heterotrimeric GTP-binding proteins. Typically, upon ligand binding, a *Bordetella pertussis*-toxin-sensitive G protein, usually of the $G\alpha_{i2}$ type, initiates a signaling cascade leading to activation of a phosphatidyl-inositol-specific phospholipase C, small GTPases, Src-family protein tyrosine kinases, and phosphatidylinositol-3-OH (PI-3) kinases.

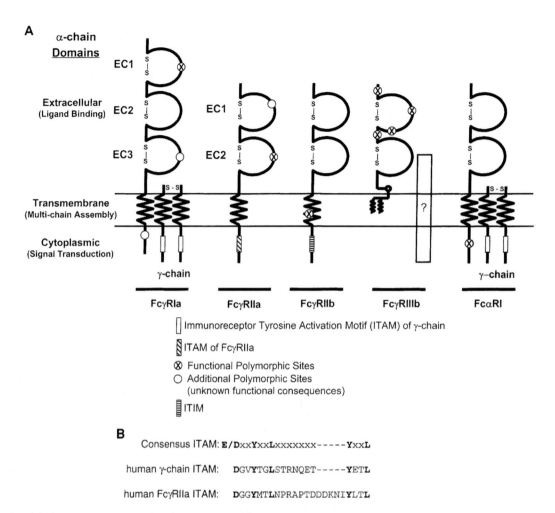

Fig. 7.1 Immunoglobulin receptors expressed on human neutrophils. (A) Human neutrophils constitutively express two receptors for IgG (FcγRIIa and FcγRIIIb) and a receptor for IgA Fc*a*RI. Upon stimulations with IFNγ or IL-10, neutrophils can also express the FcγRIa IgG receptor. These homologous receptors share certain structural and functional domains and motifs. In the extracellular ligand-binding domains, all of these receptors have two or three immunoglobulin-like domains. In the cytoplasmic domain (except FcγRIIIb), an ITAM is necessary for receptor-induced cell activation. The Fcγ receptors are most homologous and form a group of gene families on the q arm of chromosome 1. Fc*a*RI is also homologous to the Fcγ receptors but more distantly related than the Fcγ receptors are to each other. The gene for Fc*a*RI has been mapped to the q arm of chromosome 19 and it probably diverged from a common ancestor gene early in the evolution of immunoglobulin receptors. (B) The ITAM expressed in the cytoplasmic domains of γ-chain and FcγRIIa are similar but distinct. The primary sequence differences in these ITAMs can lead to distinct activation phenotypes.

Phospholipase C activation leads to the production of IP$_3$ which releases intracellular Ca^{2+}, leading to a transient rise in cytosolic Ca^{2+} concentration and diacylglycerol which activates protein kinase C. The rise in cytosolic Ca^{2+} is required for granule release and superoxide production but is probably not required for cytoskeletal reorganization. PI-3 kinases can be activated by the β/γ subunit of G proteins, small GTPases or Src-family tyrosine kinases. The small GTPases are particularly important in the formation of the oxidase complex and for regulation of cytoskeletal rearrangements involving adhesion and chemotaxis. They can also activate phospholipase D. If specificity can be achieved, therapeutic targeting of neutrophil chemotaxis and activation by IL-8, C5a, or other chemoattractants represents an attractive goal in RA.

Adhesion receptors

After initial neutrophil interaction with chemotactic agonists, adhesion receptors play an important role in altering neutrophil activation. The process of neutrophil margination in the vessel, adherence to endothelial cells, and transmigration are all active processes that are mediated by specific adhesion receptor interactions[85]. Initial interactions between neutrophils and activated endothelial cells involve binding of L selectin on the neutrophil with its receptor on endothelial cells. This interaction promotes rolling of neutrophils along the endothelial cells leading to firm adhesion mediated by the β$_2$ integrin CD11b/CD18 binding to ICAM-1 on the endothelial cell. The initial L selectin-mediated binding may also up-regulate CD11b/CD18 expression on neutrophils[86]. Engagement and cross-linking of CD11b by its counter-receptor can activate neutrophils at the same time that it leads to an enhanced rate of apoptosis through CD11b-mediated oxidant production[87,88]. This may be a mechanism by which the neutrophils can limit their own pro-inflammatory potential and suggests that interruption of the carefully orchestrated interplay of adhesion molecules may have some unanticipated results. For example murine models of arthritis in P selectin knockout mice may have a more severe, rather than less severe, phenotype[89].

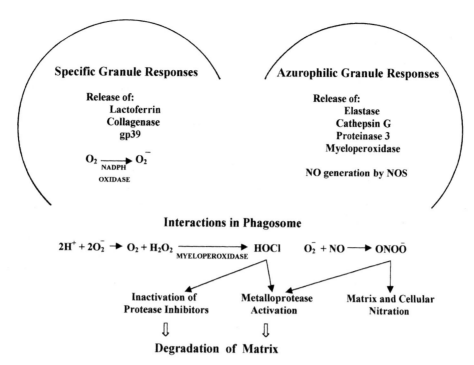

Fig. 7.2 Neutrophil responses to tissue-adherent immune complexes. Ligation of Fc receptors results in release of specific and azurophilic granule proteinases into phagolysosomes in concert with activation of oxidant-generating enzymes. Oxidative modification of enzymes and regulatory proteins by phagosome reaction products promotes the enzymatic degradation of adjacent tissue matrix. Oxidants derived from superoxide and nitric oxide may furthermore modify cellular functions or engender somatic mutations.

Receptors for immunoglobulins

Another class of receptors that are potent activators of neutrophils are the receptors for the Fc region immunoglobulin. Most important for RA are the receptors for the Fc region of IgG (FcγR) and for the Fc region of IgA (FcαR) (reviewed in Refs 50–52, 90). Neutrophils constitutively express two distinct FcγR, FcγRIIa (CD32) and FcγRIIIb (CD16), and a receptor of IgA (FcαRI) (Fig. 7.1). Activation of neutrophils can lead to the appearance of another IgG receptor (FcγRIa) and up-regulation of FcαRI. Engagement of Fc receptors, upon cross-linking by immune complexes, by ANCA or by surface-absorbed Ig, results in activation of neutrophils, triggering the respiratory burst, degranulation, and phagocytosis (or frustrated phagocytosis on surfaces) (Fig. 7.2). While the mechanisms by which each of these receptors signal are distinct, there are a number of common themes[91]. These receptors do not use G protein signaling pathways, but they do engage tyrosine kinase-dependent signaling pathways, first involving an Src-family kinase (such as fgr) and then activation of the p72 syk kinase and PI-3 kinase. Unlike FcγRIIIb, neutrophil FcγRIa and FcγRIIa receptors use an immunoreceptor tyrosine activation motif (ITAM) that is required for the initial activation steps. FcγRIIIb is an extremely interesting receptor due to its linkage to the outer leaflet of the membrane through a glycosyl–phosphatidyl–inositol (GPI) linkage and its lack of any transmembrane or cytoplasmic domains. This receptor is clearly an active participant in neutrophil activation[92,93] and current models of signaling by GPI-anchored proteins involve the partitioning of these receptors to distinct lipid domains in the membrane that are enriched for other lipid-associated Src-kinases on the inner leaflet of the membrane[94,95].

Both constitutive neutrophil Fcγ receptors are polymorphic, and the FcγRIIa-H131/R131 and FcγRIIIb-NA1/NA2 polymorphisms open the possibility of functionally different IgG-induced responses between individuals[50–52]. In fact, the polymorphisms of these receptors have been correlated with risk to certain bacterial infections (reviewed in Ref. 94). Precedent for the importance of FcγR allelic polymorphisms in human autoimmune disease has been established by association of alleles of FcγRIIa and FcγRIIIa with SLE[52,96–99]. Corresponding association studies of FcγRIIIa have been reported in patients with RA, and the allelic distribution in patients with RA may alter the magnitude or vigor of IgG-induced neutrophil activity in patients with disease.

The H131/R131 polymorphism of FcγRIIa, the result of a single nucleotide change in the second extracellular immunoglobulin-like domain changing histidine to arginine at amino acid 131, alters the binding of IgG2 (reviewed in Refs 51, 52). The H131 allele is the only FcγR that binds IgG2 and is associated with an increased risk of heparin-induced thrombocytopenia in patients with autoimmune antiphospholipid syndrome. Conversely, the R131 allele, which binds IgG2 poorly, has been associated with certain bacterial infections and with systemic lupus erythematosus (SLE) in some ethnic groups. Another polymorphic site is found at residue 27 in the first extracellular Ig-like domain and predicts a glutamine to tryptophan change, but there is no known functional significance associated with this polymorphism. A rare substitution in codon 127, changing a glutamine to lysine, restores moderate IgG2 binding in the context of the low-binding R131 allele. The H131 allele may have increased affinity for IgG3.

The two commonly recognized allelic forms of FcγRIIIb, NA1 and NA2, were originally defined serologically. More recently, sequencing of the genes encoding the alleles has revealed five polymorphic residues. Systematic analysis of FcγRIIIb sequence from donors of the two allotypes indicates that there are two predominant genotypes that differ from each other by four amino acids in the first extracellular Ig-like domain. Combinatorial grouping of these sites to yield a larger number of alleles does not occur. The NA1 and NA2 alleles have different quantitative levels of function despite comparable binding of IgG-opsonized erythrocytes (reviewed in Refs 51, 52). Donors homozygous for the NA1 allele demonstrate a larger FcγR-mediated phagocytic response owing, at least in part, to quantitative differences in the ability of this allele to elicit a larger oxidative burst and/or degranulation response. Although the molecular basis for the higher level of function of the NA1 allele has not been determined, the NA1 and NA2 alleles have different numbers of glycosylation sites and are differentially glycosylated *in vivo*. These post-translational modifications may mediate interactions between FcγRIIIb and the β2 integrin, CD11b/CD18, in the neutrophil membrane[100] and as a result alter net receptor function. The NA1/NA2 alleles appear to have clinical significance[96]. Donors homozygous for the NA1 allele are more resistant to certain bacterial infections. In addition, donors homozygous for NA2 may be more likely to have severe infection especially in the context of the low IgG2-binding R131-allele of FcγRIIa. Theoretically, these polymorphisms may govern the intensity of the neutrophil contribution to disease in patients with RA.

Complement receptors

In addition to a seven-transmembrane-domain receptor for C5a which is critical for neutrophil recruitment in inflammatory lesions[101], neutrophils express two distinct receptors for opsonic fragments of complement. Complement receptor type 1 (CR1, CD35) has highest affinity for C3b but can also bind iC3b while CR3 (CD11b/CD18) binds iC3b[102,103]. CR1 is a member of the regulator of complement activation (RCA) family. Members of this family share a common extracellular structural domain, the short consensus repeat (SCR). Multiple SCRs are grouped into larger repeating structures called long homologous repeats (LHR). In contrast to CR1, CR3 is a β2 integrin composed of two structurally distinct chains, α_M and β2. In addition to binding iC3b, CD11b/CD18 (CR3) also binds to ICAM-1, fibrinogen, β-glucan, and possibly LPS. Functionally, CR3 is important in the transendothelial migration of neutrophils and monocytes[86]. There is also increasing evidence that CR3 is associated in the membrane with many other cell surface receptors such as CD14 (receptor for LPS), CD87 (the uPA receptor) and Fcγ receptors (both FcγRIIa and FcγRIIIb)[100]. These associations may alter the biology of these receptors.

It has long been appreciated that complement opsonization of immune complexes results in more effective stimulation of neutrophils, suggesting that complement receptors and Fc receptors interact in some way[104]. The ability of CR3 to synergize with FcγR in stimulation of phagocytosis and the respiratory burst has now been directly documented[92,93] and, as mentioned above, some studies have suggested physical association in the membrane

between FcγR and CR3[100]. While association may occur between these receptor systems, distinct signaling pathways are activated[105]. Synergism might result by convergence of these pathways on common signaling intermediates. More importantly, these results demonstrate the complexity of neutrophil biology and show that analysis of single receptor systems might not reflect the full functional capacity of the cell.

More intriguing is the recent observation that engagement of CR1 selectively down-modulates IgG-induced release of azurophilic granules[48]. Treatment of cells with the protein kinase C activator PMA leads to threonine and/or serine phosphorylation of CR1[106], but the mechanism(s) by which CR1 specifically alters the azurophilic degranulation response is not well characterized. The absence of tyrosine residues in the cytoplasmic domain of CR1 suggests, at least, that tyrosine phosphorylation pathways are not important. However, the ability of CR1 to attenuate IgG-induced primary granule release indicates that the interaction between complement opsonization and Fc receptors is more complex than synergism for activation.

Cytokine receptors

Activation of neutrophils can lead to the synthesis and/or secretion of cytokines, and, given the expression of receptors for multiple cytokines by the neutrophil, both autocrine and paracrine regulation of responses are possible. Of particular importance in the pathogenesis of RA, neutrophils have receptors for cytokines such as IL-8 (discussed above), IL-1 (reviewed in Ref. 107), and TNF-α (see below).

TNF-α has attracted particular attention given the clinical efficacy of anti-TNF therapy in RA[108]. TNF-α can prime neutrophils, facilitate neutrophil adhesion through β2 integrins, induce neutrophil secretion of both IL-1b and TNF, and stimulate oxidase activity[12,109,110]. The two structurally distinct high affinity receptors for TNF-α (p55 and p75) on neutrophils may mediate different functional responses[111]. The p55 TNFRI is able to induce all of the known responses, and mAb inhibition studies indicate a role for the p75 TNFRII in the induction of the oxidative burst. TNFRII may be required for a full neutrophil response to TNF-α perhaps through cooperative binding of TNF-α by the two receptors. This observation suggests a model in which the p75 receptor is the initial TNF-α capture receptor that facilitates presentation of the cytokine to TNFRI, especially at low concentrations of TNF-α. Nonetheless, the ability of TNF-α to induce oxidase activity and cytokine secretion and to prime neutrophils for enhanced responses to other stimuli (such as chemotactic factors and IgG[112,113]) underscores the complexity of neutrophils' responses in the inflammatory milieu and demonstrates the inter-relationship between the many receptor systems that are likely to be important for neutrophils in inflammatory diseases.

Rheumatoid synovial fluid can also contain GM-CSF, which can prime neutrophils and retard apoptosis[114]. In fact, most agents that can prime neutrophils also retard the induction of apoptosis, resulting in more sustained functional responses[115]. This delay in cell death could be an important mechanism by which chronic inflammatory reactions are perpetuated. Certainly, prolonged neutrophil survival could lead to more sustained release of IL-8, IL-1b, and TNF-α, thereby facilitating cellular transmigration and infiltration.

Receptors for lipopolysaccharide

One of the most potent neutrophil activators is LPS. While this bacterial product may not be of primary importance in the pathogenesis of RA, the study of the mechanisms by which LPS activates neutrophils is nonetheless instructive. Indeed, recent studies on the mechanisms of LPS stimulation of leukocytes have led to the recognition of the importance of an entirely new receptor system, the Toll-like receptors[8-10].

LPS is a potent stimulus that can elicit cytokine secretion, adhesion, degranulation, and an oxidative burst[7,116,117]. Paradoxically, we know little about the LPS recognition system(s) at the membrane that are necessary for these varied and robust responses[7]. The ability of LPS to activate neutrophils at low concentrations of ≤ 1ng ml^{-1} is dependent on the GPI-anchored protein CD14 on the surface of the cells. However, LPS binds most effectively to CD14 after first binding to a serum lipopolysaccharide-binding protein (LBP) and/or soluble CD14. Until very recent studies of the mammalian homologues of the *Drosophila* Toll receptor protein, the mechanism of CD14 activation of the intracellular signaling events has remained unclear. Toll is directly involved in host defense in *Drosophila*, and cross-linking the mammalian Toll-like receptor can induce cell activation leading to production of proinflammatory cytokines[9,118]. There are now five known human homologs of the Toll protein, and the link between LPS binding and the Toll-like receptors has now been established[8-10]. The resultant activation is further enhanced by the addition of CD14, and while expression of Toll-like receptors in human neutrophils has not yet been examined, it is likely that the same or a similar pathway will be important. The role of the Toll-like family of receptors in chronic inflammatory diseases such as RA is now an open question and a clear reminder that much remains to be learned.

Neutrophils in rheumatoid arthritis

Neutrophils in rheumatoid synovial fluid

Neutrophils that have emigrated into rheumatoid joints retain the ability to engage immune complexes and respond to inflammatory cytokines. The constitutively expressed Fc receptors, FcγRIIa and FcγRIIIb, show some variability in expression levels, reflecting activation and shedding of FcγRIIIb[119-122], and FcγRIa is up-regulated on synovial fluid neutrophils[116,117]. In response to ligation of Fc receptors, synovial fluid-derived neutrophils produce superoxide-derived oxidants and release both specific and azurophilic granule enzymes. These cells also retain the capacity for liberation of lipid mediators such as LTB$_4$[123,124], but the extent to which IL-1, IL-8, and other inflammatory cytokines are synthesized and secreted by rheumatoid synovial fluid neutrophils has not been established[125,126].

Alteration and degradation of articular cartilage

The consequences of neutrophil activation within the joint depend upon the activating ligand(s), cytokine milieu, site of activation, and genetic factors governing the neutrophil response. In response to fluid phase ligands, release of azurophilic granule constituents including elastase, cathepsin G, and myeloperoxidase may be limited[127]. Furthermore, the abundance of proteinase inhibitors present in normal as well as inflamed synovial fluids probably inactivate proteinases released by fluid phase neutrophils. However, immunoglobulins of the IgG and IgA classes on and within the surface layers of articular cartilage[31,128] can engage neutrophil Fc receptors and result in neutrophil activation with alteration of subjacent articular cartilage[30,129].

Surface-adherent immunoglobulins are potent stimuli for the release of both specific and azurophilic granule proteinases and for the generation of oxidants such as HOCl which can activate procollagenase[127,130]. IgG and IgA-triggered production of superoxide and release of specific granule-derived metalloproteinases (including collagenase) into phagolysosomes accompanied by myeloperoxidase derived from azurophilic granules favors the generation of HOCl and activation of latent metalloproteinases[131,132]. Other azurophilic granule-derived enzymes, including cathepsin G and possibly nitric oxide synthase, are also capable of enhancing the activity of latent metalloproteinases[133-135]. Furthermore, by inactivating tissue or synovial fluid proteinase inhibitors, HOCl generated within the phagolysosome promotes the activity of neutrophil serine proteases such as cathepsin G and elastase[136]. In a variety of *in vitro* models, neutrophil engagement of immunoglobulins adherent to matrix proteins results in degradation of adjacent matrix, even within the milieu of proteinase inhibitors or synovial fluid[137,138]. This model has been extended to explants of human articular cartilage pretreated with immunoglobulins derived from RA synovial fluid, whereby degradation of collagens and proteoglycans in the explant occurs during incubation with neutrophils in synovial fluids[139].

Histological studies of rheumatoid joints and studies with cartilage explants provide compelling evidence that neutrophils engage, and are capable of altering the articular surface. Cartilage-adherent neutrophils have been observed at the cartilage–pannus interface, and neutrophils have been shown to adhere to rheumatoid cartilage explants[30,140,141]. Immunohistochemical studies, enzymatic assays, and assays for enzyme-inhibitor complexes identifying the presence of neutrophil granule constituents, including elastase in the superficial layers of rheumatoid cartilage and at sites of erosion by synovial pannus, all provide 'footprint' evidence of neutrophil activation on the articular surface of rheumatoid joints *in vivo*[131,142].

Footholds: immune responses and evolution of the synovial pannus

Degradation of the superficial layers of articular cartilage by elastase and collagenase promotes binding of immunoglobulins to articular cartilage, including the specific binding of autoantibodies to type II collagen[143]. The binding of such autoantibodies may reflect the unmasking of 'hidden' collagen epitopes, and the alteration of articular surfaces by neutrophils may be a critical early step in the pathogenesis of RA. Indeed, the presence of immunodominant T cell-activating epitopes within type II collagen peptides after degradation by neutrophil gelatinase supports the concept that neutrophil proteases acting on cartilage substrates may promote immune responses within rheumatoid joints[144]. Through reactions catalyzed by myeloperoxidase, neutrophil-derived oxidants promote covalent cross-linking of cartilage-associated immunoglobulins, rendering them relatively insoluble to extraction[145,146]. Superoxide radicals may interact with nitric oxide generated by neutrophils or adjacent chondrocytes to generate species that oxidize and cross-link immune complexes on articular surfaces[147]. Although studies in this area are still evolving, oxidative modification and nitration of articular structures may result in the generation of additional immunogenic neoepitopes, resulting in antigen-driven production of autoantibodies. Indeed, the presence of antibodies to modified lipoproteins has established the precedent for production of antibodies to oxidized proteins[148,149], and the proliferative responses to oxygen radical or peroxynitrite modified aggregates of IgG by T cells derived from RA patients suggest that oxidative as well as proteolytic modification of immune complexes and articular structures may lead to self-perpetuating immune responses and inflammation within the joint. The production and release of BLyS by neutrophils in the same environment, especially in the synovium, may amplify the acquired immune response to these modified epitopes. While normally adaptive in enhancing responses to pathogens, such a neutrophil-driven amplification loop may enhance the intensity of the disease process.

Degradation of the articular surface by neutrophils also promotes the attachment of rheumatoid synovial fibroblasts to cartilage *in vitro*[150]. Both neutrophil serine protease and metalloproteinase-mediated alterations in cartilage facilitate fibroblast attachment[144,150], which suggests that alteration of the articular surface and enhancement of synoviocyte attachment to cartilage might be a critical event in the evolution of erosive anthropathy[151].

Oxidants and synovial cell and synovial fluid biology

Neutrophil activation within inflamed joints may also impact upon the properties of synovial fluid. Oxidants such as HOCl are capable of degrading proteoglycans and hyaluronate via oxidation of N-acetyl groups on chondroitin sulfate, hyaluronic acid, and N-acetylglucosamine[152,153]. Since high molecular weight polymers of hyaluronic acid have been shown to attenuate neutrophil phagocytic responses and inhibit release of proteoglycan from cartilage explants, depolymerization and breakdown of hyaluronate mediated by neutrophil-derived oxidants may further promote the degradation of articular cartilage[154,155]. Depolymerization of hyaluronate polymers within synovial fluid may also result in heightened nociceptive processes within rheumatoid joints. Indirect evidence for increased joint pain in RA as a result of the loss of hyaluronate polymerization is provided by at least one pilot study in which sequential injection of high molecular hyaluronate (normally used for management of knee osteoarthritis) into rheumatoid knees resulted in pain relief[156].

Although the impact of neutrophil activation directly on synovial tissues has received less attention, oxidants and the release of granule constituents can create a potent, toxic microenvironment. Somatic mutations in the p53 tumor suppressor gene have recently been described in the synovial lining cells of the rheumatoid pannus[45] and mutations of this and other genes regulating cell growth and adhesion may account for the invasive/proliferative phenotype of rheumatoid pannus. Although the mechanism(s) whereby such mutations occur have not been elucidated, products of nitration reactions have demonstrated mutagenic capacity[157], and there is evidence of abundant nitration reactions occurring within rheumatoid synovium. In addition to generating chlorinated oxidants such as HOCl, myeloperoxidase released from neutrophil granules can promote nitration reactions capable of altering cellular function[16,147]. It is certainly conceivable that neutrophils activated within or adjacent to the synovium may promote +mutagenic events in the synovium by:

(1) producing superoxide, which then reacts with nitric oxide (NO) (generated by the neutrophils or adjacent monocyte/macrophages and chondrocytes) to form reactive ONOO⁻ species;

(2) generating HOCl, which can react with ONOO⁻ to form mutagenic nitrosyl chloride species; and

(3) releasing myeloperoxidase, which catalyzes nitration events.

The interplay between neutrophils, their reaction products, and synovial biology should provide a fertile area of investigation for elucidating mechanisms of disease in RA.

References

1. Steinman, L., Escape from 'horror autotoxicus': pathogenesis and treatment of autoimmune disease. *Cell* 1995; **80**: 7–10.
2. Medzhitov, R., and Janeway, C. A., Jr. Innate immunity: the virtues of a nonclonal system of recognition. *Cell* 1997; **91**: 295–8.
3. Fearon, D. T., and Locksley, R. M. The instructive role of innate immunity in the acquired immune response. *Science* 1996; **272**: 50–4.
4. Fearon, D. T. Seeking wisdom in innate immunity. *Nature* 1997; **388**: 323–4.
5. Medzhitov, R., and Janeway, C. A., Jr. Innate immunity: impact of the adaptive immune response. *Current Opinion Immunol* 1997; **9**: 4–9.
6. Matzinger, P. Tolerance, danger, and the extended family. *Annu Rev Immunol* 1994; **12**: 991–1045.
7. Ulevitch, R. J. and Tobias, P. S. Receptor-dependent mechanisms of cell stimulation by bacterial endotoxin. *Annu Rev Immunol*, 1995; **13**: 437–57.
8. Kirschning, C. J., Wesche, H., Ayres, T. M., and Rothe, M. Human Toll-like receptor 2 confers responsiveness to bacterial lipopolysaccharide. *J Exp Med* 1998; **188**: 2091–7.

9. Yang, R. B., Mark, M. R., Gray, A., Huang, A., Xie, M. H., Zhang, M. *et al*. Toll-like receptor-2 mediates lipopolysaccharide-induced cellular signaling. *Nature* 1998; **17**: 284–8.

10. Poltorak, A., He, X., Smirnova, I., Liu, M. Y., van Huffel, C., Du, X. *et al*. Defective LPS signaling in C3H/HeJ and C57L/10ScCr mice: mutations in Tlr4 gene. *Science* 1998; **282**: 2085–8.

11. Pillinger, M. H., and Abramson, S. B. The neutrophil in rheumatoid arthritis. *Rheum Dis Clin North Am* 1995; **21**: 691–714.

12. Edwards, S. W., and Hallett, M. B. Seeing the wood for the trees: the forgotten role of neutrophils in rheumatoid arthritis. *Immunol Today* 1997; **18**: 320–4.

13. Ogilvie, A. C., Hack, C. E., Wagstaff, J., van Mierlo, G. J., Erenberg, A. J., Thomsen, L. L. *et al*. IL-1 beta does not cause neutrophil degranulation but does lead to IL-6, IL-8 and nitrite/nitrate release when used in patients with cancer. *J Immunol* 1996; **156**: 389–94.

14. Evans, T. J., Buttery, L. D., Carpenter, A., Springhall, D. R., Polak, J. M., and Cohen, J. Cytokine-treated human neutrophils contain inducible nitric oxide synthase that produces nitration of ingested bacteria. *Proc Natl Acad Sci U S A* 1996; **93**: 9553–8.

15. Domigan, N. M., Charlton, T. S., Duncan, M. W., Winterbourn, C. C., and Kettle, A. J. Chlorination of tyrosyl residues in peptides by myeloperoxidase and human neutrophils. *J Biol Chem* 1995; **270**: 16542–8.

16. Eiserich, J. P., Hristova, M., Cross, C. E., Jones, A. D., Freeman, B. A., Halliwell, B., and van der Vliet, A. Formation of nitric oxide-derived inflammatory oxidants by myeloperoxidase in neutrophils. *Nature* 1998; **391**: 393–7.

17. Sampson, J. B., Ye, Y., Rosen, H., and Beckman, J. S. Myeloperoxidase and horseradish peroxidase catalyze tyrosine nitration in proteins from nitrite and hydrogen peroxide. *Arch Biochem Biophys* 1998; **356**: 207–13.

18. Gagnon, C., Leblond, F. A., and Filep, J. G. Peroxynitrite production by human neutrophils, monocytes and lymphocytes challenged with lipopolysaccharide. *FEBS Lett* 1998; **431**: 107–10.

19. Farrell, A. J., Blake D. R., Palmer, R. M. J., and Moncada, S. Increased concentrations of nitrite in synovial fluid and serum samples suggest increased nitric oxide synthesis in rheumatic diseases. *Ann Rheum Diseases* 1992; **51**: 1219–22.

20. Kaur, H., and Halliwell, B. Evidence for nitric oxide-mediated oxidative damage in chronic inflammation: nitrotyrosine in serum and synovial fluid from rheumatoid patients. *FEBS Lett* 1994; **350**: 9–12.

21. Stichtenoth, D.O., Fauler, J., Zeidler, H., and Frolich, J. C. Urinary nitrate excretion is increased in patients with rheumatoid arthritis by prednisolone. *Ann Rheum Dis* 1995; **54**: 820–4.

22. Grabowski, P. S., England, A. J., Dykhuizen, R., Copland, M., Benjamin, N., Reid, D. M., and Ralston, S. H. Elevated nitric oxide: production in rheumatoid arthritis: detection using the fasting urinary nitrate:creatinine ratio. *Arthritis Rheum* 1996; **39**: 643–7.

23. Wigand, R., Meyer, J., Busse, R., and Hecker, M. Increased serum NG-hydroxy-L-arginine in patients with rheumatoid arthritis and systemic lupus erythematosus as an index of an increased nitric oxide synthase activity. *Ann Rheum Dis* 1997; **56**: 330–2.

24. Hilliquin, P., Borderie, D., Hervann, A., Menkes, C. J., and Ekindjian, O. G. Nitric oxide as S-nitrosoproteins in rheumatoid arthritis. *Arthritis Rheum* 1997; **40**: 1512–17.

25. Sandhu, J. K., Robertson S., Birnboim H. C., and Goldstein R. Distribution of protein nitrotyrosine in synovial tissues of patients with rheumatoid arthritis and osteoarthritis. *J Rheumatol* 2003; **30**: 1173–81.

26. Okamoto, T., Akaike, T., Nagano, T., Miyajima, S., Suga, M., Ando, M. *et al*. Activation of human neutrophil procollagenase by nitrogen dioxide and peroxynitrite: a novel mechanism for procollagenase activation involving nitric oxide. *Arch Biochem Biophys* 1997; **342**: 261–74.

27. Menninger, H., Putzier, R., Mohr, W., Wessinghage, D., and Tillmann, K. Granulocyte elastase at the site of cartilage erosion by rheumatoid synovial tissue. *Z Rheumatol* 1980; **39**: 145–6.

28. Mohr, W., Westerhellweg, H., and Wessinghage, D. Polymorphonuclear granulocytes in rheumatic tissue destruction. III. An electron—microscopic study of PMNs at the pannus cartilage junction in rheumatoid arthritis. *Ann Rheum Dis* 1981; **40**: 396–9.

29. Mohr, W. Cartilage destruction via the synovial fluid in rheumatoid arthritis. *J Rheumatol* 1995; **22**: 1436–8.

30. Ugai, K., Ziff, M., and Jasin, H. E. Interaction of polymorphonuclear leukocytes with immune complexes trapped in joint collagenous tissues. *Arthritis Rheum* 1979; **22**: 353–64.

31. Ugai, K., Ishikawa, H., Hirohata, K., and Shirane, H. Interaction of polymorphonuclear leukocytes with immune complexes trapped in rheumatoid articular cartilage. *Arthritis Rheum* 1983; **26**: 1434–41.

32. Jasin, H. E. Autoantibody specificities of immune complexes sequestered in articular cartilage of patients with rheumatoid arthritis and osteoarthritis. *Arthritis Rheum* 1985; **28**: 241–8.

33. Staite, N. D., Messner, R. P., and Zoschke, D. C. Inhibition of human T lymphocyte E rosette formation by neutrophils and hydrogen peroxide: differential sensitivity between helper and suppressor T lymphocytes. *J Immunol* 1987; **139**: 2424–30.

34. Hirohata, S., Yanagida, T., Yoshino, Y., and Miyashita, H. Polymorphonuclear neutrophils enhance suppressive activities of anti-CD3 induced CD4+ suppressor T cells. *Cellular Immunol* 1995; **160**: 270–7.

35. Romani, L., Bistoni, F., and Puccetti, P. Initiation of T-helper cell immunity to Candida albicans by IL-12H: the role of neutrophils. *Chemical Immunol* 1997; **68**: 110–35.

36. Romani, L., Mencacci, A., Cenci, E., Del Sero, G., Bistoni, F., and Puccetti, P. An immunoregulatory role for neutrophils in CD4+ T helper subset selection in mice with candidiasis. *J Immunol* 1997; **158**: 2356–62.

37. Romani, L., Mencacci, A., Cenci, E., Spaccapelo, R., Del Sero, G., Nicoletti, I. *et al*. Neutrophil: production of IL-12 and IL-10 in candidiasis and efficacy of IL-12 therapy in neutropenic mice. *J Immunol* 1997; **158**: 5349–56.

38. Mencacci, A., Del Sero, G., Cenci, d'Ostiani, C. F., Bacci, A., Montagnoli, C., Kopf, M., and Romani, L. Endogenous interleukin 4 is required for development of protective CD4+ T helper type 1 cell responses to Candida albicans. *J Exp Med* 1998; **187**: 307–17.

39. Bosch, X., Llena, J., Collado, A., Font, J., Mirapeix, E., Ingelmo, M. *et al*. Occurrence of antineutrophil cytoplasmic and antineutrophil (peri)nuclear antibodies in rheumatoid arthritis. *J Rheumatol* 1995; **22**: 2038–45.

40. Braun, M. G., Csernok, E., Schmitt, W. H., and Gross, W. L. Incidence, target antigens, and clinical implications of antineutrophil: cytoplasmic antibodies in rheumatoid arthritis. *J Rheumatol* 1996; **23**: 826–30.

41. Rother, E., Schochat, T., and Peter, H. H. Antineutrophil cytoplasmic antibodies (ANCA) in rheumatoid arthritis: a prospective study. *Rheumatol Int* 1996; **15**: 231–17.

42. Volck, B., Price, P. A., Johansen, J. S., Sorensen, O., Benfield, T. L., Nielsen, H. J. *et al*. YKL-40, a mammalian member of the chitinase family, is a matrix protein of specific granules in human neutrophils. *Proc Assoc Am Physicians* 1998; **110**: 351–60.

43. Baeten, D., DeKeyser, F., Elewaut, D., Rijnders, A. M. W., Verheijden, G. F., Miltenburg, A. *et al*. HC gp-39 expression is synovial lining is correlated with joint destruction in RA. *Arthritis Rheum* 1998; **41**: S365.

44. Nakamura, N., Nakamura, K., and Yodoi, J. Redox regulation of cellular activation. *Ann Rev Immunol* 1997; **15**: 351–69.

45. Firestein, G. S., Echeverri, F., Yeo, M., Zvaifler, N. J., and Green, D. R. Somatic mutations in the p53 tumor suppressor gene in rheumatoid arthritis synovium. *Proc Natl Acad Sci U S A* 1997; **94**: 10895–900.

46. Bharadwaj, D., Stein, M. P., Volzer, M., Mold, C., and Du Clos, T. W. The major receptor for C-reactive protein on leukocytes is Fcγ Receptor II. *J Exp Med* 1999; **190**: 585–90.

47. Marnell, L. L., Mold, C., Volzer, M. A., Burlingame, R. W., and Du Clos, T. W. C-reactive protein binds to Fc gamma RI in transfected COS cells. *J Immunol* 1995; **155**: 2185–93.

48. Sambandam, T., and Chatham, W. W. Ligation of CR1 attenuates Fc receptor-mediated myeloperoxidase release and HOCl production by neutrophils. *J Leukoc Biol* 1998; **63**: 477–85.

49. Chatham, W. W. and Blackburn, W. D., Jr. Fixation of C3 to IgG attenuates neutrophil HOCl generation and collagenase activation. *J Immunol* 1993; **151**: 949–58.

50. Edberg, J. C., Salmon, J. E., and Kimberly, R. P. Functional capacity of Fc gamma receptor III (CD16) on human neutrophils. *Immunol Res* 1992; **11**: 239–51.

51. Kimberly, R. P., Salmon, J. E., and Edberg, J. C. Receptors for immunoglobulin G: molecular diversity and implications for disease. *Arthritis Rheum* 1995; **38**: 306–14.

52. Gibson, A. W., Wu, J. Edberg, J. C., and Kimberly R. P. Diversity in Fc receptors. In *Lupus: cellular and molecular pathogenesis* (Kammer, G., and Tsokos, G., eds), pp. 557–73. Totawa, NJ: Humana Press; 1999.

53. Bennett, L., Palucka, A. K., Arce, E., Cantrell, V., Borvak, J., Banchereau, J., and Pascual, V. Interferon and granulopoiesis signatures in systemic lupus erythematosus blood. *J Exp Med* 2003; **197**: 681–5.

54. Ji, H., Ohmura, K., Mahmood, U., Lee, D. M., Hofhuis, F. M., Boackle, S. A. et al. Arthritis critically dependent on innate immune system players. *Immunity* 2002; **16**: 157–68.

55. Stark, M. A., Huo, Y., Burcin, M. A., Olson, T. S., and Ley, K. Phagocytosis of apoptotic neutrophils regulates granulopoiesis via IL-23 and IL-17 *Immunity* 2005; **22**: 285–94.

56. Henson, P. M., Henson, J. E., Fittschen, C., Bratton, D. L., and Riches, D. W. H. Degranulation and secretion by phagocytic cells. In *Inflammation: basic principles and clinical correlates*, 2nd edn (Gallin, J. I., Goldstein, I. M., and Snyderman, R., eds), pp. 511–39. New York: Raven Press; 1992.

57. Abramson, J. S., and Wheeler, J. G. (1993). *The neutrophil*. IRL Press at Oxford University Press, Oxford.

58. Borregarrd, N., and Cowland, J. B. Granules of human neutrophilic polymorphonuclear leukocytes. *Blood* 1997; **89**: 3503–21.

59. Gullsberg, U., Andersson, E., Garwicz, D., Lindmark, A., and Olsson, I. Biosynthesis, processing and sorting of neutrophil proteins: insights into neutrophil granule development. *Eur J Haemat* 1997; **58**: 137–53.

60. Khanna-Gupta, A., Zibello, T., and Berliner, N. Coordinate regulation of neutrophil secondary granule protein expression. *Curr Top Microbiol Immunol* 1996; **211**: 165–71.

61. Muller-Ladner, U., Gay, R. E., and Gay, S. Molecular biology of cartilage and bone destruction. *Current Opin Rheum* 1998; **10**: 212–19.

62. Csernok, E., Trabandt, A., and Gross, W. L. Immunogenetic aspects of ANCA-associated vasculitides. *Exp Clin Immunogenet* 1997; **14**: 177–82.

63. Kocher, M., Edberg, J. C., Fleit, H. B., and Kimberly, R. P. Antineutrophil cytoplasmic antibodies preferentially engage FcγRIIIb on human neutrophils. *J Immunol* 1998; **161**: 6909–14.

64. Edberg, J. C., Wainstein, E., Wu, J., Csernok, E., Sneller, M. C., Hoffman, G. S. et al. Analysis of FcγRII gene polymorphisms in Wegener's granulomatosis. *Exp Clin Immunogenet* 1997; **14**: 183–95.

65. Scharenberg, A. M., and Kinet, J. P. The emerging field of inhibitory signaling: SHP or SHIP? *Cell* 1996; **87**: 961–4.

66. Hampton, M. B., Kettle, A. J., and Winterbourn, C. C. Inside the neutrophil phagosome: oxidants, myeloperoxidase, and bacterial killing. *Blood* 1998; **92**: 3007–17.

67. Klebanoff, S. J. Oxygen metabolites from phagocytes. In *Inflammation: basic principles and clinical correlates*, 2nd edn (Gallin, J. I., Golstein, I. M., and Snyderman, R., eds), pp. 541–88. New York: Raven Press; 1992.

68. Davies, P., and MacIntyre, D. E. Prostaglandins and inflammation. In *Inflammation: basic principles and clinical correlates*, 2nd edn (Gallin, J. I., Golstein, I. M., and Snyderman, R., eds), pp. 123–38. New York: Raven Press; 1992.

69. Tanaka, S., Edberg, J. C., Chatham, W. W., Fassina, G., and Kimberly, R. P. Fc gamma RIIIb allele-sensitive release of alpha-defensins: anti-neutrophil cytoplasmic antibody-induced release of chemotaxins. *J Immunol* 2003; **171**: 6090–6.

70. Scapini P., Carletto, A., Nardelli, B., Calzetti, F., Roschke, V., Merigo, F. et al. Proinflammatory mediators elicit secretion of the intracellular B-lymphocyte stimulator pool (BLyS) that is stored in activated neutrophils: implications for inflammatory diseases. *Blood* 2005; **105**: 830–7.

71. Tan, S. M., Xu, D., Roschke, V., Perry, J. W., Arkfeld, D. G., Ehresmann, G. R. et al. Local production of B lymphocyte stimulator protein and APRIL in arthritic joints of patients with inflammatory arthritis. *Arthritis Rheum* 2003; **48**: 982–92.

72. Cassatella, M. A. 1996. Cytokines produced by polymorphonuclear neutrophils: molecular and biological aspects. Chapman and Hall, New York.

73. Ottonello, L., Cutolo, M., Frumento, G., Arduino, N., Bertolotto, M., Mancini, M. et al. Synovial fluid from patients with rheumatoid arthritis inhibits neutrophil apoptosis: role of adenosine and proinflammatory cytokines. *Rheumatology* 2002; **41**: 1249–60.

74. Nick, J. A., Avdi, N. J., Gerwins, P., Johnson, G. L., and Worthen, G. S. Activation of a p38 mitogen-activated protein kinase in human neutrophils by lipopolysaccharide. *J Immunol* 1996; **156**: 4867–75.

75. Baggiolini, M. Chemokines and leukocyte traffic. *Nature* 1998; **392**: 565–8.

76. Baggiolini, M., Dewald, B., and Moser, B. Human chemokines: an update. *Ann Rev Immunol* 1997; **15**: 675–705.

77. Galligan, C. L., Matsuyama, W., Matsukawa, A., Mizuta, H., Hodge, D. R., Howard, O. M., and Yoshimura, T. Up-regulated expression and activation of the orphan chemokine receptor, CCRL2, in rheumatoid arthritis. *Arthritis Rheum* 2004; **50**: 1806–14.

78. Biber. K., Zuurman, M. W., Homan, H., and Boddeke, H. W. Expression of L-CCR in HEK 293 cells reveals functional responses to CCL2, CCL5, CCL7, and CCL8. *J Leukoc Biol* 2003; **74**: 243–51.

79. Lee, B., Doranz, B. J., Rana, S., Yi, Y., Mellado, M., Frade, J. M. et al. Influence of the CCR2-V64I polymorphism on human immunodeficiency virus type 1 coreceptor activity and on chemokine receptor function of CCR2b, CCR3, CCR5, and CXCR4. *J Virol* 1998; **72**: 7450–8.

80. Mummidi, S., Ahuja, S. S., Gonzalez, E., Anderson, S. A., Santiago, E. N., Stephan, K. T. et al. Genealogy of the CCR5 locus and chemokine system gene variants associated with altered rates of HIV-1 disease progression. *Nature Med* 1998; **4**: 786–93.

81. Winkler, C., Modi, W., Smith, M. W., Nelson, G. W., Wu, X., Carrington, M. et al. Genetic restriction of AIDS pathgenesis by an SDF-1 chemokine gene variant. ALIVE Study, Hemophilia Growth and Development Study (HGDS), Multicenter AIDS Cohort Study (MACS), Multicenter Hemophilia Cohort Study (MHCS), San Francisco City Cohort (SFCC). *Science* 1998; **279**: 389–93.

82. Gomez-Reino, J. J., Pablos, J. L., Carreira, P. E., Santiago, B., Serrano, L., Vicario, J. L. et al. Association of rheumatoid arthritis with a functional chemokine receptor, CCR5. *Arthritis Rheum* 1999; **42**: 989–92.

83. Philips, M. R., Pillinger, M. H., Staud, R., Volker, C., Rosenfeld, M. G., Weissmann, G., and Stock, J. B. Carboxyl methylation of Ras-related proteins during signal transduction in neutrophils. *Science* 1993; **259**: 977–80.

84. Bokoch, G. M. Chemoattractant signaling and leukocyte activation. *Blood* 1995; **86**: 1649–60.

85. Springer, T. A. Traffic signals for lymphocyte recirculation and leukocyte emigration: the multistep paradigm. *Cell* 1994; **76**: 301–14.

86. Gopalan, P. K., Smith, C. W., Lu, H., Berg, E. L., McIntire, L. V., and Simon, S. I. Neutrophil CD18-dependent arrest on intracellular adhesion molecule 1 (ICAM-1) in shear flow can be activated through L-selectin. *J Immunol* 1997; **158**: 367–75.

87. Schnitzler, N., Haase, G., Podbielski, A., Lutticken, R., and Schweizer, K. G. A co-stimulatory signal through ICAM-β2 integrin-binding potentiates neutrophil phagocytosis. *Nature Med* 1999; **5**: 231–5.

88. Coxon, A., Rieu, P., Barkalow, F. J., Askari, S., Sharpe, A. H., von Andrian, U. H. et al. A novel role for the β2 integrin CD11b/CD18 in neutrophil apoptosis: a homeostatic mechanism in inflammation. *Immunity* 1996; **5**: 653–66.

89. Bullard, D. C. Adhesion molecules in inflammatory diseases: insights from knockout mice. *Immunol Res* 2002; **26**: 27–33.

90. Hulett, M. D. and Hogarth, P. M. Molecular basis of Fc receptor function. *Adv Immunol* 1994; **57**: 1–127.

91. Daeron, M. Fc receptor biology. *Ann Rev Immunol* 1997; **15**: 203–34.

92. Edberg, J. C., and Kimberly, R. P. Modulation of Fcγ and complement receptor function by the glycosyl-phophatidylinositol-anchored form of FcγRIII. *J Immunol* 1994; **152**: 5826–35.

93. Zhou, M. J., and Brown, E. J. CR3 (Mac-1, αMβ2, CD11b/CD18) and FcγRIII cooperate in generation of a neutrophil respiratory burst: requirement for FcγRIII and tyrosine phosphorylation. *J Cell Biol* 1994; **125**: 1407–16.

94. Green, J. M., Schreiber, A. D., and Brown, E. J. Role for a glycan phosphoinositol anchor in Fcγ receptor synergy. *J Cell Biol* 1997; **139**: 1209–18.

95. Brown, D. A., and London, E. Functions of lipid rafts in biological membranes. *Ann Rev Cell Dev Biol* 1998; **14**: 111–36.

96. van der Pol, W. and van de Winkel, J. G. IgG receptor polymorphisms: risk factors for disease. *Immunogenetics*, 1998; **48**: 222–32.

97. Duits, A. J., Bootsma, R. H., Derksen, R. H. W., Spronk, P. E., Kater, L., Kallenberg, C. G. M. *et al.* Skewed distribution of IgG Fc receptor IIa (CD32) polymorphisms is associated with renal disease in systemic lupus erythematosus patients. *Arthritis Rheum* 1995; **39**: 1832–6.

98. Salmon, J. E., Millard, S., Schachter, L. A., Arnett, F. C., Ginzler, E. M., Gourley, M. F. *et al.* FcγRIIA alleles are heritable risk factors for lupus nephritis in African Americans. *J Clin Invest* 1996; **97**: 1348–54.

99. Wu, J., Edberg, J. C., Redecha, P. B., Bansal, V., Guyre, P. M., Coleman, K. *et al.* A novel polymorphism of FcγRIIIa (CD16) alters receptor function and predisposes to autoimmune disease. *J Clin Invest* 1997; **100**: 1059–70.

100. Petty, H. R., and Todd, R. F. Receptor–receptor interactions of complement receptor type 3 in neutrophil membranes. *J Leuk Biol* 1993; **54**: 492–4.

101. Grant, E. P., Picarella, D., Burwell, T., Delaney, T., Croci, A., Avitahl, N. *et al.* Essential role for the C5a receptor in regulating the effector phase of synovial infiltration and joint destruction in experimental arthritis. *J Exp Med* 2002; **196**: 1461–71.

102. Ahearn, J. M., and Fearon, D. T. Structure and function of complement receptors CR1 (CD35) and CR2 (CD21). *Adv Immunol* 1989; **46**: 183–219.

103. Ross, G. D., and Vetvicka, V. CR3 (CD11b, CD18): a phagocyte and NK cell membrane receptor with multiple ligand specificities and functions. *Clin Exp Immunol* 1993; **92**: 181–4.

104. Miller, G. W., and Nussenzweig, V. Complement as a regulator of interactions between immune complexes and cell membranes. *J Immunol* 1974; **113**: 464–9.

105. Edberg, J. C., Moon, J. M., Chang, D. J., and Kimberly, R. P. Differential regulation of human neutrophil FcγRIIa (CD32) and FcγRIIIb (CD16)-induced Ca²⁺ transients. *J Biol Chem* 1998; **273**: 8071–9.

106. Changelian, P. S., and Fearon, D. T. Tissue-specific phosphorylation of complement receptors CR1 and CR2. *J Exp Med* 1986; **163**: 101–15.

107. Dinarello, C. A. Interleukin-1, interleukin-1 receptors and interleukin-1 receptor antagonist. *Int Rev Immunol* 1998; **16**: 457–99.

108. Moreland, L. W. Soluble tumor necrosis factor receptor (p75) fusion protein (Enbrel) as a therapy of rheumatoid arthritis. *Rheum Dis Clinics N Am*, 1998; **24**: 579–91.

109. Naismith, J. H., and Sprang, S. R. Modularity in the TNF-receptor family. *Trends Biochem Sci* 1998; **23**: 74–9.

110. Darnay, B. G., and Aggarwal, B. B. Early events in TNF signaling: a story of associations and dissociations. *J Leuk Biol* 1997; **61**: 559–66.

111. Peschon, J. J., Torrance, D. S., Stocking, K. L., Glaccum, M. B., Otten, C., Willis, C. R. *et al.* TNF receptor-deficient mice reveal divergent roles for p55 and p75 in several models of inflammation. *J Immunol* 1998; **160**: 943–52.

112. Simms, H. H., Gaither, T. A., Fries L. F., and Frank M. M. Monokines released during short-term Fc gamma receptor phagocytosis up-regulate polymorphonuclear leukocytes and monocyte-phagocytic function. *J Immunol* 1991; **147**: 265–72.

113. Gresham, H. D., Zheleznyak A., Mormol J. S., and Brown E. J. Studies on the molecular mechanisms of human neutrophil Fc receptor–mediated phagocytosis: evidence that a distinct pathway for activation of the respiratory burst results in reactive oxygen metabolite-dependent amplification of ingestion. *J Biol Chem* 1990; **265**: 7819–26.

114. Wei, S., Liu, J. H., Epling-Burnette, P. K., Gamero, A. M., Ussery, D., Pearson, E. W. *et al.* Critical role of Lyn kinase in inhibition of neutrophil apoptosis by granulocyte-macrophage colony-stimulating factor. *J Immunol* 1996; **157**: 5155–62.

115. Homburg, C. H., and Roos, D. Apoptosis of neutrophils. *Curr Opin Hematol* 1996; **3**: 94–9.

116. Haslett, C., Savill, J. S., and Meagher, L. The neutrophil. *Curr Opin Immunol* 1989; **2**: 10–18.

117. Smedly, L. A., Tonnesen, M. G., Sandhaus, R. A., Haslett, C., Guthrie, L. A., Johnston, R. B. *et al.* Neutrophil-mediated injury to endothelial cells: enhancement by endotoxin and essential role of neutrophil elastase. *J Clin Invest* 1986; **77**: 1233–43.

118. Medzhiton, R., Preston-Hurlbut, P., and Janeway, C. A. A human homologue of the Drosophila Toll protein signals activation of adaptive immunity. *Nature* 1991; **388**: 394–7.

119. Quayle, J. A., Watson, F., Bucknall, R. C., and Edwards, S. W. Neutrophils from the synovial fluid of patients with rheumatoid arthritis express the high affinity immunoglobulin G receptor, FcγRI (CD64): role of immune complexes and cytokines in induction of receptor expression. *Immunology* 1997; **91**: 266–73.

120. Felzmann, T., Gadd, S., Majdic, O. *et al.* Analysis of function-associated receptor molecules on peripheral blood and synovial fluid granulocytes from patients with rheumatoid and reactive arthritis. *J Clin Immunol* 1988; **11**: 205–12.

121. Watson, F., Robinson, J. J., Phelan, M. *et al.* Receptor expression in synovial fluid neutrophils from patients with rheumatoid arthritis. *Ann Rheum Dis* 1993; **52**: 354–9.

122. Goulding, N. J., and Guyre, P. M. Impairment of neutrophil Fcγ receptor mediated transmembrane signaling in active rheumatoid arthritis. *Ann Rheum Dis* 1992; **51**: 594–9.

123. Jobin, D., Kreis, C., Gauthier, J. *et al.* Differential synthesis of 5-lipoxygenase in peripheral blood and synovial fluid neutrophils in rheumatoid arthritis. *J Immunol* 1991; **146**: 2701–7.

124. Poubelle, P. E., Bourgoin, S., McColl, S. R. *et al.* Altered formation of leukotriene B₄ in vitro by synovial fluid neutrophils in rheumatoid arthritis. *J Rheum* 1989; **16**: 280.

125. Lord, P. C. W., Wilmoth, L. M. G., Mizel, S. B. *et al.* Expression of interleukin-1α and β genes by human blood polymorphonuclear leukocytes. *J Clin Invest* 1991; **87**: 1312–21.

126. Marucha, P. T., Zeff, R. A., and Kreutzer, D. L. Cytokine regulation of IL-1b gene expression in the human polymorphonuclear leukocyte. *J Immunol* 1990; **145**: 2932–7.

127. Chatham, W. W., Turkiewicz, A., and Blackburn, W. D., Jr. Determinants of neutrophil HOCl generation: ligand-dependent responses and the role of surface adhesion. *J Leuk Biol* 1994; **56**: 654–60.

128. Vetto, A. A., Mannik, M., Zatarain-Rios, E., and Wener, M. H. Immune deposits in articular cartilage of patients with rheumatoid arthritis have a granular pattern not seen in osteoarthritis. *Rheumatol Int* 1990; **10**: 13.

129. Velvart, M., and Fehr, K. Degradation in vivo of articular cartilage in rheumatoid arthritis and juvenile chronic arthritis by cathepsin G and elastase from polymorphonuclear leukocytes. *Rheumatol Int* 1987; **7**: 195–202.

130. Henson, P. M. The immunologic release of constituents from neutrophil leukocytes. I. The role of antibody and complement on non-phagocytosable surfaces or phagocytosable particles. *J Immunol* 1971; **107**: 1535.

131. Weiss, S. J., Peppin, G., Ortiz, X., and Ragsdale, C. Oxidative autoactivation of latent collagenase by human neutrophils. *Science* 1985; **227**: 747.

132. Chatham, W. W., Heck, L. W., and Blackburn, W. D. Jr. Ligand-dependent release of active neutrophil collagenase. *Arthritis Rheum* 1990; **33**: 328.

133. Capodici, C., Mathukumaran, G., Amorosu, M., and Berg, R. A. Activation of neutrophil collagenase by cathepsin G. *Inflammation* 1989; **13**: 245–58.

134. Chatham, W. W., Blackburn, W. D. Jr., and Heck, L. W. Addictive enhancement of neutrophil collagenase by HOCl and cathepsin G. *Biochem Biophys Res Commun* 1992; **184**: 560–7.

135. Chatham, W. W., Sampson, J., Beck, J., and Blackburn, W. D. Jr. Activation of neutrophil collagenase by peroxynitrite: evidence for nitric oxide production during neutrophil activation with surface bound IgG. *Arthritis Rheum* 1996; **39**: S37.

136. Ossanua, P. J., Test, S. T., Mathesen, N. R., Regiani, S., and Weiss, S. J. Oxidative regulation of neutrophil elastase-alpha-1-proteinase inhibitor interactions. *J Clin Invest* 1986; **77**: 1939.

137. Weiss, S. J., and Regiani, S. Neutrophils degrade subendothelial matrices in the presence of alpha-1 protease inhibitor. *J Clin Invest* 1984; **73**: 1297–303.

138. Chatham, W. W., Heck, L. W., and Blackburn, W. D. Jr. Lysis of fibrillar collagen by neutrophils in synovial fluid: a role for surface bound immunoglobulins. *Arthritis Rheum* 1990; **33**: 1333–9.

139. Chatham, W. W., Swaim, R. S., Frohsin, H. Jr., Heck, L. W., Miller, E. J., and Blackburn, W. D. Jr. Degradation of human articular cartilage by neutrophils is synovial fluid. *Arthritis Rheum* 1993; **36**: 51–8.

140. Mohr, W., and Menninger, H. Polymorphonuclear granulocytes at the pannus–cartilage junction in rheumatoid arthritis. *Arthritis Rheum* 1980; **33**: 228–34.

141. Bromley, M., and Woolley, D. E. Histopathology of the rheumatoid lesion: identification of cell types at sites of cartilage erosion. *Arthritis Rheum* 1984; **27**: 857–63.

142. Momohara, S. Kashiwazaki, S., Inoue, K., Saito, S., and Nakagawa, T. Elastase from polymorphonuclear leukocytes in articular cartilage and synovial fluids of patients with rheumatoid arthritis. *Clin Rheumatol* 1997; **16**: 133–40.

143. Jasin, H. E., and Taurog, J. D. Mechanisms of disruption of the articular cartilage surface in inflammation: neutrophil elastase increases the availability of collagen type II epitopes for binding with antibody on the surface of articular cartilage. *J Clin Invest* 1991; **87**: 1531–6.

144. Van den Steen, P. E., Proost, P., Grillet, B., Brand, D. D., Kang, A. H., Van Damme, J., and Opdenakker, G. Cleavage of denatured natural collagen type II by neutrophil gelatinase B reveals enzyme specificity, post-translational modifications in the substrate, and the formation of remnant epitopes in rheumatoid arthritis. *FASEB J* 2002; **16**: 379–89.

145. Jasin, H. E. Oxidative cross-linking of immune complexes by human polymorphonuclear leukocytes. *J Clin Invest* 1988; **81**: 6.

146. Jasin, H. E. Oxidative modification of inflammatory synovial fluid immunoglobulin G. *Inflammation* 1993; **17**: 167.

147. Uesugi, M., Hayashi, T., and Jasin, H. E. Covalent cross-linking of immune complexes by oxygen radicals and nitrite. *J Immunol* 1998; **161**: 1422–7.

148. Bui, M. N., Sack, M. N., Moutsatsos, G. *et al.* Autoantibody titers to oxidized low-density lipoprotein in patients with coronary atherosclerosis. *Am Heart J* 1996; **131**: 663–7.

149. Horkko, S., Miller, E., Dudl, E. *et al.* Antiphospholipid antibodies are directed against epitopes of oxidized phospholipids: recognition of cardiolipin by monoclonal antibodies to epitopes of oxidized low density proteins. *J Clin Invest* 1996; **98**: 815–25.

150. McCurdy, L., Chatham, W. W., and Blackburn, W. D. Jr. Rheumatoid synovial fibroblast adhesion to human articular cartilage: enhancement by neutrophil proteases. *Arthritis Rheum* 1995; **38**: 1694–9.

151. Harris, E. D. Jr. Rheumatoid arthritis: pathophysiology and implications for therapy. *N Eng J Med* 1989; **322**: 1277–89.

152. Greenwarld, R. A., and Moi, W. W. Effect of oxygen-derived free radicals on hyaluronic acid. *Arthritis Rheum* 1980; **23**: 455–63.

153. Schiller, J., Arnhold, J., Sonntag, K., and Arnold K. NMR studies on human, pathologically changed synovial fluids: role of hypochlorous acid. *Magn Reson Med* 1996; **35**: 848–53.

154. Shimazu, A., Jikko, A., Iwamoto, M. *et al.* Effects of hyaluronic acid on the release of proteoglycan from the cell matrix in rabbit chondrocyte cultures in the presence and absence of cytokines. *Arthritis Rheum* 1993; **36**: 247–53.

155. Tamoto, K., Tada, M., Shimada, S. *et al.* Effects of high molecular weight hyaluronates on the functions of guinea pig polymorphonuclear leukocytes. *Semin Arthritis Rheum* 1993; **22** (Suppl.): 4–8.

156. Goto, M., Hosako, Y., Katayama, M., and Yamada, T. Biochemical analysis of rheumatoid synovial fluid after serial intra-articular injection of high molecular weight sodium hyaluronate. *Int J Clin Pharmacol Res* 1993; **13**: 161–6.

157. Nguyen, T., Brunson, D., Crespi, C. L., Penman, B. W., Wishnok, J. S., and Tannenbaum, S. R. DNA damage and mutation in human cells exposed to nitric oxide in vitro. *Proc Natl Acad Sci U S A*, 1992; **89**: 3030–4.

8 | The role of fibroblast-like synoviocytes in rheumatoid arthritis

Ulf Müller-Ladner and Steffen Gay

Introduction

The fibroblast-like synoviocyte (FLS), also termed synovial fibroblast or type B synovial fibroblast, has developed from a cell known to be involved in homeostasis within the synovium to a key pathogenic cell that mediates joint destruction in rheumatoid arthritis (RA). This evolution is based on the advances in molecular biology, which has provided novel insights into the role and function of a variety of RA synovial cells. Interestingly enough, the FLS now being characterized as driving cells in the destructive processes in the rheumatoid joint were described adequately as 'transformed-appearing' on a histological level by Fassbender decades ago[1].

This accumulation of novel experimental data addressing the function of these cells is mainly based on developments in high-resolution molecular analysis[2,3] in the different cells operative in RA synovium and the recent identification of the two main cellular pathways involved in rheumatoid joint destruction[4]. Aside from the well-known T cell-dependent pathway(s), the detailed molecular and cellular characterization of T cell-independent pathway(s) has emerged[5]. Specifically, the involvement of pattern-recognition or Toll-like receptors[4], the expression of protooncogenes[2,6], the attachment to matrix and articular cartilage, and the up-regulation of matrix-degrading enzymes at sites of synovial attachment characterized the contribution of FLS to the invasive and destructive phenotype in rheumatoid synovium[5].

The functional alterations inherent with the role of FLS in the RA synovium include also an imbalance between synovial cell proliferation and the physiological cell death (apoptosis). This property is reflected by the finding that the destructive potential of FLS is maintained for more than 220 days in the severe combined immunodeficiency (SCID) T cell-deficient mouse model of RA involving coimplantation of RA synovium or FLS with normal human cartilage under the renal capsule or the skin[7,8]. Thus, the specific properties of RA FLS as compared with other fibroblasts and resident synovial cells characterize these cells as a distinct pathophysiological entity, which is illustrated best by the functional term activated synovial fibroblast[9].

Physiological properties of fibroblast-like synoviocytes

In non-diseased synovium, FLS and synovial macrophages are the two dominant cell types of the terminal layer lining the joint cavity. The lining layer, which is usually one to three cells deep, is not separated from the underlying connective tissue and vasculature by a basement membrane or a separating cell layer, which also enables unrestricted diffusion of signaling and effector molecules, which were released by the synovial cells or which have entered the synovium from the vascular or joint cavity. In contrast, the variety of cells located in the sublining includes fibroblasts, macrophages, mast cells, (peri)vascular cells, dendritic cells, and different types of lymphocytes[10].

With regard to the phenotype, FLS resemble tissue fibroblasts. The endoplasmic reticulum is prominent and the Golgi apparatus is well developed. The nucleus is pale and usually shows a number of nucleoli. During their lifetime, the shape of the synoviocytes can vary considerably. They alter their morphologic appearance, and in a long-term setting they undergo either proliferation or apoptosis. The pivotal function of FLS, especially in the lining layer, is to provide the joint cavity and the adjacent cartilage of the two articulating bones and their resident chondrocytes with lubricating molecules such as hyaluronic acid, with nutritive plasma proteins, and with oxygen. FLS also synthesize numerous matrix components, including collagen and hyaluronan, and their capability to remodel articular matrix, cartilage, and bone is reflected by the synthesis of a variety of enzymes. Amongst these are matrix metalloproteinases (MMPs), membrane-type metalloproteinases, cathepsins, and uridine diphosphoglucose dehydrogenase, with the latter being expressed specifically in the ultimate lining cells[11]. FLS lack specific HLA DR marker molecules and cannot yet be detected by joint-specific anti-fibroblast antibodies. At present, the best markers are vimentin, prolyl-5-hydroxylase, and Thy-1. FLS interact intensively with each other, with other cells, and with the matrix by adhesion molecules and through cytokines, growth factors, and chemokines, as outlined below.

Fibroblast-like synoviocytes in histopathology

Although the absolute number of every cell type is increased in the majority of arthritides, the increase of FLS specifically in active disease is one of the predominant features of RA synovium. In early RA, however, the initial events resulting in this increase are largely unknown and may even occur before inflammation is evident, a feature which has been supported by recent findings in innate immunity[4]. The phenotype of FLS appears transformed and activated, and is closely associated with sites of destruction of adjacent cartilage and bone[5]. On a light microscopy level, FLS are characterized by large, pale nuclei containing prominent nucleoli and an abundant cytoplasm, therefore to some extent resembling semimalignant cells[1]. As mentioned above, activation of these cells is further illustrated by an enhanced expression of matrix-degrading enzymes as well as short- and long-range signaling molecules[2]. Of note, fibrosis in rheumatoid synovium, which can frequently be observed in long-term disease, appears to be mediated by differentiation of certain FLS into myofibroblast-like cells when stimulated by transforming growth factor-β[12].

Regulation of cellular activation

Triggers

As outlined above, activated FLS are characteristic for the pathophysiology of RA[5,9]. This activation, however, does not imply a largely uncontrolled proliferation but describes rather an increase in metabolic activity, which is combined with an activated cellular phenotype. In contrast to their 'normal' counterparts, activated FLS are characterized by a dense, rough, endoplasmic reticulum, numerous irregular nuclei, and changes in the normally spindle-shaped cell skeleton. Potential stimuli or triggers for this activation, which are currently being discussed, could be infectious or non-infectious agents or their respective (degradation) products[4,13,14].

For example, oncogene- or virus-derived gene sequences incorporated into the synovial fibroblast DNA, as illustrated in an experimental model[15], might be one of the primary triggers for such a phenotype. In the majority of rheumatic diseases, retroviruses have been repeatedly proposed as an etiologic factor for the induction of autoimmunity, cellular activation, and long-term proliferation[16]. In this context of a potential involvement of a retrovirus in certain forms of arthritis, the data showing a distinct association of the human T-cell lymphotropic virus (HTLV-I) with the development of a chronic arthropathy are of considerable interest. The fact, on the other hand, that cellular activation requires at least two cooperating proto-oncogenes[17,18] has been demonstrated in the retrovirus-dependent tax transgenic mouse model, in which the tax-transfected animals develop severe RA-like arthritis. In these animals, the overexpression of tax, a part of the HTLV-I viral genome, induces the up-regulation of the proto-oncogene c-fos, as well as the pro-inflammatory cytokines IL-1β, and IL-6[19]. Similarly, endogenous retroviral L1 elements in FLS result in an up-regulation of Mapkinase p38δ, an inducer of certain MMPs[13,20], which has been found to be one of the key findings supporting the idea of an important role for the innate immune system in early activation of rheumatoid FLS. Subsequently, it could be shown that bacterial peptidoglycans are able to activate FLS via stimulation of one of the basic innate immune receptor systems, the Toll-like receptors (TLRs), which resulted in an up-regulation of pro-inflammatory cytokines, adhesion molecules, and MMPs, including ICAM, IL-6, IL-8, MMP-1, MMP-3, and MMP-13[21]. On the other hand, pro-inflammatory cytokines such as IL-1 and tumor necrosis factor (TNF) were able to further enhance the expression of TLR-2 expression in FLS. Completing this vicious circle, stimulation of TLR-2 resulted also in a strong synthesis of several important chemokines in FLS, which—*in vivo*—like monocyte chemoattractant protein (MCP)-2 and gro-2 might be one of the key mechanisms of FLS-induced accumulation of inflammatory cells to the rheumatoid synovium. These findings clearly demonstrate that FLS are part of the innate immune system.

Extracellular stimuli

Growth factors

Fibroblast growth factor (FGF), transforming growth factor (TGF)-β, and platelet-derived growth factor (PDGF) are cytokines that induce cell proliferation, which includes also FLS as target cells. Of these, FGF is predominantly an autocrine growth factor for synoviocytes and vascular epithelium. FLS not only proliferate in response to this growth factor, they are conversely also able to produce FGF, thus triggering local fibroblast growth[22]. Notably, the effect of FGF-2 is not restricted to the proliferation of FLS: it also influences the maturation of osteoclasts and subsequently bone destruction[23]. TGF-β, on the other hand, is expressed in synovial tissue and produced by synovial macrophages. Its effects depend on the location and concentration within the synovium. TGF-β induces proliferation of the synovial lining and stimulates collagen production by FLS when injected directly into the joint cavity. TGF-β also stimulates IL-1 and the synthesis of MMP-1[24]. Notably, the effects of TGF-β are also linked to the (anti)apoptotic pathways—as described in detail below—by modulating the activity of phosphatidylinositol 3 (pi-3) kinase and akt in rheumatoid FLS[25]. PDGF is a strong stimulator of synovial growth, and also one of the few cytokines for which a direct proto-oncogene-triggered activation of synovial cells has been shown[26].

Cytokines

Cytokines known to be produced by FLS, either spontaneously or after stimulation, include a variety of pro-inflammatory molecules[27–42], as summarized in Table 8.1, although not all mRNAs of FLS-derived cytokines are stable[41]. Most of these cytokines can stimulate FLS to activate intracellular signaling pathways[43] and to produce other cytokines, pluripotent effector molecules such as activin and galectin[2,44,45], and matrix-degrading enzymes[46]. These effects can be further enhanced by 'associated' costimulatory molecules such as TWEAK[47], and by the crosstalk between different cytokine-dependent signaling cascades[48]. In some cases, only the receptor but not the respective cytokine can be detected in RA synovium. For example, it could be shown that the receptor for IL-21 is expressed on RA FLS but mRNA for IL-21 was neither detectable in RA synovium nor inducible by key pro-inflammatory cytokines and growth factors such as IL-1, TNF, PDGF, and TGF[49].

Cytokines are also able to influence the phenotype of FLS. For example, the synthetic PPARγ ligand troglitazone was able to induce transformation of FLS into adipocyte-like cells, an effect which was regulated by different pro-inflammatory cytokines such as IL-1 and TNF via C/EBF transcription factor activity[50]. In addition, regulation of osteoclastogenesis is also modulated by

Table 8.1 Cytokine synthesis by FLSs

Cytokine	Produced by FLS in RA	Produced by FLS in culture
IL-1	+	+
IL-2	+	−
IL-3	?	−
IL-4	−	−
IL-5	−	−
IL-6	+	+
IL-7	+	+
IL-8	+	+
IL-9	−	−
IL-10	+	+
IL-11	+	+
IL-12	+	−
IL-13	?	−
IL-15	+	+
IL-16	+	+
IL-17	+	+
IL-18	+	−
IL-21	−	−
IL-22	+	+
Interferon-α	+	−
Interferon-β	+	+
Interferon-γ	−	−
TNF-α	+	−
TNF-β	−	−

TNF-dependent osteoprotegerin synthesis in FLS[51] and by TNF and IL-1-dependent up-regulation of bone morphogenetic proteins (BMP)-2 and -6 in FLS[52]. Notably, the latter BMP protected against nitric oxide (NO)-triggered FLS apoptosis[52]. However, the majority of experiments addressing cytokine production by FLS *in vitro* are difficult to evaluate, as the rate of their synthesis depends on the individual sites of retrieval and of the culture conditions.

Prostaglandins

Pro-inflammatory prostaglandin pathways take part in synovial inflammation and joint destruction in RA. Interestingly, FLS are contributing to the overall prostaglandin production in RA synovium[53–55]. Operative in these pathways, cyclooxygenases (COX-1 and COX-2) catalyze the enzymatic activation of arachidonic acid to prostaglandins, which are the most potent mediators of inflammation. Notably, the source of COX-2 in the synovial lining appears to be the FLS, and inhibition experiments revealed a direct link between these cells and the synthesis of cyclooxygenase-2[56]. In addition, COX-2 inhibitors exert also proapoptotic effects on FLS as celecoxib was able to reduce proliferation of FLS by induction of PPAR-γ-independent apoptosis[57]. Similarly a number of non-selective and selective COX inhibitors, including ibuprofen, diclofenac, meloxicam, and rofecoxib, were able to inhibit IL-1-triggered prostaglandin E2 production in RA FLS[58].

Chemokines

FLS have been regarded as 'sentinel cells'[59], which enhance (chemo)attraction of leukocytes, and a variety of chemoattractive molecules are produced by FLS[60]. After stimulation of the CD40 ligand/CD40 system, for example by cell contact with T lymphocytes[61], FLS can release chemotactic molecules such as macrophage inflammatory protein (MIP), monocyte chemoattractant protein (MCP), RANTES, and IL-8[61,62]. FLS express MIP-3α after stimulation with IL-1β, IL-18, and TNF-α, followed by perivascular chemoattraction of mononuclear cells[63], and the release of MCP-1 by FLS is stimulated by oncostatin M[64]. On the other hand, the interaction of FLS and leukocytes via β2-integrin/VCAM-1 results in the up-regulation of MIP-1α synthesis in RA synovial fluid polymorphonuclear monocytes[65]. Similarly, hypoxia stimulated the up-regulation of ICAM-1 in FLS, which resulted in enhanced adhesiveness of FLS to lymphocytes[66].

Influx of pro-inflammatory CD4-positive T cells is also facilitated by FLS because of the production of chemoattractive IL-16[27], which is activated within the cell via a protein kinase C pathway[67], by production of stromal cell-derived factor (SDF)-1), one of the key factors for T cell pseudoemperipolesis[68]. In addition, FLS most likely are also taking part in shifting the Th1–Th2 balance towards the former by producing Th1-associated CXCR3 ligands. Even more interesting is the finding that immunoglobulins (maybe even rheumatoid factors) from RA patients, but not from osteoarthritis (OA) patients, are able to induce the up-regulation of IL-16 in FLS and therefore contribute to FLS-mediated chemoattraction of pro-inflammatory cells in RA synovium[36,69]. Chemokines such as CX3CL1 (fractalkine) can also directly act on destructive processes, as it could be shown that fractalkine was able to up-regulate MMP-2 production in FLS[70]. Conversely, IL-17, a CD4+ T cell-derived cytokine, can up-regulate cytokine production in rheumatoid FLS and further enhance the pro-inflammatory interaction cascade[28].

The impact of chemokine-related pathways on synovial pathophysiology is reflected in the costimulatory links of chemokines with cellular adhesion. FLS express constitutively the chemokine SDF-1, which can be further enhanced by hypoxia[71], but B cell pseudoemperipolesis could only be achieved after IL-4-dependent up-regulation of vascular cell-adhesion molecule-1 (VCAM-1)[72]. Moreover, recent data demonstrate that activation of FLS via the TLR-2 receptor induces the synthesis of potent chemokines, including granulocyte chemotactic peptide (GCP)-2 and MCP-2[73].

Molecular profile of RA fibroblast-like synoviocytes

The advances in molecular biology have also introduced novel techniques for analysis of gene expression and molecular mechanisms operative in RA FLS[2,3,74,75]. However, evaluation of the pathways using these highly sensitive techniques has frequently required a completely new standardization and validation procedure[76,77]. Especially in *ex vivo* settings, cultured FLS alter substantially the profile of gene expression after few (in most cases 5–6) passages, which may result in a completely different outcome of an experimental setting when higher passages are used for certain experiments[75]. Moreover, results obtained from a given level of expression, for example RNA, need to be verified by a different approach, generally on the protein level[3] and/or by double labeling. However, it needs to be mentioned that, at present, no FLS-specific marker with 100% sensitivity and specificity exists[78] and that markers (antibodies) used for labeling of non-FLS synovial cells may—to a small percentage—also mark FLS cells *in vitro*[79].

The intracellular signature: activation and proliferation vs. apoptosis

Activation and proliferation

In the past years, a large body of evidence has accumulated that a long-term imbalance between proliferation and apoptosis is operative in FLS. In addition, experimental data show that the observed cellular and metabolic alterations of synoviocytes in RA are mediated by an up-regulation of proto-oncogenes[2,6,80]. Although the distinct events leading to the initiation of fibroblast proliferation in RA are not exactly defined, the mitogenic c-sis/PDGF system was one of the first examples of a chain of defined events capable of stimulating synovial growth[26].

Early-response genes appear also to be involved in the initial steps of FLS activation. For example, the early-response gene egr-1, also named zinc finger gene Z-225, is up-regulated in RA FLS, and the increased expression of egr-1 persists over numerous passages[81]. By *in situ* hybridization, mRNA of egr-1 was detected in numerous cells of the rheumatoid synovium. The c-fos oncogene is another (inducible) gene activated in FLS in RA[82]. A major effect of the respective translated Fos proteins is the activation of tissue-degrading molecules[83] such as MMP-1 and MMP-3, which is reflected by the finding that fos and egr-1 expression is correlated with the expression of MMP-1 at sites of synovial invasion in rheumatoid joint destruction. Notably, c-fos antisense oligonucleotides were able to inhibit the expression of the related activator protein (AP)-1 protein and proliferation of FLS[84], and inhibition of AP-1 results in a down-regulation of IL-1 and IL-8[85]. Moreover, the transformed appearance of FLS is associated with the expression of the cell-activating proto-oncogenes myc and ras in RA synovium, and myc protein expression could be demonstrated in a high number of FLS at sites of cartilage and bone destruction[86,87]. Similarly, the oncogene ras is expressed predominantly in the synovial lining layer associated with the expression of the proteolytic enzyme cathepsin L at sites of invasive growth[86]. This destructive potential of ras, raf-, and myc-dependent FLS activation was further supported by gene transfer-based inhibition experiments, in which overexpression of double-negative ras, raf, and myc mutants ameliorated inflammation and reduced bone destruction in adjuvant arthritis[88], as well as cartilage destruction and FLS invasiveness in the SCID mouse model for RA[89].

Other important regulators of gene transcription are nuclear transcription factors such as nuclear factor kB (NFκB), which is expressed by FLS. It can be triggered by retroviral infection, including HTLV-I, as well as by pro-inflammatory cytokines such as IL-1[90]. Both isoforms of NF-κB can be detected in RA synovium, especially in FLS in the lining layer. With regard to pro-inflammatory pathways, NF-κB can induce the expression of COX-2 protein[91]. When exposed to TNF-α, FLS show an increased proliferation and a decreased contact inhibition[92]. Of interest, these effects are related to a TNF-α–dependent induction of egr-1[93], of NF-κB[94], and others, including members of the notch family[95].

With regard to NF-κB-dependent subsequent signaling, RANK (receptor activator of nuclear factor κB), a member of the TNF receptor family, appears to be one of the most important effector membrane receptors. RANK initiates primarily a bone-degrading pathway via its binding partner RANK ligand (RANKL) in rheumatoid synovium, and RANKL was found to be expressed strongly at sites of bone erosion. As FLS are part of this RANK/RANKL interaction system[96], they are also involved in osteoclastogenesis and bone destruction[97–99]. Of interest, rheumatoid FLS expressing higher levels of RANKL induced a higher number of osteoclast-like cells than did RA FLS expressing only low levels of RANKL, which has also been termed osteoclast differentiation factor (ODF)[98].

Owing to their role in intracellular activation of FLS, NF-κB-dependent pathways have also been a target for therapeutic approaches in the past years. This idea has been supported by the NF-κB-inhibiting effects of glucocorticoids through up-regulation of the NF-κB-inhibiting molecule IκB. IκB activity is regulated by two kinases, IκB kinase-1 and -2, also named IKK1 and IKK2. IκB, as well as IKK1 and IKK2, are present in RA synovium. In contrast TNF-α and IL-1 were found to be important activators of NF-κB[92,100]. This intracellular signalling pathway may also include the known inactivation of IκB by cytokine-dependent phosphorylation and ubiquitination. Moreover, IKK2-dominant negative mutant cell populations showed resistance to TNF-α-triggered NF-κB nuclear translocation, whereas lack of IKK1 did not affect this pathway[101]. Of note, recent experiments examining an ATP-competitive small molecule inhibitor of NF-κB revealed that the interaction with IκB in RA FLS appears to be more complex than expected, as this inhibitor not only interfered with IκB phosphorylation and degradation but also with p65 transactivation[102]. In a similar approach comparing the role of IKK in different synovial target cells, it could be shown that IKK2 regulated specifically IL-6 and IL-8 synthesis in FLS but was not essential for the synthesis of TNF[103]. Downstream NF-κB-dependent activation processes in FLS include specific Ets transcription factors such as ESE that potentially mediate pro-inflammatory stimuli at sites of inflammation[104]. Experimental inhibition of NF-κB by adenoviral overexpression of IκB also revealed novel downstream effector genes, including the antiapoptotic gene BIRC-3 and the FLICE inhibitory protein (FLIP)-like gene GG2–1[105]. In addition, antagonizing NF-κB mRNA by using antisense oligonucleotides resulted in decreased binding of NF-κB to the pro-inflammatory cyclooxygenase gene promoter[91].

Overexpression of accessory proteins that bind to nuclear receptors and subsequently suppress gene transcription and intracellular signaling kinases are also driving pro-inflammatory and autoimmune mechanisms[106] and activate FLS[56]. For example, the nuclear receptor cofactor SMRT (silencing mediator for retinoid and thyroid hormone receptors), suppresses MMP-1 promoter activity in FLS. On the other hand, the importance of mRNA stabilization in FLS has been demonstrated by the fact that IL-6 gene expression is regulated by p38 mitogen-activated protein kinase (MAPK), which enhances IL-6 mRNA stabilization[107]. p38 MAPK furthermore modulates pro-inflammatory pathways in FLS, and inhibition of p38 MAPK resulted in an inhibition of IL-1-dependent up-regulation of prostaglandin E2 and COX-2[56]. Similar to NF-κB, the MAPK such as p38 MAPK and c-jun kinases (JNKs) appear to be amongst the key mechanisms involved in regulation of matrix degradation in rheumatoid synovium: activation of p38 MAPK inhibited Ras/Raf-induced MMP-1 gene expression[108] and JNK triggered IL-1-dependent MMP-1 gene expression[109]. Conversely, the cell cycle inhibitor/tumor suppressor retinoblastoma down-regulated especially MMP-1 production by FLS via a p38-dependent pathway[110].

Recently, kinases upstream from p38 and operative in FLS have been identified. Amongst them are MKK-4 (MAP kinase kinase) and MKK-7, both of which were activated by phosphorylation following IL-1 simulation[111], as well as MKK-3 and MKK-6, two key regulators of p38 activation[110], which are induced by IL-1 and TNF[112]. Directly related kinase-dependent mechanisms operative in FLS activation include the MAPK/extracellular signal-regulated kinases (ERK) kinase kinase (MEKK)[113] with an effector side consisting at least of COX-2 and prostaglandin E2[114]. The therapeutic potential of these pathways was illustrated by the down-regulation of IL-6, IL-8, MMP-1, and MMP-3 production in FLS after application of a specific p38 MAPK inhibitor[115]. Notably, aside from cytokine-dependent pathways mediated by p38α and -β, more proof for a cytokine-independent activation of FLS is given by the involvement of p38 MAPK in TGF-dependent hyaluronan synthase 1 activation[116], the ERK/phosphatidylinositol (PI) 3-dependent up-regulation of the oncofetal H19 gene in FLS[117], and the expression of endogenous L1 elements in these cells leading to the up-regulation of p38δ, an inducer of MMP-1[13].

Other cell cycle inhibitors such as p21, which may contribute to FLS activation and growth of RA synovium, have also been identified as being dysregulated in, or even lacking[3], key compartments of human RA. Conversely, restoration of p21 expression was able to down-regulate pro-inflammatory mediators such as IL-6[118] and inhibition of histone deacetylase, which acts by histone hyperacetylation of FLS, showed a similar consecutive up-regulation of p21 combined with down-regulation of TNF and IL-1[119].

Most recently, a novel ligand-dependent transcriptional factor, the peroxisome proliferator-activated receptor-γ (PPARγ) has been added to the puzzle of synoviocyte pathophysiology. Stimulation of PPARγ results in inhibition of transcription activity of nuclear transcription factors and down-regulation of pro-inflammatory cytokines. In RA FLS, stimulation of PPARγ induces a negative regulation of NF-κB and AP-1, followed by a down-regulation of numerous cytokines, including TNF-α, IL-1, IL-6, and IL-8 as well as of matrix metalloproteinases such as MMP-1 and MMP-3[120–122].

Apoptosis

A key feature of rheumatoid synovium is that less than 3% of the activated FLS undergo apoptosis[123], which is also reflected by the fact that they are rather resistant to Fas-induced apoptosis. In addition, increasing experimental data indicate that these findings and the respective long-term proliferation of FLS and their invasive growth is due to a unbalanced regulation of the cell cycle. In this regard, it is important to note that activated rheumatoid arthritis synovial fluid (RA-SF) does not exhibit an increased rate of proliferation *in vitro* nor *in vivo*[81,124]. Nevertheless, these alterations of the cell-cycle regulation have stimulated researchers to examine the effect of inducing apoptosis in RA synovium by application of anti-Fas antibodies. In the HTLV-I tax transgenic mouse model, which exhibits RA-like destructive arthritis, intra-articular application of anti-Fas antibodies improved joint swelling and arthritis, and this effect was most likely achieved by induction of considerable apoptosis[125]. Similarly, targeting pro-apoptotic members of the TNF-family such as TNF-related apoptosis-inducing ligand (TRAIL) revealed that the sensitivity of rheumatoid FLS to apoptosis might be a highly selective process as only agonistic antibodies against TRAIL-R2 (DR5) and not TRAIL-R1 (DR4) were able to induce apoptosis in cultured FLS[126]. In addition, the respective intracellular downstream apoptosis-inducing cascade most likely requires a variety of different molecules such as caspases, cytochrome C, and mitochondria[127]. Notably, the apoptosis-inducing effect of TRAIL appears to be restricted to RA synovium as FLS derived from OA synovium rarely express DR5[128], and was accompanied by a down-regulation of MMPs and pro-inflammatory cytokines. In addition, intra-articular overexpression of TRAIL by viral gene transfer exerted a comparable effect in a rabbit arthritis model[129]. Notably, osteoprotegerin (OPG) appears to protective against TRAIL-induced apoptosis as OPG reduced the rate of apoptosis of FLS after incubation with TRAIL, an effect which could be antagonized by anti-OPG monoclonal antibody[130]. However, it needs to be stressed that some of these findings are highly controversial because Park et al.[131] could not detect an induction of apoptosis in RA FLS and Perlman et al.[132] could not observe any DR5 on the surface of RA FLS.

Human FLS, in contrast to murine FLS obtained from arthritis models[133], are also rather resistant to Fas-induced apoptosis by anti-Fas antibodies. This resistance might be due—at least in part—to the up-regulation of FLIP, which exerts an antiapoptotic effect through inhibition of the apoptosis-triggering intracellular enzyme caspase 8 in the synovial lining[134]. Conversely, down-regulation of FLIP by antisense oligonucleotides sensitized FLS to Fas-mediated apoptosis[135]. Intracellular regulation of FLIP appears to be mediated by NF-κB, as the resistance of FLS to TNF-α-triggered apoptosis is dependent on NF-κB activation[136].

A potent inhibitor of apoptosis that has also been found to be up-regulated in FLS is the proto-oncogene Bcl-2, which is located in the inner mitochondrial membrane, the endoplasmic reticulum, and the nuclear membrane. Bcl-2 inhibits one of the terminal steps of apoptosis and recent data indicate that the regulation of

Bcl-2 expression is related to the autocrine activation of IL-15 receptors by synovial fibroblast-derived antiapoptotic IL-15[137]. Other members of the Bcl family are also involved in FLS activation. Bcl-3, a known regulator of NF-κB activity, modulates IL-1-dependent synthesis of MMP-1 via NF-κB.

The lack of tumor suppressor genes such as p53, maspin[138], or PTEN[139] may also contribute to long-term survival of FLS. Although the role of p53, which is expressed in rheumatoid FLS and scattered throughout synovial tissue[140], has not been completely elucidated, especially as its presence and activity might be dependent on distinct but varying local synovial factors. Amongst them are macrophage migration inhibitory factor[141] and environmental factors including exposure to radiation[142] and genomic mutations[143,144]. Activation of the latter may also be directly linked to the alterations in the DNA mismatch repair enzyme repertoire in RA synovium and FLS[145,146]. However, the p53-associated alterations in RA synovium and in RA FLS can be used as 'model system' for examining activation pathways in FLS. For example, accumulation of intracellular p53 by proteasome inhibitors can prevent PDGF-stimulated synovial cells from progressing into the S-phase of the cell cycle. Moreover, in the collagen-induced arthritis model, p53-deficient mice showed an increased severity of arthritis lacking any indication for apoptosis, and inhibition of endogenous p53 increased the aggressiveness of RA FLS towards normal cartilage in the SCID mouse model for RA[147].

The tumor suppressor PTEN is involved in the development of various malignant diseases, and in RA the lack of PTEN in the synovial lining and at sites of invasive growth most likely contributes significantly to the longevity of activated FLS at sites of destruction[148]. This effect could be based on the PTEN-dependent effect on IκB/NFκB and other nuclear factors such as akt/protein kinase B, similar to that observed in neoplasms[149–152]. SUMO-1, a molecule that protects against Fas- and TNF-induced cell death, has also been shown to be expressed intensively in RA synovium[153].

The role of FLS in animal models

As RA appears to be a disease, which—in nature—is restricted to humans, the majority of animal models can only reflect a limited spectrum of pathways operative in their human counterpart. However, a variety of animal models have provided insights into the pathways that are involved in joint destruction[154]. One of the most intensively examined 'prototype' models of spontaneous arthritis in animals is the MRL-lpr/lpr mouse. In homozygous animals, the mutation of a single gene (lpr) triggers severe autoimmune disease, a lymphoproliferative disorder with the production of rheumatoid factors and a RA-like symmetric polyarthritis. The initial disease in these animals is characterized by a high number of FLS showing a transformed or activated appearance, as observed by Fassbender in human rheumatoid synovium[1], and to a lesser extent by inflammatory cells. Proliferation-associated proto-oncogenes ras and myc in these murine FLS are linked to the expression of cathepsins B and L, as well as to MMP-1 leading to progressive articular destruction[86,155]. At later stages, inflammatory cells appear in the subsynovial tissue, resembling the situation in human rheumatoid synovium[86]. The genomic mutation site in these animals is located in the Fas apoptosis gene. This lpr mutation is the result of a retrotransposon (endogenous retrovirus) insertion within the Fas gene[156,157].

The SCID-mouse model for RA

To explore the role of FLS in cartilage destruction and their interaction with different articular structures in detail, a model lacking the influence of the immune system has been developed in several steps. The initial experiments were performed with thymus-deficient nude mice, in which FLS derived from RA patients formed a pannus-like tissue. The following step was based on the observation that synovium can be implanted into SCID mice and maintain its phenotype for an extended period of time. This improved model consisted of co-implanting small pieces of normal human cartilage and RA synovium under the kidney capsule of SCID mice. The implants survived for more than 200 days and, similar to human disease, the synovium progressively invaded the cartilage[7]. Molecular characterization of this early stage of RA-like synovial growth demonstrated matrix-degrading proteinases in FLS at the site of cartilage destruction. In the next step, the key role of the FLS in this model was supported by the co-implantation of cultured human rheumatoid FLS with normal human cartilage, resulting in a similar invasion and cathepsin production at the sites of attachment without any involvement of human macrophages as well as B and T cells[158]. Notably, these observations were supported by findings in c-fos transgenic mice, showing also that synovial hyperplasia can occur independent of overt T cell influence, and in a similar human setting, an AIDS patient with long-term RA showed progressive joint destruction and production of matrix-degrading proteinases by FLS at the site of invasion despite lacking synovial or peripheral blood CD4+ T cells[159].

Fibroblasts as targets for novel therapeutic approaches

Based on the above-mentioned pluripotent properties of FLS in joint destruction, these cells have within the past years moved steadily into the center of interest with regard to development of novel therapeutic strategies. In parallel to the developments in molecular medicine, specific attention has been paid to cellular interaction, regulation of production of matrix-degrading enzymes, and involvement in angiogenesis.

Communication and interaction

Within the family of molecules that take part in the interaction of cells with other cells and their surrounding matrix, the 'communication ligands and receptors', a large majority of these molecules belong to adhesion molecules. They consist of integrin, selectin, and immunoglobulin supergene families[204]. Observations indicate that the production and release of matrix-degrading enzymes (e.g., MMP-1) by FLS is triggered by integrin-matrix interactions[160]. In addition, pro-inflammatory cytokines such as IL-1β are able to enhance integrin expression on FLS[161].

Increasing data show that a variety of members of the immunoglobulin gene superfamily, especially, are expressed on FLS. VCAM-1 could be found in the lining layer of proliferating RA synovium and, in particular the FLS, which are invading articular cartilage express VCAM-1 to a large extent[162]. In the synovial microvasculature, VCAM-1 binds to the lymphocyte membrane very-late activation antigen-4 (VLA-4), which serves also as ligand for an alternatively spliced form of fibronectin, CS-1. CS-1, on the other hand, is also involved in multidirectional interaction between FLS, matrix, and lymphocytes[163]. Pro-inflammatory cytokines, including TNF-α, IL-1β, and IL-18 can induce VCAM-1 expression on FLS, in some cases through different intracellular activation pathways or after interaction with T cells[164,165]. This cellular interaction can be inhibited by glucocorticoids, which may account for some of the beneficial effects observed in RA patients. Another fibronectin ligand, the integrin α5β1 (CD49e), is also up-regulated in cultured RA FLS[166], and similar observations were made for the integrin receptors for collagen type IV, laminin, and tenascin[166]. The value of these findings was supported by the inhibition of the invasion of rheumatoid FLS into bovine cartilage following application of antibodies to α4 integrins[167], and by blocking the ligand for VCAM-1, which inhibited only transendothelial migration[168]. Of note, rheumatoid FLS express also mRNA for the sensory neuropeptide substance P, which can enhance the effect of pro-inflammatory cytokines on VCAM-1 expression[169].

On cultured FLS, ICAM-1, a predominantly macrophage-derived adhesion molecule[170,171], is expressed at low levels. However, when stimulated with various cytokines such as IFN-γ, IL-1, or TNF-α, the expression of ICAM-1 on these cells can be markedly increased. The interaction of RA FLS with T lymphocytes appears to be mediated through ligation of ICAM-1 to its binding partner LFA-1. *In vivo*, ICAM-1-positive FLS are surrounded by LFA-1-positive T lymphocytes, which are associated with an up-regulation of IL-1 expression by FLS[172]. The potential importance of the role of ICAM-1 in the pathogenesis of RA has been further supported by the clinical finding that short-term treatment with monoclonal antibodies to ICAM-1 in RA patients resulted in clinical improvement of the disease in about half of the patients[173], and that pulse methylprednisolone reduced considerably the expression of synovial lining ICAM-1.

However, interaction of FLS with matrix is not only based on expression of adhesion molecules; cartilage and bone matrix proteins can also modulate adherence of FLS significantly[174,175]. Moreover, for direct interaction of FLS in the lining layer, integral membrane proteins such as cadherin-11, which could be shown to drive the formation of tissue-like sheets and lining-like structures *in vitro* and which are expressed in a tissue-restricted pattern, appear to be of utmost importance for the pannus formation in rheumatoid synovium[176].

Matrix destruction

Key players in the destruction of articular cartilage and bone are matrix metalloproteinases (MMPs) and cathepsins. MMPs include collagenases, stromelysin, gelatinases, and membrane-type (MT) MMPs. At present, MMPs 1–24 and numerous intracellular signaling pathways operative in regulation of MMP synthesis have been characterized[177,178]. MMPs can be activated by extracellular MMP inducers such as EMMPRIN[179,180] and cleave connective tissue matrix components, including collagens, glycoproteins, and proteoglycans. In RA synovium, the number of MMP-1-producing cells and the net excess of MMP-1 compared with their natural inhibitors TIMPs 1–3 (tissue inhibitors of metalloproteinases 1–3) correlated with the degree of synovial inflammation[180,181]. Of note, the invasiveness of FLS appears to be linked to a distinct MMP profile including MMP-1, MMP-3, and MMP-10[124], and direct cellular contacts and interactions within the synovial compartment are critical for the secretion of MMPs and the integrity of gap junctions[182].

The best known member of the MMP family is MMP-1, also referred to as collagenase-1. MMP-1 cleaves the collagens I, II, VII, and X. FLS at sites of invasion or within the synovial lining layer are a major source of these enzymes[183] and most likely drives RA joint destruction to a large extent[184]. With regard to its potential for novel treatment approaches, it could be shown that inhibition of MMP-1 synthesis by retroviral overexpression of ribozymes targeting MMP-1 mRNA results in a significant reduction of the invasiveness of FLS in the SCID-mouse model for RA[185] without affecting the production of other MMPs. MMP-13 (collagenase-3), on the other hand, cleaves predominantly cartilage collagen type II and is also present abundantly in the RA synovial lining[186]. A more pleiotropic member of the MMP family, MMP-9 or gelatinase B, is a marker for inflammation rather than being specific for RA. This finding is supported by the fact that MMP-9 is not restricted to FLS, but is also synthesized by endothelial cells, macrophages, and leukocytes[187,188]. Moreover, experiments addressing the regulation of MMP-2 revealed a direct link of MMP up-regulation in FLS with the PI3-kinase and akt-pathway[189].

Membrane-type MMPs are amongst the most interesting recently discovered molecules involved in, and associated with RA and FLS pathophysiology. MT1-MMP (MMP-14) and MT3-MMP (MMP-16) are able to cleave extracellular matrix components and can activate other MMPs. Abundant expression of MT1-MMP and MT3-MMP was found in RA synovium, with MT3-MMP being expressed by FLS, and MT1-MMP by FLS and CD68-positive osteoclasts and macrophages[190,191]. The respective proteolytic activity at sites of synovial attachment to cartilage was found to be mediated by a complex consisting of MT1-MMP, TIMP-2, and MMP-2, and the distinct role of MT1 and MT3-MMP in joint destruction was supported by their overexpression in RA synovium when compared to MT2-MMP (MMP-15) and MT4-MMP (MMP-17)[191].

Another family of proteolytic enzymes operative in RA synovium are cathepsins, which are also linked to the activation of numerous proto-oncogenes observed in FLS. For example, the transfection of ras oncogene into fibroblasts leads to cellular activation and the induction of cathepsin L, and the expression of cathepsin L correlates with ras expression and the metastatic potential of cells. Cathepsin L degrades collagen types I, II, IX, XI[192] and proteoglycans, and therefore contributes substantially to cartilage destruction in RA[80,86,193]. The importance of this enzyme has been further underlined by a recent approach, in which cathepsin L-specific ribozymes that block the translation of cathepsin L mRNA into active protein were able to inhibit the cathepsin L-mediated cartilage destruction in the SCID-mouse model for RA[194]. In addition, the contribution of FLS to bone degradation appears to be the production of cathepsin K[195]. Fluoromethylketones are able to inhibit this cathepsin B and L activity when administered orally in a murine arthritis model illustrating—at least to some extent—the therapeutic attractiveness of matrix-degrading enzymes[196].

Another system of matrix degradation is the plasminogen activation system, centered around the serine proteinase plasmin. Plasmin can activate matrix metalloproteinases and has direct proteolytic properties. FLS can synthesize high amounts of urokinase-plasminogen activator *in vitro* and the receptor of this activator is also expressed on the surface of FLS, and part of the matrix-degrading capabilities of RA-SF appears to be mediated by plasmin, as shown by gene transfer of a plasmin inhibitor[197] supporting the hypothesis of a substantial role of the plasminogen activation system in rheumatoid synovium. In addition, activated FLS not only contribute to osteoclastogenesis[198] but also appear to degrade bone by the expression of a proton pump[199].

With regard to FLS-targeted therapy, overexpression of TIMPs has been evaluated in various settings. TIMP-1 mRNA and protein is present in the synovial lining[200], and pro-inflammatory cytokines such as IL-1 and TNF-α—in contrast to IL-11[201]—appear not to influence the expression of TIMP-1[202]. TIMP-1 is up-regulated by early growth response genes such as egr-1[203]. Of interest, gene transfer experiments have shown that both TIMP-1 and TIMP-3, which are also inhibitors of TNF-α converting enzyme (TACE)[204], a molecule which activates TNF-α synthesis in RA synovium, can

specifically inhibit the synovial fibroblast-mediated destruction of cartilage in the SCID-mouse model[205]. These data suggest that the transfer of TIMP-3 might inhibit both the TNF-α cytokinedriven pathway and the cytokine-independent pathway of joint destruction in RA. Novel metalloproteinase inhibitors such as RECK (reversion-inducing cysteine-rich protein with Kazal motifs), which are expressed by FLS and macrophages in RA synovium, may further extend the spectrum of potential candidates for therapeutic inhibitory strategies[206].

Angiogenesis

Intensive vascularization is one of the essentials for synovial activation and joint destruction[207]. During this process, the up-regulation of the proangiogenic growth factor vascular endothelial growth factor (VEGF) appears to be a key event. VEGF mRNA and protein, as well as its respective receptor flk-1 (kinase insert domain receptor (KDR)) are present in rheumatoid synovium[208,209] and co-cultivation experiments of FLS with inflammatory cells could show that both VEGF synthesis and neovascularization were stimulated by this interaction, which included the up-regulation of specific integrins[210]. These findings were supported by the fact that virus-mediated overexpression of soluble VEGF receptor sFlt-1 was able to suppress disease activity in collagen-induced arthritis[210].

On the other hand, pro-inflammatory cytokines are also able to up-regulate proangiogenic factors in FLS. This angiogenesis-inducing effect could be shown for angiopoietin-1, which is not only present in RA synovium but was also up-regulated in FLS

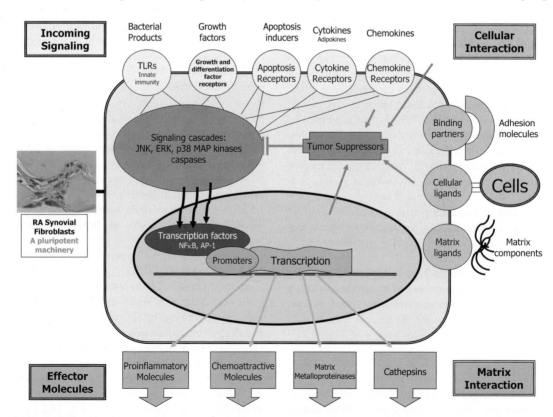

Fig. 8.1 The rheumatoid fibroblast-like synoviocyte is embedded into an extracellular 'network of activating cytokines' and plays a pivotal role in joint destruction in RA by production of numerous matrix-degrading factors specifically operative at sites of cartilage and bone destruction.

by TNF-α both on the mRNA and protein levels[211]. The expression of angiopoietin-1 and -2 in FLS appears to be linked to its respective endothelium-specific tyrosine kinase receptors Tie-1 and Tie-2 in an autocrine/paracrine manner, which also induces enhanced chemotactic migration of FLS[212]. Moreover, antagonizing pro-inflammatory cytokines such as IL-6 by anti-IL-6 receptor monoclonal therapy was able to reduce VEGF serum levels in RA[213]. Moreover, it has recently been shown that members of the thrombospondin family, that is, thrombospondin-2, can inhibit FLS-dependent vascularization as thrombospondin-2-transduced FLS were able to inhibit local vascularization and inflammation in the SCID-mouse model[214].

However, the potential stimuli for the up-regulation of proangiogenic factors in RA synovium are still under intensive investigation. Amongst a variety of potential factors, hypoxia appears to be one of the key triggers. Hypoxia not only modulates expression of chemotactic factors[215], it also contributes to up-regulation of matrix metalloproteinases such as MMP-1 and MMP-3 combined with down-regulation of TIMP-1 in FLS[216]. IL-1 appears to further enhance this effect, which includes also the up-regulation of COX-2[217]. Most recently, it was shown that hypoxia induces the expression of Id-2, which could be detected at sites of synovial invasion into cartilage and bone. In the same set of experiments, it was also demonstrated that Id-2 facilitates osteoclastogenesis[218].

FLS as drug carriers and drug targets

The potential use of FLS as drug carriers has been demonstrated impressively in the SCID-mouse model of RA, in which the metabolically active cartilage-invading FLS take up albumin conjugates (HSA-MTX) intracellularily[219]. In this specific model, MTX and HSA-MTX both inhibited cartilage invasion and degradation with comparable efficiency[220]. Similarly, it could be shown that in different animal models albumin conjugates accumulated in tumors as well as in inflamed joints of arthritis mice[221]. The molecular mechanisms that are driving these effects most likely affect FLS population doubling time[221] and the disruption of pro-inflammatory cytokine loops[222]. Although it is not yet conclusive, the active metabolite of leflunomide, A771726, is able to down-regulate MAPK signaling pathways in FLS, suggesting that thereby there occurs a significant inhibition of the production of MMP-1, MMP-3, and MMP-13[223], and also an increased synthesis of IL-1 receptor antagonist[224]. However, long-term efficacy of exogenously administered joint-protective drugs such as IL-1ra still remains a problem, which might be overcome by gene transfer in optimized settings[225].

Outlook

Distinct cellular and molecular events distinguish RA from other arthritides and RA FLS from non-RA FLS. At present the majority of data indicate a key role for these highly activated cells specifically at sites of cartilage or bone destruction. This role is continuously being extended by the detection of previously unknown pathways and mechanisms such as proinflammatory adipokines[226]. As illustrated in Fig. 8.1, this rheumatoid fibroblast-like synoviocyte, which is intrinsically activated and in addition embedded into an extracellular 'network of activating cytokines', plays a pivotal role in joint destruction in RA and is therefore a logical target for the development of novel therapeutic approaches.

Acknowledgements

The work has been supported by the German Research Society (DFG # Mu 1383/1–3, 3–4, and 10–1) and the Swiss National Science Foundation (SNF 3200–64142.00).

References

1. Fassbender, H. G. Histomorphologic basis of articular cartilage destruction in rheumatoid arthritis. *Coll Rel Res* 1983; **3**: 141–55.
2. Neumann, E., Kullmann, F., Judex, M. *et al.* Identification of differentially expressed genes in rheumatoid arthritis by a combination of complementary DNA array and RNA arbitrarily primed-polymerase chain reaction. *Arthritis Rheum* 2002; **46**: 52–63.
3. Judex, M., Neumann, E., Lechner, S. *et al.* Laser-mediated microdissection facilitates analysis of area-specific gene expression in rheumatoid synovium. *Arthritis Rheum* 2003; **48**: 97–102.
4. Ospelt, C., Neidhart, M., Gay, R. E., and Gay, S. Synovial activation in rheumatoid arthritis. *Front Biosci* 2004; **9**: 2323–34.
5. Franz, J. K., Pap, T., Müller-Ladner, U., Gay, R. E., Burmester, G. R., and Gay, S. T cell-independent joint destruction. In *T cells in arthritis* (Miossec P, van den Berg WB, Firestein GS, eds), pp. 55–74. Basel: Birkhäuser; 1998.
6. Müller-Ladner, U., Kriegsmann, J., Gay, R. E., and Gay, S. Oncogenes in rheumatoid arthritis. *Rheum Dis Clin N Am* 1995; **21**: 675–90.
7. Geiler, T., Kriegsmann, J., Keyszer, G., Gay, R. E., and Gay, S. A new model for rheumatoid arthritis generated by engraftment of rheumatoid synovial tissue and normal human cartilage into SCID mice. *Arthritis Rheum* 1994; **37**: 1664–71.
8. Judex, M., Neumann, E., Fleck, M. *et al.* 'Inverse wrap': an improved implantation technique for virus-transduced synovial fibroblasts in the SCID-mouse model for RA. *Mod Rheumatol* 2001; **11**: 145–50.
9. Firestein, G. S., and Zvaifler, N. J. How important are T cells in chronic rheumatoid synovitis? II. T cell-independent mechanisms from beginning to end. *Arthritis Rheum* 2002; **46**: 298–308.
10. Rooney, M., Condell, D., Quinlan, W. *et al.* Analysis of the histologic variation of synovitis in rheumatoid arthritis. *Arthritis Rheum* 1988; **31**: 956–63.
11. Edwards, J. C. W. Fibroblast biology: development and differentiation of fibroblasts in arthritis. *Arthritis Res Ther* 2000; **2**: 344–7.
12. Mattey, D. L., Dawes. P. T., Nixon, N. B., and Slater, H. Transforming growth factor β1 and interleukin 4 induced a smooth muscle actin expression and myofibroblast-like differentiation in human synovial fibroblasts in vitro: modulation by basic fibroblast growth factor. *Ann Rheum Dis* 1997; **56**: 426–31.
13. Neidhart, M., Rethage, J., Kuchen, S. *et al.* Retrotransposable L1 elements expressed in rheumatoid arthritis synovial tissue: association with genomic DNA hypomethylation and influence on gene expression. *Arthritis Rheum* 2000; **43**: 2634–47.
14. Mehraein, Y., Lennerz, C., Ehlhardt, S. *et al.* Latent Epstein-Barr virus (EBV) infection and cytomegalovirus (CMV) infection in synovial tissue of autoimmune chronic arthritis detemined by RNA- and DNA-in situ hybridization. *Mod Pathol* 2004; **17**: 781–9.
15. Neumann, E., Judex, M., Kullmann, F. *et al.* Inhibition of cartilage destruction by double gene transfer of IL-1ra and IL-10 is mediated by the activin pathway. *Gene Ther* 2002; **9**: 1508–1519.
16. Gay, S., and Kalden, J. R. Retroviruses and autoimmune rheumatic diseases. *Clin Exp Immunol* 1994; **98**: 1–5.
17. Carson, D. A., and Ribeiro, J. M. Apoptosis and disease. *Lancet* 1993; **341**: 1251–4.

18. Land, H., Parada, L. F., and Weinberg, R. A. Tumorigenic conversion of primary fibroblasts requires at least two cooperating oncogenes. *Nature* 1983; **304**: 596–602.

19. Nakajima, T., Aono, H., Hasunuma, T. *et al*. Overgrowth of human synovial cells driven by the human T cell leukemia virus type I tax gene. *J Clin Invest* 1991; **92**: 186–93.

20. Kuchen, S., Seemayer, C. A., Rethage, J. *et al*. The L1 retroelement-related p40 protein induces p38delta MAP kinase. *Autoimmunity* 2004; **37**: 57–65.

21. Kyburz, D., Rethage, J., Seibl, R. *et al*. Bacterial peptidoglykans but not CpG oligodeoxynucleotides activate synovial fibroblasts by toll-like receptor signaling. *Arthritis Rheum* 203; **48**: 642–50.

22. Seibl, R., Birchler, T., Loeliger, S. *et al*. Expression and regulation of Toll-like receptor 2 in rheumatoid arthritis synovium. *Am J Pathol* 2003; **162**: 1221–7.

23. Nakano, K., Okada, Y., Saito, K., and Tanaka, Y. Induction of RANKL expression and osteoclast maturation by the binding of fibroblast growth factor 2 to heparan sulfate proteoglycan on rheumatoid synovial fibroblasts. *Arthritis Rheum* 2004; **50**: 2450–8.

24. Cheon, H., Yu, S. J., Yoo, D. H. *et al*. Increased expression of pro-inflammatory cytokines and metalloproteinase-1 by TGF-β1 in synovial fibroblasts from rheumatoid arthritis and normal individuals. *Clin Exp Immunol* 2002; **127**: 547–52.

25. Kim, G., Jun, B., and Elkon, K. B. Necessary role of phosphatidylinositol 3-kinase in transforming growth factor β-mediated activation of akt in normal and rheumatoid arthritis synovial fibroblasts. *Arthritis Rheum* 2002; **46**: 1504–11.

26. Lafyatis, R., Remmers, E. F., Roberts, A. B., Yocum, D. E., Sporn, M. B., and Wilder, R. L. Anchorage independent growth regulation of synoviocytes from arthritic and normal joints: stimulation by exogenous platelet-derived growth factor and inhibition by transforming growth factor-beta and retinoids. *J Clin Invest* 1989; **83**: 1267–76.

27. Franz, J. K., Kolb, S. A., Hummel, K. M. *et al*. Interleukin-16, produced by synovial fibroblasts, mediates chemoattraction for CD4$^+$ T lymphocytes in rheumatoid arthritis. *Eur J Immunol* 1998; **28**: 2661–71.

28. Chabaud, M., Fossiez, F., Taupin, J-L., and Miossec, P. Enhancing effect of IL-17 on IL-1-induced IL-6 and leukemia inhibitory factor production by rheumatoid arthritis synoviocytes and its regulation by Th2 cytokines. *J Immunol* 1998; **161**: 409–14.

29. McInnes, I. B., and Liew, F. Y. Interleukin-15: a proinflammatory role in rheumatoid arthritis synovitis. *Immunol Today* 1988; **19**: 75–9.

30. Firestein, G. S. The T cell cometh: interplay between adaptive immunity and cytokine networks in rheumatoid arthritis. *J Clin Invest* 2004; **114**: 471–4.

31. Firestein, G. S., Alvaro-Gracia, J. M., and Maki, R. Quantitative analysis of cytokine gene expression in rheumatoid arthritis. *J Immunol* 1990; **144**: 3347–53.

32. Koch, A. E., Kunkel, S. L., Burrows, J. C. *et al*. Synovial tissue macrophage as a source of the chemotactic cytokine IL-8. *J Immunol* 1997; **147**: 2187–95.

33. Keyszer, G. M., Heer, A. H., Kriegsmann, J. *et al*. Detection of insulin-like growth factor I and II in synovial tissue specimens of patients with rheumatoid arthritis and osteoarthritis by in situ hybridization. *J Rheumatol* 1995; **22**: 275–81.

34. Lotz, M., and Guerne, P. A. Interleukin-6 induces the synthesis of tissue inhibitor of metalloproteinases-1/erythroid potentiating activity (TIMP-1/EPA). *J Biol Chem* 1991; **266**: 2017–20.

35. Alvaro-Gracia, J. M., Zvaifler, N. J., and Firestein, G. S. Cytokines in chronic inflammatory arthritis. V. Mutual antagonism between interferon-gamma and tumor necrosis factor-alpha on HLA-DR expression, proliferation, collagenase production, and granulocyte-macrophage colony-stimulating factor production by rheumatoid arthritis synoviocytes. *J Clin Invest* 1990; **86**: 1790–8.

36. Franz, J. K., Kolb, S. A., Hummel, K. M. *et al*. Interleukin-16, produced by synovial fibroblasts mediates chemo attraction for CD4+ T lymphocytes in rheumatoid arthritis. *Eur J Immunol* 1998; **28**: 2661–71.

37. Schuler, M. K., and Aicher, W. K. Interleukin-18 is regulated by G protein pathways and protein kinase signals in human fibroblasts. *Rheumatol Int* 2400; **24**: 1–8.

38. Möller, B., Paulukat, J., Nold, M. *et al*. Interferon-gamma induces expression of interleukin-18 binding protein in fibroblast-like synoviocytes. *Rheumatology* 2003; **42**: 442–5.

39. Hata, H., Sakaguchi, N., Yoshitomi, H. *et al*. Distinct contribution of IL-6, TNF-alpha, IL-1, Nad IL-10 to T cell-mediated spontaneous autoimmune arthritis in mice. *J Clin Invest* 2004; **114**: 582–8.

40. Braun, A., Takemura, S., Vallejo, A. N., Goronzy, J. J., and Weyand, C., M., Lymphotoxin beta-mediated stimulation of synoviocytes in rheumatoid arthritis. *Arthritis Rheum* 2004; **50**: 2140–50.

41. Zeisel, M. B., Neff, L. A., Randle, J. *et al*. Impaired release of IL-18 from fibroblast-like synoviocytes activated with protein I/II, a pathogen-associated molecular pattern from oral streptococci, results from defective translation of IL-18 mRNA in pro-IL-18. *Cell Microbiol* 2004; **6**: 593–8.

42. Zeisel, M. B., Druet, V. A., Wachsmann, D., and Sibilia, J. MMP-3 expression and release by rheumatoid arthritis fibroblast-like synoviocytes induced with a bacterial ligand α5β1. *Arthritis Res Ther* 7, R118–R126.

43. Hwang, S. Y., Kim, J. Y., Kim, K. W. *et al*. IL-17 induces production of IL-6 and IL-8 in rheumatoid arthritis synovial fibroblasts via NF-kappaB-and PI3-kinase/Akt-dependent pathways. *Arthritis Res Ther* 2004; **6**: R120–R128.

44. Ota, F., Maeshima, A., Yamashita, S. *et al*. Activin A induces cell proliferation of fibroblast-like synoviocytes in rheumatoid arthritis. *Arthritis Rheum* 2004; **48**: 2442–9.

45. Ohshima, S., Kuchen, S., Seemayer, C. A. *et al*. Galectin 3 and its binding protein in rheumatoid arthritis. *Arthritis Rheum* 2003; **48**: 2788–95.

46. Jeong, J. G., Kim, J. M., Cho, H. *et al*. Effects of IL-1beta on gene expression in human rheumatoid synovial fibroblasts. *Biochem Biophys Res Commun* 2004; **324**: 3–7.

47. Chicheportiche, Y., Chicheportiche, R., Sizing, I. *et al*. Proinflammatory activity of TWEAK on human dermal fibroblasts and synoviocytes: blocking and enhancing effects of anti.TWEAK monoclonal antibodies. *Arthritis Res* 2002; **4**: 126–33.

48. Deon, D., Ahmed, S., Tai, K. *et al*. Cross-talk between IL-1 and IL-6 signaling pathways in rheumatoid arthritis synovial fibroblasts. *J Immunol* 2001; **167**: 5395–403.

49. Jüngel, A., Distler, J. H., Kurowska-Stolarska, M. *et al*. Expression of interleukin-21 receptor, but not interleukin-21, in synovial fibroblasts and synovial macrophages of patients with rheumatoid arthritis. *Arthritis Rheum* 2004; **50**: 1468–76.

50. Yamasaki, S., Nakashima, T., Kawakami, A. *et al*. Cytokines regulate fibroblast-like synovial cell differentiation to adipocyte-like cells. *Rheumatology* 2004; **43**: 448–52.

51. Kubota, A., Hasegawa, K., Suguro, T., and Koshihara, Y. Tumor necrosis factor-alpha promotes the expression of osteoprotegerin in rheumatoid arthritis synovial fibroblasts. *J Rheumatol* 2004; **31**: 426–35.

52. Lories, R. J., Derese, I., Ceuppens, J. L., and Luyten, F. P. Bone morphogenetic proteins 2 and 6, expressed in arthritic synovium, are regulated by proinflammatory cytokines and differentially modulate fibroblast-like synoviocyte apoptosis. *Arthritis Rheum* 2003; **48**: 2807–18.

53. Müller-Ladner, U., Gay, R. E., and Gay, S. Signaling and effector pathways. *Curr Opin Rheumatol* 1900; **1**: 194–201.

54. Alsalameh, S., Amin, R. J., Kunisch, E. *et al*. Preferential induction of prodestructive matrix metalloproteinase-1 and proinflammatory interleukin 6 and prostaglandin E2 in rheumatoid arthritis synovial fibroblasts via tumor necrosis factor receptor-p55. *J Rheumatol* 2003; **30**: 1680–90.

55. Westman, M., Korotkova, M., af Klint, E. *et al*. Expression of microsomal prostaglandin E synthase 1 in rheumatoid arthritis synovium. *Arthritis Rheum* 2003; **50**: 1774–80.

56. Faour, W. H., He, Y., He, Q., W. *et al*. Prostaglandin E^2 regulates the level and stability of cyclooxygenase-2 mRNA through activation of p38 mitogen-activated protein kinase in interleukin-1β-treated human synovial fibroblasts. *J Biol Chem* 276: 31720–31.

57. Kusunoki, N., Yamazaki, R., and Kawai, S. Induction of apoptosis in rheumatoid synovial fibroblasts by celecoxib, but not by other selective cyclooxygenase 2 inhibitors. *Arthritis Rheum* 2002; **46**: 3159–67.

58. Kojima, F., Naraba, H., Sasaki, Y. *et al*. Prostaglandin E2 is an enhancer of interleukin-1beta-induced expression of

membrane-associated prostaglandin E synthase in rheumatoid synovial fibroblasts. *Arthritis Rheum* 2003; **48**: 2819–28.

59. Smith, R. S., Smith, T. J., Blieden, T. M., and Phipps, R. P. Fibroblasts as sentinel cells: synthesis of chemokines and regulation of inflammation. *Am J Pathol* 1997; **151**: 317–22.

60. Tolboom, T. C., Huidekoper, A. L., Kramer, I. M. *et al*. Correlation between expression of CD44 splice variant v8-v9 and invasiveness of fibroblast-like synoviocytes in an in vitro system. *Clin Exp Rheumatol* 2400; **22**: 158–64.

61. Min, D. J., Cho, M. L., Lee, S. H., *et al*. Augmented production of chemokines by the interaction of type II collagen-reactive T cells with rheumatoid synovial fibroblasts. *Arthritis Rheum* 2004; **50**: 1146–55.

62. Liu, M. F., Chao, S. C., Wang, C. R., and Lei, H. Y. Expression of CD40 and CD40 ligand among cell populations within rheumatoid synovial compartment. *Autoimmunity* 2001; **34**: 107–13.

63. Matsui, T., Akahoshi, T., Namai, R. *et al*. Selective recruitment of CCR6-expressing cells by increased production of MIP-3a in rheumatoid arthritis. *Clin Exp Immunol* 2001; **125**: 155–61.

64. Langdon, C., Leith, J., Smith, F., and Richards, C. D. Oncostatin M stimulates monocyte chemoattractant protein-1- and interleukin-1-induced matrix metalloproteinase-1 production by human synovial fibroblasts in vitro. *Arthritis Rheum* 1997; **40**: 2139–46.

65. Hanyuda, M., Kasama, T., Isozaki, T. *et al*. Activated leucocytes express and secrete macrophage inflammatory protein-1alpha upon interaction with synovial fibroblasts of rheumatoid arthritis via a beta2-integrin/ICAM-1 mechanism. *Rheumatology* 2003; **42**: 1390–7.

66. Han, M. K., Kim, J. S., Park, B. H. *et al*. NF-kappaB-dependent lymphocyte hyperadhesiveness to synovial fibroblasts by hypoxia and reoxygenation: potential role in rheumatoid arthritis. *J Leukoc Biol* 2003; **73**: 525–9.

67. Weis-Klemm, M., Alexander, D., Pap, T. *et al*. Synovial fibroblasts from rheumatoid arthritis patients differ in their regulation of IL-16 gene activity in comparison to osteoarthritis fibroblasts. *Cell Physiol Biochem* 2004; **14**: 293–300.

68. Bradfield, P. F., Amft, N., Vernon-Wilson, E. *et al*. Rheumatoid fibroblast-like synoviocytes overexpress the chemokine stromal cell-derived factor 1 (CXCL12), which supports distinct patterns and rates of CD4+ and CD8+ T cell migration within synovial tissue. *Arthritis Rheum* 2003; **48**: 2472–82.

69. Pritchard, J., Tsui, S., Horst, N., Cruikshank, W. W., and Smith, T., J. Synovial fibroblasts from patients with rheumatoid arthritis, like fibroblasts from Graves'disease, express high levels of IL-16 when treated with Igs against insulin-like growth factor-1 receptor. *J Immunol* 2004; **173**: 3564–9.

70. Blaschke, S., Koziolek, M., Schwarz, A. *et al*. Proinflammatory role of fractalkine (CX3CL1) in rheumatoid arthritis. *J Rheumatol* 2003; **30**: 1918–27.

71. Hitchon, C., Wong, K., Ma, G. *et al*. Hypoxia-induced production of stromal cell-derived factor 1 (CXCL12) and vascular endothelial growth factor by synovial fibroblasts. *Arthritis Rheum* 2002; **46**: 2587–97.

72. Burger, J. A., Zvaifler, N. J., Tsukada, N. *et al*. Fibroblast-like synoviocytes support B-cell pseudoemperipolesis via a stromal cell-derived factor-1 and CD106 (VCAM-1)-dependent mechanism. *J Clin Invest* 2001; **107**: 305–15.

73. Pierer, M., Kyburz, D., Rethage, J. *et al*. TLR2 dependent upregulation of chemokines in RA-SF. *Arthritis Rheum* 2002; **46**: S553.

74. Van der Pouw Kraan, T. C., van Gaalen, F. A., Huizinga, T. W *et al*. Discovery of distinctive gene expression profiles in rheumatoid synovium using cDNA microarray technology: evidence for the existence of multiple pathways of tissue destruction and repair. *Genes Immun* 2003; **4**: 187–96.

75. Neumann, E., Lechner, S., Tarner, H. *et al*. Evaluation of differentially expressed genes by a combination of cDNA array and RAP-PCR using the AtlasImage 2.0 software. *J Autoimmun* 2003; **21**: 161–6.

76. Firestein, G. S., and Pisetsky, D. S. DNA microarrays: boundless technology or bound by technology. Guidelines for studies using microarray technology. *Arthritis Rheum* 2002; **46**: 859–61.

77. Distler, O., Neumann, E., Müller-Ladner, U., and Gay, S. Minimum information about a microarray experiment: comment on the editorial by Firestein, GS and Pietsky, DS. *Arthritis Rheum* 2003; **48**, 861.

78. Neidhart, M., Seemayer, C. A., Hummel, K. M. *et al*. Functional characterization of adherent synovial fluid cells in rheumatoid arthritis: destructive potential in vitro and in vivo. *Arthritis Rheum* 2003; **48**: 1873–80.

79. Kunisch, E., Fuhrmann, R., Roth, A. *et al*. Macrophage specificity of three anti-CD68 monoclonal antibodies (KP1, EBM11, and PGM1) widely used for immunohistochemistry and flow cytometry. *Ann Rheum Dis* 2004; **63**: 774–84.

80. Trabandt, A., Gay, R. E., and Gay, S. Oncogene activation in rheumatoid synovium. *APMIS* 1992; **100**: 861–75.

81. Aicher, W. K., Heer, A. H., Trabandt, A. *et al*. Overexpression of zinc-finger transcription factor Z-225/egr-1 in synoviocytes from rheumatoid arthritis patients. *J Immunol* 1994; **152**: 5940–8.

82. Khoa, N. D., Nakazawa, M., Hasunuma, T. *et al*. Potential role of HOXD9 in synoviocyte proliferation. *Arthritis Rheum* 2004; **44**: 1013–21.

83. Schönthal, A., Herrlich, P., Rahmsdorf, H. J., and Ponta, H. Requirement for fos gene expression in the transcriptional activation of collagenase by other oncogenes and phorbol esters. *Cell* 1988; **54**: 325–44.

84. Morita, Y., Kashihara, N., Yamamura, M. *et al*. Antisense oligonucleotides targeting c-fos mRNA inhibit rheumatoid synovial fibroblast proliferation. *Ann Rheum Dis* 1988; **57**: 122–4.

85. Onodera, S., Nishihara, J., Koyama, Y. *et al*. Macrophage migration inhibitory factor up-regulates the expression of interleukin-8 messenger RNA in synovial fibroblasts of rheumatoid arthritis patients: common transcriptional regulatory mechanism between interleukin-8 and interleukin-1beta. *Arthritis Rheum* 2004; **50**: 1437–47.

86. Trabandt, A., Aicher, W. K., Gay, R. E. *et al*. Expression of the collagenolytic and ras-induced cysteine protease cathepsin L and proliferation-associated oncogenes in synovial cells of MRL/l mice and patients with rheumatoid arthritis. *Matrix* 2004; **10**: 349–61.

87. Case, J. P., Lafyatis, R., Remmers, E. F., Kumkumian, G. K., and Wilder, R. L. Transin/stromelysin expression in rheumatoid synovium: a activation-associated metalloproteinase secreted by phenotypically invasive synoviocytes. *Am J Pathol* 1898; **135**: 1064–9.

88. Yamamoto, A., Fukuda, A., Seto, H. *et al*. Suppression of arthritic bone destruction by adenovirus-mediated dominant-negative Ras gene transfer to synoviocytes and osteoclasts. *Arthritis Rheum* 2003; **48**: 2682–92.

89. Pap, T., Nawrath, M., Heinrich, J. *et al*. Cooperation of Ras and Myc-dependent pathways in regulating the growth and invasiveness of synovial fibroblasts in rheumatoid arthritis. *Arthritis Rheum* 2004; **50**: 2794–802.

90. Inoue, H., Takamori, M., Nagata, N. *et al*. An investigation of cell proliferation and soluble mediators induced by interleukin-1β in human synovial fibroblasts: comparative response in osteoarthritis and rheumatoid arthritis. *Inflamm Res* 2001; **50**: 65–72.

91. Crofford, L. J., Tan, B., McCarthy, C. J., and Hla, T. Involvement of nuclear factor κB in the regulation of cyclooxygenase-2 expression by interleukin-1 in rheumatoid synoviocytes. *Arthritis Rheum* 1997; **40**: 226–36.

92. Fujisawa, K., Aono, H., Hasunuma, T., Yamamoto, K., Mita, S., and Nishioka, K. Activation of transcription factor NFκB in human synovial cells in response to tumor necrosis factor-α. *Arthritis Rheum* 1996; **39**: 197–203.

93. Grimbacher, B., Aicher, W. K., Peter, H. H., and Eibel, H. TNF-α induces the transcription factor Egr-1, pro-inflammatory cytokines and cell proliferation in human skin fibroblasts and synovial lining cells. *Rheumatol Int* 1998; **17**: 185–92.

94. Gerritsen, M. E., Shen, C-P., and Perry, A. Synovial fibroblasts and the sphingomyelinase pathway: sphingomyelin turnover and ceramide generation are not signaling mechanisms for the actions of tumor necrosis factor-α. *Am J Pathol* 1998; **152**: 505–12.

95. Ando, K., Kanazawa, S., Tetsuka, T. *et al*. Induction fo Notch signaling by tumor necrosis factor in rheumatoid synovial fibroblasts. *Oncogene* 2003; **22**: 7796–803.

96. Gravallese, E. M., Manning, C., Tsay, A. *et al.* Synovial tissue in rheumatoid arthritis is a source of osteoclast differentiation factor. *Arthritis Rheum* 2000; 43: 250–8.

97. Takayanagi, H., Iizuka, H., Juji, T. *et al.* Involvement of receptor activator of nuclear factor κB ligand/osteoclast differentiation factor in osteoclastogenesis from synoviocytes in rheumatoid arthritis. *Arthritis Rheum* 2000; 43: 259–69.

98. Shigeyama, Y., Pap, T., Künzler, P. *et al.* Expression of osteoclast differentiation factor in rheumatoid arthritis. *Arthritis Rheum* 2000; 43: 2523–30.

99. Romas, E., Gillespie, M. T., and Martin, T. J. Involvement of receptor activator of NFκB ligand and tumor necrosis factor-α in bone destruction in rheumatoid arthritis. *Bone* 2002; 30: 340–6.

100. Aupperle, K. R., Bennett, B. L., Boyle, D. L. *et al.* NF-κB regulation by IκB kinase in primary fibroblast-like synoviocytes. *J Immunol* 1999; 163: 427–33.

101. Aupperle, K. R., Bennett, B. L., Han, Z. *et al.* NF-κB regulation by IκB kinase-2 in rheumatoid arthritis synoviocytes. *J Immunol* 2001; 166: 2705–11.

102. Kishore, N., Sommers, C., Mathialgan, S. *et al.* A selective IKK-2 inhibitor blocks NF-kappa B-dependent gene expression in interleukin-1 beta-stimulated synovial fibroblasts. *J Biol Chem* 2003; 278: 32861–71.

103. Andreakos, E., Smith, C., Kiriakidis, S. *et al.* Heterogeneous requirement of IkappaB kinase 2 for inflammatory cytokine and matrix metalloproteinase production in rheumatoid arthritis: implications for therapy. *Arthritis Rheum* 2003; 48: 1901–12.

104. Grall, F., Gu, X., Tan, L. *et al.* responses to the proinflammatory cytokines interleukin-1 and tumor necrosis factor alpha in cells derived from rheumatoid synovium and other joint tissues involve nuclear factor kappaB-mediated induction of the Ets transcription factor ESE-1. *Arthritis Rheum* 2003; 48: 1249–60.

105. Zhang, H. G., Hyde, K., Page, G. P. *et al.* Novel tumor necrosis factor alpha-regulated genes in rheumatoid arthritis. *Arthritis Rheum* 2004; 50: 420–31.

106. Johnson, G. L., and Lapadat, R. Mitogen-activated protein kinase pathways mediated by ERK, JNK, and protein kinases. *Science* 2002; 298; 1911–12.

107. Miyazawa, K., Mori, A., Miyata, H. *et al.* Regulation of interleukin-1β-induced interleukin-6 gene expression in human fibroblast-like synoviocytes by p38 mitogen-activated protein kinase. *J Biol Chem* 1998; 273: 24832–8.

108. Westermarck, J., Li, S. P., Kallunki, T. *et al.* p38 mitogen-activated protein kinase-dependent activation of protein phosphatases 1 and 2A inhibits MEK1 and MEK2 activity and collagenase 1 (MMP-1) gene expression. *Mol Cell Biol* 2001; 21: 2373–83.

109. Han, Z., Boyle, D. L., Chang, L. *et al.* c-Jun N terminal kinase is required for metalloproteinase expression and joint destruction in inflammatory arthritis. *J Clin Invest* 2001; 108: 73–81.

110. Bradley, K., Scatizzi, J. C., Fiore, S. *et al.* Retinoblastoma suppression of matrix metalloproteinase 1, but not interleukin-6, through a p38-dependent pathway in rheumatoid arthritis synovial fibroblasts. *Arthritis Rheum* 2004; 50: 78–87.

111. Sundarrajan, M., Boyle, D. L., Chabaud-Riou, M., Hammaker, D., and Firestein, G. S. Expression of the MAPK kinases MKK-4 and MKK-7 in rheumatoid arthritis and their role as key regulators of JNK. *Arthritis Rheum* 2003; 48: 2450–60.

112. Chabaud-Riou, M., and Firestein, G. S. Expression and activation of mitogen-activated protein kinase kinases-3 and −6 in rheumatoid arthritis. *Am J Pathol* 2004; 164: 177–84.

113. Hammaker, D. R., Boyle, D. L., Chabaud-Riou, M., and Firestein, G. S. Regulation of c-Jun N-terminal kinase by MEKK-2 and mitogen-activated protein kinase kinase kinases in rheumatoid arthritis. *J Immunol* 2004; 172: 1612–18.

114. Crofford, L. J., McDonagh, K.T., Guo, S. *et al.* Adenovirus binding to cultured synoviocytes triggers signaling through MAPK pathways and induces expression of cyclooxygenase-2. *J Gene Med.* 2005; 7: 288–96.

115. Westra, J., Limburg, P. C., de Boer, P., and van Rijswijk, M. H. Effects of RWJ 67657, a p38 mitogen activated protein kinase (MAPK) inhibitor, on the production of inflammatory mediators by rheumatoid synovial fibroblasts. *Ann Rheum Dis* 2004; 63:1453–9.

116. Stuhlmeier, K. M., and Pollaschek, C. Differential effect of transforming growth factor beta (TGF-beta) on the genes encoding hyaluronan synthases and utilization of the p38 MAPK pathway in TGF-beta-induced hyaluronan synthase 1 activation. *J Biol Chem* 2004; 279: 8753–60.

117. Stuhlmüller, B., Kunisch, E., Franz, J. *et al.* Detection of oncofetal h19 RNA in rheumatoid arthritis synovial tissue. *Am J Pathol* 2003; 163: 901–11.

118. Perlman, H., Bradley, K., Liu, H. *et al.* IL-6 and matrix metalloproteinase-1 are regulated by the cyclin-dependent kinase inhibitor p21 in synovial fibroblasts. *J Immunol* 2003; 170: 838–45.

119. Nishida, K., Komiyama, T., Miyazawa, S. *et al.* Histone deacetylase inhibitor suppression of autoantibody-mediated arthritis in mice via regulation of p16INK4a and p21 (WAF1/Cip1) expression. *Arthritis Rheum* 2004; 50: 3365–76.

120. Fahmi, H., Pelletier, J. P., Di Battista, J. A. *et al.* Peroxisome proliferator-activated receptor γ activators inhibit MMP-1 production in human synovial fibroblasts likely by reducing the binding of the activator protein 1. *Osteoarthritis Cartilage* 2002; 10: 100–8.

121. Yamasaki, S., Nakashima, T., Kawakami, A. *et al.* Functional changes in rheumatoid fibroblast-like synovial cells through activation of peroxisome proliferator-activated receptor γ-mediated signalling pathway. *Clin Exp Immunol* 2002; 129: 379–84.

122. Ji, J. D., Cheon, H., Jun, J. B. *et al.* Effects of peroxisome proliferator-activated receptor-γ?(PPAR-γ) on the expression of inflammatory cytokines and apoptosis induction in rheumatoid synovial fibroblasts and monocytes. *J Autoimmun* 2001; 17: 215–21.

123. Matsumoto, S., Müller-Ladner, U., Gay, R. E., Nishioka, K., and Gay, S. Ultrastructural demonstration of apoptosis, Fas and Bcl-2 expression of rheumatoid synovial fibroblasts. *J Rheumatol* 1996; 23: 1345–52.

124. Tolboom, T. C., Pieterman, E., van der Laan, W. H. *et al.* Invasive properties of fibroblast-like synoviocytes: correlation with growth characteristics and expression of MMP-1, MMP-3, and MMP-1. *Ann Rheum Dis* 2002; 61: 975–80.

125. Hoa, T. T. M., Hasunuma, T., Aono, H., *et al.* Novel mechanisms of selective apoptosis in synovial T cells of patients with rheumatoid arthritis. *J Rheumatol* 1996; 23: 1332–7.

126. Ichikawa, K., Liu, W., Fleck, M. *et al.* TRAIL-R2 (DR5) mediates apoptosis of synovial fibroblasts in rheumatoid arthritis. *J Immunol* 2003; 171: 1061–9.

127. Itoh, K., Hase, H., Kojima, H. *et al.* central role of mitochondria and p53 in Fas-mediated apoptosis of rheumatoid synovial fibroblasts. *Rheumatology* 2004; 43: 277–85.

128. Miranda-Carus, M. E., Balsa, A., Benito-Miguel, M. *et al.* Rheumatoid arthritis synovial fluid fibroblasts express TRAIL-R2 (DR5) that is functionally active. *Arthritis Rheum* 2004;50: 2786–93.

129. Yao, Q., Wang, S., Gambotto, A. *et al.* Intra-articular adenoviral-mediated gene transfer of trail induces apoptosis of arthritic rabbit synovium. *Gene Ther* 2003; 10: 1055–60.

130. Miyashita, T., Kawakami, A., Nakashima, T. *et al.* Osteoprotegerin (OPG) acts as an endogenous decoy receptor in tumor necrosis factor-related apoptosis-inducing ligand (TRAIL)-mediated apoptosis of fibroblast-like synovial cells. *Clin Exp immunol* 2004; 137: 430–6.

131. Park, Y. W., Ji, J. D., Lee, J. S., Ryang, D. W., and Yoo, D. H. Actinomycin D renders cultured synovial fibroblasts susceptible to tumour necrosis factor related apoptosis-inducing ligand (TRAIL)-induced apoptosis. *Scand J Rheumatol* 2003; 32: 356–63.

132. Perlman, H., Nguyen, N., Liu, H. *et al.* Rheumatoid arthritis synovial fluid macrophages express decreased tumor necrosis factor-related apoptosis-inducing ligand R2 and increased decoy receptor tumor necrosis factor related apoptosis-inducing ligand R3. *Arthritis Rheum* 2003; 48: 3096–101.

133. Hoang, T. R., Hammermuller, A., Mix, E. *et al.* A proinflammatory role for Fas in joints of mice with collagen-induced arthritis. *Arthritis Res Ther* 2004; 6: R404–R414.

134. Schedel, J., Gay, R. E., Künzler, P. *et al.* FLICE-inhibitory protein expression in synovial fibroblasts and at sites of cartilage and bone erosion in rheumatoid arthritis. *Arthritis Rheum* 2004; 46: 1512–18.

135. Palao, G., Santiago, B., Galindo, M. *et al.* Down-regulation of FLIP sensitizes rheumatoid synovial fibroblasts to Fas-mediated apoptosis. *Arthritis Rheum* 2004; 50: 2803–10.

136. Bai, S., Liu, H., Chen, K. H. *et al.* NF-kappaB-regulated expression of cellular FLIP protects rheumatoid arthritis synovial fibroblasts from tumor necrosis factor alpha-mediated apoptosis. *Arthritis Rheum* 2004; 50: 3844–55.

137. Kurowska, M., Rudnicka, W., Kontny, E. *et al.* Fibroblast-like synoviocytes from rheumatoid arthritis patients express functional IL-15 receptor complex: endogenous IL-15 in autocrine fashion enhances cell proliferation and expression of Bcl-x(L) and Bcl-2. *J Immunol* 2002; 169: 1760–7.

138. Schedel, J., Distler, O., Woenckhaus, M. *et al.* Discrepancy between mRNA and protein expression of tumour suppressor maspin in synovial tissue may contribute to synovial hyperplasia in rheumatoid arthritis. *Ann Rheum Dis* 2004; 63: 1205–11.

139. Pap, T., Franz, J. K., Hummel, K, M., *et al.* Activation of synovial fibroblasts in rheumatoid arthritis: lack of expression of the tumour suppressor PTEN at sites of invasive growth and destruction. *Arthritis Res* 2004; 2: 59–64.

140. Firestein, G. S., Nguyen, K., Aupperle, K. R., Yeo, M., Boyle, D. L., and Zvaifler, N. J. Apoptosis in rheumatoid arthritis: p53 overexpression in rheumatoid arthritis synovium. *Am J Pathol* 1990; 149: 2143–51.

141. Leech, M., Lacey, D., Xue, J. R. *et al.* Regulation of p53 by macrophage migration inhibitory factor in inflammatory arthritis. *Arthritis Rheum* 2003; 48: 1881–9.

142. Seemayer, C. A., Kuchen, S., Neidhart, M. *et al.* p53 in rheumatoid arthritis synovial fibroblasts at sites of invasion. *Ann Rheum Dis* 2003; 62: 1139–44.

143. Firestein, G. S., Echeverri, F., Yeo, M., Zvaifler, N. J., and Green, D. R. Somatic mutations in the p53 tumor suppressor gene in rheumatoid arthritis synovium. *Proc Natl Acad Sci USA* 1997; 94: 10895–900.

144. Kullmann, F., Judex, M., Neudecker, I. *et al.* Analysis of the p53 tumor suppressor gene in rheumatoid arthritis synovial fibroblasts. *Arthritis Rheum* 1999; 42: 1594–600.

145. Lee, S. H., Chang, D. K., Goel, A. *et al.* Microsatellite instability and suppressed DNA repair enzyme expression in rheumatoid arthritis. *J Immunol* 2003; 170: 2214–20.

146. Kullmann, F., Kirner, A., Judex, M. *et al.* Microsatellite instability in rheumatoid synovial fibroblasts. *Ann Rheum Dis* 2003; 59: 386–9.

147. Pap, T., Aupperle, K. R., Gay, S. *et al.* Invasiveness of synovial fibroblasts is regulated by p53 in the SCID mouse in vivo model of cartilage invasion. *Arthritis Rheum* 2001; 44: 676–81.

148. Gustin, J. A., Maehama, T., Dixon, J. E., and Donner, D. B. The PTEN tumor suppressor protein inhibits tumor necrosis factor-induced nuclear factor-κB activity. *J Biol Chem* 2003; 276: 27740–4.

149. Pianetti, S., Arsura, M., Romieu-Mourez, R. *et al.* Her-2/neu overexpression induces NF-κB via a PI3-kinase/Akt pathway involving calpain-mediated degradation of IkB-a that can be inhibited by the tumor suppressor PTEN. *Oncogene* 2001; 20: 1287–99.

150. Koul, D., Yao, Y., Abbruzzese, J. L. *et al.* Tumor suppressor MMAC/PTEN inhibits cytokine-induced NFκB activation without interfering with the IκB degradation pathway. *J Biol Chem* 2003; 276: 11402–8.

151. Zhang, H. G., Wang, Y., Xie, J. F. *et al.* Regulation of tumor necrosis factor α-mediated apoptosis of rheumatoid arthritis synovial fibroblasts by the protein kinase akt. *Arthritis Rheum* 2001; 44: 1555–67.

152. Okura, T., Gong, L., Kamitani, T. *et al.* Protection against Fas/APO-1- and tumor necrosis factor-mediated cell death by a novel protein, sentrin. *J Immunol* 1997; 157: 4277–81.

153. Franz, J. K., Pap, T., Hummel, K. M. *et al.* Expressions of sentrin, a novel antiapoptotic molecule at sites of synovial invasion in rheumatoid arthritis. *Arthritis Rheum* 2000; 43: 599–607.

154. O'Sullivan, F. X., Gay, R. E., and Gay, S. Spontaneous arthritis models. In *Mechanisms and models in rheumatoid arthritis* (Henderson, B., Pettipher, R., and Edwards, J., eds), pp. 471–83. London: Academic Press; 1995.

155. Trabandt, A., Gay, R. E., Fassbender, H. G., and Gay, S. Cathepsin B in synovial cells at the site of joint destruction in rheumatoid arthritis. *Arthritis Rheum* 1991; 34: 1444–51.

156. Wu, J., Zhou, T., He, J., and Mountz, J. D. Autoimmune disease in mice due to integration of an endogenous retrovirus in an apoptosis gene. *J Exp Med* 1993; 178: 461–8.

157. Chu, J-L., Drappa, J., Parnassa, A., and Elkon, K. B. The defect in Fas mRNA expression in MRL/lpr mice is associated with insertion of the retrotransposon. *J Exp Med* 1993; 178: 723–30.

158. Müller-Ladner, U., Kriegsmann, J., Franklin, B. N. *et al.* Synovial fibroblasts of patients with rheumatoid arthritis attach to and invade normal human cartilage when engrafted into SCID mice. *Am J Pathol* 1996; 149: 1607–15.

159. Müller-Ladner, U., Kriegsmann, J., Gay, R. E., Koopman, W. J., Gay, S., and Chatham, W. W. Progressive joint destruction in a HIV-infected patient with rheumatoid arthritis. *Arthritis Rheum* 1995; 38; 1328–32.

160. Riikonen, T., Westermarck, J., Koivisto, L., Broberg, A., Kähäri, V. M., and Heino, J. Integrin $\alpha 2\beta 1$ is a positive regulator of collagenase (MMP-1) and collagen $\alpha 1(1)$ gene expression. *J Biol Chem* 1995; 270: 13548–52.

161. Pirilä, L., and Heino, J. Altered integrin expression in rheumatoid synovial lining type B cells: in vitro cytokine regulation of $\alpha 1\beta 1$, $\alpha 6\beta 1$, $\alpha v\beta 5$ integrins. *J Rheumatol* 1996; 23: 1691–8.

162. Kriegsmann, J., Keyszer, G. M., Geiler, T., Bräuer, R., and Gay, R. E., and Gay, S. Expression of vascular cell adhesion molecule-1 mRNA and protein in rheumatoid arthritis synovium demonstrated by in situ hybridization and immunohistochemistry. *Lab Invest* 1995; 72: 209–13.

163. Müller-Ladner, U., Kriegsmann, J., Stahl, D. *et al.* Expression of alternatively spliced CS-1 fibronectin isoform and its counter-receptor VLA-4 in rheumatoid arthritis synovium. *J Rheumatol* 1997; 24: 1873–80.

164. Morel, J. C., Park, C. C., Zhu, K. *et al.* Signal transduction pathways involved in rheumatoid arthritis synovial fibroblast interleukin-18-induced vascular cell adhesion molecule-1 expression. *J Biol Chem* 2002; 277: 34679–91.

165. Möller, B., Kessler, U., Rehart, S. *et al.* Expression of interleukin-18 receptor in fibroblast-like synoviocytes. *Arthritis Res* 2002; 4: 139–44.

166. Rinaldi, N., Schwarz-Eywill, M., Leppelmann-Jansen, P. *et al.* Increased expression of integrins on fibroblast-like synoviocytes from rheumatoid arthritis in vitro correlates with enhanced binding to extracellular matrix proteins. *Ann Rheum Dis* 1997; 56: 45–51.

167. Wang, A. Z., Wang, J. C., Fisher, G. W., and Diamond, H. S. Interleukin-1β-stimulated invasion of articular cartilage by rheumatoid synovial fibroblasts is inhibited by antibodies to specific integrin receptors and by collagenase inhibitors. *Arthritis Rheum* 1997; 40: 1298–307.

168. Shang, X-Z., Lang, B. J., and Issekutz, A. C. Adhesion molecule mechanisms mediating monocyte migration through synovial fibroblast and endothelium barriers: role for CD11/CD18, very late antigen-4 (CD49d/CD29), very late antigen-5 (CD49e/CD29), and vascular cell adhesion molecule-1 (CD106). *J Immunol* 1998; 160: 467–74.

169. Lambert, N., Lescoulié, P. L., Yassine-Diab, B., Enault, G., Mazières, B., and De Préval, C. Substance P enhances cytokine-induced vascular cell adhesion molecule-1 (VCAM-1) expression on cultured rheumatoid fibroblast-like synoviocytes. *Clin Exp Immunol* 1998; 113: 269–75.

170. Hale, L. P., Martin, M. E., McCollum, D. E. *et al.* Immunohistologic analysis of the distribution of cell adhesion molecules within the inflammatory synovial microenvironment. *Arthritis Rheum* 1998; 32: 22–30.

171. Koch, A. E., Burrows, J. C., Haines, G. K., Carlos, T. M., Harlan, J. M., and Leibovich, S. J. Immunolocalization of endothelial and leukocyte adhesion molecules in human rheumatoid and osteoarthritic synovial tissues. *Lab Invest* 1991; 64: 313–20.

172. Nakatsuka, K., Tanaka, Y., Hubscher, S. *et al.* Rheumatoid synovial fibroblasts are stimulated by the cellular adhesion to T cells through lymphocyte function associated antigen-1/intercellular adhesion molecule-1. *J Rheumatol* 1997; 24: 458–64.

173. Kavanaugh, A. F., Davis, S. L., Nichols, L. A. *et al.* Treatment of refractory rheumatoid arthritis with a monoclonal antibody to intercellular adhesion molecule 1. *Arthritis Rheum* 1994; 37: 992–9.

174. Schedel, J., Wenglen, C., Distler, O. *et al.* Differential adherence of osteoarthritis and rheumatoid arthritis synovial fibroblasts to cartilage and bone matrix proteins and its implications for osteoarthritis pathogenesis. *Scand J Immunol* 2004; **60**: 514–23.

175. Neidhart, M., Zaucke, F., von Knoch, R. *et al.* Galectin-3 is induced in rheumatoid arthritis synovial fibroblasts after adhesion to cartilage oligomeric matrix protein. *Ann Rheum Dis* 2005; **64**: 419–24.

176. Valencia, X., Higgins, J. M. G., Kiener, H. P. *et al.* Cadherin-11 provides specific cellular adhesion between fibroblast-like synoviocytes. *J Exp Med* 2004; **200**: 1673–9.

177. Vincenti, M. P., and Brinckerhoff, C. E. Transcriptional regulation of collagenase (MMP-1, MMP-13) genes in arthritis: integration of complex signaling pathways for the recruitment of gene-specific transcription factors. *Arthritis Res* 2002; **4**: 157–64.

178. Smolian, H., Aurer, A., Sittinger, M. *et al.* Secretion of gelatinases and activation of gelatinase A (MMP-2) by human rheumatoid synovial fibroblasts. *Biol Chem* 2001; **382**: 1491–9.

179. Tomita, T., Nakase, T., Kaneko, M. *et al.* Expression of extracellular matrix metalloproteinase inducer and enhancement of the production of matrix metalloproteinases in rheumatoid arthritis. *Arthritis Rheum* 2002; **46**: 373–8.

180. Maeda, S., Sawai, T., Uziki, M. *et al.* Determination of interstitial collagenase (MMP-1) in patients with rheumatoid arthritis. *Ann Rheum Dis* 1995; **54**: 970–5.

181. Clark, I. M., Powell, L. K., Ramsey, S., Hazelman, B. L, and Cawston, T. E. The measurement of collagenase, TIMP, and collagenase-TIMP complex in synovial fluids from patients with osteoarthritis and rheumatoid arthritis. *Arthritis Rheum* 1993; **36**: 372–80.

182. Kolomytkin, O. V., Marino, A. A., Waddell, D. D. *et al.* IL-1β-induced production of metalloproteinases by synovial cells depends on gap junction conductance. *Am J Physiol Cell Physiol* 2002; **282**: C1254–C1260.

183. Gravallese, E. M., Darling, J. M., Ladd, A. L., Katz, J. N., and Glimcher, L. In situ hybridization studies on stromelysin and collagenase mRNA expression in rheumatoid synovium. *Arthritis Rheum* 1991; **34**: 1071–84.

184. Müller-Ladner, U., and Gay, S. MMPs and rheumatoid synovial fibroblasts: Siamese twins in joint destruction? *Ann Rheum Dis* 2002; **61**: 957–9.

185. Rutkauskaite, E., Zacharias, W., Schedel, J. *et al.* Ribozymes that inhibit the production of matrix metalloproteinase 1 reduce the invasiveness of rheumatoid arthritis synovial fibroblasts. *Arthritis Rheum* 2004; **50**: 1448–56.

186. Lindy, O., Konttinen, Y. T., Sorsa, T. *et al.* Matrix metalloproteinase 13 (collagenase 3) in human rheumatoid synovium. *Arthritis Rheum* 1997; **40**: 1391–9.

187. Ahrens, D., Koch, A. E., Pope, R. M., Stein-Picarella, M., and Niedbala, M. J. Expression of matrix metalloproteinase 9 (96-kd gelatinase B) in human rheumatoid arthritis. *Arthritis Rheum* 1996; **39**: 1576–87.

188. Gruber, B. L., Sorbi, D., French, D. L. *et al.* Markedly elevated serum MMP-9 (gelatinase B) levels in rheumatoid arthritis: a potentially useful laboratory marker. *Clin Immunol Immunopathol* 1996; **78**: 161–71.

189. Choi, Y. A., Lim, H. K., Kim, J. R. *et al.* Group IB secretory phospholipase A2 promotes matrix metalloproteinase-2-mediated cell migration via the phosphatidylinositol 3-kinase and Akt pathway. *J Biol Chem* 2004; **279**: 36579–85.

190. Mitsui, H., Nishimura, A., Yoshimura, K., Okinaga, S., Matsuta, K., and Tsuchiya, N. Expression of membrane type matrix metalloproteinases in the synovial tissue from patients with rheumatoid arthritis. *Arthritis Rheum* 1998; **42**: (Suppl.), 1710.

191. Pap, T., Shigeyama, Y., Kuchen, S. *et al.* Differential expression pattern of membrane-type matrix metalloproteinases in rheumatoid arthritis. *Arthritis Rheum* 2000; **43**: 1226–32.

192. Maciewicz, R. A., Wotton, S. F., Etherington, D. J., and Duance, V. C. Susceptibility of the cartilage collagens type II, IX and XI to degradation by the cysteine proteinases, cathepsin D and L. *FEBS Lett* 1990; **269**: 189–93.

193. Keyszer, G. M., Heer, A. H., Kriegsmann, J. *et al.* Comparative analysis of cathepsin L, cathepsin D and collagenase mRNA expression in synovial tissues of patients with rheumatoid arthritis and osteoarthritis by in situ hybridization. *Arthritis Rheum* 1995; **38**: 976–84.

194. Schedel, J., Seemayer, C. A., Pap, T. *et al.* Targeting cathepsin L (CL) by specific ribozymes decreases CL protein synthesis and cartilage destruction in rheumatoid arthritis. *Gene Ther* 2004; **11**: 1040–7.

195. Hummel, K. M., Petrow, P. K., Jeisy, E. *et al.* Cathepsin K mRNA is expressed in synovium of patients with rheumatoid arthritis (RA) at sites of bone destruction. *J Rheumatol* 1998; **25**: 1887–94.

196. Esser, R. E., Angelo, R. A., Murphey, M. D. *et al.* Cysteine proteinase inhibitors decrease articular cartilage and bone destruction in chronic inflammatory arthritis. *Arthritis Rheum* 1994; **37**: 236–47.

197. Van der Laan, W. H., Pap, T., Ronday, H. K. *et al.* Cartilage degradation and invasion by rheumatoid synovial fibroblasts is inhibited by gene transfer of a cell surface-targeted plasmin inhibitor. *Arthritis Rheum* 2000; **43**: 1710–18.

198. Pap, T., Claus, A., Ohtsu, S. *et al.* Osteoclast-independent bone resorption by fibroblast-like cells. *Arthritis Res* 2003; **5**: R163–R173.

199. Ohtsu, S., Pap, T., Shigeyama, Y. *et al.* Identification of a novel splice variant of an osteoclast-like v-ATPase BETA-1 subunit in activated fibroblasts. *Arthritis Rheum* 2000; **43**: (Suppl.), S165.

200. Firestein, G. S., and Paine, M. Expression of stromelysin and TIMP in rheumatoid arthritis synovium. *Am J Pathol* 1992; **140**: 1309–14.

201. Wahl, S. M., Allen, J. B., Wong, H. L., Dougherty, S. F., and Ellingsworth, L. R. Antagonistic and agonistic effects of transforming growth factor-beta and IL-1 in rheumatoid synovitis. *J Immunol* 1990; **145**: 2514–19.

202. MacNaul, K. L., Chartrain, N., Lark, M., Tocci, M. J., and Hutchinson, N. I. Discoordinate expression of stromelysin, collagenase, and tissue inhibitor of metalloproteinases-1 in rheumatoid human synovial fibroblasts: synergistic effects interleukin-1 and tumor necrosis factor-α on stromelysin expression. *J Biol Chem* 1990; **265**: 17238–45.

203. Aicher, W. K., Alexander, D., Haas., C. *et al.* Transcription factor early growth response 1 activity up-regulates expression of tissue inhibitor of metalloproteinases 1 in human synovial fibroblasts. *Arthritis Rheum* 2003; **48**: 348–59.

204. Ohta, S., Harigai, M., Tanaka, M. *et al.* Tumor necrosis factor-α (TNF-α) converting enzyme contributes to production of TNF-α in synovial tissues from patients with rheumatoid arthritis. *J Rheumatol* 2001; **28**, 1756–63.

205. Van der Laan, W. H., Quax, P. H., Seemayer, C. A. *et al.* (2003). Cartilage degradation and invasion by rheumatoid synovial fibroblasts is inhibited by gene transfer of TIMP-1 and TIMP-3. *Gene Ther* 2003; **10**: 234–42.

206. Van Lent, P. L., Span, P. N., Sloetjes, A. W. *et al.* (2005). Expression and localization of the metalloproteinase inhibitor RECK (reversion inducing cysteine-rich protein with Kazal motifs) in inflamed synovial membranes of patients with rheumatoid arthritis. *Ann Rheum Dis* 2005; **64**: 368–74.

207. Neidhart, M., Wehrli, R., Bruhlmann, P., Michel, B. A., Gay, R. E., 64: 368–74. Gay, S. Synovial fluid CD 146 (MUC18), a marker for synovial membrane angiogenesis in rheumatoid arthritis. *Arthritis Rheum* 1999; **12**: 622–30.

208. Kasama, T., Shiozawa, F., Kobayashi, K. *et al.* Vascular endothelial growth factor expression by activated synovial leukocytes in rheumatoid arthritis: critical involvement of the interaction with synovial fibroblasts. *Arthritis Rheum* 2001; **44**: 2512–24.

209. Giatromanolaki, A., Sivridis, E., Athanassou, N. *et al.* The angiogenic pathway 'vascular endothelial growth factor/flk-1(KDR)-receptor' in rheumatoid arthritis and osteoarthritis. *J Pathol* 2001; **194**: 101–8.

210. Afuwape, A. O., Feldmann, M., and Paleolog, E. M. Adenoviral delivery of soluble VEGF receptor 1 (sFlt-1) abrogates disease activity in murine collagen-induced arthritis. *Gene Ther* 2003; **10**: 1950–60.

211. Gravallese, E. M., Pettit, A. R., Lee, R. *et al.* Angiopoietin-1 is expressed in the synovium of patients with rheumatoid arthritis and is induced by tumour necrosis factor alpha. *Ann Rheum Dis* 2003; **62**: 100–7.

212. Takahara, K., Iioka, T., Furukawa, K. *et al.* Autokrine/paracrine role of the angiopoietin-1 and -2 /Tie2 system in cell proliferation and chemotaxis of cultured fibroblastic synoviocytes in rheumatoid arthritis. *Hum Pathol* 2004; **35**: 150–8.

213. Nakahara, H., Song, J., Sugimoto, M. *et al.* Anti-interleukin-6 receptor antibody therapy reduces vascular endothelial growth factor production in rheumatoid arthritis. *Arthritis Rheum* 2003; **48**: 1521–9.

214. Park, Y. W., Kang, Y. M., Butterfield, J. *et al.* Thrombospondin 2 functions as an endogenous regulator of angiogenesis and inflammation in rheumatoid arthritis. *Am J Pathol* 2004; **165**: 2087–98.

215. Safronova, O., Nakahama, K., Onodera, M., Muneta, T., and Morita, I. Effect of hypoxia on monocyte chemotactic protein-1 (MCP-1) gene expression induced by interleukin-1beta in human synovial fibroblasts. *Inflamm Res* 2003; **52**: 480–6.

216. Cha, H. S., Ahn, K. S., Jeon, C. H. *et al.* Influence of hypoxia on the expression of matrix metalloproteinase-1, -3 and tissue inhibitor of metalloproteinase-1 in rheumatoid synovial fibroblasts. *Clin Exp Rheumatol* 2003; **21**: 593–8.

217. Demasi, M., Cleland, L. G., Cook-Johnson, R. J., and James, M. J. Effects of hypoxia on the expression and activity of cyclooxygenase 2 in fibroblast-like synoviocytes: interactions with monocyte-derived soluble mediators. *Arthritis Rheum* 2004; **50**: 2441–9.

218. Kurowska-Stolarska, M., Distler, J., Pap, T. *et al.* The inhibitor of differentiation-2 (Id-2) induced by hypoxia promotes bone degradation in rheumatoid arthritis (RA). *Arthritis Rheum* 2004; **51**: (Suppl.), 1751.

219. Wunder, A., Müller-Ladner, U., Stelzer, E. H. *et al.* Albumin-based drug delivery as novel therapeutic approach for rheumatoid arthritis. *J Immunol* 2003; **170**: 4793–801.

220. Fiehn, C., Neumann, E., Wunder, A. *et al.* Methotrexate (MTX) and albumin coupled with MTX (MTX-HSA) suppress synovial fibroblast invasion and cartilage degradation in vivo. *Ann Rheum Dis* 2004; **63**: 884–6.

221. Lories, D. J., Derese, I., De Bari, C., and Luyten, F. P. In vitro growth rate of fibroblast-like synovial cells is reduced by methotrexate treatment. *Ann Rheum Dis* 2003; **62**: 568–71.

222. Miranda-Carus, M. E., Balsa, E., Benito-Miguel, M. *et al.* Il-15 and the initiation of cell contact-dependent synovial fibroblast-T lymphocyte cross-talk in rheumatoid arthritis: effect of methotrexate. *J Immunol* 2004; **173**: 1473–6.

223. Migita, K., Miyashita, T., Ishibashi, H. *et al.* Suppressive effect of leflunomide metabolite (A77 1726) on metalloproteinase production in IL-1beta stimulated rheumatoid synovial fibroblasts. *Clin Exp Immunol* 2004; **137**: 612–16.

224. Palmer, G., Burger, D., Mezin, F. *et al.* The active metabolite of leflunomide (A77 1726), increases the production of IL-1 receptor antagonist in human synovial fibroblasts and articular chondrocytes. *Arthritis Res Ther* 2004; **6**: R181–R189.

225. Gouze, J. N., Gouze, E., Palmer, G. D. *et al.* A comparative study of the inhibitory effects of interleukin-1 receptor antagonist following administration as a recombinant protein or by gene transfer. *Arthritis Res Ther* 2003; **5**: R301–R309.

226. Ehling, A., Schäffler, A., Tarner, I H, *et al.* The potential of adiponectin in driving arthritis. *J Immunol* 2006; in press.

9 | *The roles of B cells in rheumatoid arthritis*

Gregg J. Silverman

Introduction

Decades of intensive investigation into the pathogenesis of rheumatoid arthritis(RA) have led to the characterization of complex interactions of diverse infiltrating cell types, which are regulated by a variety of membrane-associated and secreted molecules. Many decades ago, B lymphocytes were first implicated in surveys that demonstrated immunoglobulin(Ig) complexes in joints affected by the chronic inflammatory synovitis of RA. B lymphocytes and Ig-producing plasma cells were also found to be prominent participants in the infiltrated and hyperplastic synovia, and more recent observations have indicated that these cells contribute to pathogenesis by both local Ig-dependent and independent functions. However, despite extensive efforts, there has been limited progress in proving that specific anti-self and/or anti-microbial antigenic targets are responsible for the recruitment of clonally restricted B cell sets into the rheumatoid synovium, and as a result controversies persist regarding the factors responsible for the recruitment of these B lymphocytes. In the following sections, the cumulative evidence of the roles of B-lineage cells and their products is discussed, and important recent observations are highlighted.

RA as an immune complex-mediated disease

IgG autoantibodies and immune complexes (ICs) have long been recognized as potent pathologic triggers of inflammatory responses. In the 1960s, IgG aggregates were first shown to be abundant in RA synovial fluids, and experimental models of IC disease provided a foundation for hypotheses regarding the causes of rheumatoid synovitis. With the recognition of IC-mediated inflammatory pathways, which included evidence that local IgG IC formation was postulated to trigger complement activation leading to tissue damage, many parallels were drawn between the IC-mediated processes responsible for autoimmune glomerulonephritis and for rheumatoid synovitis[1]. Despite their similarities, the pathogenesis of RA appeared to differ as the consumption of complement is generally restricted to the joints[2], while in systemic lupus erythematosus (SLE) there is often consumption of complement in the plasma and also at other sites affected by the disease.

Although other cells and pro-inflammatory pathways are believed to also contribute to pathogenesis, it has been argued that the formation of pathogenic ICs are the rate-limiting step in the development of RA. Moreover, the relative composition and solubility of ICs that form in RA are likely important in determining their tissue distribution and capacity to contribute to the chronic inflammatory process[3].

While earlier theories attributed the pathogenesis of RA to the local deposition of ICs, it remained unclear whether these complexes are generated locally. It also remains controversial as to whether there are specific foreign or self-antigens preferentially produced in joint tissues, or locally deposited from the circulation, to become the targets of over-exuberant and destructive immune responses. Alternatively, the initiation and/or perpetuation phases of RA pathogenesis may instead involve ICs that are generated elsewhere, then pass through the circulation to accumulate in the joints.

Over the years a range of exogenous and endogenous antigens have been proposed as immune targets involved in RA. These implicated antigens include the common viral pathogens cytomegalovirus (CMV) and Epstein—Barr virus (EBV), as well as gp39 and proteoglycans. Arguably the best candidate antigenic immune target is type II collagen (CII), a major component of articular cartilage. As discussed below, immunization with collagen can induce inflammatory arthritis in a number of species, including mouse, rat, and monkey. Importantly, the pathogenetic potential of these autoantibodies was documented when the passive transfer of human anti-CII antibodies, from a seronegative RA patient, induced inflammatory arthritis in mice[4]. Hence, even though autoantibodies to CII are not universally detected in all RA patients, it is likely that these autoimmune responses may at least contribute to the pathologic process in some RA patients.

More recently, the roles of human antibodies to glucose-6 phosphate isomerase (GPI)[5,6] and citrullinated proteins have also been debated. Although to date direct roles in etiopathogenesis have not been demonstrated, levels of anti-GPI antibodies are reported to correlate with disease severity[6], while the detection of citrulline-specific antibodies(i.e., anti-citrulline cyclic peptide, CCP) is a sensitive and specific biomarker for the diagnosis of RA, especially in disease of recent onset[7].

Rheumatoid factors and pathogenesis

Rheumatoid factors (RFs) are a special type of autoantibody that are specific for the constant regions of IgG, and natural RF autoantibodies are known to be induced during physiologic secondary immune responses in which they appear to be tightly regulated[8]. In contrast, high circulating levels of RFs are detectable in more than 80% of RA patients, and may also be present in a 'hidden' or complexed form in the synovial fluids of some seronegative patients. Contributing to their acknowledged role in pathogenesis, RFs efficiently fix and activate complement *in vitro* by the classical pathway[9]. *In vivo* turnover studies of radiotagged complement proteins have also demonstrated that complement consumption is greatly accelerated in seropositive RA patients, compared to control subjects, especially at extra-vascular sites of inflammation[10]. RA synovitis is clearly more severe in the majority of RA patients who systemically and locally produce high levels of RFs (reviewed in Ref. 11).

Consistent with the notion that IC formation is maximal at the synovial sites of inflammation, complement activation was shown to be much greater in RA synovial fluid than in blood[12,13]. Levels of C4 breakdown fragments at these sites also correlate with titers of circulating IgM-RFs. Notably, while IgM-RFs are most commonly found, RFs can be of any isotype, and patients with higher titers of RF often display class switched IgG-RFs. The greatest pathogenic potential is believed to be conveyed by IgG-RFs produced and deposited in the joint, as IgG-RFs have the capacity for self-association[14].

Once the complement cascade has been activated, downstream products, especially the soluble anaphylatoxin, C5a, further contribute to the pro-inflammatory milieu by both recruiting infiltrating leukocytes and enlisting other components of the membrane attack complex that can induce cell lysis[15,16]. Documenting the relevance of these pathways to pathogenesis, clinical flares of RA disease activity correlate with increased levels of RF-secreting cells, which are especially prevalent in the bone marrow and synovial fluid of RA patients[17].

IgM-RFs have been reported to account for more than 10% of local plasma cells in RA synovia[17–19]. However, infusions of RFs from RA patients into healthy individuals have been reported to cause neither sustained nor transient synovitis[20], indicating that RF autoantibodies by themselves are not pathogenic. Nevertheless, IgM-RF containing ICs may also include IgG antibodies and unidentified peptides, which could derive from self- or exogenous antigens. In addition, the recently solved crystallographic structure of a human IgM-RF-Fc co-complex revealed that contacts with IgG antigen involved only the periphery of the antigen-binding cleft of the autoantibody[21]. These findings may indicate that RA RF is capable of binding of IgG as well as other self- or foreign antigens. Thus, while RF alone is not pro-inflammatory, RF associated with IC may enhance local inflammatory processes, and extensive clinical evidence has shown the contribution of RFs to extra-articular disease.

Fc receptors and immune pathogenesis

While IC formation was long ago implicated in the pathogenesis of RA, the central importance of these observations was underappreciated until there was a better understanding of the greater range of cellular and molecular pathways by which ICs can recruit components of both the innate and adaptive immune systems into the self-perpetuating inflammatory process. Only over the past two decades have the encoding genes and functions of these proteins begun to be elucidated, and there are now known to be a growing family of cell membrane-associated receptors for Ig and IC complexes[22,23].

While unknown at the time of earlier investigations of RA, recent characterizations of the interactions between IgG containing ICs and cellular receptors for Fc regions of IgG (FcγR), and the development of relevant murine model systems, have enabled a more thorough examination of the impact of Fc-mediated pathways on pathogenesis. In the mouse, four classes of Fcγ cell surface receptors are currently known and these are heterogeneous in their binding specificities and affinities for different IgG isotypes, and in their preferences for IC versus uncomplexed IgG, with parallel findings in human Fc. Moreover, the intracellular signaling motifs of these different receptors can either activate or inhibit cellular effector functions[24] (reviewed in Ref. 22).

While mice with deficiencies in complement components typically display attenuated IC-mediated disease, the loss of activating FcγRIII can completely ablate arthritis development (discussed below). Connecting these model systems to clinical disease, *in vitro* blockade of FcγRIIIA on human macrophages was recently shown to prevent the release of tumor necrosis factor (TNF)-α and IL-1α by human macrophages[25], suggesting that FcγRIII may be an especially important mediator of IC-induced tissue damage in RA.

The pathogenic potential of ICs that arise at sites of disease may also derive in part from their size and composition (discussed in Ref. 3). It has been proposed that in RA patients, ICs are formed with RFs that are too small to be cleared by complement, but large enough to induce TNF production due to their interactions via FcγRIIIa[25]. Moreover, FcγRIIIa appears to be preferentially expressed in certain anatomic sites. In addition to synovium, FcγRIIIa is often preferentially expressed at extra-articular sites of rheumatoid disease (i.e., serosae, alveoli, sclera, bone marrow, secondary lymphoid tissue, Kuppfer cells in the RE system, and salivary glands)[26]. In more recent studies, IC-induced inflammatory disease was shown to be exacerbated by the downstream generation of C5a, which acts through the C5a receptor, while the influence of C5a also altered the ratio of activating to inhibitory FcγR on macrophages triggered by IC[27]. Together, these studies demonstrated a direct link between the C5a chemoattractant and FcγR-related mechanisms responsible for IC-triggered inflammatory responses.

Recent investigations of murine models of RA have led to a revision of our understanding of the role of secreted autoantibodies in RA. As discussed below, the host response to IC functions in the joints is critically dependent on interactions with cell surface FcγR on B cells and macrophages. Complement alone may be inadequate to sustain chronic inflammatory responses that follow IC deposition, as stimulatory and inhibitory FcγR may in fact be the primary regulators of subsequent immune responses.

Diverse functional roles of B cells

In addition to being the precursors of plasma cells, the antibody-producing factories of the body, the B cells in RA can serve several other critical functions (Tables 9.1 and 9.2). Among these other functions, B cells can act as highly efficient antigen-presenting cells (APCs), supporting the activation of autoreactive T cells. In fact, by virtue of the high affinity of their specific membrane-associated Ig for antigen, an antigen-specific B cell can take up, process, and present peptides from nominal antigen with 1000-fold or greater efficiency than 'professional' APCs[28]. Moreover, RF-bearing B cells can also take up the nominal antigen contained in IgG IC, to enable highly efficient antigen processing and presentation to CD4+ T cells[29]. In addition, activated B cells can synthesize and secrete cytokines and also display membrane-associated molecules, which provide non-specific help to adjacent T cells. Murine models have shown that B cells may play central roles in pathogenic autoimmune responses that are unrelated to autoantibody production[30]. These findings suggested that antigen-specific and RF-bearing B cells may orchestrate immune responses in lymphoid tissues, and at sites of disease, by Ig-independent pathways (discussed in Ref. 31). There is also evidence that RA synovial inflammatory tissue can breach the cortical barrier, resulting in the formation of B cell-rich aggregates in the adjacent bone marrow that is also associated with increased formation of new bone.[30a]

Relevant to the roles of RFs as cellular receptors for B lymphocytes, recent studies in RF-expressing immunoglobulin transgenic B cells have shown that these B cell receptors (BCRs) can mediate uptake of macromolecular complexes of IC containing components from dying cells, which contain ligands for cellular Toll-like receptors (TLRs)[32]. Interactions with these self-ligand-ICs can impart both BCR signals and TLR signals, providing potent RF B cell-specific stimulation. These studies have defined an emerging immunologic paradigm, which may contribute to the ongoing stimulatory stimuli for autoreactive B cells, presumably to support the survival and activation of other cell types recruited into pathologic autoimmune responses.

In recent years a greater appreciation has developed for the distinct sets of mature B cells, which vary based on their surface phenotype, anatomic localization, signaling thresholds, and functional roles in physiologic immune responses. As an important step to understanding these differences, in a recent report laser dissection microscopy was used to define gene expression profiling by cDNA microarray in the three major mature B cell types in the human spleen: mantle zone, marginal zone, and follicular B cells[33]. These studies revealed that the transcriptional program of B cells in the germinal center, the site of active B cell proliferation and antigenic selection, is dominated by up-regulation of genes associated with proliferation and DNA repair or recombination. In contrast, the mantle zone and marginal zones, the residences of heterogeneous groups of B-lineage cells that included those responsible for immunologic memory, showed increased expression of genes promoting cellular quiescence. Each of these three compartments also expressed distinct repertoires of apoptosis-associated genes, as well as differential expression of chemokines and chemokine receptors[33]. These pioneering studies will no doubt provide a foundation for investigations of B cells infiltrating ectopic lymphoid tissues in RA and other diseases, leading to a more detailed understanding of the influences responsible for these pathologic self-perpetuating processes.

The best experimental support for a direct role in RA pathogenesis of B cell functions, which are independent of antibody formation, came from studies of human RA synovial explants engrafted into severe combined immunodeficiency (SCID) mouse chimeras[34]. Treatment of these mice with rituximab, which induced CD20-mediated targeted deletion of all B cells in the xenograft, resulted in an impairment of production of IL-1 and TNF-α. As RA synovial T cells have been shown to enhance the production of inflammatory cytokine by macrophages, these studies were interpreted as evidence that T cell activation in rheumatoid synovium is B cell dependent, as APCs other than B cells could not substitute for the maintenance of T cell activation[34].

Ectopic lymphoid tissue in rheumatoid synovium

Histopathologic examinations have shown that 60% or more of the synovial samples from RA patients contain infiltrates of B and T lymphocytes. Three separate patterns of infiltrates have been described: (a) diffuse lymphocytic infiltrates with interdigitating dendritic cells and variable amounts of B cells; (b) aggregates of infiltrating B and T cells in more substantial numbers, associated with interdigitating dendritic cells in disorganized groupings; (c) T cells and B lymphocytes clustered in aggregates arrayed around interdigitating dendritic cells and associated with follicular dendritic cell (FDC) networks[35-37] (Fig. 9.1). In this latter pattern, found in less than one-third of patients, the synovial cellular infiltrates included distinct B cell follicle-like structures that appear to be organized into close spatial relationship to CD4+ T cells and CD8+ T cells[38]. Notably, these aggregates may be directly adjacent to areas of cartilage and bone destruction. In general, the histologic features of this type of RA synovial infiltrate are similar to the germinal center (GC) reactions that arise in peripheral lymphoid tissues during antigen-specific responses after

Table 9.1 Major physiologic functions of B lymphocytes

Precursors of antibody-producing plasma cells
Provide non-cognate help for T cell activation
Efficient antigen-presenting cells, especially for recall antigens
Produce cytokines (e.g., IL-4 and IL-10) that support the survival of other mononuclear cells
Generate and respond to chemotactic factors responsible for leukocyte migration and development of granulation tissue
Sustain immunologic memory

Table 9.2   Potential pathologic functions of B lymphocytes in rheumatoid arthritis

Presentation of immune-complexed antigens to autoreactive T cells
Expression of adhesion and other costimulatory molecules that promote T cell activation
Synthesis of chemokines that induce leukocyte infiltration
Production of factors that initiate and sustain angiogenesis and granulation tissue formation
Release of autoantibodies (especially RF) that are directly or indirectly (via immune complex formation) destructive to tissues
Maintenance of a memory response to autoantigens

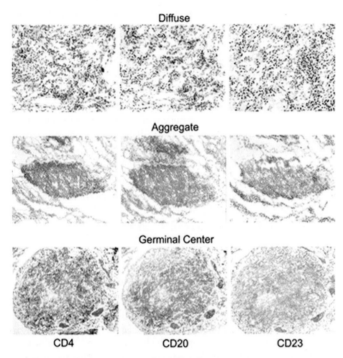

Diffuse

Aggregate

Germinal Center

CD4   CD20   CD23

Fig. 9.1   Range of ectopic lymphoid microstructures in RA synovitis. Serial sections of synovial tissues were stained with anti-CD4 (*left*), anti-CD20 (*center*), or anti-CD23 mAb (*right*). In a subset of patients, T cells and B cells were diffusely distributed throughout the tissue. Other patients formed T cell—B cell aggregates lacking FDCs and GC-like structures reactions. In the third subset of patients, T cell—B cell follicles with GC-like accumulations in the center were identified. Original magnification, ×400 (diffuse), ×200 (aggregate and GC-like). (From Ref. 37, reproduced with permission.) See also colour plate section.

immunization. As discussed in later sections, cytokines affecting lymphocyte survival may play different roles in these types of RA synovial infiltrates. While such GC-like aggregates have not been described in patients with seronegative RA (i.e., patients without detectable circulating RFs), knowledge is currently lacking on whether each of these three patterns of the organization of lymphoid infiltrates is stable over time, or whether during disease progression there is a sequential change in histologic patterns, and/or whether a specific pattern can reflect disease severity or can be used as a predictor of prognosis.

Immunohistochemical analyses have also shown that within the lymphocytic infiltrates in the RA synovial tissue, plasma cells may be organized in concentric rings around the large cellular clusters of T cells and B cells or as perivascular clusters[35]. In addition, B cells and T cells in rheumatoid synovial samples may also bear the Ki-67 cell surface antigen, which is used as a proliferation-associated cell marker in studies of malignant cells. However, in

RA synovial tissue the Ki-67 marker has been detected primarily on lymphocytes in the GC-like pattern[39], even though concurrent mitotic figures in RA synovial intima are very low, suggesting that local B or T cell proliferative expansions may be quite limited and/or that Ki-67 expression may be associated with activated, but not necessarily proliferating cells. Moreover, B cell proliferation in ectopic lymphoid infiltrates has been seen mainly in the network of the FDC, while in human tonsilar GC reactions proliferation occurs in a separate dark zone[40]. These findings suggest that ectopic GC-like structures have organizational and functional differences from their physiologic analogs. In addition, in other studies the dominant population of B cells from RA synovia have been reported to be impaired in their capacity to respond to mitogenic stimuli, suggesting they in fact act as though functionally inactive (i.e., anergic)[41].

While the diseased joints in RA patients may have organized lymphoid infiltrates that emulate physiologic peripheral lymphoid tissues, these changes do not appear to be entirely specific for RA. The affected joints of patients with ankylosing spondylitis have also been shown at times to harbor GC-like aggregates[42]. Even the synovia from osteoarthritic joints can occasionally contain infiltrates of activated B cells that display clonally related antibody gene sequences[43,44]. These findings suggest that the local B cell accumulations accumulate in ectopic lymphoid tissue by mechanisms that are common to inflammatory synovitis, but not specific for RA. Accumulations of plasma cells appear to be more specific for RA. These findings support the hypothesis that the special immunopathogenetic pathways of RA lead to abnormalities in the maturation of B lineage cells[45]. Moreover, *in vitro* studies have confirmed the special capacity of rheumatoid synoviocytes to support the terminal differentiation of plasma cells[46].

Abnormal B cell clonal representation in ectopic rheumatoid infiltrates

Advances in our understanding of the pathways responsible for the guided migration of lymphocytes to peripheral lymphoid tissues, and subsequent maintenance of their survival, have provided a different perspective on the origins of the lymphoid infiltrates of rheumatoid synovium. In peripheral lymphoid tissue, B cells constitutively express lymphotoxin-αβ (LT-αβ) which can engage LT-β receptors on stromal cells and cells of myeloid lineage, resulting in the induction of the chemokine, CXCL13 (also termed B lymphocyte chemoattractant, BLC, or B cell-attracting chemokine, BCA-1). In turn, B cells are attracted

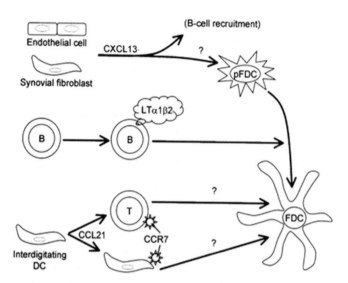

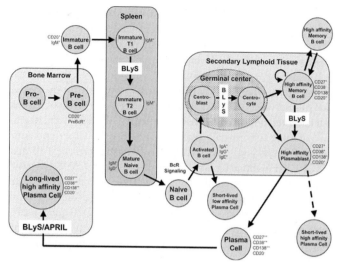

Fig. 9.2 A model of ectopic germinal center formation in the rheumatoid inflammation. GC-like reactions in the synovium are restricted to tissues containing FDC networks, assigning a checkpoint function to FDC development/maturation. Also, FDC precursors need to be recruited to this tissue site that is normally free of lymphoid structures. At least three independent pathways must contribute to this key event. Endothelial cells and synoviocytes begin to release CXCL13. The recruitment of B cells by this chemokine is unlikely to be the only function it fulfills in rheumatoid synovitis. In tissues with T cell–B cell aggregates without formation of GC-like structures, CXCL13 is lacking despite the accumulation of B cells. CXCL13 may also recruit FDC precursors as participants in the inflammatory infiltrate. LT-β is known to affect the differentiation and maturation of the FDC network, and likely also affects rheumatoid synovitis. CCL21 recruits CCR7-expressing T cells and dendritic cells (DCs), and may influence the process of FDC network generation and GC-like accumulations. Possibly, T cells and DCs responding to the chemokine CCL21 have a direct effect on FDC development and, thus, participate in lymphoid neogenesis. (From Ref. 36, reproduced with permission.)

Fig. 9.3 The roles of BLyS (also termed BAFF) in B cell development. The life of a conventional B cell is depicted from stem cells in the bone marrow, through the spleen and peripheral lymphoid tissues. The pathway reflects a composite of several defined steps from murine and human B cell development. The sites of BLyS action are shown as determined by *in vitro* activity or *in vivo* from the phenotypes of numerous mouse strains that carry mutations in BLyS, APRIL, or B receptors. Cells emerge from the bone marrow having undergone antibody gene rearrangement to produce functional antigen receptors. Cells travel through the blood or the lymphatic system. Maturation of the B cells occurs in the spleen. BLyS is essential for the T1 to T2 transition during splenic development; mice lacking BLyS have few B cells beyond this point of development. BLyS has been shown to be involved in several further maturation steps by *in vitro* activity. BCMA is up-regulated during plasma cell differentiation and BCMA-deficient animals have normal immune responses but the long-term survival of antibody-secreting plasma cells is impaired. A BCMA ligand (BLyS and/or APRIL) is therefore necessary for the survival of long-term plasma cells. PreBcR, pre-B cell receptor. (From Ref. 107, reproduced with permission.)

through their membrane expression of the chemokine receptor, CXCR5, towards the CXCL13 produced by these stromal cells. In response, these stromal cells are induced to display more LT-αβ. In parallel, T cells express the receptor, CCR7, which recognizes the chemokine ligands, CCL21 and CCL19, produced by some stroma. By these pathways, entering B cells and T cells become segregated into distinct areas of peripheral lymphoid tissue.

During their passage through the venules of affected synovial tissues, circulating lymphocytes may be preferentially directed to inflamed RA synovium in RA patients due to interactions along endothelial surfaces by a sulfotransferase termed GlcNAc6ST-2 (also known as HEC-GlcNAc6ST, GST-3, LSST, or CHST4). Moreover, both TNF-α and LT-αβ can induce the expression of GlcNAc6ST-2 in cultured human umbilical vein endothelial cells[47]. While lymphotoxin has been shown to determine the tropisms that underlie the normal development of lymphoid tissue, it also likely contributes to the inflammatory infiltrates associated with different disease states (Fig. 9.2). For instance, in the joint activated T cells produce lymphotoxin-β (LT-1β2), which acts as a downstream effector required for the development of primary B cell follicles in synovial infiltrates. In a recent report, expression of LT-1β2 and CXCL13 transcripts were found to be independent variables that correlated with the presence of GC-like lymphoid aggregates in

rheumatoid synovial biopsies[34]. Moreover, treatment with a decoy receptor that blocks LT was also shown to ameliorate disease in the collagen-induced arthritis (CIA) murine model system[48]. These observations suggest that the cytokine pathways associated with the pathogenesis of RA contribute to the induction of a vascular addressin in synovial vessels, which leads to the development of pathologic ectopic lymphoid aggregates.

Rheumatoid synovial tissues have also been found to be rich sources of CXCL12 (also termed stromal cell-derived factor, SDF-1)[49]. SDF-1 responsiveness is most marked in the early B cell precursors, pro-B and pre-B cells, and recent bone marrow immigrants and lymphocytes at the immature B cell stage, but not mature B cells. SDF-1 and also CXCL13 are produced by fibroblast-like synoviocytes (FLS) found in RA patients, which likely are important for the accumulation of B-lineage cells in ectopic lymphoid aggregates in rheumatoid synovium[34,50,51]. These interactions also contribute to the resistance of B cells to apoptosis, supporting an earlier hypothesis that specialized synovial 'nurse-like cells', peculiar to RA synovium, mediate homing and survival of B cells[50].

The B cell-specific pro-survival TNF family member BAFF (also called BLyS) has also recently been detected at high levels in rheumatoid synovial fluid, suggesting that this pro-survival factor is also locally produced in inflamed joints[52], and contributes to local lymphoid accumulations (Fig. 9.3). Notably, FLS primed with interferon-γ (IFN-γ and TNF-α was shown to induce high levels of BAFF expression, which contributed to enhanced survival of co-cultured B cells[53]. Such interactions have been proposed to protect synovial B cells from apoptosis in rheumatoid joints.

Because they are major sources of Ig/autoantibodies, there is great interest in also understanding the factors responsible for the migration and survival of plasma cells. In part, the prominence of plasma cell accumulations in rheumatoid tissues may be due to the migration of these cells toward gradients of SDF-1, CXCL9 (monokine induced by IFN-γ), CXCL10 (IFN-γ-inducible protein 10), and CXCL11 (IFN-inducible T cell α chemoattractant)[54]. SDF-1, as well as IL-5, IL-6, TNF-α, and ligands for CD44, can also prolong the longevity of plasma cells[55]. As plasma cells are devoid of several surface markers present on mature B cells (e.g., CD20 and CD22), these findings may provide a therapeutic approach for affecting the long-lived plasma cells that may contribute to the perpetuation of disease.

While the cellular processes responsible for the peripheral production of chemoattractants and survival factors remain to be fully elucidated, emerging evidence suggests that mesenchymal cells, released from the bone marrow that migrates to sites of inflammation, may be involved in the process. Stem cell-derived growth factors may play integral or even central roles in the initiation and perpetuation of the chronic inflammatory processes responsible for rheumatoid pathogenesis[56]. In fact, *in vivo* experimental models had long ago shown that peripheral immunizations led to the increased production and release of B-lineage precursors from the bone marrow[57]. Hence, even non-specific irritants, which we now suspect may act through the induction of chemokine/chemokine receptors, can induce a surge in the release of lymphocyte cells from the central compartment and migration into affected peripheral tissues. Relevant to the pathogenesis of RA, it has been shown that this process can be regulated by the peripheral production of TNF-α[58], which is known to be produced in joints affected by RA.

Atypical B cell repertoire expression in rheumatoid synovia

As lymphocytes from a B cell clone each express very similar antigen receptors (i.e., antibody or BCRs), analyses of local antibody gene sequence expression are important indicators of the clonal diversity of local B cells. Moreover, physiologic antigen-induced immune responses, which induce GC reactions in lymph nodes or spleen, are known to result in local accumulations of the progeny cells of antigen-specific B cell clones that all express highly related antigen receptor genes, varying only by one or a small number of specific point mutations.

To investigate the mechanisms responsible for the B cell accumulations in rheumatoid synovium, the antibody gene transcripts have been analyzed for restricted clonal heterogeneity at these sites. From these investigations, a great prevalence of hypermutated sequences were found with patterns of silent to replacement mutations that suggested that the infiltrating B cells include memory B cells selected based on their antigen-binding specificities (although the specific ligand is unknown)[59-61]. In fact, such studies

have shown that these RA joint samplings generally yield relatively few related sequences. These findings could indicate that in rheumatoid synovia there are clonally related daughter cells with limited survival[35], which may suggest that GC reactions do occur in RA synovium but that the associated proliferation and antigenic selection processes have limited efficiency. Alternatively, as related or identical sequences have also been found in different joints and in the blood of an individual RA patient, these findings may be most consistent with the trafficking of memory B cells that arose at other anatomic sites[62].

Antibody gene sequences recovered from RA joints also often display somatic diversification patterns uncommonly seen in healthy adults[63]. RA joints are reported to contain B cells expressing V gene rearrangement encoding for very large CDR3s, the portions in the antibody most important for determining binding specificity[64]. In healthy adults, larger immunoglobulin heavy chain CDR3s are more common in the bone marrow, the central site where B lymphogenesis continues throughout adult life. But such B cells are commonly subsequently deleted and they do not survive/persist in peripheral lymphoid tissues in healthy individuals[65,66]. Based on these observations, the accumulation of B cells with atypical BCR expression in rheumatoid synovium may suggest that such B cells are not locally generated but enter the synovium and bypass physiologic mechanisms of immunologic tolerance that weed out autoreactive clones. Hence rheumatoid synovial B cells may not be affected by the usual receptor editing (or clonal checkpoints) that normally occur in peripheral lymphoid tissue during the recruitment of peripheral repertoires. Moreover, as longer CDR3s in the VH region are correlated with broad polyreactive autoantibody activity[67], B cells expressing these atypical BCRs may be more likely to take up autoantigen(s) for processing and presentation that leads to the local recruitment of T cells into the local pro-inflammatory milieu. Of course, such B cells may also secrete polyreactive antibodies that contribute to local pathogenesis through complement and Fc mediated pathways.

While the hypermutation of antibody genes is generally accepted as marker for antigen-selected memory B cells, infiltrations of memory B cells in rheumatoid synovium do not necessarily reflect local antigenic selection in the joint based on disease-specific autoreactive responses. Instead, these cellular aggregates respond to local chemoattractants and not joint specific (auto)antigen localizations. In any event, published antibody sequence analyses support the notion that RA synovium may contain B and T cells that do not reflect classical mono-specific antigen focused B cell responses.

Accumulation of unusual B cell precursors in rheumatoid synovia

In recent studies, an unusual population of B cell precursors, which co-express conventional light chains and the surrogate light chain of pre-B cells, have been reported to accumulate in about one-third of RA samples[68,69]. Such B-lineage cells have been shown to express polyreactive BCRs[69], which are postulated to be promiscuous in antigen uptake and processing, enabling presentation of diverse autoantigens to T cells. Defects in immune tolerance, resulting in the accumulation of polyreactive mature B cells in RA synovium, might play a key step in pathogenesis. However, these findings have not yet been confirmed by other investigators and remain controversial[70]. It also remains to be determined whether such atypical B cell precursors are functionally active in the synovium. Speculatively, the skewed distribution of the B lymphoid cells that accumulate in the synovium could also largely be explained as a direct consequence of the potent B cell-specific chemoattractant activating and anti-apoptotic factors described above. Specifically, the local production of these factors at sites of inflammation in RA joints may serve as beacons to foster the accumulation of these atypical B-lineage cells, and perhaps also their local proliferation and/or differentiation. Hence, by this scenario the development of the ectopic B lymphoid infiltrates in rheumatoid joints would not require active (auto)antigen-driven GC reactions.

Roles of B cells in murine models of inflammatory arthritis

Collagen-induced arthritis murine model

More than two decades of investigations in rodent models of CIA[71] have illuminated a wide range of molecular and cellular similarities with RA[72]. Immunization with CII induces CIA in murine strains that have inherited susceptibility conveying certain major histocompatibility complex (MHC) II alleles, and both B and T cell immunity to collagen are required for the induction of disease. Like most Class II restricted autoimmune diseases, the cytokine milieu of CIA reflects a Th1-biased response, and disease associated anti-CII autoantibodies are biased to IgG2a and IgG2b subclasses.

Although T cells also play a prominent role in pathogenesis, anti-CII autoantibodies appear to be the primary mediators of immunopathogenesis. Although disease is not as comprehensive and severe as when induced by CII immunization, arthritis can also be induced in non-susceptible strains by transfer of either affinity purified anti-CII antibodies from arthritis mice, or with a mixture of monoclonal anti-CII that recognizes two or more epitopes[73], although in some reports co-treatment with lipopolysaccharide (LPS) is required[74]. In fact, arthritis can also be induced by transfer of anti-CII antibodies into mice deficient in both B cells and T cells[75]. In naive susceptible DBA/1 mice, a single anti-CII monoclonal antibody can induce persistent arthritis with massive cellular infiltrate and cartilage and bone destruction[76].

The dependence on specific IgG effector functions was clearly shown in the demonstration that arthritis was not induced by infusions of F(ab′)2 antibodies to CII[74]. Despite the induction of high levels of IgG2a anti-CII antibodies, mice of the DBA/1 background also display attenuated disease when deficient in the complement factors, C3 or factor B, and are completely resistant when deficient in C5[77]. Thus both the classical and alternative complement pathways have been implicated in the pathogenesis of CIA.

Although robust B cell and T cell responses are still induced by CII immunization, arthritis is prevented in mice deficient in genes for either the FcγRIII or the FcR common γ chain[78], despite the binding of anti-CII antibody and C3 to cartilage surface and the presence of high levels of autoantibodies to CII. Moreover, disease can even be induced by CII immunization in non-susceptible H-2(b) mice deficient in the inhibitory FcγRIIb receptor[79]. These findings highlight the contribution of FcγR to pathogenesis in this murine model of induced arthritis.

Spontaneous inflammatory arthritis in K/B×N mice

Following the development of methods for the introduction of transgenes, a mixture of gifted investigation and serendipity led to the development of the KRN/NOD murine model of autoimmune arthritis, which has been especially revealing with regard to the potential roles of B cells in spontaneous inflammatory arthritis[80,81]. In these mice, there is complete penetrance of a genetically determined, aggressive, spontaneously arising, distal joint disorder, which displays many of the key clinical, histological, and immunological features of RA in humans (reviewed in Ref. 82). Arthritic K/B×N mice are the F1 offspring from crossing KRN/C57Bl/6 tg strain with NOD strain. Like RA, K/B×N mice spontaneously develop a chronic inflammatory disease characterized by joint infiltration by mononuclear cells and destruction of cartilage and bone. Also akin to RA, this self-perpetuating disease is believed to arise from a subtle intercellular collaborative process involving different types of immune cells, with local T cell and macrophage activation contributing to a characteristic pro-inflammatory cytokine/monokine milieu. Both of these processes represent MHC allele linked responses associated with erosive synovitis with pannus formation, and TNF-α dependence, albeit K/B×N mice are RF negative and have some differences in the joints that are involved in their paws[80].

The arthritis in K/B×N mice is believed to arise because T cells express the KRN T cell receptor that recognizes a self-peptide bound to NOD-derived MHC II molecules—this inherent autoreactivity leads to the recruitment of B cells critical to the K/B×N disease, resulting in the secretion of arthritogenic Igs[83]. Development of disease involves the coordinated functions of both B cells and T cells, as infusion of non-depleting antibody to CD4 blocks disease, and mice devoid of B cells also do not develop disease[81]. The spontaneous arthritis of K/B×N mice develops in a highly predictable and almost synchronized fashion, with onset (initiation) of arthritis at 3–4 weeks, progression to an acute stage of 'robust inflammation' at 5–7 weeks, and a chronic but less aggressive stage at 8–11 weeks. Moreover, the initial development of arthritis is mirrored by the appearance of serum anti-GPI autoAb, with levels that correlate with the overall joint disease activity.

K/B×N disease is therefore believed to reflect a breach in immunologic tolerance of B cells for GPI, a ubiquitous cytoplasmic glycolytic enzyme. Even though the GPI antigen is systemically distributed, present in all cells, and detectable at substantial levels in the circulation of healthy mice(~400 ng/ml), during disease GPI can accumulate in the joints. Importantly, the anti-GPI B cell response predictably initiates in the draining lymph nodes of affected joints, and early in disease is greatest in draining nodes of affected ankles and paws, and less in spleen and other sites.

The number of B cells secreting anti-GPI autoAb becomes quite high, and comprises up to half of the total cell population by 8–11 weeks of age (i.e., 1500–2000 $\times$ 10^5 cells) in the draining lymph nodes[84]. Moreover, the pathogenetic potential of anti-GPI antibodies has been documented in studies demonstrating that infusion of as little as 100 μl of serum from an affected mouse will provoke arthritis within hours even in mice of otherwise unrelated genetic inheritance.

Significantly, arthritis is not induced by infusions of preformed anti-GPI antibody–antigen complexes[85]. This suggested that joint disease can result when autoantibodies, produced either locally or systemically, interact with antigens on synovial surfaces to develop IC *in situ*. Like the anti-collagen system, these locally formed ICs were shown to be pro-inflammatory only if they involve antibodies to two or more epitopes, and the more diverse the antibody response the more efficient the recruitment of pro-inflammatory factors[86], suggesting a complex IgG autoantigen lattice is required for the efficient recruitment of downstream inflammatory effectors.

Studies in K/B$\times$N have also highlighted the importance of mast cells. Mast cells, which are also prominent in RA synovial infiltrates[87], express membrane-associated FcR for IgE and IgG for triggering via antigen-specific (and perhaps non-specific) Ig cross-linking, to release vasoactive and chemotactic factors that facilitate the recruitment of other leukocytes to the synovial tissues. Mast cells also produce pro-inflammatory cytokines, like TNF-α and IL-1, and proteolytic enzymes at sites of cartilage erosions[87]. Demonstrating their importance, KRN/NOD mice that lack mast cells are resistant to inflammatory and erosive arthritis induced by arthritogenic serum[87]. Based on these findings, mast cells have become appreciated as links between the B cells, autoantibodies, complement, and other inflammatory mediators, that contribute to erosive arthritis.

Studies in the K/B$\times$N model have also enabled a closer dissection of the role of complement in the development of IC-mediated synovitis. Although anti-GPI antibodies are prevalent in the circulation, disease is limited to the joints, as only articular ICs may be efficient at fixing complement. Significantly, while C4-deficient KRN/NOD mice develop arthritis of the same severity as wild type mice, animals deficient in factor B of the alternative complement pathway develop attenuated disease or no arthritis at all[88,89]. In addition, a partial dependence on C3 was also demonstrated[88], which is consistent with the known role of C3 in the stabilization of IC. Hence, while RA is associated with activation of the classical complement pathway, the alternative pathway instead has been implicated in this mouse model. However, it is uncertain whether this seeming difference primarily reflects distinctions between murine and humans.

The self-sustaining nature of this murine pro-inflammatory arthritogenic disease also appears to be linked to the preferential induction of IgG1 antibodies to GPI, and to a smaller degree IgG2b anti-GPI antibodies[84,86], which reflects poorly understood cytokine and cellular regulation of the pathologic response. Consistent with the prevalence of IgG1 anti-GPI autoantibodies, deficiency in FcγRIII greatly attenuated severity of disease[88,90].

Biologic agents for RA that target B-lineage cells

Anti-CD20 therapy

Recent clinical trials have provided the best direct evidence that B-lineage cells play central roles in the pathogenesis of clinical autoimmune disease. Of these newer agents, most is known about the B cell-targeting antibody, rituximab, This antibody deletes B cells through a variety of mechanisms: apoptosis can be induced by hypercross-linking of membrane-associated CD20 molecules; antibody-dependent cytotoxicity (ADCC) can be evoked through interaction with FcγR on adjacent mononuclear cells; and recruitment by rituximab of complement-dependent cytotoxicity has also been implicated (reviewed in Ref. 91). There is also evidence that clinical responses of different B cell malignancies to rituximab vary in their dependence on specific antibody-mediated deletional pathways. These mechanisms also appear relevant to the treatment of patients with autoimmune diseases, as these afflicted individuals may have defects in these same afferent pathways, either based on inheritance of the genetic backgrounds that also predispose them to disease, or as a consequence of the inflammatory autoimmune disease process itself (discussed in Ref. 92).

The safety and efficacy of rituximab have been documented in a multiple arm, double-blinded controlled study of seropositive (i.e., rheumatoid factor positive) RA patients who had active disease despite treatment with oral methotrexate[93]. All patients also received a course of corticosteroids, although in a later clinical trial corticosteroids were shown to not enhance the efficacy of anti-CD20 treatment[94]. By week 24 of treatment, significant efficacy was demonstrated in the rituximab—methotrexate and the rituximab—cyclophosphamide combinations compared with methotrexate alone (see Chapter 40). Co-administration with cyclophosphamide or methotrexate resulted in benefits for a greater proportion of the patients compared with rituximab alone, with responses comparable to those commonly achievable with anti-TNF-α biologic agents. Even though rituximab is a chimeric antibody that contains murine-variable regions, human anti-chimeric antibodies (HACA) developed in only 4.3% in the rituximab-treated groups, although no specific clinical manifestations were observed in those patients.

The mechanism(s) by which methotrexate or cyclophosphamide contribute to enhanced responses remain unclear. While methotrexate as a second agent has been cited as reducing the development of HACA that can blunt the efficacy of a biologic therapeutic[95], this mechanism seems unlikely based on the relatively low level of HACA found in the patients who received rituximab alone. Speculatively, these second agents may suppress the local inflammation that might otherwise speed the reappearance of pathologic B lymphocytes and the immune response responsible for disease recurrence. Clearly these topics and consideration of whether the benefits of using these second agents are RA specific, or may also be relevant to the treatment of many autoimmune diseases by B cell deletion, will need to be carefully considered in the future.

In all of these RA patients, despite evidence of effective depletion of peripheral blood B cells, levels of total Ig remained within normal ranges. In contrast, rituximab treatment was associated with rapid significant decreases in RF autoantibody levels that persisted through week 24. The greatest induced decreases were in IgG-RF, which may be the most important contributor to *in vivo* pathogenesis. Significant decreases were also induced in levels of autoantibodies to cyclic citrullinated peptides (CCP)[94]. But levels of these autoantibodies never became undetectable. In contrast, levels of anti-microbial antibodies (e.g., anti-pneumococcal and tetanus toxoid) did not fall, suggesting that these protective responses may be the products of different B-lineage cell subsets[96]. More recently, blinded controlled studies have demonstrated efficacy and safety of rituximab in refractory patients who have failed or had inadequate responses to DMARDs and TNF inhibitors[96a,96b].

Anti-BAFF agents

Although detailed clinical studies have not yet been reported, recent findings in murine models suggest that agents that block the biologic actions of the TNF family member, BAFF, hold promise for treating autoimmune diseases (reviewed in Ref. 97). Along with APRIL, a closely related ligand of poorly understood function, BAFF interacts with three different membrane receptors (i.e., B-cell maturation protein (BCMA), transmembrane activator and calcium modulator and cyclophilin ligand interactor (TACI), and BR3), which are differentially displayed on mature B cells and plasma cells[98,99]. TACI is also expressed on certain T-cells. Interactions with BAFF regulate developmental checkpoints, which include the transition from B cell precursor to enter into the mature marginal zone and follicular B cell pools. BAFF also influences the survival of GC B cells and Ig-secreting plasmablasts and plasma cells, and BAFF signaling is required for homeostasis of the peripheral B cell pool[100] (see Fig. 9.3). In addition, the survival of B cell blasts that arise following encounters via their antigen receptors (i.e., BCRs), also requires signals from BAFF interactions[101].

In RA, there is a correlation with disease activity and high levels of BAFF. Moreover, the treatment of mice in the CIA model with a TACI-Ig decoy receptor agent that inhibits BAFF/APRIL provided benefits either when given before or after induction of disease[98,100]. This is particularly important, as autoreactive B cell clones have been shown to have an increased dependence on BAFF for survival[52,102]. It is therefore plausible that survival of B cells in an environment saturated in B cell survival factors, including BAFF, facilitates the development and/or exacerbation of RA by priming the T cell-driven inflammatory process. Conversely, as described above, if synovium is depleted of B cells, then T cells do not up-regulate key pro-inflammatory cytokines. Treatment of human RA synovium-SCID mouse chimeras with TACI-Fc, a decoy receptor for both the BAFF and APRIL lymphocyte survival factors, was recently reported to result in destruction of GC-like structures and inhibition of IFN-g and Ig transcript levels, while TACI-Fc treatment of chimeras with B-cell follicle or diffuse infiltrate types of synovial implants instead increased IFNg levels[102]. While currently both decoy receptors and blocking antibodies

specific for BAFF receptors are being developed for clinical usage, it is still too early to determine whether BAFF blockade will prove to be a safe and efficacious approach for the treatment of RA and other autoimmune diseases.

Therapeutic IL-6 blockade

IL-6 is a pleiotrophic cytokine system that affects many cell types, and this cytokine contributes to both local inflammatory processes and acute phase responses (Fig. 9.4). The dysregulated induction and expansion of autoantibody-producing plasma cells has been documented in patients with RA, SLE, and other autoimmune diseases. In part, interest in this pathway has developed from the recent recognition that IL-6 is important for the development of lymphoid and bone marrow 'niches' that support the long-term survival of plasma cells that otherwise do not display CD20 or CD22, making them potentially resistant to other means for targeted deletion.

In the first report of a therapeutic trial for IL-6 blockade, 164 patients with refractory RA were randomized in a multicenter, double-blind, placebo-controlled trial to receive the humanized anti-IL-6R antibody, at one of two doses or placebo[103]. At follow-up, responses were documented with the key finding of dose-dependent overall reductions of disease activity. At three months, at the higher dose 78% of patients achieved at least a 20% improvement (see Chapter 39)[103].

Due to the many biologic activities of IL-6, a wide range of potential mechanisms of action may contribute to these documented clinical responses. Considerable improvements were found in platelet counts and hemoglobin levels, as well as fibrinogen, serum amyloid A, and albumin levels. There were also significant decreases in RF levels, especially in the patients treated with the higher dose. Hence, IL-6 blockade provided beneficial for affecting a broad range of parameters of underlying inflammation, as well as possibly down-regulating the B cell activation and/or Ig secretion responsible for RA-associated autoantibody production.

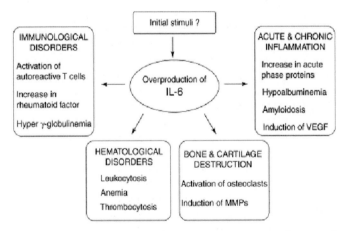

Fig. 9.4 Pleiotropic properties of IL-6. IL-6 acts on many cell types and organs throughout the body, to stimulate aspects of the innate and adaptive immune systems, and also potentially contributes to pathways of acute and chronic inflammation. MMP, matrix metalloproteinases; VEGF, vascular endothelial growth factor. (From Ref. 108, reproduced with permission.)

Concluding remarks

In the past, studies of B lymphocytes have emphasized their roles as producers of protective antibodies and autoantibodies, and/or the mechanisms by which these responses may be under T cell control. As discussed above, this overly narrow perspective has recently been revised to integrate a wide range of the potential roles by which B cells are now recognized to contribute to, or even control, immune responses.

These discoveries have also enabled a more comprehensive understanding of the pathogenetic pathways of diseases such as RA, in which accumulation of B-lineage cells, from atypical precursors and plasma cells to the organization of B cells into GC-like ectopic lymphoid tissue, may contribute to the associated inflammation and tissue destruction. As discussed above, these insights have also led to the development and application of novel B cell deletion therapies, and other approaches, including those for the targeting B cells via their surface BCR[104], CD19[105], or CD22[106] are also being evaluated. Based on recent reports, B cell-targeted therapies may provide efficacy, even in patients unresponsive to current therapeutic agents, by affecting underlying pathogenesis by means which were not even considered just a few years ago.

References

1. Zvaifler, N. J. The immunopathology of joint inflammation in rheumatoid arthritis. *Adv Immunol* 1973; **16**: 265–336.
2. Pekin, T. J. Jr., and Zvaifler, N. J. Hemolytic complement in synovial fluid. *J Clin Invest* 1964; **43**: 1372–82.
3. Edwards, J. C., and Cambridge, G. Rheumatoid arthritis: the predictable effect of small immune complexes in which antibody is also antigen. *Br J Rheumatol* 1998; **37**: 126–30.
4. Wooley, P. H., Luthra, H. S., Singh, S. K., Huse, A. R., Stuart, J. M., and David, C. S. Passive transfer of arthritis to mice by injection of human anti-type II collagen antibody. *Mayo Clin Proc* 1984; **59**: 737–43.
5. Schaller, M. M., Stohl, W., Tan, S. M., Benoit, V. M., Hilbert, D. M., and Ditzel, H. J. Elevated levels of anti-glucose-6-phosaphate isomerase (GPI) IgG in serum and synovial fluid from patients with inflammatory arthritis. *Ann Rheum Dis* 2004; **64**: 743–9.
6. Matsumoto, I., Lee, D. M., Goldbach-Mansky, R., Sumida, T., Hitchon, C. A., Schur, P. H. *et al.* Low prevalence of antibodies to glucose-6-phosphate isomerase in patients with rheumatoid arthritis and a spectrum of other chronic autoimmune disorders. *Arthritis Rheum* 2003; **48**: 944–54.
7. Goldbach-Mansky, R., Lee, J., McCoy, A., Hoxworth, J., Yarboro, C., Smolen, J. S. *et al.* Rheumatoid arthritis associated autoantibodies in patients with synovitis of recent onset. *Arthritis Res* 2000; **2**: 236–43.
8. Haberman, A. M., William, J., Euler, C., and Shlomchik, M. J. Rheumatoid factors in health and disease: structure, function, induction and regulation. *Curr Dir Autoimmun* 2003; **6**: 169–95.
9. Vaughan, J. H., and Chihara, T. Lymphocyte function in rheumatic disorders. *Arch Intern Med* 1975; **135**: 1324–8.
10. Kaplan, R. A., Curd, J. G., Deheer, D. H., Carson, D. A., Pangburn, M. K., Muller-Eberhard, H. J., and Vaughan, J. H. Metabolism of C4 and factor B in rheumatoid arthritis: relation to rheumatoid factor. *Arthritis Rheum* 1980; **23**: 911–20.
11. Dorner, T., Egerer, K., Feist, E., and Burmester, G. R. Rheumatoid factor revisited. *Curr Opin Rheumatol* 2004; **16**: 246–53.
12. Ruddy, S., Britton, M. C., Schur, P. H., and Austen, K. F. Complement components in synovial fluid: activation and fixation in seropositive rheumatoid arthritis. *Ann N Y Acad Sci* 1969; **168**: 161–72.
13. Ruddy, S., and Austen, K. F. The complement system in rheumatoid synovitis. I. An analysis of complement component activities in rheumatoid synovial fluids. *Arthritis Rheum* 1970; **13**: 713–23.
14. Brown, P. B., Nardella, F. A., and Mannik, M. Human complement activation by self-associated IgG rheumatoid factors. *Arthritis Rheum* 1982; **25**: 1101–7.
15. Goldstein, I. M., and Weissmann, G. Generation of C5-derived lysosomal enzyme-releasing activity (C5a) by lysates of leukocyte lysosomes. *J Immunol* 1974; **113**: 1583–8.
16. Borel, J. F., Keller, H. U., and Sorkin, E. Studies on chemotaxis. XI. Effect on neutrophils of lysosomal and other subcellular fractions from leukocytes. *Int Arch Allergy Appl Immunol* 1969; **35**: 194–205.
17. Fehr, K., Velvart, M., Rauber, M., Knopfel, M., Baici, A., Salgam, P., and Boni, A. Production of agglutinators and rheumatoid factors in plasma cells of rheumatoid and nonrheumatoid synovial tissues. *Arthritis Rheum* 1981; **24**: 510–19.
18. Youinou, P. Y., Morrow, J. W., Lettin, A. W., Lydyard, P. M., and Roitt, I. M. Specificity of plasma cells in the rheumatoid synovium. I. Immunoglobulin class of antiglobulin-producing cells. *Scand J Immunol* 1984; **20**: 307–15.
19. Sata, M., and Walsh, K. Oxidized LDL activates fas-mediated endothelial cell apoptosis. *J Clin Invest* 1998; **102**: 1682–9.
20. Harris, J., and Vaughan, J. H. Transfusion studies in rheumatoid arthritis. *Arthritis Rheum* 1961; **4**: 47–55.
21. Sutton, B. J., Corper, A. L., Sohi, M. K., Jefferis, R., Beale, D., and Taussig, M. J. The structure of a human rheumatoid factor bound to IgG Fc. *Adv Exp Med Biol* 1998; **435**: 41–50.
22. Ravetch, J. V., and Bolland, S. IgG Fc receptors. *Annu Rev Immunol* 2001; **19**: 275–90.
23. Davis, R. S., Ehrhardt, G. R., Leu, C. M., Hirano, M., and Cooper, M. D. An extended family of Fc receptor relatives. *Eur J Immunol* 2005; **35**: 674–80.
24. Sylvestre, D., Clynes, R., Ma, M., Warren, H., Carroll, M. C., and Ravetch, J. V. Immunoglobulin G-mediated inflammatory responses develop normally in complement-deficient mice. *J Exp Med* 1996; **184**: 2385–92.
25. Abrahams, V. M., Cambridge, G., Lydyard, P. M., and Edwards, J. C. Induction of tumor necrosis factor alpha production by adhered human monocytes: a key role for Fcgamma receptor type IIIa in rheumatoid arthritis. *Arthritis Rheum* 2000; **43**: 608–16.
26. Bhatia, A., Blades, S., Cambridge, G., and Edwards, J. C. Differential distribution of Fc gamma RIIIa in normal human tissues and co-localization with DAF and fibrillin-1: implications for immunological microenvironments. *Immunology* 1998; **94**: 56–63.
27. Shushakova, N., Skokowa, J., Schulman, J., Baumann, U., Zwirner, J., Schmidt, R. E., and Gessner, J. E. C5a anaphylatoxin is a major regulator of activating versus inhibitory FcgammaRs in immune complex-induced lung disease. *J Clin Invest* 2002; **110**: 1823–30.
28. Lanzavecchia, A. Receptor-mediated antigen uptake and its effect on antigen presentation to class II-restricted T lymphocytes. *Annu Rev Immunol* 1990; **8**: 773–93.
29. Roosnek, E., and Lanzavecchia, A. Efficient and selective presentation of antigen-antibody complexes by rheumatoid factor B cells. *J Exp Med* 1991; **173**: 487–9.
30. Chan, O. T., Hannum, L. G., Haberman, A. M., Madaio, M. P., and Shlomchik, M. J. A novel mouse with B cells but lacking serum antibody reveals an antibody-independent role for B cells in murine lupus. *J Exp Med* 1999; **189**: 1639–48.
30a. Jimenez-Boj, E., Redlich, K., Turk, B., Hanslik-Schnabel, B., Wanivenhaus, A., Chott, A., Smolen, J. S., and Schett, G. Interaction between synovial inflammatory tissue and bone marrow in rheumatoid arthritis. *J Immunol* 2005; **175**(4): 2579–88.
31. Chan, O. T., Madaio, M. P., and Shlomchik, M. J. The central and multiple roles of B cells in lupus pathogenesis. *Immunol Rev* 1999; **169**: 107–21.
32. Leadbetter, E. A., Rifkin, I. R., Hohlbaum, A. M., Beaudette, B. C., Shlomchik, M. J., and Marshak-Rothstein, A. Chromatin-IgG complexes activate B cells by dual engagement of IgM and Toll-like receptors. *Nature* 2002; **416**: 603–7.
33. Shen, Y., Iqbal, J., Xiao, L., Lynch, R. C., Rosenwald, A., Staudt, L. M. *et al.* Distinct gene expression profiles in different

B-cell compartments in human peripheral lymphoid organs. *BMC Immunol* 2004; **5**: 20.

34. Takemura, S., Klimiuk, P. A., Braun, A., Goronzy, J. J., and Weyand, C. M. T cell activation in rheumatoid synovium is B cell dependent. *J Immunol* 2001; **167**: 4710–18.

35. Schroder, A. E., Greiner, A., Seyfert, C., and Berek, C. Differentiation of B cells in the nonlymphoid tissue of the synovial membrane of patients with rheumatoid arthritis. *Proc Natl Acad Sci USA* 1996; **93**: 221–5.

36. Weyand, C. M., and Goronzy, J. J. Ectopic germinal center formation in rheumatoid synovitis. *Ann N Y Acad Sci* 2003; **987**, 140–9.

37. Takemura, S., Braun, A., Crowson, C., Kurtin, P. J., Cofield, R. H., O'Fallon, W. M. *et al.* Lymphoid neogenesis in rheumatoid synovitis. *J Immunol* 2001; **167**: 1072–80.

38. Wagner, U. G., Kurtin, P. J., Wahner, A., Brackertz, M., Berry, D. J., Goronzy, J. J., and Weyand, C. M. The role of CD8 + CD40L+ T cells in the formation of germinal centers in rheumatoid synovitis. *J Immunol* 1998; **161**: 6390–7.

39. Krenn, V., Schalhorn, N., Greiner, A., Molitoris, R., Konig, A., Gohlke, F., and Muller-Hermelink, H. K. Immunohistochemical analysis of proliferating and antigen-presenting cells in rheumatoid synovial tissue. *Rheumatol Int* 1996; **15**: 239–47.

40. Kim, H. J., Krenn, V., Steinhauser, G., and Berek, C. Plasma cell development in synovial germinal centers in patients with rheumatoid and reactive arthritis. *J Immunol* 1999; **162**: 3053–62.

41. Reparon-Schuijt, C. C., van Esch, W. J., van Kooten, C., Ezendam, N. P., Levarht, E. W., Breedveld, F. C., and Verweij, C. L. Presence of a population of CD20+, CD38- B lymphocytes with defective proliferative responsiveness in the synovial compartment of patients with rheumatoid arthritis. *Arthritis Rheum* 2001; **44**: 2029–37.

42. Voswinkel, J., Weisgerber, K., Pfreundschuh, M., and Gause, A. B lymphocyte involvement in ankylosing spondylitis: the heavy chain variable segment gene repertoire of B lymphocytes from germinal center-like foci in the synovial membrane indicates antigen selection. *Arthritis Res* 2001; **3**: 189–95.

43. Magalhaes, R., Gehrke, T., Souto-Carneiro, M. M., Kriegsmann, J., and Krenn, V. Extensive plasma cell infiltration with crystal IgG inclusions and mutated IgV (H) gene in an osteoarthritis patient with lymphoplasmacellular synovitis: a case report. *Pathol Res Pract* 2002; **198**: 45–50.

44. Shiokawa, S., Matsumoto, N., and Nishimura, J. Clonal analysis of B cells in the osteoarthritis synovium. *Ann Rheum Dis* 2001; **60**: 802–5.

45. Magalhaes, R., Stiehl, P., Morawietz, L., Berek, C., and Krenn, V. Morphological and molecular pathology of the B cell response in synovitis of rheumatoid arthritis. *Virchows Arch* 2002; **441**: 415–27.

46. Dechanet, J., Merville, P., Durand, I., Banchereau, J., and Miossec, P. The ability of synoviocytes to support terminal differentiation of activated B cells may explain plasma cell accumulation in rheumatoid synovium. *J Clin Invest* 1995; **95**: 456–63.

47. Pablos, J. L., Santiago, B., Tsay, D., Singer, M. S., Palao, G., Galindo, M., and Rosen, S. D. A HEV-restricted sulfotransferase is expressed in rheumatoid arthritis synovium and is induced by lymphotoxin-alpha/beta and TNF-alpha in cultured endothelial cells. *BMC Immunol* 2005; **6**: 6.

48. Fava, R. A., Notidis, E., Hunt, J., Szanya, V., Ratcliffe, N., Ngam-Ek, A. *et al.* A role for the lymphotoxin/LIGHT axis in the pathogenesis of murine collagen-induced arthritis. *J Immunol* 2003; **171**: 115–26.

49. Seki, T., Selby, J., Haupl, T., and Winchester, R. Use of differential subtraction method to identify genes that characterize the phenotype of cultured rheumatoid arthritis synoviocytes. *Arthritis Rheum* 1998; **41**: 1356–64.

50. Burger, J. A., Zvaifler, N. J., Tsukada, N., Firestein, G. S., and Kipps, T. J. Fibroblast-like synoviocytes support B-cell pseudoemperipolesis via a stromal cell-derived factor-1- and CD106 (VCAM-1)-dependent mechanism. *J Clin Invest* 2001; **107**: 305–15.

51. Shi, K., Hayashida, K., Kaneko, M., Hashimoto, J., Tomita, T., Lipsky, P. E. *et al.* Lymphoid chemokine B cell-attracting chemokine-1 (CXCL13) is expressed in germinal center of ectopic lymphoid follicles within the synovium of chronic arthritis patients. *J Immunol* 2001; **166**: 650–5.

52. Tan, S. M., Xu, D., Roschke, V., Perry, J. W., Arkfeld, D. G., Ehresmann, G. R. *et al.* Local production of B lymphocyte stimulator protein and APRIL in arthritic joints of patients with inflammatory arthritis. *Arthritis Rheum* 2003; **48**: 982–92.

53. Ohata, J., Zvaifler, N. J., Nishio, M., Boyle, D. L., Kalled, S. L., Carson, D. A., and Kipps, T. J. Fibroblast-like synoviocytes of mesenchymal origin express functional B cell-activating factor of the TNF family in response to proinflammatory cytokines. *J Immunol* 2005; **174**: 864–70.

54. Hauser, A. E., Debes, G. F., Arce, S., Cassese, G., Hamann, A., Radbruch, A., and Manz, R. A. Chemotactic responsiveness toward ligands for CXCR3 and CXCR4 is regulated on plasma blasts during the time course of a memory immune response. *J Immunol* 2002; **169**: 1277–82.

55. Cassese, G., Arce, S., Hauser, A. E., Lehnert, K., Moewes, B., Mostarac, M. *et al.* Plasma cell survival is mediated by synergistic effects of cytokines and adhesion-dependent signals. *J Immunol* 2003; **171**: 1684–90.

56. Sen, M. Wnt signalling in rheumatoid arthritis. *Rheumatology* (Oxford) 2005; **44**: 708–13.

57. Fulop, G. M., and Osmond, D. G., Regulation of bone marrow lymphocyte production. III. Increased production of B and non-B lymphocytes after administering systemic antigens. *Cell Immunol* 1983; **75**: 80–90.

58. Ueda, Y., Yang, K., Foster, S. J., Kondo, M., and Kelsoe, G. Inflammation controls B lymphopoiesis by regulating chemokine CXCL12 expression. *J Exp Med* 2004; **199**: 47–58.

59. Clausen, B. E., Bridges, S. L. Jr., Lavelle, J. C., Fowler, P. G., Gay, S., Koopman, W. J., and Schroeder, H. W. Jr. Clonally-related immunoglobulin VH domains and nonrandom use of DH gene segments in rheumatoid arthritis synovium. *Mol Med* 1998; **4**: 240–57.

60. Gause, A., Gundlach, K., Carbon, G., Daus, H., Trumper, L., and Pfreundschuh, M. Analysis of VH gene rearrangements from synovial B cells of patients with rheumatoid arthritis reveals infiltration of the synovial membrane by memory B cells. *Rheumatol Int* 1997; **17**: 145–50.

61. Lee, S. K., Bridges, S. L. Jr., Kirkham, P. M., Koopman, W. J., and Schroeder, H. W. Jr. Evidence of antigen receptor-influenced oligoclonal B lymphocyte expansion in the synovium of a patient with longstanding rheumatoid arthritis. *J Clin Invest* 1994; **93**: 361–70.

62. Voswinkel, J., Weisgerber, K., Pfreundschuh, M., and Gause, A. The B lymphocyte in rheumatoid arthritis: recirculation of B lymphocytes between different joints and blood. *Autoimmunity* 1999; **31**: 25–34.

63. Miura, Y., Chu, C. C., Dines, D. M., Asnis, S. E., Furie, R. A., and Chiorazzi, N. Diversification of the Ig variable region gene repertoire of synovial B lymphocytes by nucleotide insertion and deletion. *Mol Med* 2003; **9**: 166–74.

64. Bridges, S. L. Jr., Koopman, W. J., Lee, S. K., Clausen, B. E., Kirkham, P. M., Rundle, C. H., and Schroeder, H. W. Jr. Immunoglobulin gene expression in rheumatoid arthritis. *Agents Actions Suppl* 1995; **47**: 23–35.

65. Raaphorst, F. M., Raman, C. S., Tami, J., Fischbach, M., and Sanz, I. Human Ig heavy chain CDR3 regions in adult bone marrow pre-B cells display an adult phenotype of diversity: evidence for structural selection of DH amino acid sequences. *Int Immunol* 1997; **9**: 1503–15.

66. Zemlin, M., Schelonka, R. L., Bauer, K., and Schroeder, H. W. Jr. Regulation and chance in the ontogeny of B and T cell antigen receptor repertoires. *Immunol Res* 2002; **26**: 265–78.

67. Ichiyoshi, Y., and Casali, P. Analysis of the structural correlates for antibody polyreactivity by multiple reassortments of chimeric human immunoglobulin heavy and light chain V segments. *J Exp Med* 1994; **180**: 885–95.

68. Meffre, E., Davis, E., Schiff, C., Cunningham-Rundles, C., Ivashkiv, L. B., Staudt, L. M. *et al.* Circulating human B cells that express surrogate light chains and edited receptors. *Nat Immunol* 2000; **1**: 207–13.

69. Meffre, E., Schaefer, A., Wardemann, H., Wilson, P., Davis, E., and Nussenzweig, M. C. Surrogate light chain expressing human peripheral B cells produce self-reactive antibodies. *J Exp Med* 2004; **199**: 145–50.

70. Wang, Y. H., Stephan, R. P., Scheffold, A., Kunkel, D., Karasuyama, H., Radbruch, A., and Cooper, M. D. Differential surrogate light chain expression governs B-cell differentiation. *Blood* 2002; **99**: 2459–67.

71. Courtenay, J. S., Dallman, M. J., Dayan, A. D., Martin, A., and Mosedale, B. Immunisation against heterologous type II collagen induces arthritis in mice. *Nature* 1980; **283**: 666–8.

72. Brand, D. D., Kang, A. H., and Rosloniec, E. F. Immunopathogenesis of collagen arthritis. Springer Semin *Immunopathol* 2003; **25**: 3–18.

73. Terato, K., Hasty, K. A., Reife, R. A., Cremer, M. A., Kang, A. H., and Stuart, J. M. Induction of arthritis with monoclonal antibodies to collagen. *J Immunol* 1992; **148**: 2103–8.

74. Kagari, T., Tanaka, D., Doi, H., and Shimozato, T. Essential role of Fc gamma receptors in anti-type II collagen antibody-induced arthritis. *J Immunol* 2003; **170**: 4318–24.

75. Nandakumar, K. S., Backlund, J., Vestberg, M., and Holmdahl, R. Collagen type II (CII)-specific antibodies induce arthritis in the absence of T or B cells but the arthritis progression is enhanced by CII-reactive T cells. *Arthritis Res Ther* 2004; **6**: R544–R550.

76. Nandakumar, K. S., Andren, M., Martinsson, P., Bajtner, E., Hellstrom, S., Holmdahl, R., and Kleinau, S. Induction of arthritis by single monoclonal IgG anti-collagen type II antibodies and enhancement of arthritis in mice lacking inhibitory FcgammaRIIB. *Eur J Immunol* 2003; **33**: 2269–77.

77. Hietala, M. A., Nandakumar, K. S., Persson, L., Fahlen, S., Holmdahl, R., and Pekna, M. Complement activation by both classical and alternative pathways is critical for the effector phase of arthritis. *Eur J Immunol* 2004; **34**: 1208–16.

78. Diaz de Stahl, T., Andren, M., Martinsson, P., Verbeek, J. S., and Kleinau, S. Expression of FcgammaRIII is required for development of collagen-induced arthritis. *Eur J Immunol* 2002; **32**: 2915–22.

79. Yuasa, T., Kubo, S., Yoshino, T., Ujike, A., Matsumura, K., Ono, M., Ravetch, J. V., and Takai, T. Deletion of fcgamma receptor IIB renders H-2 (b) mice susceptible to collagen-induced arthritis. *J Exp Med* 1999; **189**: 187–94.

80. Kouskoff, V., Korganow, A. S., Duchatelle, V., Degott, C., Benoist, C., and Mathis, D. Organ-specific disease provoked by systemic autoimmunity. *Cell* 1996; **87**: 811–22.

81. Lou, Q., Kelleher, R. J., Sette, A., Loyall, J., Southwood, S., Bankert, R. B., and Bernstein, S. H. Germline tumor-associated immunoglobulin VH region peptides provoke a tumor specific immune response without altering the response potential of normal B-cells. *Blood* 2004; **104**: 752–9.

82. Kyburz, D., and Corr, M. The KRN mouse model of inflammatory arthritis. *Springer Semin Immunopathol* 2003; **25**: 79–90.

83. Nagaoka, H., Muramatsu, M., Yamamura, N., Kinoshita, K., and Honjo, T. Activation-induced deaminase (AID)-directed hypermutation in the immunoglobulin Smu region: implication of AID involvement in a common step of class switch recombination and somatic hypermutation. *J Exp Med* 2002; **195**: 529–34.

84. Mandik-Nayak, L., Wipke, B. T., Shih, F. F., Unanue, E. R., and Allen, P. M. Despite ubiquitous autoantigen expression, arthritogenic autoantibody response initiates in the local lymph node. *Proc Natl Acad Sci USA* 2002; **99**: 14368–73.

85. Matsumoto, I., Maccioni, M., Lee, D. M., Maurice, M., Simmons, B., Brenner, M. *et al.* How antibodies to a ubiquitous cytoplasmic enzyme may provoke joint-specific autoimmune disease. *Nat Immunol* 2002; **3**: 360–5.

86. Maccioni, M., Zeder-Lutz, G., Huang, H., Ebel, C., Gerber, P., Hergueux, J. *et al.* Arthritogenic monoclonal antibodies from K/BxN mice. *J Exp Med* 2002; **195**: 1071–7.

87. Lee, D. M., Friend, D. S., Gurish, M. F., Benoist, C., Mathis, D., and Brenner, M. B. Mast cells: a cellular link between autoantibodies and inflammatory arthritis. *Science* 2002; **297**: 1689–92.

88. Ji, H., Ohmura, K., Mahmood, U., Lee, D. M., Hofhuis, F. M., Boackle, S. A. *et al.* Arthritis critically dependent on innate immune system players. *Immunity* 2002; **16**: 157–68.

89. Waldrop, S. L., Pitcher, C. J., Peterson, D. M., Maino, V. C., and Picker, L. J. Determination of antigen-specific memory/effector CD4+ T cell frequencies by flow cytometry: evidence for a novel, antigen-specific homeostatic mechanism in HIV-associated immunodeficiency. *J Clin Invest* 1997; **99**: 1739–50.

90. Corr, M., and Crain, B. The role of FcgammaR signaling in the K/B x N serum transfer model of arthritis. *J Immunol* 2002; **169**: 6604–9.

91. Cragg, M. S., Walshe, C. A., Ivanov, A. O., and Glennie, M. J. The biology of CD20 and its potential as a target for mAb therapy. *Curr Dir Autoimmun* 2005; **8**: 140–74.

92. Silverman, G. J. Anti-CD20 therapy in SLE: a step closer to the clinic. *Arth Rheum* 2005; **52**: 371–7.

93. Edwards, J. C., Szczepanski, L., Szechinski, J., Filipowicz-Sosnowska, A., Emery, P., Close, D. R. *et al.* Efficacy of B-cell-targeted therapy with rituximab in patients with rheumatoid arthritis. *N Engl J Med* 2004; **350**: 2572–81.

94. Emery, P., Fleischmann, R. M., Filipowicz-Sosnowska, A., Schechtman, J., Ramos-Remus, C., Gomez-Reino, J. J., Hessey, E. W., Shaw, T. M., N. Li, N. F., and Agarwal, S. Rituximab in Rheumatoid Arthritis: A Double-Blind, Placebo-Controlled, Dose-Ranging Trial. *Arthritis Rheum* 2005; **52**(9): suppl. S709 (abstract).

95. Maini, R. N., Breedveld, F. C., Kalden, J. R., Smolen, J. S., Davis, D., Macfarlane, J. D. *et al.* Therapeutic efficacy of multiple intravenous infusions of anti-tumor necrosis factor alpha monoclonal antibody combined with low-dose weekly methotrexate in rheumatoid arthritis. *Arthritis Rheum* 1998; **41**: 1552–63.

96. Cambridge, G., Leandro, M. J., Edwards, J. C., Ehrenstein, M. R., Salden, M., Bodman-Smith, M., and Webster, A. D. Serologic changes following B lymphocyte depletion therapy for rheumatoid arthritis. *Arthritis Rheum* 2003; **48**: 2146–54.

96a. Cohen, S. B., Greenwald, M., Dougados, M. R., Emery, P., Furie, R., Shaw, T. M. *et al.* Efficacy and safety of rituximab in active RA patients who experienced an inadequate response to one or more anti-TNF therapies (REFLEX Study). *Arthritis Rheum* 2005; **52**(9): suppl. S677 (abstract).

96b. Emery, P., Fleischmann, R., Filipowicz-Sosnowska, A., Schechtman, J., Szczepanski, L., Kavanaugh, A. *et al.* The efficacy and safety of rituximab in patients with active rheumatoid arthritis despite methotrexate treatment: results of phase IIB randomized, double-blind, placebo-controlled, dose-ranging trial. *Arthritis Rheum* 2006; **54**: 1390–400.

97. Mackay, F., Sierro, F., Grey, S. T., and Gordon, T. P. The BAFF/APRIL system: an important player in systemic rheumatic diseases. *Curr Dir Autoimmun* 2005; **8**: 243–65.

98. Wang, H., Marsters, S. A., Baker, T., Chan, B., Lee, W. P., Fu, L. *et al.* TACI-ligand interactions are required for T cell activation and collagen-induced arthritis in mice. *Nat Immunol* 2001; **2**: 632–7.

99. Cheema, G. S., Roschke, V., Hilbert, D. M., and Stohl, W. Elevated serum B lymphocyte stimulator levels in patients with systemic immune-based rheumatic diseases. *Arthritis Rheum* 2001; **44**: 1313–19.

100. Gross, J. A., Dillon, S. R., Mudri, S., Johnston, J., Littau, A., Roque, R. *et al.* TACI-Ig neutralizes molecules critical for B cell development and autoimmune disease: impaired B cell maturation in mice lacking BLyS. *Immunity* 2001; **15**: 289–302.

101. Balazs, M., Martin, F., Zhou, T., and Kearney, J. Blood dendritic cells interact with splenic marginal zone B cells to initiate T-independent immune responses. *Immunity* 2002; **17**: 341–52.

102. Seyler, T. M., Park, Y. W., Takemura, S., Bram, R. J., Kurtin, P. J., Goronzy, J. J., and Weyand, C. M. BlyS and APRIL in rheumatoid arthritis. *J Clin Invest* 2005; **115**: 3083–92.

103. Nishimoto, N., Yoshizaki, K., Miyasaka, N., Yamamoto, K., Kawai, S., Takeuchi, T. *et al.* Treatment of rheumatoid arthritis with humanized anti-interleukin-6 receptor antibody: a multicenter, double-blind, placebo-controlled trial. *Arthritis Rheum* 2004; **50**: 1761–9.

104. Silverman, G. J., Goodyear, C. S., and Siegel D. L. On the mechanism of protein A immunomodulation. *Transfusion* 2005; **45**: 274–80.

105. Schlenzka, J., Moehler, T. M., Kipriyanov, S. M., Kornacker, M., Benner, A., Bahre, A. *et al.* Combined effect of recombinant CD19 x CD16 diabody and thalidomide in a preclinical model of human B cell lymphoma. *Anticancer Drugs* 2004; **15**: 915–19.

106. Juweid, M. Technology evaluation: epratuzumab, Immunomedics/Amgen. *Curr Opin Mol Ther* 2003; **5**, 192–8.

107. Baker, K. P. BLyS—an essential survival factor for B cells: basic biology, links to pathology and therapeutic target. *Autoimmun Rev* 2004; **3**, 368–75.

108. Nishimoto, N., and Kishimoto, T. Inhibition of IL-6 for the treatment of inflammatory diseases. *Curr Opin Pharmacol* 2004; **4**, 386–91.

10 | Innate immunity and immune complexes in rheumatoid arthritis

Peter A. Nigrovic and David M. Lee

Introduction

Prominent within the the complex histopathology of the rheumatoid synovium are cellular and soluble constituents traditionally viewed as members of the innate immune system. Support for the notion that innate immune mechanisms function pathogenically in rheumatoid arthritis (RA) derives from multiple animal models that have demonstrated a critical role for innate immune elements in the genesis of joint inflammation. In this chapter, we will introduce innate immunity generally and within the synovium and discuss how these mechanisms may participate in RA, with a focus on the potential role of immune complexes in the pathogenesis of this common and potentially disabling condition.

Innate immunity

The term **innate immune system** denotes a set of mechanisms capable of mounting a rapid immunologic defense in the absence of prior immunologic experience with particular pathogens. Innate immune effectors include soluble proteins, such as complement and anti-bacterial peptides; cells such as macrophages, neutrophils, dendritic cells, and mast cells; and cytoplasmic proteins directed against intracellular pathogens (Table 10.1). Each of these mechanisms targets pathogens through the recognition of structures common among microbes—termed pathogen-associated molecular patterns (PAMPs)—such as bacterial cell wall components (e.g. lipopolysaccharide, LPS) and distinctive protein glycosylation patterns. Innate immunity is phylogenetically much older than adaptive (B and T cell) immunity, and in higher animals the two systems have co-evolved to have frequent and important interactions with each other. Innate immune mechanisms help lymphocytes distinguish self from foreign and pathogenic from benign, while lymphocytes and their products (cytokines, antibodies) recruit innate immune mechanisms as effectors. Thus, innate immunity has three principal functions:

1. Provide a first line of defense against invading pathogens.

2. Promote and guide the initiation of antigen-specific (adaptive) immunity.

3. Participate in the effector phase of the final immune response.

While defects in innate immunity lead to more or less well-defined immunodeficiency states, excessive or aberrant triggering of these mechanisms can also contribute to inflammatory disease.

Soluble components of innate immunity

Complement

Best understood among the soluble components of innate immunity is complement (Fig. 10.1). Originally identified as a component of serum able to 'complement' antibody-induced lysis of bacteria, complement consists of a set of proteins with multiple important immunologic functions. The phylogenetically older **alternative pathway** of complement activation relies on the spontaneous hydrolysis of complement component C3. When stabilized by covalent binding to a surface devoid of complement inhibitors, such a bacterial cell wall, the C3 fragment C3b binds and cleaves factor B in a manner favored by the cofactor properdin to generate enzymatic complexes: a C3 convertase capable of accelerating the deposition of more C3b, progressing to a C5 convertase responsible for cleaving C5 and initiating the formation of the C5b–C9 membrane attack complex (MAC). Functionally similar convertases can be generated via the **classical**

Table 10.1 The innate immune system

Soluble
  Complement
    Classical pathway
    Lectin pathway
    Alternative pathway
  Pentraxins: CRP, SAP, PTX3
  Anti-microbial peptides
Cells
  Macrophages
    Monocytes
    Tissue-resident macrophages
  Neutrophils
  Dendritic cells
  Mast cells
  NK cells
  'Innate' lymphocytes
  NKT cells
  $\gamma\delta$ T cells
  B-1 B cells
  Marginal zone B cells
Intracellular
  NOD1, NOD2

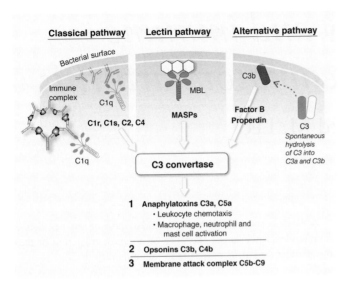

Fig. 10.1 The complement cascade. Complement may be activated through antibodies bound to antigen, lectin proteins bound to foreign carbohydrate residues, and through the covalent attachment of C3b to a favorable surface. Each of these processes leads to the formation of a C3 convertase which cleaves C3 and activates the rest of the pathway. See text for details. MBL, mannose binding lectin; MASPs, mannose-binding protein-associated serine proteases 1 and 2.

pathway, an enzymatic cascade initiated by the Fc portions of antigen-bound IgG and IgM and involving the complement proteins C1q/r/s, C4, and C2. A third pathway of complement activation, the **lectin pathway**, is homologous to the classical pathway but is activated by carbohydrate-binding proteins instead of antibodies. These lectins, including mannose binding lectin and the ficolins, are a kind of 'innate antibody' targeting characteristic microbial glycosylation patterns.

The functions of complement are diverse. The classical pathway enables immunoglobulin to recruit complement in the fight against pathogens, a classic example of the interaction between adaptive and innate immunity. Further, the covalent attachment of opsonin fragments C3b and C4b to antibody—antigen immune complexes helps to prevent deposition of these complexes in the vasculature, both by facilitating clearance via cells bearing complement receptors and by favoring the formation of smaller, less immunostimulatory aggregates (discussed further below). Classical pathway activation also plays a part in the clearance of apoptotic debris. Interestingly, deficiency of complement components in the classical pathway is associated with autoimmune disease, though elevated infection risk is generally not observed.

By contrast, deficiency of C3 and the alternative pathway is associated with pyogenic infections, confirming the importance of this mechanism in innate immune defense. Production of the MAC contributes to bacterial lysis by punching holes in the cell membrane, a function particularly important in defense against *Neisseria* species. Cleavage of C3 and C5 also results in the generation of the anaphylatoxins C3a and C5a, which are potent chemotactic and activating factors for neutrophils, macrophages, and mast cells.

Pentraxins

In addition to complement, humans produce several different innate defensive peptides classified structurally as pentraxins. These include C-reactive protein (CRP) and serum amyloid protein (SAP), generated in the liver as part of the acute phase response, and PTX3 produced in the periphery by many lineages including dendritic cells, endothelial cells, and monocytes/macrophages[1]. These proteins are natural opsonins, binding pathogen signatures (such as the pneumococcal C polysaccharide for which CRP is named) and promoting phagocytosis. Pentraxins can also bind C1q and fix complement by the classical pathway. The importance of these molecules in innate immune defense has been demonstrated in knockout animals.

Anti-microbial peptides

Mammals and most other complex multicellular organisms produce a wide range of small peptides with potent innate anti-microbial action. In humans, these include defensins, the cathelicidin LL-37, lysozyme, lactoferrin, and many others[2,3]. These peptides are expressed constitutively or inducibly at sites of frequent contact with pathogens, such as skin and the intestinal and respiratory mucosae, as well as by defensive cells such as neutrophils and cytotoxic T cells. Production in locations without regular pathogen contact, including the joint, has also been demonstrated[4,5]. Functions of these proteins are diverse and include permeabilization of bacterial membranes, sequestration of cations such as iron, and the recruitment of phagocytes, dendritic cells, and lymphocytes.

Cellular components of innate immunity

Pattern recognition by innate immune cells

A range of cell types contribute importantly to innate immune defense, including neutrophils, macrophages, and mast cells. These cells distinguish pathogen from host by a series of membrane-bound pattern recognition receptors. Foremost among these are the Toll-like receptors (TLRs), an 11–member family of transmembrane proteins hard-wired to recognize pathogen signatures such as LPS, double-stranded RNA, and undermethylated CpG repeats (Table 10.2)[6]. Many other pattern recognition receptor families also exist, including C-type lectins against microbial carbohydrates and a range of scavenger receptors[7].

Innate immune cells also express receptors that enable coordination with soluble innate pattern recognition systems. Thus, receptors for the complement cleavage components C3b, iC3b, and C4b enable macrophages to phagocytose pathogens to which these particles have become covalently attached, while receptors for C3a and C5a mediate the chemotactic and immunostimulatory functions of these soluble anaphylatoxins on neutrophils and other immune cells. The pentraxins CRP, SAP, and PTX3 also serve as opsonins, though their respective receptors remain controversial[1].

Fc receptors on innate immune cells

An important class of receptors found on all innate immune cells are the Fc receptors, which bind the Fc region of immunoglobulins (Ig). Binding of Ig to these receptors results in effects which vary

Table 10.2 The known human Toll-like receptors and their ligands

Receptor	Ligands	Notes
TLR1	See TLR2	
TLR2	Peptidoglycan, zymosan, some LPS	Functions as a heterodimer with TLR2 and 6
TLR3	dsRNA	
TLR4	LPS, lipoteichoic acid	Cofactors CD14 and MD-2
TLR5	Flagellin	
TLR6	See TLR2	
TLR7	ssRNA, imiquimod (synthetic)	
TLR8	ssRNA	
TLR9	Unmethylated CpG DNA	
TLR10	?	
TLR11	? (uropathogenic *E. coli*)	

Source: Ref. 253.

Table 10.3 The human Fcγ receptors

Receptor	Function	Cell distribution
FcγRI	Stimulatory	Macrophages; inducible in neutrophils, mast cells
FcγRII		
FcγRIIa	Stimulatory	Macrophages, neutrophils, dendritic cells, ?mast cells
FcγRIIb	Inhibitory	Macrophages, neutrophils, mast cells, dendritic cells, B cells
FcγRIII		
FcγRIIIa	Stimulatory	Macrophages, dendritic cells, NK cells, ?mast cells
FcγRIIIb	Stimulatory[a]	Neutrophils

[a]GPI-linked protein; net effect of ligation stimulatory, though transduction of a signal through the cell membrane requires coordination with other surface proteins. Cell distribution represents a partial list.

with the particular receptor and the type of cell, including stimulation or inhibition of cell activity, endocytosis, and antibody-dependent cell-mediated cytotoxicity (ADCC). Multiple receptors have been defined.

The complexity of responses mediated via Fc receptors is illustrated by the receptors for IgG (Table 10.3)[8]. In humans, five receptors are specific for this immunoglobulin. FcγRI is a high-affinity activating receptor found on macrophages and other myeloid lineage cells; ligation may trigger cell activation and receptor-mediated endocytosis. FcγRIIa and FcγRIIIa are low-affinity receptors capable of sending activating signals when cross-linked by multivalent ligands, such as immune complexes. These receptors are found on macrophages, natural killer (NK) cells, and others. Activation of these receptors triggers a number of responses depending on the cell type; examples include synthesis of cytokines, mast cell degranulation, and NK cell-mediated ADCC. These stimulatory effects are balanced by FcγRIIb, an inhibitory receptor of similar affinity to FcγRIIIa whose ligation delivers an inhibitory signal capable of blocking signals arising from activating Fc receptors. Since FcγRIIb and FcγRIIIa are generally expressed on the same cells, reciprocal modulation of expression levels by inflammatory mediators such as C5a permits rapid modulation of the sensitivity of an effector cell to immune complex stimulation[8,9]. Finally, FcγRIIIb is a low-affinity receptor expressed on neutrophils. Linked to the cell membrane via a glycan phosphoinositol (GPI) linker protein rather than a transmembrane domain, FcγRIIIb does not share activation motifs in common with the other activating receptors, yet plays an important role in recruitment of neutrophils to sites of immune complex deposition and, in concert with FcγRIIa, in the activation of neutrophils by immune complexes[10,11].

Specific cells of innate immunity

Neutrophils

Neutrophils originate in the bone marrow and circulate with a half-life of less than 12 hours. They are the primary phagocyte in the blood and predominate in many acute inflammatory infiltrates[12]. Immigration of neutrophils into inflamed tissue is mediated via adhesion molecules on both neutrophils and endothelium and occurs under the influence of a large number of pro-inflammatory and chemotactic mediators. Once in the tissues, neutrophils become activated through Fc receptor ligation, complement receptor ligation, and other signals, killing their microbial targets through phagocytosis, generation of reactive oxygen and nitrogen species, and elaboration of proteolytic enzymes and anti-microbial peptides. Neutrophils also contribute to the perpetuation of the inflammatory response by elaboration of pro-inflammatory mediators, including arachidonic acid metabolites, cytokines, and chemokines.

Macrophages

The second principal phagocyte of the innate immune system is the macrophage. Circulating as a monocyte, the cell is recruited to inflamed tissues by mechanisms analogous to those involved in neutrophil recruitment. Alternately, macrophages may reside constitutively within normal tissues, examples being Kupffer cells of the liver, microglial cells in the central nervous system (CNS), and synovial macrophages within the joint. Once at the site of inflammation, the functional phenotype assumed by the macrophage is highly sensitive to the local environment. Activated by Fc receptor ligation, anaphylatoxins, opsonins, PAMPs, and cytokines, macrophages phagocytose and kill microbes in much the same way as do neutrophils, and may produce a broad range of pro-inflammatory cytokines including TNF-α and IL-1. Under the influence of yet other stimuli, macrophages may elaborate immunomodulatory cytokines, including TGF-β[12,13]. A more detailed discussion of this lineage can be found in Chapter 5.

Mast cells

Recognized for their role in IgE-mediated allergy and anaphylaxis, mast cells also play a more general role in innate immune surveillance[14]. Mast cells arise from circulating hematopoietic progenitors and enter the tissues in an immature state, clustering around blood vessels, nerves, and near mucosal surfaces and differentiating under the influence of local conditions into a number of different phenotypes. In addition to FcεR1, the principal IgE receptor, mast cells express other receptors of importance in innate immune responses. These include receptors for C3a and C5a, TLRs, and the IgG receptors FcγRIIb and FcγRIIIa. They can phagocytose, generate reactive oxygen species, and present antigen[15]. Evidence from mice deficient in mast cells suggests that their key role in innate immune defense is to initiate the recruitment of inflammatory effector cells through the release of vasoactive and pro-inflammatory mediators including histamine, arachidonic acid metabolites, cytokines, chemokines, and proteases[16,17]. In this respect, their remarkable ability to store pre-formed mediators makes them a key player in the very early response to an inflammatory stimulus.

Dendritic cells

Dendritic cells (DCs) stand at the interface between innate and adaptive immunity[18]. Residing in the tissues in immature form, DCs sample their environment via endocytosis and a dense array of surface receptors. Induced to mature by TLR ligands, TNF-α, or other signals, DCs migrate to local lymph nodes where they present pathogenic antigens to naïve T cells in the context of costimulatory molecules and instructional cytokines. In this way, DCs initiate adaptive immunity and direct its general polarity along the Th0–Th3 spectrum. Under some conditions, mature DCs stay within the tissues, where they generate cytokines and prime local immune responses. A separate subset of DCs, called plasmacytoid DCs, circulate in the bloodstream and serve as the major source of interferon (IFN)-α and -β during viral infections before they, too, enter the tissues and function like tissue-resident DCs.

Natural killer cells

NK cells are circulating lymphocytes that lack specific antigen receptors but instead recognize cells that bear hallmarks of viral infection or neoplastic transformation. Using a set of activating and inhibitory surface receptors, NK cells attack cells that have down-regulated major histocompatability complex (MHC) class I and other 'self'-specific surface proteins or that express proteins associated with cellular stress or infection. Further, using FcγRIIIa, NK cells directly lyse cells opsonized by IgG (ADCC). This cytotoxicity is mediated by toxins including perforin and granzyme, as well as cytokines such as IFN-γ, and appears to play a role in controlling inappropriate or excessive immune responses as well as intracellular infections and malignancy[19].

Other cells involved in innate immune responses

The large majority of T and B cells await exposure to particular antigens before expanding clonally to participate in immune responses. However, within these populations are subsets of lymphocytes which appear to exhibit 'pre-programmed' receptors that enable participation in the innate response. These include CD1d-restricted NKT cells, T cells bearing the γδ T cell receptor (TCR) rather than the typical αβ TCR, B-1 B cells, and marginal zone B cells[20]. While still bearing recombined antigen receptors, these cells arise under selective pressures that result in a constrained specificity that typically includes autologous antigens, including antigens exposed by stressed cells. Such lymphocytes appear to both potentiate and regulate adaptive immune responses.

For example, 'innate' NKT cells express semi-invariant αβ TCRs that recognize host lipoproteins in the context of the MHC I-like antigen-presenting molecule CD1d. Since these cells are in regular contact with such host antigens, they circulate in a 'primed' state and are able to serve as potent amplifiers of early immune responses against pathogens[21]. They also appear to have an important regulatory function, and abnormalities in this population may promote certain autoimmune conditions[22,23]. γδ T cells express a surprisingly low TCR diversity, and appear to home to specific tissues in a receptor-dependent fashion. Under inflammatory conditions, γδ T cells are believed to participate in the regulation of both local mesenchymal cells and infiltrating αβ T cells[24]. B-1 B cells in the peritoneum and the marginal zone B cells of lymph nodes are important sources of IgM antibodies in the absence of pathogen exposure. These 'innate' antibodies frequently recognize autologous antigens, including apoptotic cell debris, and such cross-reactivity may both promote the survival of these clones and play a part in immune homeostasis[20]. The role of these and other B cells in RA is discussed in Chapter 9.

Cytoplasmic components of innate immunity

Within the last few years, a large family of intracellular mechanisms to detect and respond to infection has begun to be appreciated. The hallmark receptors of this type are NOD1 and NOD2, proteins that reside in the cytoplasm of cells and incite inflammatory responses when activated by bacterial products. A central role for these proteins in inflammatory diseases is made clear by the association of mutations in the *NOD2* gene with Crohn's disease and the familial granulomatous arthritis Blau syndrome[25]. Understanding of these pathways is still in its infancy, and their participation in inflammatory diseases remains incompletely defined.

Innate immunity in the normal joint

The articular cavity is a vulnerable potential space, essentially acellular and filled with protein-rich fluid. Animal models have documented that seeding of the joints occurs readily in experimental bacteremia with pneumococcus, staphylococcal species, and other agents[26,27]. Accordingly, the synovium requires mechanisms capable of initiating defensive responses without waiting for lymphocyte instruction. Simultaneously, the unique structural demands of the joint—in particular, the need for a broad expanse of acellular cartilage surface and for synovial fluid to lubricate and nourish the chondrocytes—appear to have imposed certain constraints on local innate immune mechanisms. In this section we will review soluble and cellular innate immune elements in normal synovium.

Complement physiology in the synovium

The synovial fluid is thought to be formed as an ultrafiltrate of the plasma supplemented with constituents synthesized by fibroblast-like synoviocytes (FLS) (e.g. lubricin, hyaluronan) (see Chapter 8). Not all proteins are found equally in plasma and synovial fluid. Complement is one example: functional levels of total hemolytic complement (CH_{50}) in fluid from normal joints are lower than serum levels and rise rapidly in inflammatory states such as gout, at least in part through increased vascular permeability allowing influx of complement from plasma[28]. Interestingly, complement components may also be produced locally by FLS, macrophages, and chondrocytes; production from these cells can be augmented by stimulation via IFN-γ, TNF-α, LPS, and immune complexes[29–31].

Complement activation in the joint, as elsewhere, is tightly regulated by soluble and membrane-bound complement inhibitors. These include inhibitors of the classical pathway, such as C1 esterase inhibitor[32]; the alternative pathway, including factor H and FHL-1[33]; both the classical and alternative pathways, such as decay accelerating factor (DAF, CD55) and membrane cofactor protein[34]; and the formation of the membrane attack complex, including CD59 (protectin)[35]. Despite this array of regulatory mechanisms, it may be that the joint remains unusually susceptible to complement fixation, particularly the surface of cartilage, which being essentially acellular lacks membrane-bound complement inhibitors. Thus, neutralization of CD59 by intra-articular injection of blocking F(ab')$_2$ fragments results in spontaneous arthritis in the rat, while mice genetically deficient in this membrane-bound protein are particularly susceptible to antigen-induced arthritis[36,37]. Further, cartilage appears to be a focus of complement fixation in RA and many animal models of arthritis (reviewed below), despite the presence of complement-inhibiting sialic acid residues on the cartilage surface[38,39]. It is interesting to speculate that this vulnerability to intra-articular complement activation provides a physiologic justification for the relative deficiency of complement components in normal synovial fluid, despite the susceptibility of this potential space to bacterial infection.

Other soluble components of innate immunity in the synovium

While relatively deficient in complement, the joint does possess other soluble mediators of innate immunity. Normal synovial membrane contains the anti-microbial peptides lysozyme, secretory phospholipase A2, lactoferrin, beta-defensin 1, and others. Both synovial macrophages and fibroblasts participate in this synthesis. Under conditions of inflammation, the profile of anti-microbial peptides changes, with augmented production of peptides including the neutrophil chemoattractant cathelicidin LL-37[4]. FLS exposed to TNF-α produce the pentraxin PTX3, while stimulated chondrocytes produce a range of anti-microbial peptides[5,40]. Though the physiologic role of these mediators remains undetermined, it has been suggested that they may shape the spectrum of pathogens causing septic arthritis[5]. Through effects on other leukocyte lineages, their contribution to intra-articular inflammation of any cause may be substantial[3].

Innate cellular populations in the normal synovium

The normal synovium consists of a thin lining layer, 1–4 cells thick, resting on a sublining of vascular loose connective tissue. Two principal cell types make up the lining layer: synovial macrophages, also called type A synoviocytes, and FLS, or type B synoviocytes. The relatively hypocellular sublining contains these two populations as well as blood vessels, nerves, mast cells, and dendritic cells[41].

Synovial macrophages

The hallmark innate immune cell in the synovium is the synovial macrophage. These cells are considered to belong to the macrophage lineage because of their phagocytic potential, bone marrow origin, and expression of the leukocyte common antigen CD45, along with characteristic markers including CD14 and CD68[42–45] (see Chapter 5). Limited direct information is available about innate receptor expression in normal human synovial macrophages, though by extension from work in other macrophage subpopulations they would be expected to express a broad range of pattern recognition receptors, including TLRs, as well as receptors for complement fragments[12]. Expression of FcγRI, II, and III at baseline has been well documented[46].

The function of synovial macrophages in joint homeostasis is incompletely defined, though they are believed to have a role in clearing the synovium of particulate matter[47]. Interestingly, *op/op* (osteopetrotic) mice carrying a mutation in M-CSF are devoid of synovial macrophages, yet have not been noted to exhibit gross joint dysfunction in the absence of further insult to the synovium[48,49]. Depletion of this population experimentally has been noted to correlate with a reduced inflammatory response to arthritogenic stimuli, though uncertainty about the selectivity of the depleting procedures complicates the interpretation of these data[50].

Mast cells

Aside from macrophages, the only other classical innate immune population substantially represented in the healthy human synovium is the mast cell. Scattered within the subsynovium in proximity to nerves and blood vessels, mast cells comprise up to 3% of cells in the normal synovium[51]. To this extent the joint resembles the peritoneum and pleural cavity, both vulnerable potential spaces whose linings also exhibit a substantial population of mast cells. The role of mast cells in normal joint physiology remains undetermined, but one important function is likely to be monitoring for early signs of bacterial infection using receptors for pathogen signatures, complement fragments and IgG. The capacity of mast cells to release pre-formed mediators and rapidly elaborate lipid

Table 10.4 Complement and immunoglobulin deposits identified by immunohistochemistry in joints from patients with RA

Study	n	RF+	Tissue	IgG%	IgM%	IgA%	C3%	C4%	IC%[a]
Fish 1966 (57)	7	57%	Synovium	100	57	0	57		57
Rodman 1967 (58)	8	75%	Synovium	100	63	13	100	100	100
Brandt 1968 (59)	10	80%	Synovium	80	80		80		80
Bonomo 1970 (60)	10	70%	Synovium	100			100		
Cooke 1975 (117)	42	69%	Cartilage	90	73	85	93		83
Ghose 1975 (254)	21	62%	Synovium	67	67	43	67		62
Ugai 1983 (122)	9	nr	Cartilage	100	67	29	100		100
Vetto 1990 (255)	34	54%	Cartilage	65	42	59	48	'Few'	> 35

RF, rheumatoid factor; nr, not reported; IC, immune complexes.
[a] Immune complexes considered present when Ig and complement colocalize. Not all tests were performed on all samples.

mediators and pro-inflammatory cytokines renders mast cells uniquely equipped to 'jump start' the immune response within the joint[52].

Other populations

Beyond macrophages and mast cells, the synovium contains other populations capable of participation in innate immune responses. Though fibroblasts are not generally considered an innate immune cell, FLS may express Toll-like receptors and respond to cytokine signals from macrophages and mast cells (e.g. TNF-α and IL-1), leading to the elaboration of a broad range of pro-inflammatory mediators[53,54]. Endothelial cells also respond directly to TLR ligands and other pro-inflammatory signals; activation of synovial vessels under inflammatory condition can contribute substantially to recruitment and activation of innate effector cells[55]. The role of local innervation in arthritis is undefined. Dendritic cells in the normal synovium remain incompletely characterized but, as might be expected, appear to belong to the myeloid subset and do not exhibit phenotypic features of activation or maturation[56].

Innate immunity in the pathogenesis of rheumatoid arthritis

Compared with the normal synovium, the rheumatoid joint exhibits marked histologic changes. These include striking hypertrophy of the synovial lining layer, accumulation of neutrophils in the joint cavity, infiltration of the subsynovium with mononuclear cells, depletion of cartilage matrix, and the development of erosive pannus. In this section we examine the contribution of innate immune elements to these pathologic changes.

Complement and immune complexes in RA

Evidence for complement fixation

Involvement of the complement system in rheumatoid arthritis has been extensively investigated. Immunohistochemical studies have documented deposition of C3 and C4 in the majority of rheumatoid joints, within the synovial lining, on the articular

cartilage, and decorating synovial blood vessels (Table 10.4)[57–60]. Though rheumatoid patients generally have normal or slightly elevated serum complement levels, levels of complement (CH_{50}) measured in synovial fluid are often substantially lower than would be expected given the usual increase in permeability and local complement synthesis accompanying the inflamed state (Fig. 10.2). This striking finding differentiates RA from conditions such as gout and psoriatic arthritis, and along with measurement of complement split products in rheumatoid serum and synovial fluid provided the first strong evidence that complement may play a role in the pathogenesis of RA[28,61–64].

Follow-up studies have provided a more differentiated view of complement consumption in the rheumatoid joint. Though as a group rheumatoid joints exhibit lower synovial fluid CH_{50} than joints affected by other arthritides, very low complement values generally occur only in patients who are rheumatoid factor positive[62,65,66]. Analysis of specific complement factors has demonstrated activation of the classical pathway, with depletion of C1, C4, and C2[62,67,68]. Alternate pathway activation has also been documented, with elevation of the cleavage products of factor B and consumption of properdin in RA synovial fluid but not in crystal-induced arthritis and osteoarthritis[63,69,70]. As would be expected whatever the mode of complement activation, the potent chemotactic anaphylatoxins C3a and C5a are frequently detectable, as are components of the C5b–C9 membrane attack complex[35,61,70,71]. Since sublethal MAC deposition can stimulate synovial fibroblasts, this latter finding is of potential interest[72,73]. Further evidence of complement fixation in rheumatoid synovium includes the presence of complement components C1q, C3, and C4, in association with large IgG and/or IgM immune complexes, within phagocytic vesicles of synovial fluid neutrophils and synovial lining macrophages[74]. Interestingly, preliminary data suggest that blockade of C5 activation has therapeutic value in established RA, as has been observed in animal models of antibody-induced arthritis[75,76].

Complement activation in patients with RA is not limited to the joints. While serum complement levels in most patients are normal or high, depressed CH_{50} may be seen in patients with active rheumatoid vasculitis, and serum evidence for activation of the classical and alternative pathways can be identified in a substantial proportion of patients[63,64,77–81]. Immunofluorescence evidence of complement fixation may be seen in rheumatoid vasculitis and in rheumatoid nodules[82,83]. In each of these situations, extra-articular complement consumption occurs most prominently (though not exclusively) in seropositive patients.

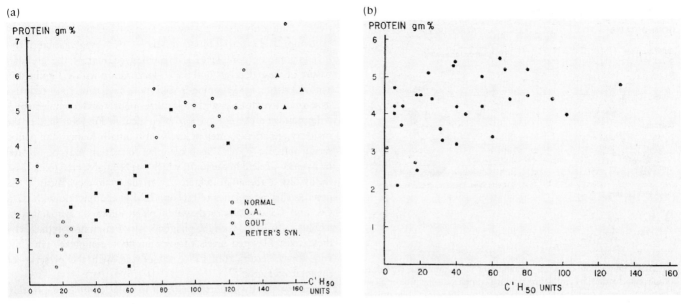

Fig. 10.2   Relative hypocomplementemia of rheumatoid synovial fluid. (a) Synovial fluid CH_{50} is low in normal joint fluid and rises proportionately to total protein in osteoarthritis, gout, and Reiter's syndrome. (b) By contrast, synovial fluid samples from patients with RA commonly show complement levels substantially lower than expected for the protein concentration, consistent with local complement consumption. A similar relationship holds between total fluid leukocyte count and CH_{50}. In this series, 27 of 31 RA patients were positive for rheumatoid factor. (From Ref. 28, reprinted with permission.)

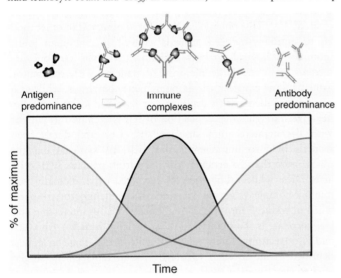

Fig. 10.3   Immune complex formation. Small immune complexes form when antigen or antibody is present in excess, while larger complexes form at equivalence. The symptoms of clinical serum sickness occur during the period of formation of the largest immune complexes.

Immune complexes in rheumatoid arthritis

Immune complex physiology

Immune complexes are the consequence of the interaction between multivalent antibodies and antigens with multiple epitopes. Crosslinking of antigens by antibodies results in the formation of lattices whose size depends on the ratio of antigen to antibody, the type of antibody involved (e.g. IgG has two antigen-binding sites while pentameric IgM has ten), and other considerations (Fig. 10.3). Complexes may form in circulation or by binding of antibody to antigen in the extravascular space. Since the largest and most pathogenic complexes are formed when antigen and antibodies are present at equivalence, hypocomplementemia and clinical symptoms in classic serum sickness occur during the brief window before rising antibody titers greatly exceed antigen load[84].

Immune complex formation is a regular event in the humoral immune response, and a multilayered system is in place to handle them. Conformational changes in IgM and IgG complexed with antigen enable complement fixation and subsequent attachment of C3b and C4b to the immune complex. This binding has important functional consequences for the immune complex (Fig. 10.4). C3b and C4b enable binding to CR1 on red blood cells, helping to prevent tissue deposition and allowing transport to phagocytes in the liver and spleen for disposal. Complement fixation also helps to destabilize larger immune complexes in favor of smaller, more soluble ones, and renders circulating immune complexes less pro-inflammatory by limiting the binding of immune complexes to Fc receptors[85–87]. Given these important interactions, an immune complex consisting of IgG1 and IgG3, isotypes that fix complement well, may behave differently than one made up of IgG2 and IgG4, which fix complement poorly.

When ineffectively cleared, immune complexes can cause tissue injury via complement fixation and activation of cells bearing Fcγ receptors (Fig. 10.5). The fate of a particular immune complex depends on its size, charge, and other characteristics. Smaller complexes remain soluble or may potentially enter directly into the tissues, while larger complexes tend to deposit in the vessels, where they trigger inflammation driven by FcγR-expressing circulating neutrophils[11,88]. Since the endothelial basement membrane is the typical site of entrapment of larger immune complexes, local accumulation of these complexes requires intravascular release of vasoactive agents to open spaces between endothelial cells and enable access to the basement membrane; hemodynamic turbulence may also contribute[89]. The charge of the antigen also plays a role in the ultimate localization of an immune complex; thus, complexes containing positively charged antigens tend to deposit (or form) on the negatively charged surface of the renal basement membrane, and a similar tendency for deposition on articular cartilage has been noted[90,91]. In this context it is interesting to note that the synovium, like the glomerulus, features capillaries and venules which are fenestrated and therefore basement membranes that are already exposed[92].

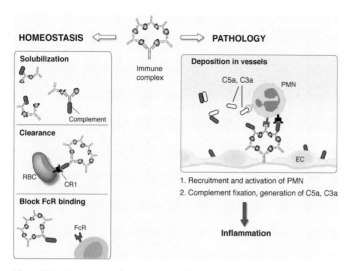

Fig. 10.4 Interaction between complement and immune complexes. Complement fixation by circulating immune complexes may protect as well as harm the host. Complement helps to neutralize large circulating immune complexes by favoring breakup into small, more soluble complexes; by opsonizing them for binding to CR1 on RBCs, allowing transport to the liver and spleen; and by hindering the binding of complexed antibody to Fc gamma receptors on inflammatory cells. Immune complexes that escape these mechanisms may deposit in the vasculature and tissues and cause inflammation via Fc receptor binding and complement activation.

Circulating immune complexes in patients with rheumatoid arthritis

Since the discovery that hypocomplementemia is a regular finding in rheumatoid joints, multiple groups have investigated the prevalence of circulating immune complexes (ICs) in patients with rheumatoid arthritis. Though technical issues hamper comparison of studies, commonly half or more of patients with RA are found to have readily demonstrable ICs in blood samples[93–95]. These complexes are of variable size, ranging from simple dimers of rheumatoid factor to much larger antigen–antibody lattices; RF is commonly but not invariably present[96]. Levels of IC have been noted to correlate inconsistently with disease activity, though these levels as well as immune complex size are typically elevated in patients with extra-articular manifestations of RA, including Felty's syndrome[95,97,98]. Indeed, immune complexes have been identified in sites of extra-articular disease, including pleura and pericardium[99,100]. Interestingly, injection of radiolabeled immune complexes and damaged autologous RBCs, as well as *in vitro* studies, have suggested alterations in reticuloendothelial function in some patients with RA that may contribute to delayed clearance and increased tissue deposition of immune complexes[101–103].

Glycosylation of antibodies in rheumatoid arthritis

Antibodies are generally substantially glycosylated, a characteristic which may play an important role in maintaining circulatory half-life and capacity to fix complement[104]. Glycosylation of circulating IgG has been noted to be abnormal in many patients with RA, resulting in an enhanced ability to fix complement via mannose-binding lectin[105–107].

Immune complexes in the rheumatoid joint

The prominence of classical pathway activation in synovial fluid suggests the involvement of complement-fixing immune complexes, and in fact these are regularly observed in the rheumatoid joint

(Table 10.2). Immunohistochemical studies of rheumatoid synovium commonly show patchy staining for IgG in the lining, subsynovium, and synovial blood vessels[41,57–60,108]. Aggregation of this IgG in immune complexes is presumed because of the granular nature of these deposits and the co-localization with C3 and C4 in synovial tissue. IgM staining is seen more sparingly, almost always in seropositive disease, and co-localizes poorly with complement[41].

Immune complexes have also been identified in joint fluid in the majority of patients, often at levels substantially higher than paired serum samples[94,109–112]. Such complex formation may be favored by hyaluronic acid in the joint, which has been observed to increase the avidity of rheumatoid factor by an uncertain mechanism[113]. As noted earlier, aggregates of IgG and IgM in conjunction with C1q, C4, and C3 are observed within phagosomes of synovial neutrophils, consistent with the phagocytosis of immune complexes by these cells. Elevated levels of joint immune complexes correlate with lower serum fluid CH_{50} values and with the presence of rheumatoid factor[74,111].

One potentially important site for immune complex deposition in the joint is the articular cartilage. Studies in a rabbit model of arthritis induced by injection of antigen into the knee have documented the preferential and prolonged attachment of antigen-antibody complexes to articular cartilage, menisci, and ligaments, whereas antigen deposited in the synovial lining is rapidly cleared[114,115]. This phenomenon has been observed in other models of antibody-induced arthritis as well as in human joints: immunohistological analysis of human articular cartilage and menisci from the large majority of patients with rheumatoid arthritis show complement-fixing immune complexes, while samples from patients with traumatic or psoriatic joint disease are negative, though some deposition of ICs is common in patients with degenerative joint disease[116–120]. Correspondingly, neutrophils bind to immune-complex rich RA synovial explants much more than to articular cartilage from patients with other arthritides, while rabbit menisci encrusted experimentally with immune complexes generate a pannus-like inflammatory response when introduced into the normal knee[121,122]. An interesting clinical correlate is the observation that patients with RA who have had synovectomy often relapse, while joints that have been debrided of all articular cartilage in joint replacement surgery tend to stay quiet[117,123–125].

It is worth emphasizing that, common though immune complex deposition is, it is not present in every patient with RA, and patients with other forms of arthritis (e.g. psoriatic arthritis) typically lack deposition of immune complexes and complement in the joints. Indeed, patients with inflammatory arthritis in the setting of congenital (Bruton's) and acquired agammaglobulinemia have been described; in some of these, complement fixation was noted in the synovium in the absence of detectable systemic or local immunoglobulin[126–128].

Immune complex composition in RA

The presence of immune complexes in the serum and synovial fluid of patients with RA has understandably stimulated considerable investigation into the antigen contained within these immune complexes. Multiple potential antigens have been identified, including DNA[129], type II collagen[119,130], fibrinogen[131], and others. Other systematic investigations of immune complexes precipitated from rheumatoid joints have disclosed little aside

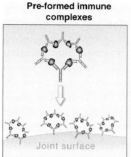
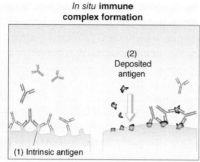

Fig. 10.5 Three potential mechanisms of immune complex deposition in the joints. Pre-formed circulating immune complexes may deposit directly or form *in situ*, where the antigen may be either intrinsic to the joint or deposited there from the circulation. Each of these three mechanisms may then be amplified by local factors, such as the relative deficiency of complement inhibitors on cartilage.

from IgG, IgM, and complement components; rheumatoid factor activity is regularly identified, suggesting that IgG may itself frequently be the antigen[131–136].

Interestingly, not all complement fixing 'immune complexes' in RA involve immunoglobulin. As discussed earlier, pentraxins are produced by multiple immune and non-immune cell types in the setting of inflammation and fix complement via C1q and the classical pathway. PTX3 is found at elevated concentrations in the rheumatoid joint, while CRP—C1q complexes circulate in many patients with RA and correlate with disease activity and serologic evidence of systemic immune activation[40,81]. The pathophysiologic significance of these findings remains undetermined.

Fc gamma receptors and RA

The presence of synovial fluid hypocomplementemia implies one pathway for the induction of tissue injury by immune complexes, yet other pro-inflammatory mechanisms are likely operative as well. As discussed earlier, immune complexes are capable of crosslinking the low-affinity Fc gamma receptors FcγRII and FcγRIII. Ligation of these receptors potently activates multiple cell types, including neutrophils, macrophages, mast cells, DCs, and NK cells. In fact, in some animal models of immune complex-mediated disease, Fc receptors appear at least as important as complement in the initiation of inflammation[137].

Evidence that this pathway is operative in RA comes from the observation that a polymorphism in FcγRIIIa resulting in enhanced IgG binding is more common in RA patients than in controls, though it has not been observed in all populations studied; the association appears strongest in nodular disease[138–142]. Interestingly, the reciprocal polymorphism is more common in systemic lupus erythematosus (SLE), suggesting a role for impaired handling of immune complexes in that disorder[143]. Macrophages from patients with RA have also been noted to express a higher level of FcγRIIIa, corresponding to enhanced production of pro-inflammatory cytokines upon stimulation via this receptor[46,144]. Data from animal models of arthritis also support a role for FcγRIIIa (see below).

A role for rheumatoid factor?

Rheumatoid factors (RF) are a heterologous group of antibodies directed against the Fc portion of IgG (see Chapter 3 for a detailed discussion). Most commonly of the IgM class, they may also be IgG, IgA, or occasionally IgE. While not specific for RA, seropositivity in rheumatoid patients correlates with more aggressive disease, and rheumatoid factors from RA patients have often undergone affinity maturation and display a higher affinity for IgG than those observed in chronic infection and other RF-associated conditions[145].

The role of rheumatoid factor in the pathogenesis of RA remains incompletely defined. Both self-aggregated (IgG) RF and RF bound to other immunoglobulins can activate complement[61,136,146,147]. Rheumatoid factor in the plasma may promote deposition of immune complexes by inhibiting the ability of complement to break up immune complexes and by directly linking smaller complexes together into larger, less soluble lattices; these effects may in part account for the observation that RF is found in most RA patients with vasculitis and depressed serum complement, and that synovial fluid neutrophils that have phagocytosed large immune complexes are found overwhelmingly in seropositive patients[74,77,148,149]. Levels of RF in synovial fluid generally exceed those in serum, suggesting local production, and indeed a large proportion of plasma cells isolated from rheumatoid synovium are capable of making RF, occasionally even in patients without measurable RF in the serum[150]. This intra-articular RF might promote complement fixation by crosslinking antibody deposited on joint surfaces, correlating with the documentation of RF in many intra-articular immune complexes and most RA patients with markedly depressed joint fluid CH_{50}, as noted earlier[62]. Thus, RF may serve as an amplifier of antibody-mediated inflammation in situations where the immune response to an antigen would not itself engender pathologic immune complexes[151].

However, the interaction of RF with immune complexes and complement is complex. When IgG immune complexes are formed in conditions of antigen excess, they are small and fix complement poorly; in this situation, crosslinking by RF substantially enhances the ability to activate the classical pathway. However, large IgG aggregates and immune complexes fix complement well, and addition of RF tends to limit complement activation, perhaps by steric interference with by C1q binding sites[147,152,153]. Further, binding of IgM RF to the Fc portion of IgG immune complexes physically inhibits binding to Fc gamma receptors, potentially limiting stimulation of innate immune cells by immune complexes[154,155]. Thus, RF may play an immunomodulatory as well as pro-inflammatory role in the rheumatoid joint.

Lessons from animal models: complement, immune complexes, and arthritis

Though the association of RA with complement fixation and immune complex deposition is compelling, intrinsic limitations in human research hamper assessment of the precise pathophysiologic contribution of these factors. By contrast, animal models provide the opportunity to dissect mechanisms of disease, particularly in the mouse where a wide variety of genetically deficient ('knockout') strains and reagents are available. Immunoglobulin and complement have been implicated in many though not all mouse models of arthritis (see Chapter 4, reviewed in Ref. 151). We will examine insights gained through these models with a focus on K/B×N arthritis.

This model was discovered fortuitously in a cross between the KRN mouse (on a C57Bl/6 background, thus K/B) and the NOD mouse. The KRN mouse bears a transgenic T cell receptor that recognizes bovine ribonuclease. By sheer chance, in the context of the NOD MHC class II molecule A^{g7}, this receptor also recognizes a peptide from the glycolytic enzyme glucose-6–phosphate isomerase (GPI). Arthritis results from the deposition or *in situ* formation of GPI+anti-GPI immune complexes in the joints, though other organ systems remain largely unaffected. This arthritis has clinical and histopathologic similarity to RA, including symmetry, a distal-to-proximal gradient of severity, formation of erosive pannus, and the accumulation of neutrophils in the joint lumen. Importantly, arthritis can be transferred to other mice via administration of K/B×N serum or sets of monoclonal anti-GPI antibodies[156–159].

This adoptive transfer variant of the K/B×N model allows experimental investigation of the effector phase of antibody-induced synovitis. Thus, though T and B cells are required to generate GPI-specific immunoglobulin, serum transfer into RAG knockout animals demonstrates that these cells play no vital role in the synovial pathophysiology. By contrast, mice deficient for components of the alternative pathway of complement (C3 and factor B) are resistant, as are mice that lack C5 and the C5a receptor, though the classical pathway of complement and the MAC are dispensable[160]. FcγRIII but not FcγRI is required, consistent with the central role of immune complexes in pathogenesis[49,160]. Largely similar dependence on both complement and Fc receptors is observed in other antibody-mediated arthritis models[151]. While these models are not phenocopies of RA—rheumatoid factor is generally not seen, and no ubiquitous target antigen has been identified in RA despite years of diligent investigation—they do suggest that immune complex deposition and complement fixation are more than mere epiphenomena in RA.

Studies in animal models have also shed important light on the mechanisms by which antibody might reach the joint. The synovial fluid is generally regarded as an ultrafiltrate of the plasma, and as seen in other areas where ultrafiltrates are generated (glomerulus, choroid plexus), the local endothelium is not continuous but fenestrated[92]. Plasma seeping through these fenestrations must cross the endothelial basement membrane before percolating through the hyaluronan-rich synovial extracellular matrix and between the synovial lining cells. Such transit occurs only to a limited degree for immunoglobulins, as evinced by the low concentration of Ig in normal synovial fluid and by studies using labeled antibodies to cartilage-specific type II collagen[161–163]. For more robust influx, a permeabilization signal is required. In K/B×N serum transfer arthritis this signal appears to be delivered by circulating anti-GPI+GPI immune complexes formed within minutes of serum administration; neutrophils, mast cells, and perhaps other cells activated via Fc receptors translate this signal into increased permeability in the synovial vasculature[163,163a]. Interestingly, in the mouse, vessels in skin and lung do not exhibit the same phenomenon, nor are all joints equally affected. Though the purpose of this striking and apparently tissue-specific reversal of vascular permeability to immunoglobulin remains unclear, it is tempting to speculate that it represents a mechanism to protect the joint from immune damage in the healthy state while allowing rapid immune access at the first sign of infection.

Murine models also highlight distinct pathways by which immune complexes may appear in the synovium. Conceptually there are three possible mechanisms: direct deposition of circulating immune complexes onto the joint surface; deposition of antibody onto antigen intrinsic to the joint; and deposition of a circulating antigen which then provides a target for antibody (Fig. 10.5). Human serum sickness may represent the first possibility, though it is unclear if immune complexes actually enter the joints or remain trapped in the joint vasculature[89]. The second appears to be the mechanism of collagen-induced arthritis (CIA), a model in which immunization of mice with allogenic type II collagen produces antibodies reactive against articular cartilage[164,165]. The third is represented by the K/B×N model, characterized by autoantibodies against a ubiquitous enzyme but with joint-specific manifestations at least in part because trace amounts of GPI deposit on the joint surface[116]. Binding of antibody to deposited antigen can result in 'antigen trapping,' with accumulation of the antigen within the joint due to delayed clearance; indeed, such accumulation is observed in K/B×N joints[116,166]. The formation, perpetuation, and pathologic effect of immune complexes arising through any of these pathways will depend substantially on factors in the synovial microenvironment, including mechanisms of immune complex clearance and the presence of local complement inhibitors.

It is worth noting that not all animal models of arthritis exhibit an antibody-dependent mechanism of inflammation[151]. Recently, a mouse strain bearing a mutation in the T cell receptor-associated signal transduction molecule zap70 has been described. This animal exhibits symmetric synovitis, serum rheumatoid factor, and other features making it an intriguing model of RA. Though these mice have hypergammaglobulinemia and circulating immune complexes, disease may be transferred to SCID mice by CD4+ T cells but not serum, suggesting that immunoglobulins may not be required[167].

Summary: complement and immune complexes in RA

Human data, supported by experimental models in animals, implicate complement and immune complexes in the pathogenesis of rheumatoid arthritis in a substantial proportion of patients. It remains unclear whether articular immune complexes deposit from the circulation or form *in situ*, and the factors favoring the joints as sites for immune complexes and complement fixation are still incompletely defined. Rheumatoid factor may contribute to pathology by linking small immune complexes together and by enabling IgG (including IgG RF) to function as an antigen. Downstream events from immune complex formation likely include stimulation of innate immune cells via Fc gamma receptors as well as pro-inflammatory effects of activated complement.

Innate cellular populations in RA

As discussed earlier, innate immune populations found constitutively within the synovium include macrophages, mast cells, and dendritic cells, while FLS and endothelial cells also participate in inflammation. In the context of synovitis, other cells are recruited and may participate in the pathophysiology of inflammation, including monocyte-derived macrophages, neutrophils, NK cells,

NKT cells, and γδ T cells. In this section, we will review the role of these cells in synovial inflammation, with an emphasis on their potential functions in immune complex-mediated disease.

Macrophages

Rheumatoid synovial tissue demonstrates dramatic expansion of the synovial macrophage population to constitute the large majority of cells in the hypertrophied synovial lining[168,169]. This expansion correlates with disease activity and progression of joint damage[170–172]. Most of this rapid increase in joint macrophages is believed to arise via recruitment of circulating precursors, as has been observed experimentally in animal models[173].

This expanded population of macrophages likely plays a pivotal role within the rheumatoid joint[12,47]. Upon activation, macrophages generate a large array of mediators with important effects on many aspects of the inflammatory process, including recruitment of other inflammatory cells, activation of synovial fibroblasts, resorption of matrix, cartilage, and bone, and the development of new blood vessels. Indeed, immunohistochemical and *in situ* hybridization studies of rheumatoid synovial macrophages have demonstrated the production of key pro-inflammatory mediators, including TNF-α and IL-1, and suggest that this lineage is the predominant population of cells producing these cytokines in synovial tissue[174–176]. Further, differentiation of CD14+ synovial monocytes into osteoclasts under the influence of receptor activator of NF-κB ligand (RANKL) may be a critical step in the generation of bone erosions in RA[177]. Finally, it remains possible that macrophages producing anti-inflammatory mediators such as IL-10 and TGF-β might play an immunomodulatory rather than inflammatory role in the joint[12,49].

Multiple pathways may be responsible for macrophage activation in the rheumatoid joint. T cell cytokines, including IFN-γ and IL-17, may have striking effects on macrophage phenotype and function[12,13]. Synovial macrophages also express receptors for complement and IgG, and enhanced expression of FcγRII and FcγRIII is noted to correlate with production of TNF-α[46,178]. Further, exogenous or endogenous TLR ligands can activate macrophages to release pro-inflammatory mediators (discussed further below).

Data from animal models are consistent with an important pathogenic role for both resident and recruited macrophages in arthritis. Depletion of phagocytes, including macrophages, from the synovial lining prior to induction of immune complex-mediated arthritis results in reduced infiltration of neutrophils and decreased cartilage damage[50]. Partial ablation of circulating monocytes with etoposide is associated with reduced severity of joint inflammation in response to intra-articular injection of bacterial DNA or experimental staphylococcal sepsis, even though synovial lining macrophages are not depleted by this therapy[179,180]. Interestingly, mice deficient in M-CSF (osteopetrotic or *op/op* mice) exhibit no synovial lining macrophages yet develop arthritis relatively normally in response to administration of K/B×N serum[48,49,181]. Though some macrophages have been observed to arrive subsequently, these data suggests that synovial macrophages are not required for the initiation of an immune

complexes-mediated inflammatory cascade. By contrast, *op/op* mice appear relatively protected from arthritis resulting from treatment with intra-articular methylated bovine serum albumin and subcutaneous IL-1[182].

Neutrophils

Neutrophils are rare in the normal joint but accumulate dramatically in rheumatoid synovial fluid, where they are the predominant cell type[162]. By contrast, they remain a variable but usually minority population within synovial tissue infiltrates in established RA[41,182a,183,184]. Neutrophils are recruited into the joint through processes similar to those involved in monocyte/ macrophage recruitment; these include up-regulated expression and affinity of adhesion molecules on endothelial cells and on the neutrophils, as well a variety of cytokines and chemokines[12]. Partition of these cells into synovial fluid rather than synovial tissues is incompletely understood, though factors chemotactic for neutrophils (e.g. IL-8, C5a, leukotriene B4) are found in elevated concentrations in joint fluid, as are factors that inhibit neutrophils apoptosis (e.g. C5a, GM-CSF)[185–187]. Since neutrophils have a life span of hours to a few days, even in inflammatory fluids, the persistence of neutrophilic joint effusions represents ongoing recruitment of neutrophils, estimated at over a billion cells per day within a single large joint[188].

Neutrophils are of great potential interest in the pathogenesis of joint disease in RA (see Chapter 7). Activated via complement or the Fc receptors FcγRIIa and FcγRIIIb, neutrophils are capable of generating a wide variety of mediators with pro-inflammatory and tissue destructive effects. These include IL-1, TNF-α, IL-8, leukotrienes, collagenase, elastase, and reactive oxygen metabolites[186]. Such cytokine production in response to immune complexes is especially robust in neutrophils 'primed' by exposure to cytokines such as TNF-α and GM-CSF, readily available in rheumatoid synovial fluid[189,190]. Not surprisingly, given the large number of these cells in direct approximation to articular cartilage, neutrophils are implicated in cartilage matrix degradation. This effect could be especially prominent if the articular surface becomes coated with immune complexes, a situation in which 'frustrated phagocytosis' leads to the release of reactive oxygen metabolites and other mediators directly onto the cartilage surface[191].

Animal models permit experimental investigation of the functional role of neutrophils in arthritis. Neutrophils contribute to joint swelling in arthritis mediated by intra-articular injection of streptococcal cell wall extract, though they appear to have a less important role in arthritis initiated via joint injection of bacterial DNA[179,192]. Experimental data from both the K/B×N serum transfer model and collagen antibody-induced arthritis have demonstrated a critical role for neutrophils in autoantibody-mediated inflammatory arthritis. In these models, arthritis is mitigated or abrogated entirely in mice depleted of neutrophils, and administration of depleting antibodies in early established disease markedly improves joint inflammation[165,193]. Interestingly, in the K/B×N model, neutrophil depletion prior to the injection of serum also limits the deposition of anti-GPI antibodies in the joints, implicating neutrophils in immune complex-mediated vascular permeability[163].

Mast cells

Mast cells are commonly noted to accumulate in sites of chronic inflammation, and the rheumatoid joint is no exception. Though patient-to-patient variability is considerable, mast cells can constitute 5% or more of the synovial cellular infiltrate, in particular in joints that are intensely inflamed[194–196]. Expanded populations may be seen in other arthritides as well, including SLE and psoriatic arthritis[195]. They are found throughout the synovial sublining as well as near sites of active erosions into cartilage and bone[197,198]. Recruitment from circulating precursors and replication of mature mast cells within the joint are thought to contribute to this expansion. Mast cell mediators, including histamine and tryptase, are frequently elevated in synovial fluid from patients with RA, consistent with local mast cell activation[199,200]. The phenotype of mast cells in the rheumatoid joint appears more heterogeneous than in the normal synovium, though the significance of this observation remains uncertain[201].

The potential contribution of mast cells to synovitis is substantial. Activated mast cells may release a wide range of pro-inflammatory mediators. These include the cytokines TNF-α, IL-1, and IL-6; vasoactive mediators such as histamine, prostaglandin D2, and the cysteinyl leukotrienes; and potent chemoattractants for neutrophils and macrophages, including leukotriene B4, IL-8, and MCP-1. Mast cells also generate factors that promote the hyperplasia and activation of synovial fibroblasts, endothelial cells (angiogenesis), and osteoclasts. Finally, mast cells synthesize mediators with immunoregulatory and anti-inflammatory functions, including IL-4, IL-10 and TGF-β (reviewed in Ref. 52). The net effect of these mediators in human arthritis is difficult to predict.

Animal data have helped to clarify certain aspects of the mast cell contribution to inflammatory arthritis. Histologic evidence of mast cell activation (degranulation) has been noted in multiple animal models of arthritis. Interestingly, mice congenitally deficient in mast cells are resistant to K/B×N serum transfer arthritis, and this susceptibility is restored by reconstitution with cultured mast cells[202,203]. Since degranulation of mast cells is one of the earliest detectable histologic changes in these mice, evident within hours of serum administration, one plausible interpretation is that mast cells serve as a primary responder to immune complexes within the joint, initiating the local inflammatory response much in the way they are believed to do in bacterial infection. To the extent that immune complexes, complement, and endogenous TLR ligands (discussed below) play a role in human RA, mast cells activated via these stimuli could well contribute in an ongoing fashion to inflammation within the joint.

Dendritic cells

While dendritic cell phenotype and function in normal human synovium remain poorly defined, multiple investigators have studied the distribution and phenotype of DCs in the rheumatoid joint. Despite the paradigm that mature DCs migrate to lymph nodes, dendritic cells bearing phenotypic markers of maturity (expression of CD86, CD83, and DC-LAMP, nuclear localization of RelB) are consistently found in the rheumatoid synovium in association with perivascular lymphocytic infiltrates and lymphoid aggregates of B and T cells[56,204–206]. Such mature DCs are seen in other inflammatory arthritides as well, including spondyloarthritis and gout, though only rarely in osteoarthritis[205]. While DCs usually migrate out of local tissues in response to an alteration in chemokine receptor expression in favor of the lymph node homing receptor CCR7, mature DCs in the synovium are found in proximity to synoviocytes expressing the CCR7 ligands CCL19 and CCL21, possibly accounting for the failure of these cells to emigrate[206]. Immature dendritic cells, assessed by expression of CD1a, are found scattered within RA synovium lining and sublining as well as in the periphery of lymphocytic infiltrates; as expected, the Langerhan's cell marker langerin is not found[206]. Plasmacytoid DCs have been documented in rheumatoid synovium as well[207].

Rheumatoid synovial fluid is also enriched with DCs compared with peripheral blood. In one study, 20–45% of all non-T mononuclear cells in rheumatoid synovial fluid were DCs[204]. These cells display an intermediate level of maturation, with lower expression of CD86, MHC class II, and cytoplasmic rather than nuclear RelB[56,204,208]. Plasmacytoid DCs have also been found in rheumatoid joint fluid[209].

Occasionally, lymphoid follicles are noted within RA synovium, consisting principally of B lymphocytes. In lymph nodes, these follicles are organized around follicular dendritic cells (FDCs), cells of non-hematopoietic lineage capable of trapping antigen on their surfaces in the form of immune complexes for presentation to B cells. Interestingly, fibroblast-like synoviocytes derived from patients with RA have been observed *in vitro* to express FDC activity[210].

The function of synovial dendritic cells in the pathogenesis of RA remains uncertain. Given the likely participation of T lymphocytes in RA pathogenesis, it is plausible that mature synovial DCs serve as an important antigen-presenting cell for memory T cells patrolling the joint, a role for which their perivascular position would be ideal. At the level of innate immunity, mature dendritic cells activate NK cells via IL-2 and produce other inflammatory markers with important local effects, including TNF-α, IL-1β, and multiple chemokines[211]. The role of DCs in arthritis has not yet been extensively explored in animal models.

NK cells

Natural killer cells have been observed in rheumatoid arthritis both within the synovium and in the joint fluid[212,213]. While most circulating NK cells express high levels of FcγRIIIa and low levels of NCAM (CD56), NK cells in the rheumatoid joint and in most other inflamed tissues are CD56[bright] and express lower levels of Fc receptors[213–215]. Cells of this phenotype are generally inefficient at cell-mediated cytotoxicity (including antibody-dependent cytotoxicity, ADCC) but tend to be excellent producers of cytokines, including IFN-γ and GM-CSF[216]. The presence of these cells in the joint may serve to amplify the local immune response via bidirectional cytokine- and contact-mediated interactions with dendritic cells and macrophages, though the pathophysiologic importance of this effect is unknown[215,217]. Experimental evidence from animal models of arthritis is limited but so far does not indicate that such an amplification loop is of critical importance[179]. The role of NK cells in the development of autoimmunity at the level of the T cell has been reviewed elsewhere[19].

NKT cells

NKT cells expressing semi-invariate CD1d-restricted T cell receptors constitute approximately 0.1% of circulating T cells, but are found in greater concentration in liver, spleen, and other sites[23]. They also accumulate in inflamed tissue under the influence of cytokines and chemokines. When activated, the principal NKT effector function is elaboration of Th1 and/or Th2 cytokines, including IFN-γ and IL-4, with resultant effects on NK cells, DCs, and other populations. NKT cells appear to be protective in certain animal models of autoimmune disease, including diabetes, encephalitis, and uveitis, but contribute to immunopathology in models of asthma and colitis[22,23]. Lower levels of functional NKT cells have been noted in the circulation of some patients with RA, though this observation is not limited to RA and is of uncertain significance[218].

Animal data diverge. In the collagen-induced arthritis model, invariant NKT-deficient (Jα281–/–) animals develop joint inflammation normally; treatment with a Th2-skewing NKT agonist affords partial protection from disease in WT but not Jα281–/– animals, and amelioration is observed when treatment is initiated after the establishment of disease[219]. These data indicate that NKT cells do not play a vital role in the generation of pathogenic anti-collagen antibodies, nor in the translation of these antibodies into joint inflammation, though under pharmacologic stimulation they may modulate this process by an undetermined mechanism. By contrast, in K/B×N serum transfer arthritis, NKT-deficient mice exhibit markedly attenuated disease, while NKT cell superactivation aggravates synovitis[220]. This pro-inflammatory effect requires production of both IL-4 and IFN-γ by NKT cells, resulting in suppressed production of the anti-inflammatory cytokine TGF-β by cells within the synovium. The relevance of these observations to human disease remains unknown.

γδ T cells

As discussed earlier, γδ T cells are a subpopulation of T cells expressing a limited diversity of TCR rearrangements and characterized by homing to specific tissues as well as a general tendency toward autoreactivity. In many but not all patients with rheumatoid arthritis, γδ T cells accumulate in the synovium and synovial fluid, where they express a TCR repertoire distinct from circulating γδ T cells consistent with receptor-driven specific homing and/or clonal expansion[221,222]. The contribution of these cells to the disease process, in terms of both the development of autoimmunity and the course of joint inflammation, remains obscure. In the collagen-induced arthritis model, administration of depleting antibody against γδ T cells prior to immunization with type II collagen delays the onset of disease, but administration near to the anticipated onset of arthritis in immunized mice induces explosive initiation of joint inflammation; by contrast, mice congenitally deficient in γδ T cells develop arthritis normally[223].

Toll-like receptors and rheumatoid arthritis

As noted previously, the Toll-like receptors are key pattern recognition receptors in innate immunity. TLRs are expressed constitutively or inducibly on macrophages, neutrophils, DCs, and mast cells, as well as other immune and mesenchymal cells. In the rheumatoid synovium, expression of both TLR2 and TLR4 (binding the Gram-positive bacterial components peptidoglycan and LPS, respectively) has been documented; interestingly, fibroblast-like synoviocytes rather than macrophages appear to be the major cell type expressing TLR2[54,224]. Correspondingly, peptidoglycan stimulation of cultured human synovial fibroblasts from patients with RA results in striking alterations in gene expression and elaboration of chemotactic and pro-inflammatory mediators[53,225]. Animal models of disease induced by systemic or intra-articular administration of bacterial extracts support the potential of synovial Toll-like receptors to participate in the onset of synovitis[179,226–230].

Since most cases of RA do not begin with overt bacterial infection, while most cases of septic arthritis do not proceed to chronic synovitis, what is the relevance of these observations to RA? First, bacterial TLR ligands have been noted in the joints of rheumatoid patients, though also in patients with other arthritides[231]. This opens the possibility that such exogenous products may be a contributory, if not sufficient, cause of joint inflammation in some patients. Second, and more intriguingly, productive engagement of TLRs may not be restricted to pathogens. Though still controversial, certain endogenous products of tissue inflammation appear to activate DCs and other cells via TLRs[232,233]. These include heat shock proteins, hyaluronic acid fragments, and fibronectin, all present in the rheumatoid joint. Support for an auxiliary role of TLR ligands in inflammatory arthritis comes from experiments in mice deficient in TLR4. Though these mice still develop arthritis when administered K/B×N serum, joint swelling is somewhat less intense and resolves more rapidly than in wild-type controls[234]. Interesting correlations in human disease include a reduced prevalence of a hyporesponsive TLR4 allele in RA patients compared to controls (albeit in one of three series) and the observation that therapeutic inhibition of TNF-α reduces TLR4 expression in cultured human dendritic cells[235–238].

Aside from stimulation of innate immune cells within the joint, TLR ligands could potentially have an important role in molding the adaptive immune response in RA. TLR stimulation of dendritic cells results in the inhibition of regulatory T cells, while ligation of TLRs on T cells may permit activation even in the absence of costimulation from antigen-presenting cells; both of these processes would promote aberrant T cell activation in the joint[239,240]. Of more direct relevance to rheumatoid arthritis is the expression of TLRs on B cells. B cells express most known TLRs, and stimulation of B cells via their membrane-bound antigen receptors in concert with a TLR ligand can lead to brisk antibody production. Immune complexes containing endogenous DNA, observed in some rheumatoid joints, can stimulate TLR9 and therefore permit B cells to escape the requirement for T cell help[241,242]. Such TLR ligand-mediated amplification of antibody production, including the production of rheumatoid factor, may contribute to the generation of pathogenic autoantibodies in the rheumatoid joint.

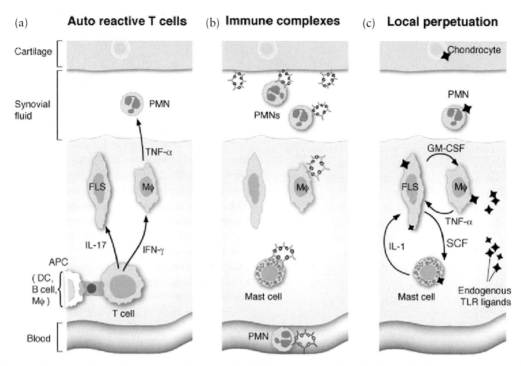

Fig. 10.6 Candidate mechanisms of innate immune recruitment in RA. (a) Orchestration of local inflammation by autoreactive T cells. (b) Deposition or *in situ* formation of immune complexes, resulting in complement fixation and Fc receptor-mediated activation of resident and recruited innate immune cells. (c) Perpetuation of inflammation via local positive feedback loops and the formation of endogenous TLR ligands. These mechanisms are not mutually exclusive. Cytokines are named as examples and not intended to represent a complete list. APC, antigen-presenting cell; Mφ;, macrophage; SCF. See text for details.

Synthesis and conclusions: innate immunity in rheumatoid arthritis

The rheumatoid synovium consists of a dense collection of synoviocytes and infiltrating inflammatory cells. Prominent within the infiltrate are T and B lymphocytes, scattered diffusely or organized into aggregates and even germinal centers. These observations, combined with the identification of the strong association of the MHC class II 'shared epitope' with the presence and severity of RA, have understandably encouraged the hypothesis that RA is a T-cell driven autoimmune disease.

While T cells undoubtedly play a central role in the pathogenesis of RA, recent findings have refocused attention on other populations within the synovium[243]. T cell-derived cytokines are found at relatively low levels in RA synovium, while the cytokine products of myeloid or fibroblast cells, including TNF-α, IL-1, and IL-6, are found in abundance and/or have been shown to play critical pathogenic roles[244,245]. Further, as reviewed above, murine models of arthritis have demonstrated that erosive, pannus-forming synovitis may arise even in the complete absence of T and B lymphocytes. Thus, independent of orchestration from adaptive immune mechanisms, cellular elements intrinsic to the joint appear capable of mounting an organized response to pro-inflammatory stimuli that replicates many of the histologic features of RA.

The question remains as to the contribution of innate immune mechanisms to human rheumatoid arthritis. At the very least it is clear that innate effector mechanisms play an important role in inflammation within the rheumatoid joint, supplying pro-inflammatory cytokines, degradative enzymes, osteoclast precursors,

and growth factors responsible for angiogenesis as well as FLS hyperplasia and activation. What remains uncertain is the mechanism by which activation of the innate immune machinery is initiated and perpetuated. Here at least three possibilities merit consideration (Fig. 10.6):

1. Direct stimulation of innate effector cells in the joint by infiltrating T lymphocytes reacting against local antigens, autologous or exogenous. Such autoreactive T cells may contribute to the the pathogenesis of collagen-induced arthritis and SKG arthritis[167,246]. The generation of antibodies under the direction of autoreactive T cells could be an important auxiliary pathway for joint injury in such a scenario.

2. Stimulation mediated via antibodies, deposited in the joint through direct targeting of a joint-specific antigen or by 'incidental' accumulation of antigen or antigen-containing immune complexes in the joint. Collagen antibody-induced arthritis and K/B×N serum transfer arthritis model these scenarios, respectively, and demonstrate little or no requirement for adaptive lymphocytes once antibodies are generated.

3. Initiation of inflammation by any of a number of triggers followed by propagation of inflammation within the joint, for example via autocrine and paracrine cytokine circuits or local generation of endogenous TLR ligands. No animal model yet convincingly demonstrates this mechanism, though the attenuation of K/B×N serum transfer arthritis in TLR4-deficient animals suggests a TLR-mediated local amplification loop[234]. Such circuits are unlikely to generate truly autonomous synovitis but may contribute substantially to inflammation induced by other mechanisms.

These three possibilities are not mutually exclusive. Thus, T cell help for RF-positive B cells may promote the formation of large immune complexes, while immune complexes taken up by antigen-presenting cells may facilitate the presentation of autoantigens to T cells[247]. TLRs can serve as non-specific promoters of antibody production by B cells while facilitating the escape of autoantigen-specific T cells from control by regulatory T cells[6,239]. It is probable that the contribution of each mechanism to synovitis differs from patient to patient, given the substantial variability in immune complex deposition and complement consumption among joints from different RA patients.

Beyond these three mechanisms, other factors will also contribute substantially to the ultimate course of inflammation within the joint. Recent work in the field of human autoinflammatory diseases and in mouse models of TNF-α and IL-1 dysregulation have highlighted the ways in which more or less subtle inter-individual variation in cytokine control pathways can contribute to inflammation in the joints and elsewhere[25,248–251]. Finally, evidence is growing that fibroblast-like synoviocytes from patients with RA demonstrate an aberrant activated phenotype[252]. By this and other mechanisms, FLS may play a role in the course of joint disease independent of innate or adaptive immunity.

References

1. Garlanda, C., Bottazzi, B., Bastone, A., and Mantovani, A. Pentraxins at the crossroads between innate immunity, inflammation, matrix deposition and female fertility. *Annu Rev Immunol* 2004.
2. Zasloff, M. Antimicrobial peptides of multicellular organisms. *Nature* 2002; **415**: 389.
3. Yang, D., and Oppenheim, J. J. Antimicrobial proteins act as 'alarmins' in joint immune defense. *Arthritis Rheum* 2004; **50**: 3401.
4. Paulsen, F., Pufe, T., Conradi, L., Varoga, D., Tsokos, M., Papendieck, J., and Petersen, W. Antimicrobial peptides are expressed and produced in healthy and inflamed human synovial membranes. *J Pathol* 2002; **198**: 369.
5. Varoga, D., Pufe, T., Harder, J., Meyer-Hoffert, U., Mentlein, R., Schroder, J. M. *et al*. Production of endogenous antibiotics in articular cartilage. *Arthritis Rheum* 2004; **50**: 3526.
6. Iwasaki, A., and Medzhitov, R. Toll-like receptor control of the adaptive immune responses. *Nat Immunol* 2004; **5**: 987.
7. Janeway, C. A., Jr., and Medzhitov, R. Innate immune recognition. *Annu Rev Immunol* 2002; **20**: 197.
8. Ravetch, J. V., and Bolland, S. IgG Fc receptors. *Annu Rev Immunol* 2001; **19**: 275.
9. Shushakova, N., Skokowa, J., Schulman, J., Baumann, U., Zwirner, J., Schmidt, R. E., and Gessner, J. E. C5a anaphylatoxin is a major regulator of activating versus inhibitory FcgammaRs in immune complex-induced lung disease. *J Clin Invest* 2002; **110**: 1823.
10. Chuang, F. Y., Sassaroli, M., and Unkeless, J. C. Convergence of Fc gamma receptor IIA and Fc gamma receptor IIIB signaling pathways in human neutrophils. *J Immunol* 2000; **164**: 350.
11. Coxon, A., Cullere, X., Knight, S., Sethi, S., Wakelin, M. W., Stavrakis, G., Luscinskas, F. W., and Mayadas, T. N. Fc gamma RIII mediates neutrophil recruitment to immune complexes: a mechanism for neutrophil accumulation in immune-mediated inflammation. *Immunity* 2001; **14**: 693.
12. Liu, H., and Pope, R. M. Phagocytes: mechanisms of inflammation and tissue destruction. *Rheum Dis Clin North Am* 2004; **30**: 19.
13. Stout, R. D., and Suttles, J. Functional plasticity of macrophages: reversible adaptation to changing microenvironments. *J Leukoc Biol* 2004; **76**: 509.
14. Galli, S. J., Maurer, M., and Lantz, C. S. Mast cells as sentinels of innate immunity. *Curr Opin Immunol* 1999; **11**: 53.
15. Marshall, J. S. Mast-cell responses to pathogens. *Nat Rev Immunol* 2004; **4**: 787.
16. Malaviya, R., Ikeda, T., Ross, E., and Abraham, S. N. Mast cell modulation of neutrophil influx and bacterial clearance at sites of infection through TNF-alpha. *Nature* 1996; **381**: 77.
17. Echtenacher, B., Mannel, D. N., and Hultner, L. Critical protective role of mast cells in a model of acute septic peritonitis. *Nature* 1996; **381**: 75.
18. Banchereau, J., Briere, F., Caux, C., Davoust, J., Lebecque, S., Liu, Y. J. *et al*. Immunobiology of dendritic cells. *Annu Rev Immunol* 2000; **18**: 767.
19. French, A. R., and Yokoyama, W. M. Natural killer cells and autoimmunity. *Arthritis Res Ther* 2004; **6**: 8.
20. Bendelac, A., Bonneville, M., and Kearney, J. F. Autoreactivity by design: innate B and T lymphocytes. *Nat Rev Immunol* 2001; **1**: 177.
21. Brigl, M., Bry, L., Kent, S. C., Gumperz, J. E., and Brenner, M. B. Mechanism of CD1d-restricted natural killer T cell activation during microbial infection. *Nat Immunol* 2003; **4**: 1230.
22. Chatenoud, L. Do NKT cells control autoimmunity? *J Clin Invest* 2002; **110**: 747.
23. Kronenberg, M. Toward an understanding of NKT cell biology: progress and paradoxes. *Annu Rev Immunol* 2005; **26**: 877.
24. Hayday, A., and Tigelaar, R. Immunoregulation in the tissues by gammadelta T cells. *Nat Rev Immunol* 2003; **3**: 233.
25. Hull, K. M., Shoham, N., Chae, J. J., Aksentijevich, I., and Kastner, D. L. The expanding spectrum of systemic autoinflammatory disorders and their rheumatic manifestations. *Curr Opin Rheumatol* 2003; **15**: 61.
26. lewis, G. W., and Cluff, L. E. Synovitis in rabbits during bacteremia and vaccination. *Bull Johns Hopkins Hosp* 1965; **116**: 175.
27. Bremell, T., Lange, S., Yacoub, A., Ryden, C., and Tarkowski, A. Experimental Staphylococcus aureus arthritis in mice. *Infect Immun* 1991; **59**: 2615.
28. Pekin, T. J., Jr., and Zvaifler, N. J. Hemolytic complement in synovial fluid. *J Clin Invest* 1964; **43**: 1372.
29. Ruddy, S., and Colten, H. R. Rheumatoid arthritis: biosynthesis of complement proteins by synovial tissues. *N Engl J Med* 1974; **290**: 1284.
30. Katz, Y., and Strunk, R. C. Synovial fibroblast-like cells synthesize seven proteins of the complement system. *Arthritis Rheum* 1988; **31**: 1365.
31. Firestein, G. S., Paine, M. M., and Littman, B. H. Gene expression (collagenase, tissue inhibitor of metalloproteinases, complement, and HLA-DR) in rheumatoid arthritis and osteoarthritis synovium: quantitative analysis and effect of intraarticular corticosteroids. *Arthritis Rheum* 1991; **34**: 1094.
32. Breitner, S., Storkel, S., Reichel, W., and Loos, M. Complement components C1q, C1r/C1s, and C1INH in rheumatoid arthritis: correlation of in situ hybridization and northern blot results with function and protein concentration in synovium and primary cell cultures. *Arthritis Rheum* 1995; **38**: 492.
33. Friese, M. A., Manuelian, T., Junnikkala, S., Hellwage, J., Meri, S., Peter, H. H. *et al*. Release of endogenous anti-inflammatory complement regulators FHL-1 and factor H protects synovial fibroblasts during rheumatoid arthritis. *Clin Exp Immunol* 2003; **132**: 485.
34. Davies, M. E., Horner, A., Loveland, B. E., and McKenzie, I. F. Upregulation of complement regulators MCP (CD46), DAF (CD55) and protectin (CD59) in arthritic joint disease. *Scand J Rheumatol* 1994; **23**: 316.
35. Konttinen, Y. T., Ceponis, A., Meri, S., Vuorikoski, A., Kortekangas, P., Sorsa T. *et al*. 1996. Complement in acute and chronic arthritides: assessment of C3c, C9, and protectin (CD59) in synovial membrane. *Ann Rheum Dis* 55: 888.
36. Mizuno, M., Nishikawa, K., Goodfellow, R. M., Piddlesden, S. J., Morgan, B. P., and Matsuo, S. The effects of functional suppression of a membrane-bound complement regulatory protein, CD59, in the synovial tissue in rats. *Arthritis Rheum* 1997; **40**: 527.
37. Williams, A. S., Mizuno, M., Richards, P. J., Holt, D. S., and Morgan, B. P. Deletion of the gene encoding CD59a in mice increases disease severity in a murine model of rheumatoid arthritis. *Arthritis Rheum* 2004; **50**: 3035.

38. Fearon, D. T. Regulation by membrane sialic acid of beta1H-dependent decay-dissociation of amplification C3 convertase of the alternative complement pathway. *Proc Natl Acad Sci U S A* 1978; **75**: 1971.

39. Laver-Rudich, Z., and Silbermann, M. Cartilage surface charge: a possible determinant in aging and osteoarthritic processes. *Arthritis Rheum* 1985; **28**: 660.

40. Luchetti, M. M., Piccinini, G., Mantovani, A., Peri, G., Matteucci, C., Pomponio G. *et al*. Expression and production of the long pentraxin PTX3 in rheumatoid arthritis (RA). *Clin Exp Immunol* 2000; **119**: 196.

41. Zvaifler, N. J. The immunopathology of joint inflammation in rheumatoid arthritis. *Adv Immunol* 1973; **16**: 265.

42. Barland, P., Novikoff, A. B., and Hamerman, D. Electron microscopy of the human synovial membrane. *J Cell Biol* 1962; **14**: 207.

43. Adam, W. S. Fine structure of synovial membrane: phagocytosis of colloidal carbon from the joint cavity. *Lab Invest* 1966; **15**: 680.

44. Edwards, J. C. The origin of type A synovial lining cells. *Immunobiology* 1982; **161**: 227.

45. Athanasou, N. A., and Quinn, J. Immunocytochemical analysis of human synovial lining cells: phenotypic relation to other marrow derived cells. *Ann Rheum Dis* 1991; **50**: 311.

46. Blom, A. B., Radstake, T. R., Holthuysen, A. E., Sloetjes, A. W., Pesman, G. J., Sweep F. G. *et al*. Increased expression of Fcgamma receptors II and III on macrophages of rheumatoid arthritis patients results in higher production of tumor necrosis factor alpha and matrix metalloproteinase. *Arthritis Rheum* 2003; **48**: 1002.

47. Burmester, G. R., Stuhlmuller, B., Keyszer, G., and Kinne, R. W. Mononuclear phagocytes and rheumatoid synovitis: mastermind or workhorse in arthritis? *Arthritis Rheum* 1997; **40**: 5.

48. Cecchini, M. G., Dominguez, M. G., Mocci, S., Wetterwald, A., Felix, R., Fleisch H. *et al*. Role of colony stimulating factor-1 in the establishment and regulation of tissue macrophages during postnatal development of the mouse. *Development* 1994; **120**: 1357.

49. Bruhns, P., Samuelsson, A., Pollard, J. W., and Ravetch, J. V. Colony-stimulating factor-1-dependent macrophages are responsible for IVIG protection in antibody-induced autoimmune disease. *Immunity* 2003; **18**: 573.

50. Van Lent, P. L., Holthuysen, A. E., Van Rooijen, N., Van De Putte, L. B., and Van Den Berg, W. B. Local removal of phagocytic synovial lining cells by clodronate-liposomes decreases cartilage destruction during collagen type II arthritis. *Ann Rheum Dis* 1998; **57**: 408.

51. Castor, W. The microscopic structure of normal human synovial tissue. *Arthritis Rheum* 1960; **3**: 140.

52. Nigrovic, P. A., and Lee, D. M. Mast cells in inflammatory arthritis. *Arthritis Res Ther* 2005; **7**: 1.

53. Kyburz, D., Rethage, J., Seibl, R., Lauener, R., Gay, R. E., Carson, D. A., and Gay, S. Bacterial peptidoglycans but not CpG oligodeoxynucleotides activate synovial fibroblasts by toll-like receptor signaling. *Arthritis Rheum* 2003; **48**: 642.

54. Seibl, R., Birchler, T., Loeliger, S., Hossle, J. P., Gay, R. E., Saurenmann T. *et al*. Expression and regulation of Toll-like receptor 2 in rheumatoid arthritis synovium. *Am J Pathol* 2003; **162**: 1221.

55. Middleton, J., Americh, L., Gayon, R., Julien, D., Aguilar, L., Amalric, F., and Girard, J. P. Endothelial cell phenotypes in the rheumatoid synovium: activated, angiogenic, apoptotic and leaky. *Arthritis Res Ther* 2004; **6**: 60.

56. Pettit, A. R., MacDonald, K. P., O'Sullivan, B., and Thomas, R. Differentiated dendritic cells expressing nuclear RelB are predominantly located in rheumatoid synovial tissue perivascular mononuclear cell aggregates. *Arthritis Rheum* 2000; **43**: 791.

57. Fish, A. J., Michael, A. F., Gewurz, H., and Good, R. A. Immunopathologic changes in rheumatoid arthritis synovium. *Arthritis Rheum* 1966; **9**: 267.

58. Rodman, W. S., Williams, Jr. R. C., Bilka, P. J., and Muller-Eberhard, H. J. Immunofluorescent localization of the third and the fourth component of complement in synovial tissue from patients with rheumatoid arthritis. *J Lab Clin Med* 1967; **69**: 141.

59. Brandt, K. D., Cathcart, E. S., and Cohen, A. S. Studies of immune deposits in synovial membranes and corresponding synovial fluids. *J Lab Clin Med* 1968; **72**: 631.

60. Bonomo, L., Tursi, A., Trizio, D., Gillardi, U., and Dammacco, F. Immune complexes in rheumatoid synovitis: a mixed staining immunofluorescence study. *Immunology* 1970; **18**: 557.

61. Zvaifler, N. J. Breakdown products of C 3 in human synovial fluids. *J Clin Invest* 1969; **48**: 1532.

62. Ruddy, S., and Austen, K. F. The complement system in rheumatoid synovitis. I. An analysis of complement component activities in rheumatoid synovial fluids. *Arthritis Rheum* 1970, **13**: 713.

63. Ruddy, S., Fearon, D. T., and Austen, K. F. Depressed synovial fluid levels of properdin and properdin factor B in patients with rheumatoid arthritis. *Arthritis Rheum* 1975; **18**: 289.

64. Nydegger, U. E., Zubler, R. H., Gabay, R., Joliat, G., Karagevrekis, C. H., Lambert, P. H., and Miescher, P. A. Circulating complement breakdown products in patients with rheumatoid arthritis: correlation between plasma C3d, circulating immune complexes, and clinical activity. *J Clin Invest* 1977; **59**: 862.

65. Hedberg, H. Studies on synovial fluid in arthritis. I. The total complement activity. II. The occurrence of mononuclear cells with in vitro cytotoxic effect. *Acta Med Scand Suppl* 1967; **479**: 1.

66. Schur, P. H., Britton, M. C., Franco, A. E., Corson, J. M., Sosman, J. L., and Ruddy, S. Rheumatoid synovitis: complement and immune complexes. *Rheumatology* 1975; **6**: 34.

67. Fostiropoulos, G., Austen, K. F., and Bloch, K. J. Total hemolytic complement and second component of complement activity in serum and synovial fluid of patients with rheumatic diseases. *Arthritis Rheum* 1964; **7**: 308.

68. Townes, A. S., and Sowa, J. M. Complement in synovial fluid. *Johns Hopkins Med J* 1970; **127**: 23.

69. El-Ghobarey, A., and Whaley, K. Alternative pathway complement activation in rheumatoid arthritis. *J Rheumatol* 1980; **7**: 453.

70. Brodeur, J. P., Ruddy, S., Schwartz, L. B., and Moxley, G. Synovial fluid levels of complement SC5b-9 and fragment Bb are elevated in patients with rheumatoid arthritis. *Arthritis Rheum* 1991; **34**: 1531.

71. Jose, P. J., Moss, I. K., Maini, R. N., and Williams, T. J. Measurement of the chemotactic complement fragment C5a in rheumatoid synovial fluids by radioimmunoassay: role of C5a in the acute inflammatory phase. *Ann Rheum Dis* 1990; **49**: 747.

72. Daniels, R. H., Houston, W. A., Petersen, M. M., Williams, J. D., Williams, B. D., and Morgan, B. P. Stimulation of human rheumatoid synovial cells by non-lethal complement membrane attack. *Immunology* 1990; **69**: 237.

73. Jahn, B., Von Kempis, J., Kramer, K. L., Filsinger, S., and Hansch, G. M. Interaction of the terminal complement components C5b-9 with synovial fibroblasts: binding to the membrane surface leads to increased levels in collagenase-specific mRNA. *Immunology* 1993; **78**: 329.

74. Britton, M. C., and Schur. P. H. The complement system in rheumatoid synovitis. II. Intracytoplasmic inclusions of immunoglobulins and complement. *Arthritis Rheum* 1971; **14**: 87.

75. Wang, Y., Rollins, S. A., Madri, J. A., and Matis, L. A. Anti-C5 monoclonal antibody therapy prevents collagen-induced arthritis and ameliorates established disease. *Proc Natl Acad Sci U S A* 1995; **92**: 8955.

76. Jain, R. I., Moreland, L. W., Caldwell, J. R., Rollins, S. A., and Mojcik, C. F. A single dose, placebo controlled, double blind, phase I study of the humanized anti-C5 antibody h5G1.1 in patients with rheumatoid arthritis. *Arthritis Rheum* 1999; **42**: S77.

77. Mongan, E. S., Cass, R. M., Jacox, R. F., and Vaughen, J. H. A study of the relation of seronegative and seropositive rheumatoid arthritis to each other and to necrotizing vasculitis. *Am J Med* 1969; **47**: 23.

78. Weinstein, A., Peters, K., Brown, D., and Bluestone. R. Metabolism of the third component of complement (C3) in patients with rheumatoid arthritis. *Arthritis Rheum* 1972; **15**: 49.

79. Versey, J. M., Hobbs, J. R., and Holt, P. J. Complement metabolism in rheumatoid arthritis. I. Longitudinal studies. *Ann Rheum Dis* 1973; **32**: 557.

80. Mollnes, T. E., Lea, T., Mellbye, O. J., Pahle, J., Grand, O., and Harboe, M. Complement activation in rheumatoid arthritis evaluated by C3dg and the terminal complement complex. *Arthritis Rheum* 1986; **29**: 715.

81. Molenaar, E. T., Voskuyl, A. E., Familian, A., van Mierlo, G. J., Dijkmans, B. A., and Hack, B. A. Complement activation in patients

with rheumatoid arthritis mediated in part by C-reactive protein. *Arthritis Rheum* 2001; **44**: 997.

82. Mellbye, O. J., Forre, O., Mollnes, T. E., and Kvarnes, L. Immunopathology of subcutaneous rheumatoid nodules. *Ann Rheum Dis* 1991; **50**: 909.

83. Kato, H., Yamakawa, M., and Ogino, T. Complement mediated vascular endothelial injury in rheumatoid nodules: a histopathological and immunohistochemical study. *J Rheumatol* 2000; **27**: 1839.

84. Lawley, T. J., Bielory, L., Gascon, P., Yancey, K. B., Young, N. S., and Frank, M. M. A prospective clinical and immunologic analysis of patients with serum sickness. *N Engl J Med* 1984; **311**: 1407.

85. Miller, G. W., and Nussenzweig, V. A new complement function: solubilization of antigen-antibody aggregates. *Proc Natl Acad Sci U S A* 1975; **72**: 418.

86. Takahashi, M., Tack, B. F., and Nussenzweig, V. Requirements for the solubilization of immune aggregates by complement: assembly of a factor B-dependent C3-convertase on the immune complexes. *J Exp Med* 1977; **145**: 86.

87. Fernandez, N., Renedo, M., Alonso, S., and Crespo, S. Release of arachidonic acid by stimulation of opsonic receptors in human monocytes: the FcgammaR and the complement receptor 3 pathways. *J Biol Chem* 2003; **278**: 52179.

88. Cochrane, C. G., and Hawkins, D. Studies on circulating immune complexes. 3. Factors governing the ability of circulating complexes to localize in blood vessels. *J Exp Med* 1968; **127**: 137.

89. Cochrane, C. G., and Koffler, D. Immune complex disease in experimental animals and man. *Adv Immunol* 1973; **16**: 185.

90. van den Berg, W. B., and van de Putte, L. B. Electrical charge of the antigen determines its localization in the mouse knee joint: deep penetration of cationic BSA in hyaline articular cartilage. *Am J Pathol* 1985; **121**: 224.

91. van den Berg, W. B., van de Putte, L. B., Zwarts, W. A., and Joosten, L. A. Electrical charge of the antigen determines intraarticular antigen handling and chronicity of arthritis in mice. *J Clin Invest* 1984; **74**: 1850.

92. Schumacher, H. R., Jr. Ultrastructure of the synovial membrane. *Ann Clin Lab Sci* 1975; **5**: 489.

93. Kunkel, H. G., Muller-Eberhard, H. J., Fudenberg, H. H., and Tomasi, T. B. Gamma globulin complexes in rheumatoid arthritis and certain other conditions. *J Clin Invest* 1961; **40**: 117.

94. Halla, J. T., Volanakis, J. E., and Schrohenloher, R. E. Immune complexes in rheumatoid arthritis sera and synovial fluids: a comparison of three methods. *Arthritis Rheum* 1979; **22**: 440.

95. Reynolds, W. J., Yoon, S. J., Emin, M., Chapman, K. R., and Klein, M. H. Circulating immune complexes in rheumatoid arthritis: a prospective study using five immunoassays. *J Rheumatol* 1986; **13**: 700.

96. Mageed, R. A., Kirwan, J. R., Thompson, P. W., McCarthy, D. A., and Holborow, E. J. Characterisation of the size and composition of circulating immune complexes in patients with rheumatoid arthritis. *Ann Rheum Dis* 1991; **50**: 231.

97. Zubler, R. H., Nydegger, U., Perrin, L. H., Fehr, K., McCormick, J., Lambert, P. H., and Miescher, P. A. Circulating and intra-articular immune complexes in patients with rheumatoid arthritis: correlation of 125I-Clq binding activity with clinical and biological features of the disease. *J Clin Invest* 1976; **57**: 1308.

98. Andreis, M., Hurd, E. R., Lospalluto, J., and Ziff, M. Comparison of the presence of immune complexes in Felty's syndrome and rheumatoid arthritis. *Arthritis Rheum* 1978; **21**: 310.

99. Halla, J. T., Schrohenloher, R. E., and Volanakis, J. E. Immune complexes and other laboratory features of pleural effusions: a comparison of rheumatoid arthritis, systemic lupus erythematosus, and other diseases. *Ann Intern Med* 1980; **92**: 748.

100. Ball, G. V., Schrohenloher, R., and Hester, R. Gamma globulin complexes in rheumatoid pericardial fluid. *Am J Med* 1975; **58**: 123.

101. Williams, B. D., Pussell, B. A., Lockwood, C. M., and Cotton, C. Defective reticuloendothelial system function in rheumatoid arthritis. *Lancet* 1979; **1**: 1311.

102. Fields, T. R., Gerardi, E. N., Ghebrehiwet, B., Bennett, R. S., Lawley, T. J., Hall R. P. *et al.* Reticuloendothelial system fc receptor function in rheumatoid arthritis. *J Rheumatol* 1983; **10**: 550.

103. Lobatto, S., Daha, M. R., Westedt, M. L., Pauwels, M. L., Evers-Schouten, J. H., Voetman A. A. *et al.* Diminished clearance of soluble aggregates of human immunoglobulin G in patients with rheumatoid arthritis. *Scand J Rheumatol* 1989; **18**: 89.

104. Rudd, P. M., Elliott, T., Cresswell, P., Wilson, I. A., and Dwek, R. A. Glycosylation and the immune system. *Science* 2001; **291**: 2370.

105. Parekh, R. B., Dwek, R. A., Sutton, B. J., Fernandes, D. L., Leung, A., Stanworth D. *et al.* Association of rheumatoid arthritis and primary osteoarthritis with changes in the glycosylation pattern of total serum IgG. *Nature* 1985; **316**: 452.

106. Sumar, N., Isenberg, D. A., Bodman, K. B., Soltys, A., Young, A., Leak A. M. *et al.* Reduction in IgG galactose in juvenile and adult onset rheumatoid arthritis measured by a lectin binding method and its relation to rheumatoid factor. *Ann Rheum Dis* 1991; **50**: 607.

107. Malhotra, R., Wormald, M. R., Rudd, P. M., Fischer, P. B., Dwek, R. A., and Sim, R. B. Glycosylation changes of IgG associated with rheumatoid arthritis can activate complement via the mannose-binding protein. *Nat Med* 1995; **1**: 237.

108. Kinsella, T. D., Baum, J., and Ziff, M. Immunofluorescent demonstration of an IgG-B1C complex in synovial lining cells of rheumatoid synovial membrane. *Clin Exp Immunol* 1969; **4**: 265.

109. Luthra, H. S., McDuffie, F. C., Hunder, G. G., and Samayoa, E. A. Immune complexes in sera and synovial fluids of patients with rheumatoid arthritis: radioimmunoassay with monocylonal rheumatoid factor. *J Clin Invest* 1975; **56**: 458.

110. Hannestad, K. Presence of aggregated gamma-G-globulin in certain rheumatoid synovial effusions. *Clin Exp Immunol* 1967; **2**: 511.

111. Winchester, R. J., Agnello, V., and Kunkel, H. G. The joint-fluid gammaG-globulin complexes and their relationship to intraarticular complement diminution. *Ann N Y Acad Sci* 1969; **168**: 195.

112. Hay, F. C., Nineham, L. J., Perumal, R., and Roitt, I. M. Intra-articular and circulating immune complexes and antiglobulins (IgG and IgM) in rheumatoid arthritis: correlation with clinical features. *Ann Rheum Dis* 1979; **38**: 1.

113. Faaber, P., van den Bersselaar, L. A., van de Putte, L. B., and van den Berg, W. B. Immune complex formation between IgM rheumatoid factor and IgG generated by hyaluronic acid. *Arthritis Rheum* 1989; **32**: 1521.

114. Cooke, T. D., and Jasin, H. E. The pathogenesis of chronic inflammation in experimental antigen-induced arthritis. I. The role of antigen on the local immune response. *Arthritis Rheum* 1972; **15**: 327.

115. Cooke, T. D., Hurd, E. R., Ziff, M., and Jasin, H. E. The pathogenesis of chronic inflammation in experimental antigen-induced arthritis. II. Preferential localization of antigen-antibody complexes to collagenous tissues. *J Exp Med* 1972; **135**: 323.

116. Matsumoto, I., Maccioni, M., Lee, D. M., Maurice, M. Simmons, B., Brenner M. *et al.* How antibodies to a ubiquitous cytoplasmic enzyme may provoke joint-specific autoimmune disease. *Nat Immunol* 2002; **3**: 360.

117. Cooke, T. D., Hurd, E. R., Jasin, H. E., Bienenstock, J., and Ziff, M. Identification of immunoglobulins and complement in rheumatoid articular collagenous tissues. *Arthritis Rheum* 1975; **18**: 541.

118. Cooke, T. D., Bennett, E. L., and Ohno, O. The deposition of immunoglobulins and complement in osteoarthritic cartilage. *Int Orthop* 1980; **4**: 211.

119. Jasin, H. E. Autoantibody specificities of immune complexes sequestered in articular cartilage of patients with rheumatoid arthritis and osteoarthritis. *Arthritis Rheum* 1985; **28**: 241.

120. Ishikawa, H., Smiley, J. D., and Ziff, M. Electron microscopic demonstration of immunoglobulin deposition in rheumatoid cartilage. *Arthritis Rheum* 1975; **18**: 563.

121. Jasin, H. E., and Cooke, T. D. The inflammatory role of immune complexes trapped in joint collagenous tissues. *Clin Exp Immunol* 1978; **33**: 416.

122. Ugai, K., Ishikawa, H., Hirohata, K., and Shirane, H. Interaction of polymorphonuclear leukocytes with immune complexes trapped in rheumatoid articular cartilage. *Arthritis Rheum* 1983; **26**: 1434.

123. Ellison, M. R., Kelly, K. J., and Flatt, A. E. The results of surgical synovectomy of the digital joints in rheumatoid disease. *J Bone Joint Surg Am* 1971; **53**: 1041.

124. Patzakis, M. J., Mills, D. M., Bartholomew, B. A., Clayton, M. L., and Smyth, C. J. A visual, histological, and enzymatic study of regenerating rheumatoid synovium in the synovectomized knee. *J Bone Joint Surg Am* 1973; 55: 287.

125. Bryan, R. S., Peterson, L. F., and Combs, Jr. J. J. Polycentric knee arthroplasty: a review of 84 patients with more than one year follow-up. *Clin Orthop* 1973; 94: 136.

126. Janeway, C. A., Gitlin, D., Craig, J. M., and Grice, D. S. Collagen disease in patients with congenital agammaglobulinemia. *Trans Assoc Am Physicians* 1956; 69: 93.

127. Good, R. A., Rotstein, J., and Mazzitello, W. F. The simultaneous occurrence of rheumatoid arthritis and agammaglobulinemia. *J Lab Clin Med* 1957; 49: 343.

128. Munthe, E., Hoyeraal, H. M., Froland, S. S., Mellbye, O. J., Kass, E., and Natvig, J. B. Evidence for complement activation by the alternate pathway in the arthritis of hypogammaglobulinemic patients. *Rheumatology* 1975; 6: 43.

129. Marcus, R. L., and Townes, A. S. The occurrence of cryoproteins in synovial fluid: the association of a complement-fixing activity in rheumatoid synovial fluid with cold-precipitable protein. *J Clin Invest* 1971; 50: 282.

130. Clague, R. B., and Moore, L. J. IgG and IgM antibody to native type II collagen in rheumatoid arthritis serum and synovial fluid: evidence for the presence of collagen-anticollagen immune complexes in synovial fluid. *Arthritis Rheum* 1984; 27: 1370.

131. Male, D., Roitt, I. M., and Hay, F. C. Analysis of immune complexes in synovial effusions of patients with rheumatoid arthritis. *Clin Exp Immunol* 1980; 39: 297.

132. Winchester, R. J., Agnello, V., and Kunkel, H. G. Gamma globulin complexes in synovial fluids of patients with rheumatoid arthritis: partial characterization and relationship to lowered complement levels. *Clin Exp Immunol* 1970; 6: 689.

133. Munthe, E., and Natvig, J. B. Characterization of IgG complexes in eluates from rheumatoid tissue. *Clin Exp Immunol* 1971; 8: 249.

134. Winchester, R. J. Characterization of IgG complexes in patients with rheumatoid arthritis. *Ann N Y Acad Sci* 256: 73.

135. Male, D. K., and Roitt, I. M. Molecular analysis of complement-fixing rheumatoid synovial fluid immune complexes. *Clin Exp Immunol* 1981; 46: 521.

136. Mannik, M., and Nardella, F. A. IgG rheumatoid factors and self-association of these antibodies. *Clin Rheum Dis* 1985; 11: 551.

137. Sylvestre, D., Clynes, R., Ma, M., Warren, H., Carroll, M. C., and Ravetch, J. V. Immunoglobulin G-mediated inflammatory responses develop normally in complement-deficient mice. *J Exp Med* 1996; 184: 2385.

138. Nieto, A., Caliz, R., Pascual, M., Mataran, L., Garcia, S., and Martin, J. Involvement of Fcgamma receptor IIIA genotypes in susceptibility to rheumatoid arthritis. *Arthritis Rheum* 2000; 43: 735.

139. Morgan, A. W., Griffiths, B., Ponchel, F., Montague, B. M., Ali, M., Gardner P. P. *et al.* Fcgamma receptor type IIIA is associated with rheumatoid arthritis in two distinct ethnic groups. *Arthritis Rheum* 2000; 43: 2328.

140. Brun, J. G., Madland, T. M., and Vedeler, C. A. Immunoglobulin G fc-receptor (FcgammaR) IIA, IIIA, and IIIB polymorphisms related to disease severity in rheumatoid arthritis. *J Rheumatol* 2002; 29: 1135.

141. Radstake, T. R., Petit, E., Pierlot, C., van de Putte, L. B., Cornelis, F., and Barrera, P. Role of Fcgamma receptors IIA, IIIA, and IIIB in susceptibility to rheumatoid arthritis. *J Rheumatol* 2003; 30: 926.

142. Morgan, A. W., Keyte, V. H., Babbage, S. J., Robinson, J. I., Ponchel, F., Barrett J. H. *et al.* FcgammaRIIIA-158V and rheumatoid arthritis: a confirmation study. *Rheumatology (Oxford)* 2003; 42: 528.

143. Koene, H. R., Kleijer, M., Swaak, A. J., Sullivan, K. E., Bijl, M., Petri M. A. *et al.* The Fc gammaRIIIA-158F allele is a risk factor for systemic lupus erythematosus. *Arthritis Rheum* 1998; 41: 1813.

144. Abrahams, V. M., Cambridge, G., Lydyard, P. M., and Edwards. J. C. Induction of tumor necrosis factor alpha production by adhered human monocytes: a key role for Fcgamma receptor type IIIa in rheumatoid arthritis. *Arthritis Rheum* 2000; 43: 608.

145. Burastero, S. E., Casali, P., Wilder, R. L., and Notkins, A. L. Monoreactive high affinity and polyreactive low affinity rheumatoid factors are produced by CD5+ B cells from patients with rheumatoid arthritis. *J Exp Med* 1988; 168: 1979.

146. Sabharwal, U. K., Vaughan, J. H., Fong, S., Bennett, P. H., Carson, D. A., and Curd, J. G. Activation of the classical pathway of complement by rheumatoid factors: assessment by radioimmunoassay for C4. *Arthritis Rheum* 1982; 25: 161.

147. Gale, R. J., Nikoloutsopoulos, A., Bradley, J., and Roberts-Thomson. P. J. Immune complex activation of neutrophils and enhancement of the activation by rheumatoid factor and complement. *J Rheumatol* 1985; 12: 21.

148. Mitchell, W. S., Naama, J. K., Veitch, J., and Whaley, K. IgM-RF prevents complement-mediated inhibition of immune precipitation. *Immunology* 1984; 52: 445.

149. Balestrieri, G., Tincani, A., Migliorini, P., Ferri, C., Cattaneo, R., and Bombardieri, S. Inhibitory effect of IgM rheumatoid factor on immune complex solubilization capacity and inhibition of immune precipitation. *Arthritis Rheum* 1984; 27: 1130.

150. Natvig, J. B., and Munthe, E. Self-associating IgG rheumatoid factor represents a major response of plasma cells in rheumatoid inflammatory tissue. *Ann N Y Acad Sci* 1975; 256: 88.

151. Monach, P. A., Benoist, C., and Mathis, D. The role of antibodies in mouse models of rheumatoid arthritis, and relevance to human disease. *Adv Immunol* 2004; 82: 217.

152. Heimer, R., Levin, F. M., and Kahn. M. F. Inhibition of complement fixation by human serum: the activity of a gamma-1M globulin and rheumatoid factor in complement fixation reactions. *J Immunol* 1963; 91: 866.

153. Schmid, F. R., Roitt, I. M., and Rocha, M. J. Complement fixation by a two-component antibody system: immunoglobulin G and immunoglobulin M anti-globulin (rheumatoid factor). Parodoxical effect related to immunoglobulin G concentration. *J Exp Med* 1970; 132: 673.

154. Messner, R. P., Laxidal, T., Quie, P. G., and Williams, Jr. R. C. Serum opsonin, bacteria, and polymorphonuclear leukocyte interactions in subacute bacterial endocarditis: anti-gamma-globulin factors and their interaction with specific opsonins. *J Clin Invest* 1968; 47: 1109.

155. Panoskaltsis, A., and Sinclair, N. R. Rheumatoid factor blocks regulatory Fc signals. *Cell Immunol* 1989; 123: 177.

156. Kouskoff, V., Korganow, A. S., Duchatelle, V., Degott, C., Benoist, C., and Mathis, D. Organ-specific disease provoked by systemic autoimmunity. *Cell* 1996; 87: 811.

157. Korganow, A. S., Ji, H., Mangialaio, S., Duchatelle, V., Pelanda, R., Martin T. *et al.* From systemic T cell self-reactivity to organ-specific autoimmune disease via immunoglobulins. *Immunity* 1999; 10: 451.

158. Matsumoto, I., Staub, A., Benoist, C., and Mathis. D. Arthritis provoked by linked T and B cell recognition of a glycolytic enzyme. *Science* 1999; 286: 1732.

159. Maccioni, M., Zeder-Lutz, G., Huang, H., Ebel, C., Gerber, P., Hergueux J. *et al.* Arthritogenic monoclonal antibodies from K/BxN mice. *J Exp Med* 2002; 195: 1071.

160. Ji, H., Ohmura, K., Mahmood, U., Lee, D. M., Hofhuis, F. M., Boackle S. A. *et al.* Arthritis critically dependent on innate immune system players. *Immunity* 2002; 16: 157.

161. Jonsson, R., Karlsson, A. L., and Holmdahl, R. Demonstration of immunoreactive sites on cartilage after in vivo administration of biotinylated anti-type II collagen antibodies. *J Histochem Cytochem* 1989; 37: 265.

162. Ropes, M. W., and Bauer, W. 1953. *Synovial fluid changes in joint disease*. Harvard University Press, Cambridge, MA.

163. Wipke, B. T., Wang, Z., Nagengast, W., Reichert, D. E., and Allen, P. M. Staging the initiation of autoantibody-induced arthritis: a critical role for immune complexes. *J Immunol* 2004; 172: 7694.

163a. Binstadt, B. A., Patel, P. R., Alencar, H., Nigrovic, P. A., Lee, D. M., Mahmood, U., Weissleder, R., Mathis, D., and Benoist, C. Particularities of the vasculature can promote the organ specificity of autoimmune attack. *Nat Immunol* 2006; 29 [Epub ahead of print].

164. Trentham, D. E., Townes, A. S., and Kang, A. H. Autoimmunity to type II collagen: an experimental model of arthritis. *J Exp Med* 1977; 146: 857.

165. Nandakumar, K. S., Svensson, L., and Holmdahl. R. Collagen type II-specific monoclonal antibody-induced arthritis in mice: description of the disease and the influence of age, sex, and genes. *Am J Pathol* 2003; **163**:1827.

166. Jasin, H. E. The mechanism of trapping of immune complexes in experimental antigen-induced arthritis. *Rheumatology* 1975; **6**:288.

167. Sakaguchi, N., Takahashi, T., Hata, H., Nomura, T., Tagami, T., Yamazaki S. *et al.* Altered thymic T-cell selection due to a mutation of the ZAP-70 gene causes autoimmune arthritis in mice. *Nature* 2003; **426**:454.

168. Poulter, L. W., Duke, O., Hobbs, S., Janossy, G., and Panayi, G. Histochemical discrimination of HLA-DR positive cell populations in the normal and arthritic synovial lining. *Clin Exp Immunol* 1982; **48**: 381.

169. Hogg, N., Palmer, D. G., and Revell, P. A. Mononuclear phagocytes of normal and rheumatoid synovial membrane identified by monoclonal antibodies. *Immunology* 1985; **56**:673.

170. Yanni, G., Whelan, A., Feighery, C., and Bresnihan, B. Synovial tissue macrophages and joint erosion in rheumatoid arthritis. *Ann Rheum Dis* 1994; **53**:39.

171. Mulherin, D., Fitzgerald, O., and Bresnihan, B. Synovial tissue macrophage populations and articular damage in rheumatoid arthritis. *Arthritis Rheum* 1996; **39**:115.

172. Tak, P. P., Smeets, T. J., Daha, M. R., Kluin, P. M., Meijers, K. A., Brand, R. *et al.* Analysis of the synovial cell infiltrate in early rheumatoid synovial tissue in relation to local disease activity. *Arthritis Rheum* 1997; **40**:217.

173. Dreher, R. Origin of synovial type A cells during inflammation: an experimental approach. *Immunobiology* 1982; **161**:232.

174. Firestein, G. S., Alvaro-Gracia, J. M., and Maki, R. Quantitative analysis of cytokine gene expression in rheumatoid arthritis. *J Immunol* 1990; **144**:3347.

175. Wood, N. C., Dickens, E., Symons, J. A., and Duff, G. W. In situ hybridization of interleukin-1 in CD14-positive cells in rheumatoid arthritis. *Clin Immunol Immunopathol* 1992; **62**:295.

176. Chu, C. Q., Field, M., Allard, S., Abney, E., Feldmann, M., and Maini, R. N. Detection of cytokines at the cartilage/pannus junction in patients with rheumatoid arthritis: implications for the role of cytokines in cartilage destruction and repair. *Br J Rheumatol* 1992; **31**:653.

177. Pettit, A. R., Ji, H., von Stechow, D., Muller, R., Goldring, Choi Y. *et al.* TRANCE/RANKL knockout mice are protected from bone erosion in a serum transfer model of arthritis. *Am J Pathol* 2001; **159**:1689.

178. Broker, B. M., Edwards, J. C., Fanger, M. W., and Lydyard. P. M., The prevalence and distribution of macrophages bearing Fc gamma R I, Fc gamma R II, and Fc gamma R III in synovium. *Scand J Rheumatol* 1990; **19**:123.

179. Deng, G. M., Verdrengh, M., Liu, Z. Q., and Tarkowski, A. The major role of macrophages and their product tumor necrosis factor alpha in the induction of arthritis triggered by bacterial DNA containing CpG motifs. *Arthritis Rheum* 2000; **43**:2283.

180. Verdrengh, M., and Tarkowski, A. Role of macrophages in Staphylococcus aureus-induced arthritis and sepsis. *Arthritis Rheum* 2000; **43**:2276.

181. Yoshida, H., Hayashi, S., Kunisada, T., Ogawa, M., Nishikawa, S., Okamura H. *et al.* The murine mutation osteopetrosis is in the coding region of the macrophage colony stimulating factor gene. *Nature* 1990; **345**:442.

182. Yang, Y. H., and Hamilton, J. A. Dependence of interleukin-1-induced arthritis on granulocyte-macrophage colony-stimulating factor. *Arthritis Rheum* 2001; **44**:111.

182a. Tak, P. P., Smeets, T. J., Daha, M. R., Kluin, P. M., Meijers, K. A., Brand, R., Meinders, A. E., and Breedveld, F. C. Analysis of the synovial cell infiltrate in early rheumatoid synovial tissue in relation to local disease activity. *Arthritis Rheum* 1997; **40**: 217–25.

183. Kulka, J. P., Bocking, D., Ropes, M. W., and Bauer, W. Early joint lesions of rheumatoid arthritis. *AMA Arch Pathol* 1955; **59**:129.

184. Schumacher, H. R., and Kitridou, R. C. Synovitis of recent onset: a clinicopathologic study during the first month of disease. *Arthritis Rheum* 1972; **15**:465.

185. Yamamoto, T., Nishiura, H., and Nishida, H. Molecular mechanisms to form leukocyte infiltration patterns distinct between synovial tissue and fluid of rheumatoid arthritis. *Semin Thromb Hemost* 1996; **22**:507.

186. Edwards, S. W., and Hallett, M. B. Seeing the wood for the trees: the forgotten role of neutrophils in rheumatoid arthritis. *Immunol Today* 1997; **18**:320.

187. Lee, A., Whyte, M. K., and Haslett, C. Inhibition of apoptosis and prolongation of neutrophil functional longevity by inflammatory mediators. *J Leukoc Biol* 1993; **54**:283.

188. Hollingsworth, J. W., Siegel, E. R., and Creasey. W. A. Granulocyte survival in synovial exudate of patients with rheumatoid arthritis and other inflammatory joint diseases. *Yale J Biol Med* 1967; **39**: 289.

189. Robinson, J. J., Watson, F., Bucknall R. C., and Edwards, S. W. Stimulation of neutrophils by insoluble immunoglobulin aggregates from synovial fluid of patients with rheumatoid arthritis. *Eur J Clin Invest* 1992; **22**:314.

190. Fossati, G., Bucknall, R. C., and Edwards, S. W. Insoluble and soluble immune complexes activate neutrophils by distinct activation mechanisms: changes in functional responses induced by priming with cytokines. *Ann Rheum Dis* 2002; **61**:13.

191. Henson, P. M. The immunologic release of constituents from neutrophil leukocytes. II. Mechanisms of release during phagocytosis, and adherence to nonphagocytosable surfaces. *J Immunol* 1971; **107**:1547.

192. Schimmer, R. C., Schrier, D. J., Flory, C. M., Dykens, J., Tung, D. K., Jacobson P. B. *et al.* Streptococcal cell wall-induced arthritis: requirements for neutrophils, P-selectin, intercellular adhesion molecule-1, and macrophage-inflammatory protein-2. *J Immunol* 1997; **159**:4103.

193. Wipke, B. T., and Allen. P. M. Essential role of neutrophils in the initiation and progression of a murine model of rheumatoid arthritis. *J Immunol* 2001; **167**:1601.

194. Crisp, A. J., Chapman, C. M., Kirkham, S. E., Schiller, A. L., and Krane, S. M. Articular mastocytosis in rheumatoid arthritis. *Arthritis Rheum* 1984; **27**:845.

195. Godfrey, H. P., Ilardi, C., Engber, W., and Graziano, F. M. Quantitation of human synovial mast cells in rheumatoid arthritis and other rheumatic diseases. *Arthritis Rheum* 1984; **27**:852.

196. Malone, D. G., Wilder, R. L., Saavedra-Delgado, A. M., and Metcalfe, D. D. Mast cell numbers in rheumatoid synovial tissues: correlations with quantitative measures of lymphocytic infiltration and modulation by antiinflammatory therapy. *Arthritis Rheum* 1987; **30**:130.

197. Bromley, M., Fisher, W. D., and Woolley, W. D. Mast cells at sites of cartilage erosion in the rheumatoid joint. *Ann Rheum Dis* 1984; **43**:76.

198. Bromley, M., and Woolley, D. E. Histopathology of the rheumatoid lesion: identification of cell types at sites of cartilage erosion. *Arthritis Rheum* 1984; **27**:857.

199. Malone, D. G., Irani, A. M., Schwartz, L. B., Barrett, K. E., and Metcalfe, D. D. Mast cell numbers and histamine levels in synovial fluids from patients with diverse arthritides. *Arthritis Rheum* 1986; **29**:956.

200. Buckley, M. G., Walters, C., Wong, W. M., Cawley, M. I., Ren, S., Schwartz, L. B., and Walls, A. F. Mast cell activation in arthritis: detection of alpha- and beta-tryptase, histamine and eosinophil cationic protein in synovial fluid. *Clin Sci (Lond)* 1997; **93**:363.

201. McNeil, H. P., and Gotis-Graham, I. Human mast cell subsets: distinct functions in inflammation? *Inflamm Res* 2000; **49**:3.

202. Lee, D. M., Friend, D. S., Gurish, M. F., Benoist, C., Mathis, D., and Brenner, M. B. Mast cells: a cellular link between autoantibodies and inflammatory arthritis. *Science* 2002; **297**:1689.

203. Corr, M., and Crain, B. The role of FcgammaR signaling in the K/B x N serum transfer model of arthritis. *J Immunol* 2002; **169**:6604.

204. Thomas, R., Davis, L. S., and Lipsky, P. E. Rheumatoid synovium is enriched in mature antigen-presenting dendritic cells. *J Immunol* 1994; **152**:2613.

205. Pettit, A. R., Ahern, M. J., Zehntner, S., Smith, M. D., and Thomas. R. Comparison of differentiated dendritic cell infiltration of autoimmune and osteoarthritis synovial tissue. *Arthritis Rheum* 2001; **44**: 105.

206. Page, G., Lebecque, S., and Miossec, P. Anatomic localization of immature and mature dendritic cells in an ectopic lymphoid organ: correlation with selective chemokine expression in rheumatoid synovium. *J Immunol* 2002; **168**: 5333.

207. Cavanagh, L. L., Boyce, A., Smith, L., Padmanabha, J., Filgueira, L., Pietschmann, P., and Thomas, R. Rheumatoid arthritis synovium contains plasmacytoid dendritic cells. *Arthritis Res Ther* 2005; **7**: R230.

208. Zvaifler, N. J., Steinman, R. M., Kaplan, G., Lau, L. L., and Rivelis. M. Identification of immunostimulatory dendritic cells in the synovial effusions of patients with rheumatoid arthritis. *J Clin Invest* 1985; **76**: 789.

209. Lande, R., Giacomini, E., Serafini, B., Rosicarelli, B., Sebastiani, G. D., Minisola G. *et al.* Characterization and recruitment of plasmacy-toid dendritic cells in synovial fluid and tissue of patients with chronic inflammatory arthritis. *J Immunol* 2004; **173**: 2815.

210. Lindhout, E., van Eijk, M., van Pel, M., Lindeman, J., Dinant, H. J., and de Groot, C. Fibroblast-like synoviocytes from rheumatoid arthritis patients have intrinsic properties of follicular dendritic cells. *J Immunol* 1999; **162**: 5949.

211. Foti, M., Granucci, F., and Ricciardi-Castagnoli, P. A central role for tissue-resident dendritic cells in innate responses. *Trends Immunol* 2004; **25**: 650.

212. Tak, P. P., Kummer, J. A., Hack, C. E., Daha, M. R., Smeets, T. J., Erkelens G. W. *et al.* Granzyme-positive cytotoxic cells are specifically increased in early rheumatoid synovial tissue. *Arthritis Rheum* 1994; **37**: 1735.

213. Dalbeth, N., and Callan, M. F. A subset of natural killer cells is greatly expanded within inflamed joints. *Arthritis Rheum* 2002; **46**: 1763.

214. Pridgeon, C., Lennon, G. P., Pazmany, L., Thompson, R. N., Christmas, S. E., and Moots, R. J. Natural killer cells in the synovial fluid of rheumatoid arthritis patients exhibit a CD56bright, CD94bright, CD158negative phenotype. *Rheumatology (Oxford)* 2003; **42**: 870.

215. Dalbeth, N., Gundle, R., Davies, R. J., Lee, Y. C., McMichael, A. J., and Callan, M. F. CD56bright NK cells are enriched at inflamma-tory sites and can engage with monocytes in a reciprocal program of activation. *J Immunol* 2004; **173**: 6418.

216. Cooper, M. A., Fehniger, T. A., Fuchs, A., Colonna, M., and Caligiuri, M. A. NK cell and DC interactions. *Trends Immunol* 2004; **25**: 47.

217. Gerosa, F., Baldani-Guerra, B., Nisii, C., Marchesini, V., Carra, G., and Trinchieri, G. Reciprocal activating interaction between natural killer cells and dendritic cells. *J Exp Med* 2002; **195**: 327.

218. Kojo, S., Adachi, Y., Keino, H., Taniguchi, M., and Sumida, T. Dysfunction of T cell receptor AV24AJ18+, BV11+ double-negative regulatory natural killer T cells in autoimmune diseases. *Arthritis Rheum* 2001; **44**: 1127.

219. Chiba, A., Oki, S., Miyamoto, K., Hashimoto, H., Yamamura, T., and Miyake, S. Suppression of collagen-induced arthritis by natural killer T cell activation with OCH, a sphingosine-truncated analog of alpha-galactosylceramide. *Arthritis Rheum* 2004; **50**: 305.

220. Kim, H. Y., Kim, H. J., Min, H. S., Kim, S., Park, W. S., Park, S. H., and Chung, D. H. NKT cells promote antibody-induced joint inflammation by suppressing transforming growth factor beta1 production. *J Exp Med* 2005; **201**: 41.

221. Holoshitz, J., Koning, F., Coligan, J. E., De Bruyn, J., and Strober. S. Isolation of CD4- CD8- mycobacteria-reactive T lymphocyte clones from rheumatoid arthritis synovial fluid. *Nature* 1989; **339**: 226.

222. Soderstrom, K., Bucht, A., Halapi, E., Lundqvist, C. Gronberg, A., Nilsson E. *et al.* High expression of V gamma 8 is a shared feature of human gamma delta T cells in the epithelium of the gut and in the inflamed synovial tissue. *J Immunol* 1994; **152**: 6017.

223. Peterman, G. M., Spencer, C., Sperling, A. I., and Bluestone. J. A., Role of gamma delta T cells in murine collagen-induced arthritis. *J Immunol* 1993; **151**: 6546.

224. Radstake, T. R., Roelofs, M. F., Jenniskens, Y. M., Oppers-Walgreen, B., van Riel, P. L., Barrera P. *et al.* Expression of toll-like receptors 2 and 4 in rheumatoid synovial tissue and regulation by proinflammatory cytokines interleukin-12 and interleukin-18 via interferon-gamma. *Arthritis Rheum* 2004; **50**: 3856.

225. Pierer, M., Rethage, J., Seibl, R., Lauener, R., Brentano, F., Wagner U. *et al.* Chemokine secretion of rheumatoid arthritis synovial fibroblasts stimulated by Toll-like receptor 2 ligands. *J Immunol* 2004; **172**: 1256.

226. Cromartie, W. J., Craddock, J. G., Schwab, J. H., Anderle, S. K., and Yang, C. H. Arthritis in rats after systemic injection of streptococcal cells or cell walls. *J Exp Med* 1977; **146**: 1585.

227. Deng, G. M., Nilsson, I. M., Verdrengh, M., Collins, L. V., and Tarkowski, A. Intra-articularly localized bacterial DNA containing CpG motifs induces arthritis. *Nat Med* 1999; **5**: 702.

228. Liu, Z. Q., Deng, G. M., Foster, S., and Tarkowski, A. Staphylococcal peptidoglycans induce arthritis. *Arthritis Res* 2001; **3**: 375.

229. Joosten, L. A., Koenders, M. I., Smeets, R. L., Heuvelmans-Jacobs, M., Helsen, M. M., Takeda K. *et al.* Toll-like receptor 2 pathway drives streptococcal cell wall-induced joint inflammation: critical role of myeloid differentiation factor 88. *J Immunol* 2003; **171**: 6145.

230. Frasnelli, M. E., Tarussio, D., Chobaz-Peclat, V., Busso, N., and So. A. TLR2 modulates inflammation in zymosan-induced arthritis in mice. *Arthritis Res* 2005; 7.

231. van der Heijden, I. M., Wilbrink, B., Tchetverikov, I., Schrijver, I. A., Schouls, L. M., Hazenberg M. P. *et al.* Presence of bacterial DNA and bacterial peptidoglycans in joints of patients with rheumatoid arthritis and other arthritides. *Arthritis Rheum* 2000; **43**: 593.

232. Johnson, G. B., Brunn, G. J., and Platt, J. L. Activation of mammalian Toll-like receptors by endogenous agonists. *Crit Rev Immunol* 2003; **23**: 15.

233. Tsan, M. F., and Gao, B. Endogenous ligands of Toll-like receptors. *J Leukoc Biol* 2004; **76**: 514.

234. Choe, J. Y., Crain, B., Wu, S. R., and Corr, M. Interleukin 1 receptor dependence of serum transferred arthritis can be circumvented by toll-like receptor 4 signaling. *J Exp Med* 2003; **197**: 537.

235. Radstake, T. R., Franke, B., Hanssen, S., Netea, M. G., Welsing, P., Barrera P. *et al.* The Toll-like receptor 4 Asp299Gly functional variant is associated with decreased rheumatoid arthritis disease susceptibility but does not influence disease severity and/or outcome. *Arthritis Rheum* 2004; **50**: 999.

236. Kilding, R., Akil, M., Till, S., Amos, R., Winfield, J., Iles, M. M., and Wilson, A. G. A biologically important single nucleotide polymorphism within the toll-like receptor-4 gene is not associated with rheumatoid arthritis. *Clin Exp Rheumatol* 2003; **21**: 340.

237. Sanchez, E., Orozco, G., Lopez-Nevot, M. A., Jimenez-Alonso, J., and Martin, J. Polymorphisms of toll-like receptor 2 and 4 genes in rheumatoid arthritis and systemic lupus erythematosus. *Tissue Antigens* 2004; **63**: 54.

238. Netea, M. G., Radstake, T., Joosten, L. A., van der Meer, J. W., Barrera, P., and Kullberg. B. J. Salmonella septicemia in rheumatoid arthritis patients receiving anti-tumor necrosis factor therapy: association with decreased interferon-gamma production and Toll-like receptor 4 expression. *Arthritis Rheum* 2003; **48**: 1853.

239. Pasare, C., and Medzhitov, R. Toll pathway-dependent blockade of CD4+CD25+ T cell-mediated suppression by dendritic cells. *Science* 2003; **299**: 1033.

240. Sobek, V., Birkner, N., Falk, I., Wurch, A., Kirschning, C. J., Wagner H. *et al.* Direct Toll-like receptor 2 mediated co-stimulation of T cells in the mouse system as a basis for chronic inflammatory joint disease. *Arthritis Res Ther* 2004; **6**: R433.

241. Leadbetter, E. A., Rifkin, I. R., Hohlbaum, A. M., Beaudette, B. C., Shlomchik, M. J., and Marshak-Rothstein, A. Chromatin-IgG complexes activate B cells by dual engagement of IgM and Toll-like receptors. *Nature* 2002; **416**: 603.

242. Krieg, A. M. A role for Toll in autoimmunity. *Nat Immunol* 2002; **3**: 423.

243. Firestein, G. S. Evolving concepts of rheumatoid arthritis. *Nature* 2003; **423**: 356.

244. Firestein, G. S., and Zvaifler, N. J. How important are T cells in chronic rheumatoid synovitis? *Arthritis Rheum* 1990; **33**: 768.

245. Firestein, G. S., and Zvaifler, N. J. How important are T cells in chronic rheumatoid synovitis? II. T cell-independent mechanisms from beginning to end. *Arthritis Rheum* 2002; **46**: 298.

246. Nandakumar, K. S., Backlund, J., Vestberg, M., and Holmdahl. R., Collagen type II (CII)-specific antibodies induce arthritis in the absence of T or B cells but the arthritis progression is enhanced by CII-reactive T cells. *Arthritis Res Ther* 2004; **6**: R544.

247. Roosnek, E., and Lanzavecchia, A. Efficient and selective presentation of antigen-antibody complexes by rheumatoid factor B cells. *J Exp Med* 1991; **173**: 487.

248. Keffer, J., Probert, L., Cazlaris, H., Georgopoulos, S., Kaslaris, E., Kioussis, D., and Kollias, G. Transgenic mice expressing human tumour necrosis factor: a predictive genetic model of arthritis. *Embo J* 1991; **10**: 4025.

249. Phillips, K., Kedersha, N., Shen, N., Blackshear, P. J., and Anderson, P. Arthritis suppressor genes TIA-1 and TTP dampen the expression of tumor necrosis factor alpha, cyclooxygenase 2, and inflammatory arthritis. *Proc Natl Acad Sci U S A* 2004; **101**: 2011.

250. Horai, R., Saijo, S., Tanioka, H., Nakae, S., Sudo, K., Okahara A. *et al*. Development of chronic inflammatory arthropathy resembling rheumatoid arthritis in interleukin 1 receptor antagonist-deficient mice. *J Exp Med* 2000; **191**: 313.

251. Xanthoulea, S., Pasparakis, M., Kousteni, S., Brakebusch, C., Wallach, D., Bauer J. *et al*. Tumor necrosis factor (TNF) receptor shedding controls thresholds of innate immune activation that balance opposing TNF functions in infectious and inflammatory diseases. *J Exp Med* 2004; **200**: 367.

252. Geiler, T., Kriegsmann, J., Keyszer, J., Gay, R. E., and Gay, S. A new model for rheumatoid arthritis generated by engraftment of rheumatoid synovial tissue and normal human cartilage into SCID mice. *Arthritis Rheum* 1994; **37**: 1664.

253. Takeda, K., Kaisho, T., and Akira. S., Toll-like receptors. *Annu Rev Immunol* 2003; **21**: 335.

254. Ghose, T., Woodbury, J. F., Ahmad, S., and Stevenson, B. Immunopathological changes in rheumatoid arthritis and other joint diseases. *J Clin Pathol* 1975; **28**: 109.

255. Vetto, A. A., Mannik, M., Zatarain-Rios, E., and Wener, M. H. Immune deposits in articular cartilage of patients with rheumatoid arthritis have a granular pattern not seen in osteoarthritis. *Rheumatol Int* 1990; **10**: 13.

11 | Angiogenesis and cell trafficking

Christopher D. Buckley, Andrew Filer, and
Costantino Pitzalis

Introduction

Histologically, the rheumatoid synovium is characterized by a number of defining factors. Critical amongst these are lining layer hyperplasia, accompanied by significant new capillary growth from existing blood vessels (angiogenesis), and infiltration of the hypertrophied synovium by specific, well-defined populations of mononuclear leukocytes. Angiogenic vessel formation occurs in the rheumatoid arthritis (RA) synovium, and is considered to be pivotal to the early development and persistence of disease, maintaining supplies of nutrients and cytokines to the expanded lining layer and pannus tissue[1]. Furthermore, the expanded endothelial cell population generated during angiogenesis performs a number of important pathological roles, including cytokine production, coagulation, antigen presentation, and leukocyte recruitment[2]. Angiogenesis is normally tightly controlled in order to supply the metabolic demands of tissues by a number of pro- and anti-angiogenic factors, the balance of which becomes abnormal in a number of pathological states, including diabetes mellitus and tumor growth. In this chapter we discuss the mechanisms controlling angiogenesis, along with the evidence implicating specific angiogenic pathways in RA.

Synovial mononuclear infiltrates have a characteristic composition and distribution, consisting mainly of T lymphocytes, macrophages, and antigen-presenting dendritic cells (DCs), with fewer B lymphocytes, plasma cells, and natural killer (NK) cells[3,4]. T lymphocyte-rich areas surrounding blood vessels comprise mainly CD4+ cells and have a high CD4+/CD8+ ratio, with transitional areas consisting mainly of CD8+ cells. Antigen-presenting cells cluster with T lymphocytes in perivascular sites and within characteristic lymphoid structures[5,6], which may vary from loosely defined lymphoid infiltrates to germinal center-like structures[7]. The latter feature, termed lymphoid neogenesis, is shared with a select group of organ-specific pathologies, including autoimmune thyroid disease, Sjögren's syndrome, and inflammatory bowel disease, and has been shown to be linked to the aberrant production of the constitutively expressed lymphoid chemokines[8]. The characteristic inflammatory infiltrate seen in RA is generated by changes in the homeostatic processes that regulate trafficking of leukocytes from the intravascular space into the tissues through an endothelial cell barrier, and their migration through, and subsequent retention within, the tissues. These processes are governed by interactions with other inflammatory and stromal cells, and extracellular matrix (ECM) components. These cell–cell or cell–matrix events are mediated by defined mechanisms, the most important of which are interactions between families of cell adhesion molecules (CAMs) and their ligands, and interactions between chemokines and their receptors. This chapter will not attempt an exhaustive description of adhesion, migration, and trafficking mechanisms, but will briefly review general mechanisms, then concentrate upon issues specific to the synovium and rheumatoid arthritis.

Angiogenesis

The process of angiogenesis is now seen as an important element in the development and persistence of rheumatoid disease. The finding by Taylor and colleagues that serum levels of vascular endothelial growth factor (VEGF), the prototypic endothelium-selective growth factor, correlated with radiological damage at one year in early arthritis patients makes a powerful argument for angiogenesis as crucial to RA disease[9]. Moreover, serum VEGF levels fall in parallel with clinical improvement following treatment with anti-TNF (tumor necrosis factor) therapy[10]. Quantitation of synovial vascularity by Doppler ultrasound techniques has linked increased intra-articular blood flow with inflammatory indices in RA and with bone erosion in early arthritis[11,12]. This evidence has been corroborated by positive findings using anti-angiogenic therapies in experimental RA systems and animal models of arthritis[9]. There have been a number of excellent reviews of the subject[2,13,14]; therefore this section will summarize basic principles in the regulation of angiogenesis, and review findings relevant to RA.

Regulation of angiogenesis

With crucial roles in growth, wound healing, and tissue repair, angiogenesis is necessarily under tight control, maintained by a strict balance between a number of pro- and anti-angiogenic factors (Table 11.1). During angiogenesis, coordinated migration and proliferation of endothelial cells occurs, with formation of capillary tubes, deposition of basement membrane, and subsequent migration and proliferation of accessory cells such as pericytes (stromal cells that line blood vessels abluminally) and smooth muscle cells. Remodeling then occurs, with regression of redundant vessels and apoptosis of superfluous endothelial cells[15]. It is important to recognize that the rheumatoid synovium is characterized not only by exuberant vessel growth, particularly within pannus tissues, but also by abnormal vascular structures which histologically resemble high endothelial venules (HEVs) and which normally act as portals of entry for lymphocytes into lymph nodes[2]. Interestingly, these vessels act as foci for aggregates of

Table 11.1 Examples of pro- and anti-angiogenic factors in RA

Pro-angiogenic	
Growth factors	Fibroblast growth factors, PDGF
Cytokines	VEGF, TGF-β, TNF-α, IL-1, IL-18, G-CSF, GM-CSF
Chemokines	ELR-containing, CXCL12 (SDF-1), CX3CL1 (fractalkine)
Soluble adhesion molecules	Soluble VCAM-1, soluble E-selectin
Non-endothelial growth factors	Angiopoietin-1
Anti-angiogenic	
Cytokines	IL-4, IL-10, IL-12, IL-1RA
Chemokines	Non-ELR containing
Peptide breakdown products	Angiostatin, endostatin
Iatrogenic	Minocycline, chloroquine, thalidomide, gold sulfasalazine, methotrexate, cyclosporin, penicillamine TNF-α inhibitors

G-CSF, granulocyte colony-stimulating factor; GM-CSF, granulocyte-macrophage colony-stimulating factor; IL, interleukin-1; IL-1RA, interleukin-1 receptor antagonist; PDGF, platelet-derived growth factor; TGF-β, transforming growth factor-β; TNF-α, tumour necrosis factor-α; VCAM, vascular cell adhesion molecule; VEGF, vascular endothelial growth factor.

lymphocytes[7]. A clear explanation for the presence of these vessels remains elusive, but it is evident that angiogenesis is not only increased, but possibly dysregulated in the RA synovium. Increased vascularity is not a universal finding throughout the RA synovium. Instead there is a heterogeneous distribution of areas of angiogenesis which may be associated with locally active inflammation. Current evidence suggests that increased vascularity only occurs within actively inflamed joints[16,17].

Factors regulating angiogenesis within the RA synovium

Vascular endothelial growth factor

VEGF is the most endothelial-specific factor so far characterized[18,19], existing in five isoforms determined by alternate gene splicing, which bind with varying affinities to a family of three receptors. Receptor binding results in angiogenesis, chemoattraction of endothelial cells, monocytes, and neutrophils, and increased vascular permeability[13]. As mentioned above, VEGF levels correlate with measures of disease activity in RA[9,20], suggesting an important role in the pathogenesis of the disease. Increased VEGF expression at the mRNA level clearly associates with increased synovial vascularity[21], and an increase in microvessels expressing VEGF receptors is seen in RA compared to osteoarthritis and normal controls[22]. At a cellular level, VEGF expression is increased in macrophages, endothelial cells, and synovial fibroblasts[23,24]. Furthermore, *in vitro* co-culture of synovial fluid monocytes and neutrophils with RA synovial fibroblasts synergistically increases expression of VEGF, a process for which integrins appear to be vital[25]. Studies using inhibition of VEGF are also compelling; a VEGF receptor-Fc construct suppressed synovial endothelial proliferation in RA synovial tissue explants[26]. In collagen-induced arthritis (CIA) models, anti-VEGF has been shown to reduce arthritis onset, severity, and joint angiogenesis, while blockade of the VEGF receptor Flt-1 (VEGF-R1) reduces synovial angiogenesis[27]. Similarly, using antibodies to VEGF-R1 and a VEGF-R1 tyrosine kinase inhibitor in the K/BxN murine arthritis model, amelioration of disease and decreased angiogenesis were observed[28].

Why is there such a close relationship between VEGF-related angiogenesis and disease activity in RA? Some of the increased VEGF expression seen in RA may relate to the decreased oxygen tension in the rheumatoid synovium[29]. The majority of gene regulation under conditions of hypoxia is now known to be under control of the HIF (hypoxia-inducible factor) and FIH (factor-inhibiting HIF) pathways. Under conditions of hypoxia HIFα subunits are stabilized[30] and FIH activity is inhibited[31,32], allowing the formation of a HIF complex which translocates to the nucleus and promotes transcription of hypoxia-responsive genes such as glycolytic enzymes and, crucially, VEGF[33]. A significant mechanism for the angiogenic effects of cytokines highly expressed in the synovium such as TGF (transforming growth factor)-β and IL-1 appears to lie in their induction of VEGF from fibroblasts and macrophages[34,35]. It has been shown that hypoxia augments VEGF production by some of these pathways[34]. In RA, the increased volume of expanded synovial tissue populated by large numbers of inflammatory leukocytes may worsen hypoxic stresses, in addition to exerting angiogenic effects more directly via cytokine and VEGF release. Lastly, inflammatory environments may induce angiogenesis by other less specific mechanisms, such as shear stress resulting from increased vascular flow, and resulting extravasation of angiogenic plasma proteins.

Chemokines and angiogenesis

The chemokine (CK) family (Table 11.2) consists of some fifty chemoattractant cytokines which bind to members of the classical G-protein-coupled receptor (GPCR) family[36]. Downstream signaling activates phospholipase C to mobilize intracellular calcium and utilizes the Rho GTPase and phosphatidylinositol-3-OH kinase (PI3K) pathways[37]. Such diverse signaling results in a variety of outcomes, including activation of leukocyte integrins and shape changes leading to chemotaxis[38,39]. CKs share a common three dimensional structure despite remarkably low sequence homology of less than 20%[36]. Structural similarity is maintained in part by the presence of a disulfide bond between two characteristic cysteine residues. Chemokines are classified according to the position of these cysteine residues, which may be adjacent, as in CCL2 (MCP-1, monocyte chemoattractant

Table 11.2 Chemokines and chemokine receptors

Inflammatory CK receptor	Inflammatory CK	Constitutive CK receptor	Constitutive CK
CCR1	CCL3 (MIP-1α), CCL5 (RANTES), CCL7 (MCP-3), CCL23 (MPIF-1)[a]	CCR4	CCL17 (TARC)[a], CCL22 (MDC)[a]
CCR2	CCL2 (MCP-1), CCL7 (MCP-3), CCL8 (MCP-2)	CCR7	CCL19 (ELC/MIP-3β), CCL21 (SLC/6ckine)
CCR3	CCL11 (eotaxin-1), CCL24 (eotaxin-2), CCL26 (eotaxin-3)	CCR9	CCL25 (TECK)
CCR5	CCL5 (RANTES), CCL3 (MIP-1α), CCL4 (MIP-1β), CCL8 (MCP-2)	CCR10	CCL27 (CTACK), CCL28 (MEC)[a]
CCR6	CCL20 (LARC/MIP-3α)	CXCR4	CXCL12 (SDF-1)[b]
CCR8	CCL1 (I-309), CCL4 (MIP-1β)	CXCR5	CXCL13 (BLC/BCA-1)
CXCR1	CXCL6 (GCP-2)[b], CXCL8 (IL-8)[b]		
CXCR2	CXCL1 (GRO-α)[b], CXCL2 (GRO-β)[b], CXCL5 (ENA78)[b], CXCL6 (GCP-2)[b], CXCL7 (NAP-2)[b], CXCL8 (IL-8)[b]		
CXCR3	CXCL9 (Mig), CXCL10 (IP10), CXCL11 (ITAC)		
CXCR6	CXCL16		
XCR1	XCL1 (lymphotactin)		
CX3CR1	CX3CL1 (fractalkine)[a,b]		

BCA-1, B cell-attracting chemokine 1; BLC, B lymphocyte chemoattractant; CTACK, cutaneous T cell-attracting chemokine; ELC, EBL-1-ligand chemokine; ENA, epithelial cell-derived neutrophil attractant; GRO, growth-related oncogene; IL, interleukin; IP10, IFN-inducible protein 10; ITAC, IFN-inducible T cell-α chemoattractant; LARC, liver- and activation-regulated chemokine; MCP, monocyte chemoattractant protein; MDC, macrophage-derived chemokine; MEC, mucosae-associated epithelial chemokine; Mig, monokine induced by IFN-γ; MIP, macrophage inflammatory protein; MPIF, myeloid progenitor inhibitory factor; NAP, neutrophil-activating peptide; SDF, stromal-derived factor; SLC, secondary lymphoid tissue chemokine; TARC, thymus- and activation-regulated chemokine; TECK, thymus-expressed chemokine.
[a] Angiogenic chemokines.
[b] Heterogeneous constitutive versus inflammatory status.
NB: some chemokines bind more than the receptors shown; not all chemokines are shown.

protein 1), or separated by a single amino acid, as in CXCL12 (stromal cell-derived factor (SDF)-1). One important structural exception to this rule is CX3CL1 (fractalkine), in which the first two cysteines are separated by three amino acids; this chemokine is unique in that it may be secreted or expressed bound to cells by a mucin-rich, transmembrane stalk[40,41]. It was Alisa Koch's group who initially discovered that IL-8, in addition to having chemoattractant effects, also demonstrated angiogenic properties[42]. Subsequently it became clear that among CKs of the CXC family, the presence of an ELR motif defined angiogenic properties. CK lacking the motif are largely angiostatic [36], a notable exception being CXCL12, which lacks an ELR motif but displays angiogenic properties[43]. Fractalkine has also been shown to be angiogenic both in membrane bound and free forms[44].

The RA synovium is characterized by the presence both of angiostatic CKs such as CXCL9 (Mig) and CXCL10 (I-TAC) and of angiogenic CKs such as CXCL5 (ENA-78), CXCL8 (IL-8), and CXCL12[45,46]. CXCL12 is of particular interest as a constitutive chemokine, as it is involved in the homeostatic trafficking of blood precursors. Pablos *et al.* reported that rheumatoid synovial fibroblasts were responsible for secreting CXCL12, demonstrating by immunohistochemistry that it colocalized on endothelial cells with the angiogenesis marker $\alpha_v\beta_3$ integrin, consistent with a role for CXCL12 in both cell recruitment and angiogenesis[47]. Synovial hypoxia may also play a role in determining chemokine expression, as both CXCL12 on synovial fibroblasts, and CXCR4 on monocytes have been shown to be up-regulated under hypoxic conditions[48,49]. Soluble fractalkine has also been shown by Alisa Koch's group to contribute to the angiogenic effects of RA synovial fluid, suggesting an important role in disease[50]. Given the degree of CK expression in the RA synovium, it appears

that CKs are important players in determining the balance between pro-angiogenic and anti-angiogenic factors in the RA synovium.

Other pro-angiogenic factors in RA

Both fibroblast growth factors (FGFs) and platelet-derived growth factor (PDGF) are produced by cells of the synovium, including fibroblasts, endothelial cells, and macrophages, and are pro-angiogenic in addition to having other growth stimulating effects[50]. No conclusive data are available from human studies of RA, but when FGF was administered by gene therapy in a rat adjuvant-induced arthritis (AIA) model, a worsening of disease and increased angiogenesis were observed, indicating a possible pathogenic role in synovial inflammation[51]. As mentioned above, a number of cytokines, including basic fibroblast growth factor (bFGF), TNF-α, IL-18, and VEGF, are able to stimulate angiogenesis, but do so by indirect means. One route is via stimulating VEGF production. Another shared mechanism occurs via integrins[50]. Integrins exist as αβ heterodimers which bind to a number of important ligands, amongst which are extracellular matrix proteins such as collagen and fibronectin (see below and Table 11.4). Integrins are vital in the regulation of infiltration, migration, and proliferation of leukocyte subpopulations, but also have wide ranging roles regulating the migration and proliferation of stromal cell types, including endothelial cells. The $\alpha_v\beta_3$ integrin heterodimer is involved in angiogenic signaling, and is significantly up-regulated in the RA synovial vasculature[52]. Use of an α_v subunit antagonist in a rabbit model of arthritis reduced both angiogenesis and joint inflammation[13]. The results of clinical

Table 11.3 Selectins and their receptor/ligand molecules

Endothelial distribution	Endothelial receptor/ligand	Leukocyte receptor/ligand	Leukocyte distribution
HEV, activated endothelium	PNAd/CD34 MAdCAM-1	L-selectin/CD62L	Lymphocyte subset, monocyte, neutrophil, eosinophil
Endothelial Weibel–Palade granules Platelet α granule	P-selectin/CD62P	PSGL-1 variants, sialyl Lewis$^{x/a}$	Lymphocyte subset, monocyte, neutrophil, NK
Activated endothelium	E-selectin/CD62E	PSGL-1 variants, sialyl Lewis$^{x/a}$	Lymphocyte subset, monocyte, neutrophil, eosinophil, basophil, NK

HEV, high endothelial venule; MAdCAM-1, mucosal addressin cell adhesion molecule-1; NK, natural killer cell; PNAd, peripheral node addressin; PSGL-1, P-selectin glycoprotein ligand-1.

Table 11.4 Integrins and their receptor/ligand molecules in leukocyte-endothelial interactions

Subunits	Alternative	Distribution	Ligand
β$_2$ integrins			
α$_L$ β$_2$	LFA-1, CD11a/CD18	B & T lymphocytes, monocytes, neutrophils	ICAM-1, ICAM-2, ICAM-3
α$_M$ β$_2$	Mac-1, CR3, CD11b/CD18	Monocytes, neutrophils, NK cells	ICAM-1, iC3b, fibrinogen, Factor X
α$_X$ β$_2$	P150, 95, CD11c/CD18	Monocytes, neutrophils, NK cells	iC3b, fibrinogen
α$_4$ integrins			
α$_4$ β$_1$	VLA-4, CD49d/CD29	B & T lymphocytes, monocytes, neural crest derived cells, fibroblasts	VCAM-1, fibronectin
α$_4$ β$_7$	CD49d	B & T lymphocyte sub-populations	MAdCAM-1, VCAM-1, fibronectin
α$_v$ integrins			
α$_v$ β$_3$	CD52/CD61, vitronectin receptor	Macrophages, osteoclasts, angiogenic endothelial cells	Vitronectin, fibronectin, osteopontin, thrombospondin-1, tenascin

ICAM, intercellular adhesion molecule; LFA, lymphocyte function-associated antigen; MAdCAM, mucosal addressin cell adhesion molecule; VCAM, vascular cell adhesion molecule; VLA, very late antigen.

trials using monoclonal antibodies to α$_v$β$_3$ are awaited[53]. A closely linked mechanism for the regulation of angiogenesis involves the shedding of soluble adhesion molecules by synovial constituents. Molecules such as E-selectin and vascular cell adhesion molecule (VCAM)-1 are shed by activated endothelial cells, and can bind in an autocrine fashion to their respective endothelial receptors (Tables 11.3 and 11.4)[50]. Interestingly, treatment with anti-TNF therapy has been shown to reduce endothelial activation and reduce levels of soluble E-selectin[54]. The angiopoietin system represents a different class of vascular growth factor compared to VEGF; angiopoietin-1 (Ang-1) does not induce proliferation or migration of endothelial cells, but instead appears to regulate downstream mechanisms, including assembly of accessory cells such as smooth muscle cells and pericytes, and formation of basement membrane[13]. Ang-1 is expressed by macrophages, endothelial cells, and synovial fibroblasts, and is expressed at high levels in RA compared to osteoarthritis synovia[55]. Furthermore, *in vitro* ang-1 expression in synovial fibroblasts is increased by TNF-α[56]. Tie-1 and Tie-2, receptors in the angiopoietin system, are similarly overexpressed in RA[50], suggesting a further, complementary mechanism underlying the pro-angiogenic balance in RA.

Anti-angiogenic factors in the RA synovium

The evidence for increased activity of pro-angiogenic factors in RA is persuasive. However, anti-angiogenic factors should also be considered, though information in this relatively novel area is scant. The presence of anti-angiogenic CK has already been mentioned. However, other cytokines such as IL-4 demonstrate anti-angiogenic properties, as shown in a rat AIA model[57]. This may account for a proportion of the anti-inflammatory effects produced by IL-4 in *ex vivo* synovial culture experiments and animal models[57,58]. Similarly, natural CK antagonists are able to inhibit angiogenesis. For instance, IL-1RA (IL-1 receptor antagonist) inhibits angiogenesis in rat AIA models[59]. An important group of angiostatic compounds comprises peptide breakdown products of larger proteins. Angiostatin is a peptide breakdown product of plasminogen which has been shown to induce endothelial apoptosis[60]. Such effects may prove useful therapeutically, as in murine CIA models angiostatin decreased both angiogenesis and arthritis severity[61]. Similarly, endostatin is a fragment of type XVIII collagen which exhibits anti-angiogenic properties, and has been shown to inhibit production of FGF and VEGF as well as ameliorate disease severity in the TNF-α transgenic murine model of arthritis[62]. Interestingly, levels of endostatin are not raised in RA compared to osteoarthritis[63], further supporting the hypothesis that the balance of pro- and anti-angiogenic factors in RA favors growth. Exogenous compounds have been developed with the aim of inhibiting angiogenesis. For instance TNP-470, a fungal derivative which suppresses angiogenesis, decreased synovial tissue volume in an *in vivo* severe combined immunodeficient (SCID) implantation model of RA[64]. It has also been shown to attenuate arthritis and reduce VEGF levels in murine models of arthritis[65]. Some of the success of existing disease-modifying treatments may also be due to the inhibition of angiogenesis. For example, drugs such as cyclosporine, gold, methotrexate, and glucocorticoids inhibit production of VEGF by synovial fibroblasts[50]. These and other drugs such as sulfasalazine and minocycline similarly have been identified as angiostatic agents[9,50]. Anti-TNF blockade reduces synovial angiogenesis, and is thought to reduce joint swelling via decreased VEGF production, leading to decreased vascular permeability[10].

In conclusion, it is clear that angiogenesis has an intimate relationship with disease activity and persistence in RA and that a strictly regulated balance is tipped in favor of angiogenesis in active disease. It remains unclear whether the degree of angiogenesis in RA is an appropriate, secondary response to the prevailing conditions in the synovium, or is pathologically up-regulated, representing a primary disease mechanism. Attenuating angiogenesis certainly restricts synovial inflammation in the models mentioned above, suggesting that further targeting of this process may offer improved outcomes via a relatively disease-specific route.

Cell trafficking

Ubiquitous mechanisms of leukocyte entry into tissues

Lymphocytes, monocytes, and neutrophils use a ubiquitous set of mechanisms to effect entry to tissues from the circulation. Extravasation is an active process, enabling cells to escape from rapid circulatory flow, read information displayed on endothelial cells and their associated proteoglycans molecules, adhere to the endothelium, and ultimately penetrate the vessel wall. Understanding of the critical steps in extravasation has grown progressively over the past 15 years as a result of both *in vitro* and *in vivo* studies of leukocyte adhesion to endothelia under flow conditions[66–68]. Such studies illustrate that leukocytes initially slow from rapid circulatory flow, and roll on endothelial monolayers, sampling the surface. A proportion of cells detach from rolling and resume physiological flow, but those which remain in contact become stationary, then undergo a shape change to a more flattened morphology. After a few minutes, leukocytes actively migrate through the endothelial monolayer (diapedesis), moving either between or directly through endothelial cells[67,69]. This process has historically been split into a four stage paradigm, making overlapping use of three families of molecules: capture receptors (selectins), activation molecules (chemokines), and adhesion molecules (integrins). Combinations of these molecules and their ligands are responsible for the four stages currently identified in the extravasation of leukocytes.

The first step, primary adhesion, involves capture of cells via selectin molecules which bind to specialized oligosaccharide ligands (Table 11.3) using multiple, transient, weak interactions. The structures of selectin ligands are still not fully understood, but all selectins bind to the tetrasaccharide sialyl Lewis^X, a characteristic which has been important in the development of selectin inhibitors. P-selectin glycoprotein ligand 1 (PSGL-1) is a major core molecule that presents selectin ligands, and is responsible for some capture of P- and L-selectins. Binding of selectins to their ligands allows cells to roll, sampling the activation status of the endothelium and presence of activating mediators[70]. Firm adhesion with arrest of rolling requires binding of leukocyte adhesion molecules of the integrin family to their complementary endothelial receptors (Table 11.4). However, in order to bind to their ligands, integrins must first be activated (triggered) from a quiescent state.

Step two, integrin activation, is therefore required in order to progress from rolling motion. This very rapid step (occurring in less than 0.2 s) is primarily mediated by chemokines[71,72]. Chemokine-receptor binding activates phospholipase C to mobilize intracellular calcium and activate protein kinase C, which in turn activates leukocyte integrins[38,39]. In order to exert chemotactic effects and achieve activation of leukocyte integrins at the endothelial surface, CKs must be immobilized on the surface of cells or within the extracellular matrix. This is achieved by binding of basic residues, shared by all CKs, to negatively charged glycosaminoglycan molecules (GAGs), allowing posting of secreted CKs on the surface of local endothelium where they can be sampled by rolling leukocytes. CKs may be expressed directly by endothelial cells, or transported across the endothelial layer from underlying tissues (a process termed transcytosis), providing an integrated readout of events within the local tissue microenvironment[72].

The third step, firm adhesion, is mediated by activated integrins binding their respective endothelial ligands of the immunoglobulin superfamily (Table 11.4). Integrins are expressed constitutively by leukocytes and many other cell types. They are expressed as heterodimers containing one α- and one β-subunit, of which at least 25 αβ combinations are known. Leukocyte-endothelium interactions principally involve binding of $\alpha_4\beta_1$ integrin to VCAM-1 or $\alpha_L\beta_2$ integrin (originally defined as lymphocyte function-associated antigen, LFA-1) and $\alpha_M\beta_2$ integrin (Mac-1) binding to intercellular adhesion molecule (ICAM)-1[73,74]. Endothelial integrin ligands are in turn characteristically up-regulated by local pro-inflammatory cytokines[73]. Firm adhesion due to activated integrin-ligand binding allows initiation of the fourth step, trans-endothelial migration (diapedesis). Cellular migration requires characteristic shape changes, creating a broad, veil-like lamellipodium at the leading edge and a rearward uropod which is retracted forwards, processes which depend upon rearrangement of the actin cytoskeleton[75]. In order to extravasate, leukocytes must migrate through or between endothelial cells, then across the basement membrane. Migration between endothelial cells requires the disruption of homophilic interactions between junctional molecules such as CD31 (PECAM-1), the junctional adhesion molecules (JAMs), and CD99[76]. Evidence suggests that integrins continue to play an active role during diapedesis via interactions with JAMs and other cell surface and matrix components, with integrin-mediated disruption of endothelial junctions and changes in cell shape and motility being signaled via Rho GTPases such as Rac[75,77]. Other factors play important roles in determining migration across the endothelium, the most significant being the movement of cells along gradients of immobilized chemokine, which may be fine-tuned by the oligomerization of chemokine molecules on extracellular matrix GAGs[72].

It is evident from the above that integrin-ligand interactions play an important role in more than one step of the extravasation process For instance, $\alpha_4\beta_1$ and $\alpha_4\beta_7$ integrins can mediate both rolling and firm adhesion on appropriate substrates *in vitro*[78,79]. This illustrates that, although fundamentally correct, the four step paradigm is somewhat simplistic as described. To summarize, extravasation is a ubiquitous but highly complex process mediated by multiple signaling and adhesion interactions, which allows multiple points of control for entry of leukocytes into tissues.

Mechanisms underlying selective accumulation of leukocytes in tissues

The mechanisms governing leukocyte trafficking need to accommodate a huge diversity of cell types, which undergo rapid cycles of activation and differentiation in response to varied inflammatory insults. A useful illustration of the mechanisms governing cell migration is provided by the prototypic pattern of T lymphocyte trafficking. Naïve T cells continuously cycle through secondary lymphoid tissues via the vascular and lymphatic circulations, gaining access to these tissues (peripheral lymph nodes, Peyer's patches, tonsils, and spleen) via specialized high endothelial venules[80]. On meeting their cognate antigen presented by professional antigen-presenting cells (APCs) in the lymph node, naïve cells differentiate into two broad classes of memory cells: central memory T cells which continue to recirculate through lymphoid tissues, and effector memory T cells which traffic through peripheral tissues[81]. Some memory T cells have been shown to recirculate to gut and skin tissues in which they were first activated[82], and there is also evidence to suggest that T cells may be directed by APCs to the site where antigen was first encountered[83]. Furthermore, CD4+ T cell responses can be seen to diverge, depending on the inflammatory stimulus, into more specialized groups, as defined by their cytokine and chemokine repertoires. In allergic reactions predominantly Th2 lymphocytes are seen along with eosinophils and basophils in the affected tissue, whereas in delayed-type hypersensitivity (DTH) reactions, Th1 T cells and macrophages predominate[84].

How is this elegant choreography of cellular movements and interactions regulated? A number of levels of regulation for

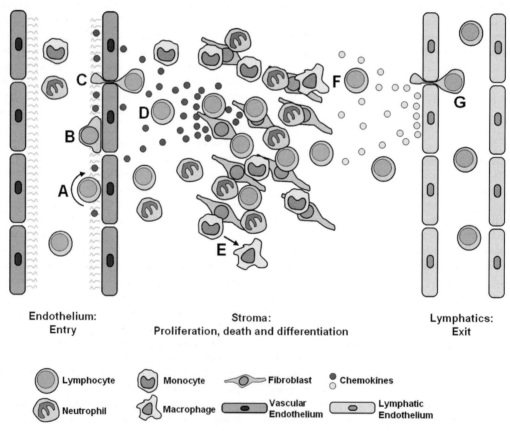

Endothelium: Stroma: Lymphatics:
Entry   Proliferation, death and differentiation   Exit

Lymphocyte   Monocyte   Fibroblast   Chemokines

Neutrophil   Macrophage   Vascular   Lymphatic
                                        Endothelium   Endothelium

Fig. 11.1 Leukocyte–stromal interactions regulate the extravasation and recirculation of leukocytes in distinct phases. The molecular basis by which leukocytes leave the circulation and migrate across endothelium has been well studied; stromal and lymphatic trafficking remain less well understood. (A) Leukocytes are captured by selectin-ligand interactions and roll, sampling the presence of chemokines and other activation markers on the endothelium and associated matrix proteins. (B) Chemokines trigger activation of integrins, enabling firm adhesion. (C) Diapedesis: leukocytes migrate through the endothelial layer. (D) Leukocytes follow chemokine gradients into the tissue stroma. Within the stroma, some cells are destined to die, such as neutrophils. (E) Others such as monocytes may differentiate into cells destined to die, such as macrophages; others may proliferate. (F) Those cells destined to recirculate must change their repertoire of chemokine receptors, following other chemokine gradients towards the lymphatic endothelium and exiting from the tissue towards draining lymph nodes (G). The endothelium regulates entry, the stroma regulates proliferation, survival, and differentiation, and the lymphatics regulate exit. See also colour plate section.

leukocyte trafficking exist to govern the selective accumulation of leukocyte subsets within specific tissues. These can be visualized as three different area codes (Fig. 11.1). Firstly, at the vascular endothelial level, interactions of leukocyte CAMs (some of them functioning as 'homing receptors') with tissue-specific microvascular endothelial counter receptors (known collectively as 'addressins'), and between CKs with their corresponding receptors expressed selectively by different classes of leukocyte. In combination these provide an address code which directs cells to cross appropriate endothelia. These two elements clearly overlap, and form part of the endothelial 'area-code' seen by leukocytes. Secondly, different microenvironments within the same tissue are responsible for selective accumulation of leukocyte subpopulations. CKs along with integrin-matrix interactions play essential roles in directional cues within tissues, while stromal cells such as fibroblasts and associated matrix are able to regulate the survival, proliferation, and differentiation of leukocyte subpopulations[85]. These allow an element of selection by matrix and chemokine-secreting stromal elements within different microenvironments, that is, a stromal area code. The best known example of this is represented by the selective localization of B and T lymphocytes in their respective areas in secondary lymphoid tissues (discussed later). Thirdly, it is important to recognize that exit from tissues is also subject to regulation. Having migrated through the endothelium, cells such as neutrophils and tissue macrophages are destined to die within the tissue. However, recirculating cells must exit from the tissue via the lymphatics in order to traffic to draining lymph nodes, that is, a lymphatic area code. CKs are known to play an important role here, lymphatic endothelium selectively expressing a profile of CKs which results in chemotaxis of cells such as T lymphocytes and dendritic cells. Subversion of some of these pathways appears to be responsible for the infiltrates seen in RA, and will be considered below.

General mechanisms of selective leukocyte-endothelium interactions

Specific adhesive interactions undoubtedly play a crucial role in determining selective recruitment of leukocytes. A ubiquitous mechanism has been described at two overlapping levels of selectin-ligand, and integrin-ligand interactions. However, some variants of these CAMs are expressed selectively by endothelia (often, as mentioned, referred to as addressins) and homing lymphocytes, allowing specialized endothelia to specifically recruit subpopulations of lymphocytes. Such addressin-CAM relationships are rarely of a simple binary nature, but some well characterized examples do exist. For instance, L-selectin on lymphocytes interacts with peripheral node addressin (PNAd/CD34) and a sialated variant of mucosal addressin cell-adhesion molecule 1 (MAdCAM-1) on endothelial cells of lymphoid tissues, directing lymphocytes to lymph nodes and intestinal Peyer's patches, respectively[80,86]. The interaction of $\alpha_4\beta_7$, preferentially expressed by lymphocytes and monocytes, with MAdCAM-1 (preferentially expressed by intestinal microvascular endothelium) is a further means by which these cell types are targeted to gut lymphoid tissues[87]. Once migrated through the mucosal endothelium, inflammatory leukocytes switch integrin α chain from α_4 to α_E, giving

a new heterodimer $\alpha_E\beta_7$, which recognizes E-cadherin expressed by gut epithelial cells[88]. Leukocytes are therefore targeted in combinatorial fashion, first to extravasate via the endothelium, then to the epithelial source of antigen. Confirmatory findings from knockout mouse models demonstrate that absence of L-selectin reduces the size of peripheral lymph nodes, while β_7-deficient mice exhibit underdeveloped gut-associated lymphoid tissue (GALT)[89,90]. Another addressin conferring some specificity is CLA (cutaneous lymphocyte antigen), a glycosylation variant of PSGL-1[91]. The receptor partner for CLA is E-selectin, ubiquitously expressed by all endothelia, but at very high density in dermal vessels, suggesting that quantitative expression can contribute to selectivity[92]. Thus addressins are in part responsible for selective pathways of skin and intestinal homing. Further variants of PSGL-1 are responsible for some of the selective recruitment seen in Th1 and Th2 diverged CD4+ lymphocytes. Both groups express PSGL-1; however, the variant expressed by Th1 cells binds both P- and E-selectin enabling traffic to sites of DTH reactions, a property absent from PSGL-1 expressed by Th2 cells[93,94]. Interestingly, rolling leukocytes shed PSGL-1, which may then interact with L-selectin, providing a means of lymphocyte recruitment in the late stages of inflammation[95].

More selectivity is seen in leukocyte trafficking than can be accounted for by adhesive interactions alone. A further, crucial element of specificity is added by chemokines and the selective expression of chemokine receptors on leukocytes. Thus trafficking leukocytes undergo not only CK-mediated activation of integrins, but also CK receptor-mediated chemotaxis on meeting endothelium-bound CKs. We now know that around 50 chemokines bind to some 20 chemokine receptors. Consequently CKs and CK receptors bind promiscuously, with receptors being activated by more than one ligand, and most CKs activating more than one receptor (Table 11.2). Others bind exclusively and monogamously as a single chemokine-receptor pair, for instance CXCL12 (SDF-1) and CXCR4. Functionally, CKs and their receptors fall into two broad functional groups: constitutive (homeostatic) and inflammatory (inducible) CKs (Table 11.2). Constitutive CKs are continuously expressed and govern basal, physiologically essential processes such as hemopoiesis and lymphocyte recirculation. In general, constitutive CKs and receptors tend to exhibit monogamous relationships, whilst those involved in inflammatory trafficking exhibit overlapping or redundant binding. Not all CKs fall easily into the two categories, but this classification is functionally useful.

Cells responding to constitutive CKs may need to change the sensitivity of their receptors to a constantly expressed level of ligand. For instance, pro- and pre-B cells are highly responsive to CXCL12, whilst dependent upon marrow stromal cells for mitogenic support, but at later stages of development lose this responsiveness[96]. By contrast, receptors for inflammatory CKs (such as CXCR1 and CXCR2, the receptors for CXCL8) must be persistently expressed by inflammatory cells such as neutrophils in order for them to be activated and chemoattracted by infrequently expressed inflammatory CKs. Regulation may therefore be achieved either at the level of ligand expression, receptor expression, or both.

In light of the above, the dramatic change in migratory characteristics of T lymphocytes undergoing the switch from

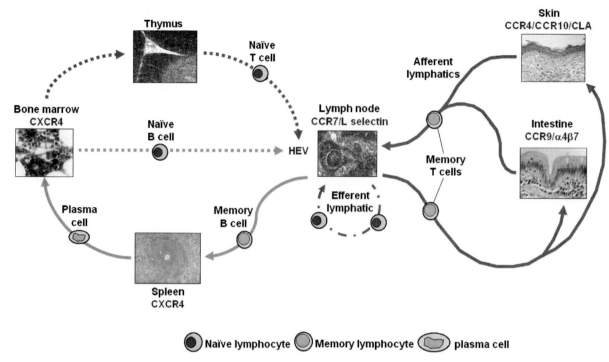

Fig. 11.2 Vascular codes regulate tissue specific homing within the immune system. During the development of an immune response, immature naïve T cells (dotted arrows) and B cells (dotted arrows) that have been educated in the thymus and bone marrow, respectively, enter lymph nodes through HEVs using the endothelial entry code CCR7 and L-selectin. Antigen-experienced B cells leave the lymph node and migrate into specific niches such as the red pulp of the spleen and the bone marrow using the endothelial entry code CXCR4. Antigen-experienced central memory T cells continue to recirculate back to lymph nodes via the efferent lymphatics and thoracic duct. Effector memory T cells preferentially recirculate to the tissue in which they were initially activated; for example if they are activated in a lymph node draining the skin they acquire the skin entry code CCR4/CCR10/CLA and if activated in a lymph node draining the gut they acquire the gut entry code CCR9/$\alpha_4\beta_7$. At the end of immune surveillance within tissues, memory T cells can recirculate back to lymph nodes via the afferent lymphatics. See also colour plate section.

naïve to memory cells can be accounted for by a change in complementary receptors for both addressins and CKs (Fig. 11.2). Naïve lymphocytes gain access to lymph nodes via high endothelial venules because they express the correct full address code: high levels of L-selectin and the CK receptor CCR7[80]. Central memory T cells retain expression of CCR7 in order to continue trafficking through lymph nodes, while effector memory cells express CCR5 and CCR2, which allows them to respond to CKs produced in inflamed tissues, such as CCL5 (regulated on activation normal T cell expressed and secreted, RANTES), CCL2 (monocyte chemoattractant protein 1, MCP-1) and CCL3 (macrophage inflammatory protein 1α, MIP-1α)[97]. In addition, recent evidence suggests that T cells are imprinted with an appropriate endothelial address code during activation in lymphoid tissues by DCs, resulting in their return to the tissues in which they were activated. For instance, only DCs taken from Peyer's patches were able to imprint CD8+ T cells with the full gut homing code, comprising $\alpha_4\beta_7$, and CCR9, the receptor for CCL25 (thymus-expressed chemokine, TECK), which is expressed exclusively in thymus and intestine[98]. Retinoic acid may be one of the signals generated by intestinal DCs which imprints this information on T cells[99]. Dudda and colleagues demonstrated that DCs injected intracutaneously could induce CLA positivity in CD8+ T cells, while intraperitoneal injection of identical DCs induced T cells expressing $\alpha_4\beta_7$[100]. Antigen presentation may therefore communicate via costimulatory information not only the nature of the antigen, but also the location in which it was encountered.

The story for skin homing T cells is less clear. Basal homing to the skin appears to rely upon interactions between CCR8 expressed by T cells and the ligand CCL1[101]. In inflammation, almost all CLA+ T cells express CCR4, explaining the predominance of CCR4+ Th1 T cells in the skin[102,103]. CCL27 (cutaneous T cell-attracting chemokine, CTACK), a CCR10 ligand, is expressed exclusively by dermal keratinocytes and post-capillary venules during inflammation[103,104], but only a fraction of CLA+ T cells expresses CCR10, the proportion varying with different types of inflammation[104,105]. Therefore, though the role of CLA appears clear, those of CKs and CK receptors such as CCL27 and CCR10 are less so. Such regulation is evidently highly complex, but the use of multiple CK-receptor pairs coupled with the redundancy inherent in CK binding allows modulation of expression of different CKs and CK receptors, giving the immune system huge flexibility to adapt to requirements for different leukocyte populations in response to diverse conditions.

CKs have a wider role in determining inflammatory cellular infiltrates appropriate to specific responses: for instance, CKs induced by interferon-γ (IFN-γ), the archetypal Th1 cytokine, CXCL11 (interferon-inducible T cell alpha chemoattractant, I-TAC), CXCL9 (monokine induced by IFN-γ, Mig) and CXCL10 (IFN-inducible protein 10, IP-10) are agonists for CXCR3, a receptor expressed along with CCR5 by Th1 differentiated T cells. However these ligands are also antagonists for CCR3, which is expressed by Th2 polarized cells[106]. Eosinophils also express CCR3, the receptor for CCL11, CCL24, and CCL26 (eotaxins 1, 2, and 3), which are released in Th2-type allergic inflammatory responses. Though eosinophils share some other chemokine receptors with monocytes, the latter express CCR5 but not CCR3. Thus CKs and CK receptor expression patterns are able to determine the selective recruitment of specific myeloid populations[107]. Other families of CKs are broadly selective for certain cell types, for instance the CXC chemokines CXCL1-8 predominantly recruit neutrophils. A further example of tissue CK profiles determining the type of inflammation seen in a microenvironment occurs during the switch from acute to chronic inflammation. Chronic inflammation, as demonstrated in DTH reactions, usually follows acute inflammation in a precisely choreographed sequence of events, and the molecular mechanisms governing this switch have recently become clearer. In a model of peritoneal inflammation, Hurst et al.[108] showed that the interaction between the cytokine IL-6 and its soluble receptor (sIL-6R) appeared to determine the switch between acute and chronic inflammatory infiltrates by shifting the chemokine repertoire of the local microenvironment. Infiltrating neutrophils produce sIL-6R, which binds IL-6 and allows signaling in the absence of membrane-anchored IL-6 receptor. This suppresses the stromal production of neutrophil-attracting CXC chemokines induced by the pro-inflammatory cytokines TNF-α and IL-1, while inducing expression of the CC chemokine CCL2 (MCP-1), which attracts a mononuclear cell population. The acute inflammatory infiltrating neutrophil population therefore directly generates the message that switches the local CK repertoire to attract a cellular population typical of chronic inflammation.

General mechanisms of leukocyte accumulation within tissue microenvironments

It has been pointed out above that there are multiple points of control present in the extravasation process. This offers the possibility of significant selection at the point of recruitment by the endothelium. However, this offers only a partial explanation for the selective accumulation of leukocyte subsets, particularly in persistent chronic inflammatory diseases such as RA[85]. Once the endothelial barrier has been crossed, cells such as neutrophils die within the tissue, but mononuclear cells may either undergo apoptosis, return to the circulation via lymphatics, or be retained in the tissue within the microenvironments. Movement into and within tissues is controlled by means of haptotaxis (movement along gradients of adhesion molecules or immobilized ligands) and chemotaxis (movement along gradients of soluble chemoattractants). Cells entering microenvironments must negotiate through ECM constituents such as collagen, laminin, fibronectin, and proteoglycans by means of adhesion molecules, principally integrins, for which these ECM molecules are ligands. Chemokine receptor interactions uniquely integrate adhesion and chemotaxis, and are the other major determinants of fate in terms of localization within tissue microenvironments. It is now clear that a succession of overlapping interactions occurs during recruitment and tissue migration, making the 'combinatorial' use of multiple pairs of CKs and CK receptors and 'vector-summing' the signals of competing CKs[109]. Leukocytes migrate across the endothelium using one receptor/agonist pair, through the interstitium using another pair, and to the target microenvironment using yet another pair. Only cells displaying all three receptors can successfully home to the target region. In the presence of high levels of an agonist, receptors may undergo homologous desensitization, or down-regulation, while up-regulating a different receptor, allowing cells to move from one environment to another. It is also known that leukocytes are able to interpret new signals in the light of memory of their recent chemokine environment[110].

The best characterized model of migration within and between tissue microenvironments is that of lymphoid tissue and its constituent DCs, T and B lymphocytes. Immature DCs are specialized for encountering antigen in inflammatory sites, to which they migrate by expressing inflammatory chemokine receptors such as CCR1, 2, 5, and 6[111], which are shared with their monocyte precursors. CCL20 (MIP-3α), a CCR6 ligand, appears to be crucial in this process as it is highly expressed by inflamed epithelia[112], and also in the sub-epithelial dome of Peyer's patches where DCs sample antigen directly[113]. Once they have encountered new antigen, DCs undergo a process of maturation under the local influence of inflammatory cytokines and bacterial and viral products. As a result inflammatory CK receptors are down-regulated, and up-regulation of the constitutive receptors CCR4, CCR7, and CXCR4 occurs, causing DCs to migrate into local draining lymphatics (which express the CCR7 ligand CCL21 (secondary lymphoid tissue chemokine, SLC)) and thereby into peripheral lymph nodes[114]. Trafficking of B and T cells is regulated by CXCL13 (BCA-1, B cell-attracting chemokine 1), its receptor CXCR5, and CCL21 and CCL19 (EBL-1-ligand chemokine, ELC), which are both CCR7 agonists. Within the lymph node CXCR5-bearing B cells are attracted to follicular areas, while T cells and DCs are maintained within parafollicular zones by local expression of CCL21 and CCL19[115,116]. Some T cells which have been successfully presented with their cognate antigen by DCs then up-regulate CXCR5, allowing them to migrate towards, and interact with B cells; those T cells destined to provide help in germinal centers maintain CXCR5 expression, and fail to express CLA, CCR7, or α4β7, implying that such germinal center T cells represent a distinct sub-population[117]. In summary, movement within tissues has parallels to the process of extravasation, in that both adhesive and chemotactic cues are integrated in overlapping and combinatorial fashion. However, within tissues preferential localization of cells occurs in the absence of flow, and the presence of diverse matrix components may influence localization within specific microenvironments.

Specific mechanisms governing leukocyte accumulation in the joint

Selective leukocyte entry

Although the idea that specific pathways regulate the recirculation of synovial lymphocytes has been recognized for a number of years, direct proof of the existence of an endothelial code or addressin specific to the joint is still lacking. However, there is indirect evidence to support this concept. Jalkanen and colleagues provided evidence to support a synovium-specific lymphocyte-endothelial recognition mechanism[118]. Differential binding of lymphocytes to frozen sections was demonstrated, with lymphoblastoid lines binding to lymphoid tissue and not synovial microvascular endothelium (MVE). Furthermore, some T cell lines derived from lymphoid, gut, and synovial tissues bound preferentially to homotypic tissue sections[119]. The greatest level of cross adhesion was seen between gut and synovium-derived cells, a finding which fits with data showing that, in common with gut but not skin lymphocytes, the majority of synovial lymphocytes express $\alpha_4\beta_7$ integrin[120,121]. This potential overlap goes well with clinical observations of a relationship between gastrointestinal and joint disease, whether in the context of infection or chronic inflammation, as in inflammatory bowel disease. However, the synovial MVE does not express the $\alpha_4\beta_7$ ligand MAdCAM-1, suggesting that this integrin is binding to alternative ligands. These may include VCAM-1, which is expressed by rheumatoid synovial (and other inflammatory) MVE and other stromal cells[122], and fibronectin peptides, which are known to be expressed on the luminal surface of synovial MVE in RA[123]. More recently, persuasive evidence that the synovial microvasculature can be specifically targeted, and hence may possess an as yet unidentified addressin code, comes from two models. In the first, Gerlag and colleagues showed that a phage displaying a peptide which binds to $\alpha_V\beta_3$ and $\alpha_V\beta_5$ could home to inflamed synovium, and ameliorate collagen-induced arthritis in mice[124]. One solution to the problems of trying to examine trafficking into inflamed RA synovial tissue *in vivo* is to implant synovial tissue into SCID mice. Using this second model, Lee and colleagues screened a library of peptide-displaying phages, demonstrating the existence of human synovial MVE-specific binding peptides, though the MVE receptor(s) itself still remains to be identified[125]. Further indirect evidence for joint-specific migration pathways comes from studies in psoriatic arthritis[126]. Here, skin infiltrating T lymphocytes expressed CLA, while those found in the joint from the same patients did not. This suggests that lymphocyte localization is governed not simply by the presence of inflammation, but also by microenvironment-specific mechanisms. Data from models using skin blisters to examine migration of leukocytes into inflammatory skin indicate that skin localization of CLA+ lymphocytes relates to active increased migration of such T cells, rather than acquisition of CLA positivity once in the microenvironment[126]. Once again, evidence for a joint-specific code remains elusive, with studies reporting promiscuous expression of markers associated non-specifically with highly activated endothelia in inflammatory sites, such as vascular adhesion protein (VAP)-1, CD44 ligands, endoglin (a member of the TGF-β receptor family), P- and E-selectins, and ICAMs 1–3[127]. Many drugs used therapeutically in RA, not least anti-TNF therapy, down-regulate expression of these markers in the synovium. However, trials using more specific inhibitors, for instance against ICAM-1, have failed to show consistent results[127]. As mentioned above, the *in vivo* phenotype of synovial MVE is unusual, with HEV-like morphology in areas where lymphoid infiltrates are more organized[2]. This has made the study of endothelial-leukocyte interactions problematic, as *in vitro* culture of synovial MVE leads to rapid loss of its specialized phenotype. It remains unclear at which time point HEVs develop in the course of lymphoid neogenesis, and whether the HEV-like phenotype is induced by local factors, or results from high numbers of infiltrating lymphocytes.

Are there sources of inflammatory CKs which could act via the endothelium to recruit inflammatory cells to the RA joint? Abundant monocytes and macrophages, and stromal elements such as synovial fibroblasts, are subject to a pro-inflammatory cytokine network and direct contact interactions with other infiltrating cells such as T lymphocytes[128,129], leading to high levels of expression of many inflammatory CKs in the rheumatoid synovium. Neutrophil-attracting CKs are expressed at high levels by monocytes and stimulated fibroblasts and include CXCL8 (IL-8), CXCL5 (ENA-78, epithelial cell-derived neutrophil attractant 78) and CXCL1 (GRO-α, growth related oncogene-α)[130–132]. Monocytes and T cells may be recruited by a range of CXC and CC chemokines found at high levels in the synovium; CXCL10 (IP-10) and CXCL9 (Mig) are highly expressed in synovial tissue and fluid[133]. CCL2 (MCP-1) is found in synovial fluid and known to be produced by synovial fibroblasts; it is considered to be a pivotal chemokine for the recruitment of monocytes[134,135]. CCL3 (Mip-1α), CCL4 (Mip-1β), and CCL5 (RANTES) are chemotactic for monocytes and lymphocytes, expressed at high levels in inflamed rheumatoid synovium and known products of synovial fibroblasts[133,136]. CCL20 (Mip-3α) is also overexpressed in the synovium, and has a similar chemoattractant profile via its specific receptor, CCR6[137,138]. CX3CL1 (fractalkine) is also widely expressed in the rheumatoid synovium[139]. A number of CK receptors have been shown to differ between peripheral blood and synovial samples, suggesting that they may arise either by selective recruitment by endothelial expressed CKs, or up-regulation by the microenvironment after recruitment. In RA patients, circulating monocytes express mainly CCR1, CCR2, and CCR4, whereas monocytes isolated from synovial fluid express higher levels of CXCR3 and CCR5[140]. Similarly, synovial CD4 T lymphocytes appear to express higher levels of CCR5, CXCR2, CXCR3, and CXCR6 than circulating cells while expressing low levels of CCR3, suggesting a Th1 selective recruitment bias[141]. Clearly such exuberant expression of CKs of an inflammatory type may be responsible for considerable recruitment of activated lymphocytes, monocytes, and neutrophils, though once again, such expression does not constitute a disease-specific profile.

Selective leukocyte survival and retention

What do we know about selective mechanisms governing accumulation of leukocytes within the synovium itself? One important clue comes from the distribution of mononuclear cells in RA. As mentioned above, antigen-presenting cells cluster with lymphocytes in perivascular sites and within characteristic lymphoid structures[5,6]. RA is unique in that synovial lymphoid infiltrates can be divided into at least three distinct histological groupings, varying from diffuse lymphocyte infiltrates to clear germinal center reactions[7]. Moreover, there is evidence that such differing histological types correlate with other serum indicators of disease activity[142,143]. This long-described feature, termed lymphoid neogenesis, relies upon inappropriate, but highly organized temporal and spatial expression by stromal cells of the same constitutive CKs, particularly CXCL13 and CCL21, which are associated with true lymphoid organogenesis (Fig. 11.3). Genesis of lymphoid follicular structures in diseases such as diabetes and RA appears to rely upon expression of these CKs, in association with the lymphotoxins-α and -β (LT-α and LT-β) and TNF-α[7,144]. In this

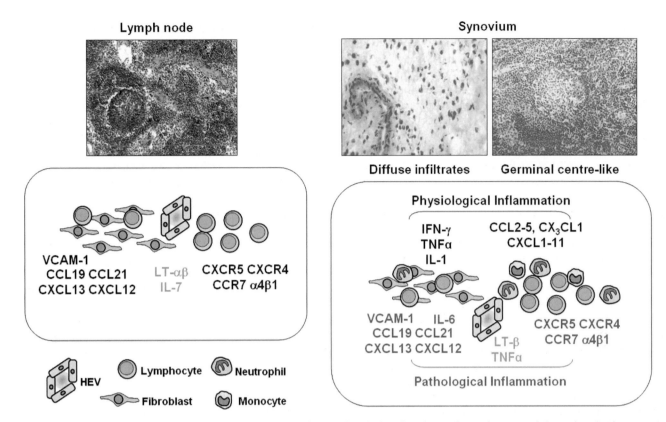

Fig. 11.3 Stromal codes regulating accumulation, differentiation and survival in the lymph node are aberrantly expressed during lymphoid neogenesis in rheumatoid arthritis. Homeostatic chemokines (CXCL12, CXCL13, CCL19, CCL21), adhesion molecules (VCAM-1), and cytokines/growth factors (IL-6, IL-7) are components of the stromal code that help define stromal niches such as the lymph node and bone marrow, governing leukocyte accumulation, differentiation, and survival. Stromal cells produce/express the appropriate cytokine/chemokine/adhesion receptor that is recognized by cognate receptors on infiltrating leukocytes. In the case of the lymph node, structure is developed and maintained as a result of lymphotoxin-α?and -β and IL-7 production by 'inducer' lymphocytes which induce the secretion of constitutive chemokines from stromal 'organizer' cells. During physiological inflammation, inflammatory chemokines (CCL2-CCL5, CX3CL1 and CXCL1-CXCL11 and inflammatory mediators such as IFN-γ, TNF-α, and IL-1 are produced by stromal cells and lead to the recruitment of inflammatory cells (lymphocytes, neutrophils, and monocytes). However, in persistent, pathological inflammation such as occurs in RA, stromal cells begin to aberrantly produce/express components of the physiological stromal code normally associated with lymphoid tissues, leading to lymphoid neogenesis. TNF-α and lymphotoxin-β are important in maintaining lymphoid structures. See also colour plate section.

context it is important to note that transgenic animals overexpressing the TNF-α gene display increased formation of focal lymphoid aggregates and develop a chronic arthritis similar to RA[145]. Clearly one of the many mechanisms of action of anti-TNF therapy may involve the dissolution of such aggregates. In transgenic mouse models, expression of CXCL13 in the pancreatic islets was sufficient for the development of T and B cell clusters, but as they lacked follicular dendritic cells, was not sufficient for true germinal center formation[146]. CCL21 does appear to be sufficient in some cases for lymph node formation; murine pancreatic islet models have demonstrated formation of lymph node-like structures in the presence of CCL21[147,148], and lymphoid infiltrates in response to CCL19 expression, a possible common pathway being the induction of lymphotoxins on infiltrating lymphocytes[114]. Lack of CCL21 signaling impairs T cell traffic into lymph node structures via high endothelial venules, and results in disorganization of T cell zones[149,150]. Weyand and colleagues used the histological heterogeneity seen in RA to identify those factors critical to formation of lymphoid microstructures, showing that transcription levels of CXCL13 and CCL21 were increased 10 to 20 times in tissues with germinal centers compared to tissues with other histological patterns. Multivariate analysis showed that LT-β

and CXCL13 were necessary, but not sufficient for lymphoid neogenesis[7]. Expression of CCL21 mRNA and protein has been clearly demonstrated in non-lymphatic endothelium, both within and outside organized lymphoid infiltrates in RA synovium[151]. It therefore seems likely that expression of lymphoid constitutive CKs contributes significantly to the entry, local organization, and exit of lymphocytes in the RA synovium.

In addition, the constitutive chemokine CXCL12 and its receptor CXCR4 have emerged as unexpected but crucial players in the accumulation of T lymphocytes within the rheumatoid synovial microenvironment. CXCR4 is expressed constitutively on naïve T cells, but not on highly differentiated CD45RO+ T cells in peripheral blood[152]. Unexpectedly, CD45RO+ T lymphocytes were found to express CXCR4 receptors at high levels in the rheumatoid synovium. Its ligand CXCL12 was highly expressed on endothelial cells at the sites of T cell accumulation[47,152,153]. In addition, stromal-cell derived TGF-β is responsible for up-regulation of CXCR4 receptors on T cells in the synovium[152]. Cross-talk between chemokine and cytokine networks may operate to reinforce the retention of T cells by CXCL12. For example, locally raised IL-1 or TNF-α levels cause synovial fibroblasts and macrophages to secrete IL-15. This cytokine also up-regulates CXCR4 on T cells, and may thus also contribute to the retention of T lymphocytes[153]. Evidence also suggests that the stability of lymphocyte infiltrates is reinforced by a positive feedback loop, whereby tissue CXCL12 promotes CD40 ligand expression on T cells, which in turn stimulates further CXCL12 production by synovial fibroblasts[153]. There is therefore clear evidence in support of the hypothesis that aberrant expression of constitutive CKs by synovial fibroblasts is responsible for retention of T cells within the RA synovium. Other cell constituents of the rheumatoid inflammatory infiltrate may be affected by the CXCL12/CXCR4 axis. Blades and colleagues showed an increased expression of CXCL12/CXCR4 by monocyte/macrophage cells in RA compared with OA. In addition, using implanted human synovial tissue in SCID mice, they demonstrated that monocytes are recruited into transplanted synovial tissue by CXCL12[154]. Contact-mediated B cell survival induced by synovial fibroblasts has been shown to depend upon a CXCL12 and CD106 (VCAM-1)-dependent mechanism which is independent of TNF-α[155]. Overexpression of CXCL12 was also identified as a distinct feature of rheumatoid, as opposed to osteoarthritis synovia using cDNA arrays[156]. Useful data validating these findings come from a CIA model in DBA/1 (IFN-γ receptor deficient) mice, where administration of the specific CXCR4 antagonist AMD3100 significantly ameliorated disease severity[157]. In another murine CIA model the small molecule CXCR4 antagonist 4F-benzoyl-TN14003 ameliorated clinical severity and suppressed DTH responses[158]. The CXCL12/CXCR4 constitutive CK pair therefore seems to play an important role in cellular retention in RA. It seems likely that CXCR4 antagonists will be of use in the therapy of rheumatoid arthritis, provided that toxicity issues due to stem cell mobilization from the bone marrow (in which CXCL12/CXCR4 interactions maintain the relationship between hemopoietic stem cells and bone marrow stromal cells) do not pose a major problem. Recent evidence suggests that the synovial microenvironment may in part be responsible for induction and continued expression of both inflammatory (CCL5 and CXCR3) and constitutive (CXCL12 and CCR7) CK receptors in synovial T cells. This provides an alternative explanation for the disproportionately high levels of some CK receptors seen on synovial T cells, and for the presence of constitutive CK receptors such as CCR7 and CXCR4 on retained lymphocytes[159]. In summary, the inappropriate temporal and spatial expression of constitutive CKs by stromal cells plays a crucial role in the accumulation of leukocytes within the synovium.

Though there is clear evidence for mechanisms orchestrating the recruitment and selection of lymphocytes and monocytes, relatively few neutrophils are seen in the RA synovium, and large numbers are found in synovial fluid, despite the production of multiple neutrophil-recruiting CKs. This is thought to result from a lack of expression of specific adhesion receptors by neutrophils for important ECM components such as collagen and fibronectin (FN). In contrast, mononuclear cells express high levels of these receptors, which belong largely to the β_1 integrin subfamily of VLA molecules. Each VLA integrin heterodimer mediates adhesion to at least one of the three major ECM glycoproteins. In addition, each ligand is recognized by multiple VLA integrins. Lymphocytes adhere to FN mainly via VLA-4 and VLA-5 integrin receptors, which recognize two different binding sites of the FN molecule. VLA-4 binds to the third connecting segment (IIICS) region[160,161], while VLA-5 recognizes the key short peptide sequence RGDS, within the central cell binding domain[162]. The collagen receptors have been identified as VLA-1,

VLA-2, and VLA-3, while the VLA-6 integrin has been shown to bind to laminin. Interestingly VLA-1 and VLA-2 are not present on resting T cells, but are expressed after long term activation *in vitro* and are found in approximately 60% of RA synovial T cells. Binding via these integrins to ECM ligands is likely to be functionally relevant, as suggested by data showing that treatment with a monoclonal antibody against VLA-1 in a rat model of arthritis ameliorated disease and reduced evidence of T cell activation[163]. The ECM provides not only a supporting physical environment for stromal and immune cells, but also guidance cues which may be read by infiltrating lymphocytes, allowing them to come into close contact with other cells such as APCs for the initiation of immune responses. ECM proteins have multiple adhesive domains that facilitate a multiplicity of interactions between cells and ECMs and provide costimulatory signals for the amplification of inflammatory cascades[164–166].

Until recently, the majority of research on leukocyte trafficking has concerned recruitment of cells via the vascular endothelium. However, a recent breakthrough in the elucidation of trafficking pathways has been the development of specific markers for lymphatic endothelium. Of these, the most specific is LYVE-1, a hyaluronan receptor expressed exclusively on draining lymphatic vessels[167]. Markers such as LYVE-1 now allow us to address some fundamental questions about differences between vascular and lymphatic vessels, and the part played by the latter in control of trafficking out of the joint. Recent work has identified gradients of expression of the constitutive chemokines CCL19 and CXCL12: in lymphoid tissue (tonsil), higher CK expression was seen on vascular than lymphoid vessels, consistent with the attraction and retention of lymphocytes. In RA synovium, by contrast, levels of chemokine expression were equally high in vascular and lymphoid vessels, suggesting that increased tissue expression of constitutive CKs plays a role in lymphocyte retention by subverting the normal CK gradient which causes egress via lymphatics towards draining lymph nodes[159].

In conclusion, no specific synovial receptors for trafficking have yet been identified, though it remains likely that selective pathways do exist which regulate the localization of sub-populations of joint-homing leukocytes. Were joint specific mechanisms of adhesion and recruitment to be elucidated, this would allow the joint to be targeted without the serious risks associated with generalized adhesion blockade. What has become evident, however, is that the rheumatoid synovium belongs to a select group of persistent inflammatory diseases characterized by subversion of the normal constitutive pathways which regulate the formation of lymphoid tissues, and trafficking of cells through them. The tissue phenotype resulting from these events is the formation of ectopic lymphoid deposits. Identifying further the mechanisms driving aberrant expression of constitutive CKs may offer new therapeutic opportunities to target inflammation in RA.

References

1. Walsh, D. A. Angiogenesis and arthritis. *Rheumatology (Oxford)* 1999; **38**: 103–12.
2. Koch, A. E. Review: angiogenesis: implications for rheumatoid arthritis. *Arthritis Rheum* 1998; **41**: 951–62.
3. Pitzalis, C., Kingsley, G., Lanchbury, J. S., Murphy, J., and Panayi, G. S. Expression of HLA-DR, DQ and DP antigens and interleukin-2

receptor on synovial fluid T lymphocyte subsets in rheumatoid arthritis: evidence for 'frustrated' activation. *J Rheumatol* 1987; **14**: 662–6.

4. Firestein, G. S. Invasive fibroblast-like synoviocytes in rheumatoid arthritis: passive responders or transformed aggressors? *Arthritis Rheum* 1996 Nov; **39**: 1781–90.

5. Itoh, J., Kinjoh, K., Ohyama, A., Nose, M., and Kyogoku, M. Application of two-color immunofluorescence staining to demonstration of T-cells and HLA-DR-bearing cells in rheumatoid synovitis. *J Histochem Cytochem* 1992 Nov; **40**: 1675–83.

6. Dinther-Janssen, A. C., Pals, S. T., Scheper, R., Breedveld, F., and Meijer, C. J. Dendritic cells and high endothelial venules in the rheumatoid synovial membrane. *J Rheumatol* 1990 Jan; **17**: 11–17.

7. Takemura, S., Braun, A., Crowson, C., Kurtin, P. J., Cofield, R. H., O'Fallon, W. M. *et al*. Lymphoid neogenesis in rheumatoid synovitis. *J Immunol* 2001 Jul 15; **167**: 1072–80.

8. Weyand, C. M., Kurtin, P. J., and Goronzy, J. J. Ectopic lymphoid organogenesis: a fast track for autoimmunity. *Am J Pathol* 2001 Sep; **159**: 787–93.

9. Taylor, P. C. VEGF and imaging of vessels in rheumatoid arthritis. *Arthritis Res* 2002; **4** (Suppl. 3): S99–107.

10. Paleolog, E. M., Young, S., Stark, A. C., McCloskey, R. V., Feldmann M., and Maini, R. N. Modulation of angiogenic vascular endothelial growth factor by tumor necrosis factor alpha and interleukin-1 in rheumatoid arthritis. *Arthritis Rheum* 1998 Jul; **41**: 1258–65.

11. Qvistgaard, E., Rogind, H., Torp-Pedersen, S., Terslev, L., Danneskiold-Samsoe, B., and Bliddal, H. Quantitative ultrasonography in rheumatoid arthritis: evaluation of inflammation by Doppler technique. *Ann Rheum Dis* 2001 Jul; **60**: 690–3.

12. Taylor, P. C., Steuer, A., Gruber, J., Cosgrove, D. O., Blomley, M. J., Marsters, P. A. *et al*. Comparison of ultrasonographic assessment of synovitis and joint vascularity with radiographic evaluation in a randomized, placebo-controlled study of infliximab therapy in early rheumatoid arthritis. *Arthritis Rheum* 2004 Apr; **50**: 1107–16.

13. Clavel, G., Bessis, N., and Boissier, M. C. Recent data on the role for angiogenesis in rheumatoid arthritis. *Joint Bone Spine* 2003 Sep; **70**: 321–6.

14. Brenchley, P. E. Antagonising angiogenesis in rheumatoid arthritis. *Ann Rheum Dis* 2001 Nov; **60** (Suppl. 3): iii71–iii74.

15. Desmouliere, A., Redard, M., Darby, I., and Gabbiani, G. Apoptosis mediates the decrease in cellularity during the transition between granulation tissue and scar. *Am J Pathol* 1995 Jan; **146**: 56–66.

16. Walsh, D. A., Wade, M., Mapp, P. I., and Blake, D. R. Focally regulated endothelial proliferation and cell death in human synovium. *Am J Pathol* 1998 Mar; **152**: 691–702.

17. FitzGerald, O., Soden, M., Yanni, G., Robinson, R., and Bresnihan, B. Morphometric analysis of blood vessels in synovial membranes obtained from clinically affected and unaffected knee joints of patients with rheumatoid arthritis. *Ann Rheum Dis* 1991 Nov; **50**: 792–6.

18. Achen, M. G., and Stacker, S. A. The vascular endothelial growth factor family: proteins which guide the development of the vasculature. *Int J Exp Pathol* 1998 Oct; **79**: 255–65.

19. Neufeld, G., Cohen, T., Gengrinovitch, S., and Poltorak, Z. Vascular endothelial growth factor (VEGF) and its receptors. *FASEB J* 1999 Jan; **13**: 9–22.

20. Sone, H., Sakauchi, M., Takahashi, A., Suzuki, H., Inoue, N., Iida, K. *et al*. Elevated levels of vascular endothelial growth factor in the sera of patients with rheumatoid arthritis correlation with disease activity. *Life Sci* 2001 Sep 7; **69**: 1861–9.

21. Ikeda, M., Hosoda, Y., Hirose, S., Okada, Y., and Ikeda, E. Expression of vascular endothelial growth factor isoforms and their receptors Flt-1, KDR, and neuropilin-1 in synovial tissues of rheumatoid arthritis. *J Pathol* 2000 Aug; **191**: 426–33.

22. Giatromanolaki, A., Sivridis, E., Athanassou, N., Zois, E., Thorpe, P. E., Brekken RA *et al*. The angiogenic pathway 'vascular endothelial growth factor/flk-1(KDR)-receptor' in rheumatoid arthritis and osteoarthritis. *J Pathol* 2001 May; **194**: 101–8.

23. Koch, A. E., Harlow, L. A., Haines, G. K., Amento, E. P., Unemori, E. N., Wong, W. L. *et al*. Vascular endothelial growth factor: a cytokine modulating endothelial function in rheumatoid arthritis. *J Immunol* 1994 Apr 15; **152**: 4149–56.

24. Fava, R. A., Olsen, N. J., Spencer-Green, G., Yeo, K. T., Yeo, T. K., Berse, B. *et al*. Vascular permeability factor/endothelial growth factor (VPF/VEGF): accumulation and expression in human synovial fluids and rheumatoid synovial tissue. *J Exp Med* 1994 Jul 1; **180**: 341–6.

25. Kasama, T., Shiozawa, F., Kobayashi, K., Yajima, N., Hanyuda, M., Takeuchi, H. T. *et al*. Vascular endothelial growth factor expression by activated synovial leukocytes in rheumatoid arthritis: critical involvement of the interaction with synovial fibroblasts. *Arthritis Rheum* 2001 Nov; **44**: 2512–24.

26. Sekimoto, T., Hamada, K., Oike, Y., Matsuoka, T., Matsumoto, M., Chosa, E. *et al*. Effect of direct angiogenesis inhibition in rheumatoid arthritis using a soluble vascular endothelial growth factor receptor 1 chimeric protein. *J Rheumatol* 2002 Feb; **29**: 240–5.

27. Miotla, J., Maciewicz, R., Kendrew, J., Feldmann, M., and Paleolog, E. Treatment with soluble VEGF receptor reduces disease severity in murine collagen-induced arthritis. *Lab Invest* 2000 Aug; **80**: 1195–205.

28. De, B. M., Ben Mahdi, M. H., Ollivier, V., Grossin, M., Dupuis, M., Gaudry, M. *et al*. Blockade of vascular endothelial growth factor receptor I (VEGF-RI), but not VEGF-RII, suppresses joint destruction in the K/BxN model of rheumatoid arthritis. *J Immunol* 2003 Nov 1; **171**: 4853–9.

29. Mapp, P. I., Grootveld, M. C., and Blake, D. R., Hypoxia. oxidative stress and rheumatoid arthritis. *Br. Med. Bull.* 1995; **51**: 419–36.

30. Jaakkola, P., Mole, D. R., Tian, Y. M., Wilson, M. I., Gielbert, J., Gaskell, S. J. *et al*. Targeting of HIF-alpha to the von Hippel-Lindau ubiquitylation complex by O2-regulated prolyl hydroxylation. *Science* 2001 Apr 20; **292**(5516): 468–72.

31. Lando, D., Peet, D. J., Whelan, D. A., Gorman, J. J., and Whitelaw, M. L. Asparagine hydroxylation of the HIF transactivation domain a hypoxic switch. *Science* 2002 Feb 1; **295**(5556): 858–61.

32. Sang, N., Fang, J., Srinivas, V., Leshchinsky, I., and Caro, J. Carboxyl-terminal transactivation activity of hypoxia-inducible factor 1 alpha is governed by a von Hippel-Lindau protein-independent, hydroxylation-regulated association with p300/CBP. *Mol Cell Biol* 2002 May; **22**: 2984–92.

33. Wenger, R. H. Cellular adaptation to hypoxia: O2-sensing protein hydroxylases, hypoxia-inducible transcription factors, and O2-regulated gene expression. *FASEB J* 2002 Aug; **16**: 1151–62.

34. Berse, B, Hunt, J. A., Diegel, R. J., Morganelli, P., Yeo, K., Brown, F. *et al*. Hypoxia augments cytokine (transforming growth factor-beta (TGF-beta) and IL-1)-induced vascular endothelial growth factor secretion by human synovial fibroblasts. *Clin Exp Immunol* 1999 Jan; **115**: 176–82.

35. Bottomley, M. J., Webb, N. J., Watson, C. J., Holt, P. J., Freemont, A. J., and Brenchley P. E. Peripheral blood mononuclear cells from patients with rheumatoid arthritis spontaneously secrete vascular endothelial growth factor (VEGF): specific up-regulation by tumour necrosis factor-alpha (TNF-alpha) in synovial fluid. *Clin Exp Immunol* 1999 Jul; **117**: 171–6.

36. Rossi, D., and Zlotnik, A. The biology of chemokines and their receptors. *Annu Rev Immunol* 2000; **18**: 217–42.

37. Curnock, A. P., Logan, M. K., Ward, S. G. Chemokine signalling: pivoting around multiple phosphoinositide 3-kinases. *Immunology* 2002 Feb; **105**: 125–36.

38. Bokoch, G. M. Chemoattractant signaling and leukocyte activation. *Blood* 1995 Sep 1; **86**: 1649–60.

39. Kunkel, E. J., and Butcher, E. C. Chemokines and the tissue-specific migration of lymphocytes. *Immunity* 2002 Jan; **16**: 1–4.

40. Bazan, J. F., Bacon, K. B., Hardiman, G., Wang, W., Soo, K., Rossi, D. *et al*. A new class of membrane-bound chemokine with a CX3C motif. *Nature* 1997 Feb 13; **385**(6617): 640–4.

41. Pan, Y., Lloyd, C., Zhou, H., Dolich, S., Deeds, J., Gonzalo, J. A. *et al*. Neurotactin, a membrane-anchored chemokine upregulated in brain inflammation. *Nature* 1997 Jun 5; **387**(6633): 611–17.

42. Koch, A. E., Polverini, P. J., Kunkel, S. L., Harlow, L. A., DiPietro, L. A., Elner V. M. *et al*. Interleukin-8 as a macrophage-derived mediator of angiogenesis. *Science* 1992 Dec 11; **258**(5089): 1798–801.

43. Szekanecz, Z., and Koch, A. E. Chemokines and angiogenesis. *Curr Opin Rheumatol* 2001 May; **13**: 202–8.

44. Volin, M. V., Woods, J. M., Amin, M. A., Connors, M. A., Harlow, L. A., and Koch, A. E. Fractalkine: a novel angiogenic chemokine in rheumatoid arthritis. *Am J Pathol* 2001 Oct; **159**: 1521–30.

45. Belperio, J. A., Keane, M. P., Arenberg, D. A., Addison, C. L., Ehlert, J. E., Burdick, M. D. *et al*. CXC chemokines in angiogenesis. *J Leukoc Biol* 2000 Jul; **68**: 1–8.

46. Koch, A. E., Volin, M. V., Woods, J. M., Kunkel, S. L., Connors, M. A., Harlow, L. A. *et al*. Regulation of angiogenesis by the C-X-C chemokines interleukin-8 and epithelial neutrophil activating peptide 78 in the rheumatoid joint. *Arthritis Rheum* 2001 Jan; **44**: 31–40.

47. Pablos, J. L., Santiago, B., Galindo, M., Torres, C., Brehmer, M. T., Blanco, F. J. *et al*. Synoviocyte-derived CXCL12 is displayed on endothelium and induces angiogenesis in rheumatoid arthritis. *J Immunol* 2003 Feb 15; **170**: 2147–52.

48. Hitchon, C., Wong, K., Ma, G., Reed, J., Lyttle, D., and El Gabalawy, H. Hypoxia-induced production of stromal cell-derived factor 1 (CXCL12) and vascular endothelial growth factor by synovial fibroblasts. *Arthritis Rheum* 2002 Oct; **46**: 2587–97.

49. Schioppa, T., Uranchimeg, B., Saccani, A., Biswas, S. K., Doni, A., Rapisarda, A. *et al*. Regulation of the chemokine receptor CXCR4 by hypoxia. *J Exp Med* 2003 Nov 3; **198**: 1391–402.

50. Koch, A. E. Angiogenesis as a target in rheumatoid arthritis. *Ann Rheum Dis* 2003 Nov; **62** (Suppl. 2): ii60–ii67.

51. Yamashita, A., Yonemitsu, Y., Okano, S., Nakagawa, K., Nakashima, Y., Irisa, T. *et al*. Fibroblast growth factor-2 determines severity of joint disease in adjuvant-induced arthritis in rats. *J Immunol* 2002 Jan 1; **168**: 450–7.

52. Johnson, B. A., Haines, G. K., Harlow, L. A., and Koch, A. E. Adhesion molecule expression in human synovial tissue. *Arthritis Rheum* 1993 Feb; **36**: 137–46.

53. Wilder, R. L. Integrin alpha V beta 3 as a target for treatment of rheumatoid arthritis and related rheumatic diseases. *Ann Rheum Dis* 2002 Nov; **61** (Suppl. 2): ii96–ii99.

54. Paleolog, E. M., Hunt, M., Elliott, M. J., Feldmann, M., Maini, R. N., and Woody, J. N. Deactivation of vascular endothelium by monoclonal anti-tumor necrosis factor alpha antibody in rheumatoid arthritis. *Arthritis Rheum* 1996 Jul; **39**: 1082–91.

55. Shahrara, S., Volin, M. V., Connors, M. A., Haines, G. K., and Koch, A. E. Differential expression of the angiogenic Tie receptor family in arthritic and normal synovial tissue. *Arthritis Res* 2002; **4**: 201–8.

56. Scott, B. B., Zaratin, P. F., Colombo, A., Hansbury, M. J., Winkler, J. D., and Jackson, J. R. Constitutive expression of angiopoietin-1 and -2 and modulation of their expression by inflammatory cytokines in rheumatoid arthritis synovial fibroblasts. *J Rheumatol* 2002 Feb; **29**: 230–9.

57. Woods, J. M., Katschke, K. J., Volin, M. V., Ruth, J. H., Woodruff, D. C., Amin, M. A. *et al*. IL-4 adenoviral gene therapy reduces inflammation, proinflammatory cytokines, vascularization, and bony destruction in rat adjuvant-induced arthritis. *J Immunol* 2001 Jan 15; **166**: 1214–22.

58. Woods, J. M., Tokuhira, M., Berry, J. C., Katschke, K. J., Jr., Kurata, H., Damergis, J. A. Jr. *et al*. Interleukin-4 adenoviral gene therapy reduces production of inflammatory cytokines and prostaglandin E2 by rheumatoid arthritis synovium ex vivo. *J Investig Med* 1999 Jul; **47**: 285–92.

59. Coxon, A., Bolon, B., Estrada, J., Kaufman, S., Scully, S., Rattan, A. *et al*. Inhibition of interleukin-1 but not tumor necrosis factor suppresses neovascularization in rat models of corneal angiogenesis and adjuvant arthritis. *Arthritis Rheum* 2002 Oct; **46**: 2604–12.

60. Claesson-Welsh, L., Welsh, M., Ito, N., Anand-Apte, B., Soker, S., Zetter, B. *et al*. Angiostatin induces endothelial cell apoptosis and activation of focal adhesion kinase independently of the integrin-binding motif RGD. *Proc Natl Acad Sci U S A* 1998 May 12; **95**: 5579–83.

61. Kim, J. M., Ho, S. H., Park, E. J., Hahn, W., Cho, H., Jeong, J. G. *et al*. Angiostatin gene transfer as an effective treatment strategy in murine collagen-induced arthritis. *Arthritis Rheum* 2002 Mar; **46**: 793–801.

62. Yin, G., Liu, W., An, P., Li, P., Ding, I., Planelles, V. *et al*. Endostatin gene transfer inhibits joint angiogenesis and pannus formation in inflammatory arthritis. *Mol Ther* 2002 May; **5** (5 Pt 1): 547–54.

63. Nagashima, M., Asano, G., and Yoshino, S. Imbalance in production between vascular endothelial growth factor and endostatin in patients with rheumatoid arthritis. *J Rheumatol* 2000 Oct; **27**: 2339–42.

64. Nagashima, M., Tanaka, H., Takahashi, H., Tachihara, A., Tanaka, K., Ishiwata, T. *et al*. Study of the mechanism involved in angiogenesis and synovial cell proliferation in human synovial tissues of patients with rheumatoid arthritis using SCID mice. *Lab Invest* 2002 Aug; **82**: 981–8.

65. De, B. M., Grossin, M., Weber, A. J., Chopin, M., Elbim, C., Pla, M. *et al*. Suppression of arthritis and protection from bone destruction by treatment with TNP-470/AGM-1470 in a transgenic mouse model of rheumatoid arthritis. *Arthritis Rheum* 2000 Sep; **43**: 2056–63.

66. Butcher, E. C. Leukocyte-endothelial cell recognition; three (or more) steps to specificity and diversity. *Cell* 1991 Dec 20; **67**: 1033–6.

67. Adams, D. H., and Shaw, S. Leucocyte-endothelial interactions and regulation of leucocyte migration. *Lancet* 1994 Apr 2; **343**(8901): 831–6.

68. Mempel, T. R., Scimone, M. L., Mora, J. R., and von Andrian, U. H. In vivo imaging of leukocyte trafficking in blood vessels and tissues. *Curr Opin Immunol* 2004 Aug; **16**: 406–17.

69. Engelhardt, B., and Wolburg, H. Mini-review: transendothelial migration of leukocytes. Through the front door or around the side of the house? *Eur J Immunol* 2004 Nov; **34**: 2955–63.

70. Lasky, L. A. Selectin-carbohydrate interactions and the initiation of the inflammatory response. *Annu Rev Biochem* 1995; **64**: 113–39.

71. Baggiolini, M. Chemokines and leukocyte traffic. *Nature* 1998 Apr 9; **392**(6676): 565–8.

72. Middleton, J., Patterson, A. M., Gardner, L., Schmutz, C., and Ashton, B. A. Leukocyte extravasation: chemokine transport and presentation by the endothelium. *Blood* 2002 Dec 1; **100**: 3853–60.

73. Hogg, N., Harvey, J., Cabanas, C., and Landis, R.C. Control of leukocyte integrin activation. *Am Rev Respir Dis* 1993 Dec; **148** (6 Pt 2): S55–S59.

74. Hogg, N., and Berlin, C. Structure and function of adhesion receptors in leukocyte trafficking. *Immunol Today* 1995 Jul; **16**: 327–30.

75. Friedl, P., Hegerfeldt, Y., and Tusch, M. Collective cell migration in morphogenesis and cancer. *Int J Dev Biol* 2004; **48**: 441–9.

76. Springer, T. A. Traffic signals for lymphocyte recirculation and leukocyte emigration: the multistep paradigm. *Cell* 1994 Jan 28; **76**: 301–14.

77. Chavakis, T., Preissner, K. T., and Santoso, S. Leukocyte transendothelial migration: JAMs add new pieces to the puzzle. *Thromb Haemost* 2003 Jan; **89**: 13–17.

78. Alon, R., Kassner, P. D., Carr, M. W., Finger, E. B., Hemler, M. E., and Springer, T. A. The integrin VLA-4 supports tethering and rolling in flow on VCAM-1. *J Cell Biol* 1995 Mar; **128**: 1243–53.

79. Berlin, C., Bargatze, R. F., Campbell, J. J., von Andrian, U. H., Szabo, M. C., Hasslen, S. R. *et al*. Alpha 4 integrins mediate lymphocyte attachment and rolling under physiologic flow. *Cell* 1995 Feb 10; **80**: 413–22.

80. Warnock, R. A., Askari, S., Butcher, E. C., and von Andrian UH. Molecular mechanisms of lymphocyte homing to peripheral lymph nodes. *J Exp Med* 1998 Jan 19; **187**: 205–16.

81. Sallusto, F., Lenig, D., Forster, R., Lipp, M., and Lanzavecchia, A. Two subsets of memory T lymphocytes with distinct homing potentials and effector functions. *Nature* 1999 Oct 14; **401**(6754): 708–12.

82. Campbell, D. J., and Butcher, E. C. Rapid acquisition of tissue-specific homing phenotypes by CD4(+) T cells activated in cutaneous or mucosal lymphoid tissues. *J Exp Med* 2002 Jan 7; **195**: 135–41.

83. Dudda, J. C., and Martin, S. F. Tissue targeting of T cells by DCs and microenvironments. *Trends Immunol* 2004 Aug; **25**: 417–21.

84. Romagnani, S. The Th1/Th2 paradigm. *Immunol Today* 1997 Jun; **18**: 263–6.

85. Buckley, C. D., Pilling, D., Lord, J. M., Akbar, A. N., Scheel-Toellner D., and Salmon, M. Fibroblasts regulate the switch from acute resolving to chronic persistent inflammation. *Trends Immunol* 2001 Apr; **22**: 199–204.

86. Von Andrian, U. H., and Mackay, C. R. T-cell function and migration: two sides of the same coin. *N Engl J Med* 2000 Oct 5; **343**: 1020–34.

87. Berlin, C., Berg, E. L., Briskin, M. J., Andrew, D. P., Kilshaw, P. J., Holzmann, B. *et al*. Alpha 4 beta 7 integrin mediates lymphocyte binding to the mucosal vascular addressin MAdCAM-1. *Cell* 1993 Jul 16; **74**: 185–95.

88. Buckley, C. D., and Simmons, D. L. Cell adhesion: a new target for therapy. *Mol Med Today* 1997 Oct; **3**: 449–56.

89. Arbones, M. L., Ord, D. C., Ley, K., Ratech, H., Maynard-Curry, C., Otten, G. *et al*. Lymphocyte homing and leukocyte rolling and migration are impaired in L-selectin-deficient mice. *Immunity* 1994 Jul; **1**: 247–60.

90. Wagner, N., Lohler, J., Kunkel, E. J., Ley, K., Leung, E., Krissansen, G. *et al*. Critical role for beta7 integrins in formation of the gut-associated lymphoid tissue. *Nature* 1996 Jul 25; **382**(6589): 366–70.

91. Fuhlbrigge, R. C., Kieffer, J. D., and Armerding, D., Kupper, T. S. Cutaneous lymphocyte antigen is a specialized form of PSGL-1 expressed on skin-homing T cells. *Nature* 1997 Oct 30; **389**(6654): 978–81.

92. Butcher, E. C., and Picker, L. J. Lymphocyte homing and home-ostasis. *Science* 1996 Apr 5; **272**(5258): 60–6.

93. Borges, E., Tietz, W., Steegmaier, M., Moll, T., Hallmann, R., Hamann, A. *et al*. P-selectin glycoprotein ligand-1 (PSGL-1) on T helper 1 but not on T helper 2 cells binds to P-selectin and supports migration into inflamed skin. *J Exp Med* 1997 Feb 3; **185**: 573–8.

94. Austrup, F., Vestweber, D., Borges, E., Lohning, M., Brauer, R., Herz, U. *et al*. P- and E-selectin mediate recruitment of T-helper-1 but not T-helper-2 cells into inflamed tissues. *Nature* 1997 Jan 2; **385**(6611): 81–3.

95. Sperandio, M., Smith, M. L., Forlow, S. B., Olson, T. S., Xia, L., McEver, R. P. *et al*. P-selectin glycoprotein ligand-1 mediates L-selectin-dependent leukocyte rolling in venules. *J Exp Med* 2003 May 19; **197**: 1355–63.

96. D'Apuzzo, M., Rolink, A., Loetscher, M., Hoxie, J. A., Clark-Lewis, I., Melchers, F. *et al*. The chemokine SDF-1, stromal cell-derived factor 1, attracts early stage B cell precursors via the chemokine receptor CXCR4. *Eur J Immunol* 1997 Jul; **27**: 1788–93.

97. Sallusto, F., Mackay, C. R., and Lanzavecchia, A. The role of chemokine receptors in primary, effector, and memory immune responses. *Annu Rev Immunol* 2000; **18**: 593–620.

98. Mora, J. R., Bono, M. R., Manjunath, N., Weninger, W., Cavanagh, L. L., Rosemblatt, M. *et al*. Selective imprinting of gut-homing T cells by Peyer's patch dendritic cells. *Nature* 2003 Jul 3; **424**(6944): 88–93.

99. Iwata, M., Hirakiyama, A., Eshima, Y., Kagechika, H., Kato, C., and Song, S.Y. Retinoic acid imprints gut-homing specificity on T cells. *Immunity* 2004 Oct; **21**: 527–38.

100. Dudda, J. C., Simon, J. C., and Martin, S. Dendritic cell immunization route determines CD8+ T cell trafficking to inflamed skin: role for tissue microenvironment and dendritic cells in establishment of T cell-homing subsets. *J Immunol* 2004 Jan 15; **172**: 857–63.

101. Schaerli, P., Ebert, L., Willimann, K., Blaser, A., Roos, R. S., Loetscher, P. *et al*. A skin-selective homing mechanism for human immune surveillance T Cells. *J Exp Med* 2004 May 3; **199**: 1265–75.

102. Kim, C. H., Rott, L., Kunkel, E. J., Genovese, M. C., Andrew, D. P., Wu, L. *et al*. Rules of chemokine receptor association with T cell polarization in vivo. *J Clin Invest* 2001 Nov; **108**: 1331–9.

103. Campbell, J. J., Haraldsen, G., Pan, J., Rottman, J., Qin, S., Ponath, P. *et al*. The chemokine receptor CCR4 in vascular recognition by cutaneous but not intestinal memory T cells. *Nature* 1999 Aug 19; **400**(6746): 776–80.

104. Homey, B., Alenius, H., Muller, A., Soto, H., Bowman, E. P., Yuan, W. *et al*. CCL27-CCR10 interactions regulate T cell-mediated skin inflammation. *Nat Med* 2002 Feb; **8**: 157–65.

105. Soler, D., Humphreys, T. L., Spinola, S. M., and Campbell, J. J. CCR4 versus CCR10 in human cutaneous TH lymphocyte trafficking. *Blood* 2003 Mar 1; **101**: 1677–82.

106. Loetscher, P., Pellegrino, A., Gong, J. H., Mattioli, I., Loetscher, M., Bardi, G. *et al*. The ligands of CXC chemokine receptor 3, I-TAC, Mig, and IP10, are natural antagonists for CCR3. *J Biol Chem* 2001 Feb 2; **276**: 2986–91.

107. Baggiolini, M. Chemokines in pathology and medicine. *J Intern Med* 2001 Aug; **250**: 91–104.

108. Hurst, S. M., Wilkinson, T. S., McLoughlin, R. M., Jones, S., Horiuchi, S., Yamamoto, N. *et al*. Il-6 and its soluble receptor orchestrate a temporal switch in the pattern of leukocyte recruitment seen during acute inflammation. *Immunity* 2001 Jun; **14**: 705–14.

109. Foxman, E. F., Campbell, J. J., and Butcher, E. C. Multistep navigation and the combinatorial control of leukocyte chemotaxis. *J Cell Biol* 1997 Dec 1; **139**: 1349–60.

110. Foxman, E. F., Kunkel, E. J., and Butcher, E. C. Integrating conflicting chemotactic signals: the role of memory in leukocyte navigation. *J Cell Biol* 1999 Nov 1; **147**: 577–88.

111. Sallusto, F., Schaerli, P., Loetscher, P., Schaniel, C., Lenig, D., Mackay, C. R. *et al*. Rapid and coordinated switch in chemokine receptor expression during dendritic cell maturation. *Eur J Immunol* 1998 Sep; **28**: 2760–9.

112. Dieu-Nosjean, M. C., Massacrier, C., Homey, B., Vanbervliet, B., Pin, J. J., Vicari, A. *et al*. Macrophage inflammatory protein 3alpha is expressed at inflamed epithelial surfaces and is the most potent chemokine known in attracting Langerhans cell precursors. *J Exp Med* 2000 Sep 4; **192**: 705–18.

113. Iwasaki, A., and Kelsall, B. L. Localization of distinct Peyer's patch dendritic cell subsets and their recruitment by chemokines macrophage inflammatory protein (MIP)-3alpha, MIP-3beta, and secondary lymphoid organ chemokine. *J Exp Med* 2000 Apr 17; **191**: 1381–94.

114. Luther, S. A., Bidgol, A., Hargreaves, D. C., Schmidt, A., Xu, Y., Paniyadi, J. *et al*. Differing activities of homeostatic chemokines CCL19, CCL21, and CXCL12 in lymphocyte and dendritic cell recruitment and lymphoid neogenesis. *J Immunol* 2002 Jul 1; **169**: 424–33.

115. Cyster, J. G. Chemokines and cell migration in secondary lymphoid organs. *Science* 1999 Dec 10; **286**(5447): 2098–102.

116. Ebisuno, Y., Tanaka, T., Kanemitsu, N., Kanda, H., Yamaguchi, K., Kaisho, T. *et al*. Cutting edge: the B cell chemokine CXC chemokine ligand 13/B lymphocyte chemoattractant is expressed in the high endothelial venules of lymph nodes and Peyer's patches and affects B cell trafficking across high endothelial venules. *J Immunol* 2003 Aug 15; **171**: 1642–6.

117. Campbell, D. J., Kim, C. H., and Butcher, E. C. Chemokines in the systemic organization of immunity. *Immunol Rev* 2003 Oct; **195**: 58–71.

118. Jalkanen, S., Steere, A. C., Fox, R. I., and Butcher, E. C. A distinct endothelial cell recognition system that controls lymphocyte traffic into inflamed synovium. *Science* 1986 Aug 1; **233**(4763): 556–8.

119. Salmi, M., Granfors, K., Leirisalo-Repo, M., Hamalainen, M., MacDermott, R., Leino, R. *et al*. Selective endothelial binding of interleukin-2-dependent human T-cell lines derived from different tissues. *Proc Natl Acad Sci U S A* 1992 Dec 1; **89**: 11436–40.

120. Lazarovits, A. I., and Karsh, J. Differential expression in rheumatoid synovium and synovial fluid of alpha 4 beta 7 integrin: a novel receptor for fibronectin and vascular cell adhesion molecule-1. *J Immunol* 1993 Dec 1; **151**: 6482–9.

121. Picker, L. J., Martin, R. J., Trumble, A., Newman, L. S., Collins, P. A, Bergstresser, P. R. *et al*. Differential expression of lymphocyte homing receptors by human memory/effector T cells in pulmonary versus cutaneous immune effector sites. *Eur J Immunol* 1994 Jun; **24**: 1269–77.

122. Sweeney, S. E., and Firestein, G. S. Rheumatoid arthritis: regulation of synovial inflammation. *Int J Biochem Cell Biol* 2004 Mar; **36**: 372–8.

123. Elices, M. J., Tsai, V., Strahl, D., Goel, A. S., Tollefson, V., Arrhenius, T. *et al*. Expression and functional significance of alternatively spliced CS1 fibronectin in rheumatoid arthritis microvasculature. *J Clin Invest* 1994 Jan; **93**: 405–16.

124. Gerlag, D. M., Borges, E., Tak, P. P., Ellerby, H. M., Bredese, D. E, Pasqualini, R. *et al*. Suppression of murine collagen-induced arthritis by targeted apoptosis of synovial neovasculature. *Arthritis Res* 2001; **3**: 357–61.

125. Lee, L., Buckley, C., Blades, M. C., Panayi, G., George, A. J., and Pitzalis, C. Identification of synovium-specific homing peptides by in vivo phage display selection. *Arthritis Rheum* 2002 Aug; **46**: 2109–20.

126. Pitzalis, C., Cauli, A., Pipitone, N., Smith, C., Barker, J., Marchesoni, A. *et al*. Cutaneous lymphocyte antigen-positive T lymphocytes preferentially migrate to the skin but not to the joint in psoriatic arthritis. *Arthritis Rheum* 1996 Jan; **39**: 137–45.

127. Szekanecz, Z., and Koch, A. E. Cell-cell interactions in synovitis: endothelial cells and immune cell migration. Arthritis Res 2000; **2**: 368–73.

128. McInnes, I. B., Leung, B. P., and Liew, F. Y. Cell-cell interactions in synovitis: interactions between T lymphocytes and synovial cells. *Arthritis Res* 2000; **2**: 374–8.

129. Dayer, J. M., and Burger, D. Cytokines and direct cell contact in synovitis: relevance to therapeutic intervention. *Arthritis Res* 1999; **1**: 17–20.

130. Koch, A. E., Kunkel, S. L., Burrows, J. C., Evanoff, H. L., Haines, G. K., Pope, R. M. *et al*. Synovial tissue macrophage as a source of the chemotactic cytokine IL-8. *J Immunol* 1991 Oct 1; **147**: 2187–95.

131. Koch, A. E., Kunkel, S. L., Harlow, L. A., Mazarakis, D. D., Haines, G. K., Burdick, M. D. *et al*. Epithelial neutrophil activating peptide-78: a novel chemotactic cytokine for neutrophils in arthritis. *J Clin Invest* 1994 Sep; **94**: 1012–18.

132. Koch, A. E., Kunkel, S. L., Shah, M. R., Hosaka, S., Halloran, M. M., Haines, G. K. *et al*. Growth-related gene product alpha: a chemotactic cytokine for neutrophils in rheumatoid arthritis. *J Immunol* 1995 Oct 1; **155**: 3660–6.

133. Patel, D. D., Zachariah, J. P., and Whichard, L. P. CXCR3 and CCR5 ligands in rheumatoid arthritis synovium. *Clin Immunol* 2001 Jan; **98**: 39–45.

134. Koch, A. E., Kunkel, S. L., Harlow, L. A., Johnson, B., Evanoff, H. L., Haines, G. K. *et al*. Enhanced production of monocyte chemoattractant protein-1 in rheumatoid arthritis. *J Clin Invest* 1992 Sep; **90**: 772–9.

135. Villiger, P. M., Terkeltaub, R., and Lotz, M. Production of monocyte chemoattractant protein-1 by inflamed synovial tissue and cultured synoviocytes. *J Immunol* 1992 Jul 15; **149**: 722–7.

136. Hosaka, S., Akahoshi, T., Wada, C., and Kondo, H. Expression of
the chemokine superfamily in rheumatoid arthritis. *Clin Exp
Immunol* 1994 Sep; **97**: 451–7.

137. Matsui, T., Akahoshi, T., Namai, R., Hashimoto, A., Kurihara, Y.,
Rana, M. *et al.* Selective recruitment of CCR6-expressing cells by
increased production of MIP-3 alpha in rheumatoid arthritis. *Clin
Exp Immunol* 2001 Jul; **125**: 155–61.

138. Chabaud, M., Page, G., and Miossec, P. Enhancing effect of IL-1,
IL-17, and TNF-alpha on macrophage inflammatory protein-3alpha
production in rheumatoid arthritis: regulation by soluble receptors
and Th2 cytokines. *J Immunol* 2001 Nov 15; **167**: 6015–20.

139. Ruth, J. H., Volin, M. V., Haines, G. K., III, Woodruff, D. C., Katschke,
K. J., Jr., Woods, J. M. *et al.* Fractalkine, a novel chemokine in rheumatoid arthritis and in rat adjuvant-induced arthritis. *Arthritis Rheum*
2001 Jul; **44**: 1568–81.

140. Katschke, K. J., Jr., Rottman, J. B., Ruth, J. H., Qin, S., Wu, L.,
LaRosa, G. *et al.* Differential expression of chemokine receptors on
peripheral blood, synovial fluid, and synovial tissue monocytes/
macrophages in rheumatoid arthritis. *Arthritis Rheum* 2001 May;
44: 1022–32.

141. Godessart, N., and Kunkel, S. L. Chemokines in autoimmune disease. *Curr Opin Immunol* 2001 Dec; **13**: 670–5.

142. Klimiuk, P. A., Sierakowski, S., Latosiewicz, R., Cylwik, J. P., Cylwik,
B., Skowronski, J. *et al.* Circulating tumour necrosis factor alpha and
soluble tumour necrosis factor receptors in patients with different patterns of rheumatoid synovitis. *Ann Rheum Dis* 2003 May; **62**: 472–5.

143. Klimiuk, P. A., Sierakowski, S., Latosiewicz, R., Cylwik, J. P.,
Cylwik, B., Skowronski, J. *et al.* Soluble adhesion molecules
(ICAM-1, VCAM-1, and E-selectin) and vascular endothelial
growth factor (VEGF) in patients with distinct variants of rheumatoid synovitis. *Ann Rheum Dis* 2002 Sep; **61**: 804–9.

144. Hjelmstrom, P., Fjell, J., Nakagawa, T., Sacca, R., Cuff, C. A., and
Ruddle, N. H. Lymphoid tissue homing chemokines are expressed
in chronic inflammation. *Am J Pathol* 2000 Apr; **156**: 1133–8.

145. Keffer, J., Probert, L., Cazlaris, H., Georgopoulos, S., Kaslaris, E.,
Kioussis, D. *et al.* Transgenic mice expressing human tumour necro-
sis factor: a predictive genetic model of arthritis. *EMBO J* 1991
Dec; **10**: 4025–31.

146. Luther, S. A., Lopez, T., Bai, W., Hanahan, D., and Cyster, J. G.
BLC expression in pancreatic islets causes B cell recruitment and
lymphotoxin-dependent lymphoid neogenesis. *Immunity* 2000
May; **12**: 471–81.

147. Fan, L., Reilly, C. R., Luo, Y., Dorf, M. E., and Lo, D. Cutting edge:
ectopic expression of the chemokine TCA4/SLC is sufficient to trigger
lymphoid neogenesis. *J Immunol* 2000 Apr 15; **164**: 3955–9.

148. Chen, S. C., Vassileva, G., Kinsley, D., Holzmann, S., Manfra, D.,
Wiekowski, M. T. *et al.* Ectopic expression of the murine
chemokines CCL21a and CCL21b induces the formation of lymph
node-like structures in pancreas, but not skin, of transgenic mice. *J
Immunol* 2002 Feb 1; **168**: 1001–8.

149. Luther, S. A., Tang, H. L., Hyman, P. L., Farr, A. G., and Cyster, J. G.
Coexpression of the chemokines ELC and SLC by T zone stromal
cells and deletion of the ELC gene in the plt/plt mouse. *Proc Natl
Acad Sci U S A* 2000 Nov 7; **97**: 12694–9.

150. Forster, R., Schubel, A., Breitfeld, D., Kremmer, E., Renner-Muller,
I., Wolf, E. *et al.* CCR7 coordinates the primary immune response
by establishing functional microenvironments in secondary lymphoid organs. *Cell* 1999 Oct 1; **99**: 23–33.

151. Weninger, W., Carlsen, H. S., Goodarzi, M., Moazed, F., Crowley,
M. A., Baekkevold E. S. *et al.* Naive T cell recruitment to nonlymphoid tissues: a role for endothelium-expressed CC chemokine lig-
and 21 in autoimmune disease and lymphoid neogenesis. *J Immunol*
2003 May 1; **170**: 4638–48.

152. Buckley, C. D., Amft, N., Bradfield, P. F., Pilling, D., Ross, E.,
Arenzana-Seisdedos, F. *et al.* Persistent induction of the chemokine
receptor CXCR4 by TGF-beta 1 on synovial T cells contributes to

their accumulation within the rheumatoid synovium. *J Immunol*
2000 Sep 15; **165**: 3423–9.

153. Nanki, T., Hayashida, K., E. l. Gabalawy, H. S., Suson, S., Shi, K.,
Girschick, H. J. *et al.* Stromal cell-derived factor-1-CXC chemokine
receptor 4 interactions play a central role in CD4+ T cell accumulation in rheumatoid arthritis synovium. *J Immunol* 2000 Dec 1; **165**:
6590–8.

154. Blades, M. C., Ingegnoli, F., Wheller, S. K., Manzo, A., Wahid, S.,
Panayi, G. S. *et al.* Stromal cell-derived factor 1 (CXCL12) induces
monocyte migration into human synovium transplanted onto SCID
Mice. *Arthritis Rheum* 2002 Mar; **46**: 824–36.

155. Burger, J. A., Zvaifler, N. J., Tsukada, N., Firestein, G. S., and
Kipps, T. J. Fibroblast-like synoviocytes support B-cell pseudoemperipolesis via a stromal cell-derived factor-1- and CD106
(VCAM-1)-dependent mechanism. *J Clin Invest* 2001 Feb; **107**:
305–15.

156. van der Pouw Kraan, T. C., van Gaalen, F. A., Kasperkovitz, P. V.,
Verbeet, N. L., Smeets, T. J., Kraan, M. C. *et al.* Rheumatoid arthritis is a heterogeneous disease: evidence for differences in the activation of the STAT-1 pathway between rheumatoid tissues. *Arthritis
Rheum* 2003 Aug; **48**: 2132–45.

157. Matthys, P., Hatse, S., Vermeire, K., Wuyts, A., Bridger, G., Henson,
G. W. *et al.* AMD3100, a potent and specific antagonist of the stromal cell-derived factor-1 chemokine receptor CXCR4, inhibits
autoimmune joint inflammation in IFN-gamma receptor-deficient
mice. *J Immunol* 2001 Oct 15; **167**: 4686–92.

158. Tamamura, H., Fujisawa, M., Hiramatsu, K., Mizumoto, M.,
Nakashima, H., Yamamoto, N. *et al.* Identification of a CXCR4
antagonist, a T140 analog, as an anti-rheumatoid arthritis agent.
FEBS Lett 2004 Jul 2; **569**: 99–104.

159. Burman, A., Haworth, O., Hardie, D. L., Amft, E. N., Siewert, C.,
Jackson, D. G. *et al.* A chemokine-dependent stromal induction
mechanism for aberrant lymphocyte accumulation and compromised lymphatic return in rheumatoid arthritis. *J Immunol* 2005
Feb 1; **174**: 1693–700.

160. Mould, A. P., Wheldon, L. A., Komoriya, A., Wayner, E. A.,
Yamada, K. M., and Humphries, M. J. Affinity chromatographic
isolation of the melanoma adhesion receptor for the IIICS region of
fibronectin and its identification as the integrin alpha 4 beta 1.
J Biol Chem 1990 Mar 5; **265**: 4020–4.

161. Wayner, E. A., Garcia-Pardo, A., Humphries, M. J., McDonald,
J. A., and Carter, W. G. Identification and characterization of the
T lymphocyte adhesion receptor for an alternative cell attachment
domain (CS-1) in plasma fibronectin. *J Cell Biol* 1989 Sep; **109**:
1321–30.

162. Ruoslahti, E., and Pierschbacher, M. D. New perspectives in cell
adhesion: RGD and integrins. *Science* 1987 Oct 23; **238**(4826):
491–7.

163. Ianaro, A., Cicala, C., Calignano, A., Koteliansky, V., Gotwals, P.,
Bucci, M. *et al.* Anti-very late antigen-1 monoclonal antibody
modulates the development of secondary lesion and T-cell
response in experimental arthritis. *Lab Invest* 2000 Jan; **80**:
73–80.

164. Matsuyama, T., Yamada, A., Kay, J., Yamada, K. M., Akiyama,
S. K., Schlossman, S. F. *et al.* Activation of CD4 cells by fibronectin
and anti-CD3 antibody: a synergistic effect mediated by the
VLA-5 fibronectin receptor complex. *J Exp Med* 1989 Oct 1;
170: 1133–48.

165. Shimizu, Y., van Seventer, G. A., Horgan, K. J., and Shaw, S.
Costimulation of proliferative responses of resting CD4+ T cells by
the interaction of VLA-4 and VLA-5 with fibronectin or VLA-6 with
laminin. *J Immunol* 1990 Jul 1; **145**: 59–67.

166. Yamada, A., Nikaido, T., Nojima, Y., Schlossman, S. F., and
Morimoto, C. Activation of human CD4 T lymphocytes: interaction
of fibronectin with VLA-5 receptor on CD4 cells induces the AP-1
transcription factor. *J Immunol* 1991 Jan 1; **146**: 53–6.

167. Jackson, D. G. The lymphatics revisited: new perspectives from the
hyaluronan receptor LYVE-1. *Trends Cardiovasc Med* 2003 Jan;
13: 1–7.

12 | Cytokine networks

William P. Arend and Cem Gabay

Concept of cytokine networks

Introduction

Cytokines are important mediators of inflammation and tissue destruction in rheumatoid arthritis (RA) (reviewed in Refs 1–10). These small molecules of cell–cell communication include interferons, interleukins, growth factors, colony-stimulating factors, chemotactic factors, and others. Cytokines seldom function alone but comprise a network of synergistic, complementary, antagonist, and inhibitory factors where the net biological response in a particular tissue depends upon the balance between the multiple factors present. These molecules may act on the same cell that produced them (autocrine effect) and adjacent cells in a tissue or organ (paracrine effect), or, less commonly, travel through the circulation to other organs (endocrine effect). In recent studies, some cytokines have been noted to remain in the synthesizing cell and influence function without ever being released, exhibiting so-called intracrine effects.

Cytokines are synthesized by a variety of cells in response to multiple stimuli, are usually secreted, and bind to specific receptors on target cells. Stimulatory cytokines, or agonists, then activate specific intracellular signal transduction pathways leading to gene transcription and production of new proteins. Inhibitory cytokines may compete with an agonist for receptor binding or may function by inducing antagonistic intracellular responses. A greater understanding of the presence and role of cytokines in rheumatoid synovitis has led to the development of new therapeutic approaches to this disease.

This chapter will first summarize the classification of cytokines, induction of cytokine production, and general mechanisms of cytokine effects. Subsequent sections will discuss the role and function of specific cytokines at different stages of RA, including in the initiation phase, in the establishment of chronic synovitis, and in the systemic manifestations of this disease. Lastly will be summarized the self-regulatory nature of the cytokine network, and new therapeutic agents for RA that interfere with cytokine production or effects.

Classification of cytokines and receptors

No classification scheme for cytokines is completely adequate as the primary function of a particular factor in rheumatoid synovitis may differ considerably from its originally described biological activity. One possible classification scheme would be to group cytokines by their interaction with a common receptor or family of receptors. However, to understand better the involvement of cytokines in the pathophysiology of rheumatoid arthritis, a more logical approach is to group cytokines around their main function in this disease process. In Table 12.1, cytokines are categorized as hematopoietic, growth and differentiation, immunoregulatory, pro-inflammatory, anti-inflammatory, and chemotactic factors. To complicate matters, a particular cytokine may exhibit functions under more than one of these categories, as detailed below.

Cytokine receptors can be grouped by structural similarities, with a further division by the use of identical molecules of signal transduction (Table 12.2). The IL-1 receptor family members share an immunoglobulin domain-like structure and the TNF receptor family is characterized by the presence of cysteine-rich regions that are repeated in the extracellular domains. Some common signal transduction molecules include: the IL-2Rγ chain, which is used by the receptors for IL-2, -4, -7, and -15; the gp130 molecule, which is utilized by the receptors for IL-6 and related

Table 12.1 Functional classification of cytokines

Family	Members
Hematopoietic	SCF, IL-3, IL-5, TPO, EPO, GM-CSF, G-CSF, M-CSF
Growth and differentiation	PDGF, EGF, FGF, IGF, TGF-β, VEGF
Immunoregulatory	TGF-β, IFN-γ, IL-2, 4, 7, 9–16, 18–21, 23–27
Pro-inflammatory	IL-1α and β, TNF-α, LT, IL-6, LIF, IL-17, IL-22
Anti-inflammatory	IL-1Ra, IL-4, IL-10, IL-13, IFN-β
Chemotactic	IL-8, MIP-1α, MIP-1β, MCP-1, 2, and 3, RANTES, GROα, ENA-78

Adapted from Refs X–X.
EGF, epidermal growth factor; ENA-78, epithelial neutrophil-activating peptide; EPO, erythropoietin; FGF, fibroblast growth factor; G-CSF, granulocyte colony-stimulating factor; GM-CSF, granulocyte–macrophage colony stimulating factor; GRO, growth-related gene product; IFN, interferon; IGF, insulin-like growth factor; IL, interleukin; IL-1Ra, interleukin-1 receptor antagonist; LIF, leukemia inhibitory factor; LT, lymphotoxin; MCP, monocyte chemoattractant protein; M-CSF, macrophage colony stimulating factor; MIP, macrophage inflammatory protein; PDGF, platelet-derived growth factor; RANTES, regulated upon activation T cell expressed and secreted; SCF, stem cell factor; TGF transforming growth factor; TNF, tumor necrosis factor; TPO, thrombopoietin; VEGF, vascular endothelial growth factor.

Table 12.2 Cytokine receptor families

Family	Members	Features
Interleukin-1	IL-1RI and II, IL-18R	Ig-like domains
Tumor necrosis factor domains	TNFRI and II, and many others	Cysteine-rich
Interferon	IFN-α, β, and γRs, IL-10R	Clustered 4 cysteines
Hematopoietin	IL-2R, IL-3R, IL-4R, IL-5R, IL-6R,	W-S-X-W-S motif in
	IL-7R, IL-9R, IL-13R, IL-15R, G-CSFR, GM-CSFR, EPOR, TPOR	C-terminus
Chemokine	IL-8RA and B, MCPR, MIPR	7-transmembrane-spanning regions
Tyrosine kinase	EGFR, PDGFR, FGFR, M-CSFR, SCFR	Tyrosine kinase

molecules (IL-11, oncostatin M, ciliary neurotrophic factor, and leukemia inhibitory factor); and the GM-CSF-β chain used by GM-CSF, IL-3, and IL-5. A common signaling domain is shared by IL-1RI, IL-18R, and the Toll-like receptors (TLRs), termed the TIR domain. The relative degree of activity of a particular cytokine may be influenced by which target cells express its receptor and by the level of receptor expression. Up-regulation or down-regulation of receptor expression may occur in response to other cytokines or to molecules released during inflammatory reactions.

Induction of cytokine production

Cytokine production can be induced by soluble factors or by direct cell–cell contact. Specific receptor binding by the soluble factor, or by membrane-bound cytokines and other molecules on inducing cells, leads to activation of signal transduction pathways in target cells. The major biological effect is stimulation of transcription, although regulation of cytokine production also can occur at other levels. The stimuli for cytokine production include other cytokines themselves, complement split products, bacterial products such as lipopolysaccharides (LPSs), viral proteins, immune complexes or adherent IgG, fragments of connective tissue proteins, insolubilized crystals, and acute phase proteins[8,9]. Many of these mechanisms may be operative in the rheumatoid synovium, as inducers of particular cytokines *in vivo* may be multiple and may vary with different stages of the disease process.

Many cytokines are found at high levels in rheumatoid synovial fluids, such as TNF-α, GM-CSF, IL-6, IL-10, IL-15, IL-18, and IL-1Ra. However, the synovial tissue may be a more important source of cytokines involved in pathophysiological processes. The cytokines that have been identified at the mRNA or protein level in rheumatoid synovial tissue are summarized in Table 12.3. The primary cells producing cytokines in the rheumatoid pannus are macrophages and fibroblasts, with smaller numbers of T cells possibly secreting immunoregulatory cytokines. The relative role of T cells and their products in the rheumatoid disease process is discussed in the other chapters in this text. However, the numbers of T cells present in the rheumatoid synovium may vary between patients and throughout the disease. Small numbers of T cells, with

Table 12.3 Cytokine and chemokine expression in rheumatoid synovial tissues

Cytokine	mRNA	Protein	Cells
IL-1α and β	Yes	Yes	Macrophages and fibroblasts
IL-1Ra	Yes	Yes	Macrophages and fibroblasts
TNF-α	Yes	Yes	Macrophages and fibroblasts
IL-6	Yes	Yes	Macrophages and fibroblasts
IL-7	Yes	Yes	Fibroblasts
IL-8	Yes	Yes	Macrophages and fibroblasts
IL-10	Yes	Yes	Macrophages and T cells
IL-12	Yes	Yes	Macrophages and dendritic cells
IL-15	Yes	Yes	Macrophages and fibroblasts
IL-16	Yes	Yes	Macrophages and fibroblasts
IL-17	Yes	Yes	T cells
IL-18	Yes	Yes	Macrophages
GM-CSF	Yes	Yes	Macrophages and fibroblasts
PDGF	Yes	Yes	Macrophages
FGF	Yes	Yes	Macrophages and fibroblasts
VEGF	Yes	Yes	Macrophages
TGF-β1	Yes	Yes	Macrophages and fibroblasts
LIF	Yes	Yes	Macrophages and fibroblasts
MCP-1	Yes	Yes	Macrophages and fibroblasts
MIP-1α	Yes	Yes	Macrophages and fibroblasts
RANTES	Yes	Yes	Macrophages and fibroblasts
ENA-78	Yes	Yes	Macrophages and fibroblasts
GRO-α	Yes	Yes	Macrophages
Fractalkine	Yes	Yes	Macrophages and fibroblasts

their secreted cytokines, may exert potent stimulatory or regulatory influences on immunological and inflammatory events.

General mechanisms of cytokine effects

After cytokine binding to specific cell membrane receptors, a series of signal transduction pathways are stimulated. These pathways consist of cascades of kinases with resultant activation and nuclear localization of specific transcription factors. The transcription factor families that have been identified as being activated in the rheumatoid synovium include AP-1 (c-*fos* and c-*jun*), nuclear factor (NF)-κB (p50 and p65), p38 MAPK (mitogen-activated protein kinase), and STAT (signal transducer and activator of transcription).

The p50 and p65 subunits of the NF-κB family have been identified in macrophages in both the lining and sublining regions of the rheumatoid synovium, as well as in endothelial cells[11,12]. In patients with early inflammatory arthritis, NF-κB components were localized at the cartilage-pannus junction, suggesting a role in mediating events of joint destruction[13]. The NF-κB family of transcription factors appears to be important in the induction of transcription of the genes for the pro-inflammatory cytokines TNF-α, IL-1, IL-6, and IL-8. Blocking NF-κB in rheumatoid synovial tissue *in vitro* inhibited the production of pro-inflammatory cytokines and of matrix metalloproteinases[14]. Furthermore, mice genetically deficient in NF-κB subunits were refractory to induction of acute and chronic models of inflammatory arthritis[15]. Recent reviews have summarized the role of NF-κB in rheumatoid synovitis and the possible approaches to inhibition of this pathway in the treatment of RA[16–18].

High DNA binding activity of activator protein (AP)-1 was found in the rheumatoid synovium in both synovial fibroblasts and macrophages, correlating with disease activity[13]. The mRNAs for the proto-oncogenes c-*fos* and c-*jun* also were localized to the synovial fibroblasts and correlated with the degree of AP-1 activation[19]. Collagenase production in rheumatoid synovitis may be due, in large part, to proteins of the AP-1 family, and the AP-1 pathway appears to be selectively activated during Fas-mediated apoptosis of rheumatoid synoviocytes[20]. Upstream kinases in the AP-1 pathway, such as c-Jun, JNK (c-Jun N-terminal kinase), and other kinases are present in rheumatoid synovial tissue fibroblasts[21]. Inhibition of the c-*fos*/AP-1 pathways through the administration of specific oligonucleotides led to a reduction in joint destruction in mice with collagen-induced arthritis (CIA), an experimental animal model with many similarities to RA[22].

Other kinase signal transduction pathways activated by cytokines in the rheumatoid synovium include the ERK (extracellular signal-regulated kinases) and p38 MAPK pathways[23]. Inhibition of the p38 MAPK pathway by small molecules is effective in treating animal models of inflammatory arthritis, and p38 inhibitors are currently being evaluated as therapeutic agents in RA[24].

A recent advance in the understanding of the cellular response to cytokines has been the identification and characterization of the Jak-STAT signal transduction pathway[3,25]. An early signaling event in response to many cytokines is activation of the receptor-associated protein tyrosine kinases of the Janus kinase (Jak) family. This leads to activation of STAT proteins, latent cytoplasmic transcription factors, which are then translocated to the nucleus with up-regulation of transcription of specific genes. STAT3 is constitutively produced by freshly isolated rheumatoid synovial fluid cells and these synovial fluids induced STAT3 expression in resting peripheral blood cells while inhibiting expression of STAT1[26]. This observation may suggest inhibition of Th1 cells with decreased IFN-γ production. However, it remains unclear whether an imbalance in the Jak-STAT pathway truly exists in RA and whether intervention in this pathway will be a feasible therapeutic approach.

Initiation of rheumatoid synovitis

Early events

Concepts about the mechanisms initiating rheumatoid synovitis have evolved over the past 20 years. The theory prevalent in the 1970s, that immune complexes were responsible for initiating the steps leading to inflammation and tissue destruction, was supported by early observations on the presence of these materials in rheumatoid synovial fluids and tissues[27]. The identification and initial characterization of T cells in the rheumatoid synovium in the 1980s, coupled with the description of the human leukocyte antigen (HLA)-DR4 association with the disease, led to the concept that T cells were responsible for the initiation of rheumatoid synovitis. The 'shared epitope' hypothesis implied that antigen-specific responses of CD4+ T cells were involved in initiation of

the disease process[28]. These stimulated T cells would then activate macrophages and other cells through both direct contact and the release of cytokines, leading to enzyme production and tissue destruction. However, extensive efforts over the past 20 years have failed to identify a common rheumatologic antigen or to find evidence for a restricted clonal response on the part of rheumatoid synovial T cells[29].

The T cell theory of the pathogenesis of RA has recently been modified to suggest that non-antigen-specific mechanisms may initiate a rather indolent disease process[30]. Antigen-specific T cell responses may be secondarily induced and are responsible for leading to an aggressive stage of perpetuation with intense inflammation, rapid tissue destruction, and extra-articular manifestations. This hypothesis states that early and episodic release of TNF-α and GM-CSF from macrophages and synovial fibroblasts may be induced by a variety of non-antigen-specific processes, such as minor trauma, infections, allergic reactions, vaccinations, or local immune complex deposition[30,31]. These cytokines then differentiate resident dendritic cells (DCs) into potent antigen-presenting cells (APCs), which may selectively present self-antigens for induction of specific T cell responses. The presence of the shared epitope on HLA-DR4 molecules may decrease the threshold for transformation of a mild reactive synovitis into a rapidly destructive synovial reaction by enhancing the presentation of self-antigens by DCs.

The purported key role of DCs in the initiation of rheumatoid synovitis, and the presumed importance of TNF-α and GM-CSF in this disease process, are supported by indirect evidence. Rheumatoid synovial fluids and tissue are enriched in differentiated myeloid DCs that abundantly express HLA-DR and -DQ molecules[32,33]. Furthermore, DCs stimulated with these cytokines up-regulate expression of the B7 family of costimulatory molecules (CD80/CD86), leading to enhanced antigen presentation. CD86 expression was observed on both macrophages and myeloid DCs in the rheumatoid synovium, with the latter cells present in both a perivascular distribution and within T cell clusters[34]. Autocrine or paracrine production of GM-CSF by DCs in the rheumatoid synovium may contribute to the enhanced expression of CD86. Whether these potent APCs are truly involved in the initiation of rheumatoid synovitis, and the nature of the self-antigens involved in the early presentation to T cells, remain to be established[35].

The localization and activation of DCs in the rheumatoid synovium have been further characterized in recent studies. Circulating myeloid DC precursors differentiate into mature cells after entry into the rheumatoid joint and express nuclear RelB, a component of the NF-κB signal transduction pathway[36]. These differentiated and activated DCs were closely associated with lymphocytes[37]. Myeloid DC precursors are also present in the rheumatoid synovial fluid and, under the influence of cytokines (GM-CSF, TNF-α, stem cell factor (SCF), and IL-4), mature into cells that preferentially activate a Th1 immune response[38]. Specific chemokines attract immature myeloid DCs into the lining layer of the rheumatoid synovium and mature cells into perivascular areas[39,40]. Lastly, collagen-pulsed mature DCs transferred into specific recipient mice induced arthritis through activation of responses in both the innate and adaptive immune systems[41]. Plasmacytoid DCs have also been localized in the rheumatoid synovium, primarily in a perivascular distribution[42]. Both types of DCs can induce production of IFN-γ, IL-10, and TNF-α by allogeneic T cells. These results suggest the possibility of treating RA through the administration of agents that selectively deplete DCs in the joint or inhibit their function.

The possible role of B lymphocytes in the pathogenesis of rheumatoid synovitis has been emphasized in recent studies[43–46]. B cells expressing membrane Ig with rheumatoid factor activity selectively and efficiently present immune complexes to T cells[47]. A hypothesis was formulated that self-perpetuating B lymphocytes may drive human autoimmune diseases such as RA[48]. A randomized, double-blind, controlled trial of a single course of a B cell-depleting monoclonal antibody, rituximab, in RA led to sustained remissions in patients who took maintenance methotrexate[49]. Further clinical trials are in progress. The possibility exists that B cell depletion is efficacious in RA not necessarily by preventing antigen presentation but by blocking the T cell-activating functions of B cells[50].

Mast cells have long been known to be present in the rheumatoid synovium with the results of recent studies suggesting an important role in pathophysiology[51–53]. The absence of mast cells prevented the development of inflammation in an immune complex-mediated experimental murine model of arthritis[54]. Mast cells are a source of IL-1 and TNF-α, and immune complexes may stimulate release of these pro-inflammatory cytokines in rheumatoid synovitis.

A possible primary role for TNF-α, GM-CSF, and IL-1 in RA was suggested by the results of early studies on rheumatoid synovial fluids and cultured synovial tissue cells. The high levels of IL-1 produced by synovial cell cultures were inhibited by antibodies to TNF-α, suggesting that TNF-α may be a major inducer of IL-1 in these cells[55]. GM-CSF production by cultured rheumatoid synovial tissue cells also was inhibited by antibodies to TNF-α[56]. High levels of TNF-α (summarized in Refs 1 and 2) and of GM-CSF[57–60] were present in rheumatoid synovial fluids and tissues. IL-1 and TNF-α both induced GM-CSF production in rheumatoid synovial fibroblasts and macrophages[60]. Mice transgenic for human TNF-α expression spontaneously developed a chronic inflammatory polyarthritis[61]. However, a neutralizing antibody to the murine IL-1R type I completely prevented the development of arthritis in the TNF-α transgenic mice, suggesting that the pathogenic effects of TNF-α were mediated through the induction of IL-1[62]. These and other observations on the presence and role of IL-1 and TNF-α in RA[1,2] have led to the development of therapeutic approaches designed to prevent the effects of these cytokines, as discussed below.

Lastly, viral or bacterial infections have long been thought to play an important role in the initiation or perpetuation of rheumatoid synovitis. However, numerous efforts to culture infectious agents from rheumatoid synovial fluid or tissue, or to identify the specific presence of viral or bacterial DNA, have led to inconclusive results. A recent hypothesis has developed an argument for a role for normal intestinal microflora combined with a genetic predisposition in the pathogenesis of RA[63]. These resident bacteria may function as an adjuvant, stimulating the innate immune system in an antigen-non-specific manner to release IL-1, TNF-α, IL-18 and other innate immune cytokines.

Role of adhesion molecules and chemokines in induction of acute inflammation

Rheumatoid synovitis may be initiated by multiple antigen-specific or non-specific mechanisms, probably operating during an early, preclinical stage of the disease. However, the earliest clinical manifestations of joint swelling, erythema, and pain are due to common inflammatory mechanisms largely driven by cytokines released from synovial macrophages and fibroblasts. Up-regulation of adhesion molecule expression on endothelial cells in the postcapillary venules, and on leukocytes with recruitment and migration of these cells into the synovium, are the most important events in this stage of acute inflammation in the joint.

The three major categories of adhesion molecules are the selectins, present primarily on leukocytes and endothelial cells, the integrins, found on a variety of blood and tissue cells, and the Ig superfamily, identified on circulating white blood cells, fibroblasts, and endothelial and epithelial cells[64–66]. IL-1 and TNF-α are the major cytokines responsible for induction of expression of these adhesion molecules on endothelial cells, macrophages, dendritic cells, synovial fibroblasts, lymphocytes, and neutrophils, although IL-8 and GM-CSF also play important roles. The multiple roles for adhesion molecules in the pathophysiology of RA include:

(1) attachment of inflammatory cells in the postcapillary venule to endothelial cells;

(2) migration of these cells across the endothelium into the synovium;

(3) perivascular interactions between the inflammatory and immune cells;

(4) retention of cells in the synovium;

(5) enhancement of antigen presentation;

(6) facilitation of angiogenesis; and

(7) shedding of soluble adhesion molecules into the synovial fluid or serum.

Recognition of the importance of adhesion molecules in rheumatoid synovitis has led to experimental therapeutic approaches designed to block their expression.

Chemokines are chemotactic 8–10 kD proteins that share between 20 and 70% homology[67–70]. Over 40 chemokines have been identified and have been classified into at least four families. The α and β families contain four cysteines and include most of the common chemokines. The α or CXC chemokines possess one amino acid between the first two cysteine residues, whereas the first two cysteine residues are adjacent in the β or CC chemokines[69]. The CXC family can be divided into two subgroups: those factors containing the sequence glutamic acid-leucine-arginine near the N terminus include IL-8 and other factors chemotactic for neutrophils, whereas CXC chemokines without this sequence act on lymphocytes. The CC chemokines also can be divided into two subgroups but all of these factors act to attract monocytes, eosinophils, basophils, and lymphocytes, although with varying

Table 12.4　Chemokines found in the synovial fluids of patients with rheumatoid arthritis

Chemokine	Type	Receptor	Responsive inflammatory cells	Reference
IL-8 (CXCL8)	CXC	CXCR1, 2	Neutrophils, T cells	71–73
ENA-78 (CXCL5)	CXC	CXCR2	Neutrophils	74
GRO-α (CXCL1)	CXC	CXCR2	Neutrophils	75
MCAF (MCP-1) (CCL2)	CC	CCR2	Monocytes, T cells	76–79
MIP-1α (CCL3)	CC	CCR1, 5	Neutrophils, macrophages, T cells	80
RANTES (CCL5)	CC	CCR1, 3, 5	Macrophages, T cells	81
Fractalkine (CX₃CL1)	CX₃C	CX₃CR1	Macrophages	82

ENA, epithelial neutrophil-activating peptide; GRO, growth-related gene product; MCAF, monocyte-chemotactic and -activating factor.

selectivity. Chemokines induce cell migration and activation by binding to a complex family of specific G protein-coupled receptors on target cells[69,70].

The chemokines found in the synovial fluids of patients with RA are summarized in Table 12.4[70]. These factors function to induce the infiltration of monocytes, neutrophils, and T cells into the synovial fluid and tissue, and are also capable of activating these cells to release various secretory products. Chemokines found in the rheumatoid joint are synthesized by both macrophages and synovial fibroblasts in response to stimulation by cytokines such as IL-1, IL-17, and TNF-α[83]. Although these factors are primarily pro-inflammatory, some chemokines may selectively attract T cell subsets into the joint, possibly contributing to the initiation or maintenance of a local immune response. IL-8 is perhaps the major chemokine in rheumatoid arthritis and intervention with its production or effects is a potential therapeutic approach to RA and other acute inflammatory diseases[84,85].

Chemokine receptors are also expressed in the rheumatoid synovium[70]. Small molecule inhibitors of specific chemokine receptors have been proposed as a novel therapeutic approach to RA[86]. CIA in rats was inhibited by administration of a monoclonal antibody to MCP-1 (CCL2)[87]. CIA in mice was inhibited by administration of an inactive form of RANTES (CCL5)[88]; a non-peptide antagonist of CCR5, which blocks binding of CCL5 and CCL3 (MIP-1α)[89]; and treatment with neutralizing antibodies to CXCL13[90]. In a similar fashion, CIA in rhesus monkeys was inhibited by a small molecular weight antagonist of CCR5[91]. A polyclonal antibody to CCL5 also blocked adjuvant-induced arthritis in rats[92], and a non-peptide antagonist of CXCR2 blocked the development of acute and chronic arthritis in two experimental models of inflammatory arthritis in rabbits[93]. A potent and selective CCR1 antagonist has been developed which competitively blocks the binding of CCL3 and CCL5 to CCR1 *in vitro*[94]. This molecule inhibited 90% of the monocyte chemotactic activity present in 11/15 rheumatoid synovial fluid samples. Paradoxically, rheumatoid factor production and CIA were

enhanced in mice rendered genetically deficient in CCR2[95]. No alteration in arthritis was observed in mice lacking CCR5. Thus, CCR2 may serve a protective role in RA with other chemokine receptors mediating monocyte egress into inflamed joints. Inhibitors of chemokines or their receptors are currently being evaluated in clinical trials in patients with RA.

Establishment of chronic synovitis

Cytokine patterns in rheumatoid synovitis

Numerous studies over the past 15 years have characterized the cytokines found in rheumatoid synovial fluids, or produced by peripheral blood mononuclear cells, in an effort to understand better the role of different cytokines in the pathophysiology of joint inflammation and destruction. However, of greater importance is the pattern of cytokines produced by synovial tissue cells since the damage to cartilage, bone, and periarticular structures is mediated primarily by cells in the proliferative synovium and adjacent cartilage. Early studies failed to identify the mRNA for either IL-2 or IL-3 in the rheumatoid synovium, although M-CSF mRNA was abundantly present[96]. A comprehensive survey for the presence of mRNAs for various cytokines in rheumatoid synovium was then carried out using *in situ* hybridization[97]. The most prominent cytokine mRNAs found were the macrophage and fibroblast products IL-6, IL-1β, TNF-α, GM-CSF, and TGF-β, whereas IFN-γ was only weakly present. These observations led to the hypothesis that T cells were less important to chronic rheumatoid synovitis[98], although this interpretation remains controversial[99].

Newer studies using highly sensitive techniques have examined the cytokine profile in relationship to the duration of the synovitis and the type of histological changes present in the rheumatoid synovium. IL-2 and IFN-γ mRNA were detected in many rheumatoid synovia using the polymerase chain reaction (PCR) method, suggesting that this was primarily a Th1 disease[100]. However, the levels of Th1 cytokines in the rheumatoid joint are far lower than in other chronic Th1 diseases, such as tuberculous pleuritis. A more detailed analysis using quantitative nested PCR examined synovial specimens from patients with early synovitis (<12 months in duration) and found abundant mRNA for IL-10, IL-15, IL-1β, TNF-α, and IFN-γ[101]. Lesser amounts of mRNA for IL-6 and IL-12 were present, with absent mRNA for IL-4 and IL-13. These results indicated that macrophage-derived and some Th1 cytokine mRNAs predominated in early rheumatoid synovitis, with decreased levels present in the tissue of patients treated with prednisone or disease-modifying drugs. Other studies suggested that Th1 cytokine production predominated in the peripheral blood and synovial fluid cells of patients with recent-onset synovitis, whereas a Th2 pattern was present in those with chronic arthritis[102].

Examination of the synovial biopsies from 21 patients with active RA led to a classification into three distinct histological subsets[103]. Synovial specimens exhibiting diffuse lymphoid infiltrates without further microarrangement demonstrated low level transcription of IFN-γ, IL-4, IL-1β and TNF-α, as determined by semiquantitative PCR. In contrast, synovia exhibiting lymphoid follicles with germinal center formation demonstrated IFN-γ and IL-10 mRNA, but not IL-4. Lastly, granulomatous synovitis, the least common pattern, was characterized by high transcription of IFN-γ, IL-4, IL-1β, and TNF-α, clearly different from the other histological patterns. Diffuse synovitis was present primarily in patients with mild seronegative RA, whereas granulomatous synovitis was observed in rheumatoid factor-positive patients with nodules. Thus, diffuse synovitis in this study corresponded with a pattern of Th0 cytokines, follicular synovitis with a Th1 pattern, and granulomatous synovitis with a mixed Th1/Th2 pattern[103].

In a recent study, cytokine expression was determined in synovial tissue obtained at arthroscopy in RA patients with active inflammation, and at the time of total joint replacement in destroyed joints[104]. Synovial tissue from arthroscopy exhibited the abundant presence of TNF-α, IL-6, and VEGF, while IL-1β predominated in the surgical samples. This result may suggest the importance of IL-1 in cartilage and bone damage in RA, an observation supported by the results of studies in experimental animal models of inflammatory arthritis[105].

Two additional cytokines recently described in the rheumatoid synovium are MIF (macrophage inhibition factor) and HMGB-1 (high mobility group box chromosomal protein 1). MIF is produced by activated T cells, macrophages, and synovial fibroblasts, and may act as a proximal cytokine inducing the production of TNF-α[106]. HMGB-1 is a nuclear protein that binds DNA but is also released from cells and functions like a cytokine to stimulate macrophages[107]. HMGB-1 was expressed in the rheumatoid synovium in nuclear, cytoplasmic, and extracellular distributions, and stimulated production of TNF-α, IL-1β, and IL-6 from synovial fibroblasts[108,109]. Thus, both MIF and HMGB-1, similar to IL-18, may be upstream cytokines in the rheumatoid synovium and their inhibition may represent a new therapeutic approach to RA.

These observations emphasize a probable heterogeneity in the pathophysiological mechanisms of rheumatoid synovitis, making the general paradigm of a Th1 predominance being harmful and Th2 helpful poorly applicable. The recognition of different subsets of RA patients, either by clinical criteria or the pattern of synovial histopathology, indicates that the therapeutic effects of cytokines or their inhibitors may vary depending on the stage of disease, and the localization and timing of their administration[110]. Recognizing this heterogeneity, the following sections will summarize the effects of cytokines on different cells and pathological events in chronic rheumatoid synovitis.

Immune cell differentiation

The synovium of patients with RA is populated with CD4+ T cells that express surface characteristics of mature memory cells (CD45RO+). Most synovial T cells carry the α/β receptor complex but some are γ/δ positive. Numerous cytokines potentially influence and modulate the activity of rheumatoid synovial T cells. The major T cell-activating cytokine IL-2 was present in only a few rheumatoid synovial fluids. High levels of soluble IL-2R were detected in both the serum and synovial fluids of patients

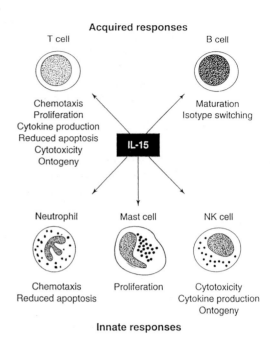

Fig. 12.1 Biological effects of IL-15 with potential relevance to rheumatoid arthritis synovitis. NK, natural killer. (Reproduced with permission from Ref. 112.)

with RA, probably secondary to release by T cells[111]. However, soluble IL-2R binds to IL-2 with low affinity and probably does not inhibit IL-2 function *in vivo*. The relative absence of IFN-γ and IL-2 in the rheumatoid synovium makes it unlikely that these cytokines are responsible for the influx of circulating T cells.

The recent description and characterization of IL-15 indicate that this cytokine may play a pivotal role in inflammatory events in the rheumatoid synovium (Fig. 12.1)[112]. IL-15 is produced by both macrophages and fibroblasts in the lining layer of the rheumatoid synovium, and in lesser amount by T cells and dendritic cells, and is found in modest concentrations in the synovial fluid[113]. IL-15 exhibits many functional similarities to IL-2, and binds to a receptor that possesses a unique α chain but utilizes the β and γ chains of the IL-2R to transduce signals in target cells. IL-15 was chemotactic for CD45RO+ T cells, and activated these cells in the rheumatoid synovium[113]. Furthermore, IL-15 directly stimulated TNF-α production in synovial T cells, and indirectly led to enhanced TNF-α production by macrophages through direct contact of these cells with IL-15-stimulated T cells[114]. The early activation molecule CD69, as well as the adhesion molecules lymphocyte function-associated antigen (LFA)-1 and intercellular adhesion molecule (ICAM)-1, were all involved in the interactions between T cells and macrophages. IL-2 had no effect in this system. IL-15 also functioned as an autocrine regulator of macrophage pro-inflammatory cytokine production, with enhanced secretion of IL-1, TNF-α, and IL-6 observed at very low concentrations of IL-15[115]. Furthermore, IL-15 was produced by endothelial cells and enhanced the migration of T cells across endothelial cells by activating the binding capacity of LFA-1 and inducing the expression of CD69[116].

It is hypothesized that IL-15 may preferentially activate T cells that have recently encountered exogenous antigens *in vivo*, or that exhibit a suboptimal response to autologous major histocompatibility complex (MHC) class II molecules[117]. In individuals with susceptible human leukocyte antigen (HLA) types who develop transient joint inflammation in response to non-specific stimuli, IL-15 may promote the adhesion and activation of memory T cells and macrophages within the synovium. Thus, IL-15 may be important in the transformation of a mild reactive synovitis into an aggressive autoimmmune reaction. The mechanisms that stimulate IL-15 production in the rheumatoid synovium are unclear, but mRNA levels for this molecule exceed production of the protein. In fact, IL-15 production is regulated primarily post-transcriptionally at the levels of translation and intracellular protein trafficking[118]. Administration of a soluble IL-15 receptor α chain prevented the development of CIA in mice, suggesting that IL-15 antagonists may be of value in treating patients with RA[119].

Other T cell cytokines may play roles in the rheumatoid synovium. The suppressed production of IL-2 and IFN-γ by synovial T cells may be secondary to the abundant presence of IL-10 in the rheumatoid synovial fluid and tissue. In addition, this cytokine exhibits anti-inflammatory effects on synovial macrophages, illustrating the self-regulatory nature of the cytokine network in this disease. Lastly, IL-12 is produced by macrophages and dendritic cells, and promotes a Th1 phenotype by enhancing IFN-γ production by CD4+ T cells and natural killer (NK) cells. However, IL-12 exhibited a dual role in CIA in mice, stimulating early arthritis expression while suppressing the chronic phase of the disease[120]. Thus, as summarized above, numerous cytokines of T cell origin or acting on T cells are present in the rheumatoid synovium with a resultant heterogeneous pattern of effects depending on many factors, including the stage of the disease.

The specific antigens that activate T cells in the rheumatoid synovium, presented in the context of class II MHC, remain unknown but may vary in type and relative importance with the stage of the disease process. In the initiation phase of synovitis, ubiquitous viral and bacterial products, or even the HLA-DR4 shared epitope itself, may be responsible. However, in chronic rheumatoid synovitis T cells may be stimulated by altered self-components such as proteoglycan and collagen fragments. Thus, once the disease becomes clinically active, the inducing agents may no longer be present and the T cells are driven by products of tissue destruction. The relative role of T cells versus autonomous macrophage and fibroblast function in the perpetuation of chronic rheumatoid synovitis is discussed briefly below, as well as in other chapters in this text.

Inflammatory cell maturation

Inflammatory cells that are involved in pathophysiological events in rheumatoid synovitis include polymorphonuclear leukocytes (neutrophils), monocytes, and macrophages. Neutrophils predominate in the synovial fluids of patients with chronic RA, and are found in the synovial tissue primarily when necrosis or secondary infection is present. Neutrophils can respond to stimulation by GM-CSF or TNF-α with secretion of small amounts of the pro-inflammatory cytokines IL-1β, TNF-α? IL-8, and GM-CSF, and of the anti-inflammatory cytokine IL-1Ra. However,

the large numbers of neutrophils that may be found in rheumatoid synovial fluids make these cells a potentially important source of IL-8 and IL-1Ra[121].

Monocytes and macrophages in the rheumatoid synovium are derived from bone marrow precursors with a constant renewal through the peripheral blood. These cells do not recirculate but are differentiated and activated in the synovium to assume new phenotypic characteristics. For example, under the influence of GM-CSF, TNF-α, IFN-γ, and IL-4, precursor myeloid cells and monocytes differentiate into potent antigen-presenting DCs. DCs not only activate lymphocytes, but may also contribute to control of immune responses through tolerizing T cells to self-antigens. The role and function of macrophages in the rheumatoid synovium have been reviewed[122]. These cells may play diverse roles in all stages of rheumatoid synovitis from initiation through chronic inflammation and tissue destruction. One of the prime functions of macrophages is phagocytosis and these cells may be important sources of bacterial and viral peptides in the non-specific process of initiation of synovitis discussed above. Macrophages are influenced by the cytokine environment in the rheumatoid synovium in multiple ways.

One of the major roles of macrophages in the pathophysiology of rheumatoid synovitis is as a source of the pro-inflammatory cytokines IL-1 and TNF-α[1,2]. Production of these cytokines may be induced in macrophages by multiple agents, including direct contact with lymphocytes, lymphocyte products, immune complexes, bacterial and viral products, and by products of damaged cartilage such as collagen fragments. IL-1 and TNF-α are thought to be key molecules in the mechanisms of tissue destruction through the induction of neutral metalloproteinase synthesis and secretion by transformed fibroblasts in the synovium and chondrocytes in the adjacent articular cartilage. In addition, these cytokines exert a net catabolic effect on articular cartilage by decreasing the production of proteoglycans and type II collagen by chondrocytes. Macrophages at the pannus-cartilage interface are also an important source of these tissue-damaging enzymes[122]. IL-1 has a catabolic effect on bone primarily through the maturation and activation of osteoclasts. This effect may be mediated in part by up-regulating the expression of receptor activator of nuclear factor κB ligand (RANKL), a member of the TNF family of cytokines that plays a major role in osteoclast maturation and activation. In addition, IL-1 induces osteoclast activation through a RANKL-independent pathway. IL-1 mediates the osteoclastogenic effect of TNF-α by enhancing the expression of RANKL by stromal cells and directly stimulating differentiation of osteoclast precursors[123]. In addition, synovial macrophages are the major source of platelet-derived growth factor (PDGF) and fibroblast growth factor (FGF), which have stimulatory effects on fibroblasts, and of GM-CSF and chemokines. Many of the current disease-modifying drugs may be effective in RA in large part because of their inhibitory effects on macrophage function[122].

IL-18 belongs to the IL-1 family of cytokines. As IL-1β, IL-18 is produced by macrophages and other cells as a propeptide that is subsequently cleaved by caspase-1 or IL-1β-converting enzyme to generate active mature IL-18. IL-18, which was originally identified as a potent IFN-γ inducing factor, acts in synergy with IL-12 to enhance IFN-γ gene expression. IL-18 is thus a cytokine that together with IL-12 promotes differentiation of Th1 cells.

However, in addition to sharing with IL-12 the property of induction of IFN-γ production, IL-18 may exhibit pro-inflammatory consequences through stimulating TNF-α production in CD4+ T cells and NK cells, with subsequent enhanced production of IL-1β and IL-8 from monocytes. Recently, the presence of macrophage-derived IL-18 was demonstrated in RA synovium and synovial fluid. IL-18 binding protein (IL-18BP) is a soluble receptor that binds IL-18 and interferes with its interaction with cell surface receptors. Human IL-18BP is expressed as four different isoforms (IL-18BPa to d) by mRNA splicing. IL-18a and c inhibit IL-18 activity at a molar excess of 2. IL-18 administration to mice with CIA facilitated the development of an erosive, inflammatory arthritis, suggesting that IL-18 can be pro-inflammatory *in vivo*[124]. In contrast, mice rendered genetically deficient in IL-18 have a reduced frequency and severity of CIA. The administration of anti-IL-18 antibodies or IL-18BP significantly reduced the clinical severity and cartilage destruction of CIA[125]. The mechanisms of mIL-18BP inhibition of CIA include reductions in cell-mediated and humoral immunity to collagen as well as decreases in production of pro-inflammatory cytokines in the spleen and joints[126].

TGF-β exerts both stimulating and inhibitory effects on monocyte/macrophage functions. TGF-β is chemotactic for monocytes and may contribute to the influx of these cells into the inflamed synovium. TGF-β stimulation of synoviocytes increases CCL2/MCP-1 production, providing an indirect mechanism for monocyte recruitment. Other potentially pro-inflammatory monocyte functions that are activated by TGF-β include induction of the third receptor for the constant region of Ig (FcγRIII, CD16), which can trigger release of superoxide anion. This cytokine also stimulates macrophage production of IL-1Ra in an autocrine and paracrine fashion through the synthesis and release of IL-1β. In addition, TGF-β pretreatment of the cells inhibited LPS-stimulated production of IL-1 and TNF-α. In contrast, cytokine production was not inhibited if the addition of TGF-β occurred after the inducing stimulus. TGF-β1 deficient mice exhibit a pronounced mononuclear leukocyte infiltration in multiple organs followed by cachexia and eventually death[127].

Monocyte differentiation is enhanced by GM-CSF, leading to increased HLA-DR expression, whereas macrophage activation occurs secondary to IFN-γ. However, given the paucity of IFN-γ in the rheumatoid synovium, it is likely that these cells are activated, at least in part, by direct contact with lymphocytes[128]. In fact, direct contact with Th1 cells preferentially induced IL-β production in human monocytes whereas Th2 cells primarily stimulated IL-1Ra synthesis. The cytokines IL-4, IL-10, and IL-13 all display anti-inflammatory effects through inhibition of IL-1 and TNF-α and enhancement of IL-1Ra production in macrophages.

T cell-derived cytokines, including IL-7 and IL-17, can stimulate monocyte/macrophage activities and participate in the pathogenesis of arthritis. Several findings indicate that IL-7 can be considered as a pro-inflammatory cytokine. Serum levels of IL-7 were significantly higher in patients with systemic juvenile idiopathic arthritis or RA[129,130]. Freshly isolated cells from RA synovium spontaneously expressed IL-7 mRNA and protein to greater amounts than cells from osteoarthritis patients. IL-7 induced the production of TNF-α, IL-1β, IL-6, and IL-8 by monocytes/macrophages[131]. IL-7 stimulated TNF-α production by synovial fluid mononuclear cells. Synovial fluid CD4+ T cells express IL-7Rα chain receptor at their cell surface and IL-7 stimulated the production of TNF-α and IFN-γ by CD4+ T cells[21]. IL-7 mRNA was expressed in RA cartilage[132]. IL-7 contributes also to bone loss and possibly to the development of joint erosions by the induction of RANKL from T cells[133].

IL-17 is a recently characterized Th1 cytokine that may play an important pro-inflammatory role in the rheumatoid synovium. IL-17 stimulated the production of IL-1β and TNF-α, as well as that of IL-6, IL-10, IL-12, and IL-1Ra, by human macrophages. In synovial fibroblasts, IL-17 stimulated the production of IL-6, IL-8, LIF, and PGE2. Although IL-1 was more potent in stimulating these responses, IL-17 could act in synergy with IL-1 and TNF-α to induce the production of cytokines and matrix metalloproteinases (MMPs)[134]. IL-17 stimulated the migration of DCs and the recruitment of T cells by inducing the production of macrophage inflammatory protein 3α (MIP-3α, also termed CCL20)[135]. IL-17 also contributed to the development of articular damage by inducing the production of MMP-3 and by decreasing the synthesis of proteoglycans by articular chondrocytes[136]. The intra-articular administration of IL-17 in normal mouse joints induced cartilage degradation. IL-17 stimulated osteoclastogenesis by increasing the expression of RANKL. Overexpression of IL-17 in the joints of mice with CIA promoted severe bone destruction accompanied by marked osteoclast activity and RANKL expression[137]. These results establish an important link between CD4+ T cells in the synovium and the development of articular inflammation with subsequent tissue damage.

Fibroblast proliferation and activation

Fibroblast-like synoviocytes play important roles at multiple levels in the pathophysiology of rheumatoid synovitis[138]. The cytokine networks in this inflamed tissue greatly influence the phenotype and functions of these cells. Both IL-1 and TNF-α induce adhesion molecule expression on synovial fibroblasts, enhancing the migration of inflammatory cells from the circulation into the joint. Under the local influence of FGF, PDGF, and other cytokines, synovial fibroblasts develop characteristics of transformed cells, such as adherence-independent growth, expression of oncogenes, and loss of contact inhibition. Furthermore, these cells are the major source in the synovium of IL-6 and angiogenic factors such as FGF, PDGF and VEGF, as well as of IL-8 and GM-CSF which may further activate macrophages. Thus, fibroblasts in the rheumatoid synovium exhibit autocrine and paracrine stimulatory interactions with nearby fibroblasts, as well as with macrophages (Fig. 12.2). These cellular interactions are mediated through cytokines and may lead to autonomous perpetuation of inflammation and tissue destruction.

A distinctive and unusual cell found at the pannus-cartilage junction in the rheumatoid synovitis has been termed 'pannocyte'. These cells exhibit characteristics of both fibroblasts and chondrocytes. Cytokine effects on pannocytes include PDGF- and TGF-β-induced proliferation and decreased growth in response to IL-1, characteristics resembling chondrocytes. However, like fibroblasts the pannocytes demonstrated constitutive production

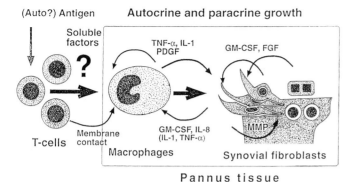

Fig. 12.2 Autocrine and paracrine mechanisms in synovial macrophage activation. MMP, matrix metalloproteinase. (Reproduced with permission from Ref. 122.)

of large amounts of collagenase, increased after stimulation with IL-1 and TNF-α. Their rapid growth and prolonged life span *in vivo* suggest that pannocytes may represent a mesenchymal cell in an earlier stage of differentiation.

Regulation of angiogenesis

The growth of new blood vessels is involved in the development of the rheumatoid pannus, and enhanced endothelial cell function is present in this tissue[139]. The importance of angiogenesis in inflammatory arthritis was emphasized by prevention of experimental models of arthritis, or suppression of the ongoing disease, by treatment with a selective angiogenesis inhibitor. Both proangiogenic factors and inhibitors, or angiostatic factors, have been found in the rheumatoid synovium with the net effect on capillary growth representing a balance between the two.

Growth factors important in promoting angiogenesis include VEGF, FGF, EGF, IGF-1, and TGF-β. VEGF is a potent angiogenic factor that possesses structural homology to PDGF and is produced by a variety of cells in sites of neovascularization. High levels of VEGF are present in rheumatoid synovial fluids, with this protein produced primarily by macrophages in the inflamed synovial tissue[140]. Both IL-1 and TNF-α stimulated VEGF production by cultured rheumatoid synovial cells[141]. The microvascular endothelial cells of synovial blood vessels strongly expressed the mRNA for VEGF receptors. The mechanism whereby VEGF and other growth factors promote angiogenesis is through stimulation of expression of members of the integrin family of adhesion molecules. Treatment of RA patients with monoclonal antibodies to TNF-α, particularly in combination with methotrexate, decreased the elevated serum levels of VEGF[141].

Many cytokines such as chemokines, interferons, and TNF-α are also involved in angiogenesis, either as stimulatory agents or as inhibitors. Chemokines have been classified into at least four different families according to their structural homology regarding the location of two or four cysteine residues. In C-X-C chemokines, the cysteines are separated by an intervening amino acid. Some C-X-Cs stimulate, while others inhibit angiogenesis. In general, chemokines carrying the glutamyl-leucyl-arginyl (ELR) motif, such as CXCL8/IL-8, CXCL1/groα, CXCL5/ENA-78, and CTAP-III/CXCL6 promote angiogenesis, while ELR-lacking chemokines

inhibit neovascularization. As an exception, CXCL12/SDF-1 lacks the ELR residues and is angiogenic[142]. CXCL8/IL-8 was angiogenic when implanted in the rat cornea and induced proliferation and chemotaxis of human umbilical vein endothelial cells. Neutralizing antibody to CXCL8/IL-8 blocked some of the angiogenic activity present in the conditioned media of rheumatoid synovial macrophages, suggesting that CXCL8/IL-8 may contribute to the angiogenesis-dependent synovial hyperplasia in arthritis[143]. While TNF-α may primarily promote endothelial cell differentiation, rather than proliferation, IL-8 stimulates angiogenesis through attracting macrophages into the synovial tissue and enhancing endothelial cell chemotaxis and proliferation.

IFNs have anti-angiogenic activity. IFN-α was the first angiogenesis inhibitor to reach clinical trial and has been successful in the treatment of life-threatening hemangiomas in children. The administration of IFN-α and IFN-β can induce endothelial cell damage, leading to necrosis of vascularized tumors[144]. IFN-β has been shown to inhibit the expression of basic fibroblast growth factor, which is considered an important angiogenic factor. The effect of IFN-γ on wound healing was evaluated in a murine model, where it was found that IFN-γ not only reduced collagen deposition but also lowered the degree of neovascularity. IFN-γ inhibits angiogenesis both through direct effects on endothelial cells and through inducing production of the angiostatic chemokines CXCL10 or IFN-γ-inducible protein (IP-10) and CXCL9 or monokine induced by IFN-γ (MIG)[139]. Thus, the cytokine network may contribute either to angiogenesis or angiostasis, depending on the balance of factors locally present in the rheumatoid synovium.

Bone destruction

The presence of activated osteoclasts is involved in the mechanism of bone destruction that occurs in established RA. Recent findings in animal models of arthritis indicate that blocking osteoclast activity prevents the development of erosions. RANKL regulates osteoclast differentiation and activity through binding to its receptor RANK[145]. Osteoprotegerin (OPG) was originally identified by sequence homology as a new member of the TNF receptor family. OPG is expressed as a soluble receptor that binds RANKL and thereby prevents the binding of this cytokine to cell surface RANK. Synovial fibroblasts and T cells from the rheumatoid synovium express RANK ligand, suggesting that this cytokine plays an important role in the development of bone erosions. The best support for the role of RANKL in the development of articular erosions was obtained with the use of OPG in experimental models of arthritis[146-148]. The administration of this RANKL inhibitor blocked the development of bone lesions but was devoid of any effect on joint inflammation.

Summary of mechanisms of tissue destruction

Numerous pro-inflammatory cytokines are involved in the pathogenesis of RA. The complexity of some of these cytokine effects on T cells, antigen-presenting cells, macrophages, endothelial cells, fibroblasts, and chondrocytes is summarized in Fig. 12.3.

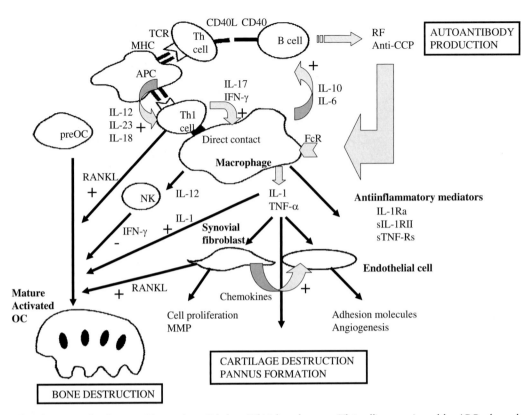

Fig. 12.3 Cells and mediators in the rheumatoid synovium. T helper (Th)1 lymphocytes (Th1 cell) are activated by APCs through peptide presentation and the release of cytokines. Activated Th lymphocytes stimulate synovial macrophages by direct cell contact and cytokines, induce the differentiation and activation of osteoclasts through the release of RANKL, and contribute to the production of autoantibodies by the release of cytokines and cognate interactions with B cells (CD40L-CD40). Autoantibodies and immune complexes can activate macrophages upon binding to FcRs. Activated macrophages release IL-1 and TNF-α, which stimulate the attraction of inflammatory cells and participate in the development of tissue damage: release of neutral MMPs, pannus formation, catabolic effect on chondrocytes (not represented in the figure), and activation of osteoclasts. Activated mast cells (not represented) are also a source of TNF-α in the rheumatoid synovium. FcR, Fc receptor; OC, osteoclast; preOC, osteoclast precursor.

These mediators of cell—cell communication may play key roles in the initiation of reactive synovitis, in the transformation of this self-limited response into an aggressive and tissue-destructive process, and in the perpetuation of chronic synovitis. In these three stages of the disease process, the same or different cytokines may play changing and complementary roles. However, the cytokine network is self-regulating and, as detailed below, other cytokines, antibodies to cytokines, and soluble cytokine receptors may all act to limit the potentially injurious effects of the pro-inflammatory members of the cytokine family.

Systemic effects and regulation of cytokine networks

Induction of the acute phase response

The acute phase response is defined as a set of biochemical, nutritional, and behavioral changes that occur in the presence of local or systemic inflammatory reaction. These changes represent adaptations by the organism in an effort to maintain essential functions and survive in the face of overwhelming infection and acute

or chronic inflammation. The acute phase proteins are plasma proteins, the levels of which are altered during the acute phase response[149]. The production of acute phase proteins by hepatocytes is regulated by different cytokines, including IL-6, IL-1, and TNF-α. In addition, these cytokines are also key mediators in the systemic manifestations of the acute phase response (Fig. 12.4).

The plasma proteins whose concentrations increase during the acute phase response are termed positive acute phase proteins and include complement factors, proteins of the coagulation and fibrinolytic system, antiproteases, transport proteins, participants in the inflammatory response, and miscellaneous proteins (Table 12.5). The most clinically useful is C-reactive protein (CRP), whose levels in plasma are generally a sensitive indicator of inflammation. The plasma levels of other proteins (negative acute phase proteins) decrease during the acute phase response (Table 12.5). IL-6 is the most important cytokine in influencing production of the acute phase proteins in the liver; IL-6 is the major inducer of CRP and serum amyloid A (SAA) production by hepatocytes, whereas IL-6 inhibits synthesis of albumin. Depending on the nature of the inflammatory condition, cytokines may exhibit a cascade of effects, where TNF-α may induce IL-1 production, which in turn stimulates IL-6 production in a variety of cells.

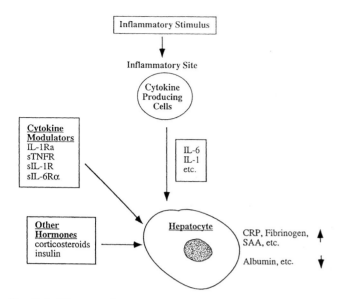

Fig. 12.4 The acute phase response is regulated both directly and indirectly by a complex network of intercellular signaling molecules involving cytokines, cytokine modulators, and other hormones. Inflammation-associated cytokines, produced by cells at the inflammatory site and probably distant cells as well, induce changes in production of acute phase proteins by hepatocytes. (Reproduced with permission from Ref. 149.)

Table 12.5   Human acute phase proteins

Proteins whose plasma concentrations increase:
Complement system: C3, C4, C9, factor B, C1-inhibitor, C4b-binding protein, mannose-binding lectin
Coagulation and fibrinolytic system: fibrinogen, plasminogen, tissue plasminogen activator, urokinase, protein S, vitronectin, plasminogen activator inhibitor-1
Antiproteases: α-1 protease inhibitor, 1-antichymotrypsin, pancreatic secretory trypsin inhibitor, inter-α-inhibitors
Transport proteins: ceruloplasmin, haptoglobin, hemopexin
Participants in inflammatory responses: secreted phospholipase A2, LPS-binding protein, IL-1 receptor antagonist, G-CSF
Others: CRP, SAA, α1-acid glycoprotein, fibronectin, ferritin, angiotensinogen, CD14

Proteins whose plasma concentrations decrease:
Albumin, transferrin, transthyretin, α-2 HS glycoprotein, α-fetoprotein, thyroxine-binding globulin, insulin-like growth factor-1, factor XII

Modified from Ref. 150.
HS, heparin sulfate.

In addition, combinations of cytokines exhibit varying patterns of stimulation of production of acute phase proteins by hepatoma cell lines, although effects on hepatocytes *in vivo* may not be the same[150]. Either IL-1 or TNF-α enhanced IL-6 induction of CRP and SAA production in these model systems, whereas TNF-α or TGF-β inhibited the stimulatory effects of IL-6 on fibrinogen production by the same cells. The combination of IL-1β and IL-6 was more potent than either cytokine alone in stimulation of IL-1Ra production by HepG2 or cultured human hepatocytes. Furthermore, both IL-4 and IL-13 amplified the stimulatory effect of IL-1β on production of IL-1Ra by these cells, whereas these cytokines exhibited no effects alone or in combination with IL-6[151]. In contrast, IL-4 inhibited the induction of other acute phase proteins by cultured primary human hepatocytes[151]. Thus, depending upon other cytokines present, the effects of IL-6 on stimulation of acute phase protein production may either be enhanced or decreased.

Serum amyloid A is the circulating precursor of AA amyloid deposits that occur in tissues of some patients with chronic inflammatory diseases. The serum levels of SAA have been reported to be very sensitive markers of inflammatory changes in patients with recent onset RA. SAA is detected in the synovium of RA patients as well as in other categories of inflammatory arthritis. Production of SAA in endothelial cells, and synovial fibroblasts, is regulated by pro-inflammatory cytokines. In addition to being a marker of disease activity, SAA may also participate in the pathophysiological pathways involved in joint damage by inducing the production of MMP-1 and MMP-3 by synovial fibroblasts[152].

Whether the net effects of IL-6 in rheumatoid synovitis are pro-inflammatory or anti-inflammatory remains controversial. IL-6 levels are increased in the serum and synovial fluid of patients with RA. Rheumatoid synovial fibroblasts constitutively produced large amounts of IL-6 *in vitro*, although synovial macrophages were also capable of producing this cytokine. Co-culture of blood monocytes on rheumatoid synovial fibroblasts led to enhanced production of IL-6, GM-CSF, LIF, and IL-8 by the synoviocytes[153]. Synoviocyte production of IL-6 in this co-culture system was inhibited by IL-1Ra, indicating the stimulatory role of endogenous IL-1, and IL-6 production was also inhibited by IL-4, IL-10, and IL-13. The monocyte appeared to be more important as an inducer of synoviocyte production of cytokines in this model, rather than as a direct source of IL-6 itself. Synoviocyte production of IL-6 was further increased by the addition of IFN-γ, IL-1β, TNF-α, or GM-CSF, thought to be secondary to the ability of these cytokines to increase the expression of adhesion molecules on both cells to enhance their interaction[153].

The anti-inflammatory potential of IL-6 is suggested by the results of many studies (reviewed in Ref. 154). The *in vivo* administration of IL-6 to humans led to enhanced circulating levels of IL-1Ra and soluble TNF receptors, but not of IL-1β or TNF-α. These and other IL-6-induced acute phase proteins have many anti-inflammatory effects. Neutralizing monoclonal antibodies to IL-6 did not reduce the proteoglycan degradation seen in antigen-induced arthritis or zymosan-induced arthritis in mice. Furthermore, proteoglycan depletion was higher in IL-6-deficient mice during zymosan-induced arthritis than in wild-type controls. This observation indicated that IL-6 may be protective for cartilage damage in this model, possibly through inducing the production of cytokine inhibitors and of tissue inhibitors of metalloproteinases (TIMP).

A pro-inflammatory role for IL-6 is suggested by its ability to activate endothelial cells to produce chemokines and express adhesion molecules, induce synovial fibroblast proliferation, and stimulate osteoclast formation and activation. Furthermore, complete protection from CIA, with an absence of inflammatory cell infiltrates in the joints, was observed in mice lacking the IL-6 gene[155]. However, IL-6 stimulated antibody production by B cells[9] and IL-6 knockout mice demonstrated reduced levels of anticollagen antibodies. Thus, IL-6 in CIA may be more important in enhancing production of autoantibodies than in acting as a local inflammatory mediator. This possibility is further substantiated by an absence of an effect on arthritis in TNF-α-transgenic mice by ablating IL-6 production[155]. However, in RA IL-6 may be responsible for some systemic manifestations such as fever, fatigue, and anorexia, as well as of osteopenia. Consistent with the experimental findings, the results of clinical trials with agents designed to block IL-6 or IL-6 signaling suggest that IL-6 exerts a pro-inflammatory effect in RA. Clinical improvement and a reduction in CRP levels were observed in patients treated with a monoclonal anti-IL-6 antibody. However, clinical improvement was only transient[156]. Recently, administration of a monoclonal anti-IL-6R antibody has proven to be efficacious in the treatment of active RA[157,158] and in children with Still's disease.

LIF, oncostatin M (OSM), and IL-11 belong to the IL-6 family of cytokines. LIF, OSM, IL-11, and IL-6 initiate signaling by inducing either the β signal transducing receptor component gp130 (in the case of IL-6) or heterodimerization between gp130 and the gp130-related LIFR-β (in the cases of LIF and OSM) or between gp130 and OSMR-β (in the case of OSM). These cytokines share some common effects on hematopoiesis, osteoclast activation, and acute phase protein production. LIF is present in the synovial fluid of patients with osteoarthritis and at higher concentrations in samples from patients with RA[159]. Cultured human synoviocytes and articular chondrocytes produced biologically active LIF after stimulation with IL-1. LIF enhanced the stimulatory effect of TNF-α on PGE2 production by synovial fibroblasts. IL-11 is expressed by synoviocytes and chondrocytes and, similar to IL-6 and OSM, it induces the production of TIMP. IL-11 is found in the synovial fluid of RA patients but its presence in the serum is variable. Exogenous addition of IL-11 inhibited the production of TNF-α, MMP-1, and MMP-3 by rheumatoid synovium. Endogenous IL-11 produced by rheumatoid synovial cells inhibited TNF-α production, particularly in combination with IL-10. IL-11 is present in the synovium of mice with CIA. The administration of recombinant human IL-11 after the onset of CIA significantly reduced the severity of arthritis and the progression of joint damage[160]. A phase I/II randomized, dose-escalating, double-blind, placebo-controlled trial with recombinant human IL-11 conducted in patients with active RA resulted in a significant reduction in the number of tender joints but did not achieve a significant improvement in the ACR20 response as compared to the placebo group[161]. OSM mRNA was detected in the joints of mice with CIA. OSM exerts pro-inflammatory effects in different experimental models. OSM stimulated the expression of adhesion molecules by endothelial cells, increased neutrophil migration through endothelial cell layer, and stimulated the expression of pro-inflammatory mediators. Intra-articular injection of adenovirus encoding murine OSM induced a severe articular inflammation with synovial hyperplasia, mononuclear cell infiltration, pannus formation, and

cartilage degradation. The administration of neutralizing anti-OSM antibodies after the onset of CIA resulted in a marked reduction of joint inflammation, and cartilage damage[162], suggesting that targeting OSM may be of potential value for the treatment of RA.

Although fever, fatigue, and muscle wasting represent some of the symptomatic effects of cytokines during acute and chronic inflammation, other systemic consequences of the acute phase response may be beneficial to the host[151]. CRP may play a role in the clearance of infectious agents, in enhancement of phagocytosis, and in prevention of neutrophil adherence to endothelial cells. CRP also inhibits the generation of superoxide anions by neutrophils and, along with other acute phase proteins, stimulates the production of IL-1Ra by monocytes. The proteinase inhibitors produced as part of the acute phase response may block the effects of some enzymes released by phagocytic cells. Lastly, the systemic manifestations of acute inflammation may reflect physiological adaptations that enhance the immune response and provide for maintenance of core organ functions, such as the central nervous system. However, failure or overwhelming of these adaptations may lead to physiological collapse, as occurs in severe endotoxemia with septic shock.

Anti-inflammatory effects of cytokines

The major cytokines that exhibit anti-inflammatory effects include IL-4, IL-10, IL-13, TGF-β, IFN-α, and IL-1Ra. In addition to their effects on T cells, IL-4, IL-10, and IL-13 all act on monocytes and macrophages to inhibit production of IL-1 and TNF-α, while enhancing production of the natural anti-inflammatory cytokine IL-1Ra. Some of the anti-inflammatory effects of IL-4 (and IL-13) may be mediated by an inhibitory effect on NF-κB activation in macrophages. IL-4 stimulates the expression of other cytokine inhibitors such as soluble IL-1 receptor type II and TNF receptors. The protective properties of IL-4 include inhibition of bone resorption, inhibition of growth factor-induced proliferation of rheumatoid synoviocytes, suppression of macrophage production of MMP, suppression of IL-1-induced production of MMP and PGE2 in human synovial fibroblasts, and a decrease in mononuclear cell recruitment to the rheumatoid synovium. In fact, continuous infusion of IL-4 led to a delay in the onset of CIA in mice and to a suppression of joint damage[163]. A most striking finding in the IL-4-treated mice was a 1000-fold decrease in the production of TNF-α by synovial cells. Overexpression of IL-4 in the joints of mice with CIA suppressed the expression of RANKL and prevented the formation of osteoclast-like cells and development of bone erosions. *In vitro* studies with bone explants from RA patients cultured in the presence of IL-4 revealed consistent suppression of type I collagen breakdown. Interestingly the protective effects of IL-4 on cartilage and bone were observed despite the persistence of severe articular inflammation and of synovial fibroblast expansion. These findings may be related to an antiapoptotic effect of IL-4.

Notably, IL-4 was not detected in RA synovial fluid and tissue[164], and thus probably does not function as a natural anti-inflammatory protein in the joint in this disease. In addition, this lack of IL-4 could contribute to the uneven Th1/Th2 balance and the chronic nature of RA. Studies in animal models of arthritis supported this characterization of IL-4 as a cytokine with antiarthritic potential. IL-4-deficient mice have a more chronic relapsing form of CIA. In proteoglycan-induced arthritis, immunization of mice lacking IL-4 or STAT6 led to more severe arthritis with a significant increase in production of IL-12, TNF-α, and IFN-γ. In arthritis induced by streptococcal cell-wall fragments, daily treatment with IL-4 suppressed the chronic, destructive phase, decreased the influx of inflammatory cells, and eliminated pannus and erosions. In CIA, IL-4 synergized with IL-10 in the protection against cartilage degradation[165].

Following the encouraging results observed with the administration of IL-4 in animal models of arthritis, a phase I dose-escalating double-blind, placebo-controlled safety study of recombinant human IL-4 was conducted in RA patients. Treatment did not produce significant benefit but was well tolerated[166].

IL-10 exhibits a similar spectrum of anti-inflammatory properties as IL-4 and IL-13 *in vitro*, but, unlike these cytokines, IL-10 is produced in the rheumatoid synovium and may suppress local inflammation. IL-10 was produced in the joints of mice with CIA and neutralization of endogenous IL-10 by prophylactic treatment with anti-IL-10 antibodies led to an earlier onset of arthritis, with increased severity. Furthermore, IL-10 administration after disease onset in murine CIA inhibited inflammation and cartilage destruction[167]. The prophylactic administration of viral IL-10 using adenoviral-mediated gene transfer inhibited the onset of collagen-induced arthritis in mice and decreased T cell proliferation *in vitro* induced by collagen type II. Although pretreatment with viral IL-10 decreased the severity of joint destruction, treatment of established disease was ineffective.

IL-10 levels are elevated in the serum and synovial fluid of patients with RA. In addition, both the mRNA and protein for IL-10 were detected in rheumatoid synovial tissue with production by macrophages and T cells[168]. Furthermore, the IL-10 was functionally important as neutralization of endogenously produced IL-10 in cultured rheumatoid synovial cells led to three-fold increases in the levels of TNF-α and IL-1β. Normal humans injected with IL-10 exhibited no adverse symptoms and inhibition of LPS-stimulated production of TNF-α and IL-1β by whole blood cells was observed. A four-week phase I trial of IL-10 in patients with RA revealed elevations in circulating levels of soluble TNF receptors and IL-1Ra, with some possible early clinical efficacy[169]. IL-10 was well tolerated despite the occurrence of reversible dose-dependent thrombocytopenia. A double-blind, dose-escalating, placebo-controlled phase II clinical trial was performed in patients with psoriatic arthritis. The administration of IL-10 was safe; whereas a positive response to treatment with IL-10 was observed for psoriasis, psoriatic arthritis did not improve[170].

TGF-β exhibited either pro-inflammatory or anti-inflammatory properties in animal models of arthritis, depending on the particular model studied, the route of delivery, and the state of differentiation of the responding cells[171]. Injection of TGF-β into joints of experimental animals generally induced acute and chronic inflammation while systemic delivery was usually anti-inflammatory. TGF-β exhibited a variety of suppressive effects on cell function *in vitro*, including inhibition of CD4+ T cell proliferation and a reduction in MHC class II expression. This cytokine was present in large amounts in the synovial fluid and tissue of patients with this disease, possibly accounting for the suppressed T cell function present in rheumatoid synovial T cells[172]. Mice rendered deficient in TGF-β production developed wasting and a mixed inflammatory cell infiltration into multiple organs with subsequent tissue necrosis. Furthermore, these mice possessed hyperproliferative lymphocytes and spontaneous production of antibodies to nuclear antigens[127]. The autoimmunity in TGF-β deficient mice appeared to be dependent upon the excessive expression of MHC class II molecules on CD4+ T cells[173]. Lastly, rats with streptococcal cell wall-induced arthritis injected with plasmid DNA for TGF-β by direct injection into muscles exhibited a marked suppression of joint inflammation and destruction.

Thus, the major effects of endogenous TGF-β in patients with rheumatoid arthritis may be to suppress fibroblast proliferation and production of tissue-damaging neutral metalloproteinases while enhancing production of the inhibitors of these enzymes[174].

IFN-β is a type I IFN predominantly produced by fibroblasts. IFN-β can exert anti-inflammatory effects by decreasing the release of TNF-α and IL-1β and enhancing the production of IL-10 and IL-1Ra. IFN-β can also inhibit T cell proliferation and migration, enhance IL-2 production by Th1 cells, up-regulate the expression of TGF-β and of its receptor on peripheral monocytes, and decrease the expression of several adhesion molecules[175]. IFN-β can also decrease the development of joint damage. IFN-β enhanced the effect of IL-1 on IL-1Ra production by cultured articular chondrocytes and synovial fibroblasts[176]. IFN-β plays a critical role in bone homeostasis by modulating the effect of RANKL on osteoclastogenesis through a negative feedback mechanism by decreasing the expression of c-Fos, an essential factor for the maturation of osteoclasts[177].

Daily injection of recombinant IFN-β in CIA decreased articular inflammation and had a protective effect on joint damage. Recombinant IFN-β was also tested in monkeys with CIA. Three monkeys with established arthritis received daily subcutaneous injection of IFN-β for one week; two exhibited significant clinical improvement with a marked decrease in CRP levels[178]. Administration of recombinant IFN-β to RA patients resulted in decreased MMP and IL-1β levels in synovial tissues but had little effect on clinical parameters of disease activity. In a recent 24-week multicenter, randomized, double blind, placebo-controlled phase II trial in patients with active RA, administration of IFN-β in combination with methotrexate did not have any clinical or radiological effect as compared to methotrexate alone[179].

IL-1Ra is a structural derivative of IL-1 that binds to IL-1 receptors with equal affinity as the agonists IL-1α and IL-1β, but fails to activate target cells[180]. The administration of IL-1Ra, either by injection of recombinant protein or by delivery through gene therapy, inhibited the development and severity of arthritis in multiple experimental animal models (reviewed in Ref. 180). Constitutive intra-articular expression of IL-1 following gene transfer to the rabbit synovium led to all of the histopathological changes of the human disease RA. Furthermore, some evidence indicated that treatments to block TNF-α in CIA in mice were primarily anti-inflammatory, whereas blocking IL-1 had a stronger inhibitory effect towards destruction of cartilage and bone[181]. Endogenous IL-1Ra was shown to be an important natural anti-inflammatory protein as neutralizing antibodies to IL-1Ra led to an exacerbation of LPS-induced arthritis in rabbits.

Collagen-induced arthritis was more severe in IL-1Ra knockout mice and was suppressed by the overexpression of IL-1Ra in transgenic mice[182]. Lastly, IL-1Ra-deficient mice bred into the BALB/cA background exhibited the spontaneous development of chronic polyarthritis with the presence of autoantibodies, thus reproducing some of the clinical and biological features of rheumatoid arthritis[183].

IL-1Ra was present in the synovial fluids of patients with rheumatoid arthritis in high levels, and the mRNA was abundantly expressed by macrophages and fibroblasts in the synovial lining, particularly at the pannus-cartilage junction. However, *in vitro* culture of rheumatoid synovial cells indicated that the amount of IL-1Ra produced was probably not sufficient to inhibit the inflammatory effects of the locally produced IL-1. The imbalance between IL-1 and IL-1Ra production by rheumatoid synovial cells could be improved in favor of IL-1Ra by culturing with IL-4, and less so with IL-10. The importance of endogenous production of IL-1Ra in patients with inflammatory arthritis was suggested by finding a high ratio of IL-1Ra to IL-1 in the knee synovial fluids of patients with Lyme arthritis who exhibited rapid spontaneous improvements, while the opposite ratio was present in the fluids of patients with more protracted courses.

The daily subcutaneous injection of recombinant IL-1Ra in a phase I clinical trial in patients with RA was more effective than weekly administration. Patients treated in this manner for six months demonstrated a moderate clinical improvement in joint inflammation with radiological evidence of a slowing in progression of joint destruction and a decrease in the rate of development of new bone lesions[184]. Patients treated with a combination of IL-1Ra and methotrexate exhibited a better clinical response with also less functional impairment than those patients receiving methotrexate alone[185]. The effect of the combination of IL-1Ra and etanercept (a fusion protein containing the extracellular domain of TNF receptor p75 and the Fc region of human IgG class 1) was studied in a randomized, double-blind, controlled study in methotrexate partial responders. The results did not show any advantage of the combination over etanercept alone but an increased proportion of infectious adverse events was observed in patients treated with the combination of cytokine inhibitors[186]. Other agents blocking the effects of IL-1 are currently being tested in clinical trials in RA patients.

Antibodies to cytokines

High affinity antibodies to native IL-1α, IL-6, IL-10, IFN-α, IFN-β, and GM-CSF are present in the sera of normal individuals, possibly developing secondary to a loss of T cell tolerance to self[187]. The antibodies against IL-1α, IL-6, IFN-α, and GM-CSF neutralized receptor binding of the respective cytokine *in vitro*. However, the physiological relevance of these naturally occurring antibodies to cytokines remains unknown. High avidity neutralizing antibodies to IFN-α, IL-1α, IL-6, and GM-CSF were found in pharmaceutical preparations of intravenous gamma globulin (IVIG), with antibody titers present *in vivo* after administration to patients. The clinical responses to IVIG may be secondary to these anticytokine antibodies, as well as to antibodies to HLA class I molecules or to anti-idiotypic antibodies also present in these preparations.

Autoantibodies to some cytokines have been described in the sera of patients with RA: IL-1α (36% of patients), IL-6 (29%), and IFN-α (12%)[188]. However, only antibodies to IL-6 and IFN-α were found in the rheumatoid sera in higher concentrations than in the sera of healthy controls. The presence and serum levels of neutralizing antibodies to IL-1α appear to be better correlated with mild polyarthritis, as was observed in patients with Sjögren's syndrome or with a self-limited polyarthritis, than with severe RA[189]. This observation suggests that the presence of antibodies to IL-1α may be protective against the development of severe destructive arthritis.

TNF-α is of major importance in the pathophysiology of RA, and treatments to block this cytokine have proven efficacious in many experimental animal models of inflammatory arthritis (reviewed in Ref. 190). In contrast to IL-1α, high avidity natural antibodies to TNF-α have not been described.

Soluble cytokine receptors

Soluble receptors to multiple cytokines are found in the sera and synovial fluids of patients with RA, generated either by proteolytic cleavage from the plasma membrane or by synthesis from alternatively spliced mRNAs[191]. It remains unclear whether the naturally occurring soluble cytokine receptors actually inhibit or prolong the action of the respective cytokine *in vivo*. Of greatest interest to RA are the soluble receptors for TNF-α, IL-1, and IL-6. Levels of soluble p55 and p75 receptors of TNF were elevated in the serum and synovial fluid of patients with RA, with higher levels in the synovial fluids suggesting local synthesis[192]. The results of clinical trials with a soluble TNFR:Fc fusion protein have been reported and will be summarized elsewhere in this text[193].

Three receptors for IL-1 exist on cell surfaces and as soluble forms. The type I IL-1 receptor (IL-1R) possesses a long cytoplasmic domain and is biologically active in stimulating intracellular signal transduction. Type II IL-1R possesses a truncated intracellular domain and fails to stimulate cells after ligand binding[194]. IL-1R accessory protein is also a member of the immunoglobulin superfamily and its extracellular sequence bears some homologies with the two other IL-1Rs. Both IL-1R type I and IL-1R accessory protein belong to the Toll-like receptor family and have some sequence homologies in their cytoplasmic domains. Soluble type I IL-1Rs were found in low levels in the synovial fluid of RA patients, and this soluble receptor preferentially bound IL-1Ra. However, high levels of soluble type II IL-1R were present in rheumatoid synovial fluids. The soluble type II IL-1R preferentially bound IL-1β and functioned as an inhibitor of IL-1 effects by preventing binding to the functional cell surface type I IL-1R. A clinical trial of subcutaneous injections of soluble type I IL-1 receptors in RA failed to show any beneficial effects. The soluble form of IL-1R accessory protein increases the binding affinity of IL-1α and IL-1β to soluble type II IL-1R by approximately 100-fold, while leaving unaltered the low binding affinity of IL-1Ra[195]. Thus, soluble IL-1R accessory protein exerts an inhibitory action on IL-1 effect. Adenoviral systemic overexpression of soluble IL-1R accessory protein markedly ameliorated CIA in mice[196].

Lastly, soluble IL-6 receptor levels are elevated in the sera of patients with juvenile arthritis[197]. The complex of IL-6 and its soluble receptor is biologically active through direct binding to cell surface gp130, the molecule responsible for mediating IL-6 effects on target cells[198].

Other levels of cytokine inhibition

Cytokine gene transcription is under the influence of both positive and negative regulatory molecules (summarized in Ref. 199). Cytokines activate cascades of signal transduction pathways with regulatory molecules modulating the biological responses to cytokines (reviewed in Ref. 9). In addition to these natural mechanisms, therapeutic agents designed to block cytokine production or effects have been developed and are being evaluated in experimental animal models of inflammatory arthritis.

Summary

This chapter has summarized some aspects of the cytokine networks in RA. Clearly, both TNF-α and IL-1 are responsible for mediating many important steps in the induction and perpetuation of tissue damage in RA, and IL-6 is a key cytokine in some of the systemic manifestations. Although pro-inflammatory cytokines may predominate in this disease process, anti-inflammatory cytokines such as TGF-β, IL-10, IL-1Ra, and soluble receptors are also produced in the rheumatoid joint and limit the local tissue injury. Thus, an imbalance between pro-and anti-inflammatory cytokines may exist to explain, at least in part, the varying course of the clinical disease. Current therapeutic efforts are designed to block the production or effects of pro-inflammatory cytokines, or to enhance the local concentration of anti-inflammatory cytokines. In addition to administration of recombinant proteins, gene therapy approaches are being employed to deliver the cDNA for anti-inflammatory cytokines to the synovium. The further discovery of new cytokines, and a characterization of their importance to pathophysiological events in the rheumatoid synovitis, may offer even more possibilities for therapeutic intervention in the future.

References

1. Arend, W. P., and Dayer, J.- M. Cytokines and cytokine inhibitors or antagonists in rheumatoid arthritis. *Arthritis Rheum* 1990; 33: 305-15.
2. Arend, W. P., and Dayer, J.- M. Inhibition of the production and effects of interleukin-1 and tumor necrosis factor α in rheumatoid arthritis. *Arthritis Rheum* 1995; 38: 151-60.
3. Ivashkiv, L. B. Cytokine expression and cell activation in inflammatory arthritis. *Adv Immunol,* 1996; 63: 337-76.
4. Feldmann, M., Brennan, F. M., and Maini, R. N. Role of cytokines in rheumatoid arthritis. *Annu Rev Immunol,* 1996; 14: 397-440.
5. Choy, E. H. S., and Panayi, G. S. Cytokine pathways and joint inflammation in rheumatoid arthritis. *N Engl J Med,* 2001; 344: 907-16.
6. Vervoordeldonk, M. J. B. M., and Tak. P. P. Cytokines in rheumatoid arthritis. *Curr Rheumatol Rep,* 2002; 4: 208-17.
7. Arend, W. P., and Gabay, C. Cytokines in the rheumatic diseases. *Rheum Dis Clin North Am,* 2004; 30: 41-67.
8. Arend, W. P. Mediators of inflammation, tissue destruction, and repair. B. Growth factors and cytokines. In *Primer on the rheumatic diseases*, 12th edn (Klippel, J. H., Crofford, L. J., Stone, J. H., and Weyand, C. M., eds), pp. 58–66. Atlanta: Arthritis Foundation; 2001.
9. Gabay, C. Cytokines and cytokine receptors. In *Arthritis and allied conditions*, 15th edn (Koopman, W. J., and Moreland, L. W., eds), pp. 423–75. Philadelphia: Lippincott Williams & Wilkins; 2005.
10. McInnes, I. B. Cytokines. In *Kelley's textbook of rheumatology*, 7th edn (Harris, E. D. Jr., Budd, R. C., Genovese, M. C., Firestein, G. S., Sargent, J. S., Sledge, C. B., and Ruddy, S. eds), pp. 379–89. Philadelphia: Elsevier Saunders; 2005.
11. Handel, M. L., McMorrow, L. B., and Gravellese, E. M. Nuclear factor-κB in rheumatoid synovium. *Arthritis Rheum* 1995; 38: 1762–70.
12. Marok, R., Winyard, P. G., Coumbe, A., Kus, M. L., Gaffney, K., Blades, K. *et al.* Activation of the transcription factor nuclear factor-κB in human inflamed synovial tissue. *Arthritis Rheum* 1996; 39: 583–91.
13. Benito, M. J., Murphy E., Murphy, E. P., van den Berg, W. B., FitzGerald O., and Bresniham, B. Increased synovial tissue NF-κB1 expression at sites adjacent to the cartilage-pannus junction in rheumatoid arthritis. *Arthritis Rheum* 2004; 50: 1781–7.
14. Bondeson, J., Foxwell, B., Brennan, F., and Feldmann, M. Defining therapeutic targets by using adenovirus: blocking NF-κB inhibits both inflammatory and destructive mechanisms in rheumatoid synovium but spares anti—inflammatory mediators. *Proc Natl Acad Sci U S A* 1999; 96: 5668–73.
15. Campbell, I. K., Gerondakis, S., O'Donnell, K., and Wicks, I. P. Distinct roles for NF-κB1 (p50) and c—Rel transcription factors in inflammatory arthritis. *J Clin Invest,* 2000; 105: 1799–806.
16. Makarov, S. S. NF-κB in rheumatoid arthritis: a pivotal regulator of inflammation, hyperplasia, and tissue destruction. *Arthritis Res* 2001; 3: 200–6.
17. Müller—Ladner, U., Gay, R. E., and Gay, S. Role of nuclear factor κB in synovial inflammation. *Curr Rheumatol Rep* 2002; 4: 201–7.
18. Firestein, G. S. NF-κB: holy grail for rheumatoid arthritis? *Arthritis Rheum* 2004; 50: 2381–6.
19. Asahara, H., Fujisawa, K., Kobata, T., Hasunuma, T., Maeda, T., Asanuma, M. *et al.* Direct evidence of high DNA binding activity of transcription factor AP-1 in rheumatoid arthritis synovium. *Arthritis Rheum* 1997; 40: 912–18.
20. Okamoto, K., Fujisawa, K., Hasunuma, T., Kobata, T., Sumida, T., and Nishioka, K. Selective activation of the JNK/AP-1 pathway in Fas—mediated apoptosis in rheumatoid arthritis synoviocytes. *Arthritis Rheum* 1997; 40: 919–26.
21. Hammaker, D. R., Boyle, D. L., Chabaud-Riou, M., and Firestein, G. S. Regulation of c-Jun N-terminal kinase by MEKK-2 and mitogen-activated protein kinase kinase kinases in rheumatoid arthritis. *J Immunol* 2004; 172: 1612–18.
22. Shiozawa, S., Shimizu, K., Tanaka, K., and Hino, K. Studies on the contribution of c-fos/AP-1 to arthritic joint destruction. *J Clin Invest* 1997; 99: 1210–16.
23. Schett, G., Tohidast-Akrad, M., Smolen, J. S., Schmid, B. J., Steiner, C.-W., Bitzan, P. *et al.* Activation, differential localization, and regulation of the stress-activated protein kinases, extracellular signal-regulated kinase, c-Jun N-terminal kinase, and p38 mitogen-activated protein kinase, in synovial tissue and cells in rheumatoid arthritis. *Arthritis Rheum* 2000; 43: 2501–12.
24. Saklatvala, J. The p38 kinase pathway as a therapeutic target in inflammatory disease. *Curr Opin Pharmacol,* 2004; 4: 372–7.
25. Finbloom, D. S., and Larner, A. C. Induction of early response genes by interferons, interleukins, and growth factors by the tyrosine phosphorylation of latent transcription factors. *Arthritis Rheum* 1995; 38: 877–89.
26. Wang, F., Sengupta, T. K., Zhong, Z., and Ivashkiv, L. B. Regulation of the balance of cytokine production and the signal transducer and activator of transcription (STAT) transcription factor activity by

cytokines and inflammatory synovial fluids. *J Exp Med*, 1995; **182**: 1825–31.

27. Zvaifler, N. J. Rheumatoid synovitis: an extravascular immune complex disease. *Arthritis Rheum*, 1974; **17**: 297–305.

28. Gregersen, P. K., Silver, J., and Winchester, R. J. The shared epitope hypothesis: an approach to understanding the molecular genetics of susceptibility to rheumatoid arthritis. *Arthritis Rheum*, 1987; **30**: 1205–13.

29. Fox, D. A. The role of T cells in the immunopathogenesis of rheumatoid arthritis. *Arthritis Rheum*, 1997; **40**: 598–609.

30. Thomas, R., and Lipsky, P. E. Presentation of self peptides by dendritic cells. *Arthritis Rheum*, 1996; **39**: 183–90.

31. Thomas, R., and Lipsky, P. E. Could endogenous self-peptides presented by dendritic cells initiate rheumatoid arthritis? *Immunol Today*, 1997; **17**: 559–64.

32. Zvaifler, N. J., Steinman, R. M., Kaplan, G., Lau, L. L., and Rivelis, M. Identification of immunostimulatory dendritic cells in the synovial effusions of patients with rheumatoid arthritis. *J Clin Invest*, 1985; **76**: 789–800.

33. Thomas, R., Davis, L. S., and Lipsky, P. E. Rheumatoid synovium is enriched in mature antigen-presenting dendritic cells. *J Immunol*, 1994; **152**: 2613–23.

34. Thomas, R., and Quinn, C. Functional differentiation of dendritic cells in rheumatoid arthritis: role of CD86 in the synovium. *J Immunol*, 1996; **156**: 3074–86.

35. Thomas, R., MacDonald, K. P. A., Pettit, A. S., Cavanagh, L. L., Padmanabha, J., and Zehntner, S. Dendritic cells and the pathogenesis of rheumatoid arthritis. *J Leukoc Biol*, 1999; **66**: 286–92.

36. Pettit, A. R., MacDonald, K. P. A., O'Sullivan, B., and Thomas, R. Differentiated dendritic cells expressing nuclear RelB are predominately located in rheumatoid synovial tissue perivascular mononuclear cell aggregates. *Arthritis Rheum*, 2000; **43**: 791–800.

37. Pettit, A. R., Ahern, M. J., Zehntner, S., Smith, M. D., and Thomas, R. Comparison of differentiated dendritic cell infiltration of autoimmune and osteoarthritis synovial tissue. *Arthritis Rheum*, 2001; **44**: 105–10.

38. Santiago-Schwarz, F., Anand, P., and Carson, S. E. Dendritic cells (DCs) in rheumatoid arthritis (RA): progenitor cells and soluble factors contained in RA synovial fluid yield a subset of myeloid DCs that preferentially activate Th1 inflammatory-type responses. *J Immunol*, 2001; **167**: 1758–68.

39. Page, G., Lebecque, S., and Miossec, P. Anatomic localization of immature and mature dendritic cells in an ectopic lymphoid organ: correlation with selective chemokine expression in rheumatoid synovium. *J Immunol*, 2002; **168**: 5333–41.

40. Lande R., Giacomini, E., Serafini, B., Rosicarelli, B., Sebastiani, G. D., Minisola, G. *et al*. Characterization and recruitment of plasmacytoid dendritic cells in synovial fluid and tissue of patients with chronic inflammatory arthritis. *J Immunol*, 2004; **173**: 2815–24.

41. Leung, B. P., Conacher, M., Hunter, D., McInnes, I. B., Liew, F. Y., and Brewer, J. M. A novel dendritic cell-induced model of erosive inflammatory arthritis: distinct roles of dendritic cells in T cell activation and induction of local inflammation. *J Immunol*, 2002; **169**: 7071–7.

42. Cavanagh, L. L., Boyce, A., Smith, L., Padmanabha, J., Filgueira, L., Pietschmann, P. *et al*. Rheumatoid arthritis synovium contains plasmacytoid dendritic cells. *Arthritis Res Ther*, 2005; **7**: R230–R240.

43. Goronzy, J. J., and Weyand, C. M. B cells as a therapeutic target in autoimmune diseases. *Arthritis Res Ther*, 2003; **5**: 131–5.

44. Silvermann, G. J., and Weisman, S. Rituximab therapy and autoimmune disorders: prospects for anti-B cell therapy. *Arthritis Rheum*, 2003; **48**: 1484–92.

45. Looney, R. J., Anolik, J., and Sanz, I. B cells as therapeutic targets for rheumatic diseases. *Curr Opin Rheumatol*, 2004; **16**: 180–5.

46. Martin, F., and Chan, A. C. Pathogenic roles of B cells in human autoimmunity: insights from the clinic. *Immunity*, 2004; **20**: 517–27.

47. Roosnek, E., and Lanzavecchia, A. Efficient and selective presentation of antigen-antibosy complexes by rheumatoid factor B cells. *J Exp Med*, 1991; **173**: 487–9.

48. Edwards, J. C. W., Cambridge, G., and Abrahams, V. M. Do self-perpetuating B lymphocytes drive human autoimmune disease? *Immunology*, 1999; **97**: 188–96.

49. Edwards, J. C. W., Szczepański, L., Szechiski, J., Filipiwicz-Sosnowska, A., Emery, P., Close, D. R. *et al*. Efficacy of B cell-targeted therapy with rituximab in patients with rheumatoid arthritis. *N Engl J Med*, 2004; **350**: 2572–81.

50. Takemura, S., Klimiuk, P. A., Braun, A., Goronzy, J. J., and Weyand, C. M. T cell activation in rheumatoid synovium is B cell dependent. *J Immunol*, 2001; **167**: 4710–18.

51. Beboist, C., and Mathis, D. Mast cells in autoimmune disease. *Nature*, 2002; **420**: 875–8.

52. Wooley, D. E. The mast cell in inflammatory arthritis. *N Engl J Med*, 2003; **348**: 1709–11.

53. Nigrovic, P. A., and Lee, D. M. Mast cells in inflammatory arthritis. *Arthritis Res Ther*, 2005; **7**: 1–11.

54. Lee, D. M., Friend, D. S., Gurish, M. F., Benoist, C., Mathis, D., and Brenner, M. B. Mast cells: a cellular link between autoantibodies and inflammatory arthritis. *Science*, 2002; **297**: 1689–92.

55. Brennan, F. M., Jackson, A., Chantry, D., Maini, R., and Feldmann, M. Inhibitory effect of TNFα antibodies on synovial cell interleukin-1 production in rheumatoid arthritis. *Lancet*, July 20; 1989: 244–7.

56. Haworth, C., Brennan, F. M., Chantry, D., Turner, M., Maini, R. N., and Feldmann, M. Expression of granulocyte-macrophage colony-stimulating factor in rheumatoid arthritis: regulation by tumor necrosis factor-α. *Eur J Immunol*, 1991; **21**: 2575–9.

57. Williamson, D. J., Begley, C. G., Vadas M. A., and Metcalf, D. The detection and initial characterization of colony-stimulating factors in synovial fluid. *Clin Exp Immunol*, 1988; **72**: 67–73.

58. Xu, W. D., Firestein, G. S., Taetle, R., Kaushansky, K., and Zvaifler, N. J. Cytokines in chronic inflammatory arthritis. II. Granulocyte-macrophage colony-stimulating factor in rheumatoid synovial effusions. *J Clin Invest*, 1989; **83**: 876–82.

59. Alvaro-Gracia, J. M., Zvaifler, N. J., and Firestein, G. S. Cytokines in chronic inflammatory arthritis. IV. Granulocyte/macrophage colony-stimulating factor-mediated induction of class II MHC antigen on human monocytes: a possible role in rheumatoid arthritis. *J Exp Med*, 1989; **179**: 865–75.

60. Alvaro-Gracia, J. M., Zvaifler, N. J., Brown, C. B., Kaushansky, K., and Firestein, G. S. Cytokines in chronic inflammatory arthritis. VI. Analysis of the synovial cells involved in granulocyte–macrophage colony–stimulating factor production and gene expression in rheumatoid arthritis and its regulation by IL-1 and tumor necrosis factor-α. *J Immunol*, 1991; **146**: 3365–71.

61. Keffer, J., Probert, L., Cazlaris, H., Georgopoulos, S., Kaslaris, E., Kioussis. *et al*. Transgenic mice expressing human tumor necrosis factor: a predictive genetic model of arthritis. *EMBO J*, 1991; **10**: 4025–31.

62. Probert, L., Plows, D., Kontogeorgos, G., and Kollias, G. The type I interleukin-1 receptor acts in series with tumor necrosis factor (TNF) to induce arthritis in TNF—transgenic mice. *European J Immunol*, 1995; **25**: 1794–7.

63. Toivanen, P. Normal intestinal microbiota in the aetiopathogenesis of rheumatoid arthritis. *Ann Rheum Dis*, 2003; **62**: 807–11.

64. Cronstein, B. N., and Weissmann, G. The adhesion molecules of inflammation. *Arthritis Rheum*, 1993; **36**: 147–55.

65. Oppenheimer-Marks, N., and Lipsky, P. E. Adhesion molecules as targets for the treatment of autoimmune diseases. *Clin Immunol Immunopathol*, 1996; **79**: 203–10.

66. Mojcik, C. F., and Shevach, E. M. Adhesion molecules: a rheumatologic perspective. *Arthritis Rheum*, 1997; **40**: 991–1004.

67. Kunkel, S. L., Lukacs, N., Kasama, T., and Streiter, R. M. The role of chemokines in inflammatory joint disease. *J Leukoc Biol*, 1996; **58**: 6–12.

68. Badolato, R., and Oppenheim, J. J. Role of cytokines, acute-phase proteins, and chemokines in the progression of rheumatoid arthritis. *Semin Arthritis Rheum*, 1996; **26**: 526–38.

69. Luster, A. D. Chemokines: chemotactic cytokines that mediate inflammation. *N Engl J Med*, 1998; **338**: 436–45.

70. Haringman, J. J., Ludikhuize, J., and Tak, P. P. Chemokines in joint disease: the key to inflammation? *Ann Rheum Dis*, 2004; **63**:1186–94.

71. Brennan, F. M., Zachariae, C. O. C., Chantry, D., Larsen, C. G., Turner, M., Maini, R. N. *et al*. Detection of interleukin 8: biological activity in synovial fluids from patients with rheumatoid arthritis and production of interleukin 8 mRNA by isolated synovial cells. *Eur J Immunol*, 1990; **20**: 2141–4.

72. Seitz, M., Dewald, B., Gerber, N., and Baggiolini, M. Enhanced production of neutrophil–activating peptide-1/interleukin-8 in rheumatoid arthritis. *J Clin Invest*, 1991; **87**: 464–9.

73. Koch, A. E., Kunkel, S. L., Burrows, J. C., Evanoff, H. L., Haines, G. K., Pope, R. M. *et al*. Synovial tissue macrophage as a source of the chemotactic cytokine IL-8. *J Immunol*, 1991; **147**: 2187–95.

74. Koch, A. E., Kunkel, S. L., Harlow, L. A., Mazarakis, D. D., Haines, G. H., Burdick, M. D. *et al*. Epithelial neutrophil activating peptide-78: a novel chemotactic cytokine for neutrophils in arthritis. *J Clin Invest*, 1994; **94**: 1012–18.

75. Koch, A. E., Kunkel, S. L., Shah, M. R., Hosaka, S., Holloran, M. M., Haines, G. K. *et al*. Growth-related gene product α: a chemotactic cytokine for neutrophils in rheumatoid arthritis. *J Immunol*, 1995; **155**: 3660–6.

76. Villiger, P. M., Terkeltaub, R., and Lotz, M. Production of monocyte chemoattractant protein-1 by inflamed synovial tissue and cultured synoviocytes. *J Immunol*, 1992; **149**: 722–7.

77. Koch, A. E., Kunkel, S. L., Harlow, L. A., Johnson, B., Evanoff, H. L., Haines, G. K. *et al*. Enhanced production of monocyte chemoattractant protein-1 in rheumatoid arthritis. *J Clin Invest*, 1992; **90**: 772–9.

78. Akahoshi, T., Wada, C., Endo, H., Hirato, K., Hosaka, S., Takagishi, K. *et al*. Expression of monocyte chemotactic and activating factor in rheumatoid arthritis: regulation of its production in synovial cells by interleukin-1 and tumor necrosis factor. *Arthritis Rheum*, 1993; **36**: 762–71.

79. Harigai, M., Hara, M., Yoshimura, T., Leonard, E. J., Inoue, K., and Kashiwazaki, S. Monocyte chemoattractant protein-1 (MCP-1) in inflammatory joint diseases and its involvement in the cytokine network of rheumatoid synovium. *Clin Immunol Immunopathol*, 1993; **69**: 83–91.

80. Koch, A. E., Kunkel, S. L., Harlow, L. A., Mazarakis, D. D., Haines, G. K., Burdick, M. D. *et al*. Macrophage inflammatory protein-1α: a novel chemotactic cytokine for macrophages in rheumatoid arthritis. *J Clin Invest*, 1994; **93**: 921–8.

81. Rathanaswami, P., Hachicha, M., Sadick, M., Schall, T. J., and McColl, S. R. Expression of the cytokine RANTES in human rheumatoid synovial fibroblasts. *J Biol Chem*, 1993; **268**: 5834–9.

82. Ruth, J. H., Volin, M. V., Haines III, G. K., Woodruff, D. C., Katschke, Jr., K. J., Woods, J. M. *et al*. Fractalkine, a novel chemokine in rheumatoid arthritis and in rat adjuvant-induced arthritis. *Arthritis Rheum*, 2003; **44**: 1568–81.

83. Chabaud, M., Page, G., and Miossec, P. Enhancing effect of IL-1, IL-17, and TNF-α on macrophage inflammatory protein-3α production in rheumatoid arthritis: regulation by soluble receptors and Th2 cytokines. *J Immunol*, 2001; **167**: 6015–20.

84. Harada, A., Mukaida, N., and Matsushima, K. Interleukin 8 as a novel target for intervention in acute inflammatory diseases. *Mol Med Today*, 1996; **2**: 482–9.

85. Kraan, M. C., Patel, D. D., Harinhman, J. J., Smith, M. D., Weedon, H., Ahern, M. J. *et al* The development of clinical signs of rheumatoid synovial inflammation is associated with increased synthesis of the chemokine CXCL8 (interleukin–8). *Arthritis Res*, 2001; **3**: 65–71.

86. Carter, P. H. Chemokine receptor antagonism as an approach to anti-inflammatory therapy: 'just right' or plain wrong? *Cur Opin Chem Biol*, 2002; **6**: 510–25.

87. Ogata, H., Takeya, M., Yoshimura, T., Takagi, K., and Takahashi, K. The role of monocyte chemoattractant protein-1 (MCP-1) in the pathogenesis of collagen-induced arthritis in rats. *J Pathol*, 1997; **182**: 106–14.

88. Plater-Zyberk, C., Hoogewerf, A. J., Proudfoot, A. E. I., Power, C. A., and Wells, T. N. C. Effect of a CC chemokine receptor antagonist on collagen-induced arthritis in DBA/1 mice. *Immunol Lett*, 1997; **57**: 117–20.

89. Yang, Y.-F., Mukai, T., Gao, P., Yamaguchi, N., Ono, S., Iwaki, H. *et al*. A non-peptide CCR5 antagonist inhibits collagen-induced arthritis by modulating T cell migration without affecting anti-collagen T cell responses. *Eur J Immunol*, 2002; **32**: 2124–32.

90. Zheng, B., Ozen, Z., Zhang, X., De Silva, S., Marinova, E., Guo, L. *et al*. CXCL13 neutralization reduces the severity of collagen-induced arthritis. *Arthritis Rheum*, 2005; **52**: 620–6.

91. Vierboom, M. P. M., Zavodny, P. J., Chou, C.-C., Tagat, J. R., Pugliese-Sivo, C., Strizki, J. *et al*. Inhibition of the development of collagen-induced arthritis in rhesus monkeys by a small molecular weight antagonist of CCR5. *Arthritis Rheum*, 2005; **52**: 627–36.

92. Barnes, D. A., Tse, J., Kaufhold, M., Owen, M., Hesselgesser, J., Strieter, R. *et al*. Polyclonal antibody directed against human RANTES ameliorates disease in the Lewis rat adjuvant-induced arthritis model. *J Clin Invest*, 1998; **101**: 2910–19.

93. Podolin, P. L., Bolognese, B. J., Foley, J. J., Schmidt, D. B., Buckley, P. T., Widdowson, K. L. *et al*. A potent and selective nonpeptide antagonist of CXCR2 inhibits acute and chronic models of arthritis in the rabbit. *J Immunol*, 2002; **169**: 6435–44.

94. Gladue, R. P., Tylaska, L. A., Brissette, W. H., Lira, P. D., Kath, J. C., Poss, C. S. *et al*. CP-481, 715, a potent and selective CCR1 antagonist with potential therapeutic implications for inflammatory diseases. *J Biol Chem*, 2003; **278**: 40473–80.

95. Qionones, M. P., Ahuja, S. K., Jimenez, F., Schaefer, J., Garavito, E., Rao, A. *et al*. Experimental arthritis in CC chemokine receptor-2 null mice closely mimics severe rheumatoid arthritis. *J Clin Invest*, 2004; **113**: 856–66.

96. Firestein, G. S., Xu, W. D., Townsend, K., Broide, D., Alvaro-Gracia, J., Glasebrook, A. *et al*. Cytokines in chronic inflammatory arthritis. I. Failure to detect T cell lymphokines (interleukin 2 and interleukin 3) and presence of macrophage colony-stimulating factor (CSF-1) and a novel mast cell growth factor in rheumatoid synovitis. *J Exp Med*, 1998; **168**: 1573–86.

97. Firestein, G. S., Alvaro-Gracia, J. M., and Maki, R. Quantitative analysis of cytokine gene expression in rheumatoid arthritis. *J Immunol*, 1990; **144**: 3347–53.

98. Firestein, G. S., and Zvaifler, N. J. How important are T cells in chronic rheumatoid synovitis? *Arthritis Rheum*, 1990; **33**: 768–73.

99. Panayi, G. S., Lanchbury, J. S., and Kingsley, G. H. The importance of the T cell in initiating and maintaining the chronic synovitis of rheumatoid arthritis. *Arthritis Rheum*, 1992; **35**: 729–35.

100. Simon, A. K., Seipelt, E., and Sieper, J. Divergent T-cell cytokine patterns in inflammatory arthritis. *Proc Nat Acad Sci U S A*, 1994; **91**: 8562–6.

101. Kotake, S., Schumacher H. R., Jr., Yarboro, C. H., Arayssi, T. K., Pando, J. A., Kanik, K. S. *et al*. In vivo gene expression of type 1 and type 2 cytokines in synovial tissues from patients in early stages of rheumatoid, reactive, and undifferentiated arthritis. *Proc Assoc Am Physicians*, 1997; **109**: 286–302.

102. Kanik, K. S., Hagiwara, E., Yarboro, C. H., Schumacher, H. R., Wilder R. L., and Klinman, D. M. Distinct patterns of cytokine secretion characterize new onset synovitis versus chronic rheumatoid arthritis. *J Rheumatol*, 1998; **25**: 16–22.

103. Klimiuk, P. A., Goronzy, J. J., Bjornsson, J., Beckenbaugh, R. D., and Weyand, C. M. Tissue cytokine patterns distinguish variants of rheumatoid synovitis. *Am J Pathol*, 1997; **151**: 1311–19.

104. Smeets, T. J. M., Barg, E. C., Kraan, M. C., Smith, M. D., Breedveld, F. C., and Tak, P. P. Analysis of the cell infiltrate and expression of proinflammatory cytokines and matrix metalloproteinases in arthroscopic synovial biopsies: comparison with synovial samples from patients with end stage destructive rheumatoid arthritis. *Ann Rheum Dis*, 2003; **62**: 635–8.

105. van den Berg, W. B., Joosten, L. A. B., and van de Loo, F. A. J. TNF α and IL-1β are separate targets in chronic arthritis. *Clin Exp Rheumatol*, 1999; **17** (Suppl. 18): S105–S114.

106. Morand, E. F., Leech, M., Weedon, H., Metz, C., Bucala, R., and Smith, M. D. Macrophage migration inhibitory factor in rheumatoid arthritis: clinical correlations. *Rheumatology*, 2002; **41**: 558–62.

107. Andersson, U., Erlandsson-Harris, H., Yang, H., and Tracey, K. J. HMGB1 as a DNA-binding cytokine. *J Leukoc Biol*, 2002; **72**: 1084–91.

108. Kokkola, R., Sundberg, E., Ulfgren, A.-K., Palmblad, K., Li, J., Wang, H. *et al*. High mobility group box chromosomal protein 1: a novel proinflammatory mediator in synovitis. *Arthritis Rheum*, 2002; **46**: 2598–603.

109. Taniguchi, N., Kawahara, K., Yone, K., Hashiguchi, Y., Yamakuchi, M., Goto, M. *et al*. High mobility group box chromosomal protein 1 plays a role in the pathogenesis of rheumatoid arthritis as a novel cytokine. *Arthritis Rheum*, 2003; **48**: 971–81.

110. Kamradt, T., and Burmester, G.-R. Cytokines and arthritis: is the Th1/Th2 paradigm useful for understanding pathogenesis? *J Rheumatol*, 1998; **25**: 6–8.

111. Symons, J. A., Wood, N. C., di Giovine, F. S., and Duff, G. W. Soluble IL-2 receptor in rheumatoid arthritis: correlation with disease activity, IL-1 and IL-2 inhibition. *J Immunol*, 1988; **141**: 2612–18.

112. McInnes, I. B., and Liew, F. Y. Interleukin 15: a proinflammatory role in rheumatoid arthritis synovitis. *Immunol Today*, 1998; **19**: 75–9.

113. McInnes, I. B., Al-Mughales, J., Field, M., Leung, B. P., Huang F.-P., Dixon, R. *et al*. The role of interleukin-15 in T-cell migration and activation in rheumatoid arthritis. *Nat Med*, 1996; **2**: 175–82.

114. McInnes, I. B., Leung, B. P., Sturrock, R. D., Field, M., and Liew, F. J. Interleukin-15 mediates T cell–dependent regulation of tumor necrosis factor–α production in rheumatoid arthritis. *Nat Med*, 1997; **3**: 189–95.

115. Alleva, D. G., Kaser, S. B., Monroy, M. A., Fenton, M. J., and Beller, D. I. IL-15 functions as a potent autocrine regulator of macrophage proinflammatory cytokine production: evidence for differential receptor subunit utilization associated with stimulation or inhibition. *J Immunol*, 1997; **159**: 2941–51.

116. Oppenheimer–Marks, N., Brezinsxhek, R. I., Mohamadzadeh, M., and Lipsky, P. E. Interleukin 15 is produced by endothelial cells and increases the transendothelial migration of T cells in vitro and in the SCID mouse-human rheumatoid arthritis model in vivo. *J Clin Invest*, 1998; **101**: 1261–72.

117. Carson, D. A. Unconventional T-cell activation by IL-15 in rheumatoid arthritis. *Nat Med*, 1997; **3**: 148–9.

118. Bamford, R. N., DeFilippis, A. P., Azimi, N., Kurys, G., and Waldmann, T. A. The 5' untranslated region, signal peptide, and the coding sequence of the carboxyl terminus of IL-15 participate in its multifaceted translational control. *J Immunol*, 1998; **160**: 4418–26.

119. Ruchatz, H., Leung, B. P., Wei, X.-Q., McInnes, I. B., and Liew, F. Y. Soluble IL-15 receptor α-chain administration prevents murine collagen-induced arthritis: a role for IL-15 in development of antigen—induced immunopathology. *J Immunol*, 1998; **160**: 5654–60.

120. Joosten, L. A. B., Lubberts, E., Helsen, M. M. A., and van den Berg, W. B. Dual role of IL-12 in early and late stages of murine collagen type II arthritis. *J Immunol*, 1997; **159**: 4094–102.

121. Beaulieu, A. D., and McColl, S. R. Differential expression of two major cytokines produced by neutrophils, interleukin-8 and the interleukin-1 receptor antagonist, in neutrophils isolated from the synovial fluid and peripheral blood of patients with rheumatoid arthritis. *Arthritis Rheum*, 1994; **37**: 855–9

122. Burmester, G. R., Stuhlmuller, B., Keyszer, G., and Kinne, R. W. Mononuclear phagocytes and rheumatoid synovitis: mastermind or workhorse in arthritis? *Arthritis Rheum*, 1997; **40**: 5–18.

123. Wei, S., Kitaura, H., Zhou, P., Ross, F. P., and Teitelbaum, S. L. Interleukin-1 mediates tumor necrosis factor-induced osteoclastogenesis. *J Clin Invest*, 2005; **115**: 282–90.

124. Gracie, J. A., Forsey, R. J., Chan, W. L., Gilmour, A., Leung, B. P., Greer, M. R. *et al*. A proinflammatory role for interleukin-18 in rheumatoid arthritis. *J Clin Invest*, 1999; **104**: 1393–401.

125. Plater-Zyberk, C., Joosten, L. A., Helsen, M. M., Sattonnet-Roche, P., Siegfried, C., Alouani, S. *et al*. Therapeutic effect of neutralizing endogenous interleukin-18 activity in the collagen-induced model of arthritis. *J Clin Invest*, 2001; **108**: 1825–32.

126. Banda, N. K., Vondracek, A., Kraus, D., Dinarello, C. A., Kim, S. H., Bendele, A. *et al*. Mechanisms of inhibition of collagen-induced arthritis by murine interleukin-18 binding protein. *J Immunol*, 2003; **170**: 2100–05.

127. Shull, M. M., Ormsby, I., Kier, A. B., Pawlowski, S., Diebold, R. J., Yin, M. *et al*. Targeted disruption of the mouse transforming growth factor-beta 1 gene results in multifocal inflammatory disease. *Nature*, 1992; **359**: 693–9.

128. Lacraz, S., Isler, P., Vey, E., Welgus, H. G., and Dayer, J. M. Direct contact between T lymphocytes and monocytes is a major pathway for induction of metalloproteinase expression. *J Biol Chem*, 1994; **269**: 22027–33.

129. De Benedetti, F., Massa, M., Pignatti, P., Kelley, M., Faltynek, C. R., and Martini, A. Elevated circulating interleukin-7 levels in patients with systemic juvenile rheumatoid arthritis. *J Rheumatol*, 1995; **22**: 1581–5.

130. van Roon, J. A., Glaudemans, K. A., Bijlsma, J. W., and Lafeber, F. P. Interleukin 7 stimulates tumour necrosis factor alpha and Th1 cytokine production in joints of patients with rheumatoid arthritis. *Ann Rheum Dis*, 2003; **62**: 113–19.

131. Alderson, M. R., Tough, T. W., Ziegler, S. F., and Grabstein, K. H. Interleukin 7 induces cytokine secretion and tumoricidal activity by human peripheral blood monocytes. *J Expe Med*, 1991; **173**: 923–30.

132. Leistad, L., Ostensen, M., and Faxvaag, A. Detection of cytokine mRNA in human, articular cartilage from patients with rheumatoid arthritis and osteoarthritis by reverse transcriptase-polymerase chain reaction. *Scand J Rheumatol*, 1998; **27**: 61–7.

133. Toraldo, G., Roggia, C., Qian, W. P., Pacifici, R., and Weitzmann, M. N. interleukin-7 induces bone loss in vivo by induction of receptor activator of nuclear factor kappa B ligand and tumor necrosis factor alpha from T cells. *Proc Natl Acad Sci U S A*, 2003; **100**: 125–30.

134. Miossec, P. Interleukin-17 in rheumatoid arthritis: if T cells were to contribute to inflammation and destruction through synergy. *Arthritis Rheum*, 2003; **48**: 594–601.

135. Chabaud, M., Page, G., and Miossec, P. Enhancing effect of interleukin-1, interleukin-17, and tumor necrosis factor-alpha on macrophage inflammatory protein-3alpha production in rheumatoid arthritis: regulation by soluble receptors and Th2 cytokines. *J Immunol*, 2001; **167**: 6015–20.

136. Lubberts, E., Joosten, L. A., van de Loo, F. A., van den Gersselaar, L. A., and van den Berg, W. B. Reduction of interleukin-17-induced inhibition of chondrocyte proteoglycan synthesis in intact murine articular cartilage by interleukin-4. *Arthritis Rheum*, 2000; **43**: 1300–6.

137. Lubberts, E., van den Bersselaar, L., Oppers-Walgreen, B., Schwarzenberger, P., Coenen-de Roo, C. J., Kolls, J. K. *et al*. Interleukin-17 promotes bone erosion in murine collagen-induced arthritis through loss of the receptor activator of NF-kappa B ligand/osteoprotegerin balance. *J Immunol*, 2003; **170**: 2655–62.

138. Firestein, G. S. Invasive fibroblast-like synoviocytes in rheumatoid arthritis: passive responders or transformed aggressors? *Arthritis Rheum*, 1996; **39**: 1781–90.

139. Koch, A. E. Review. Angiogenesis: implications for rheumatoid arthritis. *Arthritis Rheum*, 1998; **41**: 951–62.

140. Fava, R. A., Olsen, N. J., Spencer-Green, G., Yeo, K. T., Yeo, T. K., Berse, B. *et al*. Vascular permeability factor/endothelial growth factor (VPF/VEGF): accumulation and expression in human synovial fluids and rheumatoid synovial tissue. *J Exp Med*, 1994; **180**: 341–6.

141. Paleolog, E. M., Young, S., Stark, A. C., McCloskey, R. V., Feldmann, M., and Maini, R. N. Modulation of angiogenic vascular endothelial growth factor by tumor necrosis factor alpha and interleukin-1 in rheumatoid arthritis. *Arthritis Rheum*, 1998; **41**: 1258–65.

142. Szekanecz, Z., and Koch, A. E. Chemokines and angiogenesis. *Curr Opin Rheumatol*, 2001; **13**: 202–8.

143. Koch, A. E., Polverini, P. J., Kunkel, S. L., Harlow, L. A., DiPietro, L. A., Elner, V. M. *et al.* Interleukin-8 as a macrophage-derived mediator of angiogenesis. *Science*, 1992; **258**: 1798–801.

144. Dvorak, H. F., and Gresser, I. Microvascular injury in pathogenesis of interferon-induced necrosis of subcutaneous tumors in mice. *Journal of the National Cancer Institute*, 1989; **81**: 497–502.

145. Lacey, D. L., Timms, E., Tan, H. L., Kelley, M. J., Dunstan, C. R., Burgess, T. *et al.* Osteoprotegerin ligand is a cytokine that regulates osteoclast differentiation and activation. *Cell*, 1998; **93**: 165–76.

146. Kong, Y. Y., Feige, U., Sarosi, I., Bolon, B., Tafuri, A., Morony, S. *et al.* Activated T cells regulate bone loss and joint destruction in adjuvant arthritis through osteoprotegerin ligand. *Nature*, 1999; **402**: 304–9.

147. Romas, E., Sims, N. A., Hards, D. K., Lindsay, M., Quinn, J. W., Ryan, P. F. *et al.* Osteoprotegerin reduces osteoclast numbers and prevents bone erosion in collagen-induced arthritis. *Am J Pathol*, 2002; **161**: 1419–27.

148. Redlich, K., Hayer, S., Maier, A., Dunstan, C. R., Tohidast-Akrad, M., Lang, S. *et al.* Tumor necrosis factor alpha-mediated joint destruction is inhibited by targeting osteoclasts with osteoprotegerin. *Arthritis Rheum*, 2002; **46**: 785–92.

149. Gabay, C., and Kushner, I. Acute phase proteins. In *Encyclopaedia of life sciences*, 1999; London: Nature Publishing Group.

150. Gabay, C., and Kushner, I. Acute-phase proteins and other systemic responses to inflammation. *N Engl J Med*, 1999; **340**: 448–54.

151. Gabay, C., Porter, B., Guenette, D., Billir, B., and Arend, W. P. Interleukin-4 (interleukin-4) and interleukin-13 enhance the effect of interleukin-1beta on production of interleukin-1 receptor antagonist by human primary hepatocytes and hepatoma HepG2 cells: differential effect on C-reactive protein production. *Blood*, 1999; **93**: 1299–307.

152. O'Hara, R., Murphy, E. P., Whitehead, A. S., FitzGerald, O., and Bresnihan, B. Local expression of the serum amyloid A and formyl peptide receptor-like 1 genes in synovial tissue is associated with matrix metalloproteinase production in patients with inflammatory arthritis. *Arthritis Rheum*, 2004; **50**: 1788–99.

153. Chomarat, P., Rissoan, M. C., Pin, J. J., Banchereau, J., and Miossec, P. Contribution of interleukin-1, CD14, and CD13 in the increased interleukin-6 production induced by in vitro monocyte-synoviocyte interactions. *J Immunol*, 1995; **155**: 3645–52.

154. Tilg, H., Dinarello, C. A., and Mier, J. W. Interleukin-6 and APPs: anti-inflammatory and immunosuppressive mediators. *Immunology Today*, 1997; **18**: 428–32.

155. Alonzi, T., Fattori, E., Lazzaro, D., Costa, P., Probert, L., Kollias, G. *et al.* Interleukin 6 is required for the development of collagen-induced arthritis. *J Exp Med*, 1998; **187**: 461–8.

156. Wendling, D., Racadot, E., and Wijdenes, J. Treatment of severe rheumatoid arthritis by anti-interleukin 6 monoclonal antibody. *J Rheumatol*, 1993; **20**: 259–62.

157. Choy, E. H., Isenberg, D. A., Garrood, T., Farrow, S., Ioannou, Y., Bird, H. *et al.* Therapeutic benefit of blocking interleukin-6 activity with an anti-interleukin-6 receptor monoclonal antibody in rheumatoid arthritis: a randomized, double-blind, placebo-controlled, dose-escalation trial. *Arthritis Rheum*, 2002; **46**: 3143–50.

158. Nishimoto, N., Yoshizaki, K., and Miyasaka, N. A multi-center, randomized, double-blind, placebo-controlled trial of humanized anti-interleukin-6 receptor monoclonal antibody (MRA) in rheumatoid arthritis (RA). *Arthritis Rheum*, 2002; **46**: 559.

159. Lotz, M., Moats, T., and Villiger, P. M. Leukemia inhibitory factor is expressed in cartilage and synovium and can contribute to the pathogenesis of arthritis. *J Clin Invest*, 1992; **90**: 888–96.

160. Walmsley, M., Butler, D. M., Marinova-Mutafchieva, L., and Feldmann, M. An anti-inflammatory role for interleukin-11 in established murine collagen-induced arthritis. *Immunology*, 1998; **95**: 31–7.

161. Moreland, L., Gugliotti, R., King, K., Chase, W., Weisman, M., Greco, T. *et al.* Results of a phase-I/II randomized, masked, placebo-controlled trial of recombinant human interleukin-11 (rhinterleukin-11) in the treatment of subjects with active rheumatoid arthritis. *Arthritis Res*, 2001; **3**: 247–52.

162. Plater-Zyberk, C., Buckton, J., Thompson, S., Spaull, J., Zanders, E., Papworth, J. *et al.* Amelioration of arthritis in two murine

163. Horsfall, A. C., Butler, D. M., Marinova, L., Warden, P. J., Williams, R. O., Maini, R. N. *et al.* Suppression of collagen-induced arthritis by continuous administration of interleukin-4. *J Immunol*, 1997; **159**: 5687–96.

164. Miossec, P., and van den Berg, W. Th1/Th2 cytokine balance in arthritis. *Arthritis Rheum*, 1997; **40**: 2105–15.

165. Joosten, L. A., Lubberts, E., Durez, P., Helsen, M. M., Jacobs, M. J., Goldman, M. *et al.* Role of interleukin-4 and interleukin-10 in murine collagen-induced arthritis: protective effect of interleukin-4 and interleukin-10 treatment on cartilage destruction. *Arthritis Rheum*, 1997; **40**: 249–60.

166. van den Bosch, F., Russell, A., and Keystone, E. rHu interleukin-4 in subjects with active rheumatoid arthritis (RA): a phase I dose escalating safety study. *Arthritis Rheum*, 1998; **41**: 56.

167. Walmsley, M., Katsikis, P. D., Abney, E., Parry, S., Williams, R. O., Maini, R. N. *et al.* Interleukin-10 inhibition of the progression of established collagen-induced arthritis. *Arthritis Rheum*, 1996; **39**: 495–503.

168. Katsikis, P. D., Chu, C. Q., Brennan, F. M., Maini, R. N., and Feldmann, M. Immunoregulatory role of interleukin 10 in rheumatoid arthritis. *J Exp Med*, 1994; **179**: 1517–27.

169. Keystone, E., Wherry, J., and Grint, P. Interleukin-10 as a therapeutic strategy in the treatment of rheumatoid arthritis. *Rheum Dis Clin North Am*, 1998; **24**: 629–39.

170. McInnes, I. B., Illei, G. G., Danning, C. L., Yarboro, C. H., Crane, M., Kuroiwa, T. *et al.* Interleukin-10 improves skin disease and modulates endothelial activation and leukocyte effector function in patients with psoriatic arthritis. *J Immunol*, 2001; **167**: 4075–82.

171. Letterio, J. J., and Roberts, A. B. Transforming growth factor-beta: a critical modulator of immune cell function. *Clin Immunol Immunopathol*, 1997; **84**: 244–50.

172. Lotz, M., Kekow, J., and Carson, D. A. Transforming growth factor-beta and cellular immune responses in synovial fluids. *J Immunol*, 1990; **144**: 4189–94.

173. Letterio, J. J., Geiser, A. G., Kulkarni, A. B., Dang, H., Kong, L., Nakabayashi, T. *et al.* Autoimmunity associated with TGF-beta1-deficiency in mice is dependent on MHC class II antigen expression. *J Clin Invest*, 1996; **98**: 2109–19.

174. Wilder, R. L., Lafyatis, R., Roberts, A. B., Case, J. P., Kumkumian, G. K., Sano, H. *et al.* Transforming growth factor-beta in rheumatoid arthritis. *Ann N Y Acad of Sci*, 1990; **593**: 197–207.

175. van Holten, J., Plater-Zyberk, C., and Tak, P. P. Interferon-beta for treatment of rheumatoid arthritis? *Arthritis Res*, 2002; **4**: 346–52.

176. Palmer, G., Mezin, F., Juge-Aubry, C. E., Plater-Zyberk, C., Gabay, C., and Guerne, P. A. Interferon beta stimulates interleukin 1 receptor antagonist production in human articular chondrocytes and synovial fibroblasts. *Ann Rheum Dis*, 2004; **63**: 43–9.

177. Takayanagi, H., Kim, S., Matsuo, K., Suzuki, H., Suzuki, T., Sato, K. *et al.* Receptor activater of nuclear factor kB ligand maintains bone homeostasis through c-Fos-dependent induction of interferon-beta. *Nature*, 2002; **416**: 744–9.

178. Tak, P. P., Hart, B. A., Kraan, M. C., Jonker, M., Smeets, T. J., and Breedveld, F. C. The effects of interferon beta treatment on arthritis. *Rheumatology (Oxford)*, 1999; **38**: 362–9.

179. van Holten, J., Pavelka, K., Vencovsky, J., Stahl, H., Rozman, B., Genovese, M. *et al.* A multicentre, randomised, double blind, placebo controlled phase II study of subcutaneous interferon beta-1a in the treatment of patients with active rheumatoid arthritis. *Ann Rheum Dis*, 2005; **64**: 64–9.

180. Arend, W. P., Malyak, M., Guthridge, C. J., and Gabay, C. Interleukin-1 receptor antagonist: role in biology. *Annu Rev Immunol*, 1998; **16**: 27–55.

181. Joosten, L. A., Helsen, M. M., van de Loo, F. A., and van den Berg, W. B. Anticytokine treatment of established type II collagen-induced arthritis in DBA/1 mice: a comparative study using anti-tumor necrosis factor alpha, anti-interleukin-1 alpha/beta, and interleukin-1Ra. *Arthritis Rheum*, 1996; **39**: 797–809.

182. Ma, Y., Thornton, S., Boivin, G. P., Hirsh, D., Hirsch, R., and Hirsch, E. Altered susceptibility to collagen-induced arthritis in

transgenic mice with aberrant expression of interleukin-1 receptor antagonist. *Arthritis Rheum*, 1998; **41**: 1798–805.

183. Horai, R., Saijo, S., Tanioka, H., Nakae, S., Sudo, K., Okahara, A. *et al*. Development of chronic inflammatory arthropathy resembling rheumatoid arthritis in interleukin 1 receptor antagonist-deficient mice. *J Expe Med*, 2000; **191**: 313–20.

184. Bresnihan, B., Alvaro-Gracia, J. M., Cobby, M., Doherty, M., Domljan, Z., Emery, P. *et al*. Treatment of rheumatoid arthritis with recombinant human interleukin-1 receptor antagonist. *Arthritis Rheum*, 1998; **41**: 2196–204.

185. Cohen, S. B., Woolley, J. M., and Chan, W. Interleukin 1 receptor antagonist anakinra improves functional status in patients with rheumatoid arthritis. *J Rheumatol*, 2003; **30**: 225–31.

186. Genovese, M. C., Cohen, S., Moreland, L., Lium, D., Robbins, S., Newmark, R. *et al*. Combination therapy with etanercept and anakinra in the treatment of patients with rheumatoid arthritis who have been treated unsuccessfully with methotrexate. *Arthritis Rheum*, 2004; **50**: 1412–19.

187. Bendtzen, K., Hansen, M. B., Ross, C., and Svenson, M. High-avidity autoantibodies to cytokines. *Immunol Today*, 1998; **19**: 209–11.

188. Hansen, M. B., Andersen, V., Rohde, K., Florescu, A., Ross, C., Svenson, M. *et al*. Cytokine autoantibodies in rheumatoid arthritis. *Scand J Rheumatol*, 1995; **24**: 197–203.

189. Jouvenne, P., Fossiez, F., Banchereau, J., and Miossec, P. High levels of neutralizing autoantibodies against interleukin-1 alpha are associated with a better prognosis in chronic polyarthritis: a follow-up study. *Scand J Immunol*, 1997; **46**: 413–18.

190. Feldmann, M., Brennan, F., Paleolog, E., Taylor, P., and Maini, R. N. Anti-tumor necrosis factor alpha therapy of rheumatoid arthritis: mechanism of action. *Eur Cytokine Netw*, 1997; **8**: 297–300.

191. Fernandez-Botran, R., Chilton, P. M., and Ma, Y. Soluble cytokine receptors: their roles in immunoregulation, disease, and therapy. *Adv Immunol*, 1996; **63**: 269–336.

192. Roux-Lombard, P., Punzi, L., Hasler, F., Bas, S., Todesco, S., Gallati, H. *et al*. Soluble tumor necrosis factor receptors in human inflammatory synovial fluids. *Arthritis Rheum*, 1993; **36**: 485–9.

193. Moreland, L. W. Soluble tumor necrosis factor receptor (p75) fusion protein (ENBREL) as a therapy for rheumatoid arthritis. *Rheumatic Dis Clin of North Am*, 1998; **24**: 579–91.

194. Colotta, F., Dower, S. K., Sims, J. E., and Mantovani, A. The type II 'decoy' receptor: a novel regulatory pathway for interleukin 1. *Immunol Today*, 1994; **15**: 562–6.

195. Smith, D. E., Hanna, R., Della, F., Moore, H., Chen, H., Farese, A. M. *et al*. The soluble form of interleukin-1 receptor accessory protein enhances the ability of soluble type II interleukin-1 receptor to inhibit interleukin-1 action. *Immunity*, 2003; **18**: 87–96.

196. Smeets, R. L., van de Loo, F. A., Joosten, L. A., Arntz, O. J., Bennink, M. B., Loesberg, W. A. *et al*. Effectiveness of the soluble form of the interleukin-1 receptor accessory protein as an inhibitor of interleukin-1 in collagen-induced arthritis. *Arthritis Rheum*, 2003; **48**: 2949–58.

197. De Benedetti, F., Massa, M., Pignatti, P., Albani, S., Novick, D., and Martini, A. Serum soluble interleukin 6 receptor and interleukin-6/soluble interleukin-6 receptor complex in systemic juvenile rheumatoid arthritis. *J Clin Invest*, 1994; **93**: 2114–19.

198. Gabay, C., Silacci, P., Genin, B., Mentha, G., Le Coultre, C., and Guerne, P. A. Soluble interleukin-6 receptor strongly increases the production of acute-phase protein by hepatoma cells but exerts minimal changes on human primary hepatocytes. *Eur J Immunol*, 1995; **25**: 2378–83.

199. Kishimoto, T., Taga, T., and Akira, S. Cytokine signal transduction. *Cell*, 1994; **76**: 253–62.

13 | Autoantibodies in rheumatoid arthritis: prevalence and clinical significance

Günter Steiner and Josef S. Smolen

Introduction

Autoantibodies are a characteristic feature of autoimmune diseases. Although with only few exceptions autoantibodies do not appear to play important pathogenic roles, they are often very useful for diagnostic purposes. This includes various autoantibodies typical for organ-specific autoimmune diseases[1] and is likewise true for most autoantibodies that occur in autoimmune rheumatic diseases[2], such as anti-double-stranded (ds) DNA in systemic lupus erythematosus (SLE), anti-topoisomerase I (Scl-70) in scleroderma, anti-histidyl-tRNA synthetase (Jo-1) in poly/dermatomyositis, or anti-proteinase 3 in Wegener's granulomatosis. Nevertheless, some autoantibodies, such as anti-dsDNA, may also serve as indicators of disease activity.

Only few autoantibodies are truly disease-specific and their prevalence is usually below 50%. This is also true for most autoantibodies found in rheumatoid arthritis (RA) because the mere presence of rheumatoid factors (RFs), an immunological hallmark of the disease, are of rather modest specificity[3]. This has stimulated the search for novel antibodies and their respective target structures that could be useful for diagnosis of RA and in addition might enlighten our understanding of the pathogenesis of this disorder. Among the autoantibodies described in recent years there are promising candidates and some have already become part of the diagnostic repertoire (Table 13.1).

Rheumatoid factors

RFs (i.e. autoantibodies to the Fc portion of IgG) have been on the rheumatologic stage for more than 65 years and are still the best established serologic marker of RA[4,5]. They are found in 60–80% of RA patients and are thus fairly sensitive, but specificity of their mere presence is substantially lower compared to that of autoantibodies used for the diagnosis of many other rheumatic autoimmune diseases. Moreover, RFs occur less frequently in the early disease stages of RA when a clear diagnosis is often not yet possible. Apart from RA, RFs are also seen in many patients with primary Sjögren's syndrome and can be found in lower frequency (and usually also in lower titers) in all other autoimmune rheumatic diseases as well as in a number of non-autoimmune conditions such as osteoarthritis or chronic infections, and in otherwise healthy elderly individuals[3,5]. On the other hand, specificity is dependent on the concentration (titer) used as cut-off and is considerably higher at elevated titers, albeit at cost of sensitivity (Table 13.2). In fact, several investigators have observed that RFs ≤ 50 IU/mL are quite specific for RA[6–8].

As RFs are commonly of the IgM isotype, they could be conceived as constituting germ line-encoded 'natural autoantibodies'[9–11]. However, genes encoding RFs from RA patients are frequently somatically mutated[12,13]. This is similar to RFs from patients with infectious diseases, but interestingly, RFs from

Table 13.1 Autoantibodies of potential diagnostic relevance in **early** rheumatoid arthritis

Antibody (year)	Antigen (year)	Sensitivity (%)	Specificity (%)	References
Anti-perinuclear factor (1964) antikeratin (1979)/ anti-Sa (1994)	Filaggrin (1993) Deiminated arginine identified in: filaggrin (1999), fibrin (2001), vimentin (2000/2004)	40	92–99	6, 7, 23–31, 34–45
APCA/Anti-CCP (1998)		60	92–98	
Anti-RA33 (1989)	hnRNP-A2 (1993)	30	90	7, 41, 49–53
Anti-p68 (1995)	stress protein BiP (2001)	63–71	73–96	54, 55
RF (1993)	IgG	50[a]	96	3–20, 42, 43, 46, 47, 48

[a] RF ≥ 50 IU/mL.

Table 13.2 Sensitivity and specificity of rheumatoid factor[a]

Diagnosis	≤15 IU/mL	≤50 IU/mL	≤100 IU/mL
Rheumatoid arthritis	+++	++	+
Sjögren's syndrome	+++	++	+
SLE	+	+	–
MCTD	+	+	–
Scleroderma	++	+	–
Polymyositis	+	0	0
Reactive arthritis	0	0	0
Osteoarthritis	+	–	–
Healthy controls	+	0	0
Sensitivity (%)	66	46	26
Specificity (%)	72	88 (92[b])	95 (98[b])

ACPA, anti-citrullinated protein antibodies; anti-CCP, anti-cyclic citrullinated peptide; ACF, anti-citrullinated fibrinogen; APF, anti-perinuclear factor; anti-RA33, anti-RA-associated 33kD protein (hnRNP-A2); BiP, heavy chain binding protein; hnRNP, heterogeneous nuclear ribonucleoprotein; MCTD, mixed connective tissue disease; RNP, ribonucleoprotein.
–, <10%; +1, 10–35%; ++, 35–60%; +++, >60% frequency.
[a] RF was determined by nephelometry in >300 patients (. 100 patients with RA, >200 patients with other rheumatic diseases, and 30 healthy control persons).
[b] Specificity when a diagnosis of Sjögren's syndrome can be excluded.

Sjögren's syndrome patients show only little evidence of somatic hypermutation[14]. On the other hand, a broad range of immunoglobulin V genes is involved in the generation of RA RFs, which contrasts the restricted V gene usage of RF parapro-teins[15,16]. These data on somatic mutation of RF genes as well as the common presence of IgG and IGA RFs in RA patients, which is in line with an immunoglobulin class switch, indicate that RF production is T cell dependent and antigen-driven. However, the driving (auto)antigen is still unknown.

The immunoglobulin class (or isotype) of RFs may give interesting insights. Generally speaking, RFs can be of any immunoglobulin isotype. With conventional laboratory tests, such as nephelometry, primarily IgM-RF is measured (and the general term 'RF' usually means IgM-RF). Thus, the specificity of a high (≥50 IU/mL) RF level pertains to IgM-RF. On the other hand, IgG-RF (which like other isotypes can be determined by enzyme-linked immunosorbent assays (ELISA)) has been impli-cated in the pathogenesis of rheumatoid vasculitis[17], although this may not be the case in more recent cohorts of patients, where IgA-RF was prevalent[18]. Interestingly, IgA-RF may be of similar specificity as high titer IgM-RF, as it appears to be both a diag-nostic marker of RA and bears prognostic information regarding more severe erosive disease[19,20].

Importantly, as had already been shown two decades ago, occurrence of RF can precede the development of clinical symp-toms by many years[21]; in fact, RF preceded clinical manifesta-tions in 15 of 21 patients who developed RA in a prospective population study[22]. Thus, RF may have predictive power for the development of RA in otherwise healthy, younger individuals. Moreover, RF can be of prognostic value because its presence is related to the severity of RA, such as erosiveness, rapid disease progression, and unfavorable outcome[23–27]. Interestingly, the occurrence of RF is linked to the presence of the shared epitope of the human leukocyte antigen (HLA)-DR4 cluster[27,28], suggest-ing that the association between disease severity and HLA is mediated by the autoantibody. In fact, immune complexes have

been detected in RA joints, and synovial fluids of RA patients are hypocomplementemic[29,30]. Although all these observations are indicative of its pathological involvement, the role of RF in RA is still not entirely clear.

Despite this lacking proof of the mechanisms leading to RF production and the pathways of its detailed participation in the pathologic events, such involvement is further indicated by observations that RF fluctuates with disease activity: among RF-positive patients, those with high disease activity usually have higher RF levels, and effective therapy leads to decrease of RF levels such as with disease-modifying anti-rheumatic drugs (DMARDs)[31–34] or TNF-blockers[35,36]. This contrasts with other autoantibodies typical of RA, such as ACPA (see next paragraph).

Anti-citrullinated protein antibodies, antibodies to cyclic citrullinated peptide, anti-perinuclear factor, anti-keratin antibodies, anti-filaggrin antibodies (AFA), anti-citrullinated fibrinogen antibodies, and anti-Sa/vimentin antibodies

Autoantibodies to a perinuclear factor (APF) were detected already more than 40 years ago[37] and like anti-keratin antibod-ies (AKAs), which were described in 1979[38], have been repeat-edly shown to be highly specific for RA[39,40]. In 1993 an antigen targeted by APF and AKA was identified as the intermediate filament-aggregating protein filaggrin, which is expressed exclu-sively in keratinizing epithelial cells[41]. Subsequent studies showed that the APF/AKA/anti-filaggrin autoantibodies recognize epi-topes that contained the amino acid citrulline[42,43], which is generated post-translationally from arginine by the enzyme pep-tidylarginine deiminase. It was shown that these antibodies reacted with citrullinated peptides, and especially with a completely syn-thetic cyclic peptide that does not occur naturally[44]; therefore, these antibodies are now generally called anti-citrullinated protein anti-bodies (ACPA), anti-citrullinated peptide, or anti-cyclic citrulli-nated peptide (CCP) antibodies. One has to bear in mind that they recognize citrulline only when contained in a peptide which is not necessarily derived from filaggrin. Specificity of anti-citrulline antibodies is high (92–98%) and the reported sensitiv-ity of 60–70% is comparable to that of RF.

As filaggrin is an epidermal protein, it presumably does not represent the actual target of the anti-citrulline autoimmune response, which remains to be identified. A promising candidate antigen is fibrin which is present in the synovium of RA patients[45]. Since these autoantibodies, like RF, occur in the syn-ovial membrane and synovial fluid, it is conceivable that locally produced antibodies against citrullinated target structures may contribute to the inflammatory and destructive processes in the rheumatoid joint[46]. Aside from fibrin, other antigens in the synovial membrane may be present in a citrullinated form[47].

In fact, another type of autoantibody that was found to be highly specific for RA, anti-Sa, may be related to this group of anti-citrulline antibodies. Anti-Sa antibodies are directed to a 50 kD protein isolated from human tissues (spleen, placenta) and were described to occur in ~40% of patients with established RA and less frequently in patients with early disease[48,49]. Reported specificities of anti-Sa antibodies for RA range between 92% and 98%, which compares well with APF, AKA, and marker antibodies for other autoimmune diseases. Furthermore, determination of anti-Sa was shown to be of prognostic value, as the incidence of these antibodies was significantly increased in RA patients with severe destructive disease[50]. Interestingly, in a prospective study in patients with synovitis of recent onset, anti-Sa had the highest specificity and prognostic value of all autoantibodies investigated, including anti-CCP[51]. It was suggested recently that Sa is a citrullinated form of vimentin[52,53] and present in the synovial membrane[52]. However, the presence of citrullinated antigens in the synovial membrane is not specific for RA but can be found in many other disorders, including osteoarthritis[54]; this contrasts the differences regarding ACPA among those patients.

Similar to RF, the presence of ACPA has been found associated with the shared epitope of the HLA-DR4 cluster[55]. However, there may be another interesting genetic association: among Japanese patients, a gene encoding one of the four known peptidylarginine deiminases (PADIs), which are responsible for citrullination, namely PADI4, constitutes a susceptibility gene for RA[56]. The PADI4 haplotype associated with RA appears to affect the stability of PADI4 transcripts and was associated with higher serum levels of ACPA in patients with rheumatoid arthritis; whether an increase in citrullination of proteins is sufficient to induce autoimmunity remains speculative. Nevertheless, these data are of significant interest; however, they may relate mainly, if not exclusively to Asian or Japanese RA populations; currently evidence is lacking that this association is also present in Caucasians, especially since the chromosomal region containing PADI genes does not map to genome-wide linkage analyses of Caucasian RA patients.

Similar to RF, APF and AKAs have been shown to precede clinical manifestations of RA[57,58], and not surprisingly, this has recently been confirmed for ACPA[20,59,60]. Furthermore, ACPA occur in early RA patients and, like RF, appear to be associated with an increased propensity towards the development of erosions[20,51,61].

Thus, various antigens have been shown to contain citrullinated peptides and be potential targets of anti-citrulline antibodies, and the anti-CCP test exceeds the sensitivity of these tests, although a similar specificity is found using an anti-citrullinated fibrinogen assay[59]. Like RF, ACPA can be found in 'pre-RA' sera; its frequency in early RA is lower than in established RA, but it has a high sensitivity and, again similar to RF, it constitutes a good prognostic marker with respect to the development of severe, erosive disease. Nevertheless, there are a number of positive non-RA patients and up to 8% of individuals with primary Sjögren's syndrome without evidence of arthritis who have ACPA[62].

Clearly, the detection of citrullinated proteins as a target of autoantibodies in RA has been a pivotal event and the addition of this group of antibodies to citrullinated proteins/peptides, particularly ACPA, to the diagnostic and prognostic armamentarium is the most important one since the description of RF. However, these autoantibodies occur primarily (~80%) in RF positive sera and vice versa[7,10,11,44,51], and neither the sensitivity nor the prognostic value seems to exceed that of high-titer RF ($\leq$ 50 IU/mL). Just as ACPA can be positive in RF-negative individuals and then be of diagnostic and prognostic significance, RF may be positive at high levels in ACPA-negative individuals and bear a similar significance[7]. Thus, current evidence suggests that in patients with high RF levels there is no need to perform ACPA testing; rather this should be reserved for patients with arthritis and low-titered, or negative RF. Such stepwise autoantibody testing will allow optimal characterization of patients with RA in early disease stages. Moreover, as stated above, there is significant evidence that RF levels vary with disease activity, improve on DMARD therapy, and thus may even have a value during follow-up[34,63]; such evidence is currently lacking for ACPA[33,36].

Anti-A2/RA33 antibodies

These antibodies, which were first described in 1989, are directed to a nuclear protein, the heterogeneous nuclear ribonucleoprotein A2 (hnRNP-A2), which is involved in mRNA splicing and transport[64]. They occur in approximately one-third of RA patients but can be also detected in 20–30% of patients with SLE and in up to 40% of patients with the rare overlap syndrome mixed connective tissue disease (MCTD); therefore, specificity of anti-A2/RA33 antibodies for RA is only about 90%[65,66]. However, if a (rare) diagnosis of SLE (or MCTD) can be excluded, or in the absence of autoantibodies associated with SLE (such as anti-DNA or anti-Sm and anti-U1 RNP antibodies), specificity can be as high as 96%[16,65]. Frequencies of anti-RA33 may vary in different countries and, as with RF and ACPA, are lower in early than established disease. Importantly, other arthritides such as osteoarthritis, reactive arthritis, or psoriatic arthropathy are usually anti-A2/RA33 negative. Moreover, these autoantibodies may already be present in early disease, particularly in RF-negative sera[40,67]. Interestingly, these autoantibodies are also associated with an erosive type of lupus arthritis[68].

The antigen targeted is more or less ubiquitously expressed, although expression levels may differ greatly between tissues and recent data indicate that hnRNP-A2/RA33 is overexpressed in synovial membranes of RA patients where it might form a target of autoreactive B and T cells[69]. This, as well as the early presence of anti-A2/RA33 in TNF-α transgenic mice (which develop severe erosive arthritis similar to RA) and their disappearance with therapy[70] also suggests that this autoimmune response may be pathogenically involved in RA. Interestingly, among RF-negative sera there appears to be no overlap between ACPA and anti-RA33.

Anti-BiP antibodies

Autoantibodies to a ubiquituously expressed 68 kD glycoprotein were described in 1995 as occurring in more than 60% of sera from RA patients[71]. The target of these autoantibodies was identified as the stress protein BiP (immunoglobulin heavy chain binding protein), also known as grp78 (glucose-regulated protein of 78 kD), a member of the 70 kD heat shock protein family localized in the endoplasmatic reticulum[72]. Specificity of anti-BiP antibodies was initially reported to be 96%, but subsequent studies could not confirm these data since anti-BiP antibodies were also detected in other rheumatic disorders, though at somewhat lower titers than in RA[73]. Similar to hnRNP-A2/RA33 and fibrin, BiP has been shown to be highly expressed in synovial tissue[57] and data obtained in experimental animals and with human blood cells suggest that BiP reactive T cells might have immunomodulatory properties[74]. Based on these findings it has been suggested that BiP might be useful for treatment of RA[75]. On the other hand it is possible that BiP is responsible for co-eliciting autoimmune responses to other autoantigens and thus might indirectly drive the pathological autoimmune processes in RA[76].

Summary

The search for autoantigens with relevance for pathogenesis, diagnosis, and prognosis of RA has led to the characterization of several interesting novel autoantibodies in addition to RF. These antibodies can be found in 30–65% of RA patients, with reported specificities of up to 98%. However, when RF test results are interpreted correctly and only high-titer RF attributed to RA, its sensitivity, specificity, and prognostic value appear virtually unsurpassed. However, especially in sera negative for RF or with RF titers <50 IU/mL, APCA/anti-CCP/ACF is an excellent additional diagnostic and prognostic marker, while anti-RA33 has diagnostic value and is prognostic for mild disease. Thus, these antibodies are helpful as additions to RF testing. Therefore, their determination in addition to RF should be considered, particularly when RF is low or absent or when the diagnosis is uncertain. So far, commercial assays are available only for anti-citrulline and anti-A2/RA33 antibodies, but assays for anti-BiP may soon appear on the stage.

The presence of many of these autoantibodies, especially RF and ACPA, is associated with the shared epitope so characteristically linked to RA. The meaning of this association is enigmatic, although the simplest view relates to the fact that the shared epitope is involved in the presentation of antigens that lead to the respective autoantibodies, since, after all, it represents no more and no less than an immune response gene, and different immune response genes confer different responsiveness to certain (pathogenic) antigens.

To date, it is not clear whether these autoimmune responses play pathogenic roles or are consequences rather than causes of the chronic inflammatory process of RA, even if they sometimes precede the manifestation of clinical symptoms. On the other hand, there exists considerable evidence for pathogenic involvement of RF and ACPA, indicating that a potential role of autoantibodies in the disease process, at least with respect to aggravation and perpetuation of RA, should not be neglected. This is bolstered by a recently described transgenic mouse model of destructive arthritis in which an autoantibody directed to the ubiquituously expressed glycolytic enzyme glucose-6-phosphate

isomerase was sufficient to induce erosive arthritis[75–77], even though autoantibodies to this antigen play no role in RA. Thus, autoantibodies may be more than diagnostically useful epiphenomena and it will be a challenging task for the next few years to elucidate the role of these autoimmune reactions in the pathogenesis of RA, and to learn more about the best diagnostic algorithms. It will also be exciting to search for novel, even more specific markers for the disease.

References

1. Devendra, D., Yu, L., and Eisenbarth, G. S. Endocrine autoantibodies. *Clin Lab Med* 2004; **24**: 275–303.
2. Von Muhlen, C. A., and Tan, E. M. Autoantibodies in the diagnosis of systemic rheumatic diseases. *Semin Arthritis Rheum* 1995; **24**: 323–58.
3. Smolen, J. S. Rheumatoid arthritis. In *Manual of biological markers* (Maini, R. N., and van Venrooij, W. J., eds), pp. 1–18. Amsterdam: Kluwer Academic; 1996.
4. Waaler, E. On the occurrence of a factor in human serum activating the specific agglutination of sheep blood corpuscles. *Acta Pathol Microbiol Immunol Scand* 1939; **17**: 172–82.
5. Tighe, H., and Carson, D. A. Rheumatoid factors. In *Textbook of rheumatology* (Kelley W N., Harris E. D., Ruddy S., Sledge C. B, eds), pp. 241–9. Philadelphia: WB Saunders; 1997.
6. Jansen, A. L., van der Horst-Bruinsma, I., van Schaardenbzrg, D., van de Stadt, R., de Koning, M., and Dijkmans, B. A. Rheumatoid factor and antibodies to cyclic citrullinated peptide differentiate rheumatoid arthritis from undifferentiated polyarthritis in patients with early arthritis. J. *Rheumatol* 2002; **29**: 2074–6.
7. Nell, V. P. K., Machold, K. P., Eberl, G., Hiesberger, H., Hoefler, E., Smolen, J. S. *et al.* The diagnostic and prognostic significance of autoantibodies in patients with early arthritis. *Ann Rheum Dis* 2003; **62** (Suppl. 1): OP0015.
8. Sinclair, D., and Hull, D. G. Why do general practitioners request rheumatoid factor? A study of symptoms, requesting patterns and patient outcome. *Ann Clin Biochem* 2003; **30** (Pt 2): 131–7.
9. Carroll, M. C., and Prodeus, A. P. Linkages of innate and adaptive immunity. *Curr Opin Immunol* 1998; **10**: 36–40.
10. Casali, P., and Schettino, E. W. Structure and function of natural antibodies. *Curr Top Microbiol Immunol* 1998; **210**: 167–79.
11. Quintana, F. J., and Cohen, I. R. The natural autoantibody repertoire and autoimmune disease. *Biomed Pharmacother* 2004; **58**: 276–81.
12. Youngblood, K., Fruchter, L., Ding, G., Lopez, J., Bonagura, V., and Davidson, A. Rheumatoid factors from the peripheral blood of two patients with rheumatoid arthritis are genetically heterogeneous and somatically mutated. *J Clin Invest* 1994; **93**: 852–61.
13. Djavad, N., Bas, S., Shi, X., Schwager, J., Jeannet, M., Vischer, T. *et al.* Comparison of rheumatoid factors of rheumatoid arthritis patients, of individuals with mycobacterial infections and of normal controls: evidence for maturation in the absence of an autoimmune response. *Eur J Immunol* 1996; **26**: 2480–6.
14. Elagib, K. E., Borretzen, M., Jonsson, R., Haga, H. J., Thoen, D., Thompson, K. M. *et al.* Rheumatoid factors in primary Sjogren's syndrome (pSS) use diverse VH region genes, the majority of which show no evidence of somatic hypermutation. *Clin Exp Immunol* 1999; **117**: 388–94.
15. Kipps, T. J., Fong, S., Tomhave, E., Chen, P. P., Goldfien, R. J., and Carson, D. A. High-frequency expression of a conserved kappa light-chain variable-region gene in chronic lymphocytic leukemia. *Proc Natl Acad Sci U S A* 1987; **84**: 2916–20.
16. Sasso, E. H. Immunoglobulin V. genes in rheumatoid arthritis. *Rheum Dis Clin North Am* 1992; **18**: 809–36.
17. Scott, D. G., Bacon, P. A., Allen, C., Elson, C. J., and Wallington, T. IgG rheumatoid factor, complement and immune complexes in

rheumatoid synovitis and vasculitis: comparative and serial studies during cytotoxic therapy. *Clin Exp Immunol* 1981; **43**: 54–63.

18. Voskuyl, A. E., Hazes, J. M., Zwinderman, A. H., Paleolog, E. M., van der Meer, F. J., Daha, M. R. *et al*. Diagnostic strategy for the assessment of rheumatoid vasculitis. *Ann Rheum Dis* 2003; **62**: 407–13.

19. Houssien, D. A., Jonsson, T., Davies, E., and Scott, D. L. Clinical significance of IgA rheumatoid factor subclasses in rheumatoid arthritis. *J Rheumatol* 1997; **24**: 2119–22.

20. Vencovsky, J., Machacek, S., Sedova, L., Kafkova, J., Gatterova, J., Pesakova, V. *et al*. Autoantibodies can be prognostic markers of an erosive disease in early rheumatoid arthritis. *Ann Rheum Dis* 2003; **62**: 427–30.

21. Aho, K., Palosuo, T., Raunio, V, Puska, P., Aromaa, A., and Salonen, J. T. When does rheumatoid disease start? *Arthritis Rheum* 1985; **28**: 485–9.

22. Aho, K., Heliovaara, M., Maatela, J., Tuomi, T., and Palosuo, T. Rheumatoid factors antedating clinical rheumatoid arthritis. *J Rheumatol* 1991; **18**: 1282–4.

23. Scott, D. L., Symmons, D. P., Coulton, B. L., and Popert, A. J. Long-term outcome of treating rheumatoid arthritis: results after 20 years. *Lancet* 1987; **1** (8542): 1108–11.

24. Scott, D. L. Prognostic factors in early rheumatoid arthritis. *Rheumatology* (Oxford) 2000; **39** (Suppl. 11): 24–9.

25. Bukhari, M., Lunt, M., Harrison, B. J., Scott, D. G., Symmons, D. P., and Silman, A. J. Rheumatoid factor is the major predictor of increasing severity of radiographic erosions in rheumatoid arthritis: results from the Norfolk Arthritis Register Study, a large inception cohort. *Arthritis Rheum* 2002; **46**: 906–12.

26. Green, M., Marzo-Ortega, H., McGonagle, D., Wakefield, R. J., and Proudman, S. M., Conaghan, P. G. *et al*. Persistence of mild, early inflammatory arthritis: the importance of disease duration, rheumatoid factor, and the shared epitope. *Arthritis Rheum* 1999; **42**: 2184–8.

27. Mattey, D. L., Dawes, P. T., Clarke, S., Fisher, J., Brownfield A., and Thomson W *et al*. Relationship among the HLA-DRB1 shared epitope, smoking and rheumatoid factor production in rheumatoid arthritis. *Arthritis Rheum* 2002; **47**: 403–7.

28. Silman, A. J., and Pearson, J. E. Epidemiology and genetics of rheumatoid arthritis. *Arthritis Res* 2002; **4** (Suppl. 3): S265–S272.

29. Ishikawa, H., Smiley, J. D., and Ziff, M. Electron microscopic demonstration of immunoglobulin deposition in rheumatoid cartilage. *Arthritis Rheum* 1975; **18**: 563–76.

30. Neumann, E., Barnum, S. R., Tarner, I. H., Echols, J., Fleck, M., Judex, M. *et al*. Local production of complement proteins in rheumatoid arthritis synovium. *Arthritis Rheum* 2002; **46**: 934–45.

31. Olsen, N. J., Teal, G. P., and Brooks, R. H. IgM-rheumatoid factor and responses to second-line drugs in rheumatoid arthritis. *Agents Action* 1991; **34**: 169–71.

32. Spadaro, A., Riccieri, V., Sili Scavelli, A., Taccari, E., and Zoppini, A. One year treatment with low dose methotrexate in rheumatoid arthritis: effect on class specific rheumatoid factors. *Clin Rheumatol* 1993; **12**: 357–60.

33. Mikuls, T. R., O'Dell, J. R., Stoner, J. A., Parrish, L. A., Arend, W. P., Norris, J. M. *et al*. Association of rheumatoid arthritis treatment response and disease duration with declines in serum levels of IgM rheumatoid factor and anti-cyclic citrullinated peptide antibody. *Arthritis Rheum* 2004; **50**: 3776–82.

34. Paimela, L., Palosuo, T., Leirisalo-Repo, M., Helve, T., and Aho, K. Prognostic value of quantitative measurement of rheumatoid factor in early rheumatoid arthritis. *Br J Rheumatol* 2005; **34**: 1146–50.

35. Bobbio-Pallavicini, F., Alpini, C., Caporali, R., Avalle, S., Bugatti, S., Montecucco, C. *et al*. Autoantibody profile in rheumatoid arthritis during long-term infliximab treatment. *Arthritis Res Ther* 2004; **6**: R264–R267.

36. De Rycke, L., Verhelst, X., Kruithof, E., van den Bosch, F., Hoffman, I. E., Veys, E. M. *et al*. Rheumatoid factor, but not anti-cyclic citrullinated peptide antibodies, is modulated by infliximab treatment in rheumatoid arthritis. *Ann Rheum Dis* 2005; **64**: 299–302.

37. Nienhuis, R. L. F., Mandema, E., and Smids, C. A new serum factor in patients with rheumatoid arthritis, the antiperinuclear factor. *Ann Rheum Dis* 1964; **23**: 302–5.

38. Young, B. J., Mallya, R. K., Leslie, R. D., Clark, C. J., and Hamblin, T. J. Antikeratin antibodies in rheumatoid arthritis. *Br Med J* 1979; **2**: 97–9.

39. Youinou, P., and Serre, G. The antiperinuclear factor and antikeratin antibody systems. *Int Arch Allergy Immunol* 1995; **107**: 508–18.

40. Cordonnier, C., Meyer, O., Palazzo, E., de Bandt, M., Elias, A., Nicaise, P. *et al*. Diagnostic value of anti-RA33 antibody, antikeratin antibody, perinuclear factor and antinuclear antibody in early rheumatoid arthritis: comparison with rheumatoid factor. *Br J Rheumatol* 1996; **35**: 620–4.

41. Simon, M., Girbal, E., Sebbag, M., Gomes-Daudrix, V., Vincent, C., Salma, G. *et al*. The cytokeratin filament: aggregating protein filaggrin is the target of the so-called 'antikeratin antibodies', autoantibodies specific for rheumatoid arthritis. *J Clin Invest* 1993; **92**: 1387–93.

42. Girbal-Neuhauser, E., Durieux, J. J., Arnaud, M., Dalbon, P., Sebbag, M., Vincent, C. *et al*. The epitopes targeted by the rheumatoid arthritis-associated antifilaggrin autoantibodies are posttranslationally generated on various sites of (pro)filaggrin by deimination of arginine residues. *J Immunol* 1999; **162**: 585–94.

43. Schellekens, G. A., de Jong, B. A. W., van den Hoogen, F. H. J., van de Putte, L. B. A., and van Venrooij, W J. Citrulline is an essential constituent of antigenic determinants recognized by rheumatoid arthritis-specific autoantibodies. *J Clin Invest* 1998; **101**: 273–81.

44. Schellekens, G. A., Visser, H., de Jong, B. A., van den Hoogen, F. H., Hazes, J. M., Breedveld, F. C. *et al*. The diagnostic properties of rheumatoid arthritis antibodies recognizing a cyclic citrullinated peptide. *Arthritis Rheum* 2000; **43**: 155–63.

45. Masson-Bessiere, C., Sebbag, M., Girbal-Neuhauser, E., Nogueira, L., Vincent, C., Senshu, T. *et al*. The major synovial targets of the rheumatoid arthritis-specific antifilaggrin autoantibodies are deiminated forms of the alpha- and beta-chains of fibrin. *J Immunol* 2001; **166**: 4177–84.

46. Masson Bessiere, C., Sebbag, M., Durieux, J. J., Nogueira, L., Vincent, C., Girbal-Neuhauser, E. *et al*. In the rheumatoid pannus, anti-filaggrin autoantibodies are produced by local plasma cells and constitute a higher proportion of IgG than in synovial fluid and serum. *Clin Exp Immunol* 2000; **119**: 544–52.

47. Baeten, D., Peene, I., Union, A., Meheus, L., Sebbag, M., Serre, G. *et al*. Specific presence of intracellular citrullinated proteins in rheumatoid arthritis synovium: relevance to antifilaggrin autoantibodies. *Arthritis Rheum* 2001; **44**: 2255–62.

48. Després, N., Boire, G., Lopez-Longo, F. J., and Menard, H. The Sa system: a novel antigen-antibody system specific for rheumatoid arthritis. *J Rheumatol* 1994; **21**: 1027–33.

49. Hueber, W., Hassfeld, W., Smolen, J. S., and Steiner, G. Sensitivity and specificity of anti-Sa autoantibodies for rheumatoid arthritis. *Rheumatology* 1999; **38**: 155–9.

50. Hayem, G., Chazerain, P., Combe, B., Elias, A., Haim, T., Nicaise, P. *et al*. Anti-Sa antibody is an accurate diagnostic and prognostic marker in adult rheumatoid arthritis. *J Rheumatol* 1999; **26**: 7–13.

51. Goldbach-Mansky, R., Lee, J., McCoy, A., Hoxworth, J., Yarboro, C., Smolen, J. S. *et al*. Rheumatoid arthritis associated autoantibodies in patients with synovitis of recent onset. *Arthritis Res* 2000; **2**: 236–43.

52. Ménard, H. A., Lapointe, E., Rochdi, M. D., and Zhou, Z. J. Insights into rheumatoid arthritis derived from the Sa immune system. *Arthritis Res* 2000; **2**: 429–32.

53. Vossenaar, E. R., Després, N., Lapointe, E., van der Heijden, A., Lora, M., Senshu, T. *et al*. Rheumatoid arthritis specific anti-Sa antibodies target citrullinated vimentin. *Arthritis Res Ther* 2004; **6**: R142–50–R150. [First published online 5 Feb 2004]

54. Vossenaar, E. R., Smeets, T. J., Kraan, M. C., Raats, J. M., van Venrooij, W. J., and Tak, P. P. The presence of citrullinated proteins is not specific for rheumatoid synovial tissue. *Arthritis Rheum* 2004; **50**: 3485–94.

55. van Gaalen, F. A., van Aken, J., Huizinga, T. W., Schreuder, G. M., Breedveld, F. C., Zanelli, E. *et al*. Association between HLA class II genes and autoantibodies to cyclic citrullinated peptides (CCPs) influences the severity of rheumatoid arthritis. *Arthritis Rheum* 2004; **50**: 2113–21.

56. Yamada, R., Suzuki, A., Chang, X., and Yamamoto, K. Peptidylarginine deiminase type 4: identification of a rheumatoid arthritis-susceptible gene. *Trends Mol Med* 2003; **9**: 503–8.

57. Aho, K., Palosuo, T., and Kurki, P. Marker antibodies of rheumatoid arthritis: diagnostic and pathogenetic implications. *Semin Arthritis Rheum* 1994; **23**: 379–87.

58. Aho, K., von Essen, R., Kurki, P., Palosuo, T., and Heliovaara, M. Antikeratin antibody and antiperinuclear factor as markers for subclinical rheumatoid disease process. *J Rheumatol* 1993; **20**: 1278–81.

59. Nielen, M. M., van Schaardenburg, Reesink, W. H., van de Stadt, R. J., van der Horst-Bruinsma I. E., de Koning M. G. *et al*. Specific autoantibodies precede the symptoms of rheumatoid arthritis: a study of serial measurements in blood donors. *Arthritis Rheum* 2004; **50**: 380–6.

60. Rantapaa-Dahlqvist, S., de Jong, B. A., Berglin, E., Hallmans, G., Wadell, G., Stenlund, H. *et al*. Antibodies against cyclic citrullinated peptide and IgA rheumatoid factor predict the development of rheumatoid arthritis. *Arthritis Rheum* 2003; **48**: 2741–9.

61. Kroot, E. J., de Jong, B. A., van Leeuwen, M. A., Swinkels, H., van den Hoogen, F. H., van't Hof, M. *et al*. The prognostic value of anti-cyclic citrullinated peptide antibody in patients with recent-onset rheumatoid arthritis. *Arthritis Rheum* 2000; **43**: 1831–5.

62. Gottenberg, J. E., Mignot, S., Nicaise-Rolland, P., Cohen-Solal, J., Aucouturier, F., and Goetz, J. *et al*. Prevalence of anti-cyclic citrullinated peptide and anti-keratin antibodies in patients with primary Sjogren's syndrome. *Ann Rheum Dis* 2005; **64**: 114–17.

63. Olsen, N. J., Teal, G. P., and Brooks, R. H. IgM-rheumatoid factor and responses to second-line drugs in rheumatoid arthritis. *Agents Actions* 1991; **34**: 169–72.

64. Steiner, G., Hartmuth, K., Skriner, K., Maurer-Fogy, I., Sinski, A., Thalmann, E. *et al*. Purification and partial sequencing of the nuclear autoantigen RA33 shows that it is indistinguishable from the A2 protein of the heterogeneous nuclear ribonucleoprotein complex. *J Clin Invest* 1992; **90**: 1061–6.

65. Hassfeld, W., Steiner, G., Studnicka-Benke, A., Skriner, K., Graninger, W., Fischer, I. *et al*. Autoimmune response to the spliceosome: an immunological link between rheumatoid arthritis, mixed connective tissue disease and systemic lupus erythematosus. *Arthritis Rheum* 1995; **38**: 777–85.

66. Meyer, O, Tauxe, F., Fabregas, D., Gabay, C., Goycochea, M., Haim, T. *et al*. Anti-RA33 antinuclear autoantibody in rheumatoid arthritis and mixed connective tissue disease: comparison with antikeratin and antiperinuclear antibodies. *Clin Exp Rheumatol* 1993; **11**: 473–8.

67. Hassfeld, W., Steiner, G., Graninger, W., Witzmann, G., Schweitzer, H., and Smolen, J. S. Autoantibody to the nuclear antigen RA33: a marker for early rheumatoid arthritis. *Br J Rheumatol* 1993; **32**: 199–203.

68. Richter Cohen, M., Steiner, G., Smolen, J. S., and Isenberg, D. A. Erosive arthritis in systemic lupus erythematosus: analysis of a distinct clinical and serological subset. *Br J Rheumatol* 2005; **37**: 421–4.

69. Fritsch, R., Eselbock, D., Skriner, K., Jahn-Schmid, B., Scheinecker, C., Bohle, B. *et al*. Characterization of autoreactive T cells to the autoantigens heterogeneous nuclear ribonucleoprotein A2 (RA33) and filaggrin in patients with rheumatoid arthritis. *J Immunol* 2002; **169**: 1068–76.

70. Schett, G., Hayer, S., Tohidast-Akrad, M., Schmid, B. J., Lang, S., Turk, B. *et al*. Adenovirus-based overexpression of tissue inhibitor of metalloproteinases 1 reduces tissue damage in the joints of tumor necrosis factor alpha transgenic mice. *Arthritis Rheum* 2001; **44**: 2888–98.

71. Blaeß, S., Specker, C., Lakomek, H. J., Schneider, E. M., and Schwochaus, M. Novel 68 kDa autoantigen detected by rheumatoid arthritis specific antibodies. *Ann Rheum Dis* 1995; **54**: 355–60.

72. Blaeß, S., Union, A., Raymackers, J., Schumann, F., Ungethüm, U., Müller-Steinbach, S. *et al*. The stress protein BiP is overexpressed and is a major B- and T-cell target in rheumatoid arthritis. *Arthritis Rheum* 2001; **44**: 971–80.

73. Bodman-Smith, M. D., Corrigall, V. M., Berglin, E., Cornell, H. R., Tzioufas, A. G., Mavragani, C. P. *et al*. Antibody response to the human stress protein BiP in rheumatoid arthritis. *Rheumatology (Oxford)* 2004; **43**: 1283–7.

74. Corrigall, V. M., Bodman-Smith, M. D., Brunst, M., Cornell, H., and Panayi, G. S. Inhibition of antigen-presenting cell function and stimulation of human peripheral blood mononuclear cells to express an antiinflammatory cytokine profile by the stress protein BiP: relevance to the treatment of inflammatory arthritis. *Arthritis Rheum* 2004; **50**: 1164–71.

75. Panayi, G., and Corrigall, V. BiP: a new biologic immunomodulator for the treatment of rheumatoid arthritis. *Autoimmun Rev* 2004; **3** (Suppl. 1): S16–S17.

76. Purcell, A. W., Todd, A., Kinoshita, G., Lynch, T. A., Keech, C. L., and Gething, M. J. *et al*. Association of stress proteins with autoantigens: a possible mechanism for triggering autoimmunity. *Clin Exp Immunol* 2003; **132**: 193–200.

76. Matsumoto, I., Staub, A., Benoist, C., and Mathis, D. Arthritis provoked by linked T and B. cell recognition of a glycolytic enzyme. *Science* 1999; **286**: 1732–5.

77. Matsumoto, I., Lee, D. M., Goldbach-Mansky, R., Sumida, T., Hitchon, C. A., Schur, P. H. *et al*. Low prevalence of antibodies to glucose-6-phosphate isomerase in patients with rheumatoid arthritis and a spectrum of other chronic autoimmune disorders. *Arthritis Rheum* 2003; **48**: 944–54.

14 | Mechanisms of fibroblast-mediated joint destruction

Thomas Pap, Renate Gay, and Steffen Gay

Introduction

Rheumatoid arthritis (RA) is a chronic inflammatory disorder of yet unknown etiology that primarily affects the joints and results in the progressive destruction of articular cartilage and bone. The pathogenesis of RA involves complex changes which include the mutually interacting phenomena of chronic inflammation, altered immune responses, and synovial hyperplasia. The progressive destruction of cartilage and bone, however, represents a unique and most prominent feature of this disease. It clearly distinguishes RA from other arthritides and determines the outcome of disease in the majority of affected individuals[1]. Intriguingly, there is growing evidence that the pathological mechanisms of inflammation and articular damage—although overlapping—are not identical. Rather, it has been found that joint destruction may occur even when inflammation is well controlled[2], and that critical steps initiating joint destruction occur very early in the course of disease[3].

In recent years, considerable progress has been made in elucidating the molecular and cellular basis of rheumatoid joint destruction as well as in identifying potential ways to inhibit this process. Advances in molecular biology such as gene transfer technology, the utilization of novel animal models of destructive arthritis, and the observation of early stages of human disease have provided new insights into key mechanisms that ultimately lead to the destruction of extracellular matrix in RA. It has become clear that the mechanisms of rheumatoid joint destruction are linked closely to changes that occur predominantly at sites of interaction between the rheumatoid synovium and articular cartilage and bone. In this context, two phenomena have received special attention: the activation and differentiation of bone resorbing osteoclast-like cells from tissue macrophages present in the chronically inflamed RA synovium and the specific role of fibroblast-like cells in rheumatoid joint destruction. The latter cells are of particular interest because fibroblasts in the rheumatoid synovium differ significantly from normal fibroblasts and as part of a complex cellular network contribute to joint destruction by direct mechanisms as well as through interaction with neighboring cells[4,5]. Investigating the specific properties of RA synovial fibroblasts has revealed that they show features of stable cellular activation that provides the basis for both their direct and indirect effects on joint destruction (Fig. 14.1).

Composition of RA synovium

The observation that the proliferating synovial tissue, often also called 'pannus', is responsible for joint destruction in RA was recognized more than two decades ago[6,7]. Thickening of the RA synovium is largely due to a hyperplasia of the most superficial lining layer that in the course of disease grows from 2–4 layers of cells to more than 10 layers. About two-thirds of the cells in the lining layer express macrophage markers such as CD11b, CD14, CD33, CD68 as well as major histocompatibility complex (MHC) class II molecules, and can, thus, be identified as macrophages[8–12]. Macrophages constitute a major source of inflammatory cytokines in the rheumatoid synovium. About one-third of lining cells appear to originate from resident synovial cells, which have a fibroblast-like appearance and lack specific surface markers. They have been called type B synoviocytes or fibroblast-like synoviocytes and can be identified by antibodies recognizing prolyl-4-hydroxylase[13,14] or antibodies against Thy-1/CD90[15]. It is now well established that in addition to the infiltration with inflammatory cells, the increase in the numbers of synovial fibroblasts contribute significantly to

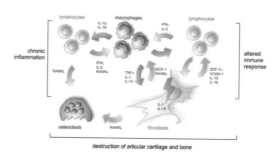

Fig. 14.1 Cellular interactions in the rheumatoid synovium. The processes of chronic inflammation, altered immune response, and progressive matrix destruction are closely linked through the interaction of different cell types. By releasing a variety of cytokines, inflammatory and immune cells (macrophages and lymphocytes), as well as resident synovial fibroblasts, create a cellular network, which ultimately leads to joint damage. Destruction of articular cartilage and bone is mediated mainly by the concerted action of fibroblasts and osteoclasts, the latter of which can differentiate directly from macrophages under the influence of RANKL (receptor activator of nuclear factor (NF)-κB ligand) and tumor necrosis factor (TNF)-α.

all aspects of synovial pathology, namely hyperplasia (particularly that of the lining layer), joint destruction, and perpetuation of chronic inflammation[16,17].

In the course of RA, the deeper sublining area of the synovium also undergoes considerable changes. These are highly variable and characterized by increased vascularization and infiltration with mononuclear cells such as T cells, B cells, and macrophages. A multitude of data suggest that both the accumulation and prolonged survival of T cells within the rheumatoid synovium can be promoted by synovial cells[18,19] and especially fibroblast-derived factors in an amplification loop[20–23]. In this context, RA synovial fibroblasts have been identified as a major source for IL-16[18,24,25] that, in addition to attracting specifically Th1-cells[26], is capable of inducing T cell anergy[27]. Underlining the specific properties of activated synovial fibroblasts in RA and promoting the concept of cellular network formation, it was demonstrated most recently that antibodies from RA patients can stimulate the production of IL-16 in RA synovial fibroblasts but not in osteoarthritis (OA) synovial fibroblasts through stimulation of the insulin-like growth factor (IGF)-1R[28]. Thus, the properties of fibroblast-derived cytokines such as IL-16 may help to explain the paradox between the abundance of T cells in the rheumatoid synovium and the lack of T cell function in the sublining of RA synovial membrane.

Increased blood vessel formation appears critical to the hyperplasia of the proliferating synovial membrane[29,30]. In addition to supplying nutrients for the hyperplastic synovial tissue, angiogenesis promotes the persistence of synovial inflammation through the influx of inflammatory cells to crate the disease-specific microenvironment in RA. Neoangiogenesis is believed to be stimulated mainly by the cells of the activated synovium[29]. Most interestingly, activated synovial fibroblasts of the lining express significant amounts of vascular cell adhesion molecule (VCAM)-1 which contribute significantly to blood vessel proliferation in the synovium but also to lymphocyte survival[31,32].

Another proangiogenic factor is angiopoietin-1 (Ang1). Ang1 is the ligand of the tyrosine kinase receptor Tie2 and is preferentially secreted by periendothelial cells such as vascular smooth muscle cells. Underlining the potential role of Ang1 for arthritis, it has been demonstrated that the systemic administration of an adenoviral construct expressing the soluble Tie2 receptor reduces the onset of arthritis in an animal model of RA and results in less severe disease. Treatment with soluble Tie2 receptor also inhibited disease progression after disease onset. These data have extended previous descriptions of Ang1 and Tie2 in the rheumatoid synovium[33–35] and confirmed animal studies demonstrating that the inhibition of angiogenesis may reduce the severity of arthritis and synovial hyperplasia[36–40]. Intriguingly, in some of these studies inhibition of angiogenesis not only reduced the inflammatory response but also affected the destruction of articular cartilage and bone[37,39,40]. This is of interest because angiogenic factors such as vascular endothelial growth factor (VEGF) may contribute to joint destruction directly by stimulating osteoclasts and osteoclast- precursors as well as indirectly by supporting synovial hyperplasia (for review see Ref. 41).

Lessons in joint destruction from animal models

Some important insights into the mechanisms of rheumatoid joint destruction have been obtained from animal models of RA. For instance, MRL-lpr/lpr mice conditionally developed an RA-like destructive arthritis, and the sequence of events resembled that in human RA. Histological studies using light and electron microscopy showed that initial joint damage in the MRL-lpr/lpr mouse model is mediated by proliferating synovial cells[42,43]. Moreover, cartilage and bone destruction occurs only at sites of synovial attachment. These observation were supported by early data demonstrating that synovial cells of MRL-lpr/lpr mice constitutively express the collagenase gene[44]. By immunohistochemistry, collagenase was detected *in situ* in proliferating synovial lining cells as well as in chondrocytes of the first stage of pathological changes in the MRL-lpr/lpr mouse arthropathy. Interestingly, collagenase-expressing synovial lining cells from these mice exhibited markedly elevated RNA levels of the c-fos proto-oncogene *in vitro*. Only after cartilage degradation was initiated were inflammatory cells observed to migrate into the synovium and accelerate the process. Although it was shown that IL-1 enhanced the onset and progression of the spontaneous arthritis in MRL-lpr/lpr mice[45], it is of particular importance that synovial lining cells mediated the initial destructive process in the absence of inflammatory cells, and that autoimmunity to collagen type II occurred as a consequence of cartilage damage rather than preceding it[46].

More recently, the TNF-α transgenic mouse model has marked an important step forward in understanding the destructive nature of human RA. It was described originally using a targeting vector that contained a genomic fragment carrying the entire human TNF-α gene[47]. In this fragment, the 3′ untranslated region (UTR) that contains important regulatory elements is replaced with the 3′ UTR of the human β-globin gene. This increases the stability of the TNF-α mRNA, and transgenic mice carrying the 3′-modified human TNF transgenes show increased expression of human TNF-α. Of interest, these mice develop a chronic inflammatory polyarthritis that is highly destructive. Treatment of the arthritic mice with a monoclonal antibody against human TNF completely prevents development of this disease. However, there is only a narrow window of time in which anti-TNF-α treatment can prevent completely the onset of arthritis, suggesting that chronic exposure of different cells to TNF-α may contribute to their stable activation. In recent years, multiple lines of TNF-α transgenic mice have been developed (for review see Ref. 48), all of which develop erosive arthritis. These lines have been used in a number of studies and particularly helped in understanding the hierarchy between TNF-α and other cytokines, the relevance of different matrix-degrading enzymes for joint destruction, and mechanisms of osteoclast-mediated bone resorption.

Injection of various antigens can also lead to the induction of erosive arthritis in rodents. Several models such as the collagen-induced arthritis (CIA) and the streptococcal-wall antigen-induced arthritis (SCW-A) have been intensively studied as animal models for human RA[49–52]. They have provided important insights into molecular mechanisms of joint inflammation and helped elucidate some key aspects of joint destruction. Thus, it could be demonstrated that induction of antigen-induced arthritis in *c-fos* transgenic mice leads to a severe destruction characterized by the predominant infiltration of fibroblast-like cells and the absence of lymphocytes[53]. Conversely, it was shown that *c-fos* deficient mice are protected completely against joint destruction in the TNF-α transgenic mouse model of RA. In this study, human TNF-α transgenic mice that develop a severe destructive arthritis were crossed with osteopetrotic, *c-fos* deficient mice. The resulting mutant mice developed a TNF-dependent arthritis in the absence of osteoclasts with all the clinical features of arthritis. However, despite the presence of severe inflammatory changes, the mice were protected against bone destruction[54].

Among the antigen-induced arthritides, the SCW-A model in Lewis rats has also been of interest, because synovial hyperplasia in this model resembles some important features of human RA. There is a tumor-like proliferation of synovial cells which express high levels of several proto-oncogene products, including *c-fos* and *c-myc* as well as matrix-degrading enzymes such as collagenase and gelatinase A[55,56]. In addition, like RA synovial fibroblasts, these cells do not show contact inhibition and can be grown under anchorage-independent conditions[57].

Notably, arthritis in each of these animal models is clearly driven by known factors. Therefore, it has not been entirely clear as to what extent their respective pathological processes resemble those of human RA, where complex interactions have been shown to occur and where all attempts to cure disease through inhibition of a single factor have failed so far. This is illustrated by studies on the induction of CIA in matrix metalloproteinase (MMP)-3 knockout mice. While MMP-3 has been assigned an important role in joint destruction (see below), it was shown that in MMP-3 knockout mice CIA does not differ significantly from that in control animals. This may indicate that MMP-3 is not intimately involved in joint destruction but more likely demonstrates the complexity of cartilage- and bone-degrading enzymes in erosive arthritis[58].

Based on the apparent lack of humanized model systems, the SCID mouse model has been developed for investigating the molecular and cellular bases of human rheumatoid joint destruction (Fig. 14.2). Since it was demonstrated that a functionally intact human immune system can survive in SCID mice recipients[59], the SCID mouse model has been widely used to study autoimmune diseases. By implanting rheumatoid synovial tissue under the renal capsule of SCID mice, it was shown that lymphocyte infiltrates disappear with time, while lining layer synoviocytes survive[60,61]. Moreover, rheumatoid fibroblast-like synoviocytes not only survived in SCID mice but maintained their characteristic biological features. Based on these observation a novel model for studying molecular mechanisms of rheumatoid joint destruction *in vivo* was developed: the SCID mouse co-implantation model for RA[62]. To imitate the situation in a rheumatoid joint in this model, human RA synovium was co-implanted with normal human cartilage under the renal capsule of SCID mice. Both RA synovial tissue and normal human cartilage could be successfully implanted into SCID mice for more than 300 days, and implanted RA synovium showed the same invasive growth and progressive cartilage destruction as in human RA joints[62]. Intriguingly, the vast majority of synovial cells found at sites of cartilage invasion resembled activated synovial fibroblasts.

To study specifically the molecular properties of these fibroblasts and their contribution to cartilage degradation, in a next step

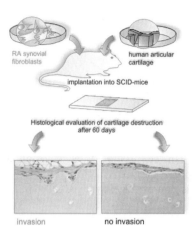

Fig. 14.2 The severe combined immunodeficient (SCID) mouse co-implantation model of rheumatoid cartilage destruction. In this model synovial fibroblasts are implanted together with normal human articular cartilage into SCID mice. Due to their non-functional immune system, these mice do not reject the human implants and allow study of the interaction of the fibroblasts with the cartilage in the absence of continuous stimulation by human inflammatory cells. While implantation of RA synovial fibroblasts results in the progressive destruction of cartilage over 60 days (*bottom left*), normal or OA synovial fibroblasts do not exhibit such destructive phenotype (*bottom right*). See also colour plate section.

normal human cartilage was implanted together with isolated synovial fibroblasts from RA patients. As the SCID mice did not reject these well-defined implants, this model has helped with the analysis of the matrix-degrading properties of RA synovial fibroblasts in the absence of both human lymphocytes and macrophages[41]. Interestingly, RA synovial fibroblasts maintained their aggressive phenotype, especially at sites of invasion. In contrast, OA synovial fibroblasts did not exhibit this invasive growth. Using *in situ* hybridization techniques to examine the presence of mRNA for matrix-degrading enzymes, a number of cartilage degrading proteases could be demonstrated[63]. In contrast, much less or none of these matrix-degrading enzymes could be found, when normal, OA synovial fibroblasts or dermal fibroblasts were examined. In addition, RA synovial fibroblasts maintained their ability to express VCAM-1 and other activation markers[63]. These results of the SCID mouse experiments indicated an active role of fibroblasts in the joint destruction of RA. Furthermore, they suggested that RA synovial fibroblasts were not just passively responding to stimuli from the inflammatory environment but also maintained their activated and aggressive phenotype in the absence of continuous stimulation with human macrophage- or lymphocyte-derived cytokines[64].

Activated synovial fibroblasts

The hypothesis that activated synovial fibroblasts are critically involved in rheumatoid joint destruction is based on observations that date back to the 1970s[65]. By analyzing large numbers of synovial specimens from RA patients it was found that invasion of cartilage and subchondral bone by synovial lining cells did not require the presence of inflammatory infiltrates. Moreover, it was shown that synovial fibroblasts from RA patients exhibit considerable morphological alterations. They have an abundant cytoplasm, a dense rough endoplasmatic reticulum, and large pale nuclei with several

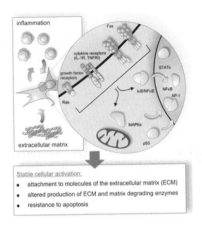

Fig. 14.3 Stable activation of RA synovial fibroblasts. RA synovial fibroblasts express a number of cell surface receptors, the stimulation of which triggers the activation different transcription factors. The respective signaling pathways show intensive cross talks. Although the mechanisms are not well understood, RA synovial fibroblasts maintain their state of activation even in the absence of continuous stimulation and show features of stable activation (for details see text).

prominent nucleoli[4,65]. Based on these morphological studies and the aforementioned SCID mouse experiments, a number of groups have set out to characterize this 'transformed-appearing' phenotype of synovial fibroblasts, and interest has focused mainly on the characteristics of this phenotype on a cellular at a molecular level, and at the mechanisms of activation with respect to their destructive properties. Their results have taught us that the stable activation of RA synovial fibroblasts is accompanied by alterations in a variety of proto-oncogenes and tumor suppressors and ultimately results in the activation of adhesion molecules, the production of matrix-degrading enzymes and changes in the susceptibility to programmed cell death (Fig. 14.3).

Increased expression of proto-oncogenes

Expression of proto-oncogenes and transcriptional factors in synovial fibroblasts has been described as a major feature indicating the activated nature of these cells[66–68].

The early response gene egr-1, a zinc finger protein having DNA binding and transcription regulatory activity, was constitutively overexpressed in RA synovial fibroblasts[69]. Interestingly, egr-1 binding sites were found in[69,70] promoter regions of several genes, which have been associated with pathomechanisms of RA. Apart from activating other proto-oncogenes, *egr-1* has been identified in collagenase-producing rheumatoid synovial fibroblasts. As shown in other studies, proto-oncogenes of the *egr* family are also involved in the activation of the cathepsin L gene[71], a matrix-degrading cysteine proteinase gene that is up-regulated highly in RA synovium. These observations are of particular interest as joint destruction in RA is largely mediated by the action of cathepsins and MMPs.

The *c-fos* proto-oncogene which is known to be co-expressed with *egr-1* has also been found in RA synovium [70,72,73]. It encodes for a basic leucine zipper transcription factor and is part of the transcriptional activator AP-1(jun/fos). The promoters of several

MMPs such as MMP-9 contain consensus binding sites for the transcription factor AP-1, and the AP-1 site has been shown to be involved in tissue-specific expression of MMPs[74,75]. However, the AP-1 site does not appear to regulate transcription of MMPs alone. Rather, there are essential interactions with other cis-acting sequences in the promoters and with certain transcription factors that bind to these sequences[75]. With respect to rheumatoid joint destruction, it is of interest that the proto-oncogene *fos* has been identified in collagenase-producing rheumatoid synovial fibroblasts[70]. These data suggest that *fos*-related proto-oncogenes play an important role in cell activation via AP-1 formation[76].

The oncogenes *ras*, *raf*, *sis*, *myb*, and *myc* have also been detected in RA patients to various extents and were predominantly up-regulated in synovial cells attaching cartilage and bone[67,68]. Binding sites for the aforementioned early response gene *egr-1* could be identified in the promoters of the oncogenes sis and ras, and about 70% of RA patients exhibit high expression of Ras and Myc proteins in synovial lining cells[70]. The cysteine proteinase, cathepsin L, which has been shown to be the major *ras*-induced protein in *ras*-transformed murine NIH 3T3 cells, was detected in 50% of the RA cases, predominantly in synovial cells[77]. Interestingly, cathepsin L in these cases was colocalized with *ras* and *myc*. Some of these proto-oncogenes appear to be involved directly in the regulation of different MMPs. Gelatinases (MMP-2 and MMP-9), together with MT1-MMP, are likely regulated by growth factors that mediate their effects through the *ras* proto-oncogene, and c-Ras plays a critical role in the increased expression and proteolytic activation of MMPs in fibroblasts[78,79]. Recently, gene transfer with dominant negative (dn) mutants of Raf-1 and dn-c-Myc demonstrated the relevance of the Ras—Raf—MAPK (mitogen-activated protein kinases) pathways for the activation and invasive behavior of RA synovial fibroblasts[80]. In this study, control fibroblasts most prominently invaded the cartilage in the SCID mouse model, while RA synovial fibroblasts transduced with dn-Raf-1 or with dn-c-Myc exhibited a marked reduction of invasion. This was accompanied by a decreased expression of MMP-1 and MMP-13 in dn-raf-1 transduced fibroblasts both *in vitro* and *in vivo*. No significant changes in apoptosis were seen in the dn-Raf-1 or dn-c-Myc transduced cell. However, RA synovial fibroblasts that were transduced with both dn-Raf-1 and dn-c-Myc rapidly underwent apoptosis. These results demonstrated that both Raf-1 and c-Myc contribute to the activation of synovial cells in RA. The clear effect of dn-Raf-1 and dn-c-Myc on the invasiveness of RA synovial fibroblasts in the SCID mouse model is in line with the concept that up-regulation of relevant signaling pathways is maintained in RA synovial fibroblasts in the absence of human inflammatory cells.

Taken together, these data suggest that pathological expression of proto-oncogenes constitutes an important step leading to the expression of matrix-degrading enzymes in RA and consecutive joint destruction.

Alterations in different tumor suppressor genes have become of growing interest in explaining some features of fibroblast activation and survival in RA. Thus, somatic mutations of the tumor suppressor gene p53 have been described in RA synoviocytes[81]. Based on additional evidence that some of these mutations can exert dominant negative effects, it has been hypothesized that the accumulation of p53 mutations may contribute to the activation of RA synovial fibroblasts. Although mutations in the p53 gene appear to show a great variability, such mutations may nonetheless constitute one mechanism that imprints the aggressive behavior into RA synovial fibroblasts. This notion is supported by data showing that inhibition of p53 in normal synovial fibroblasts results in an invasive, RA-like phenotype[82]. Consequently, RA-specific expression of p53 in the synovial tissue in both the earliest and late stages of RA has been studied. Using immunohistochemistry and Western blot techniques, it was found that synovial expression of p53 is specific for RA and can already be found in early stages of disease, particularly in cells at the site of cartilage invasion[83]. As a result of these data, it may be hypothesized that the local environment in the rheumatoid joint results in an altered expression and function of p53 at least in a subset of RA synovial fibroblasts, which in turn contributes to the stable activation of these cells[84].

It could be shown also that aggressive RA synovial fibroblasts lack the expression of mRNA for the tumor suppressor PTEN. PTEN is a tyrosine phosphatase that shows homology to the cytoskeletal proteins tensin and auxillin. Mutations in PTEN have been described in different malignancies and associate with their invasiveness and metastatic properties[85–87]. In RA, no mutations of the PTEN tumor suppressor have been found. However, *in situ* hybridization on RA synovium showed a distinct pattern of PTEN expression with negligible staining in the lining but very strong expression in the sublining[88]. Although it has been shown that down-regulation of PTEN may be caused by TGF-β, these data suggest that the lack of PTEN expression is an intrinsic feature of RA synovial fibroblasts[88]. This is of interest, because PTEN is involved in the regulation of the focal adhesion kinase[89,90] and some data indicate that PTEN is an essential mediator of FasL-mediated apoptosis through the PI 3-kinase/Akt/NF-κB pathway[91].

In this context, interesting data have come from studies of the transcriptional factor NF-κB. NF-κB is a dimeric (p65, p50), regulatory, DNA-binding protein that interacts with a number of different signal cascades. Several studies have demonstrated that NF-κB is highly activated in the synovial membrane of RA patients and constitutes a key integrating factor for intracellular as well as cytokine-mediated activation pathways[92,93]. Thus, NF-κB is a key molecule that mediates the resistance of RA synovial fibroblasts against apoptosis[94–96] and that regulates inflammatory cytokines[94,95], adhesion molecules[95,97], and matrix-degrading enzymes[95,98]. At present, the activation of NF-κB in RA synovial fibroblasts appears to constitute one important link between synovial inflammation, hyperplasia, and matrix degeneration[93,95]

Apoptosis

With respect to synovial cell proliferation it was clearly shown that synovial cells from patients with RA are activated but do not proliferate faster than those from osteoarthritis patients[69]. Using thymidine incorporation, only 1–5% of synovial cells have been found to proliferate[99], and immunohistochemistry for specific proliferation markers such as Ki-67 revealed only a very low number of positive cells[100]. Also, only 1% of fibroblast-like cells expressing proto-oncogenes such as *jun-B* and *c-fos* were positive for Ki-67, indicating that the majority of RA synovial fibroblasts do not show accelerated proliferation[101]. In contrast, recent data have provided growing evidence for changes of apoptotic pathways in RA synovium, particularly within the lining layer (for review see Ref. 102). When examined by ultrastructural methods, less than 1% of lining cells exhibit morphological features of apoptosis[103,104].

Generally, apoptosis can be induced by intrinsic, mitochondrial pathways or triggered through cell surface death receptors[102,105]. Members of the Bcl family have been identified as important regulators of mitochondrial pathways of apoptosis. Specifically, Bcl-2 has been demonstrated to exert strong anti-apoptotic effects and contribute to the pathogenesis of experimental arthritis[106]. *In situ* analysis has shown the presence of Bcl-2 in human rheumatoid arthritis synovial fibroblasts[107] and it was found that enhanced expression of Bcl-2 in RA synovial fibroblasts correlates with synovial lining thickening and inflammation[108]. Of interest, it was demonstrated that stimulation of RA synovial fibroblasts with IL-15 suppresses Bcl-2 and Bcl-x(L) mRNA[109]. Strengthening the role of Bcl family members in the regulation of fibroblast apoptosis and providing a link between cytokine-mediated stimulation of RA fibroblasts and their resistance to cell deaths, it was found in this study that apoptosis can be increased when the autocrine stimulation of RA synovial fibroblasts with IL-15 is inhibited. As mentioned above, somatic mutations of p53 tumor suppressor gene in RA synovial cells may also contribute to reduced apoptosis in these cells.

In addition to changes in mitochondrial pathways, there is evidence that RA synovial fibroblasts are also resistant to receptor-induced apoptosis such as through Fas/CD95. Several factors have been suggested to be involved in this resistance of RA synovial fibroblasts against Fas- induced cell death, but the ultimate mechanisms are incompletely understood. Elevated levels of the soluble Fas-ligand (sFasL) have been found in the synovial fluids of patients with RA[110], and based on the ability of sFasL to antagonize Fas, it has been speculated that increased expression of sFasL, as found in RA joints, may prevent Fas-induced apoptosis of synovial fibroblasts. However, as RA synovial fibroblasts maintain their resistance against Fas-induced apoptosis for extended periods of time *in vitro*, intrinsic modulation of pathways downstream of the Fas receptor most likely contributes to the resistance of RA synovial fibroblasts against apoptosis. To induce apoptosis through death receptors, specific pathways have to be activated, such as ligation of Fas to cell-bound or soluble Fas-ligand. However, some findings indicate a dual function of the Fas molecule. Apart from its pro-apoptotic function, Fas appears to be involved also in pathways leading to proliferation[111]. Therefore, intracellular signaling pathways following Fas activation may be modified by additional stimuli that determine whether the affected cell undergoes apoptosis or proliferates. These findings could also explain the fact that synovial fibroblasts are rather resistant to Fas-induced apoptosis, despite the surface expression of Fas molecules[112]. In this context, aberrant expression of FLICE-inhibitory proteins (FLIPs), the naturally occurring antagonist of proCaspase-8, has been implicated in this process[113]. Although one study did not find higher expression of

FLIPs in RA synovial fibroblasts compared to OA cells, a strong expression of FLIPs mainly at sites of cartilage destruction was found[114]. In addition, it was suggested, that the expression of FLIPs depends on the stage of disease[115]. In patients with long-term RA, increased levels of apoptosis were associated with low levels of FLIPs, while patients with short-term RA showed decreased levels of apoptosis accompanied by high expression of FLIPs. These data would suggest that resistance of RA synovial fibroblasts to apoptosis occurs early in disease.

Another molecule that modulates downstream mechanisms of the Fas signaling is sentrin-1/SUMO-1. SUMO-1 is a small ubiquitin-like protein that is 18% identical and 48% similar to human ubiquitin. In contrast to ubiquitination that leads to the degradation of proteins, SUMOylated proteins are not degraded. Rather, SUMOylation results in altered binding of modified proteins to subsequent substrates, which affects their signaling[116]. It has been demonstrated that SUMO-1 interacts also with the signal competent forms of Fas- and TNFRI-associated death domain (DD) and protects from both Fas- and TNFRI-induced cell death[117]. In the RA synovium a marked expression of SUMO-1 can be found, predominantly in RA synovial fibroblasts of the lining layer and at sites of cartilage invasion. In contrast, normal synovial tissues and synovial tissues of OA patients show only negligible expression of sentrin-1 mRNA[118]. Of note, RA synovial fibroblasts maintain their high expression of SUMO-1 when analyzed in the SCID mouse model of RA for 60 days, and most recent data suggest that the levels of SUMO-1 correlate directly with the resistance of RA synovial fibroblasts to Fas-induced apoptosis. Despite this strong association, functional data will be required to elucidate the specific effects of SUMOylation in RA synovial fibroblasts.

Taken together, these data suggest that apoptosis-suppressing signals outweigh pro-apoptotic signaling in RA, causing an imbalance of pro- and antiapoptotic pathways. This subsequently may lead to an extended life-span of synovial lining cells and result in a prolonged expression of matrix-degrading enzymes at sites of joint destruction. In addition, it appears that common mechanisms regulate the altered apoptotic response and invasive behavior of RA synovial fibroblasts[119].

Attachment

Attachment of synovial fibroblasts to the joint cartilage is one of the most prominent features involved in rheumatoid joint destruction. This process appears pivotal for RA as compared with other non-destructive forms of arthritides. Adhesion is mediated by various surface proteins. Three different families have been characterized: selectins, integrins, and the Ig superfamily.

Integrins represent a very complex family of adhesion molecules that contain heterodimers of α and β chains. So far, at least 15 different α and 8 different β chains have been described[120]. Integrins have become of general interest for RA not only because of their function as receptor molecules but also because of their interaction with several signaling pathways and cellular proto-oncogenes[121]. Thus, expression of early cell cycle genes such as *c-fos* and *c-myc* is also stimulated by integrin-mediated cell adhesion, and gene expression driven by the *fos* promoter shows strongly synergistic activation by integrin-mediated adhesion[122,123]. Different studies have demonstrated that, apart from being expressed on lymphocytes,

several β1 integrins such as VLA-3, VLA-4, and VLA-5 are highly expressed on synovial fibroblasts[124,125]. The binding of synovial fibroblasts to extracellular matrix is inhibited, at least in part, by anti-β1 integrin antibodies with the blocking efficacy being significantly higher in RA synovial fibroblasts compared with normal synovial fibroblasts[124]. As a number of integrins function as fibronectin receptors, the fibronectin-rich environment of RA cartilage surface might facilitate the adhesion of RA synovial fibroblasts to the cartilage. In addition to extracellular matrix proteins the ligands of the integrins may also be cellular surface molecules and some adhesion molecules may bind to more than one ligand. In this respect the observation that CS-1, a spliced isoform of fibronectin, is expressed highly in RA synovium[126] is of interest. CS-1 appears part of a bi-directional adhesion pathway operative in RA as it binds to the integrin VLA-4 (α4-β1,CD49d/CD29), which also ligates with VCAM-1.

VCAM-1 (CD106) is a member of the immunoglobulin gene superfamily and may contain either six or seven immunoglobulin domains of the H type[127]. Several studies have demonstrated increased VCAM-1 expression in RA synovium as compared to normal and OA synovial tissues. While some data suggested that macrophage-like cells were the major source of VCAM-1 in RA synovial tissue[128], most studies revealed high expression of VCAM-1 mainly in synovial fibroblasts. Moreover, different data suggest that VCAM-1 is particularly up-regulated in the sub-population of activated lining fibroblasts[31,129,130]. Some data demonstrated strong expression of VCAM-1 in the lining layer of RA synovium, suggesting that increased expression of VCAM-1 is associated with these aggressive cells prone to attach and subsequently invade articular cartilage[31]. Studies in the SCID mouse co-implantation model revealed increased expression of VCAM-1 in RA synovial fibroblasts, even in the absence of human inflammatory cells, for at least 60 days[63]. As mentioned above, VCAM-1 produced by RA-activated synovial fibroblasts may not only mediate the attachment to cartilage but may also contribute to T cell anergy[131,132], B cell pseudoemperipolesis[32], and the induction of angiogenesis[29].

Osteopontin, another extracellular matrix protein that promotes cell attachment, is also present in synovial fibroblast-like cells[133] and exerts a stimulatory effect on the secretion of MMP 1 in articular chondrocytes. It appears that osteopontin not only mediates attachment of synovial cells to cartilage but also contributes to perichondrocytic matrix degradation in RA. Moreover, findings demonstrating that osteopontin stimulates B cells to produce immunoglobulins[134] and is chemoattractive for macrophages[135] suggest that osteopontin produced by synovial fibroblasts might play a role in stimulating B cells to produce rheumatoid factor in the joint and to attract the influx of macrophages to the synovium in RA.

In summary, the role of adhesion molecules in RA appears to not be restricted to the attachment of synovium to cartilage and bone, but involves the recruitment of inflammatory cells as well as the induction of MMPs.

Matrix-degrading enzymes

Progressive joint destruction distinguishes RA from other inflammatory joint diseases and is mediated by the concerted action of various proteinases. The most prominent of these are MMPs and cathepsins[136,137]. The MMP family consists of more than 20 structurally related members[138]. They are characterized by a zinc molecule at the active site and include collagenases (MMP-1, MMP-13), gelatinases (MMP-2 and MMP-9), stromelysin (MMP-3), and membrane-type MMPs (MT-MMP), the latter of which are characterized by a transmembrane domain and act on the surface of cells. Two types of enzyme families are structurally related to MMPs: the ADAMs (a disintegrin and a metalloproteinase)[139] and the ADAMTS (a disintegrin and a metalloproteinase with thrombospondin motifs)[140]. These are also multidomain proteases that consist of a catalytic and a regulatory domain structurally related to MMPs. However, both families have a disintegrin domain which allows binding to cell-surface integrins. While ADAMs are bound to the cell membrane, ADAMTSs lack this transmembrane part, but contain thrombospondin type I motifs, which allows their binding to proteoglycans. The best known member of the ADAM family is TACE (ADAM-17, tumor necrosis factor converting enzyme), which cleaves membrane-bound TNF-α to a soluble form[141,142]. ADAMTS-4 and -5 are the best characterized members of the ADAMTS family. They are also known as 'aggrecanases' because they can cleave aggrecan, which is the most important proteoglycan of the cartilage.[143]

MMPs are secreted as inactive pro-enzymes and activated proteolytically by various enzymes such as trypsin, plasmin, and other proteases. MMPs differ with respect to their substrate specificities[144]: While MMP-1 degrades collagen types I, II, III, VII, and X only when they are arranged in a triple helical structure, MMP-2 can also cleave denatured collagen. MMP-3 is able to activate MMP-1 as well as to degrade proteoglycans. Several reports have implicated MMPs in rheumatoid joint destruction (for a more comprehensive review on MMPs in RA see Ref. 136).

MMP-1 is found in the synovial membranes of all RA patients but only in about 55–80% of synovial samples from trauma patients[145]. Synovial lining cells produce most MMP-1 in the diseased synovium, and MMP-1 is released from these cells immediately after production (for review see Ref. 146). As a result, expression of MMP-1 in the synovial fluid correlates with the degree of synovial inflammation[147]. However, serum concentrations of MMP-1 do not appear to reflect the levels in the synovial fluids and, therefore, measuring serum MMP-1 has not been established as a marker for disease activity.

Using different *in situ* techniques, other MMPs such as MMP-2 have been localized also to the RA synovial membrane. MMP-2 is expressed constitutively in various synovial pathologies, but increased expression of MMP-2 has been shown in RA[145]. This is true also for the second member of the gelatinase family, MMP-9[148,149]. Analyzing the expression of MMP-9 in the synovial fluids of patients with RA, OA, and other inflammatory arthritis, an association between increased levels of MMP-9 and inflammatory arthritis was found[149]. These data are of interest, because MMP-9 is expressed also in osteoclasts and has been associated with bone resorption[150].

Due to its specific properties, MMP-3 has been assigned a key role in the destruction of rheumatoid joints. This is because MMP-3 not only degrades matrix molecules but is also involved in the activation of pro-MMPs into their active forms. MMP-3 is produced abundantly by rheumatoid synovial fibroblasts when

stimulated with macrophage-conditioned medium-[151] and RA synovial fibroblasts in the lining layer are a major source of MMP-3 in the RA synovium[152]. Synovial fluids from patients with RA contain about 100-fold higher concentrations of active MMP-3 than control samples[153], and increased levels of MMP-3 have been found in the sera of patients with RA[154–157]. These increased serum levels correlate with systemic inflammation at clinical[156,158] and serological[155,157,158] levels, but the question as to whether levels of circulating MMP-3 reflect radiological damage remains unclear. No correlation between serum MMP-3 and radiological or functional scores was found in other studies[157], and it was suggested that there were no differences in the serum levels of MMP-3 between RA patients with longstanding RA that had low or high erosion scores[155]. In contrast, other data indicate that serum MMP-3 predicts joint damage at early stages of disease[159].

MMP-13 is also found expressed at the mRNA[160] and protein levels[161], especially in the lining layer of rheumatoid synovium. Due to this localization, its substrate specificity for collagen type II, and its relative resistance to known MMP inhibitors, it has been suggested that MMP-13 plays an important role in joint destruction. Of interest, expression of MMP-13 correlates with elevated levels of systemic inflammation markers[162] but studies in osteoarthritis demonstrated clearly that the expression of MMP-13 is not specific for RA. Rather, it appears that MMP-13 is associated closely with degeneration of cartilage in different pathologies.

Membrane-type matrix metalloproteinases (MT-MMPs) are also abundantly expressed in cells aggressively destroying cartilage and bone in RA[163]. Although MT1-MMP is produced constitutively by synovial fibroblasts, elevated levels have been found in RA. This is of importance, because MT1-MMP degrades extracellular matrix components, as well as activating other disease-relevant MMPs such as MMP-2 and MMP-13. In a recent study that compared the expressions of MT-MMPs in RA, it was suggested that MT1-MMP is of particular relevance to RA[163]. In this analysis, the expression of MT3-MMP mRNA was seen in fibroblasts and some macrophages particularly in the lining layer, but expression of MT2- and MT4-MMP was characterized by a scattered staining of only a few CD68 negative fibroblasts.

The expression of MMPs in RA synovial cells is regulated by several extracellular signals. These include inflammatory cytokines, growth factors, and molecules of the extracellular matrix. Among the inflammatory cytokines IL-1 and TNF-α are important inducers of MMPs. IL-1 induces the expression of a variety of MMPs, including MMP-1, -3, -8, -13, and -14 (see Ref. 136). However, as demonstrated in several studies utilizing antigen-induced arthritis in animals, IL-1 not only enhances the production of MMPs but also suppresses the synthesis of proteoglycans (PGs)[164]. In some of these studies, anti-IL-1 treatment was able to normalize chondrocyte synthetic function and reduce the activation of MMPs[165]. These data go along with the observations showing that overexpression of the IL-1 receptor antagonist (IL-1Ra) using retroviral gene transfer significantly reduces perichondrocytic matrix degradation in the SCID mouse model[166]. However, the mechanisms by which cytokines such as IL-1 induce MMPs appear to be variable and depend on the cell types. Thus, IL-1 up-regulates differentially MMP-13, via JNK and p38 protein kinase signaling[167], and MMP-1, via STAT transcription factors[168], in chondrocytes.

Other macrophage-derived inflammatory cytokines such as TNF-α have also been shown to amplify the destructive processes by stimulating the expression of some MMPs. Thus, TNF-α can stimulate the production of MMP-1 in cultured synovial cells[169,170]. However, animal models of arthritis have indicated a difference in the relative importance of TNF-α and IL-1 with respect to inflammation and joint destruction. While TNF-α appears responsible primarily for the extent of the synovitis, IL-1 seems to have a greater impact on the destruction of cartilage[171]. This hypothesis was supported mainly by data from antigen-induced arthritis and zymosan-induced arthritis in mice, where the suppression of PG synthesis seen by IL-1 was not detected with TNF-α[164]. Related studies using anti-TNF-α treatment in DBA/1 mice with CIA demonstrated efficacy only shortly after onset of the disease, and had little effect on fully established CIA[172]. In contrast, anti-IL-1 treatment ameliorated both early and full-blown CIA. This clear suppression of established arthritis was confirmed by administration of high doses of IL-1Ra[172]. Most recent data from the TNF-α transgenic mouse model of destructive arthritis, and particularly data from human trials using recombinant human IL-1Ra, have, however, challenged this view, suggesting a more complex hierarchy of cytokines in human RA synovium.

Other cytokines that regulate the expression of MMP in the RA synovium include IL-17 (MMP-1 and -9)[173] and TGF-β (MMP-13)[174]. Growth factors such as fibroblast growth factor (FGF) and platelet-derived growth factor (PDGF) are also potent inducers of MMPs and potentiate the effect of IL-1[175]. The expression of MMP can also be induced by different matrix proteins such as collagen and fibronectin. Their degradation products, especially, can activate the expression of MMPs in chondrocytes and fibroblasts, which provides the possibility for a specific activation of MMPs at sites of matrix degradation[176,177]. As a consequence, the synthesis of matrix-degrading enzymes in the inflamed joint is not only regulated by inflammatory cytokines and growth factors, but also by cleavage products of the destroyed matrix itself in an amplifying fashion.

Several signaling pathways are involved in the transcriptional activation of MMPs, and it is of particular interest that—as mentioned above—a number of factors that have been implicated in the stable activation of RA synovial fibroblasts contribute directly to the up-regulation of MMPs. The activator protein-1 (AP-1) binding site is present in the promoter region of all MMPs (except MMP-2), suggesting a central role of jun/fos transcription factor binding. Indeed, there is considerable experimental evidence that all three mitogen/stress-activated protein kinase (MAPK/SAPK) families, extracellular signal-regulated kinases (ERKs), JNK, and p38 kinase, which integrate extracellular signals upstream from jun/fos, regulate the expression of MMPs. The induction of MMP-1, -9, and -13, particularly, is mediated through MAPK/SAPK signaling[80,178,179]. The promoters of different MMPs also contain NF-κB[178,180], signal transducers and activators of transcription (STAT)[181] and ETS[182] binding sites, and it has been demonstrated that activation of these transcription factors occurs during the induction of MMP-1, -3, and -13, which is essential for joint damage in rheumatoid arthritis. Although activation of the various MAPK/SAPK and transcription factors are not tissue specific, they occur at very distinct compartments

of the rheumatoid joint, thus determining a specific pattern of MMP expression in the synovium[183]. Src-related tyrosine kinases also activate the transcription of MMP-1, as demonstrated by an inhibited increase of MMP-1 mRNA in IL-1-stimulated synovial fibroblasts using herbimycin A, an inhibitor of src-related tyrosine kinases[184]. On the other hand, tissue-specific transcription factors of MMP do exist. One example is Cbfa-1 (a runx-protein family member), which is essential for MMP-13 expression in cartilage and bone[167].

Recently, a close correlation between the expression of the MMP −1, −3, and −10 and the invasive growth of RA synovial fibroblasts has been found[185], but the specific contribution of individual MMPs to matrix degradation is only partly understood. Using gene transfer of ribozymes to MMP-1, it was demonstrated recently that the specific inhibition of MMP-1 significantly reduces the production of this enzyme in RA synovial fibroblasts and inhibits the invasiveness of the cells in the SCID mouse model[186]. In a similar study, it was shown that gene transfer of antisense RNA expression constructs against MT1-MMP, a membrane-anchored MMP, also inhibits the invasiveness of RA synovial fibroblasts. It is hoped that the use of these techniques will allow the role of individual MMPs in rheumatoid joint destruction to be clarified and result in the development of drugs targeting disease-relevant MMPs selectively.

Normally, MMP activity is balanced by the naturally occurring tissue inhibitors of metalloproteinase (TIMP-1 and TIMP-2). They interact irreversibly with MMPs such as MMP-1 and MMP-3 and are synthesized and secreted by chondrocytes, synovial fibroblasts, and endothelial cells[187–189]. *In situ* hybridization studies demonstrated striking amounts of TIMP-1 mRNA in the synovial lining of patients with RA[187]. However, the molar ratio of MMPs to TIMP, rather than the absolute levels of TIMP, is crucial for joint destruction. In RA, the amount of MMPs produced far outweighs that of the TIMPs, allowing destruction to take place. This notion has been supported by data demonstrating that the overexpression of TIMP-1 and TIMP-3 by gene transfer may result in a marked reduction in the invasiveness of RA synovial fibroblasts[190]. Of interest, TIMP-3 not only inhibits the degradation of extracellular matrix but has also been associated with a number of features that are distinct from other TIMPs. Thus, TIMP-3 has the ability to prevent shedding of cell membrane proteins such as the TNF receptor[191], the IL-6 receptor[192], and of TNF-α converting enzyme (TACE)[193]. Another interesting feature of TIMP-3 is its ability to induce apoptosis in different cell types[194–197]. In this context, it was shown recently that, in addition to its general pro-apoptotic function, TIMP-3 can sensitize RA synovial fibroblasts to Fas-ligand-induced apoptosis when expressed through adenoviral gene transfer[112]. Moreover, adenoviral delivery of TIMP-3 reverses completely the apoptosis-inhibiting effects of TNF-α in RA synovial fibroblasts. These findings indicate that overexpression of TIMP-3 in RA synovial fibroblasts may have beneficial effects both by inhibiting matrix degradation and by facilitating cell death and, therefore, may stimulate further studies on the therapeutic potential of gene transfer strategies with TIMP-3.

Cathepsins are the other major group of proteases involved in joint destruction[137]. They are classified by their catalytic mechanism and cleave cartilage types II, IX, and XI as well as proteoglycans. The cysteine proteases cathepsin B and L are up-regulated in RA synovium, especially at sites of cartilage invasion[77,198,199]. In a similar fashion to MMPs, cathepsins are activated by proto-oncogenes. Transfection of fibroblasts with the *ras* proto-oncogene leads to cellular transformation and to the induction of cathepsin L[200]. This is supported by the aforementioned *in vivo* finding of combined *ras* and cathepsin L expression. Several studies have also shown that inflammatory cytokines such as IL-1 and TNF-α can stimulate the production of cathepsins B and L by synovial fibroblast-like cells[201,202]. In this context, it was demonstrated recently that gene transfer of ribozymes to cathepsin L can inhibit significantly the fibroblast- mediated cartilage degradation both *in vitro* and *in vivo*[203].

Cathepsin K is a cysteine proteinase that plays an important role in osteoclast-mediated bone resorption. In addition, cathepsin K expression by RA synovial fibroblasts and macrophages has been reported, especially at the site of synovial invasion into articular bone, suggesting that it participates in bone destruction in RA[204].

Conclusions and perspectives

The destruction of articular structures, particularly of the cartilage surface, is a prominent and unique feature of RA. It is mediated by the concerted action of different cell types, particularly type A synoviocytes (macrophages) and type B synoviocytes (fibroblasts), with the fibroblasts of the most superficial lining layer of the rheumatoid synovium contributing most prominently to this process. Inhibition of MMPs and cathepsins, which ultimately mediate the destruction of intracellular matrix in RA, is a promising target for the treatment of RA. *In vitro* approaches as well as animal models have been used to study the exogenous administration of TIMPs and synthetic peptides that inhibit MMPs. However, given the broad array of different MMPs and cathepsins with different specificities in degrading components of extracellular matrix, as well as their regulation through different pathways, a combination of inhibitors may be required, together with a better understanding of pathways that in a disease-specific manner regulate their expression.

References

1. Gay, S., Gay, R. E., and Koopman, W. J. Molecular and cellular mechanisms of joint destruction in rheumatoid arthritis: two cellular mechanisms explain joint destruction? *Ann Rheum Dis* 1993; **52** (Suppl. 1): S39–S47.
2. Mulherin, D., Fitzgerald, O., and Bresnihan, B. Clinical improvement and radiological deterioration in rheumatoid arthritis: evidence that the pathogenesis of synovial inflammation and articular erosion may differ. *Br J Rheumatol* 1996; **35**: 1263–8.
3. Cunnane, G., Fitzgerald, O., Hummel, K. M., Gay, R. E., Gay, S., and Bresnihan, B. Collagenase, cathepsin B and cathepsin L gene expression in the synovial membrane of patients with early inflammatory arthritis. *Rheumatology (Oxford)* 1999; **38**: 34–42.
4. Pap, T., Muller-Ladner, U., Gay, R. E., and Gay, S. Fibroblast biology: role of synovial fibroblasts in the pathogenesis of rheumatoid arthritis. *Arthritis Res* 2000; **2**: 361–7.
5. Firestein, G. S. Evolving concepts of rheumatoid arthritis. *Nature* 2003; **423**: 356–61.
6. Kobayashi, I., and Ziff, M. Electron microscopic studies of the cartilage-pannus junction in rheumatoid arthritis. *Arthritis Rheum* 1975; **18**: 475–83.
7. Harris, E. D., Jr., DiBona, D. R., and Krane, S. M. A mechanism for cartilage destruction in rheumatoid arthritis. *Trans Assoc Am Physicians* 1970; **83**: 267–76.
8. Kelly, P. M., Bliss, E., Morton, J. A., Burns, J., and McGee, J. O. Monoclonal antibody EBM/11: high cellular specificity for human macrophages. *J Clin Pathol* 1988; **41**: 510–15.
9. Burmester, G. R., Stuhlmuller, B., Keyszer, G., and Kinne, R. W. Mononuclear phagocytes and rheumatoid synovitis: mastermind or workhorse in arthritis? *Arthritis Rheum* 1997; **40**: 5–18.
10. Cutolo, M., Sulli, A., Barone, A., Seriolo, B., and Accardo, S. Macrophages, synovial tissue and rheumatoid arthritis. *Clin Exp Rheumatol* 1993; **11**: 331–9.
11. Helbig, B., Gross, W. L., Borisch, B., Starz, H., and Mller-Hermelink, H. K. Characterization of synovial macrophages by monoclonal antibodies in rheumatoid arthritis and osteoarthritis. *Scand J Rheumatol Suppl* 1988; **76**: 61–6.
12. Salisbury, A. K., Duke, O., and Poulter, L. W. Macrophage-like cells of the pannus area in rheumatoid arthritic joints. *Scand J Rheumatol* 1987; **16**: 263–72.
13. Firestein, G. S. Rheumatoid synovitis and pannus. In *Rheumatology*, Vol. 1 (Klippel J. H. and Dieppe P. A., eds), pp. 5.13.1–5.13.24. London: Mosby;1998.
14. Hoyhtya, M., Myllyla, R., Piuva, J., Kivirikko, K. I., and Tryggvason, K. Monoclonal antibodies to human prolyl 4-hydroxylase. *Eur J Biochem* 1984; **141**: 472–82.
15. Zimmermann, T., Kunisch, E., Pfeiffer, R., Hirth, A., Stahl, H. D., Sack, U. *et al.* Isolation and characterization of rheumatoid arthritis synovial fibroblasts from primary culture: primary culture cells markedly differ from fourth-passage cells. *Arthritis Res* 2001; **3**: 72–6.
16. Qu, Z., Garcia, C. H., O'Rourke, L. M., Planck, S. R., Kohli, M., and Rosenbaum, J. T. Local proliferation of fibroblast-like synoviocytes contributes to synovial hyperplasia. Results of proliferating cell nuclear antigen/cyclin, c-myc, and nucleolar organizer region staining [see comments]. *Arthritis Rheum* 1994; **37**: 212–20.
17. Buckley, C. D., Pilling, D., Lord, J. M., Akbar, A. N., Scheel-Toellner, D., and Salmon, M. Fibroblasts regulate the switch from acute resolving to chronic persistent inflammation. *Trends Immunol* 2001; **22**: 199–204.
18. Franz, J. K., Kolb, S. A., Hummel, K. M., Lahrtz, F., Neidhart, M., Aicher, W. K. *et al.* Interleukin-16, produced by synovial fibroblasts, mediates chemoattraction for CD41 T lymphocytes in rheumatoid arthritis. *Eur J Immunol* 1998; **28**: 2661–71.
19. Smith, R. S., Smith, T. J., Blieden, T. M., and Phipps, R. P. Fibroblasts as sentinel cells: synthesis of chemokines and regulation of inflammation. *Am J Pathol* 1997; **151**: 317–22.
20. Buckley, C. D. Why does chronic inflammatory joint disease persist? *Clin Med* 2003; **3**: 361–6.
21. Min, D. J., Cho, M. L., Lee, S. H., Min, S. Y., Kim, W. U., Min, J. K. *et al.* Augmented production of chemokines by the interaction of type II collagen-reactive T cells with rheumatoid synovial fibroblasts. *Arthritis Rheum* 2004; **50**: 1146–55.
22. Nanki, T., Hayashida, K., El Gabalawy, H. S., Suson, S., Shi, K., Girschick, H. J. *et al.* Stromal cell-derived factor-1-CXC chemokine receptor 4 interactions play a central role in CD41 T cell accumulation in rheumatoid arthritis synovium. *J Immunol* 2000; **165**: 6590–8.
23. Salmon, M., Scheel Toellner, D., Huissoon, A. P., Pilling, D., Shamsadeen, N., Hyde, H. *et al.* Inhibition of T cell apoptosis in the rheumatoid synovium. *J Clin Invest* 1997; **99**: 439–46.
24. Weis-Klemm, M., Alexander, D., Pap, T., Schutzle, H., Reyer, D., Franz, J. K., and Aicher, W. K. Synovial fibroblasts from rheumatoid arthritis patients differ in their regulation of IL-16 gene activity in comparison to osteoarthritis fibroblasts. *Cell Physiol Biochem* 2004; **14**: 293–300.

25. Sciaky, D., Brazer, W., Center, D. M., Cruikshank, W. W., and Smith, T. J. Cultured human fibroblasts express constitutive IL-16 mRNA: cytokine induction of active IL-16 protein synthesis through a caspase-3-dependent mechanism. *J Immunol* 2000; **164**: 3806–14.

26. Lynch, E. A., Heijens, C. A., Horst, N. F., Center, D. M., and Cruikshank, W. W. Cutting edge: IL-16/CD4 preferentially induces Th1 cell migration: requirement of CCR5. *J Immunol* 2003; **171**: 4965–8.

27. Cruikshank, W. W., Lim, K., Theodore, A. C., Cook, J., Fine, G., Weller, P. F., and Center, D. M. IL-16 inhibition of CD3-dependent lymphocyte activation and proliferation. *J Immunol* 1996; **157**: 5240–8.

28. Pritchard, J., Tsui, S., Horst, N., Cruikshank, W. W., and Smith, T. J. Synovial fibroblasts from patients with rheumatoid arthritis, like fibroblasts from Graves' disease, express high levels of IL-16 when treated with Igs against insulin-like growth factor-1 receptor. *J Immunol* 2004; **173**: 3564–9.

29. Koch, A. E., Halloran, M. M., Haskell, C. J., Shah, M. R., and Polverini, P. J. Angiogenesis mediated by soluble forms of E-selectin and vascular cell adhesion molecule-1. *Nature* 1995; **376**: 517–19.

30. Clavel, G., Bessis, N., and Boissier, M. C. Recent data on the role for angiogenesis in rheumatoid arthritis. *Joint Bone Spine* 2003; **70**: 321–6.

31. Kriegsmann, J., Keyszer, G. M., Geiler, T., Brauer, R., Gay, R. E., and Gay, S. Expression of vascular cell adhesion molecule-1 mRNA and protein in rheumatoid synovium demonstrated by in situ hybridization and immunohistochemistry. *Lab Invest* 1995; **72**: 209–14.

32. Burger, J. A., Zvaifler, N. J., Tsukada, N., Firestein, G. S., and Kipps, T. J. Fibroblast-like synoviocytes support B-cell pseudoemperipolesis via a stromal cell-derived factor-1- and CD106 (VCAM-1)-dependent mechanism. *J Clin Invest* 2001; **107**: 305–15.

33. Gravallese, E. M., Pettit, A. R., Lee, R., Madore, R., Manning, C., Tsay, A. *et al.* Angiopoietin-1 is expressed in the synovium of patients with rheumatoid arthritis and is induced by tumour necrosis factor alpha. *Ann Rheum Dis* 2003; **62**: 100–7.

34. Scott, B. B., Zaratin, P. F., Colombo, A., Hansbury, M. J., Winkler, J. D., and Jackson, J. R. Constitutive expression of angiopoietin-1 and -2 and modulation of their expression by inflammatory cytokines in rheumatoid arthritis synovial fibroblasts. *J Rheumatol* 2002; **29**: 230–9.

35. Shahrara, S., Volin, M. V., Connors, M. A., Haines, G. K., and Koch, A. E. Differential expression of the angiogenic Tie receptor family in arthritic and normal synovial tissue. *Arthritis Res* 2002; **4**: 201–8.

36. Nagashima, M., Tanaka, H., Takahashi, H., Tachihara, A., Tanaka, K., Ishiwata, T., Asano, G., and Yoshino, S. Study of the mechanism involved in angiogenesis and synovial cell proliferation in human synovial tissues of patients with rheumatoid arthritis using SCID mice. *Lab Invest* 2002; **82**: 981–8.

37. de Bandt, M., Grossin, M., Weber, A. J., Chopin, M., Elbim, C., Pla, M. *et al.* Suppression of arthritis and protection from bone destruction by treatment with TNP-470/AGM-1470 in a transgenic mouse model of rheumatoid arthritis. *Arthritis Rheum* 2000; **43**: 2056–63.

38. Lu, J., Kasama, T., Kobayashi, K., Yoda, Y., Shiozawa, F., Hanyuda, M. *et al.* Vascular endothelial growth factor expression and regulation of murine collagen-induced arthritis. *J Immunol* 2000; **164**: 5922–7.

39. Sone, H., Kawakami, Y., Sakauchi, M., Nakamura, Y., Takahashi, A., Shimano, H. *et al.* Neutralization of vascular endothelial growth factor prevents collagen-induced arthritis and ameliorates established disease in mice. *Biochem Biophys Res Commun* 2001; **281**: 562–8.

40. Miotla, J., Maciewicz, R., Kendrew, J., Feldmann, M., and Paleolog, E. Treatment with soluble VEGF receptor reduces disease severity in murine collagen-induced arthritis. *Lab Invest* 2000; **80**: 1195–205.

41. Pap, T., and Distler, O. Linking angiogenesis to bone destruction in arthritis. *Arthritis Rheum* 2005; **52**: 1346–8.

42. O'Sullivan, F. X., Fassbender, H. G., Gay, S., and Koopman, W. J. Etiopathogenesis of the rheumatoid arthritis-like disease in MRL/l mice. I. The histomorphologic basis of joint destruction. *Arthritis Rheum* 1985; **28**: 529–36.

43. Tanaka, A., O'Sullivan, F. X., Koopman, W. J., and Gay, S. Etiopathogenesis of rheumatoid arthritis-like disease in MRL/1 mice: II. Ultrastructural basis of joint destruction. *J Rheumatol* 1988; **15**: 10–16.

44. Trabandt, A., Gay, R. E., Birkedal Hansen, H., and Gay, S. Expression of collagenase and potential transcriptional factors in the MRL/l mouse arthropathy. *Semin Arthritis Rheum* 1992; **21**: 246–51.

45. Hom, J. T., Cole, H., and Bendele, A. M. Interleukin 1 enhances the development of spontaneous arthritis in MRL/lpr mice. *Clin Immunol Immunopathol* 1990; **55**: 109–19.

46. Gay, S., O'Sullivan, F. X., Gay, R. E., and Koopman, W. J. Humoral sensitivity to native collagen types I-VI in the arthritis of MRL/l mice. *Clin Immunol Immunopathol* 1987; **45**: 63–9.

47. Keffer, J., Probert, L., Cazlaris, H., Georgopoulos, S., Kaslaris, E., Kioussis, D., and Kollias, G. Transgenic mice expressing human tumour necrosis factor: a predictive genetic model of arthritis. *EMBO J* 1991; **10**: 4025–31.

48. Li, P., and Schwarz, E. M. The TNF-alpha transgenic mouse model of inflammatory arthritis. *Springer Semin Immunopathol* 2003; **25**: 19–33.

49. Trentham, D. E., Townes, A. S., and Kang, A. H. Autoimmunity to type II collagen an experimental model of arthritis. *J Exp Med* 1977; **146**: 857–68.

50. Griffiths, M. M. Immunogenetics of collagen-induced arthritis in rats. *Int Rev Immunol* 1988; **4**: 1–15.

51. Holmdahl, R., Andersson, M. E., Goldschmidt, T. J., Jansson, L., Karlsson, M., Malmstrom, V., and Mo, J. Collagen induced arthritis as an experimental model for rheumatoid arthritis: immunogenetics, pathogenesis and autoimmunity. *APMIS* 1989; **97**: 575–84.

52. Wilder, R. L., Case, J. P., Crofford, L. J., Kumkumian, G. K., Lafyatis, R., Remmers, E. F. *et al.* Endothelial cells and the pathogenesis of rheumatoid arthritis in humans and streptococcal cell wall arthritis in Lewis rats. *J Cell Biochem* 1991; **45**: 162–6.

53. Shiozawa, S., Tanaka, Y., Fujita, T., and Tokuhisa, T. Destructive arthritis without lymphocyte infiltration in H2-c-fos transgenic mice. *J Immunol* 1992; **148**: 3100–4.

54. Redlich, K., Hayer, S., Ricci, R., David, J. P., Tohidast-Akrad, M., Kollias, G. *et al.* Osteoclasts are essential for TNF-alpha-mediated joint destruction. *J Clin Invest* 2002; **110**: 1419–27.

55. Case, J. P., Sano, H., Lafyatis, R., Remmers, E. F., Kumkumian, G. K., and Wilder, R. L. Transin/stromelysin expression in the synovium of rats with experimental erosive arthritis: in situ localization and kinetics of expression of the transformation-associated metalloproteinase in euthymic and athymic Lewis rats. *J Clin Invest* 1989; **84**: 1731–40.

56. Yocum, D. E., Lafyatis, R., Remmers, E. F., Schumacher, H. R., and Wilder, R. L. Hyperplastic synoviocytes from rats with streptococcal cell wall-induced arthritis exhibit a transformed phenotype that is thymic-dependent and retinoid inhibitable. *Am J Pathol* 1988; **132**: 38–48.

57. Lafyatis, R., Remmers, E. F., Roberts, A. B., Yocum, D. E., Sporn, M. B., and Wilder, R. L. Anchorage-independent growth of synoviocytes from arthritic and normal joints: stimulation by exogenous platelet-derived growth factor and inhibition by transforming growth factor-beta and retinoids. *J Clin Invest* 1989; **83**: 1267–76.

58. Mudgett, J. S., Hutchinson, N. I., Chartrain, N. A., Forsyth, A. J., McDonnell, J., Singer, I. I. *et al.* Susceptibility of stromelysin 1-deficient mice to collagen-induced arthritis and cartilage destruction. *Arthritis Rheum* 1998; **41**: 110–21.

59. Mosier, D. E., Gulizia, R. J., Baird, S. M., and Wilson, D. B. Transfer of a functional human immune system to mice with severe combined immunodeficiency. *Nature* 1988; **335**: 256–9.

60. Adams, C. D., Zhou, T., and Mountz, J. D. Transplantation of human synovium into a SCID mouse as a model for disease activity. *Arthritis Rheum* 1990; **33**: S120.

61. Rendt, K. E., Barry, T. S., Jones, D. M., Richter, C. B., McCachren, S. S., and Haynes, B. F. Engraftment of human synovium into severe combined immune deficient mice: migration of

human peripheral blood T cells to engrafted human synovium and to mouse lymph nodes. *J Immunol* 1993; **151**: 7324–36.

62. Geiler, T., Kriegsmann, J., Keyszer, G. M., Gay, R. E., and Gay, S. A new model for rheumatoid arthritis generated by engraftment of rheumatoid synovial tissue and normal human cartilage into SCID mice. *Arthritis Rheum* 1994; **37**: 1664–71.

63. Müller-Ladner, U., Kriegsmann, J., Franklin, B. N., Matsumoto, S., Geiler, T., Gay, R. E., and Gay, S. Synovial fibroblasts of patients with rheumatoid arthritis attach to and invade normal human cartilage when engrafted into SCID mice. *Am J Pathol* 1996; **149**: 1607–15.

64. Pap, T., Müller-Ladner, U., Hummel, K. M., Gay, R. E., and Gay, S. Studies in the SCID mouse model. In *Gene therapy in inflammatory diseases* (Evans C. and Robbins P., eds), pp. 35–5. Basel: Birkhäuser, 1998.

65. Fassbender, H. G. Histomorphological basis of articular cartilage destruction in rheumatoid arthritis. *Coll Relat Res* 1983; **3**: 141–55.

66. Trabandt, A., Gay, R. E., and Gay, S. Oncogene activation in rheumatoid synovium. *APMIS* 1992; **100**: 861–75.

67. Muller-Ladner, U., Gay, R. E., and Gay, S. Activation of synoviocytes. *Curr Opin Rheumatol* 2000; **12**: 186–94.

68. Müller-Ladner, U., Kriegsmann, J., Gay, R. E., and Gay, S. Oncogenes in rheumatoid synovium. *Rheum Dis Clin North Am* 1995; **21**: 675–90.

69. Aicher, W. K., Heer, A. H., Trabandt, A., Bridges, S. L., Jr., Schroeder, H. W., Jr., Stransky, G. *et al*. Overexpression of zinc-finger transcription factor Z-225/Egr-1 in synoviocytes from rheumatoid arthritis patients. *J Immunol* 1994; **152**: 5940–8.

70. Trabandt, A., Aicher, W. K., Gay, R. E., Sukhatme, V. P., Fassbender, H. G., and Gay, S. Spontaneous expression of immediately-early response genes c-fos and egr-1 in collagenase-producing rheumatoid synovial fibroblasts. *Rheumatol Int* 1992; **12**: 53–9.

71. Ishidoh, K., Taniguchi, S., and Kominami, E. Egr family member proteins are involved in the activation of the cathepsin L gene in v-src-transformed cells. *Biochem Biophys Res Commun* 1997; **238**: 665–9.

72. Asahara, H., Hasunuma, T., Kobata, T., Inoue, H., Muller Ladner, U., Gay, S. *et al*. In situ expression of protooncogenes and Fas/Fas ligand in rheumatoid arthritis synovium. *J Rheumatol* 1997; **24**: 430–5.

73. Dooley, S., Herlitzka, I., Hanselmann, R., Ermis, A., Henn, W., Remberger, K. *et al*. Constitutive expression of c-fos and c-jun, overexpression of ets-2, and reduced expression of metastasis suppressor gene nm23-H1 in rheumatoid arthritis. *Ann Rheum Dis* 1996; **55**: 298–304.

74. Himelstein, B. P., and Koch, C. J. Studies of type IV collagenase regulation by hypoxia. *Cancer Lett* 1998; **124**: 127–33.

75. Benbow, U., and Brinckerhoff, C. E. The AP-1 site and MMP gene regulation: what is all the fuss about? *Matrix Biol* 1997; **15**: 519–26.

76. Asahara, H., Fujisawa, K., Kobata, T., Hasunuma, T., Maeda, T., Asanuma, M. *et al*. Direct evidence of high DNA binding activity of transcription factor AP-1 in rheumatoid arthritis synovium. *Arthritis Rheum* 1997; **40**: 912–18.

77. Trabandt, A., Aicher, W. K., Gay, R. E., Sukhatme, V. P., Nilson, H. M., Hamilton, R. T. *et al*. Expression of the collagenolytic and Ras-induced cysteine proteinase cathepsin L and proliferation-associated oncogenes in synovial cells of MRL/I mice and patients with rheumatoid arthritis. *Matrix* 1990; **10**: 349–61.

78. Gum, R., Wang, H., Lengyel, E., Juarez, J., and Boyd, D. Regulation of 92 kDa type IV collagenase expression by the jun aminoterminal kinase- and the extracellular signal-regulated kinase-dependent signaling cascades. *Oncogene* 1997; **14**: 1481–93.

79. Korzus, E., Nagase, H., Rydell, R., and Travis, J. The mitogen-activated protein kinase and JAK-STAT signaling pathways are required for an oncostatin M-responsive element-mediated activation of matrix metalloproteinase 1 gene expression. *J Biol Chem* 1997; **272**: 1188–96.

80. Pap, T., Nawrath, M., Heinrich, J., Bosse, M., Baier, A., Hummel, K. M. *et al*. Cooperation of Ras- and c-Myc-dependent pathways in regulating the growth and invasiveness of synovial fibroblasts in rheumatoid arthritis. *Arthritis Rheum* 2004; **50**: 2794–802.

81. Firestein, G. S., Echeverri, F., Yeo, M., Zvaifler, N. J., and Green, D. R. Somatic mutations in the p53 tumor suppressor gene in rheumatoid arthritis synovium. *Proc Natl Acad Sci U S A* 1997; **94**: 10895–900.

82. Pap, T., Aupperle, K. R., Gay, S., Firestein, G. S., and Gay, R. E. Invasiveness of synovial fibroblasts is regulated by p53 in the SCID mouse in vivo model of cartilage invasion. *Arthritis Rheum* 2001; **44**: 676–81.

83. Seemayer, C. A., Kuchen, S., Neidhart, M., Kuenzler, P., Rihoskova, V., Neumann, E. *et al*. p53 in rheumatoid arthritis synovial fibroblasts at sites of invasion. *Ann Rheum Dis* 2003; **62**: 1139–44.

84. Muller-Ladner, U., and Nishioka, K. p53 in rheumatoid arthritis: friend or foe? *Arthritis Res* 2000; **2**: 175–8.

85. Li, J., Yen, C., Liaw, D., Podsypanina, K., Bose, S., Wang, S. I. *et al*. PTEN, a putative protein tyrosine phosphatase gene mutated in human brain, breast, and prostate cancer [see comments]. *Science* 1997; **275**: 1943–7.

86. Steck, P. A., Pershouse, M. A., Jasser, S. A., Yung, W. K., Lin, H., Ligon, A. H. *et al*. Identification of a candidate tumour suppressor gene, MMAC1, at chromosome 10q23.3 that is mutated in multiple advanced cancers. *Nat Genet* 1997; **15**: 356–62.

87. Teng, D. H., Hu, R., Lin, H., Davis, T., Iliev, D., Frye, C. *et al*. MMAC1/PTEN mutations in primary tumor specimens and tumor cell lines. *Cancer Res* 1997; **57**: 5221–5.

88. Pap, T., Franz, J. K., Hummel, K. M., Jeisy, E., Gay, R., and Gay, S. Activation of synovial fibroblasts in rheumatoid arthritis: lack of expression of the tumour suppressor PTEN at sites of invasive growth and destruction. *Arthritis Research* 2000; **2**: 59–64.

89. Tamura, M., Gu, J., Danen, E. H., Takino, T., Miyamoto, S., and Yamada, K. M. PTEN interactions with focal adhesion kinase and suppression of the extracellular matrix-dependent phosphatidylinositol 3-kinase/Akt cell survival pathway. *J Biol Chem* 1999; **274**: 20693–703.

90. Tamura, M., Gu, J., Matsumoto, K., Aota, S., Parsons, R., and Yamada, K. M. Inhibition of cell migration, spreading, and focal adhesions by tumor suppressor PTEN. *Science* 1998; **280**: 1614–17.

91. Di Cristofano, A., Kotsi, P., Peng, Y. F., Cordon-Cardo, C., Elkon, K. B., and Pandolfi, P. P. Impaired Fas response and autoimmunity in Pten1/– mice. *Science* 1999; **285**: 2122–5.

92. Marok, R., Winyard, P. G., Coumbe, A., Kus, M. L., Gaffney, K., Blades, S. *et al*. Activation of the transcription factor nuclear factor-kappaB in human inflamed synovial tissue. *Arthritis Rheum* 1996; **39**: 583–91.

93. Miagkov, A. V., Kovalenko, D. V., Brown, C. E., Didsbury, J. R., Cogswell, J. P., Stimpson, S. A. *et al*. NF-kappaB activation provides the potential link between inflammation and hyperplasia in the arthritic joint. *Proc Natl Acad Sci U S A* 1998; **95**: 13859–64.

94. Karin, M., and Lin, A. NF-kappaB at the crossroads of life and death. *Nat Immunol* 2002; **3**: 221–7.

95. Georganas, C., Liu, H., Perlman, H., Hoffmann, A., Thimmapaya B., and Pope R. M. Regulation of IL-6 and IL-8 expression in rheumatoid arthritis synovial fibroblasts: the dominant role for NF-kappa B but not C/EBP beta or c- Jun. *J Immunol* 2000; **165**: 7199–206.

96. Makarov, S. S. NF-kappaB in rheumatoid arthritis: a pivotal regulator of inflammation, hyperplasia, and tissue destruction. *Arthritis Res* 2001; **3**: 200–6.

97. Li, P., Sanz, I., O'Keefe, R. J., and Schwarz, E. M. NF-kappa B regulates VCAM-1 expression on fibroblast-like synoviocytes. *J Immunol* 2000; **164**: 5990–7.

98. Vincenti, M. P., Coon, C. I., and Brinckerhoff, C. E. Nuclear factor kappaB/p50 activates an element in the distal matrix metalloproteinase 1 promoter in interleukin-1beta-stimulated synovial fibroblasts. *Arthritis Rheum* 1998; **41**: 1987–94.

99. Nykanen, P., Bergroth, V., Raunio, P., Nordstrom, D., and Konttinen Y. T. Phenotypic characterization of 3H-thymidine incorporating cells in rheumatoid arthritis synovial membrane. *Rheumatol Int* 1986; **6**: 269–71.

100. Petrow, P., Theis, B., Eckard, A., Karbowski, A., Eysel, P., Salzmann, G. *et al*. Determination of proliferating cells at sites of cartilage invasion in patients with rheumatoid arthritis. *Arthritis Rheum* 1997; **40**: S251.

101. Kinne, R. W., Palombo Kinne, E., and Emmrich, F. Activation of synovial fibroblasts in rheumatoid arthritis. *Ann Rheum Dis* 1995; **54**: 501–4.

102. Baier, A., Meineckel, I., Gay, S., and Pap, T. Apoptosis in rheumatoid arthritis. *Curr Opin Rheumatol* 2003; **15**: 274–9.

103. Matsumoto, S., Muller Ladner, U., Gay, R. E., Nishioka, K., and Gay, S. Multistage apoptosis and Fas antigen expression of synovial fibroblasts derived from patients with rheumatoid arthritis. *J Rheumatol* 1996; **23**: 1345–52.

104. Nakajima, T., Aono, H., Hasunuma, T., Yamamoto, K., Shirai, T., Hirohata, K., and Nishioka, K. Apoptosis and functional Fas antigen in rheumatoid arthritis synoviocytes. *Arthritis Rheum* 1995; **38**: 485–91.

105. Pope, R. M. Apoptosis as a therapeutic tool in rheumatoid arthritis. *Nat Rev Immunol* 2002; **2**: 527–35.

106. Perlman, H., Liu, H., Georganas, C., Koch, A. E., Shamiyeh, E., Haines, G. K., III., and Pope, R. M. Differential expression pattern of the antiapoptotic proteins, Bcl-2 and FLIP, in experimental arthritis. *Arthritis Rheum* 2001; **44**: 2899–908.

107. Matsumoto, S., Muller Ladner, U., Gay, R. E., Nishioka, K., and Gay, S. Ultrastructural demonstration of apoptosis, Fas and Bcl-2 expression of rheumatoid synovial fibroblasts. *J Rheumatol* 1996; **23**: 1345–52.

108. Perlman, H., Georganas, C., Pagliari, L. J., Koch, A. E., Haines, K., III., and Pope, R. M. Bcl-2 expression in synovial fibroblasts is essential for maintaining mitochondrial homeostasis and cell viability. *J Immunol* 2000; **164**: 5227–35.

109. Kurowska, M., Rudnicka, W., Kontny, E., Janicka, I., Chorazy, M., Kowalczewski, J. *et al.* Fibroblast-like synoviocytes from rheumatoid arthritis patients express functional IL-15 receptor complex: endogenous IL-15 in autocrine fashion enhances cell proliferation and expression of Bcl-x(L) and Bcl- 2. *J Immunol* 2002; **169**: 1760–7.

110. Hasunuma, T., Kayagaki, N., Asahara, H., Motokawa, S., Kobata, T., Yagita, H., Aono, H., Sumida, T., Okumura, K., and Nishioka, K. Accumulation of soluble Fas in inflamed joints of patients with rheumatoid arthritis. *Arthritis Rheum* 1997; **40**: 80–6.

111. Freiberg, R. A., Spencer, D. M., Choate, K. A., Duh, H. J., Schreiber S. L., Crabtree G. R., and Khavari P. A. Fas signal transduction triggers either proliferation or apoptosis in human fibroblasts. *J Invest Dermatol* 1997; **108**: 215–19.

112. Drynda, A., Quax, P. H. A., Neumann, M., van der Laan, W. H., Pap, G., Drynda, S. *et al.* Gene transfer of TIMP-3 reverses the inhibitory effects of TNF-a on Fas-induced apoptosis in rheumatoid arthritis synovial fibroblasts. *J Immunol.* [In press.]. 2005.

113. Irmler, M., Thome, M., Hahne, M., Schneider, P., Hofmann, K., Steiner, V. *et al.* Inhibition of death receptor signals by cellular FLIP. *Nature* 1997; **388**: 190–5.

114. Schedel, J., Gay, R. E., Kuenzler, P., Seemayer, C., Simmen, B., Michel, B. A., and Gay, S. FLICE-inhibitory protein expression in synovial fibroblasts and at sites of cartilage and bone erosion in rheumatoid arthritis. *Arthritis Rheum* 2002; **46**: 1512–18.

115. Catrina, A. I., Ulfgren, A. K., Lindblad, S., Grondal, L., and Klareskog, L. Low levels of apoptosis and high FLIP expression in early rheumatoid arthritis synovium. *Ann Rheum Dis* 2002; **61**: 934–6.

116. Melchior, F. SUMO: nonclassical ubiquitin. *Annu Rev Cell Dev Biol* 2000; **16**: 591–626.

117. Okura, T., Gong, L., Kamitani, T., Wada, T., Okura, I., Wei, C. F. *et al.* Protection against Fas/APO-1- and tumor necrosis factor-mediated cell death by a novel protein, sentrin. *J Immunol* 1996; **157**: 4277–81.

118. Franz, J. K., Pap, T., Hummel, K. M., Nawrath, M., Aicher, W. K., Shigeyama, Y. *et al.* Expression of sentrin, a novel antiapoptotic molecule, at sites of synovial invasion in rheumatoid arthritis. *Arthritis Rheum* 2000; **43**: 599–607.

119. Pap, T., Cinski, A., Baier, A., Gay, S., and Meinecke, I. Modulation of pathways regulating both the invasiveness and apoptosis in rheumatoid arthritis synovial fibroblasts. *Joint Bone Spine* 2003; **70**: 477–9.

120. Mojcik, C. F., and Shevach, E. M. Adhesion molecules: a rheumatologic perspective. *Arthritis Rheum* 1997; **40**: 991–1004.

121. Schwartz, M. A. Integrins, oncogenes, and anchorage independence. *J Cell Biol* 1997; **139**: 575–8.

122. Dike, L. E., and Ingber, D. E. Integrin-dependent induction of early growth response genes in capillary endothelial cells. *J Cell Sci* 1996; **109**: 2855–63.

123. Dike, L. E., and Farmer, S. R. Cell adhesion induces expression of growth-associated genes in suspension-arrested fibroblasts. *Proc Natl Acad Sci U S A* 1988; **85**: 6792–6.

124. Rinaldi, N., Schwarz, E. M., Weis, D., Leppelmann, J. P., Lukoschek, M., Keilholz, U., and Barth, T. F. Increased expression of integrins on fibroblast-like synoviocytes from rheumatoid arthritis in vitro correlates with enhanced binding to extracellular matrix proteins. *Ann Rheum Dis* 1997; **56**: 45–51.

125. Ishikawa, H., Hirata, S., Andoh, Y., Kubo, H., Nakagawa, N., Nishibayashi, Y., and Mizuno, K. An immunohistochemical and immunoelectron microscopic study of adhesion molecules in synovial pannus formation in rheumatoid arthritis. *Rheumatol Int* 1996; **16**: 53–60.

126. Müller-Ladner, U., Elices, M. J., Kriegsmann, J., Strahl, D., Gay, R. E., Firestein, G. S., and Gay, S. Alternatively spliced CS-1 fibronectin isoform and its receptor VLA-4 in rheumatoid synovium demonstrated by in situ hybridization and immunohistochemistry. *J Rheumatol* 1997; **24**: 1873–80.

127. Osborn, L., Hession, C., Tizard, R., Vassallo, C., Luhowskyj, S., Chi, R. G., and Lobb, R. Direct expression cloning of vascular cell adhesion molecule 1, a cytokine-induced endothelial protein that binds to lymphocytes. *Cell* 1989; **59**: 1203–11.

128. Higashiyama, H., Saito, I., Hayashi, Y., and Miyasaka, N. In situ hybridization study of vascular cell adhesion molecule-1 messenger RNA expression in rheumatoid synovium. *J Autoimmun* 1995; **8**: 947–57.

129. Morales, D. J., Wayner, E., Elices, M. J., Alvaro, G. J., Zvaifler, N. J., and Firestein, G. S. Alpha 4/beta 1 integrin (VLA-4) ligands in arthritis: vascular cell adhesion molecule-1 expression in synovium and on fibroblast-like synoviocytes. *J Immunol* 1992; **149**: 1424–31.

130. Matsuyama, T., and Kitani, A. The role of VCAM-1 molecule in the pathogenesis of rheumatoid synovitis. *Hum Cell* 1996; **9**: 187–92.

131. Kitani, A., Nakashima, N., Izumihara, T., Inagaki, M., Baoui, X., Yu, S. *et al.* Soluble VCAM-1 induces chemotaxis of Jurkat and synovial fluid T cells bearing high affinity very late antigen-4. *J Immunol* 1998; **161**: 4931–4938.

132. Kitani, A., Nakashima, N., Matsuda, T., Xu, B., Yu, S., Nakamura, T. and Matsuyama, T. T cells bound by vascular cell adhesion molecule-1/CD106 in synovial fluid in rheumatoid arthritis: inhibitory role of soluble vascular cell adhesion molecule-1 in T cell activation. *J Immunol* 1996; **156**: 2300–8.

133. Petrow, P., Franz, J. K., Muller Ladner, U., Hummel, K. M., Gay, R. E., Prince, C., and Gay, S. Expression of osteopontin mRNA in synovial tissue of patients with rheumatoid arthritis (RA) and osteoarthritis (OA). *Arthritis Rheum* 1997; **39**: S36.

134. Lampe, M. A., Patarca, R., Iregui, M. V., and Cantor, H. Polyclonal B cell activation by Eta-1 cytokine and the development of systemic autoimmune disease. *J Immunol* 1991; **147**: 2902–6.

135. Pichler, R., Giachelli, C. M., Lombardi, D., Pippin, J., Gordon, K., Alpers, C. E. *et al.* Tubulointestinal disease in glomerulonephritis: potential role of osteopontin (uropontin). *Am J Pathol* 1994; **144**: 915–26.

136. Pap, T., Schett, G., and Gay, S. Matrix metalloproteinases. In Targeted therapies in rheumatology (Smolen J. and Lipsky P., eds), London: Martin Dunitz, 2002.

137. Müller-Ladner, U., Gay, R. E., and Gay, S. Cysteine proteinases in arthritis and inflammation. *Perspectives in Drug Discovery and Design* 1996; **6**: 87–98.

138. Nagase, H., and Woessner, J. F., Jr. Matrix metalloproteinases. *J Biol Chem* 1999; **274**: 21491–4.

139. Wolfsberg, T. G., Primakoff, P., Myles, D. G., and White, J. M. ADAM, a novel family of membrane proteins containing A Disintegrin And Metalloprotease domain: multipotential functions in cell-cell and cell-matrix interactions. *J Cell Biol* 1995; **131**: 275–8.

140. Kaushal, G. P., and Shah, S. V. The new kids on the block: ADAMTSs, potentially multifunctional metalloproteinases of the ADAM family. *J Clin Invest* 2000; **105**: 1335–7.

141. Black, R. A., Rauch, C. T., Kozlosky, C. J., Peschon, J. J., Slack, J. L., Wolfson, M. F. *et al.* A metalloproteinase disintegrin that releases tumour-necrosis factor-alpha from cells. *Nature* 1997; **385**: 729–33.

142. Moss, M. L., Jin, S. L., Milla, M. E., Bickett, D. M., Burkhart, W., Carter, H. L. *et al.* Cloning of a disintegrin metalloproteinase that processes precursor tumour-necrosis factor-alpha. *Nature* 1997; **385**: 733–6.

143. Tortorella, M. D., Burn, T. C., Pratta, M. A., Abbaszade, I., Hollis, J. M., Liu, R. *et al.* Purification and cloning of aggrecanase-1: a member of the ADAMTS family of proteins. *Science* 1999; **284**: 1664–6.

144. Krane, S. M., Conca, W., Stephenson, M. L., Amento, E. P., and Goldring, M. Mechanisms of matrix degradation in rheumatoid arthritis. *Am N Y Acad Sci* 1990; **580**: 340–54.

145. Konttinen, Y. T., Ainola, M., Valleala, H., Ma, J., Ida, H., Mandelin, J. *et al.* Analysis of 16 different matrix metalloproteinases (MMP-1 to MMP-20) in the synovial membrane: different profiles in trauma and rheumatoid arthritis. *Ann Rheum Dis* 1999; **58**: 691–7.

146. Sorsa, T., Konttinen, Y. T., Lindy, O., Ritchlin, C., Saari, H., Suomalainen, K. *et al.* Collagenase in synovitis of rheumatoid arthritis. *Semin Arthritis Rheum* 1992; **22**: 44–53.

147. Maeda, S., Sawai, T., Uzuki, M., Takahashi, Y., Omoto, H., Seki, M., and Sakurai, M. Determination of interstitial collagenase (MMP-1) in patients with rheumatoid arthritis. *Ann Rheum Dis* 1995; **54**: 970–5.

148. Gruber, B. L., Sorbi, D., French, D. L., Marchese, M. J., Nuovo, G. J., Kew, R. R., and Arbeit, L. A. Markedly elevated serum MMP-9 (gelatinase B) levels in rheumatoid arthritis: a potentially useful laboratory marker. *Clin Immunol Immunopathol* 1996; **78**: 161–71.

149. Ahrens, D., Koch, A. E., Pope, R. M., Stein, P. M., and Niedbala, M. J. Expression of matrix metalloproteinase 9 (96-kd gelatinase B) in human rheumatoid arthritis. *Arthritis Rheum* 1996; **39**: 1576–87.

150. Okada, Y., Naka, K., Kawamura, K., Matsumoto, T., Nakanishi, I., Fujimoto, N. *et al.* Localization of matrix metalloproteinase 9 (92-kilodalton gelatinase/type IV collagenase 5 gelatinase B) in osteoclasts: implications for bone resorption. *Lab Invest* 1995; **72**: 311–22.

151. Okada, Y., Takeuchi, N., Tomita, K., Nakanishi, I., and Nagase, H. Immunolocalization of matrix metalloproteinase 3 (stromelysin) in rheumatoid synovioblasts (B cells): correlation with rheumatoid arthritis. *Ann Rheum Dis* 1989; **48**: 645–53.

152. Tetlow, L. C., Lees, M., Ogata, Y., Nagase, H., and Woolley, D. E. Differential expression of gelatinase B (MMP-9) and stromelysin-1 (MMP-3) by rheumatoid synovial cells in vitro and in vivo. *Rheumatol Int* 1993; **13**: 53–9.

153. Beekman, B., van El, B., Drijfhout, J. W., Ronday, H. K., and TeKoppele, J. M. Highly increased levels of active stromelysin in rheumatoid synovial fluid determined by a selective fluorogenic assay. *FEBS Lett* 1997; **418**: 305–9.

154. Taylor, D. J., Cheung, N. T., and Dawes, P. T. Increased serum proMMP-3 in inflammatory arthritides: a potential indicator of synovial inflammatory monokine activity. *Ann Rheum Dis* 1994; **53**: 768–72.

155. So, A., Chamot, A. M., Peclat, V., and Gerster, J. C. Serum MMP-3 in rheumatoid arthritis: correlation with systemic inflammation but not with erosive status. *Rheumatology (Oxford)* 1999; **38**: 407–10.

156. Ichikawa, Y., Yamada, C., Horiki, T., Hoshina, Y., and Uchiyama, M. Serum matrix metalloproteinase-3 and fibrin degradation product levels correlate with clinical disease activity in rheumatoid arthritis. *Clin Exp Rheumatol* 1998; **16**: 533–40.

157. Manicourt, D. H., Fujimoto, N., Obata, K., and Thonar, E. J. Levels of circulating collagenase, stromelysin-1, and tissue inhibitor of matrix metalloproteinases 1 in patients with rheumatoid arthritis: relationship to serum levels of antigenic keratan sulfate and systemic parameters of inflammation. *Arthritis Rheum* 1995; **38**: 1031–9.

158. Yoshihara, Y., Obata, K., Fujimoto, N., Yamashita, K., Hayakawa, T., and Shimmei, M. Increased levels of stromelysin-1 and tissue inhibitor of metalloproteinases-1 in sera from patients with rheumatoid arthritis. *Arthritis Rheum* 1995; **38**: 969–75.

159. Yamanaka, H., Matsuda, Y., Tanaka, M., Sendo, W., Nakajima, H., Taniguchi, A., and Kamatani, N. Serum matrix metalloproteinase 3 as a predictor of the degree of joint destruction during the six months after measurement, in patients with early rheumatoid arthritis. *Arthritis Rheum* 2000; **43**: 852–8.

160. Petrow, P., Hummel, K. M., Franz, J. K., Kriegsmann, J., Müller Ladner, U., Gay, R. E., and Gay, S. In-situ detection of MMP-13 mRNA in the synovial membrane and cartilage-pannus junction in rheumatoid arthritis. *Arthritis Rheum* 1997; **40**: S336.

161. Lindy, O., Konttinen, Y. T., Sorsa, T., Ding, Y., Santavirta, S., Ceponis, A., and Lopez-Otin, C. Matrix-metalloproteinase 13 (collagenase 3) in human rheumatoid synovium. *Arthritis Rheum* 1997; **40**: 1391–9.

162. Westhoff, C. S., Freudiger, D., Petrow, P., Seyfert, C., Zacher, J., Kriegsmann, J. *et al.* Characterization of collagenase 3 (matrix metalloproteinase 13) messenger RNA expression in the synovial membrane and synovial fibroblasts of patients with rheumatoid arthritis. *Arthritis Rheum* 1999; **42**: 1517–27.

163. Pap, T., Shigeyama, Y., Kuchen, S., Fernihough, J. K., Simmen, B., Gay, R. E. *et al.* Differential expression pattern of membrane-type matrix metalloproteinases in rheumatoid arthritis. *Arthritis Rheum* 2000; **43**: 1226–32.

164. van de Loo, F. A., Joosten, L. A., van Lent, P. L., Arntz, O. J., and van den Berg, W. B. Role of interleukin-1, tumor necrosis factor alpha, and interleukin-6 in cartilage proteoglycan metabolism and destruction: effect of in situ blocking in murine antigen- and zymosan-induced arthritis. *Arthritis Rheum* 1995; **38**: 164–72.

165. van den Berg, W. B., Joosten, L. A., Helsen, M., and van de Loo, F. A. Amelioration of established murine collagen-induced arthritis with anti-IL-1 treatment. *Clin Exp Immunol* 1994; **95**: 237–43.

166. Müller-Ladner, U., Roberts, C. R., Franklin, B. N., Gay, R. E., Robbins, P. D., Evans, C. H., and Gay, S. Human IL-1Ra gene transfer into human synovial fibroblasts is chondroprotective. *J Immunol* 1997; **158**: 3492–8.

167. Mengshol, J. A., Vincenti, M. P., and Brinckerhoff, C. E. IL-1 induces collagenase-3 (MMP-13) promoter activity in stably transfected chondrocytic cells: requirement for Runx-2 and activation by p38 MAPK and JNK pathways. *Nucleic Acids Res* 2001; **29**: 4361–72.

168. Catterall, J. B., Carrere, S., Koshy, P. J., Degnan, B. A., Shingleton, W. D., Brinckerhoff, C. E. *et al.* Synergistic induction of matrix metalloproteinase 1 by interleukin-1alpha and oncostatin M in human chondrocytes involves signal transducer and activator of transcription and activator protein 1 transcription factors via a novel mechanism. *Arthritis Rheum* 2001; **44**: 2296–310.

169. Dayer, J. M., Beutler, B., and Cerami, A. Cachectin/tumor necrosis factor stimulates collagenase and prostaglandin E2 production by human synovial cells and dermal fibroblasts. *J Exp Med* 1985; **162**: 2163–8.

170. Brinckerhoff, C. E., and Auble, D. T. Regulation of collagenase gene expression in synovial fibroblasts. *Ann N Y Acad Sci* 1990; **580**: 355–74.

171. Kuiper, S., Joosten, L. A., Bendele, A. M., Edwards, C. K., Arntz, O., Helsen, M., van-de, L. F., and van-den, B. W. Different roles of TNFa and IL-1 in murine streptococcal wall arthritis. *Cytokine* 1998; **10**: 690–702.

172. Joosten, L. A., Helsen, M. M., van de Loo, F. A., and van den Berg, W. B. Anticytokine treatment of established type II collagen-induced arthritis in DBA/1 mice: a comparative study using anti-TNF alpha, anti-IL-1 alpha/beta, and IL-1Ra. *Arthritis Rheum* 1996; **39**: 797–809.

173. Jovanovic, D. V., Martel-Pelletier, J., Di Battista, J. A., Mineau, F., Jolicoeurv F. C., Benderdour, M., and Pelletier, J. P. Stimulation of 92-kd gelatinase (matrix metalloproteinase 9) production by interleukin-17 in human monocyte/macrophages: a possible role in rheumatoid arthritis. *Arthritis Rheum* 2000; **43**: 1134–44.

174. Ravanti, L., Toriseva, M., Penttinen, R., Crombleholme, T., Foschi, M., Han, J., and Kahari, V. M. Expression of human collagenase-3 (MMP-13) by fetal skin fibroblasts is induced by transforming growth factor beta via p38 mitogen-activated protein kinase. *FASEB J* 2001; **15**: 1098–100.

175. Bond, M., Fabunmi, R. P., Baker, A. H., and Newby, A. C. Synergistic upregulation of metalloproteinase-9 by growth factors

and inflammatory cytokines: an absolute requirement for transcription factor NF-kappa B. *FEBS Lett* 1998; **435**: 29–34.

176. Forsyth, C. B., Pulai, J., and Loeser, R. F. Fibronectin fragments and blocking antibodies to alpha2beta1 and alpha5beta1 integrins stimulate mitogen-activated protein kinase signaling and increase collagenase 3 (matrix metalloproteinase 13) production by human articular chondrocytes. *Arthritis Rheum* 2002; **46**: 2368–76.

177. Loeser, R. F., Forsyth, C. B., Samarel, A. M., and Im, H. J. Fibronectin fragment activation of proline-rich tyrosine kinase PYK2 mediates integrin signals regulating collagenase-3 expression by human chondrocytes through a protein kinase C-dependent pathway. *J Biol Chem* 2003; **278**: 24577–85.

178. Mengshol, J. A., Vincenti, M. P., Coon, C. I., Barchowsky, A., and Brinckerhoff, C. E. Interleukin-1 induction of collagenase 3 (matrix metalloproteinase 13) gene expression in chondrocytes requires p38, c-Jun N-terminal kinase, and nuclear factor kappaB: differential regulation of collagenase 1 and collagenase 3. *Arthritis Rheum* 2000; **43**: 801–11.

179. Han, Z., Boyle, D. L., Chang, L., Bennett, B., Karin, M., Yang, L. et al. c-Jun N-terminal kinase is required for metalloproteinase expression and joint destruction in inflammatory arthritis. *J Clin Invest* 2001; **108**: 73–81.

180. Barchowsky, A., Frleta, D., and Vincenti, M. P. Integration of the NF-kappaB and mitogen-activated protein kinase/AP-1 pathways at the collagenase-1 promoter: divergence of IL-1 and TNF-dependent signal transduction in rabbit primary synovial fibroblasts. *Cytokine* 2000; **12**: 1469–79.

181. Li, W. Q., Dehnade, F., and Zafarullah, M. Oncostatin M-induced matrix metalloproteinase and tissue inhibitor of metalloproteinase-3 genes expression in chondrocytes requires Janus kinase/STAT signaling pathway. *J Immunol* 2001; **166**: 3491–8.

182. Westermarck, J., Seth, A., and Kahari, V. M. Differential regulation of interstitial collagenase (MMP-1) gene expression by ETS transcription factors. *Oncogene* 1997; **14**: 2651–60.

183. Schett, G., Tohidast-Akrad, M., Smolen, J. S., Schmid, B. J., Steiner, C. W., Bitzan, P. et al. Activation, differential localization, and regulation of the stress-activated protein kinases, extracellular signal-regulated kinase, c-JUN N-terminal kinase, and p38 mitogen-activated protein kinase, in synovial tissue and cells in rheumatoid arthritis. *Arthritis Rheum* 2000; **43**: 2501–12.

184. Vincenti, M. P., Coon, C. I., White, L. A., Barchowsky, A., and Brinckerhoff, C. E. src-related tyrosine kinases regulate transcriptional activation of the interstitial collagenase gene, MMP-1, in interleukin-1-stimulated synovial fibroblasts. *Arthritis Rheum* 1996; **39**: 574–82.

185. Tolboom, T. C., Pieterman, E., van der Laan, W. H., Toes, R. E., Huidekoper, A. L., Nelissen, R. G. et al. Invasive properties of fibroblast-like synoviocytes: correlation with growth characteristics and expression of MMP-1, MMP-3, and MMP-10. *Ann Rheum Dis* 2002; **61**: 975–80.

186. Rutkauskaite, E., Zacharias, W., Schedel, J., Muller-Ladner, U., Mawrin, C., Seemayer, C. A. et al. Ribozymes that inhibit the production of matrix metalloproteinase 1 reduce the invasiveness of rheumatoid arthritis synovial fibroblasts. *Arthritis Rheum* 2004; **50**: 1448–56.

187. Firestein, G. S., and Paine, M. M. Stromelysin and tissue inhibitor of metalloproteinases gene expression in rheumatoid arthritis synovium. *Am J Pathol* 1992; **140**: 1309–14.

188. Clark, I. M., Powell, L. K., Ramsey, S., Hazelman, B. L., and Cawston, T. E. The measurement of collagenase, TIMP and collagenase-TIMP complex in synovial fluids from patients with osteoarthritis and rheumatoid arthritis. *Arthritis Rheum* 1993; **36**: 372–80.

189. DiBattista, J. A., Pelletier, J. P., Zafarullah, M., Fujimoto, N., Obata, K., and Martel, P. J. Coordinate regulation of matrix metalloproteases and tissue inhibitor of metalloproteinase expression in human synovial fibroblasts. *J Rheumatol Suppl* 1995; **43**: 123–8.

190. van der Laan, W. H., Quax, P. H., Seemayer, C. A., Huisman, L. G., Pieterman, E., Grimbergen, J. M. et al. Cartilage degradation and invasion by rheumatoid synovial fibroblasts is inhibited by gene transfer of TIMP-1 and TIMP-3. *Gene Ther* 2003; **10**: 234–42.

191. Smith, M. R., Kung, H., Durum, S. K., Colburn, N. H., and Sun, Y. TIMP-3 induces cell death by stabilizing TNF-alpha receptors on the surface of human colon carcinoma cells. *Cytokine* 1997; **9**: 770–80.

192. Hargreaves, P. G., Wang, F., Antcliff, J., Murphy, G., Lawry, J., Russell, R. G., and Croucher, P. I. Human myeloma cells shed the interleukin-6 receptor: inhibition by tissue inhibitor of metalloproteinase-3 and a hydroxamate-based metalloproteinase inhibitor. *Br J Haematol* 1998; **101**: 694–702.

193. Amour, A., Slocombe, P. M., Webster, A., Butler, M., Knight, C. G., Smith, B. J. et al. TNF-alpha converting enzyme (TACE) is inhibited by TIMP-3. *FEBS Lett* 1998; **435**: 39–44.

194. Ahonen, M., Baker, A. H., and Kahari, V. M. Adenovirus-mediated gene delivery of tissue inhibitor of metalloproteinases-3 inhibits invasion and induces apoptosis in melanoma cells. *Cancer Res* 1998; **58**: 2310–15.

195. Baker, A. H., Zaltsman, A. B., George, S. J., and Newby, A. C. Divergent effects of tissue inhibitor of metalloproteinase-1, -2, or -3 overexpression on rat vascular smooth muscle cell invasion, proliferation, and death in vitro: TIMP-3 promotes apoptosis. *J Clin Invest* 1998; **101**: 1478–87.

196. Baker, A. H., George, S. J., Zaltsman, A. B., Murphy, G., and Newby, A. C. Inhibition of invasion and induction of apoptotic cell death of cancer cell lines by overexpression of TIMP-3. *Br J Cancer* 1999; **79**: 1347–55.

197. Majid, M. A., Smith, V. A., Easty, D. L., Baker, A. H., and Newby, A. C. Adenovirus mediated gene delivery of tissue inhibitor of metalloproteinases-3 induces death in retinal pigment epithelial cells. *Br J Ophthalmol* 2002; **86**: 97–101.

198. Keyszer, G., Redlich, A., Haupl, T., Zacher, J., Sparmann, M., Engethum, U. et al. Differential expression of cathepsins B and L compared with matrix metalloproteinases and their respective inhibitors in rheumatoid arthritis and osteoarthritis: a parallel investigation by semiquantitative reverse transcriptase-polymerase chain reaction and immunohistochemistry. *Arthritis Rheum* 1998; **41**: 1378–87.

199. Keyszer, G. M., Heer, A. H., Kriegsmann, J., Geiler, T., Trabandt, A., Keysser, M. et al. Comparative analysis of cathepsin L, cathepsin D, and collagenase messenger RNA expression in synovial tissues of patients with rheumatoid arthritis and osteoarthritis, by in situ hybridization. *Arthritis Rheum* 1995; **38**: 976–84.

200. Joseph, L., Lapid, S., and Sukhatme, V. The major ras induced protein in NIH3T3 cells is cathepsin L. *Nucleic Acids Res* 1987; **15**: 3186.

201. Huet, G., Flipo, R. M., Colin, C., Janin, A., Hemon, B., Collyn, d. H. M. et al. Stimulation of the secretion of latent cysteine proteinase activity by tumor necrosis factor alpha and interleukin-1. *Arthritis Rheum* 1993; **36**: 772–80.

202. Lemaire, R., Huet, G., Zerimech, F., Grard, G., Fontaine, C., Duquesnoy, B., and Flipo, R. M. Selective induction of the secretion of cathepsins B and L by cytokines in synovial fibroblast-like cells. *Br J Rheumatol* 1997; **36**: 735–43.

203. Schedel, J., Seemayer, C. A., Pap, T., Neidhart, M., Kuchen, S., Michel, B. A. et al. Targeting cathepsin L (CL) by specific ribozymes decreases CL protein synthesis and cartilage destruction in rheumatoid arthritis. *Gene Ther* 2004; **11**: 1040–7.

204. Hummel, K. M., Petrow, P. K., Franz, J. K., Muller-Ladner, U., Aicher, W. K., Gay, R. E. et al. Cysteine proteinase cathepsin K mRNA is expressed in synovium of patients with rheumatoid arthritis and is detected at sites of synovial bone destruction. *J Rheumatol* 1998; **25**: 1887–94.

15 | Pain mechanisms in rheumatoid arthritis

Bruce L. Kidd

Introduction

Pain is the most prevalent symptom in rheumatoid arthritis (RA) and the source of its greatest misery. Whilst some patients have trivial complaints despite intense inflammation others are incapacitated by relatively minor disease. It is apparent that many factors operate to produce symptoms in this disorder.

This chapter will show that in the face of persistent disease the normally straightforward relationship between injury and pain is abandoned as the body strives to mount a coordinated and effective response. Hitherto suppressed inputs from both somatic and environmental sources substantially modify pain processing at multiple levels and there is a strong bi-directional interaction between the nervous system and inflammatory/immune responses.

Pain concepts/neuroplastic pain

Historical perspective

The earliest recorded descriptions were concerned mostly with the character and consequences of pain. Prerequisite conditions for perception of unpleasant sensations were first identified by Galen and included an organ to receive outside impressions, an organizational center to transform sensation into a conscious perception, and a connective pathway between them[1]. By the seventeenth century the role of sensory nerve fibers had been established although their activity was still likened by Descartes in *Principles of Philosophy* to a rope attached to a bell alerting the mind to bodily injury.

The concept of a fixed, immutable system for transmitting noxious information was challenged in the late nineteenth century by detailed clinical observations performed by Sherrington, Lewis, and others. More recent work has led to the concept of neural 'plasticity', characterized by dramatic alterations to sensory function, involving increased sensitivity and amplified responses to both noxious and non-noxious stimuli[2].

Present day pain studies feature three different approaches. At a population level, epidemiological observations have defined the incidence and prevalence of painful conditions. The inter-relationship between pain and various personal and environmental factors has been studied by clinical scientists, whereas basic scientists have focused largely on neural pathways. The challenge remains to reconcile these three approaches. Although pain classifications based on mechanisms identified from basic studies have been proposed[3], the clinical value of such schemes has yet to be fully realized.

Definitions

Pain is ultimately a personal experience that is associated with a number of secondary consequences, including communication of distress to the outside world and disability. Nociception, on the other hand, may be thought of as the neurophysiological process that underlies this phenomenon (Box 15.1).

Traditionally, pain has been regarded as being either nociceptive (i.e. arising in response to tissue injury) or neuropathic (i.e. arising in response to nerve injury). Whilst this distinction has had some therapeutic utility, it has served to maintain the

---

Box 15.1   Some useful definitions

Pain: an unpleasant sensory and emotional experience associated with actual or potential tissue damage, and described in terms of such damage.

Nociception: the detection of noxious stimuli and the subsequent transmission of encoded information to, and analysis by, the brain.

Suffering: perception of serious threat or damage to oneself. May develop in presence of a discrepancy between expectation and functional ability.

Hyperesthesia (hypersensitivity): increased sensitivity to stimulation, excluding the special senses.

Hyperalgesia: increased pain in response to a noxious stimulus.

Allodynia: pain due to a stimulus that does not normally produce pain.

Referred pain: pain perceived in an area of the body topographically distinct from the region in which the actual source of the pain is located.

Radicular pain: pain perceived as arising in a limb or the trunk caused by ectopic activation of nociceptive afferent fibers or other neuropathic mechanism.

Abridged from Ref. 4

Cartesian concept of a fixed immutable nociceptive system. The emerging recognition of nociceptive plasticity has led to an appreciation that ultimately chronic pain depends not simply on tissue or neural injury but also on sensitization within nociceptive pathways. Whilst some have used the term 'inflammatory pain' to describe such symptoms[5], the alternative expression 'neuroplastic pain' is to be preferred as it is quite clear that nociceptive plasticity, and hence pain, can arise in the absence of an overt inflammatory component.

Assessment

Pain

Despite its critical importance, pain assessment remains difficult, largely because the pain experience is subjective. Furthermore, pain is as strongly influenced by a range of personal, cultural, social, demographic, and environmental factors as it is by the character of the underlying disease. It follows that both the context in which symptoms occur and the underlying nociceptive process need to be taken into account when assessing a individual's report of pain (see Box 15.2).

Despite obvious differences between various musculoskeletal disorders, attempts to differentiate them using verbal descriptions alone have proved unrewarding. Individuals with both RA and osteoarthritis choose words such as 'aching' and 'throbbing' to describe symptoms, interspersed by activity-related episodes of 'sharp' and stabbing' pain[6,7]. Whilst inflammatory pain is generally most severe in the mornings and again towards the end of the day, this pattern varies widely and may not serve as a useful distinguishing feature in every case.

Efforts by health professionals to estimate pain through objective measures have proved useful in clinical research but not in clinical care[8]. Self-report questionnaires permit pain to be recorded in a quantitative fashion and allow for standardized assessments. The most robust quantitative pain measure in both clinical and research environments remains the 10-cm visual analogue scale (VAS). Other instruments such as the McGill pain questionnaire offer the opportunity to study additional components but have not found widespread utility in clinical practice.

Nociception

Reported pain is an unreliable guide of underlying neurophysiological mechanisms. Quantitative sensory testing and related procedures attempt to overcome this shortcoming by using psychophysical methods to assess nociceptive activity[9]. Pressure pain thresholds in response to mechanical stimuli have been shown to be reduced over both diseased joints and control sites in RA compared to controls[10]. Interestingly, no such reduction was observed in patients with ankylosing spondylitis[11] and abnormalities were shown to be more marked in RA patients than in a similar group with psoriatic arthritis matched for disease severity[12].

Capsaicin is the active ingredient in hot chilli peppers and has proved a useful tool for nociceptive research as it selectively excites unmyelinated sensory fibers concerned with nociceptive transmission. Pinprick hyperalgesia induced by intradermal capsaicin is substantially greater over the forearms of RA patients compared to normal controls[13] (Fig. 15.1). Additional studies employing mechanical rather than chemical stimuli have reported similar changes[14,15]. Taken together these studies are highly suggestive of altered nociceptive processing at both peripheral and central levels in RA. There is some evidence that these effects may be time dependent, becoming more apparent with prolonged disease[14].

Pain pathways

Joints

With probable exception of cartilage, all tissues comprising the musculoskeletal system receive an extensive sensory nerve supply. Encapsulated sensory receptors are associated with rapidly conducting Aβ fibers (conduction velocities greater than 30 m/s) and are found mainly in fibrous periarticular structures, includingligaments, tendons, and joint capsule. They are activated by non-noxious stimuli and for the most part are mechanoreceptors/proprioreceptors. In contrast, small diameter fibers are normally activated by high intensity stimuli and have been regarded as nociceptors. They include thinly myelinated Aδ fibers (conduction velocities 2.5–30 m/s) and unmyelinated C fibers (conduction velocities less than 2.5 m/s), which generally have free nerve endings and are more widely distributed in synovium, fibrous capsules, adipose tissues, ligaments, menisci, and periosteum[16].

Quantitative studies of articular nerve bundles arising from mammalian joints have established that nearly 90% of sensory fibers within these bundles are C fibers. Highly relevant observations made by Schaible and colleagues in the 1980s demonstrated that, under normal conditions, the vast majority of these fibers

---

Box 15.2   Yellow flags: predictors of enhanced pain reporting and disability

Duration of symptoms

Intensity of symptoms

History of numerous painful episodes

Anxiety

Depression

External locus of control

Catastrophizing

Activity intolerance

Dependence on passive therapies

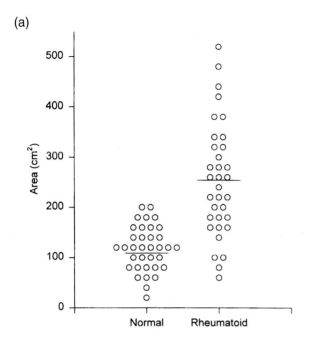

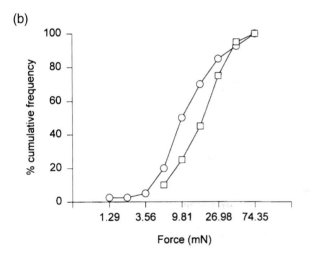

Fig. 15.1 (a) Comparison of the area of capsaicin-induced pinprick hyperalgesia in normal and rheumatoid subjects (solid line indicates mean value) demonstrating enhanced central nociceptive (pain) processing. (b) Comparison of sensory thresholds for pinprick stimuli using von Frey hairs of increasing force in normal (circles) and rheumatoid subjects (*n* = 35 each group), illustrating similar peripheral nociceptive processing at control sites over the forearm. (Reproduced from Ref. 13 with permission.)

are non-responsive to mechanical and thermal stimuli in both the physiological and noxious range[17]. The terms 'sleeping' or 'silent' nociceptors were coined to describe these fibers, which were subsequently shown to be sensitive to a range of chemical mediators[18].

Bones

The periosteal layers of bone have traditionally been regarded as possessing an extensive nerve supply whereas deeper layers were thought to have a much sparser innervation. More recent studies have challenged this view by reporting the presence of unmyelinated and thinly myelinated sensory fibers throughout the bone marrow, mineralized bone, and the periosteum. While the periosteum was shown to be the most densely innervated tissue, when the total volume of each tissue was considered, the bone marrow received the greatest total number of sensory fibers, followed by mineralized bone and then periosteum[19].

Dorsal root ganglia

The cell bodies of peripheral sensory fibers are located within the dorsal root ganglia, with large diameter cells giving rise to myelinated Aβ fibers and a proportion of more thinly myelinated Aδ fibers. In contrast, small diameter cells give rise to mainly unmyelinated axons. These can be differentiated histochemically into two distinct populations, including those cells which constitutively synthesise neuropeptides (including substance P and calcitonin gene-related peptide) and those which bind the isolectin IB4 (*Bandeiraea simplicifolia*). Whilst IB4-binding neurones are associated with cutaneous tissues, retrograde nerve tracing studies have so far failed to identify IB4-binding neurones arising from either articular tissues[20] or bone[19].

Central connections

Unmyelinated sensory fibers terminate in the spinal cord and synapse either with rapidly conducting nociceptive projection neurones or more slowly conducting interneurones. The projection neurones cross the midline, with the majority entering the contralateral spinothalamic tract, which is the major pathway for ascending nociceptive transmission[21].

Spinothalamic tract neurones divide into lateral and medial branches as they approach the thalamus. Information transmitted in the lateral branches is relayed rapidly to the somatosensory cortex, lending support to the view that the lateral system is primarily concerned with sensory—discriminative aspects of pain. This includes both localization and identification of noxious stimuli.

The more medial branches terminate in the intralaminar nuclei of the thalamus. This structure integrates information from a variety of inputs, including the brainstem reticular formation, and projects widely to the limbic and prefrontal cortices. Available data suggest that the medial pain system is concerned mainly with motivational–affective components of the pain response[22].

Accumulating evidence suggests that there is no single or 'ultimate' pain center. In keeping with other modalities, pain sensations appear to be processed in parallel networks or matrices distributed within cortical and subcortical structures[23].

Nociceptive plasticity

Peripheral mechanisms

Substances present within the extracellular space act to augment or inhibit activity in peripheral sensory neurones in a number of

(a)

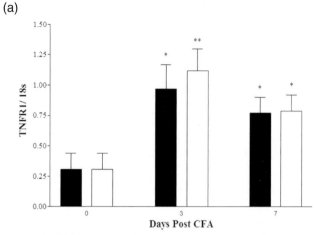

(b)

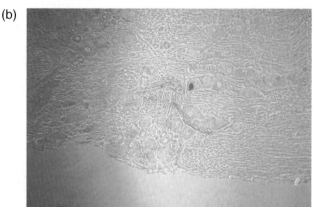

(c)

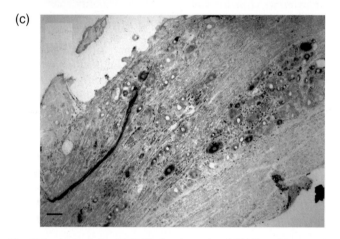

Fig. 15.2 (a) Real-time RT-PCR showing a threefold bilateral increase in TNF receptor 1 (TNFR1) mRNA in the rat dorsal root ganglia (DRG) following induction of experimental peripheral inflammation (ipsilateral side: black bars; contralateral side: white bars). (b) *In situ* mRNA hybridization, showing no detectable TNFR1 in the naïve DRG, whereas in (c) TNFR1 is detected on neuronal cells seven days after induction of inflammation. Adapted from Ref. 29 with permission.

ways. In acute situations, some mediators such as bradykinin contribute to pain by directly activating nociceptors via specific cell surface receptors whereas others are generally considered to be sensitizing agents[24]. Within the joint, experimental application of

prostaglandin E2 has been shown to sensitize nociceptors to mechanical and other stimuli with a time course that matches the development of pain-related behaviour in awake animals[18,25]. Other mediators such as the endogenous opioids and cannabinoids act at peripheral sites to reduce nociceptor activity[26].

Phosphorylation and other immediate effects on existing receptors and ion channels are important in acute situations, whereas in disorders associated with persistent disease transcriptional up-regulation of receptors and secondary signaling become more important[5]. The presence of receptors on articular sensory afferents for neurotrophin growth factors, including nerve growth factor, is important in this regard[27]. These mediators exert a global influence on nociceptor activity by regulating the expression of neuropeptides, receptors, and ion channels[28].

More profound changes in the receptor profile of nociceptive neurones have also been reported in experimental models and serve to explain the substantial anti-hyperalgesic properties of biological agents used in RA[29]. Joint inflammation is associated with increased expression of receptors for tumor necrosis factor (TNF) on DRG cells that is maintained through the time course of the model (Fig. 15.2). This is consistent with the observation that anti-TNF therapies have no intrinsic analgesic effects in normal individuals but exert a profound anti-hyperalgesic effect in patients with RA and other inflammatory conditions.

Spinal mechanisms

As is the case in the periphery, acute and longer-term mechanisms can be discerned to be operating at a spinal level in response to musculoskeletal pathology. Acute joint inflammation with resultant activation of peripheral neurones results in functional expression of N-methyl-D-aspartate (NMDA) on channel receptors (via phosphorylation and removal of a magnesium 'block') by second order spinal neurones[30]. Activation of these receptors increases intracellular calcium concentration with resultant changes in cellular excitability known collectively as 'central sensitization'[2].

A series of studies by Watkins and others have highlighted the importance of glial cells as powerful modulators of nociception within central pathways[31]. Activated glia produce cytokines such as IL-1 and IL-6 which in turn initiate a cascade of events leading to the release of mediators such as nitric oxide, prostaglandins, and growth factors. The parallel with inflammatory reactions in musculoskeletal tissues leading to peripheral sensitization is obvious.

The appreciation that central sensitization can be modulated by inflammatory agents such as prostaglandins has led to a reappraisal of the site of action of many of the anti-inflammatory/ analgesic agents commonly used in musculoskeletal practice[32]. It is now well established that the majority of spinal neurones and surrounding glia constitutively express high levels of cyclooxygenase (COX)-2 protein. Inhibition of spinal COX-2 reduces injury-induced activation of nociceptive neurones as well as the mechanical and thermal hyperalgesia that normally occurs after peripheral tissue injury[33,34].

Neurogenic inflammation

Neuroimmune interactions

A close relationship exists between the three classical defensive systems of the body; the immune, endocrine, and nervous systems. Neural tissues influence immune responses at different levels, including the brain (neuroendocrine functions), spinal cord (reflexes), and periphery (neurogenic inflammation)[35]. The influence of the latter process is well documented in disorders affecting the respiratory[36] and gastrointestinal systems[37] and evidence for an effect on the clinical features of many rheumatic disorders is also apparent[35].

Neurogenic inflammation is mediated by sensory neuropeptides, including the tachykinins, substance P (SP) and neurokinin A (NKA), as well as by the more recently identified virokinin and hemokinin. Other biologically active peptides likely to be relevant in the pathophysiology of RA include calcitonin gene-related peptide, neuropeptide tyrosine, vasoactive intestinal polypeptide, and somatostatin[36,38].

The bi-directional character of the neuroimmune relationship is well illustrated by a series of observations of the effects of opioid peptides on peptidergic sensory nerves. During inflammation, immune cells secrete endogenous opioid peptides. These then occupy peripheral opioid receptors on sensory terminals and not only produce analgesia by inhibiting neurone excitability but also exert an anti-inflammatory effect by inhibiting the release of pro-inflammatory neuropeptides[39].

Substance P

Substance P was the first of the classical neuropeptides to be identified and has received the greatest attention to date. In common with other neuropeptides, it is produced by small diameter sensory nerves and released from both central and peripheral terminals. Although initially considered to be exclusively synthesized by sensory neurones, it is now clear that immune cells, including resident macrophages and circulating leukocytes, are a second major source of this peptide[40].

Substance P stimulates the release of IL-1, IL-6, and TNF from human monocytes and also mediates mast cell degranulation and production of PGE_2 and collagenase from synoviocytes (for a review see Ref. 41). It is chemotactic for a number of cells including neutrophils, eosinophils, monocytes, and, more recently, lymphocytes[42]. The expression of vascular endothelial cell adhesion molecules is also up-regulated[43].

Tissue effects

Although the true potential of neurally released peptides to influence the natural history of human arthropathies remains uncertain, their contribution to the pathogenesis of experimental arthritis in a number of models has been examined[44–46]. Mice with a disruption of the NK-1 receptor for substance P (NK-1R) have significantly less footpad swelling and mechanical hyperalgesia than wild type animals in a Freund's complete adjuvant (FCA) arthritis model[45] (Fig. 15.3). Histological and radiological scores were markedly reduced in the knockout group, with effects on synovial hyperplasia and inflammatory cell infiltrate being particularly noticeable. In a similar fashion, disruption of the NK-1R gene protects against the injury induced by antigen–antibody complex formation in respiratory tissues[47].

A neurogenic role in the production of symmetrical joint disease has been suggested following the observation that inflammation in one joint can result in a neurogenically mediated response in the contralateral joint[48].

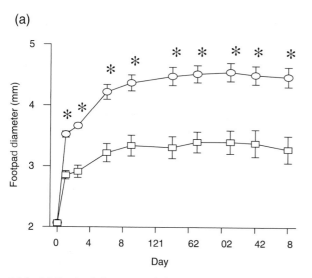
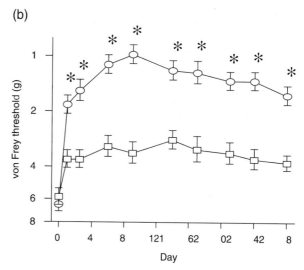

Fig. 15.3 (a) Foodpad diameter and (b) mechanical hyperalgesia in wild type (circles) and NK-1 knockout mice following adjuvant-induced inflammation (10 mg/ml) demonstrating pro-inflammatory effects of substance P during persistent disease. * indicates significant differences ($P < 0.05$). (Reproduced from Ref. 45 with permission.)

Table 15.1 Classification of musculoskeletal pain

Category	Principal mechanism	Neurophysiological effects	Modifiers	Physical effects
Level one pain	Peripheral sensitization	↑ responses to noxious stimuli Activation by novel stimuli	Inflammatory mediators	Localized pain/tenderness
Level two pain	Spinal sensitization (central sensitization)	↑ responses to noxious stimuli ↑ receptive field size Activation by convergent inputs	Somatic inputs	Referred pain/tenderness
Level three pain	Cortical sensitization (central sensitization)	↑ responses to noxious stimuli ↑ receptive field size Activation by convergent inputs	Environmental inputs	Hypervigilance Diffuse pain Behavioral change

Causes of pain in rheumatoid arthritis

Level one neuroplastic pain

Pain arising in consequence of RA may be characterized as being neuroplastic insofar as signs and symptoms are influenced not only by tissue pathology but also by nociceptive plasticity. In the first instance, mediators released from inflamed synovium will induce sensitization of articular nociceptive fibers (see Table 15.1). Consistent with this, capsaicin-induced skin flares have been shown to be enhanced over inflamed RA joints but not at reference points over non-inflamed tissues[49]. A contribution from bone-derived mediators is possible but remains unproven.

In experimental situations, inflammation is associated with increased excitability of previously high threshold and silent nociceptors such that they become responsive to benign mechanical stimuli such as walking or standing[18]. The overall level of activity within an individual fiber no doubt reflects the net balance of excitatory and inhibitory mediators present within the extracellular space to which the fiber is exposed.

The clinical correlate of peripheral sensitization is that musculoskeletal symptoms will be localized, with a relatively close relationship to mechanical stimuli such as walking or standing. Treatment with topical therapies designed to reduce inflammatory mediators might be expected to have a beneficial effect, which is in accord with clinical experience[50].

Level two neuroplastic pain

In chronic conditions such as RA, neural sensitization will not be confined to the periphery. The finding of increased areas of punctate hyperalgesia in patients with RA after topical application of capsaicin is in accord with increased excitability of spinal neurones in this condition[13].

Sensitization of spinal neurones following experimental joint inflammation results in exaggerated responses to normal stimuli, expansion of receptive field size, and reduction of the threshold for activation by novel inputs[51]. Clinically this leads to enhanced pain perception at the site of injury (primary hyperalgesia), development of pain, and tenderness in normal tissues both adjacent to (secondary hyperalgesia) and removed from (referred pain) the primary site.

Spinal nociceptive processing in RA patients is under the influence of descending inhibitory controls and inputs from other somatic structures[14]. Previous pain episodes as well as genetic factors are also likely to heavily influence activity at a spinal level. The multiplicity of mediators involved provides an opportunity for therapeutic intervention and many of the commonly used preparations, including non-steroidal anti-inflammatory drugs as well as weaker opioid drugs, are likely to be exerting analgesic effects at a spinal level.

Level three neuroplastic pain

It is abundantly clear from epidemiological studies that there is a far from straightforward relationship between RA and pain. In broad terms, psychological and social factors have been shown to be the most important predictors of both the presence and severity of pain in a range of disorders, including RA, osteoarthritis, and persistent low back pain[52]. It seems logical to assume, but remains unproven, that these external factors influence nociceptive processing at a supra-spinal or cortical level[9].

Evidence from sensory testing and function brain imaging studies supports the presence of enhanced cortical sensitization in musculoskeletal disease[53,54]. RA patients have substantially damped cortical and subcortical responses compared to control groups in response to painful stimuli, with particular differences in the prefrontal and cingulate areas[55]. Changes in central opioid receptor binding in RA patients have also been reported[56].

Cortical sensitization results in enhanced pain perception as well as increased pain reporting and behavioural change, including disability. Receptors for COX-2 are constitutively expressed in cortical tissues and it is likely that non-steroidal anti-inflammatory drugs exert effects at this level. Non-pharmaceutical approaches, including cognitive behavioural therapy, have also proved effective.

Conclusions

RA is associated with sensitization of nociceptive neurones at peripheral, spinal, and supra-spinal levels. Within each of these three cellular compartments sensitization has predictable consequences for nociceptive activity and resultant symptoms.

Sensitization at any level will serve to amplify afferent inputs and enhance perception of pain. A second and equally important effect is the integration of extraneous inputs, vital for a coordinated and appropriate response to acute or ongoing tissue pathology. Multiple somatic inputs are integrated at a spinal level, whereas cortical sensitization will inevitably be influenced by external inputs, consistent with the importance of environmental factors on pain perception and disability. Finally, pre-existing personal factors are likely to affect the overall level of reactivity. Whether such factors as anxiety and depression are risk factors for the development of pain or simply highlight a hyper-reactive nervous system remains to be seen.

Key challenges remain. The further characterization of the array of chemical mediators that underlie neural sensitization accompanying musculoskeletal conditions is an ongoing concern for both academics and the pharmaceutical industry alike. Identification of individual risk factors for the development of sensitization (yellow flags) remains a priority. Finally, much work remains to be done in overcoming outmoded dualistic concepts of pain and highlighting the importance of neural plasticity to pain in RA and other musculoskeletal conditions.

References

1. Rey, R. *History of Pain*. Harvard University Press; Cambridge, MA: 1993.
2. Melzack, R., Coderre, T. J., Katz, J., and Vaccarino, A. L. Central neuroplasticity and pathological pain. *Ann N Y Acad Sci* 2001; **933**: 157–74.
3. Woolf, C. J., and Max, M. B. Mechanism-based pain diagnosis: issues for analgesic drug development. *Anesthesiology* 2001; **95**: 241–9.
4. Merskey, H., and Bogduk, N. (eds). *Classification of Chronic Pain*, 2nd edn. pp. 209–13. Seattle: IASP Press; 1994.
5. Woolf, C. J., and Costigan, M. Transcriptional and posttranslational plasticity and the generation of inflammatory pain. *Proc Natl Acad Sci U S A* 1999; **96**: 7723–30.
6. Wagstaff, S., Smith, O. V., and Wood, P. H. N. Verbal pain descriptors used by patients with arthritis. *Ann Rheum Dis* 1985; **44**: 262–5.
7. Farrell, M., Gibson, S., and McMeeken, J., and Helme, R. Pain and hyperalgesia in osteoarthritis of the hands. *J Rheumatol* 2000; **27**: 441–7.
8. Sokka, T. Assessment of pain in patients with rheumatic diseases. *Best Pract Res Clin Rheumatol* 2003; **17**: 427–49.
9. Gracely, R. H., Eliav, E., and Hanson, P. Quantitative sensory testing: clinical considerations and new methods. *Proceedings of the 10th World Congress on Pain*. Progress in Pain Research and Management, Vol. 24 (Dostrovsky, J. O., Carr, D. B., Koltzenburg, M., eds). Seattle: IASP Press; 2003.
10. Fredriksson, L., Alstergren, P., and Kopp, S. Pressure pain thresholds in the craniofacial region of female patients with rheumatoid arthritis. *J Orofac Pain* 2003; **17**: 326–32.
11. Incel, N. A., Erdem, H. R., Ozgocmen, S., Catal, S. A., and Yorcancioglu, Z. R. Pain pressure threshold values in ankylosing spondylitis. *Rheumatol Int* 2002; **22**: 148–50. [First published online, 19 June 2002.]
12. Buskila, D., Langevitz, P., Gladman, D. D., Urowitz, S., and Smythe, H. A. Patients with rheumatoid arthritis are more tender than those with psoriatic arthritis. *J Rheumatol* 1992; **19**: 1115–19.
13. Morris, V. H., Cruwys, S. C., and Kidd, B. L. Characterisation of capsaicin-induced mechanical hyperalgesia as a marker for altered nociceptive processing in patients with rheumatoid arthritis. *Pain* 1997; **712**: 179–86.
14. Leffler, A. S., Kosek, E., Lerndal, T., Nordmark, B., and Hansson, P. Somatosensory perception and function of diffuse noxious inhibitory controls (DNIC) in patients suffering from rheumatoid arthritis. *Eur J Pain* 2002; **6**: 161–76.
15. Hendiani, J. A., Westlund, K. N., Lawand, N., Goel, N., Lisse, J., and McNearney T. Mechanical sensation and pain thresholds in patients with chronic arthropathies. *J Pain* 2003; **4**: 203–11.
16. Mapp, P. I., Kidd, B. L., Gibson, S. J., Terry, J. M., Revell, P. A., and Ibrahim, N. B. N. *et al.* Substance P- calcitonin-related peptide- and C-flanking peptide of neuropeptide Y-immunoreactive fibres are present in normal synovium but depleted in patients with rheumatoid arthritis. *Neuroscience* 1990; **37**: 143–53.
17. Grigg, P., Schaible, H., and Schmidt, R. F. Mechanical sensitivity of group III and IV afferents from posterior articular nerve in normal and inflamed cat knee. *J Neurophysiol* 1986; **554**: 635–43.
18. Schaible, H., and Grubb, B. D. Afferent and spinal mechanisms of joint pain. *Pain* 1993; **55**: 5–54.7.
19. Mach, D. B., Rogers, S. D., Sabino, M. C., Luger, N. M., Schwei, M. J., and Pomonis, J. D. *et al.* Origins of skeletal pain: sensory and sympathetic innervation of the mouse femur. *Neuroscience* 2002; **113**: 155–66.
20. Ivanavicius, S. P., Blake, D. R., Chessell, I. P., and Mapp, P. I. Isolectin B4 binding neurons are not present in the rat knee joint. *Neuroscience* 2004; **128**: 555–60.
21. Fields, H. L. *Pain*. pp. 41–79. New York: McGraw-Hill; 1987.
22. Jones, A. K P., and Derbyshire, S. W. G. Cerebral mechanisms operating in the presence and absence of inflammatory pain. *Ann Rheum Dis* 1996; **55**: 411–20.
23. Loeser, J. D., and Melzack, R. Pain: an overview. *Lancet* 1999; **353**: 1607–9. [Review.]
24. Cunha, T. M., Verri, W. A. Jr., Silva, J. S., Poole, S., Cunha, F. Q., and Ferreira, S. H. A cascade of cytokines mediates mechanical inflammatory hypernociception in mice. *Proc Natl Acad Sci U S A* 2005; **102**: 1755–60. [First published online, 21 Jan 2005.]
25. Khasar, S. G., Ho, T., Green, P. G., and Levine, J. D. Comparison of prostaglandin E1- and prostaglandin E2-induced hyperalgesia in the rat. *Neuroscience* 1994; **62**: 345–50.
26. Stein, C., Schafer, M., and Machelska, H. Attacking pain at its source: new perspectives on opioids. *Nat Med* 2003; **9**: 1003–8.
27. McMahon, S. B., and Jones, N. G. Plasticity of pain signaling: role of neurotrophic factors exemplified by acid-induced pain. *J Neurobiol* 2004; **61**: 72–87.
28. Kidd, B. L., and Urban, L. A. Mechanisms of inflammatory pain. *Br J Anaesth* 2001; **87**: 1–9.
29. Inglis, J. J., Nissim, A., Lees, D. M., Hunt, S. P., Chernajovsky, Y., and Kidd, B. L. The differential contribution of tumour necrosis factor to thermal and mechanical hyperalgesia during chronic inflammation. *Arthritis Res Ther.* 2005: 7(4): 807–16.
30. Brenner, G. J., Ji R. R., Shaffer, S., and Woolf, C. J. Peripheral noxious stimulation induces phosphorylation of the NMDA receptor NR1 subunit at the PKC-dependent site, serine-896, in spinal cord dorsal horn neurons. *Eur J Neurosci* 2004; **20**: 375–84.
31. Wieseler-Frank, J., Maier, S. F., and Watkins, L. R. Glial activation and pathological pain. *Neurochem Int* 2004; **45**: 389–95.
32. Diaz-Reval, M. I., Ventura-Martinez, R., Deciga-Campos, M., Terron, J. A., Cabre, F., and Lopez-Munoz, F. J. Evidence for a central mechanism of action of S-(1)-ketoprofen. *Eur J Pharmacol* 2004; **483**: 241–8.
33. You, H. J., Morch, C. D., Chen, J., and Arendt-Nielsen, L. Differential antinociceptive effects induced by a selective cyclooxygenase-2 inhibitor (SC-236) on dorsal horn neurons and spinal withdrawal reflexes in anesthetized spinal rats. *Neuroscience* 2003; **121**: 459–72.
34. Ghilardi, J. R., Svensson, C. I., Rogers, S. D., Yaksh, T. L., and Mantyh, P. W. Constitutive spinal cyclooxygenase-2 participates in the initiation of tissue injury-induced hyperalgesia. *J Neurosci* 2004; **24**: 2727–32.
35. Schaible, H. G., Del Rosso, A., and Matucci-Cerinic, M. Neurogenic aspects of inflammation. *Rheum Dis Clin North Am* 2005; **31**: 77–101.
36. Groneberg, D. A., Quarcoo, D., Frossard, N., and Fischer, A. Neurogenic mechanisms in bronchial inflammatory diseases. *Allergy* 2004; **59**: 1139–52.
37. Frieri, M. Neuroimmunology and inflammation: implications for therapy of allergic and autoimmune diseases. *Ann Allergy Asthma Immunol* 2003; **90** (Suppl. 3): 34–40.

38. Carlton, S. M., Du, J., Davidson, E., Zhou, S., and Coggeshall, R. E. Somatostatin receptors on peripheral primary afferent terminals: inhibition of sensitized nociceptors. *Pain* 2001; **90**: 233–44.

39. Puehler, W., and Stein, C. Controlling pain by influencing neurogenic pathways. *Rheum Dis Clin North Am* 2005; **31**: 103–13.

40. Joos, G. F., and Pauwels, R. A. Pro-inflammatory effects of substance P: new perspectives for the treatment of airways disease? *TIPS* 2000; **21**: 131–3.

41. Maggi, C. A. The effects of tachykinins on inflammatory and immune cells. *Regul Pept* 1997; **70**: 75–90.

42. Hood, V., Cruwys, S., Urban, L., and Kidd, B. Differential role of neurokinin receptors in human lymphocyte and monocyte chemotaxis. *Regul Pept* 2000; **96**: 17–21.

43. Quinlan, K. L., Song, I. S., Nouk, S. M., Letran, E. L., Olerud, J. E., and Bunnett, N. W. *et al*. VCAM expression on human dermal microvascular cells is directly and specifically up-regulated by substance P. *Am J Immunol* 1999; **162**: 1656–61.

44. Cruwys, S. C., Garrett, N. E., and Kidd, B. L. Sensory denervation with capsaicin attenuates inflammation and nociception in arthritic rats. *Neurosci Lett* 1995; **193**: 205–7.

45. Kidd, B. L., Inglis, J. J., Vetsika, E., Hood, V. C., De Felipe, C., and Bester, H. *et al*. Inhibition of inflammation and hyperalgesia in NK-1 receptor knock-out mice. *Neuroreport* 2003; **14**: 2189–92.

46. Keeble, J., Blades, M., Pitzalis, C., Castro da Rocha, F. A., and Brain, S. D. The role of substance P in microvascular responses in murine joint inflammation. *Br J Pharmacol* 2005, 7 Feb; [published online ahead of print].

47. Chavolla-Calderon, M., Bayer, M. K., and Fontan, J. J. Bone marrow transplantation reveals an essential synergy between neuronal and hemopoietic neurokinin production in pulmonary inflammation. *J Clin Invest* 2003; **111**: 973–80.

48. Kidd, B. L., Cruwys, S. C., Garrett, N. E., Mapp, P. I., Jolliffe, V. A., and Blake, D. R. Neurogenic influences on contralateral responses during rat monarthritis. *Brain Res* 1995; **688**: 72–6.

49. Jolliffe, V. A., Anand, P., and Kidd, B. L. Assessment of cutaneous sensory and autonomic axon reflexes in rheumatoid arthritis. *Ann Rheum Dis* 1995; **54**: 251–5.

50. Mason, L., Moore, R. A., Edwards, J. E., Derry, S., and McQuay, H. J. Topical NSAIDs for chronic musculoskeletal pain: systematic review and meta-analysis. *BMC Musculoskelet Disord* 2004; **5**: 28.

51. Woolf, C. J. Evidence for a central component of postinjury pain hypersensitivity. *Nature* 1983; **306**: 686–8.

52. Gran, J. T. The epidemiology of chronic generalized musculoskeletal pain. *Best Pract Res Clin Rheumatol* 2003; **17**: 547–61. [Review.]

53. Giesecke, T., Gracely, R. H., Grant, M. A., Nachemson, A., Petzke, F., Williams, D. A., and Clauw, D. J. Evidence of augmented central pain processing in idiopathic chronic low back pain. *Arthritis Rheum* 2004; **50**: 613–23.

54. Berglund, B., Harju, E. L., Kosek, E., and Lindblom, U. Quantitative and qualitative perceptual analysis of cold dysesthesia and hyperalgesia in fibromyalgia. *Pain* 2002 Mar; **96**[1–2]: 177–87.

55. Jones, A. K., and Derbyshire, S. W. Reduced cortical responses to noxious heat in patients with rheumatoid arthritis. *Ann Rheum Dis* 1997; **56**: 601–7.

56. Jones, A. K., Cunningham, V. J., Ha-Kawa, S., Fujiwara, T., Luthra, S. K., Silva, S., Derbyshire, S., and Jones, T. Changes in central opioid receptor binding in relation to inflammation and pain in patients with rheumatoid arthritis. *Br J Rheumatol* 1994; **33**: 909–16.

16 | The stress system and the hypothalamic–pituitary–adrenal axis in rheumatoid arthritis

George P. Chrousos and Gregory A. Kaltsas

Introduction

The neuroendocrine and immune systems communicate with each other via a number of shared regulatory mediators (steroid hormones, neuropeptides, and cytokines) and receptors, and play major roles in maintenance of homeostasis and adaptation[1,2]. Exposure to inflammatory stimuli is followed by an integrated response from the site of inflammation via the release of specific cytokines, the key ones being interleukin (IL) IL-1, tumor necrosis factor-alpha (TNF-α), and IL-6, and via activation of neural afferent autonomic sensory fibers[2,3]. These cytokines and afferent nerves lead to the secretion of acute phase proteins by the liver, and initiate a non-specific response via the stimulation of the hypothalamic-pituitary-adrenal (HPA) axis and the systemic/adrenomedullary sympathetic nervous systems (SNS)[2,3]. This leads to systemic elevations of glucocorticoids and catecholamines (Cas), which aim at regulating the inflammation at the site of initiation[1,2]. Rheumatoid arthritis (RA) is a paradigmatic, multifactorial autoimmune disease that is derived from the patient's *excessive* immune and inflammatory response[4]. In this chapter, the current understanding of interactions of the stress and immune systems and their physiologic and pathophysiologic implications in the initiation/perpetuation of the inflammatory component in RA will be discussed. The use of potential therapeutic means based on the presence of such alterations will also be raised.

Organization and function of the stress system

The HPA axis and the SNS are the peripheral limbs of the stress system[2]. The central components are located in the hypothalamus and brainstem and include the paraventricular nuclei (PVN) that release corticotrophin-releasing hormone (CRH) and arginine-vasopressin (AVP), and the locus ceruleus, mostly noradrenergic (NA) cell groups of the medulla and pons (the LC-NA system) (Fig. 16.1). Activation of the stress system leads to CRH-induced secretion of adrenocorticotropin (ACTH) by the corticotrophs of the anterior pituitary; AVP exerts a potent synergistic action with CRH[2]. Circulating ACTH is the key regulator of glucocorticoid (cortisol) secretion by the adrenal glands[2]; it also stimulates adrenal androgen secretion, mainly dehydroepiandrosterone (DHEA) and its sulphate (DHEAS)[5]. The SNS gives rise to preganglionic efferent fibers that terminate in ganglia located in the paravertebral chains. From these ganglia, postganglionic sympathetic fibers run to innervate tissues. Most postganglionic sympathetic fibers release Cas, primarily norepinephrine (NE), and other active substances, including CRH, neuropeptide Y (NPY), and adenosine, that also exert immunomodulatory effects[1,2]. The adrenal medulla is considered part of the sympathetic system, secreting more epinephrine (E) than NE[2].

Role of the stress system in maintaining homeostasis

The stress system has a baseline, circadian activity, but also responds to physical and emotional stressors through the secretion of CRH, AVP, glucocorticoids, and Cas, in order to maintain homeostasis[1,2]. Functionally, the CRH and LC-NE systems participate in a positive feedback loop, so that activation of one system leads to activation of the other; both systems receive stimulatory and inhibitory inputs from other neuronal systems of the brain[1,2]. The increased secretion of glucocorticoids and E/NE induces changes in cardiovascular function, intermediary metabolism, and produces modulation of the immune and inflammatory reaction[6]. In addition, the E/NE, CRH, and NPY that are released from the adrenal medulla and the postganglionic sympathetic nerve fibers exert an immunomodulatory role[2,7] (Fig. 16.2). The sensory afferent fibers not only send signals to the central nervous system (CNS), but also secrete pro-inflammatory (substance P) or anti-inflammatory (somatostatin) substances at the site of inflammation[2,7].

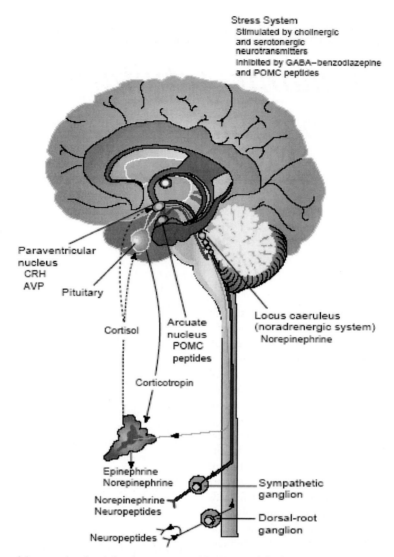

Figure 16.1 Major components of the central and peripheral stress system. The PVN and the locus caeruleus/noradrenergic (LC-NE) system are shown along with their peripheral limbs, the pituitary-adrenal axis, and the adrenomedullary and systemic sympathetic systems. The hypothalamic CRH and central noradrenergic neurones mutually innervate and activate each other, while they exert presynaptic autoinhibition through collateral fibers. AVP from the PVN synergizes with CRH on ACTH secretion. The cholinergic and serotonergic neurotransmitter systems stimulate both components of the central stress system, while the gamma aminobutyric acid/benzodiazepine (GABA/BZD) and arcuate nucleus pro-opiomelanocortin (POMC) peptide systems inhibit it. (Reproduced from Ref. 2 with permission.)

Interactions between the inflammatory reaction and the stress system

Effectors, mediators, and messenger systems

Adrenocortical hormones

The anti-inflammatory and immunosuppressive properties of glucocorticoids are exerted via ubiquitous intracellular glucocorticoid receptors[8,9]. Glucocorticoids suppress the immune activation of circulating or tissue leukocytes and inhibit the production of pro-inflammatory cytokines, mainly TNF-α, IL-1, and IL-12, by monocytes/macrophages/dendritic and T helper 1 (Th1) cells, thus suppressing innate and cellular immunity and favoring a Th2-type response[3,10]. Glucocorticoids also inhibit the expression of adhesion molecules on the surface of immune and other cells and potentiate the acute-phase reaction mainly by the liver and other tissues[2]. The activated glucocorticoid receptor also inhibits the pro-inflammatory activity of many growth factors and cytokines by directly interacting with and blocking the third messenger systems for these hormones such as the transcription factors, nuclear factor (NF)-κB and activating protein-1 (AP-1)[11,12]. Like cortisol, the secretion of adrenal androgens follows the circadian pattern of ACTH secretion, and exerts also a small immunomodulatory effect[13].

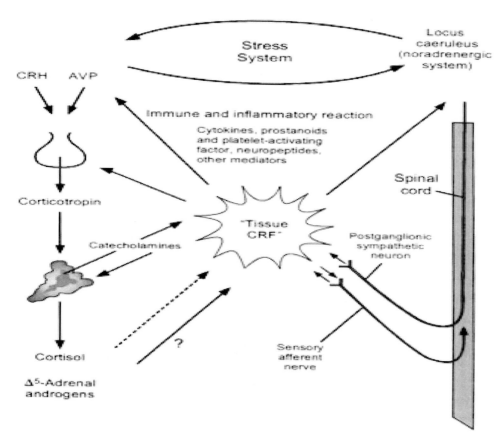

Figure 16.2 Major components and events of inflammation. In inflamed tissue, activated leukocytes and endothelial cells express adhesion molecules and create a chemokine gradient at the focus of inflammation. They attract activated circulating cells, migrant cells, and local immune accessory cells, and peripheral nerves secrete cytokines, prostanoids, platelet activating factor, neuropeptides, and other mediators of inflammation. Some of these substances, such as the inflammatory cytokines TNF-α, IL-1, and IL-6, escape into the systemic circulation, causing systemic symptoms and activating the HPA axis and the SNS. Because of such effects, these substances were historically referred to as 'tissue corticotropin releasing factor (CRF)'. (Reproduced from Ref. 2 with permission.)

Catecholamines

Lymphocyte traffic and circulation are under the influence of the SNS and Cas[2]. Cas inhibit NK cell activity, phagocytosis, and the release of lysosomal enzymes from neutrophils. Epinephrine, NE, and the sympathetic neurotransmitter adenosine (after conversion from adenosine triphosphate (ATP)) exhibit dual immunomodulatory roles through their binding to G-protein-coupled receptor subtypes[7]. Epinephrine interacts with β-adrenoreceptors, exerting stimulatory activity via G-stimulatory proteins (Gs) at low concentrations, whereas at high concentrations it also binds to the G-inhibitory (Gi)-coupled α-adrenoreceptors[3,7]. Noradrenaline and adenosine at low concentrations bind to Gi-coupled α-adrenoreceptors, whereas at high concentrations they bind to Gs-coupled β-adrenoreceptors[7]; this leads to an increase of intracellular cAMP that exerts a mainly anti-inflammatory effect[3,14]. In conjunction with their ability to suppress IL-12 secretion, Cas inhibit the development of Th1-type cells, while promoting Th2 cell differentiation[10,15].

Local effects of neuropeptides

Besides substance P, CRH is also secreted peripherally at inflammatory sites (peripheral or immune CRH) by sympathetic postganglionic or sensory afferent nerves, and influences the immune system directly, through local modulatory actions[2]. Immunoreactive CRH has been identified in inflamed human tissues from patients with various autoimmune/inflammatory diseases, including RA[2,16]. Peripheral CRH has pro-inflammatory actions which are exerted via mast cell degranulation. This effect is blocked by a CRH type 1 receptor antagonist[16]. Thus, a number of locally active substances are produced at peripheral sites, the responses of which may be different from the systemic ones[3] (Fig. 16.2).

Consequences of cytokine and neuropeptide secretion

Inflammatory cytokines reach the hypothalamic CRH and AVP neurones either in a cascade-like fashion and/or via a special transport system and/or through a breach of the blood-brain barrier[15]. In addition to their acute effects on the hypothalamus, they can directly stimulate pituitary ACTH and adrenal cortisol secretion[2,6]. Chronic activation of the HPA axis leads to a relative decrease in the production of Δ5-adrenal androgens which may counteract some of the immunosuppressive effects of Cas, thus promoting Th1 activity[17]. In addition, overall inflammatory stress is associated with reproductive quiescence[17] (Fig. 16.3).

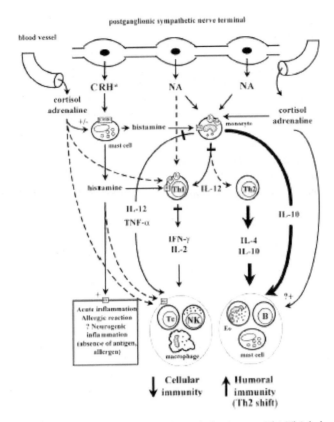

Figure 16.3 Effect of CRH–mast cell–histamine axis, glucocorticoid, and catecholamines on Th1/Th2 balance. Stress and CRH influence immune/ inflammatory and allergic responses by stimulating glucocorticoid, catecholamines, and peripheral (immune) CRH secretion, and by altering the production of key regulatory cytokines and histamine. *CRH is also released from sensory nerves upon their activation. Solid lines represent stimulation, dashed lines inhibition. CRH, peripheral (immune) corticotropin-releasing hormone; NA, noradrenaline; NK, natural killer cell; GR, glucocorticoid receptor; T, T cell; B, B cell; Tc, T cytotoxic cell; Eo, eosinophil; IFN, interferon (Reproduced from Ref. 10 with permission.)

Counter-regulators of HPA axis activation

There are several pieces of *in vitro* and *in vivo* evidence suggesting counter-regulation of activation of the stress system and particularly of the HPA axis during inflammation[5,17,18]. CRH increases the production of macrophage inhibiting factor (MIF) from the pituitary[18]. Centrally and at the site of inflammation MIF counteracts the effects of glucorticoids on pro-inflammatory cytokine production, thus maintaining the immune tone[5,17,18]. MIF levels are detected not only in the circulation but also within inflamed synovia of patients with RA[19]. Inflammatory stimuli can increase hypothalamic levels of substance P, which in turn can inhibit the activity of CRH-secreting neurones[20]. In addition, cytokines may block the stimulatory effects of CRH and ACTH on the pituitary gland and adrenal cortex[17,21], or induce resistance of their target tissues to glucocorticoids[2,8]. Prolactin (PRL) also potentiates the immune and inflammatory reaction *in vitro* and in rodents[22]. Patients with RA have been shown to have increased nocturnal PRL levels, possibly favoring a pro-inflammatory profile[23].

Rheumatoid arthritis and immune response

RA is a multifactorial disease that results in severe destruction of the microenvironment of the synovial tissue, cartilage, and juxta-articular bone[7]. Pro-inflammatory cytokines are released

in the circulation from the local inflammatory site and activate cells that circulate throughout the body[4]. In addition, primary sensory afferent nerve fibers are activated and release neuropeptides in the vicinity of nerve terminals. All these mechanisms announce a pro-inflammatory situation to the CNS and other organs such as the liver[4,7]. The CNS reacts by activating the HPA axis and the SNS in an attempt to dampen inflammation at the periphery via the anti-inflammatory action of cortisol and anti-inflammatory neurotransmitters, respectively. Both axes have a stronger anti-inflammatory impact when acting in parallel[4,7]. However, there is evidence that in RA these axes may be altered, leading to a loss of anti-inflammatory influence on local articular inflammation, thus contributing to the pathogenesis and protracted clinical manifestations of RA[3,7].

The stress system in experimental animal models

The importance of the stress system and HPA axis responses to inflammation is evident in humans by the profound morbidity and mortality of infections or inflammations in patients with unreplaced Addison's disease[24]. Animal studies and certain clinical observations support the hypothesis that suboptimal cortisol production is involved in the onset and/or progression of RA. In the obese strain (OS) of chicken the development of spontaneous Hashimoto's thyroiditis appears to be due to failure of the hypothalamus to secrete CRH and thus promote cortisol secretion from the adrenal glands[25]. The Lewis rat is susceptible to the induction of arthritis[26], encephalomyelitis[27], and other autoimmune-inflammatory states following the administration of streptococcal cell wall (SCW) extract, myelin basic protein (MBP), or other antigens. In contrast, the Fischer rat, which is histocompatible to the Lewis rat, is resistant to the induction of such diseases[24].

It appears that the difference between susceptibility and resistance in these highly inbred strains lies in the ability to mount an adequate corticosterone response able to prohibit the development of the disease, which is impaired in Lewis rats but moderately hyperactive in Fischer rats[26]. This event can be prevented by the administration of glucocorticoids to Lewis rats, while Fischer rats may develop a chronic form of arthritis if given the glucocorticoid receptor inhibitor RU 486[26]. The defect in the Lewis rat was localized to the hypothalamic CRH neurone, which was globally defective in its response to all stimulatory neurotransmitters. The overall HPA axis response to stress was decreased in the Lewis rat, which also exhibited chronic compensatory elevations of vasopressin[3]. Furthermore, it seems that the SNS exerts a protective role in RA or its experimental models in animals[3]. In the arthritis prone Lewis rat, sympathectomy enhances the severity of arthritis, whereas the β2 adrenergic receptor agonist salbutamol is a potent suppressor of arthritis[3,28]. These findings raise the possibility that the integrity of the HPA axis and the SNS is a contributory factor to the pathogenesis of RA[29].

The stress system in rheumatoid arthritis

Do the abnormalities in Lewis rats have parallels in humans? A subgroup of patients with active RA might qualify, as a poor response of the HPA axis to the stress associated with major surgery, despite dramatic postoperative elevations of IL-1 and IL-6, has been demonstrated[1,2,15]. Similarly to Lewis rats, these patients also have consistently elevated AVP levels and markedly elevated concentrations of immunoreactive CRH at inflamed joints[30,31]. In addition, several clinical observations, such as the diurnal pattern of disease activity in RA, which is dependent on the diurnal rhythm of cortisol secretion[24], and the clinical response of patients with RA to glucocorticoids, support the presence of a defective HPA axis[3,16,17,24,29]. Despite significantly elevated IL-1, TNF-α, and IL-6 levels in patients with RA, the overall activity of the HPA axis remains inappropriately normal and apparently insufficient to inhibit ongoing inflammation in both untreated and treated patients[30,32]. The finding of normal or even elevated levels of glucocorticoid receptors in peripheral blood monocytes in patients with RA supports further the concept of inadequate secretion of cortisol in RA[33], which could be due to a defect at the hypothalamic, pituitary and/or adrenal level[3,7].

HPA axis activation and dysfunction in rheumatoid arthritis

Changes at the central level of hypothalamus and pituitary gland

Acute administration of IL-6 or other pro-inflammatory cytokines results in marked ACTH secretion. However, the long-term administration of such cytokines results in a blunted ACTH response in humans[3,16,34]. Chronic inflammation has been associated with low

hypothalamic CRH and high AVP levels, indicating adaptive changes when cytokine levels are elevated in a sustained, chronic fashion[35,36]. Such a situation may lead to relatively low secretion of CRH and ACTH despite elevated levels of cytokines in patients with chronic inflammatory disorders[3,16]. Several studies have demonstrated that the ACTH response to CRH in patients with RA is not altered whereas ACTH responses may be reduced[32], suggesting a mainly hypothalamic defect[30,35].

Changes at the peripheral level of adrenal steroids

In RA, cortisol secretion is inappropriately low with respect to serum concentrations of pro-inflammatory cytokines and general inflammation[7,37–39]. A decrease in adrenal glucocorticoid production is frequently observed even when the effect of suboptimal ACTH secretion is eliminated, suggesting that the hyporesponsiveness of the HPA axis also affects the adrenal[32]. Similarly, there is a decrease of adrenal androgens. However, definitely low-DHEA(S) levels appear to be a long-term predictor of developing RA in a minority of younger female patients[7,28]. A similar effect has also been observed in other chronic inflammatory conditions[7,28,40], suggesting that reduced adrenal steroid output may not be disease-specific but rather related to the extent and duration of systemic inflammation[7]. Glucocorticoid receptor levels remain normal or even elevated in peripheral blood monocytes in untreated patients with RA, whereas glucocorticoid treated-patients show a strongly decreased receptor density probably reflecting a functional dysregulation of the HPA axis[12,33]. Recent evidence has revealed that there may also be a sub-population of patients with RA who may have impaired glucocorticoid feedback, as these patients are able to escape dexamethasone suppression and mount a cortisol response to CRH stimulation[41].

A key question about human RA is whether the hyporesponsiveness of the HPA axis is genetic, secondary to a particular type of chronic inflammation, or both[5]. To date, the data point to a genetic disturbance that defines increased susceptibility following the demonstration of impaired regulation of CRH secretion and biosynthesis at the hypothalamic level[5,32]. An impaired modulation of the central regulator of the HPA axis, particularly a genetic defect of the CRH locus in the 5' regulatory unit, seems to be crucial for the onset of the disease[14,42]. Sequencing of that particular area has revealed a number of polymorphisms that, although not present in every patient with RA, suggest a distortion in the distribution of the alleles among RA patients and other ethnically matched populations[14]. Although no specific mutation in that particular region was identified, a significant linkage with a particular haplotype on chromosome 8 with RA was found[43].

Changes at the peripheral level of the sympathetic and sensory nervous systems

Sympathetic nervous system

The sympathetic nervous system exerts a dual role as stimulation of β-adrenoreceptors and Gs increases intracellular cAMP, which inhibits the production of inflammatory cytokines. In contrast, stimulation of α2-adrenoreceptors and Gi promotes inflammation, as shown in animal models of arthritis[44–46] (Table 16.1). The involvement of the nervous system in the pathogenesis of the disease is suggested further by the clinical observation that, following stroke or

Table 16.1   Immunomodulation exerted from adrenal (cortisol, DHEA(S)), sympathetic, and afferent sensory hormones

Hormones or neurotransmitters	Modulation of immune function
Cortisol	Inhibition of oxidative products, phagocytosis, antigen presentation, collagenase production, IL-1, IL-2, IL-6, IL-12, IFN-γ, TNF, NF-κB
DHEA(S)	Inhibition of oxygen radicals, IL-1, IL-6, TNF ?
Adenosine	(A1) Inhibition of intracellular cAMP
	(A2) Inhibition of oxygen radicals, phagocytosis, NK cell activity, IL-8, IL-12, TNF
Norepinephrine (α2)	Inhibition of intracellular cAMP (increase of TNF)
Norepinephrine (β)	Inhibition of oxygen radicals, phagocytosis, NK cell activity, HLA class II expression, IL-2, IL-12, IFN-γ, TNF (increases Th2 pathways)
Substance P	Stimulation of oxygen radicals, phagocytosis, chemotaxis of monocytes, NK cell activity, IL-1, IL-2, IL-4, IL-8, IL-10, IL-12, INF, immunoglobulin production, prostaglandin E$_2$
Immune-CRH	Stimulation of oxygen radicals, phagocytosis, chemotaxis of monocytes, IL-2, IL-4, IL-8, IL-10, IL-12, INF

peripheral nerve injuries, the development of RA is either prevented or ameliorated in the affected limb[45]. Patients with RA have significantly reduced sympathetic nerve fibers in synovial tissues, which is dependent on the degree of inflammation[3,7]. It is probable that the reduction of sympathetic nerve fibers may lead to low concentrations of sympathetic neurotransmitters (the physiologic β2-adrenergic is shifted to an α-adrenergic response), thus promoting a pro-inflammatory environment in the area of the synovial lying layer[7,47].

The sensory afferent nervous system

The role of this system is more clear, as its major neurotransmitter, substance P, exerts a potent pro-inflammatory role, as the administration of substance P antagonist reduces the severity of inflammation (Table 16.1)[7]. Although substance P fibers may be reduced in patients with RA, there is a considerable preponderance compared to sympathetic fibers, which may lead to an unfavorable pro-inflammatory situation[7,48]. As a result, there are nearly normal levels of substance P-positive nerve fibers during long-term disease, but low numbers of sympathetic nerve fibers[7].

Therapeutic considerations

HPA axis deficiency correction

Due to inappropriately low cortisol levels in RA, glucocorticoids and agents that potentiate their actions are attractive therapeutic options. Low-dose cortisol replacement (<7.5 mg prednisolone/day) is one of the most common successful therapeutic modalities used[7]. Following the recently genetically determined reactivity of an individual's HPA axis, therapy with steroids in RA might be better planned based on the identification of patients that exhibit a hypoactive HPA axis[14]. Antagonists of pro-inflammatory peptides, such as substance P and CRH, may also help control the inflammatory processes in which these peptides have a primary pathogenic role. The non-peptidic CRH receptor type 1 antagonist, antalarmin, suppressed acute neurogenic and chronic

autoimmune inflammation (adjuvant-induced arthritis) in rodents[49,50]. Long-term therapy with anti-TNF normalizes the HPA axis and improves adrenal androgen secretion in patients who have not received glucocorticoids[51]. The immunopotentiating effects of Δ^5-adrenal androgens on Th1 cells may be useful in the treatment of RA and may exert glucocorticoid-sparing effects[52]. However, this was not the case in an open-label but short duration study of patients with RA[7].

Substitution of sympathetic neurotransmitters

Correction of a local sympathetic tone defect involves enhancement of intracellular cAMP levels in target immune cells by increasing local NE and adenosine levels (Table 16.1). This may well be the case in therapy with low-dose methotrexate[53] and salicylates[54]. Another possible immunosuppressive effect of cAMP is shown by the therapeutic inhibition of the degrading enzyme (adenosine deaminase) of adenosine[7]. In addition, local substitution of opioid agonists and β-adrenergic agonists, as well as inhibition of the pro-inflammatory neurotransmitter substance P, should be considered for the local control of RA[28].

Simultaneous activation of the HPA axis and the SNS could result in increased cortisol, NE, and cAMP levels in various tissues[7]. In addition, cortisol enhances NE production from the sympathetic nerve terminals and adrenal medulla by stimulating synthesizing enzymes[55]. This suggests that both anti-inflammatory systems, the HPA axis and the SNS, must be simultaneously activated to exert a full effect and that uncoupling of this mechanism might be of importance in RA.

Suppression of other pro-inflammatory pathways

Recently, it was shown that glucocorticoids exert much of their anti-inflammatory action by blocking the activity of the NF-κB and AP-1 pro-inflammatory transcription factors by direct interaction of the glucocorticoid receptor with the DNA bound

NF-κB or AP-1 heterodimers[11]. The anti-rheumatic drug leflunomide inhibits the activation of NF-κB and the TNF-α-dependent activation of AP-1[11]. The cytokines involved in the clinical manifestations of RA, such as TNF-α and IL-6, have been therapeutic targets[28]. The antagonism by MIF of glucocorticoid anti-inflammatory effects[18,19] highlights a specific potential role for anti-MIF strategies in RA, particularly in glucocorticoid-resistant states[19]. This is reinforced further as monoclonal anti-MIF antibodies dramatically inhibit the expression of disease in animal models of arthritis[56].

Conclusions

Local inflammation at the joints in RA leads to a quantitatively inadequate activation of the stress system. Thus, endogenous control of the inflammation cannot be achieved, as the HPA axis and SNS produce inappropriately low amounts of anti-inflammatory steroids and sympathetic system hormones. This may be compounded by the low number of anti-inflammatory sympathetic nerve fibers at the inflamed joints, thus allowing perpetuation of the inflammation. In the future, it may be possible to interfere with the inflammatory process in RA by an exactly timed and quantified neuroendocrine intervention right at or even before the onset of the disease.

References

1. Chrousos, G. P., and Gold, P. W. The concepts of stress and stress system disorders: overview of physical and behavioral homeostasis. *JAMA* 1992; **267**: 1244–52.
2. Chrousos, G. P. The hypothalamic-pituitary-adrenal axis and immune-mediated inflammation. *N Engl J Med* 1995; **332**: 1351–62.
3. Elenkov, I. J., and Chrousos, G. P. Stress hormones, proinflammatory and antiinflammatory cytokines, and autoimmunity. *Ann N Y Acad Sci* 2002; **966**: 290–303.
4. Cutolo, M. The role of the hypothalamus-pituitary-adrenocortical and -gonadal axis in rheumatoid arthritis. *Clin Exp Rheumatol* 1998; **16**: 3–6.
5. Crofford, L. J. The hypothalamic-pituitary-adrenal axis in the pathogenesis of rheumatic diseases. *Endocrinol Metab Clin North Am* 2002; **31**: 1–13.
6. Papanicolaou, D. A., Petrides, J. S., Tsigos, C. *et al.* Exercise stimulates interleukin-6 secretion: inhibition by glucocorticoids and correlation with catecholamines. *Am J Physiol* 1996; **271** (3 Part 1): E601–E605.
7. Straub, R. H., and Cutolo, M. Involvement of the hypothalamic-pituitary-adrenal/gonadal axis and the peripheral nervous system in rheumatoid arthritis: viewpoint based on a systemic pathogenetic role. *Arthritis Rheum* 2001; **44**: 493–507.
8. Bamberger, C. M., Schulte, H. M., and Chrousos, G. P. Molecular determinants of glucocorticoid receptor function and tissue sensitivity to glucocorticoids. *Endocr Rev* 1996; **17**: 245–61.
9. Morand, E. F., and Goulding, N. J. Glucocorticoids in rheumatoid arthritis: mediators and mechanisms. *Br J Rheumatol* 1993; **32**: 816–19.
10. Elenkov, I. J., and Chrousos, G. P. Stress hormones, Th1/Th2 patterns, pro/anti-inflammatory cytokines and susceptibility to disease. *Trends Endocrinol Metab* 1999; **10**: 359–68.
11. Neeck, G., Renkawitz, R., and Eggert, M. Molecular aspects of glucocorticoid hormone action in rheumatoid arthritis. *Cytokines Cell Mol Ther* 2002; **7**: 61–9.
12. Neeck, G., Kluter, A., Dotzlaw, H., and Eggert, M. Involvement of the glucocorticoid receptor in the pathogenesis of rheumatoid arthritis. *Ann N Y Acad Sci* 2002; **966**: 491–5.
13. Masi, A. T., Chatterton, R. T., Aldag, J. C., and Malamet, R. L. Perspectives on the relationship of adrenal steroids to rheumatoid arthritis. *Ann N Y Acad Sci* 2002; **966**: 1–12.
14. Wahle, M., Krause, A., Pierer, M., Hantzschel, H., and Baerwald, C. G. Immunopathogenesis of rheumatic diseases in the context of neuroendocrine interactions. *Ann N Y Acad Sci* 2002; **966**: 355–64.
15. Elenkov, I. J., Papanicolaou, D. A., Wilder, R. L., and Chrousos, G. P. Modulatory effects of glucocorticoids and catecholamines on human interleukin-12 and interleukin-10 production: clinical implications. *Proc Assoc Am Physicians* 1996; **108**: 374–81.
16. Elenkov, I. J., Webster, E. L., Torpy, D. J., and Chrousos, G. P. Stress, corticotropin-releasing hormone, glucocorticoids, and the immune/inflammatory response: acute and chronic effects. *Ann N Y Acad Sci* 1999; **876**: 1–11.
17. Chikanza, I. C., and Grossman, A. B. Reciprocal interactions between the neuroendocrine and immune systems during inflammation. *Rheum Dis Clin North Am* 2000; **26**: 693–711.
18. Calandra, T., and Bucala, R. Macrophage migration inhibitory factor: a counter-regulator of glucocorticoid action and critical mediator of septic shock. *J Inflamm* 1995; **47**: 39–51.
19. Leech, M., Metz, C., Hall, P. *et al.* Macrophage migration inhibitory factor in rheumatoid arthritis: evidence of proinflammatory function and regulation by glucocorticoids. *Arthritis Rheum* 1999; **42**: 1601–8.
20. Larsen, P. J., Jessop, D., Patel, H., Lightman, S. L., and Chowdrey, H. S. and Substance P. inhibits the release of anterior pituitary adrenocorticotrophin via a central mechanism involving corticotrophin-releasing factor-containing neurons in the hypothalamic paraventricular nucleus. *J Neuroendocrinol* 1993; **5**: 99–105.
21. Hu, Y., Dietrich, H., Herold, M., Heinrich, P. C., and Wick, G. Disturbed immuno-endocrine communication via the hypothalamo-pituitary-adrenal axis in autoimmune disease. *Int Arch Allergy Immunol* 1993; **102**: 232–41.
22. Wilder, R. L. Neuroimmunoendocrinology of the rheumatic diseases: past, present, and future. *Ann N Y Acad Sci* 2002; **966**: 13–19.
23. Zoli, A., Ferlisi, E. M., Lizzio, M. *et al.* Prolactin/cortisol ratio in rheumatoid arthritis. *Ann N Y Acad Sci* 2002; **966**: 508–12.
24. Panayi, G. S. A defect in the neuroendocrine axis in rheumatoid arthritis: pathogenetic implications. *Clin Exp Rheumatol*; 1993; **11** (Suppl. 8): S83–S85.
25. Brezinschek, H. P., Faessler, R., Klocker, H. *et al.* Analysis of the immune-endocrine feedback loop in the avian system and its alteration in chickens with spontaneous autoimmune thyroiditis. *Eur J Immunol* 1990; **20**: 2155–9.
26. Sternberg, E. M., Young, W. S., III, Bernardini, R. *et al.* A central nervous system defect in biosynthesis of corticotropin-releasing hormone is associated with susceptibility to streptococcal cell wall-induced arthritis in Lewis rats. *Proc Natl Acad Sci U S A* 1989; **86**: 4771–5.
27. Mason, D., MacPhee, I., and Antoni, F. The role of the neuroendocrine system in determining genetic susceptibility to experimental allergic encephalomyelitis in the rat. *Immunology* 1990; **70**: 1–5.
28. Straub, R. H., Vogl, D., Gross, V., Lang, B., Scholmerich, J., and Andus, T. Association of humoral markers of inflammation and dehydroepiandrosterone sulfate or cortisol serum levels in patients with chronic inflammatory bowel disease. *Am J Gastroenterol* 1998; **93**: 2197–202.
29. Chikanza, I. C., Petrou, P., Kingsley, G., Chrousos, G., and Panayi, G. S. Defective hypothalamic response to immune and inflammatory stimuli in patients with rheumatoid arthritis. *Arthritis Rheum* 1992; **35**: 1281–8.
30. Crofford, L. J., Kalogeras, K. T., Mastorakos, G. *et al.* Circadian relationships between interleukin (IL)-6 and hypothalamic-pituitary-adrenal axis hormones: failure of IL-6 to cause sustained hypercortisolism in patients with early untreated rheumatoid arthritis. *J Clin Endocrinol Metab* 1997; **82**: 1279–83.
31. Chikanza, I. C., Petrou, P., and Chrousos, G. Perturbations of arginine vasopressin secretion during inflammatory stress: pathophysiologic implications. *Ann N Y Acad Sci* 2000; **917**: 825–34.

32. Dekkers, J. C., Geenen, R., Godaert, G. L. *et al.* Experimentally challenged reactivity of the hypothalamic pituitary adrenal axis in patients with recently diagnosed rheumatoid arthritis. *J Rheumatol* 2001; **28**: 1496–504.

33. Sanden, S., Tripmacher, R., Weltrich, R. *et al.* Glucocorticoid dose dependent downregulation of glucocorticoid receptors in patients with rheumatic diseases. *J Rheumatol* 2000; **27**: 1265–70.

34. Mastorakos, G., Chrousos, G. P., and Weber, J. S. Recombinant interleukin-6 activates the hypothalamic-pituitary-adrenal axis in humans. *J Clin Endocrinol Metab* 1993; **77**: 1690–4.

35. Harbuz, M. S., and Jessop, D. S. Is there a defect in cortisol production in rheumatoid arthritis? *Rheumatology (Oxford)* 1999; **38**: 298–302.

36. Rovensky, J., Bakosova, J., Koska, J., Ksinantova, L., Jezova, D., and Vigas, M. Somatotropic, lactotropic and adrenocortical responses to insulin-induced hypoglycemia in patients with rheumatoid arthritis. *Ann N Y Acad Sci* 2002; **966**: 263–70.

37. Templ, E., Koeller, M., Riedl, M., Wagner, O., Graninger, W., and Luger, A. Anterior pituitary function in patients with newly diagnosed rheumatoid arthritis. *Br J Rheumatol* 1996; **35**: 350–6.

38. Cutolo, M., Foppiani, L., Prete, C. *et al.* Hypothalamic-pituitary-adrenocortical axis function in premenopausal women with rheumatoid arthritis not treated with glucocorticoids. *J Rheumatol* 1999; **26**: 282–8.

39. Kanik, K. S., Chrousos, G. P., Schumacher, H. R., Crane, M. L., Yarboro, C. H., and Wilder, R. L. Adrenocorticotropin, glucocorticoid, and androgen secretion in patients with new onset synovitis/rheumatoid arthritis: relations with indices of inflammation. *J Clin Endocrinol Metab* 2000; **85**: 1461–6.

40. Johnson, E. O., Vlachoyiannopoulos, P. G., Skopouli, F. N., Tzioufas, A. G., and Moutsopoulos, H. M. Hypofunction of the stress axis in Sjogren's syndrome. *J Rheumatol* 1998; **25**: 1508–14.

41. Harbuz, M. S., Korendowych, E., Jessop, D. S. *et al.* Hypothalamo-pituitary-adrenal axis dysregulation in patients with rheumatoid arthritis after the dexamethasone/corticotrophin releasing factor test. *J Endocrinol* 2003; **178**: 55–60.

42. Baerwald, C. G., Panayi, G. S., and Lanchbury, J. S. Corticotropin releasing hormone promoter region polymorphisms in rheumatoid arthritis. *J Rheumatol* 1997; **24**: 215–16.

43. Fife, M. S., Steer, S., Fisher, S. A. *et al.* Association of familial and sporadic rheumatoid arthritis with a single corticotrophin-releasing hormone genomic region (8q12.3) haplotype: multipoint linkage analysis of a candidate gene locus in rheumatoid arthritis demonstrates significant evidence of linkage and association with the corticotropin-releasing hormone genomic region. *Arthritis Rheum* 2002; **46**: 75–82.

44. Malfait, A. M., Malik, A. S., Marinova-Mutafchieva, L. *et al.* The beta2-adrenergic agonist salbutamol is a potent suppressor of established collagen-induced arthritis: mechanisms of action. *J Immunol* 1999; **162**: 6278–83.

45. Baerwald, C. G., and Panayi, G. S. Neurohumoral mechanisms in rheumatoid arthritis. *Scand J Rheumatol* 1997; **26**: 1–3.

46. Wiegmann, K., Muthyala, S., Kim, D. H., Arnason, B. G., and Chelmicka-Schorr, E. Beta-adrenergic agonists suppress chronic/relapsing experimental allergic encephalomyelitis (CREAE) in Lewis rats. *J Neuroimmunol* 1995; **56**: 201–6.

47. Baerwald, C. G., Burmester, G. R., and Krause, A. Interactions of autonomic nervous, neuroendocrine, and immune systems in rheumatoid arthritis. *Rheum Dis Clin North Am* 2000; **26**: 841–57.

48. Miller, L. E., Justen, H. P., Scholmerich, J., and Straub, R. H. The loss of sympathetic nerve fibers in the synovial tissue of patients with rheumatoid arthritis is accompanied by increased norepinephrine release from synovial macrophages. *FASEB J* 2000; **14**: 2097–107.

49. Webster, E. L., Lewis, D. B., Torpy, D. J., Zachman, E. K., Rice, K. C., and Chrousos, G. P. In vivo and in vitro characterization of antalarmin, a nonpeptide corticotropin-releasing hormone (CRH) receptor antagonist: suppression of pituitary ACTH release and peripheral inflammation. *Endocrinology* 1996; **137**: 5747–50.

50. Bornstein, S. R., Webster, E. L., Torpy, D. J. *et al.* Chronic effects of a nonpeptide corticotropin-releasing hormone type I receptor antagonist on pituitary-adrenal function, body weight, and metabolic regulation. *Endocrinology* 1998; **139**: 1546–55.

51. Straub, R. H., Pongratz, G., Scholmerich, J. *et al.* Long-term anti-tumor necrosis factor antibody therapy in rheumatoid arthritis patients sensitizes the pituitary gland and favors adrenal androgen secretion. *Arthritis Rheum* 2003; **48**: 1504–12.

52. van Vollenhoven, R. F., Engleman, E. G., and McGuire, J. L. Dehydroepiandrosterone in systemic lupus erythematosus: results of a double-blind, placebo-controlled, randomized clinical trial. *Arthritis Rheum* 1995; **38**: 1826–31.

53. Cronstein, B. N. The mechanism of action of methotrexate. *Rheum Dis Clin North Am* 1997; **23**: 739–55.

54. Cronstein, B. N., Montesinos, M. C., and Weissmann, G. Salicylates and sulfasalazine, but not glucocorticoids, inhibit leukocyte accumulation by an adenosine-dependent mechanism that is independent of inhibition of prostaglandin synthesis and p105 of NFkappaB. *Proc Natl Acad Sci U S A* 1999; **96**: 6377–81.

55. Ehrhart-Bornstein, M., Hinson, J. P., Bornstein, S. R., Scherbaum, W. A., and Vinson, G. P. Intraadrenal interactions in the regulation of adrenocortical steroidogenesis 11. *Endocr Rev* 1998; **19**: 101–43.

56. Leech, M., Metz, C., Santos, L. *et al.* Involvement of macrophage migration inhibitory factor in the evolution of rat adjuvant arthritis. *Arthritis Rheum* 1998; **41**: 910–17.

17 | *Examination of the synovium and synovial fluid*

Paul-Peter Tak

Introduction

The synovium lines the non-cartilaginous surfaces of the synovial joints and provides nutrients to avascular structures such as cartilage. Synovial tissue is also found in tendon sheaths and bursae[1,2]. Since rheumatoid arthritis (RA) is an inflammatory disease that primarily targets the synovium, examination of synovial tissue might provide insight into the pathogenesis of the disease. Thus, descriptive studies of rheumatoid synovium contribute to an understanding of the events that take place *in vivo* and complement experimental animal studies and *in vitro* studies. There has been an enormous upsurge in investigations of the pathological changes of the rheumatoid synovium because of the availability of new methods to obtain synovial biopsy specimens and because of the development of immunohistological methods, *in situ* hybridization, the polymerase chain reaction, and microarray analysis for examination of the tissue.

Systematic comparison of RA synovial tissue with tissue from patients with other forms of arthritis has made it possible to identify specific features of the cell infiltrate in RA. This chapter will describe these pathological changes in early and in chronic RA. The main focus is to define the cell infiltrate *in situ* to provide a morphological background for understanding the role of various cell types in the pathogenesis of RA. Furthermore, the relationship between characteristics of the synovium and disease activity and the diagnostic value of synovial tissue analysis will be discussed.

Studies of synovial tissue are increasingly the subject of scientific communication and synovial tissue analysis might become a diagnostic tool in clinical practice. Since standardization of the methodology is mandatory, several questions need to be answered; for instance questions concerning the optimal technique to obtain synovial biopsy specimens, sampling errors, the most efficient and reliable systems to evaluate the sections, and quality control. Therefore, the methods to obtain and to evaluate synovial biopsy specimens will be reviewed briefly.

Synovial fluid is in direct contact with the synovium and the articular cartilage. Examination of synovial fluid is generally less relevant than synovial tissue analysis except for the evaluation of neutrophils and platelets. However, by examination of its characteristics one can learn about the cellular events within the synovium and near the cartilage. Synovial fluid analysis may also provide information about the presence of soluble mediators at the site of inflammation. Moreover, synovial fluid analysis plays an important role in the diagnostic work-up of patients with arthritis. Hence, this chapter will also deal with some of the features of RA synovial fluid, although this will not be the main focus.

Rheumatoid synovial tissue

The synovium consists of the intimal lining layer or synovial lining layer, which comprises normally only 1–3 cell layers without an underlying basal membrane, and the synovial sublining or subsynovium, which merges with the joint capsule (Fig. 17.1). The intimal lining layer consists mainly of intimal macrophages and fibroblast-like synoviocytes (FLS). The intimal macrophages are sometimes referred to as macrophage-like synoviocytes or type A synoviocytes, while the FLS are also called type B synoviocytes. The synovial sublining is normally relatively acellular, containing scattered blood vessels, lymphatic vessels, fat cells, and fibroblasts. Since the intimal lining layer is discontinuous, synovial fluid is in direct contact with cells in both the intimal lining layer and the synovial sublining.

In RA, the synovium is hypertrophic and edematous (Fig. 17.2). Villous projections of synovial tissue protrude into

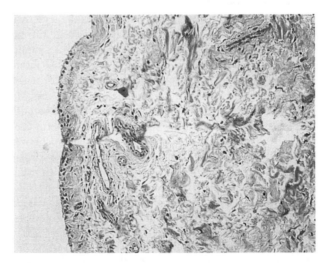

Fig. 17.1 Normal synovial tissue consisting of the intimal lining layer of 1–3 cell layers and the synovial sublining that contains scattered blood vessels, fat cells, and fibroblasts. See also Plate 11.

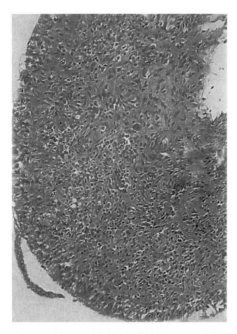

Fig. 17.2 Rheumatoid synovial tissue, showing intimal lining hyperplasia and infiltration of the synovial sublining by mononuclear cells. See also Plate 12.

Table 17.1 The cell infiltrate in rheumatiod synovial tissue

Intimal lining layer
Intimal macrophages
Fibroblast-like synoviocytes

Synovial sublining
Macrophages
T cells
plasma cells
B cells
Interdigitating dendritic cells
Follicular dendritic cells
Natural killer cells
Mast cells
Neutrophils

the joint cavity, where it overgrows and invades the underlying cartilage and bone. Proliferating synovial tissue near the synovium—cartilage junction is often referred to as pannus. Rheumatoid synovial tissue is characterized by marked intimal lining layer hyperplasia and by accumulation of T cells, plasma cells, macrophages, B cells, mast cells, natural killer cells, and dendritic cells in the synovial sublining (Table 17.1)[3]. In addition, low numbers of neutrophils may be present, often in fibrin depositions. There is large variability of synovial inflammation between individuals[4–6] and within joints[7,8]. At the pannus—cartilage junction, so-called pannocytes have been identified, which exhibit phenotypic and functional features of both FLS and chondrocytes[9,10]. These cells, with characteristics of mesenchymal precursor cells, have distinctive rhomboid morphology and very strong expression of vascular cell adhesion molecule (VCAM)-1. In addition, cells with features of osteoclasts have been identified at the synovium—cartilage junction[11]. These cells are probably derived from the monocyte/macrophage lineage[12].

Recruitment of inflammatory cells, local retention, and cell proliferation contribute to the increased cellularity of the rheumatoid

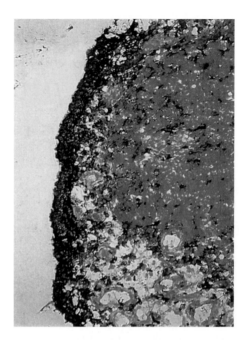

Fig. 17.3 CD68+ macrophages (red-brown) in the intimal lining layer and in the synovial sublining of rheumatoid synovial tissue. See also Plate 13.

synovium. In addition, impaired apoptosis (or programmed cell death) may enhance hyperplasia in rheumatoid synovial tissue[13]. Very few apoptotic cells are found in the synovium of RA patients[14,15], despite the presence of fragmented DNA in the intimal lining layer[13,14]. Thus, increased cellularity could be the result of immunological factors that enhance the influx of inflammatory cells into the synovium and of non-immunological factors, such as genotoxic changes due to the inflammatory microenvironment[16] and overexpression of anti-apoptotic proteins[17], which could cause reduced apoptosis.

The intimal lining layer

The thickened intimal lining layer in RA consists mainly of intimal macrophages (Fig. 17.3) and FLS (Fig. 17.4). Two-thirds or more of the synoviocytes are macrophages (Fig. 17.3). Hyperplasia of the intimal lining layer is often focal. Both intimal macrophages and FLS appear highly activated and secrete a variety of cytokines as well as matrix metalloproteinases[3]. FLS can also produce other factors such as proteoglycans and arachidonic acid metabolites[18]. Other cells that can occasionally be detected in association with the intimal lining layer include multinucleated giant cells, which form as a consequence of fusion of macrophages[19], and T cells in case of severe hyperplasia of the intimal lining layer[20]. The multinucleated cells may represent precursors of osteoclasts[21].

Fibroblast-like synoviocytes

The FLS are peculiar to synovium and have secretory features as well as an active Golgi apparatus. They appear to be of mesenchymal origin[22], although the relationship with fibroblasts in the synovial sublining and with other fibroblasts is unclear. In addition, it has been suggested that CD34 + cells derived from the bone marrow could differentiate into cells with fibroblast-like morphology[23]. It is quite likely that the FLS cell population

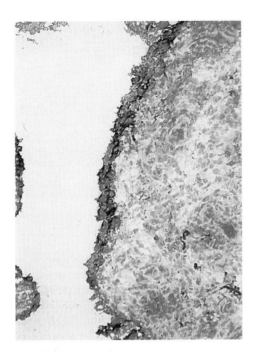

Fig. 17.4 CD55+ fibroblast-like synoviocytes (red-brown) in the intimal lining layer of rheumatoid synovial tissue. See also Plate 14.

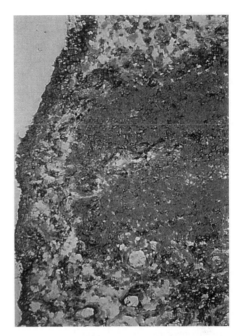

Fig. 17.5 Rheumatoid synovial tissue stained with a monoclonal antibody directed against CD97. Note prominent staining (red-brown) on intimal macrophages and on leukocytes in the synovial sublining. See also Plate 15.

consists of different subsets[24] that might differ in their origin. The increased number of FLS in RA synovium is thought to be caused in part by impaired apoptosis[15,25]; the overall frequency of morphologically defined apoptotic fibroblasts in rheumatoid synovial tissue is only about 3% of the synovial sublining fibroblasts, and the intimal lining layer FLS do not show any signs of apoptosis at all[15]. *In situ* proliferation also contributes to some extent, although rates of cell division within the intimal lining layer are low[26,27]. Furthermore, it is conceivable that synovial fibroblasts migrate towards the intimal lining layer, as a result of activation of the chemokine system and other factors[28]. Recent work has shown that cadherin-11, a molecule involved in intercellular adhesion, may be involved in the specific retention of FLS in the intimal lining layer, resulting in its specific organization[29].

FLS can be distinguished from other fibroblasts by the marked expression of CD55 or complement decay accelerating factor (DAF) (Fig. 17.4)[30,31] and VCAM-1[32,33]. CD55 is a regulatory protein of the complement cascade that protects cells from complement-mediated damage by inhibiting C3 convertases[34]. Of interest, CD55 can also act as a cellular ligand for the epidermal growth factor-TM7 (EGF-TM7) receptor CD97[35], which is expressed by nearly all intimal macrophages (Fig. 17.5)[31]. The microarchitecture of the intimal lining layer suggests that intimal macrophages and FLS may specifically interact via the CD97/CD55, the VCAM-1/α4β1 integrin, and the intercellular adhesion molecule (ICAM)-1/lymphocyte function antigen (LFA)-1 ligand pairs[31,33,36]. Other molecules, such as CD40 and β1 integrins, can also be detected on FLS, but at lower levels. Of interest is the finding that, unlike most other fibroblasts, FLS express the α6β1 integrin that serves as a receptor for laminin[37]. Laminin is an extracellular matrix molecule observed in the vicinity of FLS. In addition, FLS exhibit increased activity of the enzyme uridine diphosphoglucose dehydrogenase (UDPGD)[36], which converts UDP-glucose into UDP-glucuronate. This is one of the substrates for hyaluronan polymer synthesis. FLS exhibit relatively low human leukocyte antigen (HLA) class II expression compared with macrophages[38,39], but there is clear expression of the Toll-like receptor-2 (TLR-2), especially at the site of invasion into cartilage and bone[40].

Intimal macrophages

Macrophages are present in the intimal lining layer, particularly in the more superficial parts[41], and in the synovial sublining (Fig. 17.3). The intimal macrophages have phagocytic capacity and endocytic vacuoles. The increased number of intimal macrophages in RA is mainly the result of recruitment of bone marrow-derived mononuclear phagocytes. The circulating monocytes are thought to pass through endothelial cells and enter the synovial sublining[42]. Relatively little is known about the factors that influence the subsequent migration into the intimal lining layer. The macrophages can be identified immunohistochemically on the basis of their strong expression of CD68, a marker probably associated with lysosomes and the high activity of non-specific esterase[41]. FLS can also express CD68, but at lower levels. Of interest, intimal macrophages exhibit stronger expression of CD16 (FcγRIIIa), non-specific esterase, CD86 (B7–2) and CD97, and lower expression of CD14, than macrophages in the synovial sublining, illustrating the highly activated phenotype of the intimal macrophages in rheumatoid synovial tissue[31,41–43]. The CD16+ intimal macrophages may also express TLR-2[44]. Although monocytes could be activated prior to entry into the joint[45], these data suggest that further activation of macrophages also takes place within the synovium. In addition to the markers mentioned above, synovial macrophages may exhibit marked expression of HLA class II molecules, ICAM-1, CD11b, and myeloid-related proteins (MRP8/MRP14)[46].

Table 17.2 Lymphocyte aggregates in rheumatoid synovial tissue

T cell (mainly CD4+ CD45RO+ CD27+)
Dendritic cells and macrophages
Interdigiating B cells
Follicular dendritic cells

The synovial sublining

Edema, blood vessel proliferation, and increased cellularity of the second layer of the synovium, the synovial sublining, lead to a marked increase in synovial tissue volume in RA. The predominant cell types are T cells, plasma cells, and macrophages. Lymphocyte aggregates (Table 17.2) are observed in 50–60% of RA patients and can be surrounded by coronas of plasma cells[4]. In addition, the areas between the lymphocyte aggregates, often referred to as the diffuse leukocyte infiltrate, are infiltrated mainly by macrophages and lymphocytes[4]. In some patients, areas with granulomatous necrobiosis are apparent[5]. These areas are characterized by regions with fibrinoid necrosis lined by a collar of epithelioid histiocytes and granulation tissue. Moreover, fibrin deposition and fibrosis are often observed.

Sublining macrophages

The sublining contains large numbers of cells capable of antigen presentation, including macrophages, interdigitating dendritic cells, B cells, and other cells that express HLA class II molecules[47,48]. It is as yet a matter of debate as to which cells may serve as primary antigen-presenting cells in the synovium. The macrophages, which are derived from circulating monocytes and can be identified on the basis of their strong expression of CD68, often constitute the majority of the inflammatory cells in rheumatoid synovial tissue[4]. A substantial proportion of the synovial macrophages also express CD14 as well as the cysteine-rich scavenger receptor CD163[49]. Of interest, most cells in areas where synovial cells display tumor-like morphology are macrophages[50]. They have an activated phenotype and secrete a variety of cytokines and other pro-inflammatory mediators[4,51–53]. The accumulation of macrophages in the synovium is related to the expression of a range of adhesion molecules[54] and chemotactic factors[55,56]. In addition, the interaction between EGF-TM7 receptors, including CD97 and EMR2, which are expressed by activated synovial macrophages, and their ligand dermatan sulfate may facilitate the retention of macrophages in the synovial sublining[57].

Interdigitating dendritic cells

Interdigitating dendritic cells (DCs) are the most potent subset of antigen-presenting cells. The advent of relatively specific markers, such as RFD1, in combination with markers to exclude macrophages, made it possible to detect substantial numbers of DCs in rheumatoid synovial tissue. There are multiple interdigitating DC subsets present in RA synovium, located in proximity to CD4+ T cells in the perivascular lymphocyte aggregates and near the intimal lining layer[47,58]. Cytokines, including granulocyte–macrophage colony-stimulating factor (GM-CSF) and tumor necrosis factor (TNF-α), play an important role in the differentiation

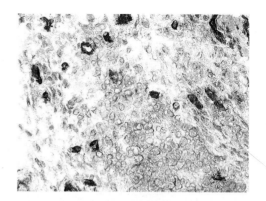

Fig. 17.6 BDCA4+ plasmacytoid dendritic cells in rheumatoid synovial tissue. See also Plate 16.

of precursor cells from the myeloid lineage into the mature and activated DCs that are observed in the rheumatoid synovium[59,60]. Differentiated DCs have been identified in the synovium by the expression of nuclear RelB and HLA-DR[61]. In addition, recent work has shown the presence of RelB-negative, CD123+ plasmacytoid dendritic cells (Fig. 17.6) in the perivascular regions, representing a distinct DC sub-population with the capacity for potent antigen-presenting function[62]. In addition to HLA class II molecules, the costimulatory molecules CD40, CD80, and CD86 are expressed by synovial DCs[63]. Thus, the morphological data suggest that DCs can undergo full functional differentiation in the cytokine milieu of the rheumatoid synovium, where they might present antigen to CD4+ T cells, especially in the perivascular lymphocyte aggregates. Whether this involves mainly endogenous auto-antigens[64], or exogenous agents such as bacteria[65] and viruses[66], remains to be elucidated. Finally, the DC-specific C-type lectin DC-SIGN has recently been detected on a subset of CD83- DCs[67]. Interestingly, ICAM-3+ T cells, which are known to bind DC-SIGN, are found in their close proximity[67]. These data may suggest that there is also a functional interaction between immature DCs and T cells in rheumatoid synovial tissue. The role of these immature cells in the synovium is at present unclear.

Follicular dendritic cells

Follicular dendritic cells (FDCs) play an important role in the accumulation of B cells by stimulatory effects on migration and proliferation and by inhibition of apoptosis. Moreover, they are thought to play a crucial role in isotype switching and final differentiation of B cells towards plasma cells or memory B cells. The origin of the synovial FDCs is at present unclear, but they may be derived from fibroblastic cells[68–70]. Of interest, these cells are observed in the synovium in proximity to proliferating B cells in lymphocyte aggregates and close to B cells near the intimal lining layer[63,71]. The microenvironment suggests a close functional relationship between FDCs and B cells in RA synovium, allowing activation and maturation of the humoral immune response. When the perivascular lymphocyte aggregates are large, substantial numbers of B cells (Fig. 17.7) can be found in close association with CD4+ cells (Fig. 17.8) and FDCs[4,72]. These areas may be surrounded by large fields of plasma cells (Fig. 17.9). The aggregates of mainly CD4+ T cells and B cells with some scattered CD8+ T cells may resemble germinal centers in up to 25%

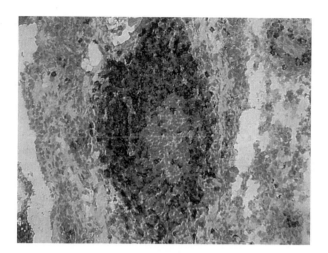

Fig. 17.7 CD22+ B cells (red-brown) in a lymphocyte aggregate in rheumatoid synovial tissue. See also Plate 17.

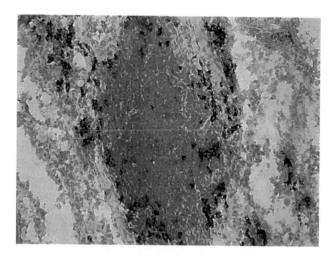

Fig. 17.9 CD38+ plasma cells (red-brown) surrounding a lymphocyte aggregate in rheumatoid synovial tissue. See also Plate 19.

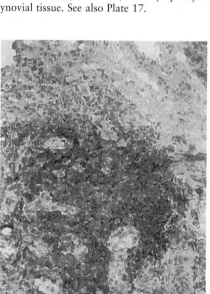

Fig. 17.8 CD4+ T cells (red-brown) in a lymphocyte aggregate in rheumatoid synovial tissue. See also Plate 18.

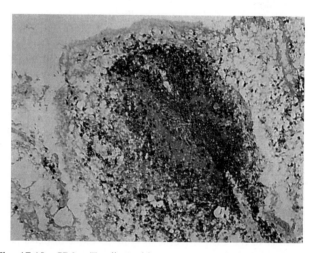

Fig. 17.10 CD3+ T cells (red-brown) in a perivascular lymphocyte aggregate and in the diffuse leukocyte infiltrate in rheumatoid synovial tissue. See also Plate 20.

of the RA patients[73], although they are morphologically not completely identical to germinal centers in lymphatic organs[74,75]. The presence of CD23+, CD21L+ FDCs in the synovium is the most distinguishing feature of the germinal center formation[76]. Chemokines are involved in the formation of these structures, as illustrated by the observation that synovial tissues with germinal centers produce markedly higher levels of the chemokines CXCL13 (a potent chemoattractant of B cells) and CCL21 (attracting naïve T cells and DCs)[73] than synovial tissues without germinal center formation.

T cells

Large numbers of T cells are present in rheumatoid synovium (Fig. 17.10). Compared with peripheral blood, the overall CD4/CD8 ratio in synovial tissue is increased[77], but this ratio differs depending on the area within the synovium[78]. There are two basic patterns of T cell infiltration. First, perivascular lymphocyte aggregates can be found, as discussed above. These aggregates consist predominantly of CD4+ cells in association with B cells, few CD8+ cells, and dendritic cells[58,77]. The endothelial cells of the post-capillary venules adjacent to the aggregates tend to be tall and may resemble high endothelial venules[79]. The second pattern of T cell infiltration is the diffuse infiltrate of T cells scattered throughout the synovium; in particular CD8+ T cells have this diffuse distribution at the periphery of the lymphocyte aggregates. Based on the overall paucity of CD8+ cells compared to CD4+ cells, the resultant lack of suppressor activity could contribute to increased stimulation of B cells and immunoglobulin synthesis in the synovium.

CD4+ T cells can be divided into two largely reciprocal subsets: CD45RA+CD45RO—naïve cells and CD45RA—CD45RO+ memory cells[80]. Synovial T cells are primarily of the CD4+CD45RO+ subset[81], which suggests previous antigen exposure. These cells exhibit greater migratory capacity than CD45RO—T cells, resulting in the accumulation at the site of inflammation[82]. The preferential recruitment of memory cells may largely explain the presence of the multitude of T cells in the synovium, where only minimal proliferating T cells are found[83,84]. The CD45RO+ cells in rheumatoid synovial tissue consist mainly of the CD45RO+CD45RB[dim] subset, which is more differentiated than the CD45RO+CD45RB[bright] early memory cells[85]. These mature memory cells have enhanced capacity to provide B cell help. Based on the marked expression of receptor activator of NF-κB ligand (RANKL)[86], they may also be involved in promoting osteoclast activation and differentiation.

The CD4+CD45RO+ memory cells can also be divided on the basis of the surface expression of activation and differentiation antigen CD27, a member of the TNF-receptor superfamily[87]. Differentiation of CD4+ T cells is reflected by the change from the CD45RO—CD27+ phenotype via CD45RO+CD27+ to the CD45RO+CD27—phenotype. The interaction between CD27 and its ligand, CD70, plays a role in T cell proliferation[88] and in expansion and differentiation of B cells[89]. Interestingly, the large majority of the CD4+ T cells in the lymphocyte aggregates, where the T cells can be found in close association with B cells and FDCs, are CD27+ memory cells[90]. This supports the view that these regions play an important part in the activation and maturation of antibody-producing cells. In line with this notion, there is a positive correlation between the levels of soluble CD27 in synovial fluid (produced by CD27+ cells) and the levels of rheumatoid factors in serum and synovial fluid of RA patients[90]. In the diffuse leukocyte infiltrate[90] and in the synovial fluid[90,91] there is a relative increase in the percentage of terminally differentiated CD8+CD27—memory T cells, which may represent terminally differentiated effector cells[92].

A subset of the CD4+ T cells in synovial tissue displays phenotypic evidence of prior activation, as indicated by the decreased density of CD3 and CD4 and the increased expression of activation antigens such as HLA class II antigens, very late activation antigen-1 (VLA-1), CD69, and CD27[90,93]. A subset of synovial T cells express CD28[94], but an expansion of CD4+CD28—T cells with characteristics of natural killer (NK) cells has also been described[95]. Many of the T cells are small and few of them express activation molecules such as transferrin and the interleukin (IL)-2 receptor[84,93]. Moreover, the percentage of interferon (IFN)-γ-producing T cells[84,96] and the detectable levels of T cell receptor (TCR)-ζ protein[97] are significantly lower in RA synovium than in a chronic T cell-mediated immunological reaction, such as tonsillitis or tuberculous pleuritis. Together, the morphological data indicate that T cells in RA synovium represent a heterogeneous population and many T cells are in a peculiar activation state.

B cells and plasma cells

B cells constitute a small proportion of the total amount of lymphocytes in rheumatoid synovium. When the perivascular lymphocyte aggregates are large, substantial numbers of B cells can be found in close association with CD4+ cells (Figs 17.7 and

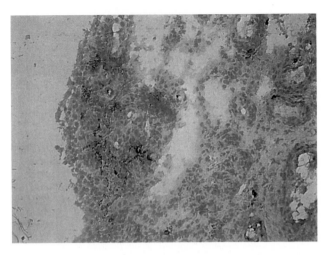

Fig. 17.11 Granzyme B+ cytotoxic cells (red-brown) in rheumatoid synovial tissue. See also Plate 21.

17.8)[72]. As noted above in the discussion of FDCs and T cells, interactions between CD4+ cells and B cells might be involved in B cell help in these areas and thus in the production of immunoglobulins. Presumably, the B cells migrate from the circulation into the synovium, where they differentiate into plasma cells[98]. Numerous plasma cells, often surrounding the lymphocyte aggregates (Fig. 17.9), may be present throughout the synovium, sometimes exceeding the number of infiltrating T cells[4]. These plasma cells may contain two or more nuclei[99]. A considerable number of the plasma cells synthesize and secrete rheumatoid factors, antibodies against citrullinated antigens, and other autoantibodies[100,101]. In keeping with these findings, the levels of rheumatoid factors and anti-cyclic citrullinated peptide (anti-CCP) antibodies are higher in synovial fluid than in peripheral blood[102,103]. The B cell response seems to be, at least in part, antigen-driven[71,104]. Thus, the rheumatoid synovium is a potent autoantibody-producing organ. The antibodies may form immune complexes in the joint leading to complement fixation and macrophage activation. In addition, B cells may be involved in the pathogenesis of synovial inflammation due to their capability for antigen-presentation and cytokine production.

Natural killer cells

Relatively little is known about the presence of NK cells in rheumatoid synovial tissue. Morphological and functional studies revealed varying results[105,106]. In addition to NK cells, CD4+ T cells expressing the NK cell receptor CD161 have been described within lymphocyte aggregates[95]. One of the difficulties in studying NK cells resides in the heterogeneity in expression of surface markers present within NK cell populations. Some NK cell markers may be lost from the surface following activation[107,108]. An alternative approach for the detection of activated NK cells is the use of functional markers for cytotoxic cells, such as granzymes, which are present in specialized granules in NK cells and cytotoxic T cells[109,110]. The use of these functional markers for killer cells offers the advantage of detecting cells that lack conventional NK cell markers. The number of granzyme-positive cells, which are present in both the intimal lining layer and the synovial sublining, is increased in RA synovial tissue compared

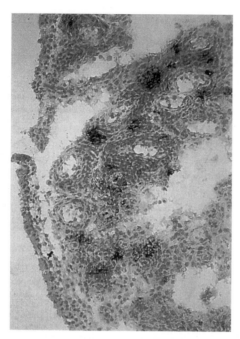

Fig. 17.12 Mast cells (red-brown) in rheumatoid synovial tissue. See also Plate 22.

with other forms of arthritis (Fig. 17.11)[111-113]. Two cell populations can be detected: large cells with a granular cytoplasm, abundant granzyme expression, and down-regulated NK cell markers; and smaller cells with diffuse cytoplasmic granzyme distribution co-expressing CD16 and CD56[7]. The notion that cytotoxic cells are active participants in the pathogenesis of RA is underscored by the markedly elevated levels of soluble granzymes in the synovial fluid of RA patients[114,115].

Mast cells

Although the number of mast cells is relatively small compared with the numbers of macrophages, T cells, and plasma cells, there is an increase in mast cells in RA synovium (Fig. 17.12)[4,116,117]. These cells can also be detected at the pannus—cartilage junction[116,118]. Mast cells containing tryptase only are observed in the more superficial part of the synovial sublining, whereas mast cells containing both tryptase and chymase are observed in the deeper layers[117]. They can be in close contact with nerves where mast cells might be activated by neuropeptides, such as substance P[119]. There is also often a close association with blood vessels[116,117], where the production of angiogenic cytokines by mast cells, such as basic fibroblast growth factor[120], could be relevant for the stimulation of angiogenesis. Synovial mast cells express a wide range of cell surface membrane antigens, complement-related antigens (e.g., the C5a receptor (CD88)), cytokine and chemokine receptors, and adhesion molecules, as well as corticotropin-releasing hormone receptor type 1[121-123]. They are activated and can produce a variety of inflammatory mediators, including vasoactive amines like histamine, arachidonic acid metabolites (including prostaglandins and leukotrienes), proteinases, cytokines, and chemokines[124]. Thus, mast cells produce and release an exceptionally wide range of effector molecules. In addition, they may play a critical role in attracting

other inflammatory cells to the synovial compartment[125], as well as in stimulating the production of pro-inflammatory cytokines and metalloproteinases by neighboring cells[126].

Neutrophils

Only a few neutrophils are found in rheumatoid synovial tissue, in part in fibrin deposits[4,33]. However, large numbers of neutrophils traffic into the synovial fluid[127] under the influence of immune complexes, chemotactic factors like C5a, and chemokines such IL-8 and growth-related gene product α[128,129]. The discrepancy between the findings in synovial tissue and synovial fluid might perhaps be explained by the expression of adhesion molecules on the endothelium that could facilitate the ingress of neutrophils, such as P-selectin and E-selectin[33], whereas other adhesion molecules on neutrophils could mediate migration through the synovial tissue into the synovial fluid[130]. The precise mechanism regulating neutrophil migration in the synovial compartment remains to be elucidated.

Synovial tissue in early rheumatoid arthritis

There is large variability of synovial inflammation between individual patients in all phases of RA[4-6,131]. Therefore, systematic comparison with the pathological changes in synovial tissue from RA patients with longstanding disease is essential to reach any conclusion about the specific features of the synovium in early RA. Comparison of infiltration by the major cell types revealed that the immunohistologic features of synovial tissue are not dependent on disease duration[4,132,133]. Moreover, the expression of cytokines[4,84,134,135], chemokines[136], matrix metalloproteinases[136], and adhesion molecules[33] is, on average, similar when synovial tissue from patients with early RA is compared with that from patients with longstanding RA. This could be explained by the fact that a phase characterized by asymptomatic synovial inflammation precedes clinically manifest arthritis[137-140]. Therefore, so-called early RA represents already a chronic phase of the disease.

Rheumatoid synovial tissue in relation to disease activity

Local disease activity is particularly associated with the number of macrophages and the expression of cytokines, such as TNF-α and IL-6, in synovial tissue (Fig. 17.13)[4]. Of interest, regression analysis revealed a negative correlation between the total number of T cells and disease activity (Fig. 17.13)[4]. It appears likely that the relationship between the number of T cells in the synovium and the clinical expression of the disease depends on the subsets involved. Specific subsets of T cells could have pro-inflammatory effects, whereas others, such as regulatory T cells, could have an anti-inflammatory effect. Studies on the tissue response to treatment provide further insight into the relationship between pathological changes in the synovium and clinical signs of the disease. These studies confirm that reduced numbers of macrophages and decreased expression of macrophage-derived cytokines are associated with clinical improvement[141-143].

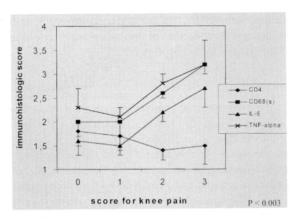

Fig. 17.13 Mean ± SEM semiquantitative scores for the number of CD4+ T cells and CD68+ sublining macrophages and the expression of IL-6 and TNF-α in the synovial tissue of 62 patients with rheumatoid arthritis in relation to the scores for knee pain. (Reproduced with permission from Lippincott Williams & Wilkins; *Arthritis Rheum* 1997, 40: 217–25.) See also Plate 23.

Diagnostic value of examination of synovial biopsy specimens

In most cases it is possible to make a diagnosis on the basis of clinical examination, routine laboratory tests, radiographic examination, and synovial fluid analysis. Examination of synovial tissue may help, however, to make a diagnosis in some relatively rare infectious, infiltrative, and deposition diseases of joints. Synovial tissue analysis in early phases of the disease could help to establish an early diagnosis in patients presenting with arthritis of recent onset. Unfortunately, many of the pathological changes in the rheumatoid synovium, such as vascular congestion, intimal lining hyperplasia, mononuclear cell infiltration, and fibrin depositions commonly occur in disorders other than RA. Still, synovial tissue analysis might have diagnostic potential in distinguishing RA from other forms of arthritis. Multivariate models can predict a diagnosis of RA solely on the basis of examination of synovial biopsy specimens with an accuracy of 85% when massive infiltration by plasma cells and macrophages in the synovial sublining are present and a diagnosis other than RA in 97% of the cases characterized by minimal infiltration by these cells[144]. The detection of lymphocyte aggregates would also support a diagnosis of RA, although their presence is not specific for the disease. The specificity of the presence of germinal centers characterized by the presence of FDCs remains to be determined. Citrullinated proteins have been detected in RA synovial tissue, but also in other forms of arthritis[103]. It is conceivable, however, that particular citrullinated proteins will be identified that are specific for RA, but this remains to be demonstrated. It has recently been suggested that the presence of HLA-DR shared epitope—human cartilage glycoprotein 39[263–275] complexes may be specific for RA synovium, but the sensitivity is low (40–50%)[64]. Taken together, the role of synovial biopsy in differential diagnosis is still limited and mainly involves the exclusion of relatively uncommon conditions.

Methods to obtain synovial biopsy specimens

Synovial tissue may be obtained either at surgery, by blind needle biopsy, or at arthroscopy. At present mainly the blind needle biopsy technique and needle arthroscopy are used. The first is a safe, well-tolerated, and technically easy way to acquire synovial tissue in a high percentage of patients with RA[145]. A limitation of this method is that in clinical practice its use is restricted to the suprapatellar pouch of the knee joint. In addition, this method is not always successful in obtaining tissue samples from clinically quiescent joints. Arthroscopic sampling of synovial tissue under direct vision is a similarly safe and well-tolerated procedure, but more complicated and expensive[145]. However, it is always possible to obtain tissue in adequate amounts and arthroscopy allows access to most joints and to most regions within the joint, including the cartilage—pannus junction.

Microscopic analysis of synovial tissue

There are essentially three methods to quantify the features of synovial inflammation: semiquantitative analysis, quantitative analysis, and computer-assisted analysis. Semiquantitative analysis involves assigning one of a limited number of scores, quantitative analysis involves counting of cells, and image analysis uses computerized digital image processing techniques to extract numerical information from visual images.

Because semiquantitative analysis is time-efficient, it offers the opportunity to evaluate sections from many biopsy specimens, which minimizes sampling error, and from many patients. This is an important advantage in light of the variation of synovial inflammation that can be found within the joint[7,8,146] and between individuals within one diagnostic group[4,5,131]. Reliable results can be obtained by evaluating sections from six different biopsy specimens, which results in a variance of less than 10%[147]. A disadvantage of this approach is that it has lower sensitivity to change than quantitative microscopic evaluation or computer-assisted analysis.

Quantitative analysis appears to be accurate, but is more laborious and time-consuming than semiquantitative analysis. Reliable quantitative microscopic measurement may be obtained from a limited number of microscopic fields, which makes it more practical[148]. However, a complete evaluation of one patient with this limited quantitative analysis takes about four times longer than with semiquantitative methods. A cross-sectional comparison of semiquantitative with quantitative analysis showed a highly significant correlation between the two methods for the evaluation of infiltration by macrophages and T cells[149,150]. This suggests that both methods can be used for the analysis of the cell infiltrate.

Computer-assisted image analysis is more sophisticated than semiquantitative analysis or quantitative microscopic analysis[149,150]. Digital image analysis has improved the analysis of multiple histological sections in a reliable, reproducible, and time-efficient way allowing the analysis of high numbers of samples, as in randomized clinical trials, including synovial tissue biomarkers. A major advantage is the ability to quantify the

Table 17.3 Examples of cytokines, chemokines, soluble cytokine-induced adhesion molecules, and soluble activation-related molecules that are elevated in rheumatoid synovial fluid

Cytokines/chemokines	Surface membrane antigens
IL-1β	IL-2 receptor
TNF-α	CD27
IL-6	CD97
IL-8	CD80
IL-12	CD14
IL-15	CD163
IL-16	HLA-DR
IL-22	
TGF-β	
HMGB-1	
RANTES	
Adhesion molecules	**Serine and cysteine proteinases**
ICAM-1	Granzyme A
VCAM-1	Granzyme B
E-selectin	Cathepsin B
	Cathepsin S

HMGB-1, high mobility group box-1; RANTES, regulated upon activation, normal T cell expressed, and presumably secreted.

concentration of the antigen of interest, which may be important, for instance in the evaluation of cytokine expression.

Rheumatoid synovial fluid

Synovial fluid is in direct contact with the synovium and the articular cartilage. The fluid contains a significant amount of extravasated plasma supplemented with high molecular molecules, in particular hyaluronan, which accounts for the viscoelastic features of synovial fluid. Synovial fluid analysis plays an important role in the diagnostic work-up in patients with arthritis, because it is easily accessible for aspiration and may help to differentiate between inflammatory and non-inflammatory arthropathies. Such a distinction is mainly made according to its appearance at the time of aspiration and the cell count. Synovial fluid analysis is important to exclude infections and crystal-induced arthritis.

Many different cell types, such as neutrophils, plasma cells, lymphocytes, macrophages, fibroblasts, and platelets, are found in rheumatoid synovial fluid. In contrast with their paucity in the synovium, neutrophils are the predominant cell type. Neutrophil counts in RA synovial fluid are variable, but can exceed $10^5/mm^3$. The turnover rate can be more than a billion cells per day. These neutrophils are activated and contain a variety of proteinases and other enzymes, such as collagenase, elastase, gelatinase, and myeloperoxidase. They also release proteins, such as fibronectin, and cytokines, such as IL-1. Thus, neutrophils can be of primary importance in the inflammation and destruction of the joint. As noted above, plasma cells in the synovium produce autoantibodies and the immune complexes formed by these antibodies may activate complement. This leads to generation of C5a, which serves as a chemotactic factor for neutrophils. Of interest, the articular cartilage of RA patients contains immune complexes[151] that could enhance adherence and invasion by neutrophils. Adhesion molecules, chemokines, and cytokines, as discussed elsewhere in this book, also influence the migration of neutrophils.

Platelets are also a potent source of many soluble mediators[152]. The mean platelet count in rheumatoid synovial fluid is about 15 000/mm³ and may be as high as 65 000/mm³ [153]. During platelet activation vasoactive, chemotactic, and bactericidal substances can be released into the fluid. In addition, cell membrane-derived metabolites from arachidonic acid, platelet activating factor (PAF), and growth factors, such as platelet-derived growth factor (PDGF) and transforming growth factor-β (TGF-β), may be derived from platelets[152]. Thus, platelets can be considered as inflammatory cells that are capable of enhancing synovial inflammation.

Many cytokine-inducible adhesion molecules and other activation-related molecules are released from the cell surface and can be measured in soluble form in synovial fluid (Table 17.3). RA patients have, for instance, high levels of soluble ICAM-1, VCAM-1, E-selectin, CD27, IL-2 receptor, CD80 (B7–1), granzymes A and B, CD97, and CD14. The increased levels of these molecules in synovial fluid represent activation of various cell types, such as T cells, macrophages, and cytotoxic cells, in the synovium. In addition, almost every known cytokine has been detected in synovial fluid from RA patients. In line with the observations of rheumatoid synovial tissue, high levels of cytokines derived from macrophages and FLS, such as IL-1β, TNF-α, IL-6, IL-8, and TGF-β are present in the fluid. The levels of T cell-derived cytokines such as IL-2, IL-4, and IFN-γ are much lower.

The levels of molecules involved in the kallikrein—kinin system are also elevated in rheumatoid synovial fluid[154]. Activation of this system by, for example, coagulation pathways and immune complexes, could cause release of other mediators, such as prostaglandins, histamine, and pro-inflammatory cytokines. This system is probably involved in the development of pain and swelling of the joints.

Recent work has shown the presence of small membrane-bound vesicles, termed microparticles, in the synovial fluid of patients with RA as well as other arthritides[155]. Their release from inflammatory cells is increased during activation and apoptosis and they are thought to contribute to local hypercoagulation and stimulate FLS to produce pro-inflammatory cytokines, chemokines, and matrix metalloproteinases (MMPs)[155–157]. Finally, joint matrix molecules or fragments of the matrix molecules can be released into the synovial fluid[158]. Measurement of these molecular markers may provide insights into the mechanisms underlying the process of destruction of bone and articular cartilage and could be used as biomarkers of joint destruction.

References

1. Henderson, B., and Pettipher, E. R. The synovial lining cell: biology and pathobiology. *Semin Arthritis Rheum* 1985; **15**: 1–32.
2. Palmer, D. G. The anatomy of the rheumatoid lesion. *Br Med Bull* 1995; **51**: 286–95.
3. Tak, P. P., and Bresnihan, B. The pathogenesis and prevention of joint damage in rheumatoid arthritis: advances from synovial biopsy and tissue analysis. *Arthritis Rheum* 2000; **43**: 2619–33.
4. Tak, P. P., Smeets, T. J. M., Daha, M. R., Kluin, P. M., Meijers, K. A. E., Brand, R. *et al*. Analysis of the synovial cellular infiltrate in early rheumatoid synovial tissue in relation to local disease activity. *Arthritis Rheum* 1997; **40**: 217–25.

5. Klimiuk, P. A., Goronzy, J. J., Bjornsson, J., Beckenbaugh, R. D., and Weyand, C. M. Tissue cytokine patterns distinguish variants of rheumatoid synovitis. *Am J Pathol* 1997; **151**: 1311–19.

6. van der Pouw Kraan, T. C., van Gaalen, F. A., Kasperkovitz, P. V., Verbeet, N. L., Smeets, T. J., Kraan, M. C. et al. Rheumatoid arthritis is a heterogeneous disease: evidence for differences in the activation of the STAT-1 pathway between rheumatoid tissues. *Arthritis Rheum* 2003; **48**: 2132–45.

7. Lindblad, S., and Hedfors, E. Intraarticular variation in synovitis: local macroscopic and microscopic signs of inflammatory activity are significantly correlated. *Arthritis Rheum* 1985; **28**: 977–86.

8. Rooney, M., Condell, D., Daly, L., Whelan, A., Feighery, C., and Bresnihan, B. Analysis of the histologic variation of synovitis in rheumatoid arthritis. *Arthritis Rheum* 1988; **31**: 956–63.

9. Zvaifler, N. J., Tsai, V., Alsalameh, S., Vonkempis, J., Firestein, G. S., and Lotz, M. Pannocytes: distinctive cells found in rheumatoid arthritis articular cartilage erosions. *Am J Pathol* 1997; **150**: 1125–38.

10. Xue, C., Takahashi, M., Hasunuma, T., Aono, H., Yamamoto, K., Yoshino, S. et al. Characterisation of fibroblast-like cells in pannus lesions of patients with rheumatoid arthritis sharing properties of fibroblasts and chondrocytes. *Ann Rheum Dis* 1997; **56**: 262–7.

11. Gravallese, E. M., Harada, Y., Wang, J. T., Gorn, A. H., Thornhill, T. S., and Goldring, S. R. Identification of cell types responsible for bone resorption in rheumatoid arthritis and juvenile rheumatoid arthritis. *Am J Pathol* 1998; **152**: 943–51.

12. Danks, L., Sabokbar, A., Gundle, R., and Athanasou, N. A. Synovial macrophage-osteoclast differentiation in inflammatory arthritis. *Ann Rheum Dis* 2002; **61**: 916–21.

13. Firestein, G. S., Yeo, M., and Zvaifler, N. J. Apoptosis in rheumatoid arthritis synovium. *J Clin Invest* 1995; **96**: 1631–8.

14. Nakajima, T., Aono, H., Hasunuma, T., Yamamoto, K., Shirai T., and Hirohata, K. et al. Apoptosis and functional Fas antigen in rheumatoid arthritis synoviocytes. *Arthritis Rheum* 1995; **38**: 485–91.

15. Matsumoto, S., Muller-Ladner, U, Gay, R. E., Nishioka, K., and Gay, S. Ultrastructural demonstration of apoptosis, Fas and Bcl-2 expression of rheumatoid synovial fibroblasts. *J Rheumatol* 1996; **23**: 1345–52.

16. Tak, P. P., Zvaifler, N. J., Green, D. R., and Firestein, G. S. Rheumatoid arthritis and p53: how oxidative stress might alter the course of inflammatory diseases. *Immunol Today* 2000; **21**: 78–82.

17. Baier, A., Meineckel, I., Gay, S., and Pap, T. Apoptosis in rheumatoid arthritis. *Curr Opin Rheumatol* 2003; **15**: 274–9.

18. Cisar, L. A., Schimmel, R. J., and Mochan, E. Interleukin-1 stimulation of arachidonic acid release from human synovial fibroblasts: blockade by inhibitors of protein kinases and protein synthesis. *Cell Signal* 1991; **3**: 189–99.

19. Weinberg, J. B., Wortham, T. S., Misukonis, M. A., Patton, K L., and Chitneni, S. R. Synovial mononuclear phagocytes in rheumatoid arthritis and osteoarthritis: quantitative and functional aspects. *Immunol Invest* 1993; **22**: 365–74.

20. Itoh, J., Kinjoh, K., Ohyama, A., Nose, M., and Kyogoku, M. Application of two-color immunofluorescence staining to demonstration of T-cells and HLA-DR-bearing cells in rheumatoid synovitis. *J Histochem Cytochem* 1992; **40**: 1675–83.

21. Gravallese, E. M., Harada, Y., Wang, J. T., Gorn, A. H., Thornhill, T. S., and Goldring, S. R. Identification of cell types responsible for bone resorption in rheumatoid arthritis and juvenile rheumatoid arthritis. *Am J Pathol* 1998; **152**: 943–51.

22. Barland, P., Novikoff, A. B., and Hamerman, D. Electron microscopy of the human synovial membrane. *J Cell Biol* 1982; **14**: 207–20.

23. Hirohata, S., Yanagida, T., Nagai, T., Sawada, T., Nakamura, H., Yoshino, S. et al. Induction of fibroblast-like cells from CD34(1) progenitor cells of the bone marrow in rheumatoid arthritis. *J Leukoc Biol* 2001; **70**: 413–21.

24. Kasperkovitz, P. V., Timmer, T. C., Smeets, T. J., Verbeet, N. L., Tak, P. P., van Baarsen, L G. et al. Fibroblast-like synoviocytes derived from patients with rheumatoid arthritis show the imprint of synovial tissue heterogeneity: evidence of a link between an increased myofibroblast-like phenotype and high-inflammation synovitis. *Arthritis Rheum* 2005; **52**: 430–41.

25. Firestein, G. S. Invasive fibroblast-like synoviocytes in rheumatoid arthritis: passive responders or transformed aggressors? *Arthritis Rheum* 1996; **39**: 1781–90.

26. Lalor, P. A., Mapp, P. I., Hall, P. A., and Revell, P. A. Proliferative activity of cells in the synovium as demonstrated by a monoclonal antibody, Ki67. *Rheumatol Int* 1987; **7**: 183–6.

27. Qu, Z. H., Garcia, C. H., O'Rourke, L. M., Planck, S. R., Kohli, M., and Rosenbaum, J. T. Local proliferation of fibroblast-like synoviocytes contributes to synovial hyperplasia: results of proliferation cell nuclear antigen/cyclin, C-myc, and nucleolar organizer region staining. *Arthritis Rheum* 1994; **37**: 212–20.

28. Garcia-Vicuna, R., Gomez-Gaviro, M. V., Dominguez-Luis, M. J., Pec, M. K., Gonzalez-Alvaro, I., Alvaro-Gracia, J. M. et al. CC and CXC chemokine receptors mediate migration, proliferation, and matrix metalloproteinase production by fibroblast-like synoviocytes from rheumatoid arthritis patients. *Arthritis Rheum* 2004; **50**: 3866–77.

29. Valencia, X., Higgins, J. M., Kiener, H. P., Lee, D. M., Podrebarac, T. A., Dascher, C. C. et al. Cadherin-11 provides specific cellular adhesion between fibroblast-like synoviocytes. *J Exp Med* 2004; **200**: 1673–9.

30. Edwards, J. C. W., Blades, S., and Cambridge, G. Restricted expression of Fc gamma RIII (CD16) in synovium and dermis: implications for tissue targeting in rheumatoid arthritis (RA). *Clin Exp Immunol* 1997; **108**: 401–6.

31. Hamann, J., Wishaupt, J. O., Van Lier, R. A. W., Smeets, T. J. M., Breedveld, F. C., and Tak, P. P. Expression of the activation antigen CD97 and its ligand CD55 in rheumatoid synovial tissue. *Arthritis Rheum* 1999; **42**: 650–8.

32. Morales Ducret, J., Wayner, E., Elices, M. J., Alvaro-Gracia, J. M., Zvaifler, N. J., and Firestein, G. S. Alpha 4/beta 1 integrin (VLA-4) ligands in arthritis: vascular cell adhesion molecule-1 expression in synovium and on fibroblast-like synoviocytes. *J Immunol* 1992; **149**: 1424–31.

33. Tak, P. P., Thurkow, E. W., Daha, M. R., Kluin, P. M., Smeets, T. J. M., Meinders, A. E. et al. Expression of adhesion molecules in early rheumatoid synovial tissue. *Clin Immunol Immunopathol* 1995; **77**: 236–42.

34. Lublin, D. M., and Atkinson, J. P. Decay-accelerating factor: biochemistry, molecular biochemistry, and function. *Annu Rev Immunol* 1989; **7**: 35–58.

35. Hamann, J., Vogel B., Van Schijndel, G. M. W., and Van Lier, R. A. W. The seven-span transmembrane receptor CD97 has a cellular ligand (CD55, DAF). *J Exp Med* 1996; **184**: 1185–9.

36. Edwards, J. C. W. Synovial intimal fibroblasts. *Ann Rheum Dis* 1995; **54**: 395–7.

37. Pirila, L., Aho, H., Roivainen, A., Konttinen, Y. T., Pelliniemi, L J., and Heino, J. Identification of alpha6beta1 integrin positive cells in synovial lining layer as type B synoviocytes. *J Rheumatol* 2001; **28**: 478–84.

38. Henderson, B., Revell, P. A., and Edwards, J. C. Synovial lining cell hyperplasia in rheumatoid arthritis: dogma and fact. *Ann Rheum Dis* 1988; **47**: 348–9.

39. Cicuttini, F. M., Martin, M., and Boyd, A. W. Cytokine induction of adhesion molecules on synovial type B cells. *J Rheumatol* 1994; **21**: 406–12.

40. Seibl, R., Birchler, T., Loeliger, S., Hossle, J. P., Gay, R. E., Saurenmann, T. et al. Expression and regulation of Toll-like receptor 2 in rheumatoid arthritis synovium. *Am J Pathol* 2003; **162**: 1221–7.

41. Broker, B. M., Edwards, J. C., Fanger, M. W., and Lydyard, P. M. The prevalence and distribution of macrophages bearing Fc gamma R. I., Fc gamma R. II, and Fc gamma R. III in synovium. *Scand J Rheumatol* 1990; **19**: 123–35.

42. Athanasou, N. A. Synovial macrophages. *Ann Rheum Dis* 1995; **54**: 392–4.

43. Balsa, A., Dixey, J., Sansom, D. M., Maddison, P. J., and Hall, N. D. Differential expression of the costimulatory molecules B7.1 (CD80) and B7.2 (CD86) in rheumatoid synovial tissue. *Br J Rheumatol* 1996; **35**: 33–7.

44. Iwahashi, M., Yamamura, M., Aita, T., Okamoto, A., Ueno, A., Ogawa, N. *et al.* Expression of Toll-like receptor 2 on CD161 blood monocytes and synovial tissue macrophages in rheumatoid arthritis. *Arthritis Rheum* 2004; **50**: 1457–67.

45. Schultze-Koops, H., Davis, L. S, Kavanaugh, A. F., and Lipsky, P. E. Elevated cytokine messenger RNA levels in the peripheral blood of patients with rheumatoid arthritis suggest different degrees of myeloid cell activation. *Arthritis Rheum* 1997; **40**: 639–47.

46. Youssef, P., Roth, J., Frosch, M., Costello, P., FitzGerald, O., Sorg, C. *et al.* Expression of myeloid related proteins (MRP) 8 and 14 and the MRP8/14 heterodimer in rheumatoid arthritis synovial membrane. *J Rheumatol* 1999; **26**: 2523–8.

47. Klareskog, L., Forsum, U., Scheynius, A., Kabelitz, D., and Wigzell, H. Evidence in support of a self-perpetuating HLA-DR-dependent delayed-type cell reaction in rheumatoid arthritis. *Proc Natl Acad Sci U S A* 1982; **79**: 3632–6.

48. Viner, N. J. Role of antigen presenting cells in rheumatoid arthritis. *Br Med Bull* 1995; **51**: 359–67.

49. Fonseca, J. E., Edwards, J. C., Blades, S., and Goulding, N. J. Macrophage subpopulations in rheumatoid synovium: reduced CD163 expression in CD41 T lymphocyte-rich microenvironments. *Arthritis Rheum* 2002; **46**: 1210–16.

50. Sack, U., Stiehl, P., and Geiler, G. Distribution of macrophages in rheumatoid synovial membrane and its association with basic activity. *Rheumatol Int* 1994; **13**: 181–6.

51. Firestein, G. S., Alvaro-Gracia, J. M., and Maki, R. Quantitative analysis of cytokine gene expression in rheumatoid arthritis. *J Immunol* 1990; **144**: 3347–53.

52. Chu, C. Q., Field, M., Allard, S., Abney, E., Feldmann, M., and Maini, R. N. Detection of cytokines at the cartilage/pannus junction in patients with rheumatoid arthritis: implications for the role of cytokines in cartilage destruction and repair. *Br J Rheumatol* 1992; **31**: 653–61.

53. Burmester, G. R., Stuhlmuller, B., Keyszer, G., and Kinne, R. W. Mononuclear phagocytes and rheumatoid synovitis: mastermind or workhorse in arthritis? *Arthritis Rheum* 1997; **40**: 5–18.

54. Mojcik, C. F., and Shevach, E. M. Adhesion molecules: a rheumatologic perspective. *Arthritis Rheum* 1997; **40**: 991–1004.

55. Haringman, J. J., Ludikhuize, J., and Tak, P. P. Chemokines in joint disease: the key to inflammation? *Ann Rheum Dis* 2004; **63**: 1186–94.

56. Koch, A. E. Chemokines and their receptors in rheumatoid arthritis: future targets? *Arthritis Rheum* 2005; **52**: 710–21.

57. Kop, E. N., Kwakkenbos, M. J., Teske, G. J., Kraan, M. C., Smeets T. J., Stacey M. *et al.* Identification of the epidermal growth factor-TM7 receptor EMR2 and its ligand dermatan sulfate in rheumatoid synovial tissue. *Arthritis Rheum* 2005; **52**: 442–50.

58. Duke, O., Panayi, G. S., Janossy, G., and Poulter, L. W. An immunohistological analysis of lymphocyte subpopulations and their microenvironment in the synovial membranes of patients with rheumatoid arthritis using monoclonal antibodies. *Clin Exp Immunol* 1982; **49**: 22–30.

59. Witmer-Pack, M. D., Olivier, W., Valinsky, J., Schuler, G., and Steinman, R. M. Granulocyte/macrophage colony-stimulating factor is essential for the viability and function of cultured murine epidermal Langerhans cells. *J Exp Med* 1987; **166**: 1484–98.

60. Thomas, R., and Lipsky, P. E. Dendritic cells: origin and differentiation. *Stem Cells* 1996; **14**: 196–206.

61. Pettit, A. R., MacDonald, K. P., O'Sullivan, B., and Thomas R. Differentiated dendritic cells expressing nuclear RelB are predominantly located in rheumatoid synovial tissue perivascular mononuclear cell aggregates. *Arthritis Rheum* 2000; **43**: 791–800.

62. Cavanagh, L. L., Boyce, A., Smith, L., Padmanabha, J., Filgueira, L., Pietschmann, P. *et al.* Rheumatoid arthritis synovium contains plasmacytoid dendritic cells. *Arthritis Res Ther* 2005; **7**: R230–R240.

63. Balsa, A., Dixey, J., Sansom, D. M., Maddison, P. J., and Hall, N. D. Differential expression of the costimulatory molecules B7.1 (CD80) and B7.2 (CD86) in rheumatoid synovial tissue. *Br J Rheumatol* 1996; **35**: 33–7.

64. Steenbakkers, P. G., Baeten, D., Rovers, E., Veys, E. M., Rijnders, A. W., Meijerink, J. *et al.* Localization of MHC class II/human cartilage glycoprotein-39 complexes in synovia of rheumatoid arthritis patients using complex-specific monoclonal antibodies. *J Immunol* 2003; **170**: 5719–27.

65. Schrijver, I. A., Melief, M. J., Tak, P. P., Hazenberg, M. P., and Laman, J. D. Antigen-presenting cells containing bacterial peptidoglycan in synovial tissues of rheumatoid arthritis patients coexpress costimulatory molecules and cytokines. *Arthritis Rheum* 2000; **43**: 2160–8.

66. Takahashi, Y., Murai, C., Shibata, S., Munakata, Y., Ishii, T., Ishii, K. *et al.* Human parvovirus B19 as a causative agent for rheumatoid arthritis. *Proc Natl Acad Sci U S A* 1998; **95**: 8227–32.

67. Van Lent, P. L., Figdor, C. G., Barrera, P., van Ginkel, K., Sloetjes, A., Van den Berg, W. B. *et al.* Expression of the dendritic cell-associated C-type lectin DC-SIGN by inflammatory matrix metalloproteinase-producing macrophages in rheumatoid arthritis synovium and interaction with intercellular adhesion molecule 3-positive T cells. *Arthritis Rheum* 2003; **48**: 360–9.

68. Imai, Y., and Yamakawa, M. Morphology, function and pathology of follicular dendritic cells. *Pathol Int* 1996; **46**: 807–33.

69. Bofill, M., Akbar, A. N., and Amlot, P. L. Follicular dendritic cells share a membrane-bound protein with fibroblasts. J. *Pathol* 2000; **191**: 217–26.

70. Lindhout, E., Van Eijk, M., Van Pel, M., Lindeman, J., Dinant, H. J., and de Groot. C. Fibroblast-like synoviocytes from rheumatoid arthritis patients have intrinsic properties of follicular dendritic cells. *J Immunol* 1999; **162**: 5949–56.

71. Schroder, A. E., Greiner, A., Seyfert, C., and Berek, C. Differentiation of B cells in the nonlymphoid tissue of the synovial membrane of patients with rheumatoid arthritis. *Proc Natl Acad Sci U S A* 1996; **93**: 221–5.

72. Yanni, G., Whelan, A., Feighery, C., and Bresnihan, B. Analysis of cell populations in rheumatoid arthritis synovial tissues. *Semin Arthritis Rheum* 1992; **21**: 393–9.

73. Goronzy, J. J., and Weyand, C. M. Rheumatoid arthritis. *Immunol Rev* 2005; **204**: 55–73.

74. Krenn, V., Schalhorn, N., Greiner, A., Molitoris, R., Konig, A., Gohlke, F. *et al.* Immunohistochemical analysis of proliferating and antigen-presenting cells in rheumatoid synovial tissue. *Rheumatol Int* 1996; **15**: 239–47.

75. Randen, I., Mellbye, O. J., Forre, O., and Natvig, J. B. The identification of germinal centres and follicular dendritic cell networks in rheumatoid synovial tissue. *Scand J Immunol* 1995; **41**: 481–6.

76. Takemura, S., Braun, A., Crowson, C., Kurtin, P. J., Cofield, R. H., O'Fallon, W. M. *et al.* Lymphoid neogenesis in rheumatoid synovitis. *J Immunol* 2001; **167**: 1072–80.

77. Janossy, G., Panayi, G. S., Duke, O., Bofill, M., Poulter, L W., and Goldstein, G. Rheumatoid arthritis: a disease of T-lymphocyte/macrophage immunoregulation. *Lancet* 1981; **2**: 839–42.

78. Kurosaka, M., and Ziff, M. Immunoelectron microscopic study of the distribution of T cell subsets in rheumatoid synovium. *J Exp Med* 1983; **158**: 1191–210.

79. Iguchi, T., and Ziff, M. Electron microscopic study of rheumatoid synovial vasculature: intimate relationship between tall endothelium and lymphoid aggregation. *J Clin Invest* 1986; **77**: 355–61.

80. Terry, L. A., Brown, M. H., and Beverley, P. C. The monoclonal antibody, UCHL1, recognizes a 180,000 MW component of the human leucocyte-common antigen, CD45. *Immunology* 1988; **64**: 331–6.

81. Potocnik, A. J., Kinne, R., Menninger, H., Zacher, J., Emmrich, F., and Kroczek, R. A. Expression of activation antigens on T cells in rheumatoid arthritis patients. *Scand J Immunol* 1990; **310**: 213–24.

82. Cush, J. J., Pietschmann, P., Oppenheimer Marks, N., and Lipsky, P. E. The intrinsic migratory capacity of memory T cells contributes to their accumulation in rheumatoid synovium. *Arthritis Rheum* 1992; **35**: 1434–44.

83. Cush, J. J., and Lipsky, P. E. Cellular basis for rheumatoid inflammation. *Clin Orthop* 1991; **265**: 9–22.

84. Smeets, T. J. M., Dolhain, R. J. E. M., Miltenburg, A. M. M., de Kuiper, R., Breedveld, F. C., and Tak, P. P. Poor expression of T cell-derived cytokines and activation and proliferation markers in early rheumatoid synovial tissue. *Clin Immunol Immunopathol* 1998; **88**: 84–90.

85. Thomas, R., Mcilraith, M., Davis, L. S., and Lipsky, P. E. Rheumatoid synovium is enriched in CD45RBdim mature memory

T cells that are potent helpers for B cell differentiation. *Arthritis Rheum* 1992; **35**: 1455–65.

86. Haynes, D. R., Crotti, T. N., Loric, M., Bain, G. I., Atkins, G. J., and Findlay, D. M. Osteoprotegerin and receptor activator of nuclear factor kappaB ligand (RANKL) regulate osteoclast formation by cells in the human rheumatoid arthritic joint. *Rheumatology (Oxford)* 2001; **40**: 623–30.

87. Hintzen, R. Q., De Jong, R., Lens, S. M. A., Van Lier, R. A. W. CD27: marker and mediator of T-cell activation? *Immunol Today* 1994; **15**: 307–9.

88. Bigler, R. D., Bushkin, Y., and Chiorazzi, N. S152 (CD27): a modulating disulfide-linked T cell activation antigen. *J Immunol* 1988; **141**: 21–8.

89. Arens, R., Nolte, M. A., Tesselaar, K., Heemskerk, B., Reedquist, K A., Van Lier, R. A. *et al.* Signaling through CD70 regulates B cell activation and IgG production. *J Immunol* 2004; **173**: 3901–8.

90. Tak, P. P., Hintzen, R. Q., Teunissen, J. J. M., Smeets, T. J. M., Daha, M. R., Van Lier, R. A. W. *et al.* Expression of the activation antigen CD27 in rheumatoid arthritis. *Clin Immunol Immunopathol* 1996; **80**: 129–38.

91. Kohem, C. L., Brezinschek, R. I., Wisbey, H., Tortorella, C., Lipsky, P. E., and Oppenheimer-Marks, N. Enrichment of differentiated CD45RB(dim), CD27– memory T cells in the peripheral blood, synovial fluid, and synovial tissue of patients with rheumatoid arthritis. *Arthritis Rheum* 1996; **39**: 844–54.

92. Hamann, D., Roos, M. T., and Van Lier, R. A. Faces and phases of human CD8 T-cell development. *Immunol Today* 1999; **20**: 177–80.

93. Firestein, G. S., and Zvaifler, N. J. How important are T cells in chronic rheumatoid synovitis? II. T cell-independent mechanisms from beginning to end. *Arthritis Rheum* 2002; **46**: 298–308.

94. Shimoyama, Y., Nagafuchi, H., Suzuki, N., Ochi, T., and Sakane, T. Synovium infiltrating T cells induce excessive synovial cell function through CD28/B7 pathway in patients with rheumatoid arthritis. *J Rheumatol* 1999; **26**: 2094–101.

95. Warrington, K. J., Takemura, S., Goronzy, J. J., and Weyand, C. M. CD41, CD28– T cells in rheumatoid arthritis patients combine features of the innate and adaptive immune systems. *Arthritis Rheum* 2001; **44**: 13–20.

96. Firestein, G. S., Xu, W. D., Townsend, K., Broide, D., Alvaro-Gracia, J. M., Glasebrook, A. *et al.* Cytokines in chronic inflammatory arthritis. I. Failure to detect T cell lymphokines (interleukin 2 and interleukin 3) and presence of macrophage colony-stimulating factor (CSF-1) and a novel mast cell growth factor in rheumatoid synovitis. *J Exp Med* 1988; **168**: 1573–86.

97. Maurice, M. M., Lankester, A. C., Bezemer, A. C., Geertsma, M. F., Tak, P. P., Breedveld, F. C. *et al.* Defective TCR-mediated signaling in synovial T cells in rheumatoid arthritis. *J Immunol* 1997; **159**: 2973–8.

98. Kim, H. J., Krenn, V., Steinhauser, G., and Berek, C. Plasma cell development in synovial germinal centers in patients with rheumatoid and reactive arthritis. *J Immunol* 1999; **162**: 3053–62.

99. Perry, M. E., Mustafa, Y., Wood, S. K., Cawley, M. I. D., Dumonde, D. C., and Brown, K A. Binucleated and multinucleated forms of plasma cells in synovia from patients with rheumatoid arthritis. *Rheumatol Int* 1997; **17**: 169–74.

100. Hakoda, M., Ishimoto, T., Hayashimoto, S., Inoue, K., Taniguchi, A., Kamatani, N. *et al.* Selective infiltration of B cells committed to the production of monoreactive rheumatoid factor in synovial tissue of patients with rheumatoid arthritis. *Clin Immunol Immunopathol* 1993; **69**: 16–22.

101. Masson-Bessiere, C., Sebbag, M., Durieux, J. J., Nogueira, L., Vincent, C., Girbal-Neuhauser, E. *et al.* In the rheumatoid pannus, anti-filaggrin autoantibodies are produced by local plasma cells and constitute a higher proportion of IgG than in synovial fluid and serum. *Clin Exp Immunol* 2000; **119**: 544–52.

102. Otten, H. G., Dolhain, R. J., de Rooij, H. H., and Breedveld, F. C. Rheumatoid factor production by mononuclear cells derived from different sites of patients with rheumatoid arthritis. *Clin Exp Immunol* 1993; **94**: 236–40.

103. Vossenaar, E. R., Smeets, T. J., Kraan, M. C., Raats, J. M., van Venrooij, W. J., and Tak, P. P. The presence of citrullinated proteins is not specific for rheumatoid synovial tissue. *Arthritis Rheum* 2004; **50**: 3485–94.

104. Van Esch, W. J., Reparon-Schuijt, C. C., Hamstra, H. J., Van Kooten, C., Logtenberg, T., Breedveld, F. C. *et al.* Human IgG Fc-binding phage antibodies constructed from synovial fluid CD381 B cells of patients with rheumatoid arthritis show the imprints of an antigen-dependent process of somatic hypermutation and clonal selection. *Clin Exp Immunol* 2003; **131**: 364–76.

105. Combe, B., Pope, R., Darnell, B., and Talal, N. Modulation of natural killer cell activity in the rheumatoid joint and peripheral blood. *Scand J Immunol* 1984; **20**: 551–8.

106. Thoen, J., Waalen, K., and Forre, O. Natural killer (NK) cells at inflammatory sites of patients with rheumatoid arthritis and IgM rheumatoid factor positive polyarticular juvenile rheumatoid arthritis. *Clin Rheumatol* 1987; **6**: 215–25.

107. Mueller, C., Gershenfeld, H. K., Lobe, C. G., Okada, C. Y., Bleackley, R. C., and Weissman, I. L. A high proportion of T lymphocytes that infiltrate H-2-incompatible heart allografts in vivo express genes encoding cytotoxic cell-specific serine proteases, but do not express MEL-14-defined lymph node homing receptor. *J Exp Med* 1988; **167**: 1124–36.

108. Hendrich, C., Kuipers, J. G., Kolanus, W., Hammer, M., and Schmidt, R. E. Activation of CD161 effector cells by rheumatoid factor complex: role of natural killer cells in rheumatoid arthritis. *Arthritis Rheum* 1991; **34**: 423–31.

109. Griffiths, G. M., and Isaaz, S. Granzymes A and B are targeted to the lytic granules of lymphocytes by the mannose-6-phosphate receptor. *J Cell Biol* 1993; **120**: 885–96.

110. Froelich, C. J., Dixit, V. M., Yang, X. H., and Yang, X. Lymphocyte granule-mediated apoptosis: matters of viral mimicry and deadly proteases. *Immunol Today* 1998; **19**: 30–6.

111. Tak, P. P., Kummer, J. A., Hack, C. E., Daha, M. R., Smeets, T. J. M., and Erkelens, G. W. *et al.* Granzyme positive cytotoxic cells are specifically increased in early rheumatoid synovial tissue. *Arthritis Rheum* 1994; **37**: 1735–43.

112. Smeets, T. J., Dolhain, R. J., Breedveld, F. C., and Tak, P. P. Analysis of the cellular infiltrates and expression of cytokines in synovial tissue from patients with rheumatoid arthritis and reactive arthritis. *J Pathol* 1998; **186**: 75–81.

113. Muller-Ladner, U, Kriegsmann, J., Tschopp, J., Gay, R. E., and Gay, S. Demonstration of granzyme A and perforin messenger RNA in the synovium of patients with rheumatoid arthritis. *Arthritis Rheum* 1995; **38**: 477–84.

114. Tak, P. P., Spaeny-Dekking, L., Kraan, M. C., Breedveld, F. C., Froelich, C. J., and Hack, C. E. The levels of soluble granzyme A and B are elevated in plasma and synovial fluid of patients with rheumatoid arthritis (RA). *Clin Exp Immunol* 1999; **116**: 366–70.

115. Goldbach-Mansky, R., Suson, S., Wesley, R., Hack, E., El Gabalawi, H. S., and Tak, P. P. Raised granzyme B levels are associated with erosions in patients with early rheumatoid factor positive rheumatoid arthritis. *Ann Rheum Dis* 2005; **64**: 715–21.

116. Crisp, A. J., Chapman, C. M., Kirkham, S. E., Schiller, A. L., and Krane, S. M. Articular mastocytosis in rheumatoid arthritis. *Arthritis Rheum* 1984; **27**: 845–51.

117. Gotis-Graham, I., and McNeil, H. P. Mast cell responses in rheumatoid synovium: association of the MCtc subset with matrix turnover and clinical progression. *Arthritis Rheum* 1997; **40**: 479–89.

118. Bromley, M., and Woolley, D. E. Histopathology of the rheumatoid lesion: identification of cell types at sites of cartilage erosion. *Arthritis Rheum* 1984; **27**: 857–63.

119. De Paulis, A., Marino, I, Ciccarelli, A., De Crescenzo, G., Concardi, M., and Verga, L. *et al.* Human synovial mast cells. 1. Ultrastructural in situ and in vitro immunologic characterization. *Arthritis Rheum* 1996; **39**: 1222–33.

120. Qu, Z. H., Huang, X. N., Ahmadi, P., Andresevic, J., Planck, S. R., and Hart, C. E. *et al.* Expression of basic fibroblast growth factor in synovial tissue from patients with rheumatoid arthritis and degenerative joint disease. *Lab Invest* 1995; **73**: 339–46.

121. Kiener, H. P., Baghestanian, M., Dominkus, M., Walchshofer, S., Ghannadan, M., and Willheim, M. *et al.* Expression of the C5a receptor (CD88) on synovial mast cells in patients with rheumatoid arthritis. *Arthritis Rheum* 1998; **41**: 233–45.

122. Ruschpler, P., Lorenz, P., Eichler, W., Koczan, D., Hanel, C., and Scholz, R. *et al.* High CXCR3 expression in synovial mast cells

associated with CXCL9 and CXCL10 expression in inflammatory synovial tissues of patients with rheumatoid arthritis. *Arthritis Res Ther* 2003; **5**: R241–R252.

123. McEvoy, A. N., Bresnihan, B., FitzGerald, O., and Murphy, E. P. Corticotropin-releasing hormone signaling in synovial tissue from patients with early inflammatory arthritis is mediated by the type 1 alpha corticotropin-releasing hormone receptor. *Arthritis Rheum* 2001; **44**: 1761–7.

124. Woolley, D. E. The mast cell in inflammatory arthritis. *N Engl J Med* 2003; **348**: 1709–11.

125. Ott, V. L., Cambier, J. C., Kappler, J., Marrack, P., and Swanson, B. J. Mast cell-dependent migration of effector CD81 T cells through production of leukotriene B4. *Nat Immunol* 2003; **4**: 974–81.

126. Woolley, D. E., and Tetlow, L. C. Mast cell activation and its relation to proinflammatory cytokine production in the rheumatoid lesion. *Arthritis Res* 2000; **2**: 65–74.

127. Youssef, P. P., Cormack, J., Evill, C. A., Peter, D. T., Roberts-Thomson, P. J., and Ahern, M. J. *et al.* Neutrophil trafficking into inflamed joints in patients with rheumatoid arthritis, and the effects of methylprednisolone. *Arthritis Rheum* 1996; **39**: 216–25.

128. Koch, A. E., Kunkel, S. L., Burrows, J. C., Evanoff, H. L., Haines, G. K., and Pope, R. M. *et al.* Synovial tissue macrophage as a source of the chemotactic cytokine IL-8. *J Immunol* 1991; **147**: 2187–95.

129. Koch, A. E., Kunkel, S. L., Shah, M. R., Hosaka, S., Halloran, M. M., and Haines, G. K. *et al.* Growth-related gene product alpha: a chemotactic cytokine for neutrophils in rheumatoid arthritis. *J Immunol* 1995; **155**: 3660–6.

130. Gao, J. X., and Issekutz, A. C. The beta 1 integrin, very late activation antigen-4 on human neutrophils can contribute to neutrophil migration through connective tissue fibroblast barriers. *Immunology* 1997; **90**: 448–54.

131. Ulfgren, A. K., Grondal, L., Lindblad, S., Khademi, M., Johnell, O., and Klareskog, L. *et al.* Interindividual and intra-articular variation of proinflammatory cytokines in patients with rheumatoid arthritis: potential implications for treatment. *Ann Rheum Dis* 2000; **59**: 439–47.

132. Baeten, D., Demetter, P., Cuvelier, C., Van Den, B. F., Kruithof, E., and Van Damme, N. *et al.* Comparative study of the synovial histology in rheumatoid arthritis, spondyloarthropathy, and osteoarthritis: influence of disease duration and activity. *Ann Rheum Dis* 2000; **59**: 945–53.

133. Zvaifler, N. J., Boyle, D., and Firestein, G. S. Early synovitis: synoviocytes and mononuclear cells. *Semin Arthritis Rheum* 1994; **23**: 11–16.

134. Tak, P. P., Thurkow, E. W., Verweij, C. L., Smeets, T. J. M., Van Lavieren, R. F., and Kluin, P. M. *et al.* Analysis of the synovial infiltrate and expression of cytokines in rheumatoid arthritis compared with Yersinia-induced arthritis patients. 1995. [Submitted.]

135. Muller-Ladner, U., Judex, M., Ballhorn, W., Kullmann, F., Distler, O., and Schlottmann, K. *et al.* Activation of the IL-4 STAT pathway in rheumatoid synovium. *J Immunol* 2000; **164**: 3894–901.

136. Katrib, A., Tak, P. P., Bertouch, J. V., Cuello, C., McNeil, H. P., and Smeets, T. J. *et al.* Expression of chemokines and matrix metalloproteinases in early rheumatoid arthritis. *Rheumatology (Oxford)* 2001; **40**: 988–94.

137. Kraan, M. C., Versendaal, H., Jonker, M., Bresnihan, B., Post, W., and 't Hart, B. A. *et al.* Asymptomatic synovitis precedes clinically manifest arthritis. *Arthritis Rheum* 1998; **41**: 1481–8.

138. Rantapaa-Dahlqvist, S., de Jong, B A., Berglin, E., Hallmans, G., Wadell, G., and Stenlund, H. *et al.* Antibodies against cyclic citrullinated peptide and IgA rheumatoid factor predict the development of rheumatoid arthritis. *Arthritis Rheum* 2003; **48**: 2741–9.

139. Nielen, M. M., van Schaardenburg, D., Reesink, H. W., Twisk, J. W., van de Stadt, R. J., and van der Horst-Bruinsma, I. E. *et al.* Increased levels of C-reactive protein in serum from blood donors before the onset of rheumatoid arthritis. *Arthritis Rheum* 2004; **50**: 2423–7.

140. Nielen, M. M., van Schaardenburg, D., Reesink, H. W., van de Stadt, R. J., van der Horst-Bruinsma, I. E., and de Koning, M. H. *et al.* Specific autoantibodies precede the symptoms of rheumatoid

arthritis: a study of serial measurements in blood donors. *Arthritis Rheum* 2004; **50**: 380–6.

141. Gerlag, D. M., Haringman, J. J., Smeets, T. J., Zwinderman, A. H., Kraan, M. C., and Laud, P. J. *et al.* Effects of oral prednisolone on biomarkers in synovial tissue and clinical improvement in rheumatoid arthritis. *Arthritis Rheum* 2004; **50**: 3783–91.

142. Haringman, J. J., Gerlag, D. M., Zwinderman, A. H., Smeets, T. J., Kraan, M. C., and Baeten, D. *et al.* Synovial tissue macrophages: highly sensitive biomarkers for response to treatment in rheumatoid arthritis patients. *Ann Rheum Dis* 2005; **64**: 834–8.

143. Smith, M. D., Kraan, M. C., Slavotinek, J., Au, V., Weedon, H., and Parker, A. *et al.* Treatment-induced remission in rheumatoid arthritis patients is characterized by a reduction in macrophage content of synovial biopsies. *Rheumatology (Oxford)* 2001; **40**: 367–74.

144. Kraan, M. C., Haringman, J. J., Post, W. J., Versendaal, J., Breedveld, F. C., and Tak, P. P. Immunohistological analysis of synovial tissue for differential diagnosis in early arthritis. *Rheumatology* 1999; **38**: 1074–80.

145. Gerlag, D. M., and Tak, P. P. Synovial biopsy. *Bailleres Best Pract Res Clin Rheumatol* 2005; **19**: 387–400.

146. Hutton, C. W., Hinton, C., and Dieppe, P. A. Intra-articular variation of synovial changes in knee arthritis: biopsy study comparing changes in patellofemoral synovium and the medial tibiofemoral synovium. *Brit J Rheumatol* 1987; **26**: 5–8.

147. Dolhain, R. J. E. M., Terhaar, N. T., Dekuiper, R., Nieuwenhuis, I. G., Zwinderman, A. H., and Breedveld, F. C. *et al.* Distribution of T cells and signs of T-cell activation in the rheumatoid joint: implications for semiquantitative comparative histology. *Brit J Rheumatol* 1998; **37**: 324–30.

148. Bresnihan, B., Cunnane, G., Youssef, P. P., Yanni, G., FitzGerald, O., and Mulherin, D. Microscopic measurement of synovial membrane inflammation in rheumatoid arthritis: proposals for the evaluation of tissue samples by quantitative analysis. *Br J Rheumatol* 1998; **37**: 636–42.

149. Youssef, P. P., Smeets, T. J. M., Bresnihan, B., Cunnane, G., FitzGerald, O., and Breedveld, F. C. *et al.* Microscopic measurement of cellular infiltration in the rheumatoid arthritis synovial membrane: a comparison of semiquantitative and quantitative analysis. *Br J Rheumatol* 1998; **37**: 1003–7.

150. Kraan, M. C., Haringman, J. J., Ahern, M. J., Breedveld, F. C., Smith, M. D., and Tak, P. P. Quantification of the cell infiltrate in synovial tissue by digital image analysis. *Rheumatology (Oxford)* 2000; **39**: 43–9.

151. Jasin, H. E. Autoantibody specificities of immune complexes sequestered in articular cartilage of patients with rheumatoid arthritis and osteoarthritis. *Arthritis Rheum* 1985; **28**: 241–8.

152. Endresen, G. K., and Forre, O. Human platelets in synovial fluid: a focus on the effects of growth factors on the inflammatory responses in rheumatoid arthritis. *Clin Exp Rheumatol* 1992; **10**: 181–7.

153. Farr, M., Wainwright, A., Salmon, M., Hollywell, C. A., and Bacon, P. A. Platelets in the synovial fluid of patients with rheumatoid arthritis. *Rheumatol Int* 1984; **4**: 13–17.

154. Sharma, J. N., and Buchanan, W. W. Pathogenic responses of bradykinin system in chronic inflammatory rheumatoid disease. *Exp Toxicol Pathol* 1994; **46**: 421–33.

155. Berckmans, R. J., Nieuwland, R., Tak, P. P., Boing, A. N., Romijn, F. P., and Kraan, M. C. *et al.* Cell-derived microparticles in synovial fluid from inflamed arthritic joints support coagulation exclusively via a factor VII-dependent mechanism. *Arthritis Rheum* 2002; **46**: 2857–66.

156. Distler, J. H., Jungel, A., Huber, L C., Seemayer, C. A., Reich, C. F., III, and Gay, R. E. *et al.* The induction of matrix metalloproteinase and cytokine expression in synovial fibroblasts stimulated with immune cell microparticles. *Proc Natl Acad Sci U S A* 2005; **102**: 2892–7.

157. Berckmans, R. J., Nieuwland, R., Kraan, M. C., Schaap, M. C. L., Pots, D., and Smeets, T. J. M. *et al.* Synovial microparticles from arthritic patients modulate chemokine and cytokine release by synoviocytes. *Arthritis Res Ther* 2005; **7**: R536–R544.

158. Saxne, T. Differential release of molecular markers in joint disease. *Acta Orthop Scand Suppl* 1995; **266**: 80–3.

SECTION 3 | *Clinical aspects*

18 | Clinical aspects of rheumatoid arthritis

Nathan J. Zvaifler

Introduction

Rheumatoid arthritis (RA) is a chronic, inflammatory, systemic disease with its primary manifestations in the synovial lining of diarthrodial joints. The disease is ubiquitous, occurs in both sexes at any age, (favoring women 3:1) and has been observed worldwide. The prevalence in most cohorts approximates 1%[1,2] Rural populations seem to be less severely affected than urban dwellers and the disease may be worse in developed countries. The prevalence of RA increases with age. It begins most commonly in the fourth and fifth decades of life with a peak onset between the ages of 35 and 50 years[3]. Variability is found not only in populations, but also in individuals. In the absence of treatment those patients with serologic reactions to immunoglobulins (rheumatoid factors, RFs) and cyclic citrullinated proteins (Chapter 13) and a particular genetic predisposition (shared human leukocyte antigen (HLA)-DRβ1 epitopes—see Chapter 1) have the prototypic severe, unrelenting, progressive, destructive, disabling disease we recognize as RA. Individuals lacking these genetic and serologic features have an arthritis that is often milder, with less characteristic bilateral symmetrical synovitis, and fewer systemic manifestations. It has been argued that these are different diseases, but in this chapter they will be considered the same, unless additional features suggest an alternative rheumatic disease (see differential diagnosis below).

Clinical features

Complaints like malaise, fatigue, mild temperature elevations, sweats, and weight loss are frequent accompaniments of RA, especially at its inception. Many patients suffer depression. The rapid amelioration of these symptoms following anti-tumor necrosis factor therapy confirms their relationship to the underlying disease (Chapter 27). Persistent stiffness in and around the joints upon arising from sleep is a consistent complaint. Such morning stiffness lasts hours, may improve midday, but usually returns in the late afternoon or evening[4]. It is aggravated by inactivity ('gelling') and improves with motion ('warming up')[5].

Systemic manifestations can initially obscure joint pain and tenderness, which are the symptoms of synovitis. Careful questioning, however, will reveal difficulty in making a tight fist, lifting heavy objects, wringing out wash cloths, opening doorknobs,

or removing caps from jars, and an avoidance of handshakes. Women comment that their shoe size has enlarged and they avoid standing as much as possible.

RA usually begins insidiously, over weeks or months; but in ~10% of patients it has an explosive onset[6]. Disease activity can be intermittent at first, but with time becomes sustained. Spontaneous remissions are uncommon (~10% of patients), occur most often in patients without detectable serum RF, and are not likely after two years of persistent disease[7,8]. Occasionally patients will report antecedent episodes of bursitis, carpal tunnel syndrome, meniscal disease in a knee joint, or a 'Morton's neuroma', which likely represents unrecognized rheumatoid synovitis

The hallmark of RA is bilateral, symmetrical polyarthritis (Table 18.1). Characteristically both wrists and the second and third metacarpal phalangeal (MCP) joints are swollen and tender. Less easily appreciated are similar abnormalities in the metatarsal phalangeal (MTP) joints of the feet, especially the 4th and 5th MTPs. Although swelling of the proximal interphalangeal (PIP) joints of the fingers is common at an early stage of the disease, the same joints in the toes are rarely involved[9]. Larger articulations, such as knees, ankles, and subtalar and elbow joints are eventually involved in a symmetrical fashion, but if only a single joint is affected then other conditions must be considered, especially infectious arthritis. Disease of the hip and shoulder joints is more difficult to ascertain and usually detected later in RA. Less appreciated is chronic synovitis of the temperomandibular and sternoclavicular joints (Fig. 18.1). A rare, but

Table 18.1 1987 revised American College of Rheumatology criteria for the classification of rheumatoid arthritis[92]

1. Stiffness in and around the joints lasting ≥ 1 h before maximal improvement
2. Arthritis of ≥ 3 joint areas, simultaneously
3. Arthritis of the proximal interphalangeal, metacarpal phalangeal, and wrist joints
4. Symmetrical arthritis
5. Rheumatoid nodules
6. A positive test for serum rheumatoid factor
7. Radiographic changes characteristic of rheumatoid arthritis (erosions and/or periarticular osteopenia in hand and/or wrist joints

A person can be classified as having rheumatoid arthritis if ≥ 4 criteria are present at any time.
Criteria 1–4 must be present for at least 6 weeks.
Criteria 2–5 must be observed by a physician.

RHEUMATOID ARTHRITIS

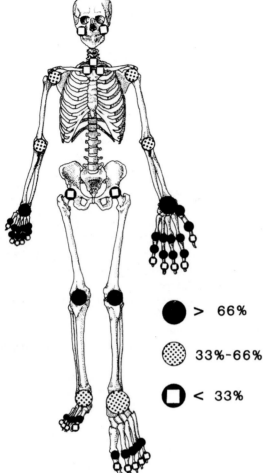

> ●   > 66%

> ▦   33%–66%

> ▢   < 33%

Fig. 18.1 Typical pattern of joints involved in adult rheumatoid arthritis. Bilateral, symmetrical swelling of both the small joints (hands and feet) and large joints (wrists, knees, ankles) with sparing of the axial skeleton, except for the cervical spine. The relative frequency of disease in individual joints is shown.

dangerous manifestation of RA because it can produce stridor and asphyxia, is cricoarytenoid arthritis[10,11]. Inflammatory arthritis in the small joints of the toes, the distal interphalangeal joints of the fingers, the lumbar spine, or sacroiliac joints are all uncommon in RA and should prompt consideration of alternative rheumatic diseases. Cervical spine disease, an important component of RA, will be addressed separately below.

Joint examination in early rheumatoid arthritis

Recognition of RA at or near its inception is of increasing importance because that is the time when the disease might be most amenable to treatment (Chapter 20). RA can usually be diagnosed, even in its early stages, by a careful history and joint examination. The proper techniques of joint evaluation are presented in a number of publications (reviewed in Refs 12 and 13) Misdiagnosis most often results from reliance on laboratory tests and imaging studies in the absence of characteristic joint findings. Likewise, patients with continuous and longstanding musculoskeletal complaints (more than a year) whose joints appear normal on careful examination do not have RA and are not likely to develop RA.

Characteristics that should be considered in the evaluation of individual joints include swelling, tenderness, and limitation in the normal range of motion. Deformity and soft tissue atrophy are usually only seen in later stages of RA. Joint tenderness is elicited by direct palpation. Tenderness thresholds vary among patients, so the examiner must learn the amount of force needed to evoke a response. Synovitis is less likely when equal pressure over a joint and the adjacent bone produces the same amount of discomfort.

Joint swelling has several causes: synovial tissue enlargement, effusion within the joint space, or bony enlargement. The later, a hallmark of degenerative arthritis, feels firm or hard and the deformity is irregular because of the unequal growth of periarticular osseous structures (osteophytes). Inflamed synovium feels spongy or doughy. Soft tissue swelling is best appreciated in the small joints of the hands. Joint margins are obscured. Mild flexion of the fingers discloses a loss of the valleys between the second, third, and fourth MCP joints. Palpation reveals fullness in the PIP joints. Their spindle-shaped (fusiform) appearance reflects the synovial attachments at the PIP joints, which only allow lateral swelling. Combined side to side and top to bottom enlargement of a PIP joint (centripetal swelling) is more characteristic of processes that inflame the bone or enthesis, as seen with psoriatic arthritis or Reiter's disease. The distal interphalangeal (DIP) finger joints are occasionally tender, but rarely swollen or inflamed. Asking the patient to make a tight fist provides a rapid assessment of the second through fifth finger joints. The fingertips will touch the proximal palmar crease if the DIP, PIP, and MCP joints achieve their normal 90° of flexion. Abnormal joints are easily isolated by this procedure (Fig. 18.2).

Examination of the dorsum of the hands in more advanced RA discloses atrophy of the interosseous muscles, secondary to MCP disease, and appearing as depressions between the metacarpal bones.

Inflammation and/or pain limits joint motion. This limitation is often the earliest finding of disease in the wrists. Normally the wrist moves ~90° in flexion and 70° in extension, but this range decreases with synovitis in the radio-carpal and ulno-carpal joints. Active motion is generally more restricted than passive motion. Gentle palpation with the fingertips on the back of the hand often reveals gritty soft tissue swelling in the groove between the forearm and the carpal bones. Swelling of the extensor carpi-ulnaris tendon sheath at the ulnar aspect of the wrist is characteristic of RA. Tenosynovitis of the common extensor digitorum communis sheath appears as a large cystic swelling on the dorsum of the wrist.

Normal extension at the elbow is 180°. Even small amounts of inflammation in the elbow joint compromise full extension. Synovial swelling or effusion is best appreciated by palpation in the grooves on either side of the olecranon process. Since the olecranon bursa is external to the joint it does not interfere with full

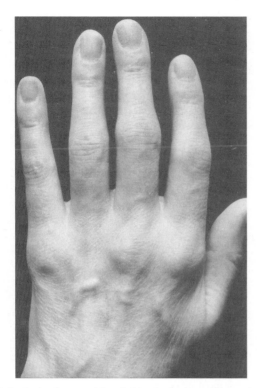

Fig. 18.2 Early rheumatoid arthritis. Red, shiny skin and fusiform swelling of the proximal interphalangeal joints of the fingers. The ill-defined joint margins of the MCP joints is due to synovial swelling. Sparing of the fourth metacarpal joint is not uncommon.

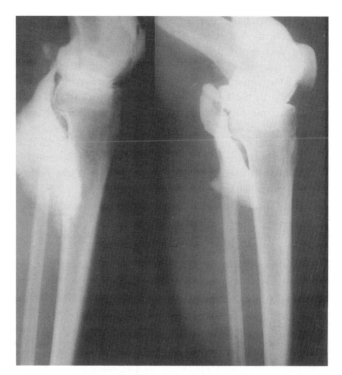

Fig. 18.3 Arthrogram of the knee joint in a lateral projection. Contrast medium introduced into the suprapatellar pouch traverses posteriorly into the semimembranosus bursa (Baker's cyst). Further extension or rupture of the cyst produces symptoms in the lower leg and ankle.

extension, even when inflamed, which allows for discrimination between arthritis (particularly septic arthritis) and bursitis.

Symptoms from disease in the shoulders are common in RA, and include tenderness, a characteristic deep aching nocturnal pain, and limited motion. The shoulder joint is complex, consisting of the gleno-humeral, acromio-clavicular, and scapulo-thoracic articulations and their attendant muscles, tendons and bursa. Warmth, joint swelling, and effusions are difficult to detect, so limitation of motion often provides the only clue to shoulder involvement. While facing the patient the examining physician should press down on the shoulder with one hand and elevate the ipsilateral arm with the opposite hand. This maneuver blocks any motion in the scapulo-thoracic articulation and isolates the gleno-humeral joint, which is the usual site of synovial inflammation.

Pain and limitation of motion are hallmarks of hip disease. The problem, however, is that correctly interpreting complaints of hip pain requires an appreciation of the localization of the symptoms. Synovitis in the femoral-acetabular articulation typically produces pain and tenderness in the groin or occasionally in the buttock. This can be confirmed by finding limitation in hip flexion and/or external rotation. Occasionally pain in the hip is referred to the knee of the same leg, especially in children.

The knee has three synovial lined joints enclosed in a common capsule. As a rule all three—the lateral femoral-tibial, medial femoral-tibial, and the patello-femoral articulations—are simultaneously involved in RA (tri-compartment disease). Normally the knee feels cooler than the tissues around it, because the most

superficial structure, the patella, is avascular. Thus, when the temperature of the knee is the same as the surrounding tissues inflammation should be suspected. Inspection often discloses atrophy of the quadriceps muscles and loss of the normal contours of the knee due to joint effusion or synovial hypertrophy. Pathological enlargement of the normal gastrocnemius-semimembranosus bursa (Baker's cyst) posterior to the knee can be seen from the rear with the patient standing and confirmed by palpating behind the slightly flexed knee. Compression of structures in the popliteal space by an expanding bursa will cause discomfort or edema of the leg from obstruction of venous return. Sometimes a Baker's cyst dissects into the tissues around the gastrocnemius muscle or ruptures, producing signs and symptoms that mimic acute thrombophlebitis[14]. Contrast arthrography (Fig. 18.3) or magnetic resonance imaging (MRI) will confirm the diagnosis and should be performed in any patient with RA who develops acute unilateral tenderness, warmth or edema of the lower leg (pseudothrombophlebitis), because anticoagulation is contraindicated in this situation.

Gross knee effusions appear as a loss of normal knee joint contours and fullness on either side of the patella or in the suprapatellar pouch. Large effusions are appreciated by ballotment of the patella. Smaller accumulations can be demonstrated by eliciting a 'bulge sign'. With the subject lying down with the leg extended the medial-anterior aspect of the knee is compressed by the examiner's hand. This is followed immediately by a sweeping motion on the outside of the joint. If fluid is present in the joint a bulge will appear in the soft tissue on the medial-anterior aspect of the knee as the effusion returns into the medial aspect of the joint.

The ankle is a hinge joint. Limited flexion and extension of the foot reflects disease in the mortise (talo tibial fibular) joint. Swelling over the medial or antero-lateral aspect of the ankle indicates synovial disease, whereas swelling posterior to the malleoli more often reflects tendon sheath inflammation.

Anatomically the foot can be divided into three segments: the hind-, mid-, and forefoot. In the hindfoot subtalar involvement impairs inversion and eversion. Pain on forced extension of the foot can be due to bursitis beneath the insertion of the Achilles tendon into the calcaneus. Plantar fasciitis causes discomfort on the underside of the heel. Pain on compression of the midfoot indicates inflammation in the tarsal joints.

Among the earliest findings in RA is swelling and pain in the MTP joints. Swelling causes a subtle spreading of the toes, which is best appreciated by standing at the head of the examining table and looking at the dorsum of the feet of the patient who is lying on his/her back. Normally the toes are in apposition, but with swelling light can be seen between them. Pain in the MTP joints is elicited by squeezing the toes together. Swelling and pain are also detected by deep palpation of individual MTP joints. Unfortunately most examiners feel just beneath the web of the toes. However, the MTP joints are located further up the foot. Their true location is appreciated best by comparing the dorsum of the foot to the palm of the hand. The MCP joints are not seen, but they can be felt at the level of the palmar crease, not at base of the fingers. Subluxations of the MTP heads, hallux valgus, and lateral deviation and clawing of the toes develop later as the disease progresses.

The atlantoaxial, zygoapophyseal (facet), uncovertebral, and intervertebral articulations comprise the joints of the cervical spine. All but the last are diarthrodial and covered by synovium. The majority of patients with early RA complain of neck pain; some have an accompanying occipital headache. Examination of the neck reveals muscle spasm and some limitation of lateral bending or rotary motion. Flexion and extension are usually well preserved. Later the neck can develop a number of serious complications, as described below

Joint examination in established RA

As RA progresses chronic inflammation, distension of joint capsules, stretching and disruption of periarticular soft tissue structures, and invasion of joint cartilage and bone by aggressive granulomatous synovium (pannus) give rise to a panoply of abnormalities. For instance a characteristic feature in the hands of patients with longstanding RA is volar subluxation of the phalanges over the metacarpals with ulnar deviation of the fingers. In most cases there is an accompanying radial deviation at the wrist ('zigzag' deformity), which is an attempt to keep the normal alignment between the finger extensors and the radius[16,17]. If the extensor tendons tear away from the top of the MCP joint capsule they will slip laterally into the clefts between the MCP joints, exaggerating the normal ulnar attitude of the power grip. The resultant mechanical factors produce a typical 'seal fin' deformity (Fig. 18.4).

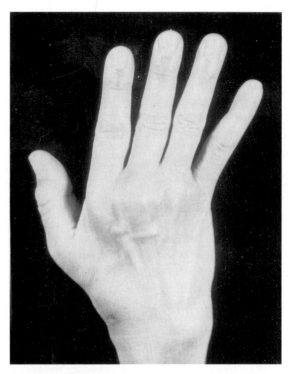

Fig. 18.4   Advanced rheumatoid arthritis. Shiny thin skin, atrophy of interosseous muscles, synovial proliferation, and swelling of the MCP joints, especially the 2nd and 3rd. At this stage fusiform swelling is no longer present in the PIP joints. Note the radial rotation of the carpus on the distal radius (radial deviation) and the ulnar deviation of fingers (zig-zag deformity).

Flexion at a MCP joint with hyperextension of the contiguous PIP joint and flexion at the DIP generates a 'swan neck' deformity; whereas a 'boutonniere' deformity of a finger results from hyper-extension at the MCP with hyperflexion at the PIP and hyperextension of the DIP joint. Biomechanical forces responsible for these complex abnormalities are discussed in most orthopedic surgery texts. Flexor tenosynovitis can interfere with flexion of the fingers and lead to fixed extension. Thickening or nodule formation in the tendon or tenosynovial proliferation sometimes causes locking or 'triggering' of the digit. Tendons attenuated by synovial pannus or rubbing on the irregular end of an eroded bone can rupture tendons (especially the extensors for the fourth and fifth fingers at the ulnar styloid).

Normally the radial-carpal, radial-ulnar, and midcarpal joints do not communicate, but with chronic inflammation their boundaries are compromised. Later with collapse of the carpal bones and subluxation at the carpal-metacarpal joints the dorsum of the wrist assumes a 'step-down' appearance. Loss of the integrity of the ulnar collateral ligament causes dorsal subluxation of the ulnar head (caput ulna), which springs up and can be depressed volarly. This has been likened to pushing down on a piano key and sets the stage for a subsequent painless rupture of the lateral extensor tendon.

Other causes of loss of extension of the ring and fifth fingers need to be considered. One is an extreme ulnar drift of the digits with lateral displacement of the extensor tendons into the intermetacarpal cleft. Another is a neuropathy due to compression of the ulnar nerve in the cubital tunnel at the elbow, or in Guyon's canal at the wrist. Combined sensory and motor deficits favor ulnar nerve entrapment at the wrist.

The median nerve passes under the volar transverse ligament and enters the hand along with nine flexor tendons through the rigid carpal tunnel. Patients with RA may complain of decreased sensation in the palmar aspect of the thumb, index, and long fingers and later weakness and thenar muscles atrophy. Tingling in the hands often begins at night, awakening the patient from sleep. The symptoms clear when the hands are shaken vigorously, only to recur early the next morning. Similar neurological complaints can be reproduced by percussion over the median nerve at the wrist (Tinel's sign) or by holding the hand in forced flexion (Phalen's sign). Nerve conduction studies will confirm the diagnosis of carpal tunnel syndrome.

A number of lesions can cause loss of function in the thumb, including: a boutonniere-like deformity due to stretching of the MCP joint capsule; volar subluxation of the first MCP during contraction of the adductor hollicus; and exaggerated adduction and flexion at the first MCP and DIP joint hyperextension in an attempt to regain pinch.

Problems in the shoulder often arise outside the gleno-humeral articulation. RA can produce chronic changes in the rotator cuff, the acromio-clavicular joint, and a number of the tendons and muscles of the shoulder joint. Tears or attrition in the cuff are indicated by distortions of normal motion. Resistance to shoulder abduction is a subtle indication of rotator cuff degeneration. With further damage or in the presence of complete tears, there is supero-lateral displacement of the humerus.

Supraspinatus tendonitis or subdeltoid bursitis causes pain whenever these structures are forced against the undersurface of the acromium ('impingement syndrome'). Chronic impingement can disrupt elements of the rotator cuff[19]. Dissolution of the acromio-clavicular ligament, which is less common, is recognized either by direct palpation or by an anterior and superior displacement of the clavicle with shoulder motion. Tenderness over the bicipital groove suggests tendonitis, and rupture of the tendon is evident by bunching up of the lateral muscle belly in the upper arm with resisted elbow flexion. Ultrasonography can be an important procedure for evaluating all the structures that make up the shoulder (Chapter 19).

The articulations of the pelvis include the lumbo-sacral, sacral-iliac, pubic symphysis, and hip joints. Hip disease in RA is ordinarily a late manifestation. An additional confusion comes from the possibility that radiographic evidence of femoral head destruction reflects corticosteroid-induced avascular necrosis, rather than RA. The patient's gait often provides clues to chronic hip problems. There are two cycles (stance and swing) in normal walking. The stance phase begins with heel strike and ends with toe off. At that moment the hip loads three times the body weight. Patients with pain in the hip shorten their stance phase to unload the extremity as quickly as possible. This results in an 'antalgic' gait. Advanced hip disease produces an apparent shortening of the extremity because the leg is held in flexion, abduction, and external rotation; a position that relaxes the joint capsule and reduces intra-articular pressure. To compensate for the abduction deformity the patient will tilt the pelvis and elevate the uninvolved extremity, resulting in a functional shortening of the affected limb.

In the knee joint the femoral and tibial condyles articulate with each other; interposed between them are fibro-cartilagenous menisci. By themselves these structures are inadequate to allow for the normal flexion, extension, and rotation of the knee. Stability and motion come from the quadriceps muscle acting through the patella and its attachments and the cruciate and collateral ligaments that arise from the joint capsule. When any of them are compromised, by chronic synovitis, effusions, and/or stretching of the joint capsule, quadriceps muscle atrophy, flexion contracture, and a valgus deformity (angulation away from the midline) eventuate. Varus deformities ('knock knee') are less common and usually result from destruction of the cartilage and bone of the medial femoral condyle by rheumatoid pannus

Ligamentous tears or stress fracture of the fibula can be a source of persistent pain in the ankle. As a rule, ankle joint involvement is usually accompanied by distortions in the midfoot and MTP joints. Weight bearing superimposed on chronic synovitis produces several different deformities of the foot[20]. Posterior tibialis tendon disease or rupture causes subtalar subluxation and eversion and the talus migrates laterally[21]. Hindfoot involvement results in a flat foot (planovalgus) deformity. In the forefoot, because of constant weight bearing, a valgus deformity of the great toe develops, followed by subluxations or dislocations of the lesser metatarsal phalangeal joints. Dorsal subluxations or dislocations of the phalanges and compensatory flexion at the PIP joints caused by the fixed length of the flexor tendons produce typical hammer toe or claw foot deformities. Accompanying this is atrophy and displacement of the soft tissue pads beneath the MTP heads, which causes them to protrude and become an unprotected weight-bearing surface. Constant friction leads to callus formation. Patients will complain of 'walking on marbles'.

Cervical spine disease is a special case because serious complications can occur with little or no physical findings. Conversely, extensive changes seen on routine radiographs may have only minimal neurological consequences. In general, the extent of cervical spine abnormalities parallels the magnitude of erosions in the hands and wrists[22]. Disk space narrowing in the upper cervical segments (usually in the absence of osteophytes), multiple anterior subluxations of vertebrae with forward flexion of the neck ('step-laddering'), zygo-apophyseal joint erosions and sclerosis, and, rarely, collapse of the lateral mass of the first cervical vertebrae are all consequences of rheumatoid synovitis and pannus[23,24]. But most profound, and quite particular to RA, are changes in the relationship between the odontoid process of C2 and the atlas (C1), which is affixed to the base of the skull[25]. These two work as a unit to support axial rotation of the head and are held in close approximation by two strong ligaments. Backward movement is blocked by impaction of the anterior arch of the atlas against the odontoid. Forward slippage is prevented by the transverse ligament, which arises from the lateral masses of the atlas, passes behind the odontoid process, and forms a synovial lined joint between itself and a facet on the back of the odontoid. The powerful alar ligaments, which run from each side of the odontoid to the lateral margins of the foramen magnum, also prevent distraction of the head from the axis.

Lateral radiograms of the normal cervical spine in flexion and extension show the close association between the odontoid and the arch of the atlas (normally less than 3 mm in full flexion)[26]. Destruction of the stabilizing ligaments decreases the anterior-posterior width of the cervical canal, potentially compromising the spinal cord. Severe neck pain and/or occipital headache can be consequences of either subluxation or nerve entrapment. Typical findings of cervical myelopathy, such as muscle weakness in the extremities, tingling or numbness in the fingers, or reflex changes in the knees or ankles, are often overlooked or incorrectly ascribed to the underlying RA. MRI is usually needed to define the soft tissues and anatomy in this area.[27] Imaging studies may also show that the spinal cord has been spared from compression because rheumatoid granulation tissue has eroded or fractured the odontoid. Destruction of the lateral atlantoaxial joints, often in association with loss of bone in the foramen magnum, causes settling of the cranium (platybasia) on the dens[28]. Vertical subluxation of the odontoid can impinge on the brainstem (basilar invagination), producing drop attacks, nystagmus, or life-threatening cardiopulmonary events. Surgical treatment can be required in the presence of neurologic signs or symptoms[29].

Rheumatoid nodules

A hallmark of RA is juxta-articular subcutaneous nodules[30,31]. These vary in size from a few millimeters to several centimeters. The smaller lesions (<2–3 mm) are firm or hard and often confused with mineral deposits or tophi. Larger nodules feel softer, rubbery, or occasionally cyst-like. Nodules often appear and disappear abruptly, although the longer they remain the less likely it is that they will clear. RA nodules occur at pressure sites: typically on the extensor surface of the forearm an inch or so below the tip of the elbow or in the olecranon bursa; in the feet beneath the metatarsal heads or at sites of rubbing from footwear, including the Achilles tendon; over the PIP or MCP joints; and in the soft tissues of the palm and finger pulps. Although nodules are usually freely movable in soft tissues, they can be tightly bound to the underlying bone or affixed to tendons. Histologically similar nodules are found throughout the viscera (rheumatoid granulomas) in systemic rheumatoid disease often associated with

a vasculitis of medium- and large-sized blood vessels (see below). Rheumatoid nodules are detected at some time in the course of RA in 20–25% of patients; usually they have serum rheumatoid factor (>95%), the RA susceptibility haplotype, and a more severe disease course. Very rarely patients are seen with widespread nodules and positive RF tests, but little or no synovitis or joint damage (rheumatoid nodulosis)[32]. A paradoxical finding is enhanced or accelerated development of rheumatoid nodules in patients treated with methotrexate.[33]

Extra-articular complications

RA has numerous complications. Many are listed in Table 18.2. While usually cataloged according to the organs affected (e.g. heart, lungs, etc.), they are easier understood in pathophysiological terms. Some are merely extensions of the processes affecting the joints. Examples include compression neuropathies (carpal or tarsal tunnel syndromes), spinal cord impingement (atlantoaxial dissociation), synovial outpouching (Baker's cyst, pseudothrombophlebitis), or tendon rupture. Others, like anemia, muscle wasting, osteopenia, and amyloid disease are consequences of chronic inflammation and persistent exposure to deleterious cytokines[34]. Synovitis has its counterpart at other serosal surfaces, accounting for pleuritis and pericarditis[35]. Episcleritis and some forms of keratitis probably have a similar pathogenesis[36]. But the majority of side-effects can be ascribed to immunological phenomena: (a) rheumatoid granulomata (cardiopulmonary disease, nodular scleritis—see Fig. 18.5); (b) lymphocytic infiltration (Sjogren's syndrome); (c) autoantibodies (Felty's syndrome); and (d) a spectrum of immune complex-mediated vascular disorders, ranging from a mild Raynaud's phenomenon, to digital and periungual micro-infarcts (Fig. 18.6), often with an accompanying mild peripheral sensory neuritis, to a lethal necrotizing vasculitis. The micro-vasculitis was common in past years before effective therapy was available, developing in 15–30% of RA patients with longstanding disease. This process, which is increasingly uncommon, is benign, with little associated morbidity[37]. Pathological examination of the small terminal digital vessels shows only intimal proliferation with minimal inflammatory

Table 18.2 Extra-articular features of RA

	Manifestations	Prevalence % (post-mortem studies)
Entrapment, extension	Carpal/tarsal tunnel syndrome; popliteal cysts, pseudophlebitis	
Nodule formation	Skin, lung, myocardium	20 (20–40)
Serositis	Pleurisy, pericarditis, effusions	10–25 (75)
Vasculitis	Periungual micro-infarcts, digital gangrene, mononeuritis, leg ulcers	1–10 (15–25)
Felty's syndrome	Neutropenia, splenomegaly, infection	1 (2)
Complications of chronic inflammation	Weight loss, fever, sweats, fatigue	10–20
Anemia	Pallor, dyspnea	75
Lymphadenopathy	Axillary, epitrochlear nodes	
Amyloidosis	Renal, cardiac, any organ	(5–15)
Osteoporosis	Bone fractures	–

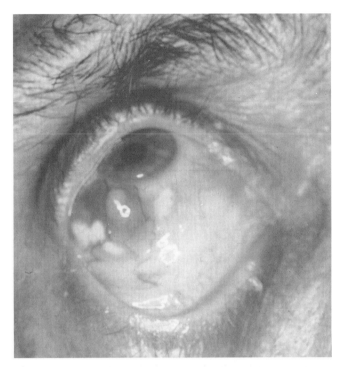

Fig. 18.5 Nodular scleritis in a patient with rheumatoid arthritis. Local atrophy produces a thin blue sclera (scleromalacia) and exposes the underlying uvea.

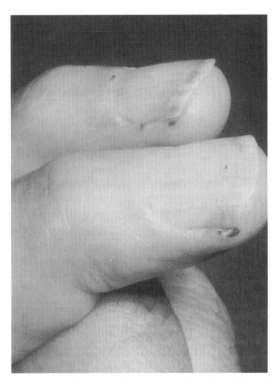

Fig. 18.6 Periungual micro-infarcts are produced by a bland intimal vascular occlusion of terminal arterioles at the nail edge.

damage[37]. Contrast this with the rare, severe, often lethal, necrotizing vasculitis of small- and medium-sized muscular arteries that resembles polyarteritis nodosa[38]. The typical patient is an older male with rheumatoid nodules and high titers of serum rheumatoid factors. Necrotic skin lesions, digital infarcts, bowel ischemia, or mononeuritis multiplex can develop acutely, often after an abrupt change in glucocorticosteroid dose, and can be fatal[39]. The serum of these patients contains cold precipitable complexes (cryoglobulins) of rheumatoid factors, immunoglobulins, and complement components[40]. Systemic rheumatoid vasculitis, while always uncommon, has become increasingly rare. Not all problems in RA patients are related to their underlying disease. It is important to recognize complications due to treatments or concomitant diseases.

Investigations

Blood tests have many uses in RA, to (a) quantify local or systemic inflammation; (b) confirm a clinical impression of RA; (c) judge the response to treatment; (d) predict its course. Most RA patients have a normocytic, hypochromic anemia that correlates with disease activity, acute phase proteins, and elevated erythrocyte sedimentation rate (ESR) or C reactive protein (CRP). The majority of RA patients have features of an anemia of chronic disease (ACD), but in a quarter the anemia responds to iron treatment (IDA)[41,42]. With an ACD the hemoglobin level is usually inversely proportional to the ESR; serum iron is low and ferritin is higher than IDA. Normal iron stores are present in the bone marrow and hemoglobin and hematocrit values return towards normal with disease control. A hemoglobin value of less than 10 g/dL suggests that blood loss is complicating ACD or some other intercurrent problem.

Thrombocytosis also reflects high disease activity, occasionally vasculitis, and increased platelet counts are associated with low hemoglobin levels[43]. Similar correlations exist with eosinophils in RA[44]. Cytokines like IL-6 elaborated by inflammatory cells cause hepatic production of a group of proteins, known as 'acute phase reactants'. These include fibrinogen, serum amyloid A and P proteins, haptoglobin, ferritin, ceruloplasmin, and several others, of which the best known is the CRP (Chapter 12). In general, there is a good correlation between the ESR and CRP and long-term time-integrated studies of the latter predict erosions on joint roentgenograms and disability and mortality[45].

Two serum antibodies—the anti-immunoglobulins called RFs and antibodies to cyclic citrullinated proteins (anti-CCPs)—should be measured at the initial evaluation of all patients suspected of having RA (Chapter 13). This is not because RF tests are needed to diagnose RA. In fact they are of limited specificity and are positive in numerous other diseases, and in 10–20% of normal individuals, where they are found to increase in frequency and amount with age. Rather, it is because RFs are confirmatory in 65–80% of patients with a clinical picture of RA and predict a more severe, destructive disease course. Anti-CPP antibodies are present in only 70–80% of RA patients, and may be more specific than RFs. Thus, they are important in differential diagnosis. Anti-CCP antibodies also predict an erosive and progressive disease. The observation that RFs and anti-CCP antibodies can be detected together in the serum of individuals destined to develop RA is likely to be important for understanding RA pathogenesis[46].

Synovial fluid (SF) analysis is occasionally helpful in establishing the diagnosis of RA and excluding infections and crystal-induced processes (Chapter 17). The fluid in RA appears turbid, and is an exudate with protein concentrations that are half to two-thirds of their serum levels. Normal SF white cell counts are usually <500 mm/^{3}; whereas RA effusions typically have white cell counts of 2000–20 000/mm^3, occasionally going as high as 50 000/mm^3. At least two-thirds are polymorphonuclear leukocytes, but the leukocytosis rarely exceeds the 90% commonly seen in septic arthritis.

The complement components (C$'$) detected in synovial fluid are derived from serum and are also locally produced by the inflamed synovium. Their concentrations are generally proportional to other proteins that enter the joint. This is true for most forms of inflammatory arthritis, but RA is different. Although RA effusions are inflammatory and have increased levels of serum proteins, both the values for total hemolytic complement and C$'$ components are often reduced to less than one-third of simultaneously determined serum values, reflecting local C$'$ consumption[47,48].

Conventional radiographs are of limited diagnostic value at the inception of RA, although ultrasonography and MRI can be helpful. However, roentgenograms remain the gold standard for assessing disease progression and response to treatment (detailed in Chapter19).

Assessing disease activity

The expression of RA varies greatly between individuals and even in the same patient at different times. Quantification of these differences is necessary for evaluating treatment. Two simple sets of disease activity criteria have been validated for use in drug trials and clinical practice (Table 18.3). They evaluate different aspects of the rheumatoid process: inflammation, pain, physical disability, and health status. Many methods have been used to quantify articular inflammation, including the total number of joints affected, area of joint involvement (small joints vs. large joints), or disease severity. For example, the American College of Rheumatology (ACR) core set[49] evaluates 68 joints, including the DIP joints of the hands and the PIP joints of the feet. These were eliminated in the European League Against Rheumatism (EULAR) core set[50] because osteoarthritis (OA) can confound

evaluation of the DIP joints and assessing the PIPs of the toes is difficult. Scoring just 28 joints (10 PIPs, 10 MCPs, 2 wrists, 2 elbows, 2 shoulders, and 2 knees) did not compromise the swollen and tender joint counts.

A simple visual analog scale (VAS) is used to grade the pain of RA. The subject is asked to indicate her/his current status by marking an X on a 0–10 cm horizontal scale with 'no pain' at one end and 'worst possible pain' at the other. A global assessment of disease activity is expressed the same way; the patient and the physician evaluating the patient's answer the question 'How well are you (the patient) doing today considering all the ways your arthritis affects you?' by placing an X on separate VAS horizontal scales. A patient's function or disability is usually based on a self-reporting questionnaire. The Health Assessment Questionnaire (HAQ) and the Arthritis Impact Measurement Score (AIMS) are two popular validated instruments sensitive to clinical changes[51,52].

Radiographs of selected involved joints should be obtained at the initial evaluation of a patient to confirm the diagnosis of RA and to assess its severity. Scoring methods developed by Sharp[53] and Larsen[54] quantify both joint space narrowing (cartilage loss) and bone erosions. The earliest structural changes often occur in the 4th and 5th MTP joints of the feet, but the hands and wrists are more convenient to measure. Radiographic changes in large joints, like the knees, appear later in the disease and are of less utility. Follow-up X-rays, done at one- or two-year intervals, can determine whether the current treatment is influencing joint damage or only controlling inflammation, since these two parameters are not synonymous.

Course and prognosis of RA

Ideas about the 'natural history' of RA (i.e. in the absence of effective therapy) are based on observations made prior to the 1950s (see Ref. 55), before serologic tests for RF, genetic analysis, and sophisticated imaging techniques were available. Indeed, there was not even universal agreement on the classification of inflammatory polyarthritis. Yet the investigators were remarkably prescient. At that time ~15 of any 100 patients diagnosed with RA had a short-lived joint disease that remitted without sequelae. Another 15–25% persisted for a time and then cleared leaving only moderate joint damage. Fifty percent of patients had a chronic, progressive disease, punctuated by remissions and exacerbations, which invariably resulted in deformities and significant disability. The remaining 10% were unresponsive to treatment and eventually developed complete disability, and confinement to a chair or bed.

Features that portend a favorable or dismal outcome have been identified (Table 18.4). Remissions rarely occur after the first year of disease. Men fare better than women, and young women do least well. More than half the patients who become pregnant improve, usually after the first trimester, but synovitis returns 2–3 months postpartum[56]. Disease that begins after age 50 has a better prognosis. It is axiomatic that the longer a progressive disease continues, the poorer the outcome. Complicating necrotizing vasculitis is associated with a particularly dismal prognosis[57].

Table 18.3 Core set of variables to assess disease activity in RA

Disease activity measure	Core sets	
	EULAR	**ACR**
Tender joint count	28 joints scored	68 joints scored
Swollen joint count	28 joints scored	68 joints scored
Pain on visual analog scale	YES	YES
Physician's global assessment of disease activity		YES
Patient's global assessment of disease activity		YES
Physical function	YES	YES
Radiographic analysis	YES	YES
Acute phase reactant	YES	YES

Adapted from Refs 49, 50.

Table 18.4 Factors that portend a poor outcome in rheumatoid arthritis

Clinical	Laboratory
Large number of inflamed joints (> 14)	Elevated ESR or CRP
Extra-articular manifestations	High titers of rheumatoid factor (IgM)
Rheumatoid nodules	RA 'susceptibility' haplotype
Continuous disease activity	Juxta-articular bone erosions

Patients rarely die from RA, although systemic vasculitis and atlantoaxial subluxation can be lethal. In the past they succumbed to the same diseases as age matched cohorts—cardiovascular events, cancer, and infections—except 5–10 years sooner. More recently that difference has narrowed, probably reflecting better control of inflammation[58-60].

Differential diagnosis

Arthritis is a symptom and joint complaints can develop in the course of more than 100 diseases[61]. A cause can usually be elucidated by a careful history and physical examination and confirmed by appropriate laboratory tests and imaging techniques[62]. Determining the origin of the patient's musculoskeletal complaints is the first step. Do they arise from soft tissue structures around the joint (periarthritis) or from within the joint (arthritis)? In periarthritis, such as tendonitis, bursitis, or fibrositis, the process tends to involve only one or a few of the larger joints, is generally not symmetrical, and spares the hands, wrists, and feet that are so often involved in true arthritic disorders. Exceptions are symptoms of pain and stiffness about the shoulder and pelvic girdle in elderly patients with polymyalgia rheumatica (PMR) and the ubiquitous pains of fibromyalgia. Clues that suggest arthritis are distortions in normal joint anatomy, signs of inflammation, and limited joint motion.

After establishing that a patient has arthritis, defining the pattern of joint disease then becomes important. Is it monoarticular (1 joint), pauciarticular (2–4 joints), or polyarticular? Is the process inflammatory (characterized by warmth, redness, and boggy synovial swelling) or non-inflammatory (hard, irregular, or bony)? What is the distribution of the arthritis? Examples include symmetrical vs. asymmetrical, axial (spinal) vs. peripheral, or large vs. small joint disease. The duration of symptoms provides important clues. Are the symptoms acute, episodic, or chronic (usually defined as continuous for more than 6–8 weeks)? Pain for many months or years in the absence of obvious joint disease is inconsistent with RA and highly suggestive of a pain syndrome, such as fibromyalgia.

Employing this method the physician can develop a profile that allows recognition of a great number of arthritic disorders. Thus, RA would be described as a chronic, inflammatory polyarthritis that involves both large and small joints in a symmetrical fashion. In contrast, the arthritis accompanying inflammatory bowel disease is more often episodic, affecting a few large joints (pauciarticular) in an asymmetrical fashion with a predilection for articulations in the lower extremities. Likewise, gouty arthritis tends to be an acute, inflammatory monoarthritis, abrupt in onset, but short-lived, often affecting the bunion joint of the great toe. Chronicity is important. For example, either rubella, parvovirus B19, or hepatitis B can present with a symmetrical polyarthritis of large and small joints that mimics RA. However, the short duration of the joint symptoms, the accompanying skin lesions, and the abbreviated course are distinguishing features.

Inflammatory polyarthritis has many causes[61]. In some situations, such as RA, the joint disease is the dominant feature, whereas in others it is only one manifestation of a systemic process. Examples might include hemophilic arthropathy, hemochromatotic joint disease, or familial Mediterranean fever. Prominent among the chronic diseases that mimic RA are the connective tissue disorders, especially systemic lupus erythematosus (SLE). In general the less destructive joint disease and the associated systemic features—distinctive skin rashes, serositis, hematological and renal abnormalities—point the way to the correct diagnosis. Likewise, scleroderma in its fully developed form with thick skin, Raynaud's phenomenon, sclerodactylia, telangectasias, and esophageal and gastrointestinal disturbance are easily recognized, but these features may only become evident after an antecedent inflammatory polyarthritis of the hands. When confronted by a patient with a chronic, inflammatory polyarthritis, examine the skin for palpable purpura, which may be the clue to a hypersensivity angiitis or cryoglobulinemia complicating a hepatitis C infection. The painful, red, pretibial lesions of erythema nodosum are associated with arthritis and are seen in a number of systemic conditions, such as sarcoidosis, some fungal infections, and inflammatory bowel disease. Erythema chronicum migrans is the hallmark of Lyme arthritis. Clubbed fingers or inflamed ears should alert the physician to hypertrophic osteoarthropathy and polychondritis, respectively.

The seronegative (RF) spondyloarthropathies, as the name implies, are a group of diseases that have in common arthritis of the axial skeleton and an asymmetrical inflammatory, destructive, oligo- or polyarthritis that favors the large joints of the lower extremities. Sacroiliitis and inflammation of the apophyseal joints of the lumbar, thoracic, and cervical spine are distinguishing features. Synovial histology is similar to RA, but the spondyloarthropathies share another attribute, namely inflammation at the site of insertions of ligaments and tendons (enthesitis) into bone, especially the Achilles tendon and plantar fascia, which makes it appear that the joint is involved beyond its synovial attachments. These entities have a distinct epidemiology and family history. Men are more often afflicted than women, rheumatoid factor serology is negative, and there is a strong association with the class I major histocompatibility gene HLA B27[63,64]. Members of this group include patients with Reiter's disease, reactive arthritis, various forms of inflammatory bowel disease, and a greater than expected number of patients with psoriasis. Iritis complicates 20% of cases[65]. A classical symptom is deep aching pain in the lower back that awakens the patient from sleep in the early morning. Arising and stretching briefly allows a return to sleep[66].

In addition to spondylitis, patients with psoriatic skin lesions can have either a symmetrical seronegative (RF) polyarthritis that mimics RA, or an asymmetrical oligoarthritis that favors lower extremity joints, or rarely, a severely destructive polyarthritis. A distinguishing feature of each is DIP joint disease. Almost invariably the contiguous nail shows psoriatic changes, which distinguishes it from the inflammatory (erosive) form of generalized osteoarthritis (GOA)[67]. Periostitis, a characteristic radiographic appearance, is often seen along the shaft of digits and has its counterpart in the beefy swollen toes ('dactylitis' or 'sausage digits') noted in patients with either Reiter's disease or psoriatic arthritis, and less frequently with enteropathic joint disease.

Variants of rheumatoid arthritis

In 1987 the American College of Rheumatology proposed criteria for the diagnosis Of RA (Table 18.1). These criteria are most useful for categorizing patients in epidemiological studies or drug trials; they are of less help in individual cases, especially at or near the disease inception. According to these criteria 65–80% of patients have a classical, seropositive (for RF) form of RA. After careful exclusion of other confounding rheumatic diseases the remainder are designated seronegative RA. Generally these patients have a milder disease and a better outcome (68). In addition, several other conditions are probably variants of RA.

Elderly onset rheumatoid arthritis

Although RA can begin at any age, the peak incidence is in the fifth and sixth decades of life. There are, however, a small number of patients, usually men, whose disease starts in their 60s or later[69]. Their arthritis is often abrupt in onset and constitutional symptoms are prominent. Frequently the large joints, especially the shoulders, are involved, resulting in a confusion with either PMR or RS3PE (see below), The presence of RF and the HLA-DR 'susceptibility' haplotype confirms the diagnosis of RA, but half the subjects lack these findings[70,71]. In their absence the condition is milder, the incidence and extent of radiographic abnormalities is less, and joint disease is very responsive to corticosteroid therapy. Whether this seronegative condition is really RA remains moot.

Felty's syndrome

The combination of splenomegaly, leukopenia, and RA, usually in patients with the HLA-DR 'susceptibility haplotype', is called Felty's syndrome. Additional features include skin hyperpigmentation, chronic leg ulcers, thrombocytopenia, and positive antinuclear antibody (ANA) tests[72,73]. Leukopenia is a misnomer because the hematologic condition is really a profound neutropenia. As a consequence, susceptibility to infection is common. Multiple causes for the hematologic findings have been advocated[74]. A typical patient with Felty's syndrome has long-standing, seropositive, nodular RA and destructive joint disease. During periods of neutropenia, however, the arthritis often becomes quiescent. Methotrexate treatment usually succeeds in elevating the white blood cell count. Responses to colony-stimulating factors (G-CSF and GM-CSF) are robust, but usually short-lived,

and joint inflammation returns in response to a rising neutrophil count. Splenectomy quickly increases the neutrophil count, which is sustained in 75% of patients[75].

A chronic T cell lymphoproliferative disorder with circulating large granular lymphocytes, neutropenia, and splenomegaly has been described[76,77]. Approximately 25–50% of these patients also have RA; some consider this entity a variant of Felty's syndrome.

Sjogren's syndrome (kerato-conjunctivitis sicca)

The classical signs and symptoms of Sjogren's syndrome (Fig. 18.7) include dry eyes, dry mucous membranes of the mouth, respiratory tract, and vagina, and enlargement of the parotid and submaxillary glands[78]. Small lip biopsies allow evaluation of the minor salivary glands and show multifocal, predominantly periductal, dense lymphocytic (CD4 T cells) infiltration, hyperplasia of ductal lining cells, and acinar atrophy[79]. Similar changes are seen in lacrimal, salivary, and exocrine glands. Common ocular symptoms are a foreign body sensation (gritty feeling), diminished tearing, conjunctival inflammation, and photosensitivity. Slit lamp examination discloses a filamentary keratitis and Shirmer's test reveals decreased lacrimation. Salivary gland insufficiency is manifest as xerostomia (a need to drink large amounts of water at meals or during the night), difficulty in chewing, dysphagia, ulcerations of the tongue, and rampant dental caries. Spicy foods or sour candies cause pain in the parotid glands. Diminished salivary gland flow rates, contrast sialography, or technetium scans are employed to confirm xerostomia.

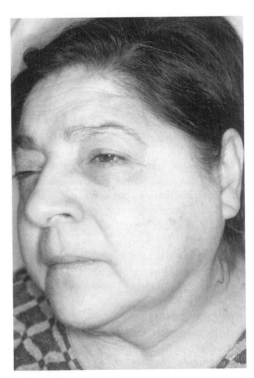

Fig. 18.7 Sjogren's syndrome. The inflamed eyes and the puffy, matted appearance of the eyelids are characteristic, as is the parotid gland enlargement.

Patients with Sjogren's syndrome are usually middle-aged women. Approximately half have RA or another connective tissue disease, but only 10–15% of patients with RA have Sjogren's. The remainder have a primary condition that represents an autoimmune exocrine glandopathy[80]. Primary Sjogren's is often associated with a mild, non-destructive polyarthritis, renal tubular acidosis, peripheral and central nervous system complaints, and lymphoproliferative disorders[81]. The latter range from focal salivary gland lymphocytic infiltrations, to widespread lymphadenopathy ('pseudolymphoma'), to a malignant lymphoma [82]. Waldenstom's macroglobulinemia may supervene.

Laboratory findings include diffuse hypergammaglobulinemia, most marked in primary Sjogren's, and autoantibodies including RF (>90%) antinuclear antibodies, and antibodies to thyroglobulin, salivary duct, or extractable nuclear antigens in about 50% of cases. Two common Sjogren's autoantibodies, called Ro/SS-A and La/SSB, are directed against ribonuclear antigens. These are detected in about 50% of cases, but are also found in other connective tissue diseases, especially SLE.

Palindromic rheumatism

Palindromes are words or sentences that read the same forward or backward. Palindromic rheumatism describes recurrent, afebrile episodes of acute pauci-arthritis that last hours to a few days, then clear without leaving residua, only to return again within the following six months[83]. Pain is sometimes severe enough to confine the patient to bed. Symptoms recur in an irregular fashion, without any identifiable cause. Any joint can be involved; most often the MCPs, PIPs, and wrists. Marked soft tissue swelling, resembling angioedema, sometimes accompanies the attacks and occasionally pea-sized nodules develop over tendons and in the thumb pad. Histological examination of the nodules shows non-specific changes without the characteristic central fibrinoid necrosis and palisading mononuclear cells seen in classical rheumatoid nodules[31]. Men and women are equally affected and the disease usually begins between the third and sixth decades of life. No laboratory abnormalities are found during attacks, other than an elevated ESR. Tests for RF become positive over time in about one-third of individuals. A review of the literature[84] suggests that at long-term follow-up a third of patients develop a chronic arthritis, indistinguishable from RA; half continue with palindromes; 15% go into remission, and a few develop other conditions. There are no HLA associations and no markers that predict the outcome.

Remitting seronegative symmetrical synovitis (RS3) with pitting edema (PE)

An inflammatory arthritis that develops abruptly in elderly (>50 years) males associated with marked swelling of the dorsum of the hands and wrists and flexor tenosynovitis, together with pitting edema of the feet and ankles was described by McCarty with the acronym RS3PE[85]. In general, the arthritis responds well to small doses of prednisone (<7.5 mg/day) or a combination of hydroxychloroquine and non-steroidal anti-inflammatory drugs (NSAIDs). Tests for RF are negative and radiographs show no bone erosions. Except for the few patients whose symptoms are part of a paraneoplastic syndrome, the prognosis is excellent[86]. The disease usually clears by one year. Mild residual flexion contractures of the fingers are common.

Adult-onset Still's disease (AOSD)

George Still described a severe form of arthritis accompanied by systemic features in young children[87]. Manifestations of this systemic-onset form of juvenile rheumatoid arthritis include once (quotidian) or twice daily high spiking fevers (up to 40°C), occurring most often in the early evening; a characteristic 'salmon pink', evanescent skin rash, that usually erupts during the temperature elevations; and serositis, lymphadenopathy, hepato-splenomegaly, and leukocytosis (>20 000/mm³). Bywaters recognized that the same features are occasionally seen in adults (AOSD), frequently presenting as a fever of unknown origin[88]. Mainly large joints are involved. Sore throat is a characteristic clinical feature and anemia, a high white blood cell count, and abnormal liver function tests are the rule[89,90]. Very high serum ferritin levels (>1000 ng/L) are detected in most AOSD patients, unlike what is found in any other form of inflammatory arthritis[91]. ANA and RF tests are seldom (<10%) positive. The outcome is highly variable although this entity may respond to anti-cytokine therapy.

References

1. Gabriel, S. E., Crowson, C. S., and O'Fallon, W. M. The epidemiology of rheumatoid arthritis in Rochester, Minnesota, 1955–1985. *Arthritis Rheum* 1999; **42**: 415–20.
2. Hailwood, S. J., Barrett, E. M., Symmons, D. P. M., and Scott, D. G. I. Extra articular features of early rheumatoid arthritis in a community based population. *Brit J Rheumatol* 1998; **37** (Suppl. 1): 102. [Abstract.]
3. Silman, A., and Hochberg, M. C. *Epidemiology of the rheumatic diseases*, 2nd edn. New York: Oxford University Press; 2001.
4. Hazes, J. M., Hayton, R., and Silman, A. J. A reevaluation of the symptom of morning stiffness. *J Rheumatol* 1993; **20**: 1138–42.
5. Bellamy, N., Sothern, R. B., Campbell, J., and Buchanan, W. W. Circadian rhythm in pain, stiffness, and manual dexterity in rheumatoid arthritis: relation between discomfort and disability. *Ann Rheum Dis* 1991; **50**: 243–8.
6. Luukkainen, R., Isomaki, H., and Kajander, A. Prognostic value of the type of onset of rheumatoid arthritis. *Ann Rheum Dis* 1983; **42**: 274–5.
7. Wolfe, F., and Hawley, D. J. Remission in rheumatoid arthritis. *J Rheumatol* 1985; **12**: 245–52.
8. Eberhardt, K. B., Rydgren, L. C., Pettersson, H., and Wollheim, F. A. Early rheumatoid arthritis: onset, course, and outcome over 2 years. *Rheumatol Int* 1990; **10**: 135–42.
9. Buchanan, W. W., and Tugwell, P. Traditional assessments of articular diseases. *Clin Rheum Dis* 1983; **9**: 515–29.
10. Leicht, M. J., Harrington, T. M., and Davis, D. E. Cricoarytenoid arthritis: a cause of laryngeal obstruction. *Ann Emerg Med* 1987; **16**: 885–8.
11. Lawry, G. V., Finerman, M. L., Hanafee, W. N., Mancuso, A. A., Fan, P. T., and Bluestone, R. Laryngeal involvement in rheumatoid arthritis: a clinical, laryngoscopic, and computerized tomographic study. *Arthritis Rheum* 1984; **27**: 873–82.
12. Grahame, R. Examination of the patient. In *Rheumatology*, 2nd edn (Klippel J. H., and Dieppe, P. A. eds), pp. 2.1–2.16. New York: Mosby; 1998.

13. El Gabalawy, H. Evaluation of the patient: history and physical examination. In *Primer of the rheumatic diseases*, 12th edn (Klippel J. H., ed.), p. 25. Atlanta: Arthritis Foundation; 2001.

14. Katz, R. S., Zizic, T. M., Arnold, W. P., and Stevens, M. B. The pseudothrombophlebitis syndrome. *Medicine (Baltimore)* 1977; 56: 151–64.

15. Paimela, L., Laasonen, L., Kankaanpaa, E., and Leirisalo-Repo, M. Progression of cervical spine changes in patients with early rheumatoid arthritis. *J Rheumatol* 1997; 24: 1280–4.

16. Pekin, T. J., and Zvaifler, N. J. Navicular displacement in rheumatoid arthritis: its recognition and significance. *Arthritis Rheum* 1963; 6: 292. [Abstract.]

17. Smith, E. M., Juvinall, R. C., Bender, L. F., and Pearson, J. R. Flexor forces and rheumatoid metacarpophalangeal deformity: clinical implications. *JAMA* 1966; 198: 130–4.

18. Di Benedetto, M. R., Lubbers, L. M., and Coleman, C. R. Relationship between radial inclination angle and ulnar deviation of the fingers. *J Hand Surg [Am]* 1991; 16: 36–9.

19. Neer, C. S. Impingement lesions. *Clin Orthop* 1983; 2: 70–7.

20. Spiegel, T. M., and Spiegel, J. S. Rheumatoid arthritis in the foot and ankle: diagnosis, pathology, and treatment. The relationship between foot and ankle deformity and disease duration in 50 patients. *Foot Ankle* 1982; 2: 318–24.

21. Michelson, J., Easley, M., Wigley, F. M., and Hellmann, D. Posterior tibial tendon dysfunction in rheumatoid arthritis. *Foot Ankle Int* 1995; 16: 156–61.

22. Rasker, J. J., and Cosh, J. A. Radiological study of cervical spine and hand in patients with rheumatoid arthritis of 15 years' duration: an assessment of the effects of corticosteroid treatment. *Ann Rheum Dis* 1978; 37: 529–35.

23. Komusi, T., Munro, T., and Harth, M. Radiologic review: the rheumatoid cervical spine. *Semin Arthritis Rheum* 1985; 14: 187–95.

24. Kauppi, M., Sakaguchi, M., Konttinen, Y. T., Hamalainen M., and Hakala M. Pathogenetic mechanism and prevalence of the stable atlantoaxial subluxation in rheumatoid arthritis. *J Rheumatol* 1996; 23: 831–4.

25. Meyers, K. A. E., Cats, A., Kremer, H. P. H., Luijendijk, W., Onulec, G. J., and Thomser, R. T. Cervival myelopathy in rheumatoid arthritis. *Clin Exp Rheumatol* 1980; 2: 239–45.

26. Reijnierse, M., Bloem, J. L., Dijkmans, B. A. *et al.* The cervical spine in rheumatoid arthritis: relationship between neurologic signs and morphology of MR imaging and radiographs. *Skeletal Radiol* 1996; 25: 113–18.

27. Breedveld, F. C., Algra, P. R., Vielvoye, C. J., and Cats, A. Magnetic resonance imaging in the evaluation of patients with rheumatoid arthritis and subluxations of the cervical spine. *Arthritis Rheum* 1987; 30: 624–9.

28. Casey, A. T., Crockard, H. A., Geddes, J. F., and Stevens, J. Vertical translocation: the enigma of the disappearing atlantodens interval in patients with myelopathy and rheumatoid arthritis. Part I. Clinical, radiological, and neuropathological features. *J Neurosurg* 1997; 87: 856–62.

29. Crockard, H. A., Essigman, W. K., Stevens, J. M., Pozo, J. L., Ransford, A. O., and Kendall, B. E. Surgical treatment of cervical cord compression in rheumatoid arthritis. *Ann Rheum Dis* 1985; 44: 809–16.

30. Ziff, M. The rheumatoid nodule. *Arthritis Rheum* 1990; 33: 761–7.

31. Stevens, M. B. Rheumatoid nodules. In *Rheumatoid arthritis etiology, diagnosis, management* (Utsinger, P. D., Zvaifler, N. J., Ehrlich, G. E., eds), pp. 487–94. Philadelphia: Lipincott; 1985.

32. Ginsberg, M. H., Genant, H. K., Yu, T. F., and McCarty, D. J. Rheumatoid nodulosis: an unusual variant of rheumatoid disease. *Arthritis Rheum* 1975; 18: 49–58.

33. Kerstens, P. J., Boerbooms, A. M., Jeurissen, M. E., Fast, J. H., Assmann, K. J., and van de Putte, L. B. Accelerated nodulosis during low dose methotrexate therapy for rheumatoid arthritis: an analysis of ten cases. *J Rheumatol* 1992; 19: 867–71.

34. Arend, W. P. Cytokines and cellular interactions in inflammatory arthritis. *J Clin Invest* 2001; 107: 1081–2.

35. Saag, K. G., Kolluri, S., Koehnke, R. K. *et al.* Rheumatoid arthritis lung disease: determinants of radiographic and physiologic abnormalities. *Arthritis Rheum* 1996; 39: 1711–19.

36. McGavin, D. D., Williamson, J., Forrester, J. V. *et al.* Episcleritis and scleritis: a study of their clinical manifestations and association with rheumatoid arthritis. *Br J Ophthalmol* 1976; 60: 192–226.

37. Watts, R. A., Carruthers, D. M., and Scott, D. G. Isolated nail fold vasculitis in rheumatoid arthritis. *Ann Rheum Dis* 1995; 54: 927–9.

38. Scott, D. G., Bacon, P. A., and Tribe, C. R. Systemic rheumatoid vasculitis: a clinical and laboratory study of 50 cases. *Medicine (Baltimore)* 1981; 60: 288–97.

39. Voskuyl, A. E., Zwinderman, A. H., Westedt, M. L., Vandenbroucke, J. P., Breedveld, F. C., and Hazes, J. M. Factors associated with the development of vasculitis in rheumatoid arthritis: results of a case-control study. *Ann Rheum Dis* 1996; 55: 190–2.

40. Weisman, M., and Zvaifler, N. Cryoglobulinemia: significance in serum of patients with rheumatoid arthritis. *J Clin Invest* 1975; 56: 725–39.

41. Vreugdenhil, G., and Swaak, A. J. Anaemia in rheumatoid arthritis: pathogenesis, diagnosis and treatment. *Rheumatol Int* 1990; 9: 243–57.

42. Peeters, H. R., Jongen-Lavrencic, M., Vreugdenhil, G., and Swaak, A. J. Effect of recombinant human erythropoietin on anaemia and disease activity in patients with rheumatoid arthritis and anaemia of chronic disease: a randomized placebo controlled double blind 52 weeks clinical trial. *Ann Rheum Dis* 1996, 55: 739–44.

43. Farr, M., Scott, D. L., Constable, T. J., Hawker, R. J., Hawkins, C. F., and Stuart, J. Thrombocytosis of active rheumatoid disease. *Ann Rheum Dis* 1983; 42: 545–9.

44. Winchester, R. J., Litwin, S. D., and Koffler, D., and Kunkel, H. G. Observations on the eosinophilia of certain patients with rheumatoid arthritis. *Arthritis Rheum* 1971; 14: 650–6.

45. Wolfe, F., and Sharpe, J. T. Radiologic outcome of recent onset. Rheumatoid arthritis: a 19 year study of radiographic progression. *Arthritis Rheum* 1998; 4: 1571–82.

46. Berglin, E., Padyukov, L., Sundin, U. *et al.* A combination of auto-antibodies to cyclic citrullinated peptide (CCP) and HLA-DRB1 locus antigens is strongly associated with future onset of rheumatoid arthritis. *Arthritis Res Ther* 2004; 6: R303–8.

47. Pekin, T. J. Jr., and Zvaifler, N. J. Hemolytic complement in synovial fluid. *J Clin Invest* 1964; 43: 1372–82.

48. Zvaifler, N. J. The immunopathology of joint inflammation in rheumatoid arthritis. *Adv Immunol* 1973; 16: 265–336.

49. Felson, D. T., Anderson, J. J., Boers, M. *et al.* The American College of Rheumatology preliminary core set of disease activity measures for rheumatoid arthritis clinical trials. The Committee on Outcome Measures in Rheumatoid Arthritis Clinical Trials. *Arthritis Rheum* 1993; 36: 729–40.

50. van Riel, P. L. Provisional guidelines for measuring disease activity in clinical trials on rheumatoid arthritis. *Br J Rheumatol* 1992: 31, 793–4.

51. Fries, J. F., Spitz, P., Kraines, R. G., and Holman, H. R. Measurement of patient outcome in arthritis. *Arthritis Rheum* 1980, 23: 137–45.

52. Meenan, R. F., Gertman, P. M., and Mason, J. H. Measuring health status in arthritis: the arthritis impact measurement scales. *Arthritis Rheum* 1980; 23: 146–52.

53. Sharp, J. T., Lidsky, M. D., Collins, L. C., and Moreland, J. Methods of scoring the progression of radiologic changes in rheumatoid arthritis: correlation of radiologic, clinical and laboratory abnormalities. *Arthritis Rheum* 1971; 14: 706–20.

54. Larsen, A. How to apply Larsen score in evaluating radiographs of rheumatoid arthritis in long-term studies. *J Rheumatol* 1995; 22: 1974–5.

55. Short, C. L., Bauer, W., and Reynolds, W. E. *Rheumatoid arthritis*. Cambridge, MA: Harvard University Press; 1957.

56. Persellin, R. H. The effect of pregnancy on rheumatoid arthritis. *Bull Rheum Dis* 1976; 27: 922–7.

57. Voskuyl, A. E., Zwinderman, A. H., Westedt, M. L., Vandenbroucke, J. P., Breedveld, F. C., and Hazes, J. M. The mortality of rheumatoid

vasculitis compared with rheumatoid arthritis. *Arthritis Rheum* 1996; **39**: 266–71.

58. Wolfe, F., Mitchell, D. M., Sibley, J. T. *et al.* The mortality of rheumatoid arthritis. *Arthritis Rheum* 1994; **37**: 481–94.

59. Symmons, D. P., Jones, M. A., Scott, D. L., and Prior, P. Long term mortality outcome in patients with rheumatoid arthritis: early presenters continue to do well. *J Rheumatol* 1998; **25**: 1072–7.

60. Reilly, P. A., Cosh, J. A., Maddison, P. J., Rasker, J. J., and Silman, A. J. Mortality and survival in rheumatoid arthritis: a 25 year prospective study of 100 patients. *Ann Rheum Dis* 1990; **49**: 363–9.

61. Blumberg, B. S., Bunim, J. J., Calkins, E., Pirani, C. L., and Zvaifler, N. J. Nomenclature and classification of arthritis and rheumatism. (Tentative). Accepted by the American Rheumatism Association. *Bull Rheum Dis* 1964; **14**: 339–40.

62. Zvaifler, N. J. Evaluation of joint complaints. In *Internal medicine*, 5th edn (Stein J. H., ed.), pp. 1198–2000. St Louis: Mosby; 1988.

63. Khan, M. A., and van der Linden, S. M. Ankylosing spondylitis and other spondyloarthropathies. *Rheum Dis Clin North Am* 1990; **16**: 551–79.

64. Kellner, H., and Yu, D. The pathogenetic aspects of spondylo-arthropathies from the point of view of HLA-B27. *Rheumatol Int* 1992; **12**: 121–7.

65. Rosenbaum, J. T. Acute anterior uveitis and spondyloarthropathies. *Rheum Dis Clin North Am* 1992; **18**: 143–51.

66. Amor, B., Dougados, M., and Mijiyawa, M. [Criteria of the classification of spondylarthropathies.] French. *Rev Rheum Mal Osteoartic* 1990; **57**: 85–9.

67. Veal, D. S., Rogers, S., and Fitzgerald, O. Classification of clinical subsets in psoriatic arthritis *Brit J Rheumatol* 1994; **33**: 133–8.

68. Mongan, E. S., and Atwater, E. C. A comparison of patients with seropositive and seronegative rheumatoid arthritis. *Med Clin North Am* 1968; **52**: 533–8.

69. Corrigan, A. B., Robinson, R. G., Terenty, T. R. *et al.* Rheumatoid arthritis of the elderly. *BMJ* 1974; **1**: 444–6.

70. Terkeltaub, R. T., Decory, R., and Esdiale, J. An immunogenetic study of older age onset in rheumatoid arthritis. *J Rheumatol* 1984; **11**: 147–52.

71. Pease, C. T., Bhakta, B. B., Devlin, J. *et al.* Does the age of onset of rheumatoid arthritis influence phenotype? A prospective study of outcome and prognostic factors. *Rheumatology (Oxford)* 1999; **38**: 228–34.

72. Rosenstein, E. D., and Kramer, N. Felty's and pseudo-Felty's syndromes. *Semin Arthritis Rheum* 1991; **21**: 129–42.

73. Campion, G., Maddison, P. J., Goulding, N. *et al.* The Felty syndrome: a case-matched study of clinical manifestations and outcome, serologic features, and immunogenetic associations. *Medicine (Baltimore)* 1990; **69**: 69–80.

74. Abdou, N. I. Heterogeneity of bone marrow directed mechanisms in the pathogenesis of the neutropenia of Felty's syndome. *Arthritis Rheum* 1983; **26**: 947–53.

75. Rashba, E. J., Rowe, J. M., and Packman, C. H. Treatment of the neutropenia of Felty syndrome. *Blood Rev* 1996; **10**: 177–84.

76. Starkebaum, G., Loughran, T. P., Jr., Gaur, L. K., Davis, P., and Nepom, B. S. Immunogenetic similarities between patients with Felty's syndrome and those with clonal expansions of large granular lymphocytes in rheumatoid arthritis. *Arthritis Rheum* 1997, **40**: 624–6.

77. Dhodapkar, M. V., Lust, J. A., and Phyliky, R. L. T-cell large granular lymphocytic leukemia and pure red cell aplasia in a patient with type I autoimmune polyendocrinopathy: response to immuno-suppressive therapy. *Mayo Clin Proc* 1994; **69**: 1085–8.

78. Vitali, C., Bombardieri, S., Jonsson, R. *et al.* Classification criteria for Sjogren's syndrome: a revised version of the European criteria proposed by the American-European Consensus Group. *Ann Rheum Dis* 2002; **61**: 554–8.

79. Daniels, T. E., and Fox, P. C. Salivary and oral components of Sjogren's syndrome. *Rheum Dis Clin North Am* 1992; **18**: 571–89.

80. Fox, R. I., Tornwall, J., and Michelson, P. Current issues in the diagnosis and treatment of Sjogren's syndrome. *Curr Opin Rheumatol* 1999; **11**: 364–72.

81. Goules, A., Masouridi, S., Tzioufas, A. G., Ioannidis, J. P., Skopouli, F. N., and Moutsopoulos, H. M. Clinically significant and biopsy-documented renal involvement in primary Sjogren's syndrome. *Medicine (Baltimore)* 2000; **79**: 241–9.

82. Voulgarelis, M., Dafni, U. G., Isenberg, D. A., and Moutsopoulos, H. M. Malignant lymphoma in primary Sjogren's syndrome: a multicenter, retrospective, clinical study by the European Concerted Action on Sjogren's Syndrome. *Arthritis Rheum* 1999; **42**: 1765–72.

83. Hench, P. S. and Rosenberg, E. F. Palandromic rheumatism. *Arch Int Med* 1944; **73**: 293–321.

84. Guerne, P. A., and Weisman, M. H. Palindromic rheumatism: part of or apart from the spectrum of rheumatoid arthritis. *Am J Med* 1992; **93**: 451–60.

85. McCarty, D. J., O'Duffy, J. D., Pearson, L., and Hunter, J. B. Remitting seronegative symmetrical synovitis with pitting edema: RS3PE syndrome. *JAMA* 1985; **254**: 2763–7.

86. Sibilia, J., Friess, S., Schaeverbeke, T. *et al.* Remitting seronegative symmetrical synovitis with pitting edema (RS3PE): a form of paraneoplastic polyarthritis? *J Rheumatol* 1999; **26**: 115–20.

87. Still, G. F. On a form of chronic joint disease in children. *Med Chir Trans* 1897; **80**: 47–50.

88. Bywaters, E. G. L. Still's disease in the adult. *Ann Rheum Dis* 1971; **30**: 121–3.

89. Cassidy, J. T. Miscellaneous conditions associated with arthritis in children. *Pediatr Clin North Am* 1986; **33**: 1033–52.

90. Pouchot, J., Sampalis, J. S., Beaudet, F. *et al.* Adult Still's disease: manifestations, disease course, and outcome in 62 patients. *Medicine (Baltimore)* 1991; **70**: 118–36.

91. Schwarz-Eywill, M., Heilig, B., Bauer, H., Breitbart, A., and Pezzutto, A. Evaluation of serum ferritin as a marker for adult Still's disease activity. *Ann Rheum Dis* 1992; **51**: 683–5.

92. Arnett, F. C., Edworthy, S. M., Bloch, D. A. *et al.* The American Rheumatism Association revised criteria for the classification of rheumatoid arthritis. *Arthritis Rheum* 1988; **31**: 315–24.

19 | *Imaging in rheumatoid arthritis*

Mikkel Østergaard, Marcin Szkudlarek, and Bo Jannik Ejbjerg

Introduction

For decades, imaging in rheumatoid arthritis (RA) has been synonymous with conventional radiography (CR). However, new imaging modalities such as magnetic resonance imaging (MRI) and ultrasonography (US) have dramatically increased the information obtainable by imaging. Concurrently, an explosion in RA drug development and in data on the importance of early aggressive therapy has fueled the search for more efficient approaches than conventional clinical and radiographical methods for diagnosis, monitoring, and prognostication of RA. Of these new approaches, MRI and US appear highly promising.

Possible purposes for using imaging in RA patients include establishing or confirming the diagnosis, determining the extent of disease, monitoring change in disease activity or structural damage, selecting patients for specific therapies (e.g. surgery or injections), identifying complications of the disease or of treatments, and assessing therapeutic efficacy in trials. These entirely different contexts may favor different imaging approaches.

CR, although able to visualize structural joint damage in patients with established disease, is not sensitive in detecting early disease manifestations as soft tissue changes and bone damage at its earliest stages[1-3]. In contrast, MRI and US allow direct visualization of early inflammatory and destructive joint changes in RA[2-6], and may, consequently, be superior objective tools for the detection and monitoring of joint and soft tissue inflammation and bone damage in RA.

This chapter outlines the virtues of CR and describes its current major importance in diagnosis and follow-up of RA, but also stresses that RA management has entered a time of exciting and expanding therapeutic, as well as imaging, possibilities. Imaging of hands, wrists, and feet will be emphasized, because these joints are most frequently involved in RA and, consequently, are generally used in the process of diagnosing and monitoring RA. Aspects of imaging of other peripheral joints, the cervical spine, and extra-articular manifestations are also briefly addressed. For a detailed description of the technical aspects of the different imaging modalities, the reader is kindly referred to textbooks of musculoskeletal radiology[7].

Conventional radiography

Imaging of RA patients almost inevitably starts with CR. CR is the traditional gold standard for assessment of joint damage in RA[1,8], and a key element of RA management in clinical practice as well as trials[9,10].

CR depicts the time-integrated cumulative record of joint damage. Disadvantages of CR include projectional superimposition due to the two-dimensional representation of a three-dimensional pathology, use of ionizing radiation, a relative insensitivity to early bone damage, and a total insufficiency for assessment of soft tissue changes, including synovitis (see details below)[11-13]. However, it is favored by low costs, high availability, possibility of standardization and blinded centralized reading, reasonable reproducibility, and existence of validated assessment methods (see below)[14]. Furthermore, CR is helpful in differentiating from other joint conditions, including osteoarthritis, psoriatic arthritis, and neoplasms[8].

Consequently, high-quality radiographs of properly positioned joints may for several purposes render other imaging approaches superfluous.

Technical aspects

Radiographs of hands, wrists, and forefeet, often supplemented with selected other affected joints, are generally used to determine the radiographic state and/or progression of disease in clinical practice (Figs 19.1 and 19.2)[9]. High-resolution images are best suited to detecting early erosive disease, and appropriate screen–film combinations should be applied, preferably single-emulsion films used with single screens. Ideal are 'rare earth phosphor' screens, which convert X-rays to light more efficiently and, therefore, require less X-ray exposure.

Digital techniques, by which computers develop the image information, have replaced the classical film–screen combination method in many radiological departments. Digital radiography has the disadvantage of having limited resolution compared to conventional films, but allows reduction of radiation exposure, post-imaging-processing (increasing image quality), and easier storage and access to radiographs through PACS (Picture Archiving and Communication System). Available data suggest that the ability to visualize small early erosions is not affected by using digital radiography[15].

Specific guidelines on proper positioning and recommended views when imaging different joints can be found in textbooks of musculoskeletal radiology[7]. As with any bone disorder, appropriate evaluation includes at least two views of the bone involved. For imaging of the RA hand, the posterior–anterior projection

(a)
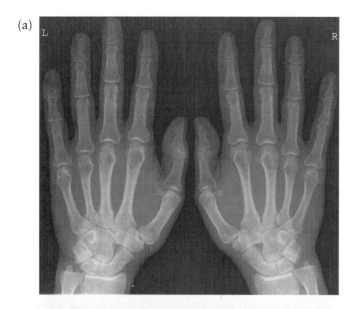

(b)
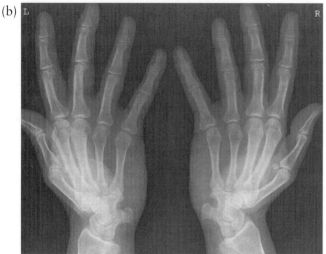

Fig. 19.1　Conventional radiographs of normal hands and wrists, in the (a) posterior–anterior and (b) supinated–oblique (Nørgaard) projections.

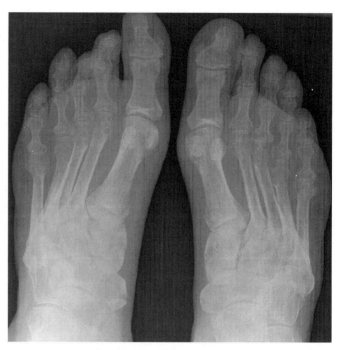

Fig. 19.2　Conventional radiograph of the feet of an RA patient. Advanced RA with joint space narrowing, numerous periarticular cysts, and bone erosions in the bones of the MTP joints.

should be supplemented with a Nørgaard, or supinated-oblique, view (Fig. 19.1)[16].

Radiographic findings in RA

The earliest radiographic changes in the hand are soft tissue changes, such as fusiform swelling around the involved joints, juxta-articular osteoporosis, and erosions of the 'bare' areas of bone, that is, areas without articular cartilage (Fig. 19.3). Traditionally, it was claimed that CR was useful for detection of soft tissue swelling, but comparisons with MRI have shown that CR is insufficient for RA soft tissue assessment[3,12,17,18].

In the course of the disease joint space narrowing, reflecting cartilage loss, and cystic lesions in the subchondral bone are frequently seen. Furthermore, malalignment and subluxation of joints may occur as a result of damage to the tendons, ligaments, and joint capsule (Figs 19.3 and 19.4). Features of secondary osteoarthritis, such as subchondral sclerosis and osteophyte formation, may become prominent (Figs 19.4 and 19.5). Complete destruction of the joint, either with lysis of the bone ends (e.g. 'pencil in a cup' appearance) or fusion of bones (ankylosis) (Fig. 19.3) may occur[18].

Standardization and reliability

In RA routine clinical management and in clinical trials, X-ray evaluation focuses on joint space narrowing and bone erosions[9,19,20]. Validated scoring methods of radiographical damage are available and extensively used in clinical trials[14,19,20]. In early disease, CR status is not related to functional outcome measures like the Health Assessment Questionnaire (HAQ) score, while in established disease (5–8 years' disease duration), the radiographical damage and functional status are statistically significantly correlated (correlation coefficient 0.3–0.5), that is, changes visualized by CR explain ~25% of disability in established RA[21]. It is likely that other structural factors, potentially detectable with other imaging modalities, such as tendon involvement and loosening of the capsule and subsequent subluxation, may also contribute to long-term disability.

Diagnosis

The presence of characteristic radiographic findings is one of the American College of Rheumatology 1987 classification criteria for RA. The criterion is defined as 'Radiographic changes typical of RA on posterior–anterior hand and wrist radiographs, which

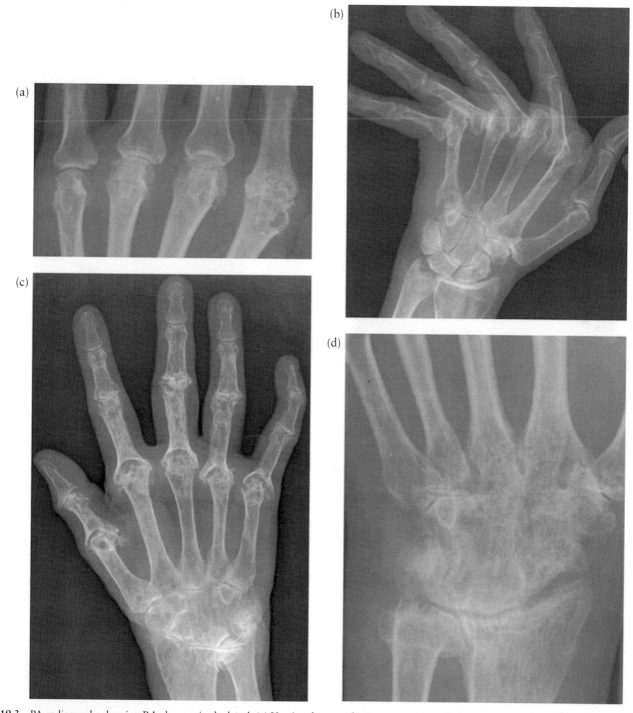

Fig. 19.3 PA-radiographs showing RA changes in the hand. (a) Varying degrees of joint space narrowing, bone erosion, and cystic lesions in the MCP joints. (b) Severe subluxation and ulnar deviation of the MCP joints. (c) Severe MCP joint bone destruction with 'pencil in a cup' appearances. (d) Ankylosis of the carpal bones.

must include erosions or unequivocal bony decalcification localized in or most marked adjacent to the involved joints'[22].

In the differential diagnostic process, the distribution of the involved joints is of major importance. RA can affect most peripheral joints, often with a symmetrical pattern, as well as the temporomandibular joints and the cervical spine. However, the distal interphalangeal (DIP) joints are spared in RA patients, in contrast to patients with psoriatic arthritis and osteoarthritis, while proximal interphalangeal (PIP) and metacarpo-phalangeal (MCP) joints are most frequently involved.

Other differential diagnostic clues are whether new bone formation occurs (or not) and whether synovial, cartilage, or entheseal involvement dominates. In RA there is generally no new bone formation except in the case of secondary osteoarthritis (Fig. 19.4), and synovial rather than entheseal involvement is seen[8].

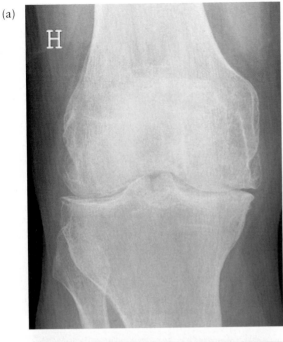

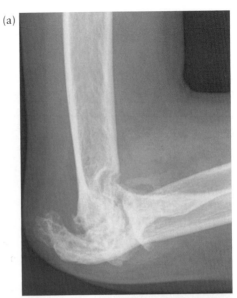

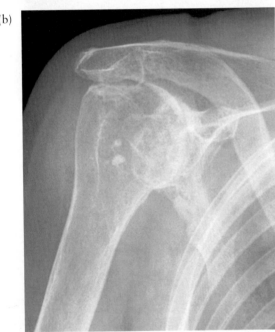

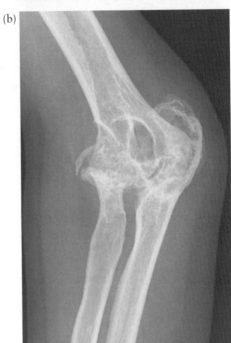

Fig. 19.4 (a) Anteroposterior radiograph of the knee in a patient with RA. Uniform joint space narrowing, generalized halisteresis, and modest secondary osteoarthritis, with marginal osteophytes. (b) Severe glenohumeral involvement in RA with joint space narrowing, secondary subcortical sclerosis, and cystic lesions.

Prognostic value

In RA, early bone erosion is correlated with poor long-term radiographical and functional outcome[23–28], and in early undifferentiated arthritis, presence of radiographic erosion increases the risk of developing persistent arthritis[29]. However, radiographic erosions are only present in a minority of patients with early RA, with prevalences of 8–40% at six months[2,30–33], and X-ray is not

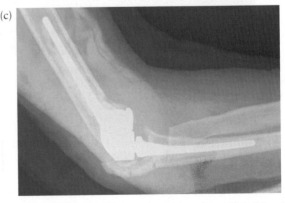

Fig. 19.5 (a) Lateral and (b) anteroposterior radiographs of the elbow showing complete destruction of the elbow. (c) Lateral view of the elbow after total joint replacement.

effective for identifying future 'non-progressors', that is, patients who will not show increasing structural joint damage (see also similar paragraph in the MRI section, below)[34]. Thus, presence of radiographic erosions in early RA is of prognostic value, while their absence is not a reliable predictor of a favorable disease course.

Monitoring of the disease course

In RA routine clinical management and in clinical trials, CR is the main measure of progression of structural joint damage. CR is internationally recommended as obligatory in clinical trials with a duration ≥ 1 year[10]. When CR is used as outcome measure the focus is on joint space narrowing (JSN) and bone erosions[9,19,20]. Validated scoring methods of radiological damage are available and extensively used in clinical trials[14,19,20,35,36]. Whether these scores, or just ascertainment of presence/absence of erosive disease and of 'progression since the last examination', are used in clinical practice varies from department to department, but using a systematic approach should be encouraged.

The Larsen method and its modifications[20,35,37] are mainly based on assessment of bone erosions and involve scoring by comparison with standard reference films, while the Sharp method and its modifications[19,36,38,39] score JSN and bone erosions separately, providing more detailed assessment and a better sensitivity to change at the expense of being considerably more time-consuming[14]. Except the original Larsen score, which also assessed large joints, all these methods evaluate hands and wrists, and some methods also the forefeet. The currently prevailing method, the van der Heijde modification of the Sharp method, scores bone erosions (22 locations, 0–5 in hands/wrists, 0–10 in feet) and JSN (22 locations; 0–4) in hands (MCP, PIP, 1st interphalangeal (IP) joints), wrists and forefeet (metatarso-phalangeal (MTP) and 1st IP), giving a total score range of 0–448[36].

CR has a limited sensitivity to change compared to MRI[11,13,40,41](see below), and in trials it requires a relatively long follow-up period (≥ 6 months) to evaluate therapy effectiveness.

The cervical spine

Cervical spine involvement is common in RA, mainly after several years of disease in rheumatoid factor positive patients with severe peripheral RA, and may cause severe pain, instability, and, ultimately, medullary compression[42–45]. Prevalences of radiological cervical affection of up to 70% have been reported[46,47], but are much lower in recent studies[45,48], in accordance with the fact that intensive disease-modifying anti-rheumatic drug (DMARD) therapy has been shown to reduce cervical radiological progression[48].

Affection of the upper cervical region predominates, although abnormalities throughout the cervical spine are frequent. Upper cervical changes include odontoid process (dens) erosion and atlantoaxial subluxations (anterior, vertical (known as cranial settling), lateral and posterior), while subaxial affections include abnormalities of apophyseal and discovertebral joints, subluxations, and dislocations.

Adequate radiographic evaluation of the cervical spine requires anterior–posterior and lateral views in extension and flexion, and should be performed in all RA patients with neck pain. The latter allows demonstration of atlantoaxial subluxation.

Atlantoaxial subluxation is caused by laxity or rupture of the transverse ligament. The characteristic finding is anterior subluxation (Fig. 19.6), that is, abnormal separation between the anterior arch of the atlas and the odontoid process of the axis. The exact lower limit of abnormal distance is not unambiguously reported, but an abnormal condition must be considered in case the distance is above 2.5 mm, or if the distance changes significantly between extension and flexion[7,49]. Cranial settling is diagnosed by radiographic measurement of the relationship between the tip of the odontoid process and landmarks at the base of the skull[7]. It may lead to protrusion of the dens through the foramen magnum and medullar compression. Significant atlantoaxial subluxations require surgery.

Subaxial involvement (Fig. 19.6) is also frequent, and involves varying degrees of the facet joint bone erosion, joint space narrowing, and subluxation, as well as disc space narrowing and spinous process erosions. Subaxial subluxations may also lead neurological deficits[7].

MRI is useful for gaining supplementary information on cervical spine affection, including spinal cord compression (see MRI section).

(a) 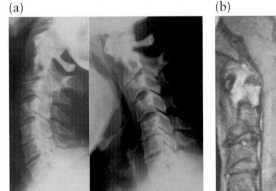 (b) 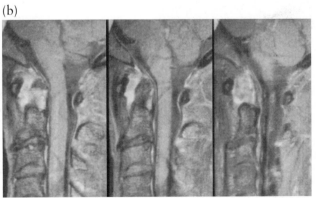 (c)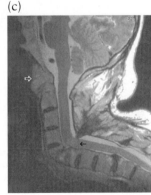

Fig. 19.6 Cervical RA changes. (a) Lateral radiograph in extension and in flexion (*right image*) shows anterior atlantoaxial subluxation with reduced distance between the odontoid process and the posterior arch of the atlas during flexion. (b) Sagittal T1-weighted fat-suppressed MR images after intravenous Gd contrast shows enhancing (vascularized) pannus at the odontoid process, without distortion of the medulla. (c) Sagittal T2-weighted MR image of a patient with C5/C6 instability. Spinal canal narrowing and intramedullar signal alteration (*black arrow*). Pannus is seen anteriorly to the odontoid process (*open arrow*). (Reprinted from Ugeskrift for Laeger 2001; **163**: 6891–6 with permission from Ugeskrift for Laeger.)

(a)

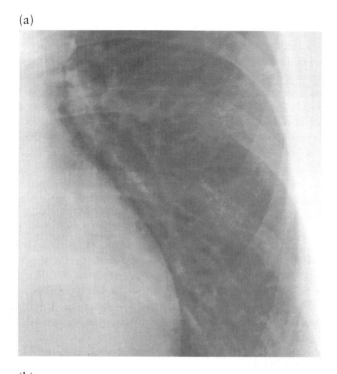

(b)

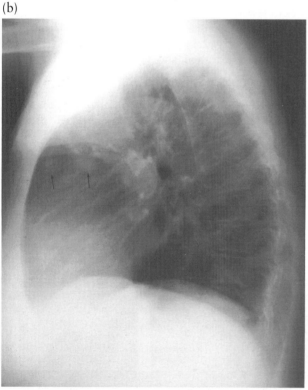

Fig. 19.7 Chest radiographs of two RA patients, (a) Anteroposterior projection shows diffuse interstitial pulmonary fibrosis. (b) Lateral projection shows parenchymal pulmonary nodules (*black arrows*). (Courtesy of Dr Jurik, Department of Radiology, Aarhus Hospital, Denmark.)

Pulmonary involvement

The respiratory system is frequently involved in RA patients[50–53]. As musculoskeletal imaging is the main focus of this chapter, imaging of the lungs will only be briefly addressed. Pulmonary involvement may be related to the disease or to therapy (particularly methotrexate pneumonitis)[54]. CR features of pulmonary involvement in RA include rheumatoid nodules, diffuse interstitial fibrosis, bronchiolitis obliterans organizing pneumonia (BOOP), and pleural inflammation with or without effusion (Fig. 19.7). Conventional chest X-ray is the primary examination, while high-resolution CT (HRCT) is the method of choice for obtaining more detailed information on parenchymal disease[51,53,55].

Practical aspects and future perspectives

Despite the mentioned limitations of the method, the costs, availability, and information value of CR are so favorable that CR will probably remain important for differentiating early RA from other joint conditions, for providing prognostic information, and possibly for monitoring RA progression in clinical practice. If thus employed, repeated assessments, for example every six months in early RA and in case of therapeutic alterations, while thereafter annually, are suggested.

However, for clinical trials and for detailed assessment of disease status and therapeutic response in early RA, it is likely that other imaging methods with a capability of visualizing synovitis and a higher sensitivity to early bone damage will gradually come to be preferred. This is to some extent already the case in proof of concept / phase II trials, while CR is still the only imaging modality accepted by drug approval authorities for registration of reduced structural joint damage in Phase III trials.

Magnetic resonance imaging

MRI allows assessment of all the structures involved in arthritic disease, that is, synovial membrane, intra- and extra-articular fluid collections, cartilage, bone, ligaments, tendons, and tendon sheaths (Figs 19.8–19.10). MRI has been shown to be more sensitive than clinical examination and X-ray for detection of inflammatory (Figs 19.9, 19.10) and destructive (Figs 19.8, 19.10) joint changes in RA[2,4,56–59].

The majority of MRI studies in RA have investigated knee, wrist, and finger joints. While the knee joint is an excellent model joint for methodological studies, the clinical value of MRI is mainly dependent on its power to evaluate wrists, hands, and feet, which are also the primary focus of this chapter. Reports on other peripheral joints are few and not essentially different[60–65]. MRI of the cervical spine is an important issue, addressed below.

For use of MRI in clinical practice, safety, availability, acceptable costs, and acceptable durations of examination and evaluation are required. MRI is very safe. It involves no ionizing radiation or increased risk of malignancies, and allergic reactions to the contrast agents are very rare. Disadvantages of MRI include higher costs and lower availability than radiography, longer examination times, and restriction to evaluation of few joints per session. The time needed to evaluate an MRI examination should also be considered, favoring the quick scoring methods compared to laborious quantitative methods[66].

The mentioned limitations are continuously decreasing. Costs of MRI in general have decreased. Dedicated extremity MRI

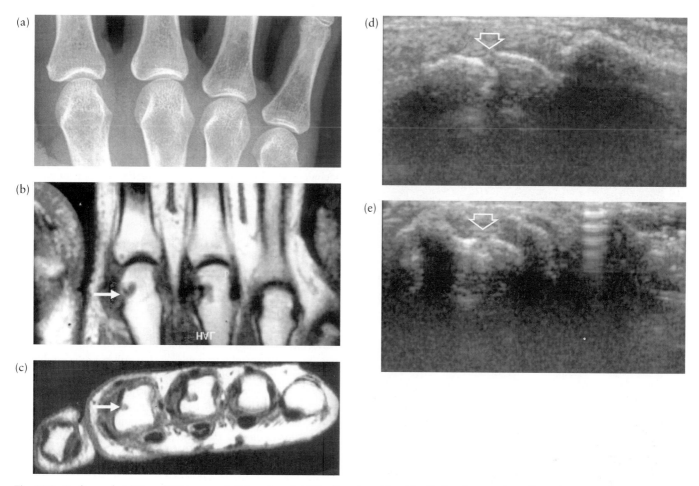

Fig. 19.8 Radiograph, MRI, and US in an early RA patient. (a) CR of hands and feet (the displayed image shows the 2nd to 5th MCP joints) is without arthritic joint changes. (b) Coronal and (c) axial T1-weighted spin echo MRI images show bone erosions in the radial aspect of the 2nd (*arrow*) and the 3rd metacarpal head. US in the (d) longitudinal and (e) transverse planes of the radial aspect of the 2nd metacarpal head demonstrates the same bone erosion as shown on MRI. (Reprinted from *Scand J Rheumatol* 2003; **32**: 63–73 with permission from Taylor & Francis.)

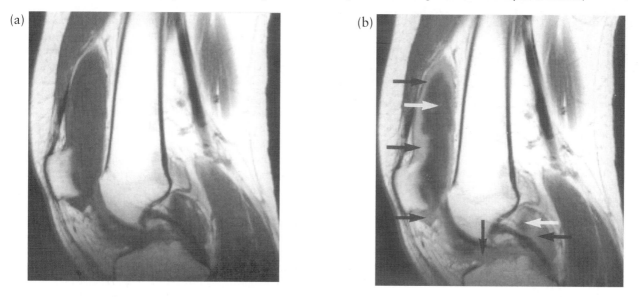

Fig. 19.9 MRI of knee joint of an RA patient. Sagittal T1-weighted spin echo images (a) before and (b) after intravenous Gd contrast, showing synovitis (*black arrows*) and joint effusion (*white arrows*). (Reprinted from Ugeskrift for Laeger 2001; **163**: 6886–90 with permission from Ugeskrift for Laeger.)

(a)
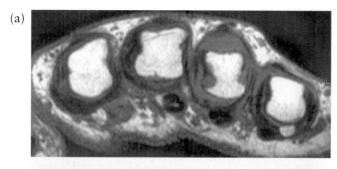

(b)
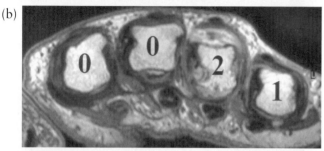

(c)
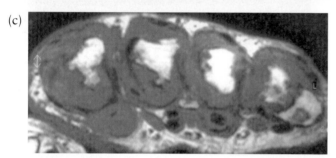

(d)
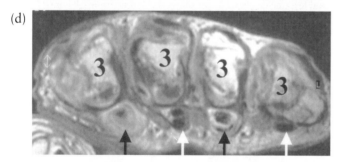

Fig. 19.10 MRI of the 2nd to 5th MCP joints of two RA patients. Axial T1-weighted spin echo images (a, c) before and (b, d) after intravenous Gd contrast. Synovitis scores, according to the OMERACT RA-MRI scoring system synovitis scores are provided. Tenosynovitis is seen at the 2nd and 4th (*black arrows*), but not the 3rd and 5th (*white arrows*) flexor tendon sheaths. (Reprinted from *Scand J Rheumatol* 2003; **32**: 63–73 with permission from Taylor & Francis.)

units, which are increasingly used, involve lower costs and less patient discomfort[5,67–69]. Costs of MRI are only a small fraction of the cost of biological RA treatment or of the indirect costs of sick leaves and early retirements. Thus, as there is evidence that MRI in early RA can help differentiate patients with aggressive disease, allowing targeting of expensive therapies to those with a poor prognosis[40,70–72], the downstream effect of using MRI could be to reduce the overall cost of care for RA patients.

Technical aspects

MRI hardware

MRI of the peripheral joints can be performed with whole-body MRI units or dedicated extremity MRI (E-MRI) units. Most studies have used whole-body MRI-units. Low-field E-MRI units have been commercially available for a few years[5,67,73] and, as machines are getting continuously smaller, transportable units are now available[69], increasing the potential for widespread rheumatological use. The advantages of E-MRI units compared with whole-body units include markedly lower costs, more comfortable patient positioning, and elimination of claustrophobia, a considerable problem in the whole-body units[74]. The disadvantages of E-MRI include a smaller field of view, longer imaging times, and a reduced number of possible imaging techniques compared with the whole-body units. In particular, spectral fat saturation sequences cannot be acquired due to the low field strength (see below).

Available data suggest that some E-MRI units may provide information on synovitis and bone destructions not markedly inferior to what is obtained by standard sequences on high-field units (Fig. 19.11)[5,67,68,73,75], but it should be considered that the performance of different machines may be very different, stressing the need for careful testing[5,67–69]. It is still not fully established to what extent the higher image quality and resolution available with the high-field units allows clinically relevant changes not visualized with E-MRI to be picked up. Nevertheless, the ease and economics, and the potential for examination of more joint regions due to quicker patient repositioning, may compensate for the fewer details from the individual joints[73].

MRI sequence selection

T1-weighted (T1w) imaging sequences are favored by relatively short imaging times, good anatomical detail, and the ability to visualize the inflamed synovium after intravenous contrast (paramagnetic gadolinium compounds, Gd) injection. Accordingly, pre- and post-Gd T1w imaging have been included in the great majority of studies. Fat and Gd-enhanced tissues have a high signal intensity on T1w images, and as Gd uptake depends on tissue vascularity and perfusion, the highly vascularized and perfused inflamed synovium is easily recognizable (Figs 19.9, 19.10).

T2-weighted (T2w) images depict both fat and fluid/edematous tissues with a high signal intensity. These are particularly useful when fat-saturation (FS) techniques, in which the signal from fat is suppressed, are applied. This increases detection of edematous tissue/fluid located in areas with fatty tissue, for example bone marrow edema (Fig. 19.12). On T1w post-Gd images, FS increases the contrast between the inflamed synovium and adjacent structures[76]. This makes inflammatory changes easily recognizable, but whether it truly gives otherwise unachievable information is questionable. FS requires a homogeneous field and a high magnetic field strength[77], not available on low field E-MRI units. The only fat-suppressed sequence possible on E-MRI, the STIR (Short Tau Inversion Recovery) technique, based on relaxation time differences, can provide comparable information on bone marrow edema[75], even though with less detail, and could be used if T2w FS imaging is not available[78].

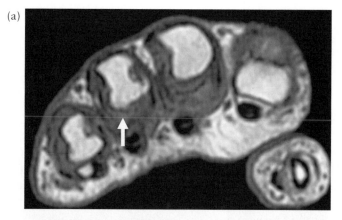

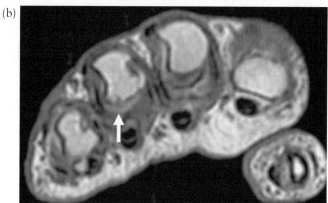

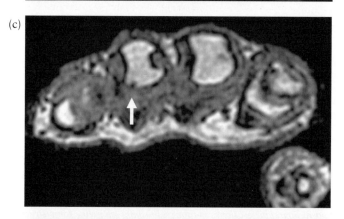

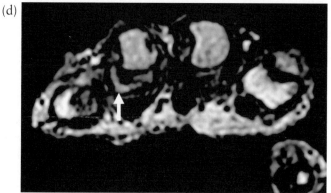

Fig. 19.11 MRI of the 2nd to 5th MCP joints, obtained on high-field and low-field MRI systems. (a, b) High-field and (c, d) low-field axial images of the 2nd to 5th MCP joints, (a, c) before and (b, d) after intravenous contrast injection show low-grade synovitis (arrows) on both MRI systems.

Omitting contrast injection would decrease imaging times and remove the only invasive element. Preliminary data suggest that unenhanced T1w plus T2FS/STIR MRI will give comparable information on erosions and bone edema, but is less accurate on synovitis, when compared to Gd-enhanced MRI (Fig. 19.12)[73,79]. Improved MRI sequences for unenhanced visualization of the synovium have been investigated[79–81]. However, most authors, including the OMERACT-MRI study group (Table 19.1), recommend using Gd-enhanced MRI if detailed assessment of synovitis is considered important[78,82,83]. If fewer details are needed, a T2w FS or STIR sequence is possibly sufficient. However, the clinical significance of the fewer details presumably achieved with unenhanced imaging has not yet been definitively clarified.

MRI findings in RA

Synovitis

MRI allows quantitative as well as less detailed evaluation of synovitis. The inflammatory activity can be estimated by quantifying the early synovial membrane signal intensity increase after intravenous injection of gadolinium contrast[84–87]. Moreover, the volume of inflamed synovial membrane (the 'inflammatory load') can be quantified[12,88–95]. These measures have been shown in knee joints to be closely correlated with histopathological findings[12,84,91,96].

Semiquantitative 'scoring' of synovitis, which is considerably less time-consuming, may replace these quantitative measures, when maximally detailed information is not needed, as the available studies[12,90,94,95] have found a relatively close correlation between the methods. In MCP joints, in early and established RA patients, a close correlation between semiquantitative assessments of synovitis obtained by mini-arthroscopy and MRI has been demonstrated[97].

Changes resembling mild synovitis or small bone erosions are occasionally found in joints of healthy controls[98], stressing the importance of searching for the optimal parameters and cut-offs to differentiate low-grade arthritis from normal.

Bone erosions

MRI detects more bone erosions in early RA than X-ray (Fig. 19.8)[2,4,5,99]. In an established RA follow-up study, 78% of new radiographic erosions could be visualized by MRI 1–5 years (median 2 years) earlier[40]. Bone erosions should be visible in two planes with a cortical break seen in at least one plane to be registered, in order to avoid misinterpretations due to partial volume artifacts[78].

In early RA populations, 45–72% of patients with < 6 months disease duration are reported to have MRI bone erosions[2,5], while corresponding values for CR erosions are 8–40%[2,30–33].

Studies that carry out comparisons with reliable gold standard references are scarce. In MCP joints in early and established RA patients, bone damage as detected by MRI could be confirmed by mini-arthroscopy[97].

(a)   (b)   (c)

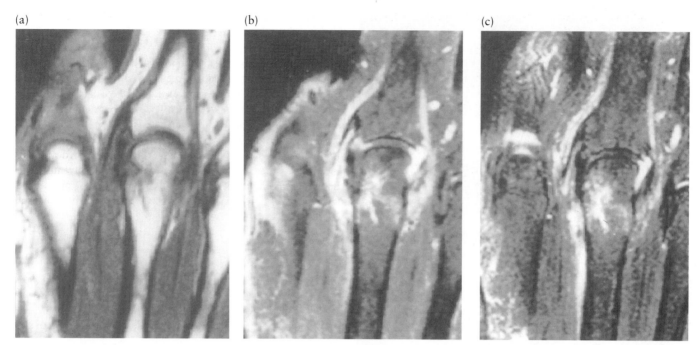

Fig. 19.12 MRI of 2nd and 3rd MCP joints of an RA patient with and without the use of contrast agent. (a) T1-weighted pre-contrast image depicts an erosion in the 3rd metacarpal head. (b) On a post-contrast T1-weighted MRI with fat saturation, the bone marrow signal is eliminated and an increased signal intensity is observed in the synovium (indicating synovitis) as well as in the bone erosion and the adjacent bone marrow (suggesting activity). (c) A pre-contrast T2-weighted fat-saturated image is remarkably similar, suggesting that RA joint pathologies can be assessed without the use of contrast agent. (Reprinted from *Scand J Rheumatol* 2003; **32**: 63–73 with permission from Taylor & Francis.)

Table 19.1   Clinical situations where use of MRI and/or US can be suggested

---

MRI and US
- Suspected, but not certain, inflammatory joint disease, to determine presence or absence of synovitis, tenosynovitis, enthesitis, and/or bone erosions
  Comment: Demonstration/exclusion of joint-related imaging signs of inflammation and/or destruction in patients without a clear clinical presentation may be helpful in ruling out/verifying inflammatory disease and in choosing the follow-up/therapeutic strategy.
- Early, unclassified inflammatory joint disease, to assist in the differential diagnostic process
  Comment: There is no definite evidence on a differential diagnostic value of MRI alone, and no data on US, but some pathologies, which are detectable by MRI and US, are known to be more frequent in some diseases than other (e.g. enthesitis in spondyloarthritides). Thus MRI or US may be a useful element in the diagnostic process.
- Clinically difficult RA cases, to assess disease activity
  Comment: Demonstrating absence or presence of signs of inflammation (MRI or US), and/or erosive progression (MRI), can be useful to confirm/exclude a satisfactory therapeutic response in clinically difficult cases with uncertain disease activity as assessed by conventional methods.

MRI
- Early RA, for prognostication and for establishing baseline for destruction
  Comment: For prognostication in early RA, particularly in patients without radiographic erosions, and for establishing a baseline for destruction, in case the efficacy of therapies or presence of erosive progression need to be assessed at a later time point.

US
- Patients with an indication for puncture of joints, bursae, or tendon sheaths
  Comment: To guide aspirations and injections, when this is considered necessary.

Bone oedema

Presence of MRI signs of increased water content in the bone marrow compartment is frequently detected[11,58,100]. This reversible phenomenon, generally referred to as bone edema, or by some authors as osteitis, even though the exact histological correlate is not known, can be seen alone or surrounding bone erosions (Fig. 19.12). As bone edema has been shown to be associated with subsequent erosive damage, it is considered to be a 'forerunner' of erosions[11,71,100].

Cartilage

Cartilage imaging is another strength of MRI. Direct cartilage visualization is more specific than indirect evaluation by assessing radiographic joint space narrowing. A number of morphological and compositional MRI markers of cartilage integrity have been studied, but almost exclusively in large joints such as the knee[101,102]. The cartilage of small joints is very thin. It can be depicted by MRI[103], but requires high-end equipment and acquisition of pulse sequences that do not delineate synovial and bone abnormalities so well, adding to imaging time, costs, and patient discomfort[104]. Moreover, the optimal cartilage evaluation methods for small joints have not been established. Accordingly, systematic studies of small joint cartilage are not available. Cartilage evaluation is generally not included in the scoring systems of RA hand, wrist, and foot joints.

Enthesitis and tenosynovitis

Enthesitis, that is, inflammation at capsular and ligamentous insertions, is a characteristic feature in seronegative spondyloarthritides[105], but does also occur in RA. Enthesitis is visualized on T2w FS and T1w post-Gd images as local high signal intensity[106–109]. The same is true for tenosynovitis (Fig. 19.10), which is common in RA, but may also occur secondary to other arthritides or as a consequence of overuse[2,4,56,110]. The tendon itself may appear normal, or it may be involved with thickening, irregularity, and/or increased signal intensity within the tendon on T2w and STIR images (tendonitis), or with complete or incomplete tears[110].

Standardization and reliability

Issues of standardization and reliability have been addressed by international initiatives under Outcome Measures in Rheumatoid Arthritis Clinical Trials (OMERACT) and European League Against Rheumatism (EULAR)[78,79,111–113] banners. Consensus MRI definitions of important joint pathologies (synovitis, bone edema, and bone erosion) and a 'core set' of basic' MRI sequences have been suggested[78]. These include imaging in two planes with T1w images before and after intravenous Gd contrast, supplemented with a T2w fat-saturated sequence or, if this is not available, a STIR sequence[78]. Based on data from iterative multicenter studies[78,79,111–113], an OMERACT RA MRI scoring system has been developed for assessment of synovitis, bone erosions, and bone edema in RA hands and wrists (Fig. 19.13)[78]. To improve the consistency of the MRI scoring among different centers and different studies, a EULAR–OMERACT reference image set for the scoring system has recently been developed[114–117]. The atlas enables scoring of MR images for inflammatory and destructive changes guided by standard reference images, similar to the method used for scoring radiographs according to the Larsen method. Validity data, including data on criterion and discriminant validity, are briefly given elsewhere in this chapter, and in more detail elsewhere[66,118].

Diagnosis

The ability of MRI to contribute in the process of diagnosing RA or other inflammatory joint diseases can be divided into two

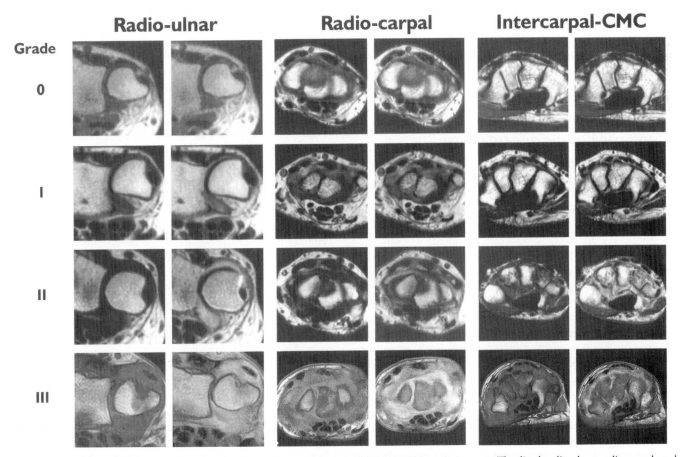

Fig. 19.13 Examples of wrist joint synovitis scores, according to the OMERACT RA-MRI scoring system. The distal radio-ulnar, radio-carpal, and intercarpal-carpometacarpal joint areas are scored separately on a scale from 0 to 3. For each grade, axial T1-weighted images before (*left*) and after (*right*) intravenous contrast injection are shown. (Reprinted from *Best Pract Res Clin Rheumatol* 2004; **18**: 861–79 with permission from Elsevier Ltd.)

fundamentally different aspects: (a) the ability to correctly detect various joint pathologies, for example synovitis or erosions (described above); and (b) the ability to correctly diagnose specific types of arthritides, for example RA or psoriatic arthritis; that is, a differential diagnostic value.

Studies of the ability of MRI to diagnose specific arthritides are few. It has been suggested that incorporation of MRI signs of synovitis in the American College of Rheumatology (ACR) 1987 revised criteria for RA, which are known not to be sufficiently sensitive in early RA[119], would increase their accuracy, leading to an earlier diagnosis of some RA patients[57,120]. Of particular interest, a prospective study of early polyarthritis patients suspected for early RA, which used clinical follow-up diagnoses as the 'gold standard' reference, found that inclusion of the MRI criterion 'bilateral joint enhancement' in the classification tree format of the ACR criteria increased the baseline sensitivity for RA from 77 to 96% and the diagnostic accuracy from 83 to 94%[57].

Early MRI erosions have been suggested as only occurring in patients with RA[4], but MRI bone erosions have also been found in other inflammatory arthritides[3,100] and changes resembling small erosions in healthy controls, too[98].

Small studies have shown that in RA, MRI signs of inflammation are more frequent in the synovial membrane than at the insertions of ligaments and tendons (enthesitis), while the opposite is true for seronegative spondyloarthropathies such as psoriatic arthritis[106–108].

MRI may be valuable in the diagnosis of specific arthritides, including early RA, but its sensitivity, specificity, etc. are not yet known. Even though it will probably never be possible to assign specific diagnoses with MRI alone, the method can be a very useful addition in the differential diagnostic process. Further testing in patients with early suspected or unclassified arthritis is needed.

Monitoring of the disease course

As MRI directly visualizes both the inflammatory and the destructive aspects of arthritic disease with unprecedented detail, it has the potential for accurate monitoring of treatment efficacy.

MRI assessment methods are quantitative (measuring), semi-quantitative (scoring), or qualitative (presence or absence), and the setting and question asked markedly influence which method should be selected[66]. The quantitative synovitis measures (early post-contrast synovial enhancement and synovial membrane volume) are sensitive to therapy-induced changes[85,121–126]. In knee joints, therapy-induced changes are 3–6 times the smallest detectable difference (SDD)[12], documenting that the reproducibility of these measures is sufficient to allow registration of changes in clinically relevant situations[12]. Volumes of erosions can also be estimated[95,127]. Unfortunately, volume quantification is very time-consuming.

Semiquantitative 'scoring' is considerably less time-consuming. The currently best validated scoring system is the OMERACT RA MRI score, which has been developed and tested through international multicenter cooperation[111–113]. A recent study confirms that longitudinal changes in synovitis scores exceed the SDD, that is, the scores are sensitive to change[73]. Good correlations between synovitis volumes and scores, including the OMERACT score,

have been reported[12,94,95]. OMERACT erosion scores and erosion volumes have been shown to correlate closely[95].

Several studies have documented that MRI is also more sensitive than X-ray for monitoring erosive progression in the individual joint region[4,11,13]. This is also true when the reproducibility is taken into account, that is, when only changes above the SDD are considered[73,128]. To be truly superior to CR for monitoring bone destruction in trials and practice, MRI of a number of joint regions feasible for imaging in one session needs to be more sensitive to change in bone destruction than X-rays of both hands, wrists, and forefeet. In a recent study of established RA, MRI of unilateral MCP joints was less sensitive to erosive progression than radiographs of both hands and wrists[128]. Another recent study found MRI of two joint regions (unilateral wrist and MCP joints or both wrists) more sensitive to change than X-rays of both hands, wrists, and forefeet (Sharp/van der Heijde scoring), both with and without adjustment for the SDD[41]. This indicates that MRI of just two joint regions, for example unilateral wrist and MCP joints, is required to improve the sensitivity to change achieved with radiographs of hands, wrists, and feet. The advantage of MRI would be expected to be higher in early RA, but no similar data from early RA patients are available.

Prognostic value

There is solid evidence that MRI findings (synovitis, bone edema, and MRI bone erosions) predict subsequent radiographic erosive progression[11,100,124,124,129]. A study of established RA wrists found a positive predictive value of 80% of high synovial membrane volumes for erosive progression the following year, while the negative predictive value of low volumes was >95%[124]. Accordingly, a recent one-year study of 40 early RA patients found no erosive progression in joints without synovitis[130]. Long-term follow-up studies have reported that MRI bone changes (erosions and/or edema) have prognostic value with respect to the 5–6-year radiographical outcome in established[40] as well as early[71] RA. In a recent study of 114 early RA patients, Tanaka *et al.* found that a high baseline combined score of wrist joint MRI erosions and synovitis was the best predictor (odds ratio 3.59) of severe radiological erosive progression in both hands, wrists, and feet as assessed by the Sharp/van der Heijde method during the next 10 years[131]. Serum-CRP (C-reactive protein) and rheumatoid factor were also significantly correlated to radiological progression, with odds ratios of 2.86 and 2.03, respectively[131]. The paper did not allow separation of the predictive value of MRI bone erosions and synovitis. Also recently, a significant relation between baseline MRI findings and long-term functional disability has been documented for the first time[72].

It is of particular importance to identify the approximately 30% of early RA patients that will not show progressive disease[34,132], in clinical trials (non-progressors dilute statistical power for showing therapeutic effect on structural progression) as well as in clinical practice (non-progressors may not require such aggressive treatment). Paulus *et al.* have found that only 41% of non-progressors can be identified by X-ray at six months[34]. In comparison, McQueen found that 82% of patients without MRI erosions at baseline had no radiographic erosions

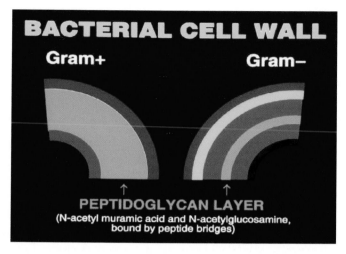

Plate 1 Comparison of Gram-positive and Gram-negative bacterial cell walls. In the Gram-positive cell wall the peptidoglycan consists of up to 70 layers, comprising a continuous net of two alternating amino sugars (N-acetylglucosamine and N-acetylmuramic acid), which are linked to each other by β-1,4-glycosidic bonds. The amino sugar layers are bound to each other by peptides attached to the muramic acid moieties.

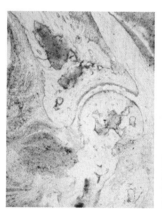

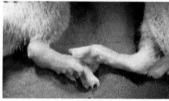

Erosive arthritis in peripheral diarthrodial, cartilagenous joints

Plate 2 Collagen induced arthritis in a DBA/1 mouse. The histology section is from the ankle, showing an inflamed talocrval joint stained with antibodies to MHC class II. The photo demonstrates the clinical occurence of CIA in the hind pain in the mouse to the left.

50-100% DBA/1 males spontaneously develop arthropathy with simlaritis with psoriasis arthritis The disease is enhanced by grouping of several males in each cage

Enthesopathy leading to ankylosis ina a PIP joint

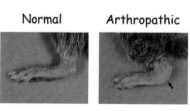

Normal   Arthropathic

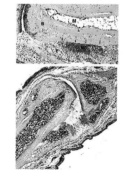

Plate 3 The polygenic control of PIA as determined from genetic segregation analysis of E3×DA crosses. The Pia designation represents the quantitative trait loci controlling different phases of the disease. The Pia4 locus has been identified as controlled by Ncf1 polymorphism.

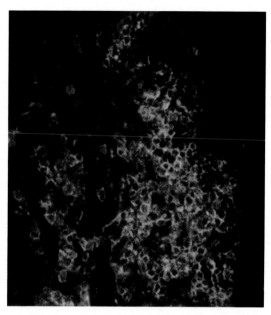

Plate 4 Immunoflourescent micrograph of a frozen section of RA synovial tissue showing a perivascular cluster of T lymphocytes (green fluorescence). The section has been stained with antibody to the CD3 complex, which is associated with the T cell antigen receptor. (Reprinted with permission from Ref. 9).

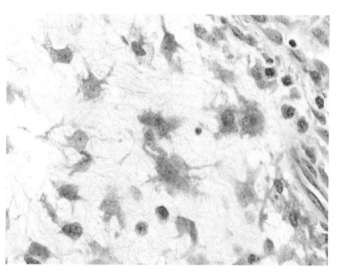

Plate 5 High-power view of a section of fixed, parrafin-embedded synovial tissue, showing T lymphocytes (smaller, rounded cells), in proximity to, and interacting with various antigen-presenting cells, including dendritic cells, macrophages, and fibroblasts. (Reprinted with permission from *Laboratory Investigation* 1995; 73: 334).

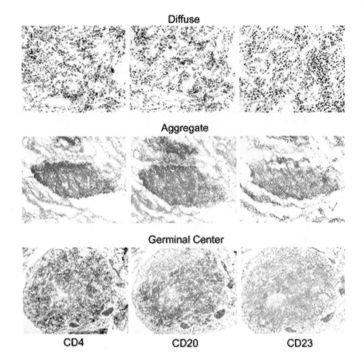

Diffuse

Aggregate

Germinal Center

CD4   CD20   CD23

Plate 6 Range of ectopic lymphoid microstructures in RA synovitis. Serial sections of synovial tissues were stained with anti-CD4 (*left*), anti-CD20 (*center*), or anti-CD23 mAb (*right*). In a subset of patients, T cells and B cells were diffusely distributed throughout the tissue. Other patients formed T cell—B cell aggregates lacking FDCs and GC-like structures reactions. In the third subset of patients, T cell—B cell follicles with GC-like accumulations in the center were identified. Original magnification, ×400 (diffuse), ×200 (aggregate and GC-like). (From Ref. 37, reproduced with permission.)

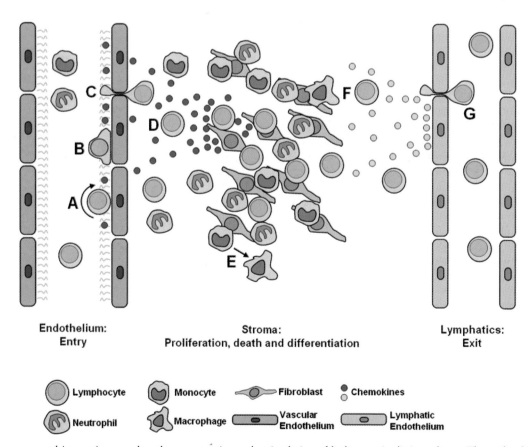

Endothelium: Entry

Stroma: Proliferation, death and differentiation

Lymphatics: Exit

Lymphocyte   Monocyte   Fibroblast   Chemokines

Neutrophil   Macrophage   Vascular Endothelium   Lymphatic Endothelium

Plate 7 Leukocyte–stromal interactions regulate the extravasation and recirculation of leukocytes in distinct phases. The molecular basis by which leukocytes leave the circulation and migrate across endothelium has been well studied; stromal and lymphatic trafficking remain less well understood. (A) Leukocytes are captured by selectin-ligand interactions and roll, sampling the presence of chemokines and other activation markers on the endothelium and associated matrix proteins. (B) Chemokines trigger activation of integrins, enabling firm adhesion. (C) Diapedesis: leukocytes migrate through the endothelial layer. (D) Leukocytes follow chemokine gradients into the tissue stroma. Within the stroma, some cells are destined to die, such as neutrophils. (E) Others such as monocytes may differentiate into cells destined to die, such as macrophages; others may proliferate. (F) Those cells destined to recirculate must change their repertoire of chemokine receptors, following other chemokine gradients towards the lymphatic endothelium and exiting from the tissue towards draining lymph nodes (G). The endothelium regulates entry, the stroma regulates proliferation, survival, and differentiation, and the lymphatics regulate exit.

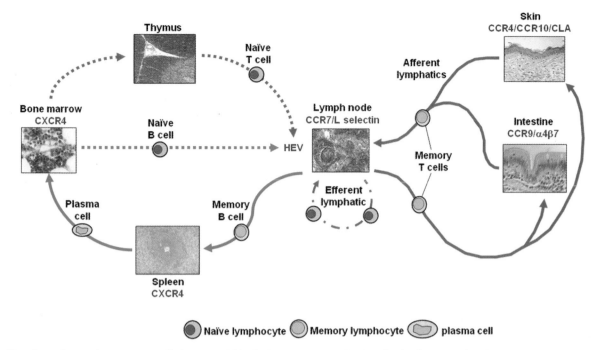

Plate 8 Vascular codes regulate tissue specific homing within the immune system. During the development of an immune response, immature naïve T cells (dotted arrows) and B cells (dotted arrows) that have been educated in the thymus and bone marrow, respectively, enter lymph nodes through HEVs using the endothelial entry code CCR7 and L-selectin. Antigen-experienced B cells leave the lymph node and migrate into specific niches such as the red pulp of the spleen and the bone marrow using the endothelial entry code CXCR4. Antigen-experienced central memory T cells continue to recirculate back to lymph nodes via the efferent lymphatics and thoracic duct. Effector memory T cells preferentially recirculate to the tissue in which they were initially activated; for example if they are activated in a lymph node draining the skin they acquire the skin entry code CCR4/CCR10/CLA and if activated in a lymph node draining the gut they acquire the gut entry code CCR9/$\alpha_4\beta_7$. At the end of immune surveillance within tissues, memory T cells can recirculate back to lymph nodes via the afferent lymphatics.

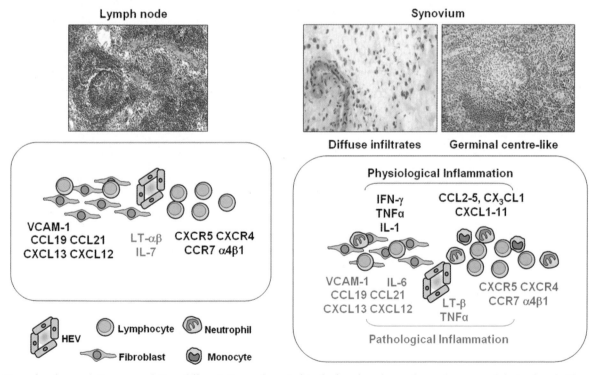

Plate 9 Stromal codes regulating accumulation, differentiation and survival in the lymph node are aberrantly expressed during lymphoid neogenesis in rheumatoid arthritis. Homeostatic chemokines (CXCL12, CXCL13, CCL19, CCL21), adhesion molecules (VCAM-1), and cytokines/growth factors (IL-6, IL-7) are components of the stromal code that help define stromal niches such as the lymph node and bone marrow, governing leukocyte accumulation, differentiation, and survival. Stromal cells produce/express the appropriate cytokine/chemokine/adhesion receptor that is recognized by cognate receptors on infiltrating leukocytes. In the case of the lymph node, structure is developed and maintained as a result of lymphotoxin-α?and -β and IL-7 production by 'inducer' lymphocytes which induce the secretion of constitutive chemokines from stromal 'organizer' cells. During physiological inflammation, inflammatory chemokines (CCL2-CCL5, CX3CL1 and CXCL1-CXCL11 and inflammatory mediators such as IFN-γ, TNF-α, and IL-1 are produced by stromal cells and lead to the recruitment of inflammatory cells (lymphocytes, neutrophils, and monocytes). However, in persistent, pathological inflammation such as occurs in RA, stromal cells begin to aberrantly produce/express components of the physiological stromal code normally associated with lymphoid tissues, leading to lymphoid neogenesis. TNF-α and lymphotoxin-β are important in maintaining lymphoid structures.

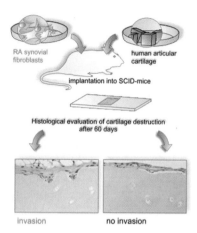

invasion   no invasion

Plate 10 The severe combined immunodeficient (SCID) mouse co-implantation model of rheumatoid cartilage destruction. In this model synovial fibroblasts are implanted together with normal human articular cartilage into SCID mice. Due to their non-functional immune system, these mice do not reject the human implants and allow study of the interaction of the fibroblasts with the cartilage in the absence of continuous stimulation by human inflammatory cells. While implantation of RA synovial fibroblasts results in the progressive destruction of cartilage over 60 days (*bottom left*), normal or OA synovial fibroblasts do not exhibit such destructive phenotype (*bottom right*).

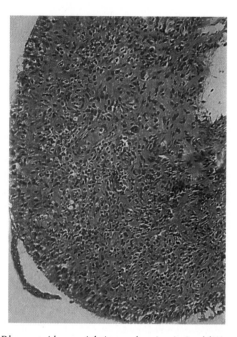

Plate 12 Rheumatoid synovial tissue, showing intimal lining hyperplasia and infiltration of the synovial sublining by mononuclear cells.

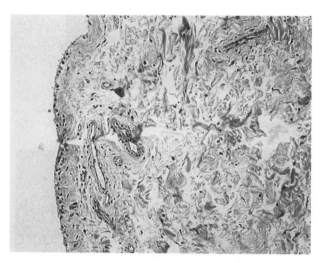

Plate 11 Normal synovial tissue consisting of the intimal lining layer of 1–3 cell layers and the synovial sublining that contains scattered blood vessels, fat cells, and fibroblasts.

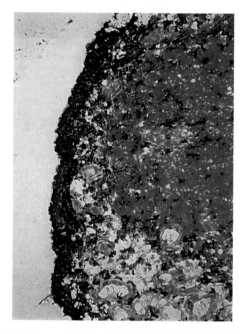

Plate 13 CD68+ macrophages (red-brown) in the intimal lining layer and in the synovial sublining of rheumatoid synovial tissue.

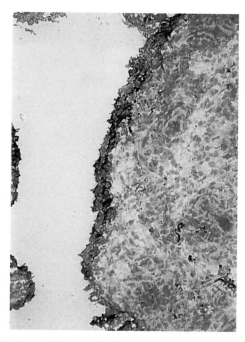

Plate 14 CD55+ fibroblast-like synoviocytes (red-brown) in the intimal lining layer of rheumatoid synovial tissue.

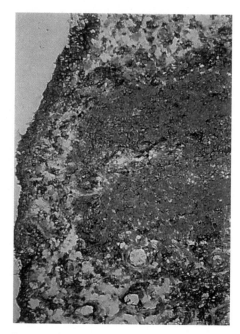

Plate 15 Rheumatoid synovial tissue stained with a monoclonal antibody directed against CD97. Note prominent staining (red-brown) on intimal macrophages and on leukocytes in the synovial sublining.

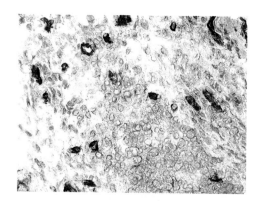

Plate 16 BDCA4+ plasmacytoid dendritic cells in rheumatoid synovial tissue.

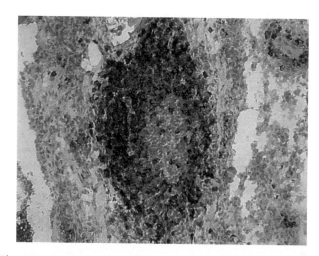

Plate 17 CD22+ B cells (red-brown) in a lymphocyte aggregate in rheumatoid synovial tissue.

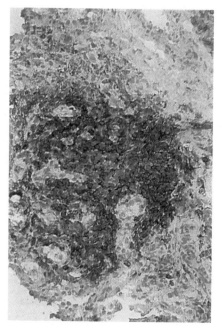

Plate 18 CD4+ (red-brown) in a lymphocyte aggregate in rheumatoid synovial tissue.

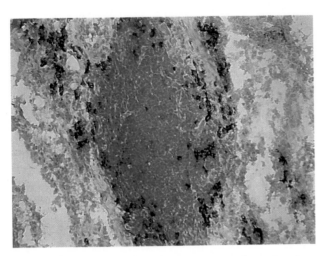

Plate 19 CD38+ plasma cells (red-brown) surrounding a lymphocyte aggregate in rheumatoid synovial tissue.

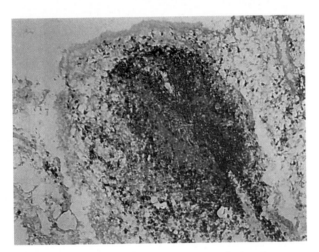

Plate 20 CD3+ T cells (red-brown) in a perivascular lymphocyte aggregate and in the diffuse leukocyte infiltrate in rheumatoid synovial tissue.

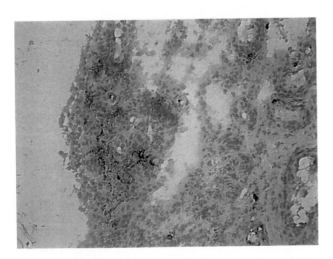

Plate 21 Granzyme B+ cytotoxic cells (red-brown) in rheumatoid synovial tissue.

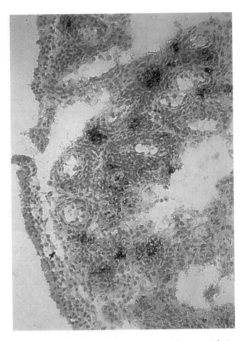

Plate 22 Mast cells (red-brown) in rheumatoid synovial tissue.

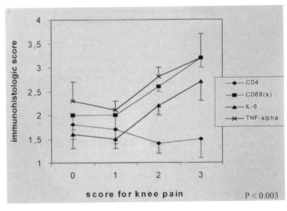

Plate 23 Mean ± SEM semiquantitative scores for the number of CD4+ T cells and CD68+ sublining macrophages and the expression of IL-6 and TNF-α in the synovial tissue of 62 patients with rheumatoid arthritis in relation to the scores for knee pain. (Reproduced with permission from Lippincott Williams & Wilkins; *Arthritis Rheum* 1997, 40: 217–25.)

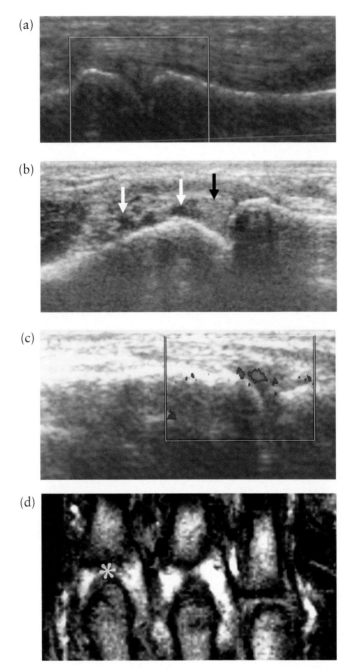

Plate 24   (a) US of a normal 2nd MCP joint, in the longitudinal plane. Power Doppler is applied in the marked rectangle, but no flow is observed. (b) US of the 2nd MCP joint of an RA patient, in the longitudinal plane. Gray-scale US shows synovial membrane thickening (*black arrow*) and joint effusion (*white arrows*). Power Doppler is not applied. (c) US of the 2nd MCP joint of another patient with RA, in the longitudinal plane. Power Doppler signal is visible in the synovium, indicating synovitis. (d) Coronal T1-weighted gradient echo MR image of the same 2nd MCP joint, acquired 50 s after intravenous contrast injection (dynamic MRI) shows, in accordance with US findings, increased signal intensity of the synovium (*asterisk*), indicating synovitis. Synovitis is also seen in the 3rd but not the 4th MCP joint. (Reprinted from *Scand J Rheumatol* 2003; **32**: 63–73 with permission from Taylor & Francis.)

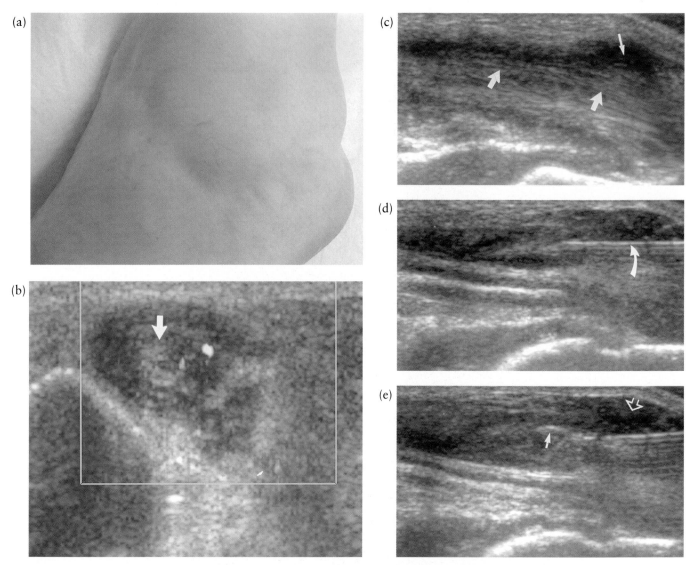

Plate 25 RA patient with tenosynovitis at the peroneous longus tendon. (a) Clinical image shows swelling of the lateral retromalleolar region. (b) US of the tendon (*arrow*), in the transverse plane, which has an irregular contour and a heterogeneous echostructure. Power Doppler signal is shown inside the tendon, indicating tendonitis. The tendon is surrounded by a hypoechoic rim, indicating tenosynovitis. (c–e) US of the same tendon as above, in the longitudinal plane, (c) before and (d) during needle insertion, and (e) during steroid injection in the tendon sheath. The thick arrows point at the tendon, the long thin arrow at the widened tendon sheath, the short arrow at air bubbles injected to verify the position of the needle tip, and the open arrow the increased post-injection fluid volume within the tendon sheath. (Reprinted from *Scand J Rheumatol* 2003; **32**: 63–73 with permission from Taylor & Francis.)

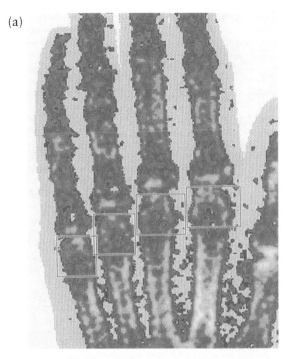

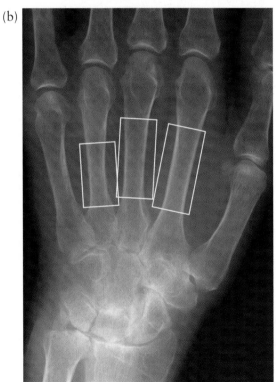

Plate 26 Dual X-ray absorptiometry (DXA) and digital X-ray radiogrammetry (DXR) in a hand of an RA patient. (a) Hand bone densitometry. The BMD measurement is performed in the juxta-articular distal 1.5 cm of the metacarpal bone (*boxes*). (b) DXR. The regions of interest used for calculation of the BMD estimate are shown (*boxes*). In the metacarpals, the cortical thickness is determined on both the radial and ulnar sides. (Courtesy of Dr Jensen, Department of Endocrinology, Copenhagen University Hospital at Hvidovre, Denmark.)

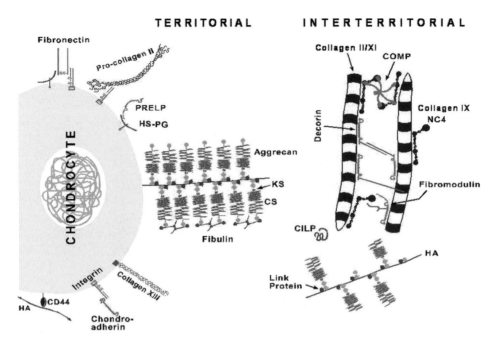

Plate 27 Schematic illustration of the constituents of cartilage matrix. The spatial relationships of the various constituents to the chondrocyte, that is, their presence in the territorial (close to the cell) or interterritorial matrix (furthest away from the cell) are shown and the macromolecular organization of matrix molecules is indicated. CILP, cartilage intermediate layer protein; HA, hyaluronan; KS, keratan sulfate; CS, chondroitin sulfate; PRELP, proline arginine-rich end leucine-rich protein; HS-PG, heparan sulfate proteoglycan.

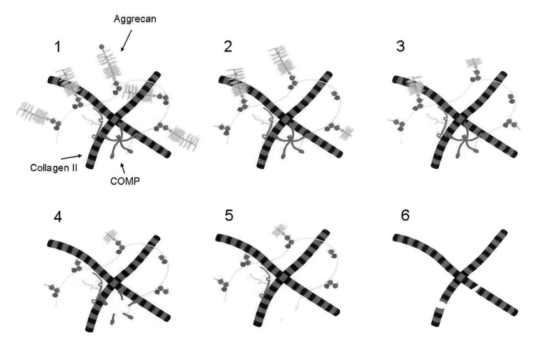

Plate 28 Schematic illustration of a suggested sequence of events in the cartilage matrix during progressive cartilage damage resulting in sequential release of matrix macromolecules. Initially aggrecan molecules are degraded and released. This step is potentially reversible. Then other non-collagenous matrix macromolecules, for example COMP, are fragmented and released. This eventually leads to instability in the collagen network and a step of irreversibility when this network is disrupted and fragments of collagen are being released. At this stage molecules at the cartilage–bone interface, for example bone sialoprotein, may also be released.

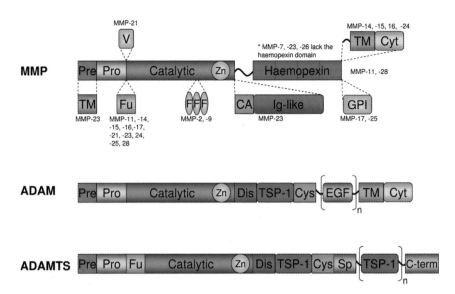

Plate 29 Domain structures of metalloproteinases. MMPs, ADAMs, and ADAMTSs have a domain structure, with several common domains across the family. All have a zinc binding domain and propeptide that preserves latency. Other domains influence the behavior of the protein; the transmembrane (TM) domain anchors the proteinase onto the membrane surface whilst other domains bind to different components of the extracellular matrix. The MMPs were originally classified according to their substrate specificity but are now more commonly grouped according to their domain structure. All MMPs have a catalytic domain containing the active site zinc (Zn). Some MMPs contain a furin recognition motif (Fu) that allows intracellular activation by furin-like proteinases. Apart from MMP -7, -26, and -23, all MMPs contain a hemopexin domain that often determines substrate specificity. Other domains found within the MMPs are the fibronectin-like domains (F) in MMP-2 and -9 and the vitronectin-like domain (v) in MMP-21. Some MMPs are anchored to the cell surface via a TM with cytoplasmic tail (Cyt) or via a GPI anchor. MMP-23 is structurally unique amongst the MMPs and contains an N-terminal TM (actually an N-terminal signal anchor), a cysteine array (CA), and an immunoglobulin-like domain (Ig-like) (adapted from Ref. 10). The ADAMs and ADAMTSs contain a disintegrin and a metalloprotease domain. The metalloprotease domains of ADAMs can induce ectodomain shedding and cleave ECM proteins. The ADAMs disintegrin (Dis) and cysteine-rich (Cys) domains have adhesive activities. All ADAMs contain a TM and their activities may be controlled in part via phosphorylation of their cytoplasmic tails (Cyt). The ADAMTSs uniquely contain a thrombospondin type-1 (TSP-1) repeat, then a Cys domain and one or more additional TSP-1 repeats (except ADAMTS-4). This is frequently followed by a C-terminal domain often containing a recently described protease and lacunin motif[34].

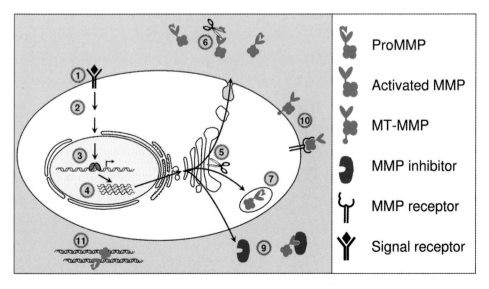

Plate 30 Control of MMP activity. Cytokines and growth factors can up-regulate or down-regulate MMP expression (1). Different intracellular signalling pathways combine (2) to activate or suppress transcription (3). RNA can be unstable and rapidly processed (4). ProMMPs can be activated intracellularly by furin (5) or after they have left the cell (6). Some MMPs are stored in granules within the cell (7) prior to secretion. All active MMPs can be inhibited by TIMPs (9). Secreted MMPs can be expressed on the cell surface, bound to cell surface receptor proteins or sequestered by ECM proteins (10). Other control mechanisms include secretion to specific regions of the plasma membrane, proteolytic processing and inactivation of MMPs, and endocytosis and lysosomal breakdown.

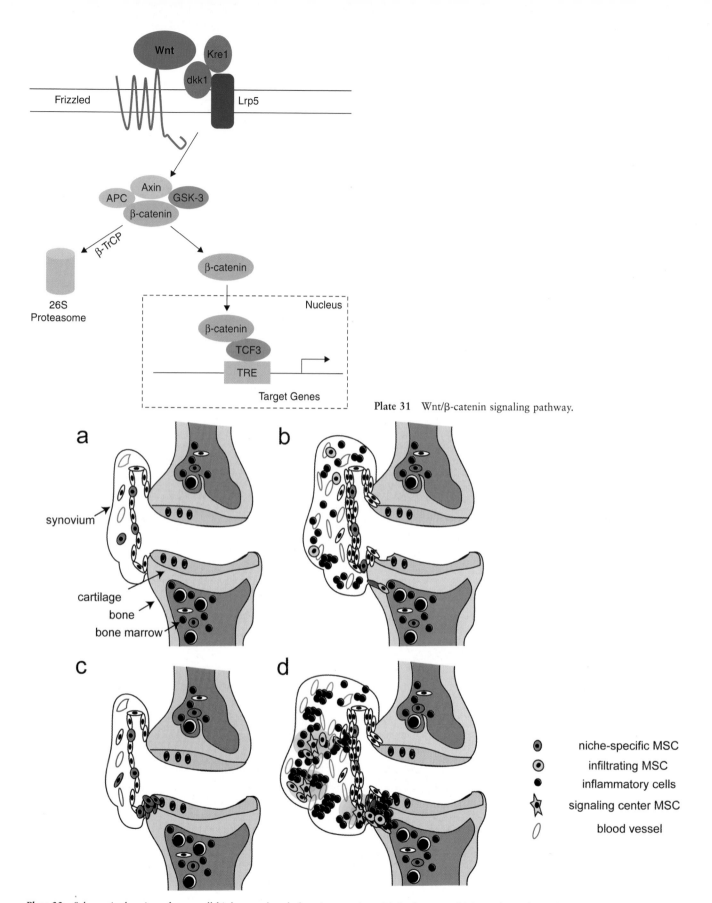

Plate 31 Wnt/β-catenin signaling pathway.

Plate 32 Schematic drawing of stem cell biology and pathology in synovium. (a) In the normal joint, a limited number of 'niche' MSCs are present in the synovial lining, the interstitium, and other joint-associated tissues, as well as the subchondral bone marrow. They contribute to the maintenance of joint homeostasis. (b) Upon joint 'injury', regardless of the type of injury, MSC recruitment (infiltrating MSCs) and proliferation (niche or infiltrating MSCs) takes place, and cell differentiation. This tissue response is considered an attempt to repair. (c) A 'successful' tissue response results in proper tissue repair and the restoration of joint homeostasis. (d) However, this process may go wrong and lead to the accumulation of 'developmental' fibroblasts with MSC characteristics, generated locally by proliferation or recruited from a distance, some of them undergoing a process of dedifferentiation or transdifferentiation. This may induce the formation of new 'signaling centers', creating gradients of signals (e.g. chemokines) attracting inflammatory cells and enhanced angiogenesis. At some point, this becomes an irreversible alteration of the stromal environment, and leads to chronic disease.

at two years' follow-up, that is, were non-progressors. This indicates a superiority of MRI, compared to X-ray, for identifying future non-progressors.

Cervical spine

All joints, tendons, and ligaments of the cervical spine can be involved in RA, leading to spine instability or subluxations (see section on CR—cervical spine, for details). Proliferating pannus (Fig. 19.6)[42,44] from the synovial joints and anatomical malalignments can in turn lead to secondary medullary compression.

The primary imaging modality is CR, but MRI can provide detailed information on bone and soft tissue abnormalities, which can be a valuable supplement to radiographic evaluation (Fig. 19.6)[43,133–138]. MRI is able to directly visualize the pannus tissue, for example around the odontoid process (Fig. 19.6). Cord compression on MRI seems a better predictor for deterioration than initial clinical and plain radiographic features, supporting that MRI is the imaging method of choice for evaluation of spinal cord affection in RA[139].

Practical aspects and future perspectives

Considering the available data on validity and prognostic value, it appears justified to recommend the introduction of MRI on specific indications in the routine clinical management of patients with diagnosed or suspected inflammatory joint diseases. Besides the evident benefit of using MRI for examination of the cervical spine in patients with neurological symptoms, clinical situations, where the use of MRI can be suggested, are mentioned in Table 19.1.

In future clinical practice, MRI may acquire an important role in the differential diagnosis of early unclassified polyarthritis, in the sensitive monitoring of therapeutic response (e.g. quick determination of whether a treatment satisfactorily suppresses joint inflammation or treatment modification is needed), and in the prognostication of patients (e.g. in order to stratify patients to different therapeutic regimens). Physicians who will use MRI may potentially make quicker, more optimal decisions due to the availability of more accurate information.

Ultrasonography

The technological advances of the last two decades have made US a useful imaging method for assessment of RA patients. While acceptable US assessment was previously confined to large joints[140–144], high-frequency linear array transducers now allow high-resolution imaging of such superficially located structures as the joints of hands and feet. US can visualize inflammatory as well as destructive RA changes. Effusion can be detected in joints, bursae, and tendon sheaths. Tendons and ligaments, including inflammation at their insertions (enthesitis), can be evaluated.

The assessment of joints with US is limited by the fact that sound (at the diagnostic frequencies) cannot penetrate bone. Therefore, the weight-bearing surfaces of the joints, as well as structures covered or 'shadowed' by bones, cannot be evaluated.

US holds several advantages. It has low running costs, is patient-friendly, easily accessible, portable, dynamic, interactive with the patient, and quick to perform. The examination involves no ionizing radiation, is multiplanar, and visualizes structures in real-time. Doppler examination provides hemodynamic information on the examined tissue. US enables quick examination of several joints in different body regions at one session and is easy to repeat, making follow-up examinations convenient and comfortable for the patient. There is no known risk associated with the use of diagnostic ultrasound.

Technical aspects

Human hearing operates between 20 Hz and 20 kHz and sounds with a frequency over 20 kHz are called ultrasounds. Imaging with ultrasound is accomplished with a pulse-echo technique. The transducer array of an ultrasound unit both generates the ultrasound pulses and receives the returning echoes from organ boundaries and from within tissues. The ultrasound unit processes the echoes and presents them as visible dots, forming the anatomic image on the screen. The examined areas on B-mode (brightness-modulated) or grey-scale US can be anechoic (echo-free or black), hypoechoic (echo-poor or dark), hyperechoic (echo-rich or bright), or isoechoic (with the same echogenicity as the surrounding tissue).

The diagnostic ultrasound frequencies lie between 2 and 20 MHz. The imaging depth (penetration) decreases with frequency, as attenuation (weakening of sound as it propagates in the tissues) increases with frequency. Higher frequencies provide higher image resolution; because of their limited imaging depth they are only used for superficial applications. Frequencies of 5–7.5 MHz are used for big and/or deep-lying joints and structures, and those above 10 MHz for superficially located structures.

Doppler US operates in accordance with the principle (called the Doppler effect) that there is change in frequency when an emitted ultrasound wave is scattered by moving blood cells. The difference in frequency between the emitted and received ultrasound signal is proportional to the velocity of the scatterers (the blood cells) and can be displayed on the screen with color pixels (color Doppler (CDUS) or power Doppler US (PDUS)). In contrast to CDUS, no information on the direction or velocity of flow is received with PDUS. Movement artefacts are also more frequently recorded. However, at least in theory, PDUS is more sensitive to low volume flow and independent of the insonation angle.

Contrast agents in US, which have gained their place primarily in assessment of vessel and oncological pathology, are liquid suspensions of encapsulated microbubbles administered intravenously, developed to increase echogenicity of the examined vessels or blood-supplied areas. US contrast agents may increase the sensitivity of Doppler US, but also imply considerable additional costs, time, and invasiveness. The future role of US contrast media in early RA, if any, is not yet clear, particularly as both new contrast agents and novel ultrasound equipment with improved flow sensitivities, even without contrast use, and improved B-mode imaging, are being developed. A recent study visualized Doppler signal in healthy joints, illustrating that physiological joint flow can be displayed with high-end units[145].

Three-dimensional US, which until now has mostly been used in obstetrics, is generated by obtaining sequential two-dimensional images over a given volume of tissue and computer-reprocessing the images. The method has a large potential as volume of inflamed tissue, erosions, and vessels may be evaluated quantitatively.

Ultrasonographic findings in RA

Synovitis

US allows assessment of synovitis, both by detection of thickening of the synovial membrane of inflamed joints, bursae, or tendon sheaths by gray-scale US and by Doppler techniques (Figs 19.14, 19.15), in which moving objects, as the blood cells, generate the signal. Doppler US can detect[142,146,147] and potentially quantify[148,149] the increased synovial blood flow occurring in joint inflammation. In knee and hip joints, power Doppler signal has been found to correlate well with the histological assessment of synovial membrane microvascular density[144,150]. No similar data from small joints are available. The high concordance between Doppler US and Gd-enhanced MRI for detection of synovitis in RA wrist and finger joints indicates that both examinations reflect similar physiological phenomena[146,151].

Bone erosions

US has been reported to be more sensitive for visualizing bone erosions in the finger joints than X-ray and comparable to MRI (Fig. 19.8)[3,152]. Recent data indicate similar findings in the MTP joints (Fig. 19.16)[153,154]. Another US, MRI, and CR study, however, found US inferior to MRI for detection and follow-up of erosions in wrists and hands[59]. A marked site-dependency of the US sensitivity for bone erosions has been observed, undoubtedly related to the fact that US cannot penetrate bone. When compared with MRI, US performance is very good in easily accessible joints such as the 2nd and 5th MCP joints and the PIP joints (three or four views possible), slightly lower for the 3rd and 4th MCP joints (where only dorsal and palmar views are available), and poor in anatomically complicated joints such as the wrist[152]. A similar pattern of site-dependency of visualization of bone erosions has been observed in RA MTP joints[154]. A study analyzing MCP joints, and radiocarpal and ulnocarpal regions of the wrist joints of patients without radiographic destructive changes, showed a significantly higher number of erosions visualized with US, in comparison with MRI[155].

It is possible to assess the vascularity inside erosions[147], potentially allowing estimation of erosion activity. Furthermore, assessment of volume of erosions should be possible with three-dimensional US, but no systematic studies on the subject have been published yet.

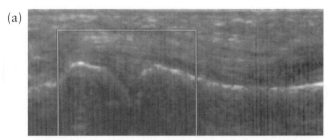

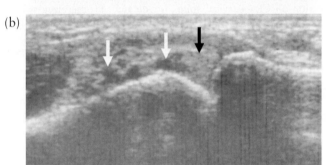

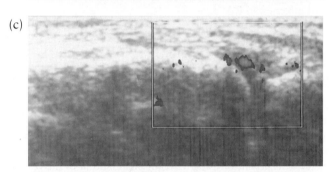

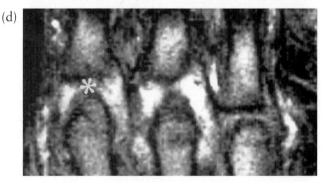

Fig. 19.14 (a) US of a normal 2nd MCP joint, in the longitudinal plane. Power Doppler is applied in the marked rectangle, but no flow is observed. (b) US of the 2nd MCP joint of an RA patient, in the longitudinal plane. Gray-scale US shows synovial membrane thickening (*black arrow*) and joint effusion (*white arrows*). Power Doppler is not applied. (c) US of the 2nd MCP joint of another patient with RA, in the longitudinal plane. Power Doppler signal is visible in the synovium, indicating synovitis. (d) Coronal T1-weighted gradient echo MR image of the same 2nd MCP joint, acquired 50 s after intravenous contrast injection (dynamic MRI) shows, in accordance with US findings, increased signal intensity of the synovium (*asterisk*), indicating synovitis. Synovitis is also seen in the 3rd but not the 4th MCP joint. (Reprinted from *Scand J Rheumatol* 2003; **32**: 63–73 with permission from Taylor & Francis.) See also colour plate section.

Cartilage

The cartilage can be visualized with US[156], but as ultrasound cannot penetrate bone, many joint surfaces, and consequently cartilage

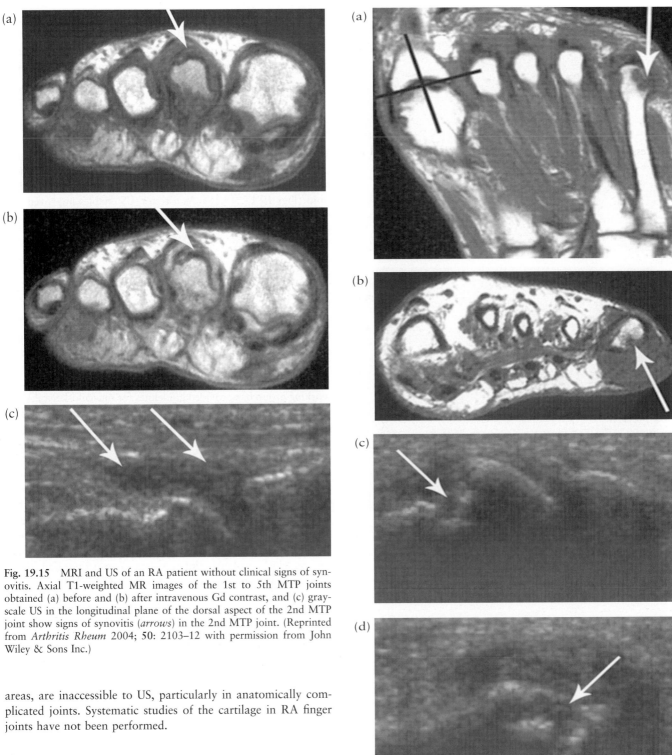

Fig. 19.15 MRI and US of an RA patient without clinical signs of synovitis. Axial T1-weighted MR images of the 1st to 5th MTP joints obtained (a) before and (b) after intravenous Gd contrast, and (c) grayscale US in the longitudinal plane of the dorsal aspect of the 2nd MTP joint show signs of synovitis (*arrows*) in the 2nd MTP joint. (Reprinted from *Arthritis Rheum* 2004; 50: 2103–12 with permission from John Wiley & Sons Inc.)

areas, are inaccessible to US, particularly in anatomically complicated joints. Systematic studies of the cartilage in RA finger joints have not been performed.

Cystic structures

Cystic structures, such as Baker's cysts (Fig. 19.17), are easily visualized with US. They were also the first among the musculoskeletal structures to be examined with US[157]. US allows differentiation from other pathologies, for example deep vein thrombosis, and is thus helpful in the differential diagnostic process. Other, smaller effusion collections around the joints or in the bursae are likewise easy to detect with US, enabling guided therapeutic interventions.

Fig. 19.16 Foot of a patient with early RA. A bone erosion in the head of the 5th metatarsal bone is seen on (a) coronal and (b) axial T1-weighted spin-echo MR images, and by US in (c) longitudinal and (d) transverse planes (*arrows*). The erosion was not visualized with CR. The 1st MTP joint, which also shows erosive changes on MRI (only one plane shown), is marked with a grid. (Reprinted from *Arthritis Rheum* 2004; 50: 2103–12 with permission from John Wiley & Sons Inc.)

(a)

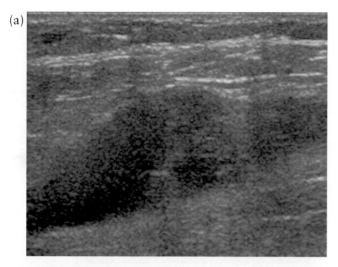

(b)

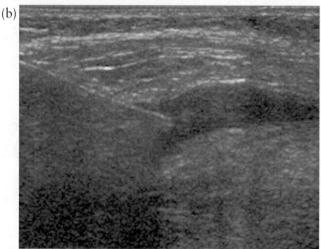

Fig. 19.17   US of a Baker's cyst. US in the longitudinal plane of the posteromedial aspect of the knee shows a popliteal cyst (a) before and (b) during an US-guided aspiration.

Tendons

US easily visualizes synovial proliferation and effusion around tendons[158]. US may be helpful in demonstrating focal or diffuse tendonitis. These features, and the possibility of dynamic evaluation of the tendon, enable precise placement of injections (Fig. 19.18).

Doppler US may potentially help in grading tenosynovitis and in differentiating tendonitis from tendinosis.

For non-RA patient groups it has been shown that US is equivalent to MRI in detecting complete rotator cuff tears (Fig. 19.19)[159]. Likewise, a small study of RA patients, including comparison with MRI, found that partial finger tendon tears can be examined with good accuracy with US[160]. US is more sensitive in detection of enthesitis than clinical examination[161,162]. Apart from B-mode findings, such as thickened entheses, adjacent bursitis and bone erosions and enthesophytes, increased power Doppler signal is proposed as an important sign of enthesitis[161].

Rheumatoid nodules

Differentiation of rheumatoid nodules from other subcutaneous structures such as gouty tophi, bursitis, or tumors may in certain clinical situations be of significance, and can be performed with US[163].

Guided intervention

Visualization of both superficial structures, such as small joints of the extremities, popliteal cysts, other distended bursae, or deep structures, like the hip joint, enables precise punctures and injections (Figs 19.17, 19.18). As a result, US enables improved success rates for diagnostic or therapeutic aspirations and injections[162,164,165].

Standardization and reliability

No consensus on the methodology of joint evaluation with US exists, making comparison of study results difficult[166]. Furthermore, the intra- and interobserver variations of the used measures have only been tested in a minority of studies[152,162,167,168], and the interscanner variation remains untested.

Recent years have brought advances in this area. A EULAR working group has provided guidelines for musculoskeletal US in rheumatology, addressing technical issues, training, and standardization of image acquisitions, but not evaluation methods[169]. A US self-training approach has been described[170]. Wakefield and coworkers have proposed a definition and a scoring system for erosions, and reported good intraobserver agreement rates when using it[152]. Ribbens et al. described the reproducibility and sensitivity to change of several measures of synovitis[167], while Szkudlarek et al. in a series of studies have suggested definitions of important joint pathologies (assessed by gray-scale and power Doppler US), and a corresponding scoring system for hands and feet, on which available validation data so far include high agreement rates between observers and with MRI[146,154,168,171,172]. Yet, no longitudinal data are so far available, and the system has not been tested by other groups, precluding final conclusions on its usefulness. An OMERACT/EULAR working group on US in RA has recently been formed, with the aim of addressing validity issues, hopefully leading to a higher degree of international consensus on techniques, joint pathology definitions, and scoring systems for use of US in RA[173].

Diagnosis

So far, no studies have investigated the diagnostic value of US in RA. A few studies have described differences in findings among particular arthritides. A study by Frediani et al. suggested, in agreement with comparable MRI studies, that in RA US signs of inflammation are more frequent in the joint than at the tendon insertions (enthesitis), while the opposite is true for psoriatic arthritis[174]. Similarly, other studies report that US signs of peripheral enthesitis are frequent in seronegative spondyloarthropathies, but not in RA[162].

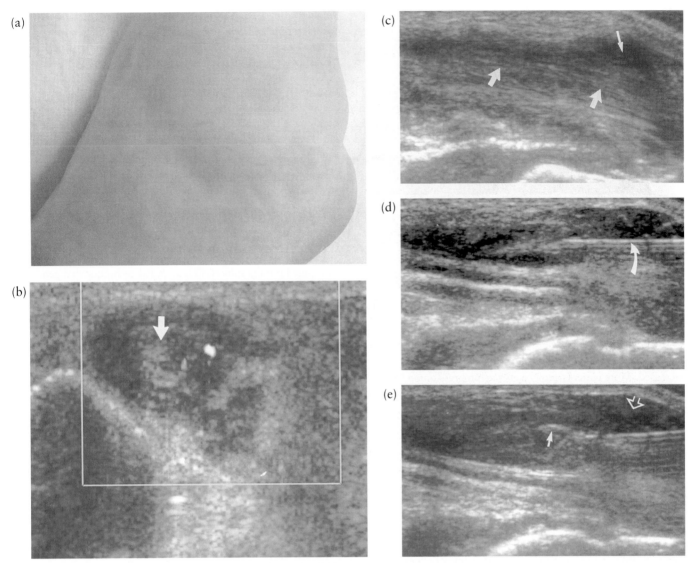

Fig. 19.18 RA patient with tenosynovitis at the peroneous longus tendon. (a) Clinical image shows swelling of the lateral retromalleolar region. (b) US of the tendon (*arrow*), in the transverse plane, which has an irregular contour and a heterogeneous echostructure. Power Doppler signal is shown inside the tendon, indicating tendonitis. The tendon is surrounded by a hypoechoic rim, indicating tenosynovitis. (c–e) US of the same tendon as above, in the longitudinal plane, (c) before and (d) during needle insertion, and (e) during steroid injection in the tendon sheath. The thick arrows point at the tendon, the long thin arrow at the widened tendon sheath, the short arrow at air bubbles injected to verify the position of the needle tip, and the open arrow the increased post-injection fluid volume within the tendon sheath. (Reprinted from *Scand J Rheumatol* 2003; **32**: 63–73 with permission from Taylor & Francis.) See also colour plate section.

It can be expected that the ability of US to visualize intra- as well extra-articular changes would translate into US assisting in some cases in the clinical process of diagnosing a specific rheumatological condition, but this is not scientifically verified.

Monitoring of the disease course

Follow-up data have revealed that US measures of synovitis (Doppler signal and B-mode synovial membrane thickness) decrease when glucocorticoids[142,149] or tumour necrosis factor alpha (TNF-α)-antagonists[167,175,176] are administered, in parallel with similar changes in clinical and laboratory measures of disease activity. This is in accordance with the expectations of markers of synovial inflammation exposed to effective anti-inflammatory drugs.

Only one US study of RA wrist, finger, or toe joints includes both reproducibility and longitudinal data[167], albeit not calculating the SDD. The SDD was not determined, but infliximab therapy changed the synovial thickness more than the coefficient of variance in the majority of joints, suggesting that this measure is sensitive to change in clinically relevant situations.

Thus, US may be a valid method for monitoring of synovitis, but data on sensitivity to change are needed.

Two studies have systematically followed the course of US bone erosions[13,59]. Backhaus *et al.*, in a two-year follow-up wrist, MCP, and PIP joint study, found that MRI and US signs of synovitis decreased, while the number of bone erosions on MRI and US

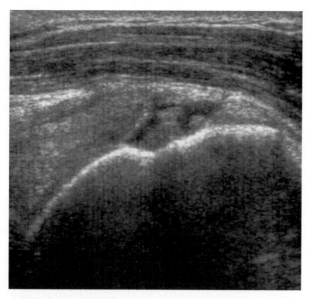

Fig. 19.19   US of a complete rotator cuff tear. Longitudinal US image shows an effusion inside a focal discontinuity in the supraspinatus tendon, with an intact deltoid muscle above it. (Courtesy of Dr Court-Payen, Department of Diagnostic Radiology, Copenhagen University Hospital at Herlev, Denmark.)

increased. More patients showed erosive progression on US compared to radiography, suggesting a higher sensitivity to change. Hoving and coworkers found a similar number of patients with progression on CR and US in a six-month follow-up study of RA wrist, MCP, and PIP joints[59]. In both studies, MRI detected progression more frequently than US and CR did. However, as the reproducibility was not evaluated in any of the studies, it is not known how often the erosive progression noted exceeded SDD.

Prognostic value

The only study addressing the prognostic value of US in RA is a randomized controlled trial of anti-TNF-α therapy in early RA[176]. Baseline US-determined synovial thickening and the degree of vascularity assessed with PDUS in the MCP joints correlated with the radiographic joint damage in the following year in patients receiving methotrexate and placebo, but not in patients treated with methotrexate and a TNF-α antagonist. Thus, it is not yet clarified whether US findings are of predictive value for later radiographic or functional status in RA.

Practical aspects and future perspectives

Further validation is needed within most areas of potential use of US in RA. Data on monitoring of joint inflammation and destruction, diagnostic value, and prognostic value are still very limited. However, there are solid data indicating that US can visualize a number of joint pathologies, including synovitis and tenosynovitis. Furthermore, it is established that US can be used to guide punctures of joints, bursae, and tendon sheaths, with following improved success rates of diagnostic or therapeutic aspirations and injections. Even though the scientific evidence for the clinical

value of using US in early RA is very limited, we feel it is justified to suggest use of US in some clinical situations in clinical practice (Table 19.1). Obviously, this requires that the ultrasonographer, being a radiologist or rheumatologist, is sufficiently trained.

US, as a more accessible, cheaper, and more patient-friendly method than MRI, is likely to become a routinely used bedside tool for the rheumatologist in the near future, gaining a place as the 'extended hand of the rheumatologist'. A prerequisite for this is sufficient training of rheumatologists, for example as part of specialty or subspecialty training. This is already the case in many European countries.

Other imaging modalities

Computed tomography

Computed tomography (CT) is an X-ray technique that generates images by measuring X-ray absorption by a detector array, circulating around the patient simultaneously with the X-ray tube. The measurements are then transformed, stored, and reconstructed as two- or, with the latest CT units, three-dimensional images.

In comparison with conventional radiography, CT is favored by its tomographic viewing perspective. This obviates projectional superimposition, which can obscure erosions and mimic joint space narrowing on conventional radiographs.

Cortical bone is easily visible, being a dense and highly absorbing structure. Thus, CT clearly delineates bone erosions from the soft tissues. Accordingly, Yu *et al.*, assessing wrists of 30 RA patients, showed that CT is more sensitive than conventional radiography for the detection of bone erosions[177]. However, CT, like conventional radiography, involves ionizing radiation and its sensitivity to RA soft tissue changes is markedly inferior to MRI and US[60,178]. Accordingly, systematic studies of CT peripheral joints in RA patients have not been performed and the modality is very rarely used in RA clinical practice.

Given the advantages of other imaging modalities, the potential of peripheral joint CT in the clinical management and clinical trials of RA patients seems minimal. However, it may be a valuable reference method for validation of bone damage observed on MRI and US[66,178,179].

High-resolution CT (HRCT) is valuable for ascertainment of pulmonary involvement in RA, including interstitial fibrosis, pulmonary nodules, and pneumonitis (see section on CR)[51,53,55].

The previous role of CT in the evaluation of the RA cervical spine has largely been taken over by MRI, due to its superior visualization of soft tissues and spinal cord compression (see section on MRI).

Nuclear medicine

Nuclear imaging provides not only morphological but also physiological information regarding the metabolic state of tissues[180,181]. Following injection of a radionuclide, gamma radiation emitted from the patient is measured by a gamma camera

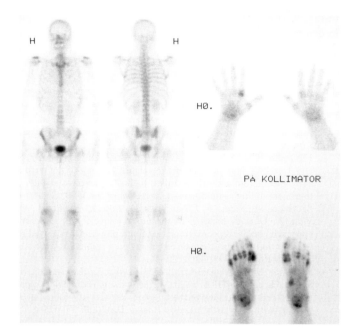

Fig. 19.20 Bone scintigraphy of an RA patient. Anterior and posterior whole-body images, with magnifications of hands and feet, are presented. Increased focal uptake of Tc-99m methylene-diphosphonate (MDP) is seen in multiple MTP joints, the right calcaneus and the right 2nd MCP joint.

and transformed into a two-dimensional image. A wide range of radionuclides are available, with the most commonly used being technetium-99m. In the classical bone scintigraphy ('bone scan'), which is the only one to be discussed here, technetium-99m is chelated to diphosphonates[180,181]. Recent inflammation-targeting radiopharmaceuticals, such as radiolabelled leukocytes and polyclonal human immunoglobulins, allow scintigraphical imaging of synovitis[180,182–184], but are currently purely experimental and will not be addressed further. Please also see elsewhere for information on single photon emission computer tomography (SPECT) and positron emission tomography (PET)[180].

Bone scintigraphy can be performed as a static or a dynamic procedure. The dynamic three-phase scintigraphy involves a radionuclide angiography (flow phase), a blood pooling phase, and the standard static late images. In the latter (Fig. 19.20), in which imaging is performed 2–4 h after technetium-99m-disphosphonate injection, increased tracer accumulation reflects increased osteoblastic activity. Bone scintigraphy has a low spatial resolution and is non-specific, as increased tracer accumulation is seen in the course of most pathological bone processes, including trauma, infection, neoplastic changes, and joint inflammation[3,4,180,185,186]. Bone scintigraphy is generally reported to be sensitive[180,181,186]. However, comparisons with MRI and US have found both MRI and US to be markedly more sensitive to joint inflammation than bone scintigraphy[3,4,13]. This indicates that scintigraphy is inferior to MRI and US for detection and monitoring of joint inflammation in RA. It may, however, be useful for excluding other differential diagnoses.

(a)

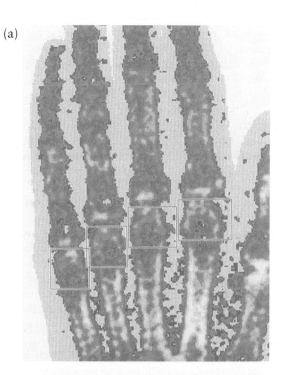

(b)

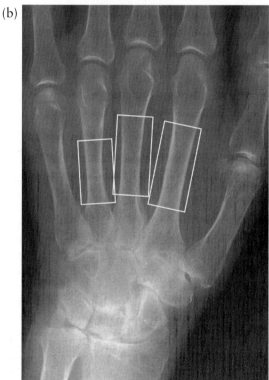

Fig. 19.21 Dual X-ray absorptiometry (DXA) and digital X-ray radiogrammetry (DXR) in a hand of an RA patient. (a) Hand bone densitometry. The BMD measurement is performed in the juxta-articular distal 1.5 cm of the metacarpal bone (*boxes*). (b) DXR. The regions of interest used for calculation of the BMD estimate are shown (*boxes*). In the metacarpals, the cortical thickness is determined on both the radial and ulnar sides. (Courtesy of Dr Jensen, Department of Endocrinology, Copenhagen University Hospital at Hvidovre, Denmark.) See also colour plate section.

Dual X-ray absorptiometry and digital X-ray radiogrammetry

Bone mineral content is routinely measured by dual X-ray absorptiometry (DXA). The method allows measurement of bone density in different areas of the skeleton, including the hand (Fig. 19.21).

Digital X-ray radiogrammetry (DXR) differs from DXA by measuring the geometrics of bones on conventional or digitized radiographs. When applied to the hand, it measures cortical thickness and width of the 2nd to 4th metacarpal bones (Fig. 19.21). Changes in cortical thickness predominantly reflect the endosteal resorption. The measurements can also be applied to other peripheral bones, such as the radius and the ulna[187–190].

In a recent early RA study, Jensen *et al.* showed that DXR, but not DXA, allowed detection of a significant decrease in bone mineral density (BMD) within a six-months follow-up period. The BMD changes were associated with disease activity and erosive disease[188]. In accordance with this, Haugeberg *et al.* found hand BMD strongly correlated with radiographic hand joint damage in patients with long-lasting RA[189]. Furthermore, Stewart *et al.* have suggested that changes in DXR BMD during the first year of follow-up in early RA patients may predict which patients will have radiographic erosions three years later[190].

Although not yet definitely established, DXR may have a clinical role in diagnosis and follow-up of periarticular osteoporosis in RA patients and as a prognostic factor for erosive disease.

Summary and perspectives

Efficient methods for diagnosis, monitoring, and prognostication are essential in early RA. Conventional radiography has important roles in the differential diagnosis of inflammatory arthritides and for providing prognostic information in early RA. Furthermore, it is currently the prevailing method for monitoring structural joint damage/disease progression in clinical practice and trials. However, it only visualizes the late signs of preceding disease activity. There is evidence for MRI and US being highly sensitive for early inflammatory and destructive changes in RA joints, and for MRI findings being sensitive to change and of predictive value for future progressive radiographic damage. On this basis the use of MRI and US for detecting arthritic joint pathologies and MRI for monitoring and prognostication of early RA can be suggested (Table 19.1). Other imaging methods can be useful on specific indications, as described above.

A number of important research issues still need to be addressed. Among these are the adequacy of less costly MRI approaches, such as extremity MRI units and MRI without use of contrast injection, standardization and validation of US, and the value of MRI and US in the differential diagnosis in suspected and undifferentiated inflammatory joint disease.

It is exciting that, with MRI and US, rheumatoid activity and damage can be imaged and measured in entirely new ways. The perspectives for clinical practice include earlier and more accurate diagnoses, targeted therapies, and precise evaluation of therapeutic response, providing optimal possibilities for total disease control and thereby the most favorable short- and long-term outcome.

References

1. Brower, A. C. Use of the radiograph to measure the course of rheumatoid arthritis: the gold standard versus fool's gold. *Arthritis Rheum* 1990; **33**: 316–24.
2. McQueen, F. M., Stewart, N., Crabbe, J., Robinson, E., Yeoman, S., and Tan, P. L. J. *et al.* Magnetic resonance imaging of the wrist in early rheumatoid arthritis reveals a high prevalence of erosion at four months after symptom onset. *Ann Rheum Dis* 1998; **57**: 350–6.
3. Backhaus, M., Kamradt, T., Sandrock, D., Loreck, D., Fritz, J., and Wolf, K. J. *et al.* Arthritis of the finger joints: a comprehensive approach comparing conventional radiography, scintigraphy, ultrasound, and contrast-enhanced magnetic resonance imaging. *Arthritis Rheum* 1999; **42**: 1232–45.
4. Klarlund, M., Østergaard, M., Jensen, K. E., Madsen, J. L., Skjødt, H., and the TIRA group. Magnetic resonance imaging, radiography, and scintigraphy of the finger joints: one year follow up of patients with early arthritis. *Ann Rheum Dis* 2000; **59**: 521–8.
5. Lindegaard, H., Vallø, J., Hørslev-Petersen, K., Junker, P., and Østergaard, M. Low field dedicated magnetic resonance imaging in untreated rheumatoid arthritis of recent onset. *Ann Rheum Dis* 2001; **60**: 770–6.
6. Grassi, W., Tittarelli, E., Pirani, O., Avaltroni, O., and Cervini, C. Ultrasound examination of metacarpophalangeal joints in rheumatoid arthritis. *Scand J Rheumatol* 1993; **22**: 243–7.
7. Resnick, D. *Diagnosis of bone and joint disorders*, 4th edn. Philadelphia: W. B. Saunders; 2002.
8. Watt, I. Basic differential diagnosis of arthritis. *Eur Radiol* 1997; **7**: 344–51.
9. American College of Rheumatology Subcommittee on Rheumatoid Arthritis Guidelines. Guidelines for the management of rheumatoid arthritis: 2002 Update. *Arthritis Rheum* 2002; **46**: 328–46.
10. Tugwell, P., and Boers, M. OMERACT conference on outcome measures in RA clinical trials: conclusion. *J Rheumatol* 1993; **20**: 590.
11. McQueen, F. M., Stewart, N., Crabbe, J., Robinson, E., Yeoman, S., and Tan, P. L. J. *et al.* Magnetic resonance imaging of the wrist in early rheumatoid arthritis reveals progression of erosions despite clinical improvement. *Ann Rheum Dis* 1999; **58**: 156–63.
12. Østergaard, M. Magnetic resonance imaging in rheumatoid arthritis. Quantitative methods for assessment of the inflammatory process in peripheral joints (thesis). *Dan Med Bull* 1999; **46**: 313–44.
13. Backhaus, M., Burmester, G. R., Sandrock, D., Loreck, D., Hess, D., and Scholz, A. *et al.* Prospective two year follow up study comparing novel and conventional imaging procedures in patients with arthritic finger joints. *Ann Rheum Dis* 2002; **61**: 895–904.
14. van der Heijde, D. M. F. M. Plain X-rays in rheumatoid arthritis: overview of scoring methods, their reliability and applicability. *Baillieres Clin Rheumatol* 1996; **10**: 435–53.
15. van der Jagt, E. J., Hofman, S., Kraft, B. M., and van Leeuwen, M.A. Can we see enough? A comparative study of film-screen vs digital radiographs in small lesions in rheumatoid arthritis. *Eur Radiol* 2000; **10**: 304–7.
16. Nørgaard, F. Earliest roentgenological changes in polyarthritis of the rheumatoid type: rheumatoid arthritis. *Radiology* 1965; **85**: 325–9.
17. McGonagle, D., Conaghan, P. G., Wakefield, R., and Emery, P. Imaging the joints in early rheumatoid arthritis. *Best Pract Res Clin Rheumatol* 2001; **15**: 91–104.
18. Klarlund, M. Magnetic resonance imaging of wrist and finger joints in rheumatoid arthritis and healthy controls. PhD dissertation, University of Copenhagen 2000.
19. Sharp, J. T., Young, D. Y., Bluhm, G. B., Brook, A., Brower, A. C., and Corbett, M. *et al.* How many joints in the hands and wrists should be included in a score of radiologic abnormalities used to assess rheumatoid arthritis? *Arthritis Rheum* 1985; **28**: 1326–35.

20. Larsen, A., Dale, K., and Eek, M. Radiographic evaluation of rheumatoid arthritis and related conditions by standard reference films. *Acta Radiol Diagn (Stockh)* 1977; **18**: 481–91.

21. Scott, D. L., Pugner, K., Kaarela, K., Doyle, D. V., Woolf, A., Holmes, J. *et al.* The links between joint damage and disability in rheumatoid arthritis. *Rheumatology (Oxford)* 2000; **39**: 122–32.

22. Arnett, F. C., Edworthy, S. M., Bloch, D. A., McShane, D. J., Fries, J. F., and Cooper, N. S. *et al.* The American Rheumatism Association 1987 revised criteria for the classification of rheumatoid arthritis. *Arthritis Rheum* 1988; **31**: 315–24.

23. Fleming, A., Crown, J. M., and Corbett, M. Prognostic value of early features in rheumatoid disease. *BMJ* 1976; **1**: 1243–5.

24. Kaarela, K. Prognostic factors and diagnostic criteria in early rheumatoid arthritis. *Scand J Rheumatol* 1985; **14** (Suppl. 57): 1–54.

25. Woolf, A. D., Hall, N. D., Goulding, N. J., Kantharia, B., Maymo, J., and Evison, G. *et al.* Predictors of the long-term outcome of early synovitis: a 5-year follow-up study. *Br J Rheumatol* 1991; **30**: 251–4.

26. van der Heijde, D. M. F. M., van Riel, P. L. C. M., van Leeuwen, M. A., van't Hof, M. A., van Rijswijk, M. H., and van de Putte, L. B. A. Prognostic factors for radiographic damage and physical disability in early rheumatoid arthritis: a prospective follow-up study of 147 patients. *Br J Rheumatol* 1992; **31**: 519–25.

27. van Leeuwen, M. A., van Rijswijk, M. H., van der Heijde, D. M. F. M., te Meerman, G. J., van Riel, P. L. C. M., and Houtman, P. M. *et al.* The acute-phase response in relation to radiographic progression in early rheumatoid arthritis: a prospective study during the first three years of the disease. *Br J Rheumatol* 1993; **32** (Suppl. 3): 9–13.

28. van der Heide, A., Remme, C. A., Hofman, D. M., Jacobs, J. W. G., and Bijlsma, J. W. J. Prediction of progression of radiologic damage in newly diagnosed rheumatoid arthritis. *Arthritis Rheum* 1995; **38**: 1466–74.

29. Visser, H., le Cessie, S., Vos, K., Breedveld, F. C., and Hazes, J. M. How to diagnose rheumatoid arthritis early: a prediction model for persistent (erosive) arthritis. *Arthritis Rheum* 2002; **46**: 357–65.

30. Nissilä, M., Isomaki, H., Kaarela, K., Kiviniemi, P., Martio, J., and Sarna, S. Prognosis of inflammatory joint diseases: a three-year follow-up study. *Scand J Rheumatol* 1983; **12**: 33–8.

31. Möttönen, T. T. Prediction of erosiveness and rate of development of new erosions in early rheumatoid arthritis. *Ann Rheum Dis* 1988; **47**: 648–53.

32. van der Heijde, D. M. F. M., van Leeuwen, M. A., van Riel, P. L. C. M., Koster, A. M., van't Hof, M. A., and van Rijswijk, M. H. *et al.* Biannual radiographic assessments of hands and feet in a three-year prospective followup of patients with early rheumatoid arthritis. *Arthritis Rheum* 1992; **35**: 26–34.

33. van der Heijde, D. M. F. M. Joint erosions and patients with early rheumatoid arthritis. *Br J Rheumatol* 1995; **34** (Suppl. 2): 74–8.

34. Paulus, H. E., Oh, M., Sharp, J. T., Gold, R. H., Wong, W. K., and Park, G. S. *et al.* Correlation of single time-point damage scores with observed progression of radiographic damage during the first 6 years of rheumatoid arthritis. *J Rheumatol* 2003; **30**: 705–13.

35. Scott, D. L., Houssien, D. A., and Laasonen, L. Proposed modification to Larsen's scoring methods for hand and wrist radiographs. *Br J Rheumatol* 1995; **34**: 56.

36. van der Heijde, D. How to read radiographs according to the Sharp/van der Heijde method. *J Rheumatol* 1999; **26**: 743–5.

37. Rau, R., and Herborn, G. A modified version of Larsen's scoring method to assess radiologic changes in rheumatoid arthritis. *J Rheumatol* 1995; **22**: 1976–82.

38. Sharp, J. T., Lidsky, M. D., Collins, L. C., and Moreland, J. Methods for scoring the progression of radiologic changes in rheumatoid arthritis. *Arthritis Rheum* 1971; **14**: 706–20.

39. Genant, H. K. Methods of assessing radiographic change in rheumatoid arthritis. *Am J Med* 1983; **75**: 35–47.

40. Østergaard, M., Hansen, M., Stoltenberg, M., Jensen, K. E., Szkudlarek, M., and Pedersen-Zbinden, B. *et al.* New radiographic bone erosions in the wrists of patients with rheumatoid arthritis are detectable with magnetic resonance imaging a median of two years earlier. *Arthritis Rheum* 2003; **48**: 2128–31.

41. Ejbjerg, B., Vestergaard, A., Jacobsen, S., Thomsen, H. S., and Østergaard, M. The smallest detectable and sensitivity to change of MRI and radiographic scores of structural joint damage in rheumatoid arthritis finger, wrist and toe joints—a comparison of the OMERACT RA MRI score applied on different joint combinations and the Sharp/van der Heijde radiographic score. *Arthritis Rheum* 2005; **52**: 691–6.

42. Zoli, A., Priolo, F., Galossi, A., Altomonte, L., Di Gregorio, F., and Cerase, A. *et al.* Craniocervical junction involvement in rheumatoid arthritis: a clinical and radiological study. *J Rheumatol* 2000; **27**: 1178–82.

43. Oostveen, J. C., Roozeboom, A. R., van de Laar, M. A., Heeres, J., den Boer, J. A., and Lindeboom, S. F. Functional turbo spin echo magnetic resonance imaging versus tomography for evaluating cervical spine involvement in rheumatoid arthritis. *Spine* 1998; **23**: 1237–44.

44. Halla, J. T., and Hardin, J. G., Jr. The spectrum of atlantoaxial facet joint involvement in rheumatoid arthritis. *Arthritis Rheum* 1990; **33**: 325–9.

45. Neva, M. H., Myllykangas-Luosujarvi, R., Kautiainen, H., and Kauppi, M. Mortality associated with cervical spine disorders: a population-based study of 1666 patients with rheumatoid arthritis who died in Finland in 1989. *Rheumatology (Oxford)* 2001; **40**: 123–7.

46. Halla, J. T., Hardin, J. G., Vitek, J., and Alarcon, G. S. Involvement of the cervical spine in rheumatoid arthritis. *Arthritis Rheum* 1989; **32**: 652–9.

47. Kauppi, M., Sakaguchi, M., Konttinen, Y. T., Hamalainen, M., and Hakala, M. Pathogenetic mechanism and prevalence of the stable atlantoaxial subluxation in rheumatoid arthritis. *J Rheumatol* 1996; **23**: 831–4.

48. Neva, M. H., Kauppi, M. J., Kautiainen, H., Luukkainen, R., Hannonen, P., Leirisalo-Repo, M. *et al.* Combination drug therapy retards the development of rheumatoid atlantoaxial subluxations. *Arthritis Rheum* 2000; **43**: 2397–401.

49. Jackson, H. The diagnosis of minimal atlanto-axial subluxation. *Br J Radiol* 1950; **23**: 672–4.

50. Anaya, J. M., Diethelm, L., Ortiz, L. A., Gutierrez, M., Citera, G., and Welsh, R. A. *et al.* Pulmonary involvement in rheumatoid arthritis. *Semin Arthritis Rheum* 1995; **24**: 242–54.

51. Dawson, J. K., Fewins, H. E., Desmond, J., Lynch, M. P., and Graham, D. R. Fibrosing alveolitis in patients with rheumatoid arthritis as assessed by high resolution computed tomography, chest radiography, and pulmonary function tests. *Thorax* 2001; **56**: 622–7.

52. Jurik, A. G., Davidsen, D., and Graudal, H. Prevalence of pulmonary involvement in rheumatoid arthritis and its relationship to some characteristics of the patients: a radiological and clinical study. *Scand J Rheumatol* 1982; **11**: 217–24.

53. Tanaka, N., Kim, J. S., Newell, J. D., Brown, K. K., Cool, C. D., and Meehan, R. *et al.* Rheumatoid arthritis-related lung diseases: CT findings. *Radiology* 2004; **232**: 81–91.

54. Hacking, J. C., and Flower, C. D. Causes and investigation of increasing dyspnoea in rheumatoid arthritis. *Ann Rheum Dis* 1995; **54**: 17–19.

55. Cortet, B., Flipo, R. M., Remy-Jardin, M., Coquerelle, P., Duquesnoy, B., Remy, J. *et al.* Use of high resolution computed tomography of the lungs in patients with rheumatoid arthritis. *Ann Rheum Dis* 1995; **54**: 815–19.

56. Rominger, M. B., Bernreuter, W. K., Kenney, P. J., Morgan, S. L., Blackburn, W. D., and Alarcon, G. S. MR imaging of the hands in early rheumatoid arthritis: preliminary results. *Radiographics* 1993; **13**: 37–46.

57. Sugimoto, H., Takeda, A., and Hyodoh, K. Early stage rheumatoid arthritis: prospective study of the effectiveness of MR imaging for diagnosis. *Radiology* 2000; **216**: 569–75.

58. McGonagle, D., Conaghan, P., O'Connor, P., Gibbon, W., Green, M., and Wakefield, R. J. *et al.* The relationship between synovitis and bone changes in early untreated rheumatoid arthritis: a controlled magnetic resonance imaging study. *Arthritis Rheum* 1999; **42**: 1706–11.

59. Hoving, J. L., Buchbinder, R., Hall, S., Lawler, G., Coombs, P., McNealy, S. *et al.* A comparison of magnetic resonance imaging, sonography, and radiography of the hand in patients with early rheumatoid arthritis. *J Rheumatol* 2004; **31**: 663–75.

60. Alasaarela, E., Suramo, I., Tervonen, O., Lähde, S., Takalo, R., and Hakala, M. Evaluation of humoral head erosions in rheumatoid arthritis: a comparison of ultrasonography, magnetic resonance imaging, computed tomography and plain radiography. *Br J Rheumatol* 1998; **37**: 1152–6.

61. Hermann, K. G., Backhaus, M., Schneider, U., Labs, K., Loreck, D., Zuhlsdorf, S. *et al.* Rheumatoid arthritis of the shoulder joint: comparison of conventional radiography, ultrasound, and dynamic contrast-enhanced magnetic resonance imaging. *Arthritis Rheum* 2003; **48**: 3338–49.

62. Melchiorre, D., Calderazzi, A., Maddali, B. S., Cristofani, R., Bazzichi, L., Eligi, C. *et al.* A comparison of ultrasonography and magnetic resonance imaging in the evaluation of temporomandibular joint involvement in rheumatoid arthritis and psoriatic arthritis. *Rheumatology (Oxford)* 2003; **42**: 673–6.

63. Lehtinen, A., Paimela, L., Kreula, J., Leirisalo-Repo, M., and Taavitsainen, M. Painful ankle region in rheumatoid arthritis: analysis of soft-tissue changes with ultrasonography and MR imaging. *Acta Radiol* 1996; **37**: 572–7.

64. Østergaard, M., Gideon, P., Henriksen, O., and Lorenzen, I. Synovial volume: a marker of disease severity in rheumatoid arthritis? Quantification by MRI. *Book of Abstracts European Society for Magnetic Resonance in Medicine and Biology* 1994; 381.

65. Forslind, K., Larsson, E. M., Eberhardt, K., Johansson, A., and Svensson B. Magnetic resonance imaging of the knee: a tool for prediction of joint damage in early rheumatoid arthritis? *Scand J Rheumatol* 2004; **33**: 154–61.

66. Østergaard, M., Duer, A., Møller, U., and Ejbjerg, B. Magnetic resonance imaging of peripheral joints in rheumatic diseases. *Best Pract Res Clin Rheumatol* 2004; **18**: 861–79.

67. Savnik, A., Malmskov, H., Thomsen, H. S., Bretlau, T., Graff, L. B., Nielsen, H. *et al.* MRI of the arthritic small joints: comparison of extremity MRI (0.2 T) vs high-field MRI (1.5 T). *Eur Radiol* 2001; **11**: 1030–8.

68. Taouli, B., Zaim, S., Peterfy, C. G., Lynch, J. A., Stork, A., and Guermazi, A. *et al.* Rheumatoid arthritis of the hand and wrist: comparison of three imaging techniques. *AJR Am J Roentgenol* 2004; **182**: 937–43.

69. Crues, J. V., Shellock, F. G., Dardashti, S., James, T. W., and Troum, O. M. Identification of wrist and metacarpophalangeal joint erosions using a portable magnetic resonance imaging system compared to conventional radiographs. *J Rheumatol* 2004; **31**: 676–85.

70. McQueen, F. M., Benton, N., Crabbe, J., Robinson, E., Yeoman, S., McLean, L. *et al.* What is the fate of erosions in early rheumatoid arthritis? Tracking individual lesions using x rays and magnetic resonance imaging over the first two years of disease. *Ann Rheum Dis* 2001; **60**: 859–68.

71. McQueen, F. M., Benton, N., Perry, D., Crabbe, J., Robinson, E., Yeoman, S. *et al.* Bone edema scored on magnetic resonance imaging scans of the dominant carpus at presentation predicts radiographic joint damage of the hands and feet six years later in patients with rheumatoid arthritis. *Arthritis Rheum* 2003; **48**: 1814–27.

72. Benton, N., Stewart, N., Crabbe, J., Robinson, E., Yeoman, S., and McQueen, F. MRI of the wrist in early rheumatoid arthritis can be used to predict functional outcome at 6 years. *Ann Rheum Dis* 2004; **63**: 555–61.

73. Ejbjerg, B. Magnetic resonance imaging in rheumatoid arthritis: a study of aspects of joint selection, contrast agent use and type of MRI unit. PhD dissertation. University of Copenhagen, 2005.

74. Peterfy, C. G., Roberts, T., and Genant, H. K. Dedicated extremity MR imaging: an emerging technology. *Radiol Clin North Am* 1997; **35**: 1–20.

75. Ejbjerg, B., Narvestad, E., Jacobsen, S., Thomsen, H. S., and Østergaard M. Optimised, low cost, low field dedicated extremity MRI is highly specific and sensitive for synovitis and bone erosions in rheumatoid arthritis wrist and finger joints: a comparison with conventional high-field MRI and radiography. *Ann Rheum Dis* 2005; **64**: 1280–7.

76. Nakahara, N., Uetani, M., Hayashi, K., Kawashara, Y., Matsumoto, T., and Oda, J. Gadolinium-enhanced MR imaging of the wrist in rheumatoid arthritis: value of fat suppression pulse sequences. *Skeletal Radiol* 1996; **25**: 639–47.

77. Rinck, P. A., Jones, R. A., Kvaerness, J., and Southon, T. E. In *Magnetic resonance in medicine: the basic textbook of the European Magnetic Resonance Forum*, 3rd edn (Rinck, P. A., ed.), pp. 1–241. Oxford: Blackwell Scientific; 1993.

78. Østergaard, M., Peterfy, C., Conaghan, P., McQueen, F., Bird, P., and Ejbjerg, B. *et al.* OMERACT Rheumatoid Arthritis Magnetic Resonance Imaging Studies: core set of MRI acquisitions, joint pathology definitions, and the OMERACT RA-MRI scoring system. *J Rheumatol* 2003; **30**: 1385–6.

79. Østergaard, M., Conaghan, P., O'Connor, P., Ejbjerg, B., Szkudlarek, M., and Peterfy, C. *et al.* Reducing costs, duration and invasiveness of magnetic resonance imaging in rheumatoid arthritis by omitting intravenous gadolinium injection: does it affect assessments of synovitis, bone erosions and bone edema? [Abstract.] *Ann Rheum Dis* 2003; **62** (Suppl. I): 67.

80. Peterfy, C. G., Majumdar, S., Lang, P., van Dijke, C. F., Sack, K., and Genant, H. K. MR imaging of the arthritic knee: improved discrimination of cartilage, synovium, and effusion with pulsed saturation transfer and fat-suppressed T1-weighted sequences. *Radiology* 1994; **191**: 413–19.

81. Rand, T., Imhof, H., Czerny, C., Breitenseher, M., Machold, K., Turetschek, K. *et al.* Discrimination between fluid, synovium, and cartilage in patients with rheumatoid arthritis: contrast enhanced spin echo versus non-contrast enhanced fat-suppressed gradient echo MR imaging. *Clin Radiol* 1999; **54**: 107–10.

82. Conaghan, P., McGonagle, D., Wakefield, R., and Emery, P. New approaches to imaging of early rheumatoid arthritis. *Clin Exp Rheumatol* 1999; **17** (Suppl. 18): 37–42.

83. Jevtic, V., Watt, I., Rozman, B., Kos-Golja, M., Praprotnik, S., Logar, D. *et al.* The value of contrast enhanced magnetic resonance imaging in evaluation of drug therapy in rheumatoid arthritis: a prospective study on hand joints in 65 patients. *Acta Pharm* 1993; **43**: 267–76.

84. König, H., Sieper, J., and Wolf, K. J. Rheumatoid arthritis: evaluation of hypervascular and fibrous pannus with dynamic MR imaging enhanced with gd-DTPA. *Radiology* 1990; **176**: 473–7.

85. Østergaard, M., Stoltenberg, M., Henriksen, O., and Lorenzen, I. Quantitative assessment of synovial inflammation by dynamic gadolinium-enhanced magnetic resonance imaging: a study of the effect of intra-articular methylprednisolone on the rate of early synovial enhancement. *Br J Rheumatol* 1996; **35**: 50–9.

86. Østergaard, M., Stoltenberg, M., Løvgreen-Nielsen, P., Volck, B., Sonne-Holm, S., and Lorenzen, I. Quantification of synovitis by MRI: correlation between dynamic and static gadolinium-enhanced magnetic resonance imaging and microscopic and macroscopic signs of synovial inflammation. *Magn Reson Imaging* 1998; **16**: 743–54.

87. Klarlund, M., Østergaard, M., Rostrup, E., Skjødt, H., and Lorenzen, I. Dynamic magnetic resonance imaging of the metacarpophalangeal joints in rheumatoid arthritis, early unclassified polyarthritis, and healthy controls. *Scand J Rheumatol* 2000; **29**: 108–15.

88. Østergaard, M., Gideon, P., Henriksen, O., and Lorenzen, I. Synovial volume: a marker of disease severity in rheumatoid arthritis? Quantification by MRI. *Scand J Rheumatol* 1994; **23**: 197–202.

89. Østergaard, M., Stoltenberg, M., Henriksen, O., and Lorenzen, I. The accuracy of MRI-determined synovial membrane and joint effusion volumes in arthritis: a comparison of pre- and post-aspiration volumes. *Scand J Rheumatol* 1995; **24**: 305–11.

90. Østergaard, M., Hansen, M., Stoltenberg, M., and Lorenzen, I. Quantitative assessment of the synovial membrane in the rheumatoid wrist: an easily obtained MRI score reflects the synovial volume. *Br J Rheumatol* 1996; **35**: 965–71.

91. Østergaard, M., Stoltenberg, M., Løvgreen-Nielsen, P., Volck, B., Jensen, C. H., and Lorenzen I. Magnetic resonance imaging-determined synovial membrane and joint effusion volumes in

rheumatoid arthritis and osteoarthritis: comparison with the macroscopic and microscopic appearance of the synovium. *Arthritis Rheum* 1997; **40**: 1856–67.

92. Polisson, R. P, Schoenberg, O. I., Fischman, A., Rubin, R., Simon, L. S., and Rosenthal, D. *et al*. Use of magnetic resonance imaging and positron emission tomography in the assessment of synovial volume and glucose metabolism in patients with rheumatoid arthritis. *Arthritis Rheum* 1995; **38**: 819–25.

93. Palmer, W. E., Rosenthal, D. I., Schoenberg, O. I., Fischman, A. J., Simon, L. S., Rubin, R. H. *et al*. Quantification of inflammation in the wrist with gadolinium-enhanced MR imaging and PET with 2-[F-18]-fluoro-2-deoxy-D-glucose. *Radiology* 1995; **196**: 647–55.

94. Klarlund, M., Østergaard, M., and Lorenzen, I. Finger joint synovitis in rheumatoid arthritis: quantitative assessment by magnetic resonance imaging. *Rheumatology (Oxford)* 1999; **38**: 66–72.

95. Bird, P., Lassere, M., Shnier, R., and Edmonds, J. Computerized measurement of magnetic resonance imaging erosion volumes in patients with rheumatoid arthritis: a comparison with existing magnetic resonance imaging scoring systems and standard clinical outcome measures. *Arthritis Rheum* 2003; **48**: 614–24.

96. Gaffney, K., Cookson, K., Blades, S., Coumbe, S., and Blake, S. Quantitative assessment of the rheumatoid synovial microvascular bed by gadolinium-DTPA enhanced magnetic resonance imaging. *Ann Rheum Dis* 1998; **57**: 152–7.

97. Ostendorf, B., Peters, R., Dann, P., Becker, A., Scherer, A., Wedekind, F. *et al*. Magnetic resonance imaging and miniarthroscopy of metacarpophalangeal joints: sensitive detection of morphologic changes in rheumatoid arthritis. *Arthritis Rheum* 2001; **44**: 2492–502.

98. Ejbjerg, B., Narvestad, E., Rostrup, E., Szkudlarek, M., Jacobsen, S., Thomsen, H. S. *et al*. Magnetic resonance imaging of wrist and finger joints in healthy subjects occasionally shows changes resembling erosions and synovitis as seen in rheumatoid arthritis. *Arthritis Rheum* 2004; **50**: 1097–106.

99. Corvetta, A., Giovagnoni, A., Baldelli, S., Ercolani, P., Pomponio, G., Luchetti, M. M. *et al*. MR imaging of rheumatoid hand lesions: comparison with conventional radiology in 31 patients. *Clin Exp Rheumatol* 1992; **10**: 217–22.

100. Savnik, A., Malmskov, H., Thomsen, H. S., Graff, L. B., Nielsen, H., Danneskiold-Samsøe, B. *et al*. MRI of the wrist and finger joints in inflammatory joint diseases at 1-year interval: MRI features to predict bone erosions. *Eur Radiol* 2002; **12**: 1203–10.

101. Gold, G. E., and Beaulieu, C. F. Future of MR imaging of articular cartilage. *Semin Musculoskelet Radiol* 2001; **5**: 313–27.

102. Burstein, D., Bashir, A., and Gray, M. L. MRI techniques in early stages of cartilage disease. *Invest Radiol* 2000; **35**: 622–38.

103. Peterfy, C. G., van Dijke, C. F., Lu, Y., Nguyen, A., Connick, T. J., and Kneeland, J. B. *et al*. Quantification of the volume of articular cartilage in the metacarpophalangeal joints of the hand: accuracy and precision of three-dimensional MR imaging. *Am J Roentgenol* 1995; **165**: 371–5.

104. Peterfy, C. G. MRI in rheumatoid arthritis: current status and future directions. *J Rheumatol* 2001; **28**: 1134–42.

105. McGonagle, D., Gibbon, W., and Emery, P. Classification of inflammatory arthritis by enthesitis. *Lancet* 1998; **352**: 1137–40.

106. Jevtic, V., Watt, I., Rozman, B., Kos-Golja, M., Demsar, F., and Jarh, O. Distinctive radiological features of small hand joints in rheumatoid arthritis and seronegative spondyloarthritis by contrast-enhanced (Gd-DTPA) magnetic resonance imaging. *Skeletal Radiol* 1995; **24**: 351–5.

107. Giovagnoni, A., Grassi, W., Terelli, F., Blasetti, P., Paci, E., Ercolani, P. *et al*. MRI of the hand in psoriatic and rheumatical arthritis. *Eur Radiol* 1995; **5**: 590–5.

108. McGonagle, D., Gibbon, W., O'Connor, P., Green, M., Pease, C., and Emery, P. Characteristic magnetic resonance imaging entheseal changes of knee synovitis in spondylarthropathy. *Arthritis Rheum* 1998; **41**: 694–700.

109. Offidani, A., Cellini, A., Valeri, G., and Giovagnoni, A. Subclinical joint involvement in psoriasis: magnetic resonance imaging and X-ray findings. *Acta Derm Venereol* 1998; **78**: 463–5.

110. Rubens, D. J., Blebea, J. S., Totterman, S. M. S., and Hooper, M. M. Rheumatoid arthritis: evaluation of wrist extensor tendons with clinical examination versus MR imaging. A preliminary report. *Radiology* 1993; **187**: 831–8.

111. Østergaard, M., Klarlund, M., Lassere, M., Conaghan, P., Peterfy, C., McQueen, F. *et al*. Interreader agreement in the assessment of magnetic resonance images of rheumatoid arthritis wrist and finger joints: an international multicenter study. *J Rheumatol* 2001; **28**: 1143–50.

112. Conaghan, P., Lassere, M., Østergaard, M., Peterfy, C., McQueen, F., O'Connor, P. *et al*. OMERACT Rheumatoid Arthritis Magnetic Resonance Imaging Studies. Exercise 4: an international multice ter longitudinal study using the RA-MRI Score. *J Rheumatol* 2003; **30**: 1376–9.

113. Lassere, M., McQueen, F., Østergaard, M., Conaghan, P., Shnier, R., Peterfy, C. *et al*. OMERACT Rheumatoid Arthritis Magnetic Resonance Imaging Studies. Exercise 3: an international multicenter reliability study using the RA-MRI Score. *J Rheumatol* 2003; **30**: 1366–75.

114. Østergaard, M., Edmonds, J., McQueen, F., Peterfy, C., Lassere, M., Ejbjerg, B. *et al*. An introduction to the EULAR-OMERACT rheumatoid arthritis MRI reference image atlas. *Ann Rheum Dis* 2005; **64** (Suppl. 1): i3–i7.

115. Bird, P., Conaghan, P., Ejbjerg, B., McQueen, F., Lassere, M., Peterfy, C. *et al*. The development of the EULAR-OMERACT rheumatoid arthritis MRI reference image atlas. *Ann Rheum Dis* 2005; **64** (Suppl. 1): i8–i10.

116. Conaghan, P., Bird, P., Ejbjerg, B., O'Connor, P., Peterfy, C., McQueen, F. *et al*. The EULAR-OMERACT rheumatoid arthritis MRI reference image atlas: the metacarpophalangeal joints. *Ann Rheum Dis* 2005; **64** (Suppl. 1): i11–i21.

117. Ejbjerg, B., McQueen, F., Lassere, M., Haavardsholm, E., Conaghan, P., O'Connor, P. *et al*. The EULAR-OMERACT rheumatoid arthritis MRI reference image atlas: the wrist joint. *Ann Rheum Dis* 2005; **64** (Suppl. 1): i23–i47.

118. Østergaard, M., and Ejbjerg, B. Magnetic resonance imaging of the synovium in rheumatoid arthritis. *Semin Musculoskelet Radiol* 2004; **8**: 287–99.

119. Huizinga, T. W., Machold, K. P., Breedveld, F. C., Lipsky, P. E., and Smolen, J. S. Criteria for early rheumatoid arthritis: from Bayes' law revisited to new thoughts on pathogenesis. *Arthritis Rheum* 2002; **46**: 1155–9.

120. Sugimoto, H., Takeda, A., Masuyama, J., and Furuse, M. Early-stage rheumatoid arthritis: diagnostic accuracy of MR imaging. *Radiology* 1996; **198**: 185–92.

121. Østergaard, M., Stoltenberg, M., Gideon, P., Wieslander, S., Sonne-Holm, S., Kryger, P. *et al*. Effect of intraarticular osmic acid on synovial membrane volume and inflammation, determined by magnetic resonance imaging. *Scand J Rheumatol* 1995; **24**: 5–12.

122. Østergaard, M., Stoltenberg, M., Gideon, P., Sørensen, K., Henriksen, O., and Lorenzen, I. Changes in synovial membrane and joint effusion volumes after intraarticular methylprednisolone: quantitative assessment of inflammatory and destructive changes in arthritis by MRI. *J Rheumatol* 1996; **23**: 1151–61.

123. Kalden-Nemeth, D., Grebmeier, J., Antoni, C., Manger, B., Wolf, F., and Kalden, J. R. NMR monitoring of rheumatoid arthritis patients receiving anti-TNF-alpha monoclonal antibody therapy. *Rheumatol Int* 1997; **16**: 249–55.

124. Østergaard, M., Hansen, M., Stoltenberg, M., Gideon, P., Klarlund, M., Jensen, K. E. *et al*. Magnetic resonance imaging-determined synovial membrane volume as a marker of disease activity and a predictor of progressive joint destruction in the wrists of patients with rheumatoid arthritis. *Arthritis Rheum* 1999; **42**: 918–29.

125. Huang, J., Stewart, N., Crabbe, J., Robinson, E., McLean, L., Yeoman, S. *et al*. A 1-year follow-up study of dynamic magnetic resonance imaging in early rheumatoid arthritis reveals synovitis to be increased in shared-epitope patients and predictive of erosions at 1 year. *Rheumatology* 2000; **39**: 407–16.

126. Reece, R. J., Kraan, M. C., Radjenovic, A., Veale, D. J., O'Connor, P. J., Ridgway, J. P. *et al*. Comparative assessment of leflunomide and methotrexate for the treatment of rheumatoid arthritis, by dynamic

enhanced magnetic resonance imaging. *Arthritis Rheum* 2002; **46**: 366–72.

127. Bird, P., Ejbjerg, B., McQueen, F., Østergaard, M., Lassere, M., and Edmonds, J. OMERACT Rheumatoid Arthritis Magnetic Resonance Imaging Studies. Exercise 5: an international multicenter reliability study using computerized MRI erosion volume measurements. *J Rheumatol* 2003; **30**: 1380–4.

128. Bird, P., Kirkham, B., Portek, I., Shnier, R., Joshua, F., Edmonds, J. *et al.* Documenting damage progression in a two-year longitudinal study of rheumatoid arthritis patients with established disease (the DAMAGE study cohort): is there an advantage in the use of magnetic resonance imaging as compared with plain radiography? *Arthritis Rheum* 2004; **50**: 1383–9.

129. Lindegaard, H., Hørslev-Petersen, K., Vallø, J., Junker, P., and Østergaard M. Baseline MRI erosions in early rheumatoid arthritis MCP- and wrist joint bones markedly increase the risk of radiographic erosions at 1 year follow-up. *Arthritis Rheum* 2002; **46**: S521.

130. Conaghan, P. G., O'Connor, P., McGonagle, D., Astin, P., Wakefield, R. J., Gibbon, W. W. *et al.* Elucidation of the relationship between synovitis and bone damage: a randomized magnetic resonance imaging study of individual joints in patients with early rheumatoid arthritis. *Arthritis Rheum* 2003; **48**: 64–71.

131. Tanaka, N., Sakahashi, H., Ishii, S., Sato, E., Hirose, K., and Ishima, T. Synovial membrane enhancement and bone erosion by magnetic resonance imaging for prediction of radiologic progression in patients with early rheumatoid arthritis. *Rheumatol Int* 2004. [First published online].

132. Paulus, H. E., van der Heijde, D. M., Bulpitt, K. J., and Gold, R. H. Monitoring radiographic changes in early rheumatoid arthritis. *J Rheumatol* 1996; **23**: 801–5.

133. Modic, M. T., Weinstein, M. A., Pavlicek, W., Boumphrey, F., Starnes, D., and Duchesneau, P. M. Magnetic resonance imaging of the cervical spine: technical and clinical observations. *Am J Roentgenol* 1983; **141**: 1129–36.

134. Bundschuh, C., Modic, M. T., Kearney, F., Morris, R., and Deal, C. Rheumatoid arthritis of the cervical spine: surface-coil MR imaging. *Am J Roentgenol* 1988; **151**: 181–7.

135. Pettersson, H., Larsson, E. M., Holtås, S., Cronqvist, S., Egund, N., Zygmunt, S. *et al.* MR imaging of the cervical spine in rheumatoid arthritis. *AJNR Am J Neuroradiol* 1988; **9**: 573–7.

136. Nagata, K., Kiyonaga, K., Ohashi, T., Sagara, M., Miyazaki, S., and Inoue, A. Clinical value of magnetic resonance imaging for cervical myelopathy. *Spine* 1990; **15**: 1088–96.

137. Stiskal, M. A., Neuhold, A., Szolar, D. H., Saeed, M., Czerny, C., Leeb, B. *et al.* Rheumatoid arthritis of the craniocervical region by MR imaging: Detection and characterization. *Am J Roentgenol* 1995; **165**: 585–92.

138. Laiho, K., Soini, I., Kautiainen, H., and Kauppi, M. Can we rely on magnetic resonance imaging when evaluating unstable atlantoaxial subluxation? *Ann Rheum Dis* 2003; **62**: 254–6.

139. Hamilton, J. D., Johnston, R. A., Madhok, R., and Capell, H. A. Factors predictive of subsequent deterioration in rheumatoid cervical myelopathy. *Rheumatology (Oxford)* 2001; **40**: 811–15.

140. van Holsbeeck, M., van Holsbeeck, K., Gevers, G., Marchhal, G., van Steen, A., Favril, A. *et al.* Staging and follow-up of rheumatoid arthritis of the knee: comparison of sonography, thermography, and clinical assessment. *J Ultrasound Med* 1988; **7**: 561–6.

141. Østergaard, M., Court-Payen, M., Gideon, P., Wieslander, S., Cortsen, M., Henriksen, O. *et al.* The value of ultrasonography in arthritis of the knee: a comparison with magnetic resonance imaging. *Scand J Rheumatol* 1994; **Suppl. 98**: 19.

142. Newman, J. S., Laing, T. J., McCarthy, T. J., and Adler, R. S. Power Doppler sonography of synovitis: assessment of therapeutic response. Preliminary observations. *Radiology* 1996; **198**: 582–4.

143. Fiocco, U., Cozzi, L., Rubaltelli, L., Rigon, C., de Candia, A., Tregnaghi, A. *et al.* Long-term sonographic follow-up of rheumatoid and psoriatic proliferative knee joint synovitis. *Br J Rheumatol* 1996; **35**: 155–63.

144. Walther, M., Harms, H., Krenn, V., Radke, S., Faehndrick, T.-P., and Gohlke, F. Correlation of power Doppler sonography with vascularity of synovial tissue of the knee joint in patients with osteoarthritis and rheumatoid arthritis. *Arthritis Rheum* 2001; **44**: 331–8.

145. Terslev, L., Torp-Pedersen, S., Qvistgaard, E., von der Recke, P., and Bliddal, H. Doppler ultrasound findings in healthy wrists and finger joints. *Ann Rheum Dis* 2004; **63**: 644–8.

146. Szkudlarek, M., Court-Payen, Strandberg, C., Klarlund, M., Klausen, T., and Østergaard, M. Power Doppler ultrasonography for assessment of synovitis in the metacarpophalangeal joints of patients with rheumatoid arthritis: a comparison with dynamic magnetic resonance imaging. *Arthritis Rheum* 2001; **44**: 2018–23.

147. Hau, M., Schultz, H., Tony, H.-P., Keberle, M., Jahns, R., Haerten, R. *et al.* Evaluation of pannus and vascularization of the metacarpophalangeal and proximal interphalangeal joints in rheumatoid arthritis by high-resolution ultrasound (multidimensional linear array). *Arthritis Rheum* 1999; **42**: 2303–8.

148. Qvistgaard, E., Røgind, H., Torp-Pedersen, S., Terslev, L., Danneskiold-Samsøe, B., and Bliddal, H. Quantitative ultrasonography in rheumatoid arthritis: evaluation of inflammation by Doppler technique. *Ann Rheum Dis* 2001; **60**: 690–3.

149. Terslev, L., Torp-Pedersen, S., Qvistgaard, E., Danneskiold-Samsøe, B., and Bliddal, H. Estimation of inflammation by Doppler ultrasound: quantitative changes after intra-articular treatment in rheumatoid arthritis. *Ann Rheum Dis* 2003; **62**: 1049–53.

150. Walther, M., Harms, H., Krenn, V., Radke, S., Kirschner, S., and Gohlke, F. Synovial tissue of the hip at power Doppler US: correlation between vascularity and power Doppler US signal. *Radiology* 2002; **225**: 225–31.

151. Terslev, L., Torp-Pedersen, S., Savnik, A., von der Recke, P., Qvistgaard, E., Danneskiold-Samsøe, B. *et al.* Doppler ultrasound and magnetic resonance imaging of synovial inflammation of the hand in rheumatoid arthritis: a comparative study. *Arthritis Rheum* 2003; **48**: 2434–41.

152. Wakefield, R. J., Gibbon, W. W., Conaghan, P. G., O'Connor, P., McGonagle, D., Pease, C. *et al.* The value of sonography in the detection of bone erosions in patients with rheumatoid arthritis. *Arthritis Rheum* 2000; **43**: 2762–70.

153. Lopez-Ben, R., Bernreuter, W. K., Moreland, L. W., and Alarcon, G. S. Ultrasound detection of bone erosions in rheumatoid arthritis: a comparison to routine radiographs of the hands and feet. *Skeletal Radiol* 2004; **33**: 80–4.

154. Szkudlarek, M., Narvestad, E., Klarlund, M., Court-Payen, M., Thomsen, H. S., and Østergaard, M. Ultrasonography of the metatarsophalangeal joints in rheumatoid arthritis, compared with magnetic resonance imaging, conventional radiography and clinical examination. *Arthritis Rheum* 2004; **50**: 2103–12.

155. Magnani, M., Salizzoni, E., Mule, R., Fusconi, M., Meliconi, R., and Galletti, S. Ultrasonography detection of early bone erosions in the metacarpophalangeal joints of patients with rheumatoid arthritis. *Clin Exp Rheumatol* 2004; **22**: 743–8.

156. Grassi, W., Lamanna, G., Farina, A., and Cervini, C. Sonographic imaging of normal and osteoarthritic cartilage. *Semin Arthritis Rheum* 1999; **28**: 398–403.

157. McDonald, D. G., and Leopold, G. R. Ultrasound B-scanning in the differentiation of Baker's cyst and thrombophlebitis. *Br J Radiol* 1972; **45**: 729–32.

158. Grassi, W., Tittarelli, E., Blasetti, P., Pirani, O., and Cervini, C. Finger tendon involvement in rheumatoid arthritis: evaluation with high-frequency ultrasound. *Arthritis Rheum* 1995; **38**: 786–94.

159. Swen, W. A., Jacobs, J. W., Algra, P. R., Manoliu, R. A., Rijkmans, J., Willems, W. J. *et al.* Sonography and magnetic resonance imaging equivalent for the assessment of full-thickness rotator cuff tears. *Arthritis Rheum* 1999; **42**: 2231–8.

160. Swen, W. A. A., Jacobs, J. W. G., Hubach, P. C. G., Klasens, J. H., Algra, P. R., and Bijlsma, J. W. J. Comparison of sonography and magnetic resonance imaging for the diagnosis of partial tears of finger extensor tendons in rheumatoid arthritis. *Rheumatology* 2000; **39**: 55–62.

161. d'Agostino, M. A., Said-Nahal, R., Hacquard-Bouder, C., Brasseur, J. L., Dougados, M., and Breban, M. Assessment of peripheral

enthesitis in the spondylarthropathies by ultrasonography combined with power Doppler: a cross-sectional study. *Arthritis Rheum* 2003; **48**: 523–33.

162. Balint, P. V., Kane, D., Wilson, H., McInnes, I. B., and Sturrock, R. D. Ultrasonography of entheseal insertions in the lower limb in spondyloarthropathy. *Ann Rheum Dis* 2002; **61**: 905–10.

163. Kotob, H., and Kamel, M. Identification and prevalence of rheumatoid nodules in the finger tendons using high frequency ultrasonography. *J Rheumatol* 1999; **26**: 1264–8.

164. Grassi, W., Farina, A., Filippucci, E., and Cervini, C. Sonographically guided procedures in rheumatology. *Semin Arthritis Rheum* 2001; **30**: 347–53.

165. Grassi, W., Farina, A., Filippucci, E., and Cervini, C. Intralesional therapy in carpal tunnel syndrome: a sonographic-guided approach. *Clin Exp Rheumatol* 2002; **20**: 73–6.

166. Østergaard, M., and Szkudlarek, M. Ultrasonography: a valid method for assessment of rheumatoid arthritis? [Editorial.] *Arthritis and Rheumatism* 2005; **52**: 691–6.

167. Ribbens, C., Andre, B., Marcelis, S., Kaye, O., Mathy, L., Bonnet, V. *et al*. Rheumatoid hand joint synovitis: gray-scale and power Doppler US quantifications following anti-tumor necrosis factor-alpha treatment: pilot study. *Radiology* 2003; **229**: 562–9.

168. Szkudlarek, M., Court-Payen, Strandberg, C., Klarlund, M., Klausen, T., and Østergaard, M. Contrast-enhanced power Doppler ultrasonography of the metacarpophalangeal joints in rheumatoid arthritis. *Eur Radiol* 2003; **13**: 163–8.

169. Backhaus, M., Burmester, G. R., Gerber, T., Grassi, W., Machold, K. P., Swen, W. A. *et al*. Guidelines for musculoskeletal ultrasound in rheumatology. *Ann Rheum Dis* 2001; **60**: 641–9.

170. Filippucci, E., Unlu, Z., Farina, A., and Grassi, W. Sonographic training in rheumatology: a self teaching approach. *Ann Rheum Dis* 2003; **62**: 565–7.

171. Szkudlarek, M., Court-Payen, Jacobsen, S., Klarlund, M., Thomsen, H. S., and Østergaard, M. Interobserver agreement in ultrasonography of the finger and toe joints in rheumatoid arthritis. *Arthritis Rheum* 2003; **48**: 955–62.

172. Szkudlarek, M., Court-Payen, Strandberg, C., Klarlund, M., Klausen, T., and Østergaard, M. Contrast-enhanced power Doppler ultrasonography of the metacarpophalangeal joints in rheumatoid arthritis: reply to letter by Klauser *et al*. [Letter.] *Eur Radiol* 2003. [First published online, 18 July 2002.]

173. Scheel, A. K., Schmidt, W. A., Hermann, K. G., Bruyn, G. A., d'Agostino, M. A., Grassi, W. *et al*. Interobserver reliability of rheumatologists performing musculoskeletal ultrasonography: results from a EULAR 'Train the Trainers' course. *Ann Rheum Dis* 2005. [First published online, 7 Jan.]

174. Frediani, B., Falsetti, P., Storri, L., Allegri, A., Bisogno, S., Baldi, F. *et al*. Ultrasound and clinical evaluation of quadricipital tendon enthesitis in patients with psoriatic arthritis and rheumatoid arthritis. *Clin Rheumatol* 2002; **21**: 294–8.

175. Hau, M., Kneitz, C., Tony, H. P., Keberle, M., Jahns, R., and Jenett, M. High resolution ultrasound detects a decrease in pannus vascularisation of small finger joints in patients with rheumatoid arthritis receiving treatment with soluble tumour necrosis factor alpha receptor (etanercept). *Ann Rheum Dis* 2002; **61**: 55–8.

176. Taylor, P. C., Steuer, A., Gruber, J., Cosgrove, D. O., Blomley, M. J., Marsters, P. A. *et al*. Comparison of ultrasonographic assessment of synovitis and joint vascularity with radiographic evaluation in a randomized, placebo-controlled study of infliximab therapy in early rheumatoid arthritis. *Arthritis Rheum* 2004; **50**: 1107–16.

177. Yu, W., Xie, Y. Z., Jiang, M., Zheng, W. F., Wang, L. H., Wang, Y. Z. *et al*. CT detection of wrist bone erosion in rheumatoid arthritis. *Chin Med J (Engl)* 1993; **106**: 509–13.

178. Perry, D., Stewart, N., Benton, N., Robinson, E., Yeoman, S., Crabbe, J. *et al*. Detection of Erosions in the rheumatoid hand: a comparative study of multidetector computerized tomography versus magnetic resonance scanning. *J Rheumatol* 2005; **32**: 256–67.

179. Goldbach-Mansky, R., Woodburn, J., Yao, L., and Lipsky, P. E. Magnetic resonance imaging in the evaluation of bone damage in rheumatoid arthritis: a more precise image or just a more expensive one? *Arthritis Rheum* 2003; **48**: 585–9.

180. Colamussi, P., Prandini, N., Cittanti, C., Feggi, L., and Giganti, M. Scintigraphy in rheumatic diseases. *Best Pract Res Clin Rheumatol* 2004; **18**: 909–26.

181. Manger, B. New developments in imaging for diagnosis and therapy monitoring in rheumatic diseases. *Best Pract Res Clin Rheumatol* 2004; **18**: 773–81.

182. Al Janabi, M. A., Jones, A. K., Solanki, K., Sobnack, R., Bomanji, J., Al Nahhas, A. A. *et al*. 99Tcm-labelled leucocyte imaging in active rheumatoid arthritis. *Nucl Med Commun* 1988; **9**: 987–91.

183. Berna, L., Torres, G., Diez, C., Estorch, M., Martinez-Duncker, D., and Carrio, I. Technetium-99m human polyclonal immunoglobulin G studies and conventional bone scans to detect active joint inflammation in chronic rheumatoid arthritis. *Eur J Nucl Med* 1992; **19**: 173–6.

184. de Bois, M. H., Tak, P. P., Arndt, J. W., Kluin, P. M., Pauwels, E. K., and Breedveld, F. C. Joint scintigraphy for quantification of synovitis with 99mTc-labelled human immunoglobulin G compared to histological examination. *Clin Exp Rheumatol* 1995; **13**: 155–9.

185. Mottonen, T. T., Hannonen, P., Toivanen, J., Rekonen, A., and Oka, M. Value of joint scintigraphy in the prediction of erosiveness in early rheumatoid arthritis. *Ann Rheum Dis* 1988; **47**: 183–9.

186. van de Wiele, C., van den Bosch, F., Mielants, H., Simons, M., Veys, E. M., and Dierckx, R. A. Bone scintigraphy of the hands in early stage lupus erythematosus and rheumatoid arthritis. *J Rheumatol* 1997; **24**: 1916–21.

187. Jensen, T. Regional bone loss in rheumatoid arthritis: a marker of disease activity and irreversible bone damage? PhD dissertation, 2003.

188. Jensen, T., Klarlund, M., Hansen, M., Jensen, K. E., Pødenphant, J, Hansen, T. M. *et al*. Bone loss in unclassified polyarthritis and early rheumatoid arthritis is better detected by digital x ray radiogrammetry than dual x ray absorptiometry: relationship with disease activity and radiographic outcome. *Ann Rheum Dis* 2004; **63**: 15–22.

189. Haugeberg, G., Lodder, M. C., Lems, W. F., Uhlig, T., Orstavik, R. E., Dijkmans, B. A. *et al*. Hand cortical bone mass and its associations with radiographic joint damage and fractures in 50–70 year old female patients with rheumatoid arthritis: cross sectional Oslo-Truro-Amsterdam (OSTRA) collaborative study. *Ann Rheum Dis* 2004; **63**: 1331–4.

190. Stewart, A., Mackenzie, L. M., Black, A. J., and Reid, D. M. Predicting erosive disease in rheumatoid arthritis. A longitudinal study of changes in bone density using digital X-ray radiogrammetry: a pilot study. *Rheumatology (Oxford)* 2004; **43**: 1561–4.

20 | Susceptibility, prognosis, and mortality

Marjatta Leirisalo-Repo

Introduction

Rheumatoid arthritis is a chronic systemic disease in which both environmental and genetic factors are proposed to play a role. There is evidence of a long-term immune aberration in individuals that later develop the clinical picture of rheumatoid arthritis. This is nicely demonstrated by the presence of rheumatoid factor and antifilaggrin antibodies (see Ref. 1) and anti-cyclic citrullinated peptide (anti-CCP) antibodies[2] in asymptomatic individuals even years prior to the diagnosis of rheumatoid arthritis. However, there are a few environmental factors known to be associated with the development of the disease. Of these, smoking is the only factor strongly associated with the risk for the development of seropositive rheumatoid arthritis in several populations (see Refs 1, 3).

Genetic factors have a role in the susceptibility. The concordance of rheumatoid arthritis in monozygotic twins is 12–15%, and computed heritability is as high as 60% (reviewed in Refs 1, 4). Of the genetic markers, human leukocyte antigen (HLA)-DRB1 gene has been demonstrated to be associated with the disease in different populations.

After the onset of clinical disease, the patients usually continue to have persistent and progressive disease; the severity and progression rate is, however, hard to predict. The determination of long-term prognosis of patients with rheumatoid arthritis depends on the patient populations studied, on the follow-up time, and on the therapeutic interventions applied during the follow-up period. The natural course is hard to determine, because the majority of patients will be exposed to therapeutic measures which may modify the progression.

In previous population studies on patients fulfilling the American Rheumatology Association (ARA) criteria for, possible, probable, or definite rheumatoid arthritis[5], many of the subjects had no evidence of chronic disease when studied a few years later[6]. These studies cannot easily be applied to the present situation because diagnostic criteria for rheumatoid arthritis were less strict. In particular, patients with possible rheumatoid arthritis might have had other more benign forms of arthritis such as reactive arthritis, psoriasis arthritis, arthritis in association with viral infections such as parvovirus, or other self-limiting arthritides of unknown etiology. However, recent studies have also shown that population cohorts with rheumatoid arthritis have a less severe course of disease compared with patients collected from specialist clinics[7,8].

Reports from many countries have also shown that a considerable proportion of patients with rheumatoid arthritis are only treated in primary care and do not seek or are not referred to specialist units. Up to 50% of patients with rheumatoid arthritis have been reported to be treated exclusively in primary care in Sweden[9,10]. In Hannover, Germany, only 16% of rheumatoid arthritis patients had consulted a rheumatologist or internist during the previous 12 months[11]. In a primary care-based registry of incident cases of inflammatory polyarthritis with disease duration of less than 12 weeks, 80% of whom fulfilled the American College of Rheumatology (ACR) diagnostic criteria[12] during the first year, 35% of the patients were treated solely by the general practitioner[13].

Unselected patients with inflammatory polyarthritis studied prospectively have a benign disease, with a majority recovering within the first two years[14,15]. By contrast, the subgroup of patients with early rheumatoid arthritis, mostly rheumatoid factor (RF) positive, have progressive arthritis, with a rate of remission during the first three years of disease of 6.5–19%[16–18].

This chapter will discuss the outcome and mortality of patients with rheumatoid arthritis, addressing the question from information available from population and hospital studies and from prospective cohort studies. In addition, the contributing effect of treatment modalities on the outcome and mortality will be discussed. As all these end points are highly dependent on the time course, only studies on patients with disease duration of at least five years will be included.

Population and hospital studies

Functional disability

Most of the reports are on patients with persistent rheumatoid arthritis, either cross-sectional or with varying information on the course of the disease (either retrospective or prospective). Of patients with rheumatoid arthritis treated at specialist clinics, 36–80% have functional disability of Steinbrocker class III–IV after 9–20 years from onset of the disease (Table 20.1). Only 10% do not develop significant disability[19]. Deterioration of functional capacity seems to be progressive and starts within the first years of the disease (Fig. 20.1). The figures are for patients surviving at least 12 years[19]. The slopes would be even steeper if all patients presenting with early disease were included prospectively, because the most severely handicapped are probably missing due to increased mortality[22,23]. Measured by a Health Assessment Questionnaire (HAQ), patients with persistent rheumatoid arthritis who attended a private practice rheumatic disease clinic in 1977–88 were estimated to reach the disability score of 1 (difficulty in activities of daily living) at a median time of 10 years, score 2 (great difficulty in activities of daily living/need of assistance) at 21 years, and score 2.5 (severe disability) at 35 years after the onset of the disease[24].

Cases selected from the general population do best: about 20% of patients selected from the general population are moderately

Table 20.1 Development of disability in patients with rheumatoid arthritis

Reference	Entry years	Number of patients	Disease duration at entry (years)	Follow-up time (years)	Cohort	Intervention[a]	Steinbrocker I/II/III/IV (%)	% with III/IV	HAQ
98	NG[b]	500	233: ≤2	. . .[c]	Hospital outpatients, retrospective	NG	NG	18	NG
		403	127: 2–5	1–5				26	
		387	140: ≥6	6–10				42	
		246		11–15				50	
		176		≥16				55	
31	1948–51	307	6–7	9	Hospital patients, active/poor function at entry, prospective	NG	20/40/27/13	40	NG
78, 80	NG	100	<1	20	Early consecutive hospital admissions, prospective	NG		45	NG
				25		NG	31/43/17/9	26	NG
41	1973	75	11	9	Hospital patients, drug trial, Retrospective	In 1973 intra-articular thiotepa Later therapy NG	16/12/34/8	42	0.96 (MHAQ)[d]
19	1966–74	681	10	12	Outpatient clinic, cross-sectional	NG	17/47/20/16	36	NG
25	1965–67	239	NG	17	Population survey, prospective	NG	16/62/15/6	21	NG (MHAQ)[d]
75	1964–86	112	64% <5	20	Clinical patients, prospective	DMARD[e]/steroids 100%	Modified:I/II 28 I:III 43IV/V 29	72	NG
35	1966–74	292	9	6	Multicenter prospective	NG	NG	NG	1.20
127	1983–88	574	10	5	Rheumatology practices, prospective, observational	100% intramuscular gold	NG		1.00
97	1981	209	12	8	Population study	NG		NG	1.16
74	1988–89	129	Newly diagnosed	6	Multiple centers, elderly, retrospective	77% DMARD	4/63/27/6	33	NG
20, 23	1966–71	102	<1	15	Hospital referrals, prospective	During first three years: 64% DMARD, 15% steroids	0/58/28/4	42	0.95
101	NG	127	5	7	Hospital referrals, prospective	100% DMAsRD	20/50/27/3	30	1.63
115	1982–86	132	1.6	6	Clinical patients, female, 20–50 years, prospective	75% DMARD	45/45/10/0	10	0.82
26	1989	103	30: ≤10	. . .	Population survey, cross-sectional	97% DMARD	0/67/33/0	33	
			44: 11–20				0/45/55/0	55	0.85
			28: ≥20				0/28/61/4	65	
8	1985	128	<1	6–7	Inception cohort, retrospective	85% DMARD	NG	NG	0.49 (MHAQ)
131	NG	2888	8–11	10	Multicenter prospective	84% DMARD 64% Steroids	NG	NG	1.18–1.60
73	1983–89	142	0.7	6	Hospital inception cohort, prospective	100% DMARD 35% Steroids	9/29/21/3	24	0.64
21	NG	200	11	. . .	Outpatient clinic, cross-sectional	70% DMARD 10% Steroids	NG	NG	1.30
71	1985–87	106	1	7	Hospital inception cohort, prospective	65% DMARD	8/90/2/0	2	1.3
121	1986–90	440	106: 0–2	5	Clinical patients, prospective	100% intramuscular gold gold	NG	NG	1.25
			93: >2–5			0% steroids			1.81
			235: >5						2.13

[a] Treatment received some time during follow-up.
[b] Not given.
[c] Not applicable.
[d] Modified HAQ.
[e] Disease-modifying anti-rheumatic drug.

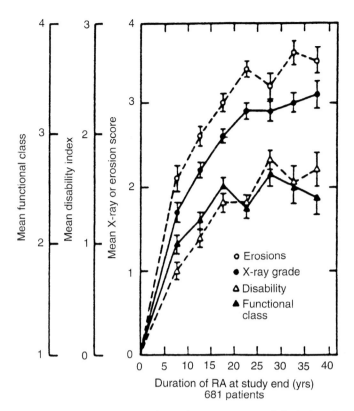

Fig. 20.1 Cross-sectional analysis of erosion score, radiological grade, disability index, and functional class in 681 rheumatoid arthritis patients. (Reproduced from Ref. 19: Sherrer YS, Bloch DA, Mitchell DM, Young DY, Fries JF (1986). The development of disability in rheumatoid arthritis. *Arthritis and Rheumatism* **29**: 494–500, with permission of Lippincott Williams and Wilkins.)

or severely incapacitated after 20 years[25]. With increasing duration of disease, a high proportion of patients have developed at least moderate disability but severe functional handicap is rare[26].

Work disability

Rheumatoid arthritis has a major impact on the work capacity of patients. Most of the studies on work disability have been performed on patients in gainful employment while the work disability in homemakers has been analyzed less frequently.

Mäkisara and Mäkisara[27] analyzed the work disability of patients treated at the Heinola Rheumatism Foundation Hospital in the 1970s. They observed a steady decrease in work capacity of patients with increasing duration of the disease. Thus, work disability was 40% in patients with duration of disease of 5 years, 50% in those with disease duration of 10 years, and 67% in those with disease duration of 15 years. The figure reported 20 years later for patients during the first 4 years of the disease in the Netherlands, 42%, is not remarkably different from the Finnish report[28].

A long-term study of a cohort of patients with persistent rheumatoid arthritis collected in 1948–51 and prospectively followed up for nine years ended up with lower figures, 12–20%, for work disability during 2–9 years of follow-up (Table 20.2).

These figures are not representative of the whole patient population because they were based only on the available subgroup of patients in gainful employment at various periods[29–31].

The risk of losing work capacity has been prospectively analyzed by two groups. Out of 75 patients fully employed during the first year of the disease, 37% were disabled at the end of six-year follow-up[32]. The figure is similar in another group of patients treated for established rheumatoid arthritis by rheumatologists in the United States. Of those fully employed at the start of the study, 34% were not able to work after five years[33]. The work ability decreased most rapidly during the first three years of the disease (Fig. 20.2).

Radiological damage

Joint damage is a hallmark of rheumatoid arthritis and few patients escape from it. In cross-sectional studies of patients with persistent rheumatoid arthritis, more than 90% of the patients had erosive changes[34]. The progression of the changes is considered to be more rapid during the first years (Fig. 20.1) but the destruction usually continues with increased duration of the disease[19,35]. About 5–6% of the joints show new erosions annually during the first years of the disease[34].

Most of the studies on long-term radiological outcome of patients with rheumatoid arthritis are cross-sectional. Therefore, it is hard to determine whether there are any changes in the outcome in patients acquiring the disease in different decades. However, Heikkilä and Isomäki[36] addressed this question by analyzing hand and feet radiographs of four cohorts of female patients aged 45–64 years, RF positive, and with disease duration between 10 and 15 years but admitted to hospital in 1962, 1972, 1982, and 1992. Interestingly, during the 30-year span, the proportion of intact joints in fingers rose from 53.5 to 70.4%, in

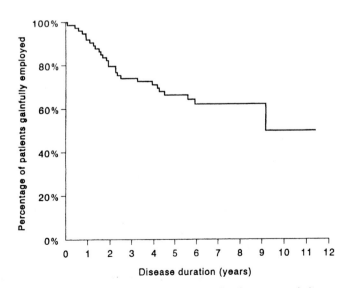

Fig. 20.2 Loss of work capacity during the first years of disease. (Reproduced from Ref.32: Mau W, Bornmann M, Weber H, Weidemann HF, Hecker H, Raspe HH (1996). Prediction of permanent work disability in a follow-up study of early rheumatoid arthritis: results of a tree structured analysis using RECPAM. *British Journal of Rheumatology* **35**: 652–9, with permission of the British Society for Rheumatology.)

Table 20.2 Work disability of patients with rheumatoid arthritis

Reference	Number of patients	Disease duration (years)	Follow-up time (years)	Cohort	Work disability at entry (%)	Work disability at outcome (%)
29	307	6–7	...	Hospital patients, active disease/poor function	8	...
			2		12	
30		6		18		
31		9		20		
98	500	233: ≤2	...	Hospital outpatients, retrospective	28	...
	403	127: 2–5	1–5		24	
	387	140: ≥6	6–10		27	
	246		11–15		29	
	176		≥ 16		32	
27	405	144: 5	...	Hospital patients, cross-sectional	40	...
		131: 10			50	
		130: 15			67	
41	75	11	9	Hospital patients, drug trial	60	85
81	84	1	2	Hospital inception cohort, prospective	32	47
71	106	1	7	0	42	37
28	119	≤ 4	...	Early rheumatoid arthritis, interview	42	...
33	392	61% >5	5	Rheumatologists' patients, prospective interview	0	34
32	75	≤1	6	Early rheumatoid arthritis, all gainfully employed, prospective	0	37

wrists from 14.0 to 29.0%, and in feet from 29.8 to 40.0%. The improved outcome may reflect that the disease has become more benign, or that earlier and more aggressive therapy has favorably affected the course, but we like to favor the latter interpretation.

Mortality

A vast majority of studies have reported that patients with rheumatoid arthritis have an increased risk for mortality compared with populations without rheumatoid arthritis (Figs 20.3–20.7). This can be estimated by the standardized mortality ration (SMR) (Table 20.3). The median life expectancy is 4–7 years shorter for male, and 3–10 years shorter for female patients[37–39]. The mortality figures depend on the age of the cohorts, follow-up time, entry selection criteria, and also on the criteria for diagnosis for rheumatoid arthritis. Some studies have included only patients with RF positive rheumatoid arthritis[40], with or without a definite laboratory abnormality[37], previously participating in a drug trial[41,42], or those of a cohort collected by

previous mail survey[43]. The interpretation of these seemingly conflicting results is an open question. Earlier studies included patients with mild and transient disease that may not have been rheumatoid arthritis[6,25].

There have been three population studies, two of which showed increased risk for mortality[45,46], while the third study observed no increased mortality rates compared with the background population[44]. This was a population study of incidence and prevalence of rheumatoid arthritis in Rochester, Minnesota, which also included patients with probable rheumatoid arthritis. In an extensive analysis of long-term prognosis of different patient cohorts by Wolfe et al.[47], patients belonging to a community-based cohort also had increased mortality risk (SMR 2.18).

Because of the heterogeneity of the studies, it is hard to analyze the contribution of the duration of the disease to the increased risk of mortality. However, there seems to be no major trend for an increase in the SMR with the duration of the disease (Table 20.3).

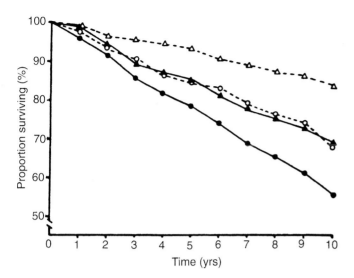

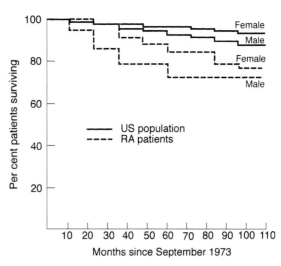

Fig. 20.3 Survival of patients with rheumatoid arthritis treated at the Rheumatism Foundation Hospital, Finland in 1959–68 and control population. Circles, men; triangles, women; closed symbols, patients; open symbols, controls. (Reproduced from Ref. 52: Mutru O, Laakso M, Isomäki H, Koota K (1985). Ten year mortality and causes of death in patients with rheumatoid arthritis. *British Medical Journal* **290**: 1979–9, with permission of the British Medical Journal.)

Fig. 20.5 Survival of patients with rheumatoid arthritis participating in a drug trial in 1973 at Vanderbilt University, United States, compared with population figures. (Reproduced from Ref. 42, Pincus T, Callahan LF, Vaughn WK (1987). Questionnaire, walking time and button test measures of functional capacity as predictive markers for mortality in rheumatoid arthritis. *Journal of Rheumatology* **14**: 240–51, with permission of the Journal of Rheumatology.)

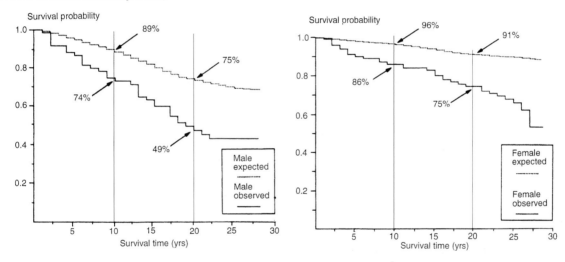

Fig. 20.4 Survival of patients with rheumatoid arthritis with disease onset between 1964 and 1978 treated at the Queen Elizabeth Hospital, Birmingham, England compared with population figures. (Reproduced from Ref. 56: Symmons DPM, Jones MA, Scott DL, Prior P (1998). Long-term outcome in patients with rheumatoid arthritis: early presenters continue to do well. *Journal of Rheumatology* **25**: 1072–7, with permission of the Journal of Rheumatology.)

The causes for increased mortality can be divided into three categories: (a) mortality due to rheumatoid arthritis; (b) mortality due to intervening illness; and (c) mortality caused by the treatment. Rheumatoid arthritis has been reported as a primary or underlying cause of mortality in 0–11%[39,43,46,48]. This is, however, not reliable, because in most studies which are based on analysis of death certificates, rheumatoid arthritis is underreported as a cause or as a contributing factor[49,50].

The shortening of life expectancy is evident after five years of the disease[51], and is mainly due to increased frequency of infections and cardiovascular, renal, and pulmonary diseases[14,50]. Amyloidosis has contributed to excess renal mortality, especially in Finland[39,52]. Mortality figures due to cancer are not higher than

that of the general population, but there is an increased frequency of hematological malignancies[40,47,53–56]. The hematological malignancies are usually lymphomas, but myeloma patients have increased frequency of rheumatoid arthritis compared with matched population controls[57,58]. Risk for mortality due to lymphoma increases with the duration[59] and high inflammatory activity of the disease[60].

In recent years, the role of drugs used to treat rheumatoid arthritis and the morbidity/mortality of patients has been analyzed in detail. While the evaluation of causes of mortality with respect to complications of the disease or to treatment is not always easy, as pointed out by Symmons[61], about 10% of all deaths have been attributed to the use of drug therapies[38,62].

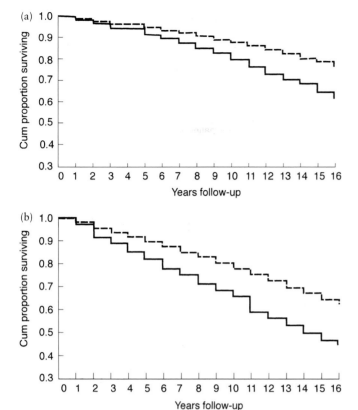

Fig. 20.6 Survival of patients with seropositive rheumatoid arthritis (solid lines). (a) Figures for females treated at the Department of Rheumatology, University of Umeå, Sweden, in 1979 compared with population figures (dashed lines). (b) Figures for males. (Reproduced from Ref. 40: Wållberg-Jonsson S, Öhman M-L, Rantapää Dahlqvist S (1997). Cardiovascular morbidity and mortality in patients with seropositive rheumatoid arthritis in Northern Sweden. *Journal of Rheumatology* **24**: 445–51, with permission of the Journal of Rheumatology.)

Disease-modifying anti-rheumatic drugs (DMARDs) are associated with frequent side-effects, some of which can be serious. However, fatal complications caused by the use of DMARDs are very rare, and have been estimated to contribute to the patient's death in less than 1% of cases[63]. In the thorough analysis of 1666 patients with rheumatoid arthritis who died in 1989, the death of 6 patents (0.4%) could be attributed to the use of DMARDs[62].

There is evidence that immunosuppressive therapy, especially azathioprine, may play a role in the increased risk of hematopoetic malignancies[64,65]. However, other studies found no association between the use of cytotoxic drugs and such malignancies[53,54]. An extensive analysis of four patient cohorts, including 3501 patients followed for up to 35 years, showed no increased mortality in patients treated with azathioprine[47]. The report of an increased frequency of lymphoma observed in a population of rheumatoid arthritis, only a few of whom had received any DMARDs, also speaks against the role of treatment as a contributing factor[60]. On the contrary, continuing high inflammatory activity was a major risk factor[60]. Methotrexate is increasingly used in the treatment of rheumatoid arthritis. While there is a report of increased mortality due to infections, but not to malignant

diseases, observed during a 10-year follow-up time in patients treated initially with methotrexate[66], another large prospective study presented evidence that methotrexate may provide a substantial survival benefit[67]; the benefit was most distinct in the reduction of cardiovascular mortality.

Contrary to the low risk of excess mortality due to DMARDs, there is increasing evidence that the use of non-steroidal anti-inflammatory drugs (NSAIDs)[38,48,62] and systemic glucocorticosteroids are associated with fatal complications. Gastrointestinal bleeding is the most frequent side-effect caused by NSAIDs, with a risk of death of 0.19% per year[68]. Other less common side-effects are kidney failure and hematological complications. About 2% of the deaths are attributed to the use of NSAIDs[62]. With these facts in mind, great expectations were addressed to the selective inhibitors of cyclo-oxygenase-2 enzyme and the introduction of coxibs as safer drugs for patients with increased risks for gastrointestinal bleeding. However, the recent observation that rofecoxib is associated with increased thromboembolic complications is worrying[69], and has led to the, at least, temporary withdrawal of rofecoxib from the market. The cardiovascular safety of other coxibs, and non-selective NSAIDs is now under close surveillance.

The use of glucocorticoids in association with NSAIDs enhances the risk for gastrointestinal complications[68]. In many studies, the mortality of patients treated with glucocorticoids has been higher compared with those who had not received such a treatment[23,42,47]. The impact on the mortality, however, is hard to estimate because the studies have not been randomized, with a bias to more severe disease in those treated with glucocorticoids. However, there is increasing evidence that glucocorticoids are an independent risk factor for cardiovascular mortality[70,71]. In addition to arteriosclerosis, glucocorticoids can increase the risk for infections and osteoporotic fractures, both of which can contribute to increased mortality. In the nation-wide analysis of mortality of patients with rheumatoid arthritis, 0.7% of deaths were associated with glucocorticoids[62].

In conclusion, the mortality of patients with rheumatoid arthritis treated at hospitals is increased. Rheumatoid arthritis as a contributing factor is usually underestimated. Cardiovascular, hematological, nephrological, and gastrointestinal causes are increased. Part of the excess mortality is related to the NSAID treatment.

Early rheumatoid arthritis cohorts

Functional disability

Ideally, the best information would be achieved on an unselected patient cohort attending a prospective study at an early phase of disease followed up by the same team with structured questionnaires for 20–30 years. However, most of the studies available have some limitations and have been running less than 10 years. In five prospective studies on patients with early rheumatoid

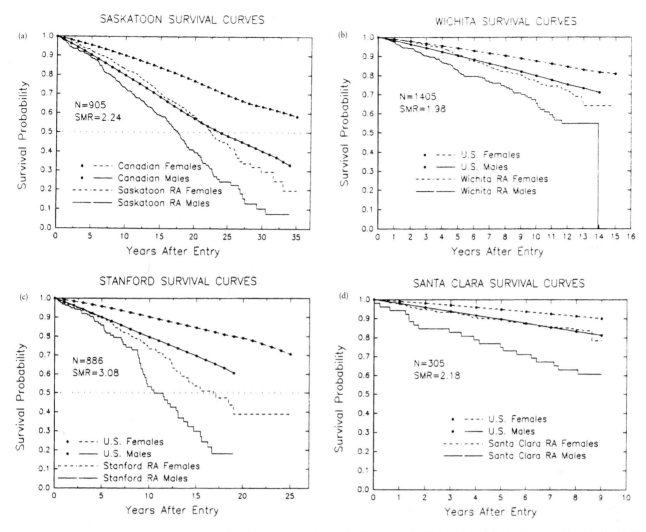

Fig. 20.7 Survival patients with rheumatoid arthritis treated for early disease at the University of Saskatchewan, Canada in 1966–1974 (A), of consecutive patients treated at an outpatient rheumatology clinic in Wichita, USA in 1973–90 (B), of consecutive patients treated at Stanford University, USA in 1965–90 (C), and of population-based cohort of patients who were identified by an advertisement in Santa Clara County, USA in 1979–1979 (D). Respective expected survival curve for each population is also given. (Reproduced from Ref. 47: Wolfe F, Mitchell DM, Sibley JT *et al.* (1994). The mortality of rheumatoid arthritis. *Arthritis and Rheumatism* **37**: 481–94, with permission of Lippincott Williams and Wilkins.)

arthritis (entry into the study within the first two years of symptoms), functional disability analyzed either by Steinbrocker or HAQ seems to vary greatly (Table 20.1). Part of this variation depends on the follow-up time but other factors such as age and functional stage of the patients at entry, treatment with DMARDs and glucocorticoids, and orthopaedic surgery, cannot be ruled out.

Contrary to cross-sectional studies, in prospective studies on patients with early rheumatoid arthritis a decrease in the functional capacity with time is less obvious. There are some prospective studies on patients with early disease followed up for 5–15 years. In a study from Sweden, median HAQ changed during 5 years non-significantly from 0.8 to 0.9[72], but increased to 1.3 during the next 3 years[73]. At 10-year follow-up, with 92% of the patients available at the study, the median HAQ was 1.1[74]. A study from Finland showed a change in mean HAQ from 0.28 to 0.64 within the first 6 years[75]. After 15 years of disease, patients followed from early disease in the United Kingdom still

had a mean HAQ of 0.95[23]. A non-significant progression from Steinbrocker class II toward class III was observed in a cohort of patients with late-onset, seropositive, erosive disease[76]. Patients with early rheumatoid arthritis seem to get better or stay at least stable during the first 10 years of the disease, but start to lose functional capacity during the second decade of the disease[77].

Results from one early cohort with reports on the functional outcome at various intervals[78–82] show that there seems to be a decrease in the severity of disability with time. However, this may be explained by the report of functional outcome being made only for patients who attended follow-up—with increasing time, the numbers of patients dying between follow-up visits increases. Patients with high functional disability have an increased risk for mortality[45,77]. Rasker and Cosh[22] have also shown that the functional capacity of patients who died during a prospective study of long-term outcome was lower at last review than in those who survived for 20–25 years (Table 20.4).

Table 20.3 Mortality in patients with rheumatoid arthritis

Reference	Entry years	Cohort	Number of patients	Age at entry	Disease duration at entry (years)	Follow-up time (years)	Mortality (%)	SMR
98	NG	Hospital outpatients, retrospective	500	NG	233: ≤2 127: 2–5 140: ≥6	13	20	NG
31	1948–51	Hospital admissions due to active disease/poor function	307	51	6–7	9	24	'Increased'
44	1950–74	Population study	521	Median 40–50	0.6	NG	27	1.16
45	1965–67	Population questionnaire, prospective	293	NG	NG	11	29	Males: 1.92 Females: 1.18
41, 42	1973	Hospital patients, drug trial	75	55	11	9	36	1.32
37	1954–57	Hospital patients	209	54	8	25	79	Males: 1.38 Females: 1.05
52	1959–68	Hospital patients	1000	55	NG	10	36	Males: 1.44 Female: 2.03
19	1966–74	Hospital patients	1043	40	10	12	27	NG
77	1964–66	Hospital patients	112	Median 40–50	72: <5 40: ≥5	20	35	NG
43	1978–81	Mail survey	279	58	NG	5	13	1.19
22	NG	Early consecutive hospital admissions, prospective	100	51	<1	25	65	NG
23	1966–71	Early rheumatoid arthritis, hospital patients, prospective	102	51	<1	12	28	1.13
48	1980–86	Various age cohorts retrospective	130	60	0.7	6	18	1.69
46	1965–89	Longitudinal population survey	172	NG	NG	. . .	46	1.28
47	Various periods	Various patients cohorts	3501	53	9	8	26	2.26
92	1973–75	Population cohort, prospective	121	NG	<0.5	20	29	1.09
39	1989	Cross-sectional population study	1666	75	16	. . .	100	Males: 1.41 Females: 1.37
40	1979	Seropositive patients treated in hospitals	606	54–56	16	13	44	Males: 1.47 Females: 1.64
56	1968–74	Various hospital cohorts	448	48	252: ≤5 196: >5	22	59	2.7

Abbreviations as in Table 20.1.

Work disability

Work disability is observed early in the disease course: in the Swedish cohort of early rheumatoid arthritis, during the first two years after entry 47% of 84 patients, and, during seven years, 37% of 106 patients were unable to work[73,83]. Importantly, 70% of those who had stopped working had done so during the first year of the disease, that is, often before having been referred to specialist care[83].

Radiological destruction

In prospective studies on cohorts of early rheumatoid arthritis, erosive changes at entry (mean duration of symptoms less than 12 months) have been detected in about 8[84], 4[85], and 47%[75,76] of the

Table 20.4 Functional capacity (%) of patients in a prospective study of early rheumatoid arthritis, functional capacity measured at 20 and 25 years in survivors and at latest review in deceased

Functional capacity (Steinbrocker)	Survivors		Dead at latest visit
	at 20 years	at 25 years	
I	24	35	26
II	31	40	15
III	39	16	24
IV	6	8	35

Reproduced from Ref. 22: Rasker JJ, Cosh JA (1992). Long-term effects of treating rheumatoid arthritis. *Baillières Clinical Rheumatology* 6: 141–60, by permission of the publisher, WB Saunders Company Limited.

patients. During the next few years, most of the patients who were non-erosive at entry developed erosions. Plant *et al.*[87] have followed up prospectively a selected cohort of patients with early (symptoms less that three years) rheumatoid arthritis without erosions at entry: 70% of the patients developed erosions during the next eight years. Erosions developed in 73% of patients with early (symptoms less than one year) rheumatoid arthritis, followed prospectively for a mean of nine years at the Middlesex Hospital[88]. Initial studies showed that the progression was most advanced during the first two years of follow-up[34,84,86,87]. However, an extensive prospective study of the early arthritis cohort in Heinola revealed that destruction is continuing up to 20 years[89]. While individual progression during the first eight years varies[87,90] (Fig. 20.8), the average radiological destruction shows continuing progression (Fig. 20.9).

Mortality

Of patients with early rheumatoid arthritis in 1966–71, followed up at the Middlesex Hospital, 28% (SMR 1.13) died during a mean of 13 years of follow-up[23]. A patient cohort with very early rheumatoid arthritis (duration of symptoms less than six months at entry), recruited from the population in 1973–75 and followed up prospectively at the Rheumatism Foundation Hospital in Heinola, had no increased risk for mortality during the next 20 years (SMR 1.09)[90]. The figures are comparable to the population study by Linos *et al.*[44] in the United States (Table 20.3), but they are lower compared with other reports on patient cohorts with established rheumatoid arthritis in prospective or cross-sectional studies (Table 20.3). The recruitment of patients from the community might be one explanation for the low mortality risk in these two studies with the lowest mortality ratios since patients not referred routinely to specialist care have a milder disease[91]. In a population study from Sweden, the mortality was not increased in those patients who had not been hospitalized during the observation period[45]. The role of early treatment, medical, vocational, and orthopedic, cannot be ruled out as patients referred for treatment within the next five years of the disease seem to have a better prognosis than those with a longer duration of disease before referral[56].

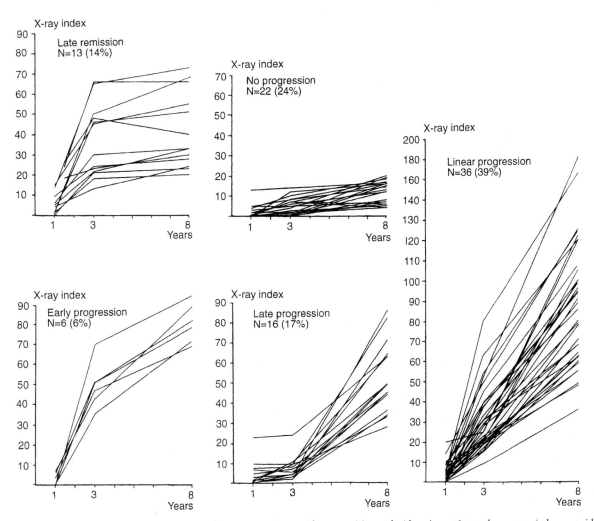

Fig 20.8 Patterns of development of radiological destruction in patients with seropositive early (duration <6 months at entry) rheumatoid arthritis. Joint destruction analyzed by Larsen score 0–200 (Ref. 91). (Reproduced from Ref. 90, Isomäki H (1992). Long-term outcome of rheumatoid arthritis. *Scandinavian Journal of Rheumatology* **21** (Suppl. 95): 3–8, with permission of the *Scandinavian Journal of Rheumatology*.)

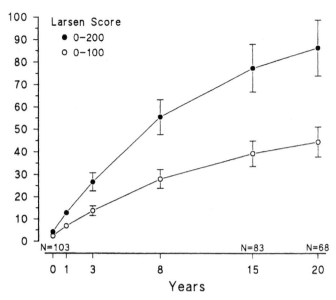

Fig. 20.9 Development of radiological destruction (means and 95% confidence limits) in patients with seropositive early (duration <6 months at entry) rheumatoid arthritis analyzed by Larsen score (0–200; Ref. 91), and a modification by Kaarela (score 0–100; Ref. 89). (Reproduced from Ref. 89: Kaarela K, Kautiainen H (1997). Continuous progression of radiological destruction in seropositive rheumatoid arthritis. *Journal of Rheumatology* **24**: 1285–7, with permission of the *Journal of Rheumatology*.)

Can one predict the outcome in rheumatoid arthritis?

Clinical features of the disease

Some clinical features of patients with rheumatoid arthritis which predict poor outcome have been identified. These include early loss of function, female sex, low education level, and persistent active disease with clinical and laboratory evidence of continuous inflammation[63,94]. Most of the information is, however, based on studies on patients with persistent rheumatoid arthritis with varying disease duration and follow-up time. Information on such patient cohorts can be biased, with only the most severe ones and those from early arthritis cohorts followed up prospectively from disease onset. The results of two such studies show that inflammatory activity at entry is a strong predictor for future prognosis. In a study from Sweden, none of the conventional variables had predictive value on radiological progression during the first 5 years of follow-up[86], but when the same patients were followed up till 10 years, high inflammatory activity (mean erythrocyte sedimentation rate (ESR) during the first three months) and positive RF were the only predictive factors[95]. A prospective study from Finland observed that active disease at inclusion predicted disability and radiological progression during the next six years[96].

Risk factors for work disability are remarkably similar in various reports from different countries. Active disease, RF positivity, erosive disease, poor functional status at entry, duration of the disease, low educational level, and older age predict the loss of work capacity[27,28,32,33,73,81,97]. Social and work-related factors also have a substantial effect on work disability[33,93,98,99].

Risk factors for increased mortality are increasing age[37,40,42,46,48], male sex[40,46,47], poor function at study entry[22,23,42,45,47,100], and poor level of general health by self-reported questionnaire[43]. Poor function evaluated by HAQ predicted mortality during the next eight years in a community cohort[99].

Features directly related to the activity of the disease, such as a high number of involved joints[42,47], high inflammatory activity[47], extra-articular manifestations[47,101], and RF positivity[45–48], also predict mortality. In some studies, the increased risk is observed only in RF positive patients[46,48]. The presence of joint destruction and extra-articular features is also reflected in the increased mortality of patients with classical versus definite rheumatoid arthritis[22]. Other factors, less directly associated with the rheumatoid disease, have also been associated with decreased life span, such as low level of education[42,47], hypertension, and previous cardiovascular event[40].

Laboratory markers

There is an increasing interest in the search for laboratory markers which would predict the functional and radiological outcome of patients. Of the conventional markers, high sedimentation rate, high C-reactive protein, low hemoglobin level, and high platelet counts are all markers of active disease[102]. Low hemoglobin and high sedimentation rate present at entry predict the six-year radiological outcome of patients with early rheumatoid arthritis[96]. Also, persistent elevation of erythrocyte sedimentation rate or C-reactive protein levels are associated with more severe joint destruction[87,103,104]. Rheumatoid factor is a hallmark for rheumatoid arthritis. Nearly all studies available agree that it is also a marker for more severe disease and predicts both joint destruction and functional disability. The level, as well as a persistently positive value, of rheumatoid factor during the early years of the disease is also associated with progressive radiological destruction (Fig. 20.10). Other autoantibodies, such as antibodies directed against antinuclear, antikeratin, antiperinuclear factor, anti-RA 33, and CCP have been analyzed in the context of predicting joint destruction. The presence of antikeratin and anti-CCP antibodies have been associated with an increased risk for severe radiological damage during the first 5–10 years of the disease[106–108].

In addition to markers measuring or associated with inflammation, much interest has been focused on the search for biochemical markers reflecting inflammation in the synovium, or changes in the metabolism of cartilage or underlying bone, as predictors of joint destruction. A persistently high serum level of hyaluronan is associated with increased radiological destruction during early rheumatoid arthritis[109]. It has a similar predictive value to a high sedimentation rate or C-reactive protein[110]. This reflects the correlation between these markers on inflammation. Interestingly, serum levels of a cartilage-derived protein, cartilage oligomeric protein (COMP), were elevated in a subgroup of patients with early rheumatoid arthritis who subsequently developed rapid destruction of hip joints[111], but the serum levels of COMP did not predict the radiological destruction of the small joints[110]. A marker of collagen I breakdown, carboxyterminal

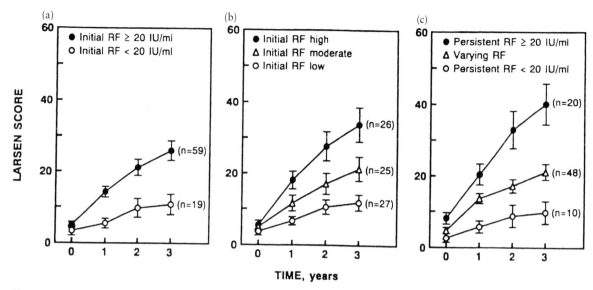

Fig. 20.10 (a) Mean Larsen score in patients with early rheumatoid arthritis divided into initially RF positive and RF negative patients. (b) Mean Larsen score in patients divided into subgroups according to the initial RF levels by tertile distribution. (c) mean Larsen score in patients divided into persistently positive, persistently negative, and variably positive and negative patients. (Reproduced from Ref. 105: Paimela L, Palosuo T, Leirisalo-Repo M, Helve T, Aho K (1995). Prognostic value of quantitative measurement of rheumatoid factor in early rheumatoid arthritis. *British Journal of Rheumatology* **34**: 1146–50, with permission of the British Society for Rheumatology.)

telopeptide (ICTP), in serum is associated with active disease and radiological erosions in early rheumatoid arthritis[112]. Serum levels of ICTP correlate both with inflammation[111] and destruction of knee joints[114], and predict radiological destruction during the first three years of the disease[113]. The markers of synovium, cartilage, and bone predict radiological destruction when analyzed in patient cohorts but they cannot be used in clinical practice to predict the radiological destruction in the small joints of a single patient. Their value in monitoring destruction of large joints has to be studied further.

Genetic markers

While the frequency of HLA-DR4, and especially the HLA-DRB1 alleles encoding the shared epitope (HLA-DRB1*01, -DRB1*04, and -DRB1*10) is higher in rheumatoid arthritis patients compared with the population as a whole, the role of genetic factors in determining the course of the disease is controversial. The presence of the shared epitope has been shown to predict the development of erosive arthritis in a population attending an early arthritis clinic[115]. Patients with established, chronic rheumatoid arthritis with severe articular damage also had higher frequency of HLA-DRB1 alleles compared with control patients with limited destruction[104]. However, the groups were not comparable. The patients with more extensive joint destruction also more often had systemic and extra-articular manifestations, positive rheumatoid factor, and more active disease compared with the rest of the patients. Prospective studies on early rheumatoid arthritis have found no significant contribution by HLA-DRB1 alleles, or the shared epitope on the radiological destruction or functional outcome of the patients during the following 5–9 years[75,88,116]. Interestingly, however, patients homozygous for the

shared epitope had about three times greater risk of undergoing joint replacement[116]. In a prospective study of patients followed up since the first five years of the disease, the number of swollen joints, rheumatoid factor, and erosion score worked well as predictors of the number of inflamed joints, radiological destruction, and functional outcome of the patients. The presence of HLA-DRB1 contributed little or no additional information[117]. Although genetics is intimately linked to the pathogenesis of rheumatoid arthritis, the association with clinical features in individual patients has not turned out to be useful in disease management.

Can the outcome and mortality in rheumatoid arthritis be modified?

Long-term effects of pharmacological therapy

Controlled studies have shown that patients treated with DMARDs have decreased joint inflammation. Some of the studies have also shown an effect on the radiological progression[118]. As discussed by Pincus[119], most of the studies are of short duration, extending only up to 2–3 years. These studies are too short to tell whether the long-term outcome of the patients would be influenced by such a treatment.

The effect of DMARDs with respect to functional outcome, work disability, or mortality is hard to estimate in the many observational studies reported. Many such studies include either no information on the drug therapies or only give information on the numbers of patients receiving DMARDs for some time during the study. In addition, the treatment has been empirical and mostly limited to patients with more active disease (see Table 20.1).

However, there is some uncontrolled evidence in favor of the role of early treatment. Radiological destruction was less frequent if gold treatment was started within the first three years of the disease[120]. Early treatment, if it resulted in decrease of C-reactive protein, has been shown to result in a fall in functional disability measured by HAQ during the subsequent two years[121]. DMARD therapy, if started within the initial two years of the disease, resulted in improved functional outcome[122,123]. Such an effect is not reached if the treatment is delayed beyond that time[123]. Individually tailored, continuous DMARD therapy started within the initial two years of symptoms cannot prevent radiological progression but most of the patients preserve their functional capacity. During the next six years, 77% of patients have normal or only slightly decreased functional capacity, but 3% end up with severe handicap[75]. In recent years a considerable amount of evidence has been presented that early institution of DMARD therapy is more effective with respect to preservation of function and retardation of joint damage compared with a more conservative approach (see Ref. 124). There is also increasing evidence in favor of combination therapy, especially of triple therapy with methotrexate, sulfasalazine, hydroxychloroquine, and low-dose prednisolone, compared to single DMARDs in patients with both early (see Refs 125, 126) and established rheumatoid arthritis[127]. The window of opportunity, that is, the time period from the onset of symptoms to the start of DMARDs, can be very narrow: in a recent analysis there was only about 3–4 months in which to start therapy with single DMARD[128].

In addition to early institution, the duration of DMARD therapy might be important in determining long-term outcome. The functional disability and number of painful joints were unchanged during the 10-year course of disease of patients with persistent rheumatoid arthritis treated with parenteral gold for at least two consecutive years[129]. This was true both for patients with persistent disease and those in whom the treatment was started within the initial two years of the disease. However, the survival of patients first treated at the Rheumatism Foundation Hospital in Heinola in 1961–66 was best in those who had been treated with parenteral gold for at least 10 years and lowest in those who had never received gold[130]. Results from England on patients followed up for a period of 10 years from the time of prescription of the initial DMARD favor the conclusion by the Heinola group since patients remaining on DMARD showed significant improvement while those not on treatment at the final analysis had deteriorated in function[131]. During follow-up, patients were also treated with multidisciplinary care, with 71% of the patients having had joint surgery as part of the treatment. Only 20% of the patients had died and 3% had become wheelchair-bound. The outcome can be compared to the results of a community-based survey by Hakala *et al.*[26], who explain the good functional outcome by early and active treatment with DMARDs, prescribed to 97% of the patients, multidisciplinary care, and by the high number of orthopedic operations[132]. Use of DMARDs also predicted survival in a community survey[99] and reduction of long-term disability in a large, multicenter databank analysis[133]. The results suggest up to 30% reduction in the

long-term disability with consistent use of DMARDs. Data on early inception cohorts on patients followed prospectively since the 1980s and early 1990s also show that, for patients treated individually with DMARDs, if indicated by disease activity[134], or with early institution and individually tailoring of DMARDs[135], the 10-year mortality is not increased compared with the background population.

Patients treated with corticosteroids seem to be at increased risk for mortality[40,42,47]. The significance of this information is biased by the indications used for the treatment. A case-controlled study on the use of prednisone showed no increased mortality but the outcome by 10 years was slightly worse with more complications due to prednisone treatment[136]. An extensive review on the use of low-dose corticosteroids in rheumatoid arthritis concluded that corticosteroids are equivalent or slightly better than placebo and active controls in improving disease activity[137]. The side-effects in long-term use of the treatment were also evident in this analysis.

In addition to physical handicap, social and work-related factors and support available by the community contribute to the subjective work disability. Yelin *et al.*[98] showed that work disability was effected by stage and duration of the disease but not by therapies received by the patient. This conclusion is based on a very conservative approach to the therapy. Recently, by applying active individual treatment strategies with combinations of DMARDs, and by individually modifying the treatments according to clinical response, it has become evident that in early rheumatoid arthritis aggressive initial therapy can save work disability days[138]. Also, the induction of early remission during the first six months of therapy is cost effective and saves the patient from work disability during subsequent five years[139]. If only ACR20 response was achieved, 21% of the patients became permanently work disabled. Even if patients reached ACR50 response, a result generally appreciated as a very good clinical result, the treatment response was not different from that of ACR20 response with respect to the work capacity[139].

The emergence of biological therapies has been a breakthrough in the management of severe rheumatoid arthritis. In addition to a rapid clinical response, tumor necrosis factor (TNF) inhibitors seem to be able to halt the progressive joint damage. However, it is too early to fully assess their impact on the long-term outcome.

In conclusion, there is a great amount of evidence showing that early diagnosis and early start of therapy with DMARD(s) has an impact on the long-term prognosis of the patients. The skilful use of combinations of DMARDs and individual monitoring and treatment of patients even with a chronic disease[140] is effective with respect to the clinical activity and the progression of joint damage. The goal to treatment should be induction and maintenance of remission. The persistence of residual disease activity, even if there is a partial response of the magnitude of ACR50, induces more costs to society and reduces the work ability compared with the situation of achieved remission[139].

Role of orthopedic surgery

Despite active medical treatment and rehabilitation procedures, joint destruction proceeds in most patients. The frequency of total joint replacement varies in different prospective studies. The lowest figure is from the Heinola study: during the first eight years of disease, 20% of patients with rheumatoid arthritis had radiological evidence of hip involvement, mostly asymptomatic; 1% had been operated on[141]. During 25 years, 21% of the patients had had large joint replacements[142]. In another prospective study of early rheumatoid arthritis from Sweden, 13% of the patients had undergone hip arthroplasty during the first seven years of disease[143]. A third prospective cohort study reported 7% for all major joint prosthesis during a mean of seven years of disease[69]. Different populations and varying resources for orthopedic surgery can influence the results. A large database of 1600 patients with persistent rheumatoid arthritis in the United States showed that, within the first 20 years, about 25% of the patients will undergo total joint replacement[144]. The figure is similar to that reported by Scott *et al.*[77] from England. Laboratory markers of inflammation and poor function increase the likelihood of joint surgery. While it is an indicator of failure of conservative treatment, the availability of prosthetic surgery is an important contribution to the well-being of the patients. An operation improves, often dramatically, the quality of life of the patient and prevents the patient entering a lower functional class.

Conclusion

- Rheumatoid arthritis patients usually develop a chronic disease.
- Rheumatoid arthritis patients often end up with decreased function.
- Rheumatoid arthritis patients have increased risk of mortality.
- Rheumatoid arthritis patients treated at specialist centres usually have more advanced and severe disease and their prognosis is usually worse compared with population cohorts.
- Rheumatoid arthritis patients in early cohorts followed up prospectively have a better prognosis.
- Predictors of poor outcome and increased mortality include early destruction, early functional handicap, and persistent inflammation.
- Early institution of DMARDs, multidisciplinary intervention with rehabilitation, and orthopedic surgery can postpone the functional deterioration in most rheumatoid arthritis patients.

References

1. Aho, K., and Heliövaara, M. Risk factors for rheumatoid arthritis. *Ann Med* 2004; **36**: 242–51.
2. Rantapää-Dahlqvist, S., de Jong, B. A., Berglin, E. *et al*. Antibodies against cyclic citrullinated peptide and IgA rheumatoid factor predict the development of rheumatoid arthritis. *Arthritis Rheum* 2003; **48**: 2741–9.
3. Klareskog, L., Alfredsson, L., Rantapää-Dahlqvist, S., Berglin, E., Stolt, P., and Padyukov, L. What precedes development of rheumatoid arthritis? *Ann Rheum Dis* 2004; **63** (Suppl. II): ii28–ii31.
4. Newton, J. L., Harney, S. M. J., Wordsworth, B. P., and Brown, M. A. A review of the MHC genetics of rheumatoid arthritis. *Genes and Immunity* 2004; **5**: 151–7.
5. Ropes, M. V., Bennett, G. A., Cobb, S., Jacos, R., and Jessar, R. A. 1958 revision of diagnostic criteria for rheumatoid arthritis. *Bull Rheum Dis* 1958; **9**: 175–6.
6. Mikkelsen, W. M., and Dodge, H. A four year follow-up of suspected rheumatoid arthritis: the Tecumseh, Michigan, community health study. *Arthritis Rheum* 1969; **12**: 87–91.
7. Hochberg, M. C. Predicting the prognosis of patients with rheumatoid arthritis: is there a crystal ball? *J Rheumatol* 1993; **20**: 1265–7.
8. Suarez-Almazor, M. E., Soskolne, C. L., Saunders, D., and Russell, A. S. Outcome in rheumatoid arthritis: a 1985 inception cohort study. *J Rheumatol* 1994; **21**: 1438–46.
9. Allebeck, P., and Lindberg, G. Rheumatic diseases in a health interview survey and in in-patient care. *Scand J Soc Med* 1984; **12**: 147–54.
10. Recht, L., Brattström, M., and Lithman, T. Chronic arthritis: prevalence, severity and distribution between primary care and referral centres in a defined rural population. *Scand J Rheumatol* 1989; **18**: 205–12.
11. Wasmus, A., Kindel, P., and Raspe, H. H. Epidemiologie der Behandlung bei an chronischer Polyarthritis Erkrankten in Hannover. *Z Rheumatol* 1989; **48**: 236–42.
12. Arnett, F. C., Edworthy, S. M., and Bloch, D. A. *et al*. The American Rheumatism Association 1987 revised criteria for the classification of rheumatoid arthritis. *Arthritis Rheum* 1988; **31**: 315–24.
13. Harrison, B. J., Symmons, D. P. M., Brennan, P., Barrett, E. M., and Silman, A. J. Natural remission in inflammatory polyarthritis: issues of definition and prediction. *Br J Rheumatol* 1996; **35**: 1096–100.
14. Wolfe, F., Ross, K., Hawley, D. J., Roberts, F. K., and Cathey, M. A. The prognosis of rheumatoid arthritis and undifferentiated polyarthritis syndrome in the clinic: a study of 1141 patients. *J Rheumatol* 1993; **20**: 2005–9.
15. Wolfe, F. The natural history of rheumatoid arthritis. *J Rheumatol* 1996; **23** (Suppl. 44): 13–22.
16. Nissilä, M., Isomäki, H., Kaarela, K., Kiviniemi, P., Martio, J., and Sarna, S. Prognosis of inflammatory joint diseases: a three-year follow-up study. *Scand J Rheumatol* 1983; **21**: 33–8.
17. Young, A. Short-term outcomes in recent-onset rheumatoid arthritis. *Br J Rheumatol* 1995; **34** (Suppl. 2): 79–86.
18. Harrison, B. J., Symmons, D. P. M., Brennan, P. *et al*. Inflammatory polyarthritis in the community is not a benign disease: predicting functional disability one year after presentation. *J Rheumatol* 1996; **23**: 1326–31.
19. Sherrer, Y. S., Bloch, D. A., Mitchell, D. M., Young, D. Y., and Fries, J. F. The development of disability in rheumatoid arthritis. *Arthritis Rheum* 1986; **29**: 494–500.
20. Young, A., Corbett, M., Winfield, J. *et al*. A prognostic index for erosive changes in the hands, feet, and cervical spine in early rheumatoid arthritis. *Br J Rheumatol* 1988; **27**: 94–101.
21. Houssein, D. A., McKenna, S. P., and Scott, D. L. The Nottingham Health Profile as a measure of disease activity and outcome in rheumatoid arthritis. *Br J Rheumatol* 1997; **36**: 69–73.
22. Rasker, J. J., and Cosh, J. A. Long-term effects of treating rheumatoid arthritis. *Bailliéres Clin Rheumatol* 1992; **6**: 141–60.
23. Corbett, M., Dalton, S., Young, A., Silman, S., and Shipley, M. Factors predicting death, survival, and functional outcome in a prospective study of early rheumatoid disease over fifteen years. *Br J Rheumatol* 1993; **32**: 717–23.
24. Wolfe, F., and Cathey, M. A. The assessment and prediction of functional disability in rheumatoid arthritis. *J Rheumatol* 1991; **18**: 1298–306.
25. Isacson, J., Allander, E., and Broström, H. L. -Å. A seventeen-year follow-up of a population survey of rheumatoid arthritis. *Scand J Rheumatol* 1987; **16**: 145–52.
26. Hakala, M., Nieminen, P., and Koivisto, O. More evidence from a community based series of better outcome in rheumatoid arthritis: data on the effect of multi-disciplinary care on the retention of functional ability. *J Rheumatol* 1994; **21**: 1432–7.

27. Mäkisara, G. L., and Mäkisara, P. Prognosis of functional capacity and work capacity in rheumatoid arthritis. *Clin Rheumatol* 1982; **1**: 117–25.

28. Doeglas, D., Suurmeijer, T., Krol, B., Sanderman, R., van Leeuwen, M., and Rijswijk, M. Work disability in early rheumatoid arthritis. *Ann Rheum Dis* 1995; **54**: 455–60.

29. Duthie, J. J. R., Thompson, M., Weir, M. M., and Fletcher, W. B. Medical and social aspects of the treatment of rheumatoid arthritis with special reference to factors affecting prognosis. *Ann Rheum Dis* 1955; **14**: 133–49.

30. Duthie, J. J. R., Brown, P. E., Know, J. D. E., and Thompson, M. Course and prognosis in rheumatoid arthritis. *Ann Rheum Dis* 1957; **16**: 411–24.

31. Duthie, J. J. R., Brown, P. E., Truelove, L. H., Baragar, F. D., and Lawrie, A. J. Course and prognosis in rheumatoid arthritis: a further report. *Ann Rheum Dis* 1964; **23**: 193–204.

32. Mau, W., Bornmann, M., Weber, H., Weidemann, H. F., Hecker, H., and Raspe, H. H. Prediction of permanent work disability in a follow-up study of early rheumatoid arthritis: results of a tree structured analysis using RECPAM. *Br J Rheumatol* 1996; **35**: 652–9.

33. Reisine, S., McQuillan, J., and Fifield, J. Predictors of work disability in rheumatoid arthritis patients: a five-year follow-up. *Arthritis Rheum* 1995; **38**: 1630–7.

34. van der Heijde, D. M. F. M. Joint erosions and patients with early rheumatoid arthritis. *J Rheumatol* 1993; **34** (Suppl 2): 74–8.

35. Sharp, J. T., Wolfe, F., Mitchell, D. M., and Bloch, D. A. The progression of erosion and joint space narrowing scores in rheumatoid arthritis during the first twenty-five years of disease. *Arthritis Rheum* 1991; **34**: 660–8.

36. Heikkilä, S., and Isomäki, H. Long-term outcome of rheumatoid arthritis has improved. *Scand J Rheumatol* 1989; **23**: 13–15.

37. Vandenbroucke, J. P., Hazevoet, H. M., and Cats, A. Survival and cause of death in rheumatoid arthritis: a 25-year prospective follow-up. *J. Rheumatol* 1984; **11**: 158–61.

38. Mitchel, D. M., Spitz, P. W., Young, D. Y., Bloch, D. A., McShane, D. J., and Fries, J. F. Survival, prognosis, and causes of death in rheumatoid arthritis. *Arthritis Rheum* 1986; **29**: 706–14.

39. Myllykangas-Luosujärvi, R., Aho, K., Kautiainen, H., and Isomäki, H. Shortening of life span and causes of excess mortality in a population-based series of subjects with rheumatoid arthritis. *Clin Exp Rheumatol* **13**: 149–53.

40. Wållberg-Jonsson, S., Öhman, M. -L., and Rantapää Dahlqvist, S. Cardiovascular morbidity and mortality in patients with seropositive rheumatoid arthritis in northern Sweden. *J Rheumatol* 1997; **24**: 445–51.

41. Pincus, T., Callahan, L. F., Sale, W. G., Brooks, A. L., Payne, L. E., and Vaughn, W. K. Severe functional declines, work disability, and increased mortality in seventy-five rheumatoid arthritis patients studied over nine years. *Arthritis Rheum* 1984; **27**: 864–72.

42. Pincus, T., Callahan, L. F., and Vaughn, W. K. Questionnaire, walking time and button test measurers of functional capacity as predictive markers for mortality in rheumatoid arthritis. *J Rheumatol* 1987; **14**: 240–51.

43. Kazis, L. E., Anderson, J. J., and Meenan, R. F. Health status as a predictor of mortality in rheumatoid arthritis: a five year study. *J Rheumatol* 1990; **17**: 609–13.

44. Linos, A., Worthington, J. W., O'Fallon, W. M., and Kurland, L. T. The epidemiology of rheumatoid arthritis in Rochester, Minnesota: a study of incidence, prevalence, and mortality. *Am J Epidemiol* 1980; **111**: 87–98.

45. Allebeck, P., Ahlbom, A., and Allander, E. Increased mortality among persons with rheumatoid arthritis, but where RA does not appear on death certificate. *Scand J Rheumatol* 1981; **10**: 301–6.

46. Jacobsson, L. T. H., Knowler, W. C., Pillemer, S. *et al.* Rheumatoid arthritis and mortality: a longitudinal study in Pima Indians. *Arthritis Rheum* 1993; **36**: 1045–53.

47. Wolfe, F., Mitchell, D. M., Sibley, J. T. *et al.* The mortality of rheumatoid arthritis. *Arthritis Rheum* 1994; **37**: 481–94.

48. van Schaardenburg, D., Hazes, J. W., de Boer, A., Zwinderman, A. H., Meijers, K. A. E., and Breedveld, F. C. Outcome of rheumatoid arthritis in relation to age and rheumatoid factor at diagnosis. *J Rheumatol* 1993; **20**: 45–52.

49. Pincus, T. The paradox of effective therapies but poor long-term outcomes in rheumatoid arthritis. *Semin Arthritis Rheum* 1992; **21** (Suppl. 3): 2–15.

50. Myllykangas-Luosujärvi, R. A., Aho, K., and Isomäki, H. Mortality in rheumatoid arthritis. *Semin Arthritis Rheum* 1995; **25**: 193–202.

51. Young, A., and van der Heijde, D. M. F. M. Can we predict aggressive disease? *Baillieres Clin Rheumatol* 1997; **11**: 27–48.

52. Mutru, O., Laakso, M., Isomäki, H., and Koota, K. Ten year mortality and causes of death in patients with rheumatoid arthritis. *Br Med J* 1985; **290**: 1797–9.

53. Laakso, M., Mutru, O., Isomäki, H., and Koota, K. Cancer mortality in patients with rheumatoid arthritis. *J Rheumatol* 1986; **13**: 522–6.

54. Matteson, E. L., Hickey, A. R., Maquire, L., Tilson, H. H., and Urowitz, M. B. Occurrence of neoplasia in patients with rheumatoid arthritis enrolled in DMARD registry: rheumatoid arthritis azathioprine registry steering committee. *J Rheumatol* 1991; **18**: 809–14.

55. Myllykangas-Luosujärvi, R., Aho, K., and Isomäki, H. Mortality from cancer in patients with rheumatoid arthritis. *Scand J Rheumatol* 1995; **24**: 76–8.

56. Symmons, D. P. M., Jones, M. A., Scott, D. L., and Prior, P. Long-term mortality outcome in patients with rheumatoid arthritis: early presenters continue to do well. *J Rheumatol* 1998; **25**: 1072–7.

57. Isomäki, H. A., Hakulinen, T., and Joutsenlahti, U. Excess risk of lymphomas, leukemia and myeloma in patients with rheumatoid arthritis. *J Chron Dis* 1978; **31**: 691–6.

58. Eriksson, M. Rheumatoid arthritis as a risk factor for multiple myeloma: a case-control study. *Eur J Cancer* 1993; **29A**: 259–63.

59. Myllykangas-Luosujärvi, R., Aho, K., and Isomaki, H. Mortality from cancer in patients with rheumatoid arthritis. *Scand J Rheumatol* 1995; **24**: 76–8.

60. Bäcklund, E., Ekbom, A., Sparén, P., Feltelius, N., and Klareskog, L. Disease activity and risk of lymphoma in patients with rheumatoid arthritis: nested case-control study. *Br Med J* 1998; **317**: 180–1.

61. Symmons, D. Excess mortality in rheumatoid arthritis: is it the disease or the drugs? *J Rheumatol* 1995; **22**: 2200–2.

62. Myllykangas-Luosujärvi, R., Aho, K., and Isomäki, H. Death attributed to antirheumatic medication in a nation-wide series of 1666 patients with rheumatoid arthritis who have died. *J Rheumatol* 1995; **22**: 1121–7.

63. Pincus, T., and Callahan, L. F. The 'side effects' of rheumatoid arthritis: joint destruction, disability, and early mortality. *Br J Rheumatol* 1993; **32** (Suppl. 1): 28–37.

64. Silman, A. J., Petrie, J., Haxleman, B., and Evans, S. J. Lymphoproliferative cancer and other malignancy in patients with rheumatoid arthritis treated with azathioprine: a 20 year follow up study. *Ann Rheum Dis* 1988; **47**: 988–92.

65. Jones, M., Symmons, D., Finn, J., and Wolfe, F. Does exposure to immunosuppressive therapy increase the 10 year malignancy and mortality risks in rheumatoid arthritis? A matched cohort study. *Br J Rheumatol* 1996; **35**: 738–45.

66. Alarcón, G. S., Tracy, I. C., Strand, G. M., Singh, K., and Macaluso, M. Survival and drug discontinuation analyses in a large cohort of methotrexate treated rheumatoid arthritis patients. *Ann Rheum Dis* 1995; **54**: 708–12.

67. Choi, H. K., Hernan, M. A., Seeger, J. D., Robins, J. M., and Wolfe, F. Methotrexate and mortality in patients with rheumatoid arthritis: a prospective study. *Lancet* 2002; **359**: 1173–7.

68. Fries, J. F., Williams, C. A., Bloch, D. A., and Michel, B. A. Nonsteroidal anti-inflammatory drug-associated gastropathy: incidence and risk factor models. *Am J Med* 1991; **91**: 213–22.

69. Yopol, E. J. Failing the public health: rofecoxib, Merck, and the FDA. *N Engl J Med* 2004; **351**: 1707–9.

70. Maxwell, S. R. J., Moots, R. J., and Kendall, M. J. Corticosteroids: do they damage the cardiovascular system? *Postgrad Med* 1994; **70**: 863–70.

71. Raynaud, J. P. Cardiovascular mortality in rheumatoid arthritis: how harmful are corticosteroids? *J Rheumatol* 1997; **24**: 415–16.

72. Eberhardt, K. B., and Fex, E. Functional impairment and disability in early rheumatoid arthritis: development over 5 years. *J Rheumatol* 1995; **22**: 1037–42.

73. Fex, E., Larsson, B. -M., Nived, K., and Eberhardt, K. Effect of rheumatoid arthritis on work status and social and leisure time activities in patients followed 8 years from onset. *J Rheumatol* 1998; **25**: 44–50.

74. Lindqvist, E., Saxne, T., Geborek, P., and Eberhardt, K. Ten year outcome in a cohort of patients with early rheumatoid arthritis: health status, disease process, and damage. *Ann Rheum Dis* 2002; **61**: 1055–9.

75. Möttönen, T., Paimela, L., Ahonen, J., Helve, T., Hannonen, P., and Leirisalo-Repo, M. Outcome in patients with early rheumatoid arthritis treated according to the 'sawtooth' strategy. *Arthritis Rheum* 1996; **39**: 996–1005.

76. Lance, N. J., and Curran, J. J. Late-onset, seropositive, erosive rheumatoid arthritis. *Semin Arthritis Rheum* 1993; **23**: 177–82.

77. Scott, D. L., Symmons, D. P. M., Coulton, B. L., and Popert, A. J. Long-term outcome of treating rheumatoid arthritis: results after 20 years. *Lancet* 1987; **i**: 1108–11.

78. Jacoby, R. K., Jayson, M. IV., and Cosh, J. A. Onset, early stages, and prognosis of rheumatoid arthritis: a clinical study of 100 patients with 11-year follow-up. *Br Med J* 1973; **2**: 96–100.

79. Rasker, J. J., and Cosh, J. A. Cause and age of death in a prospective study of 100 patients with rheumatoid arthritis. *Ann Rheum Dis* 1981; **40**: 115–20.

80. Cosh, J. A., and Rasker, J. J. A 20-year follow-up of 100 patients with rheumatoid arthritis (RA). *Ann Rheum Dis* 1982; **41**: 317.

81. Rasker, J. J., and Cosh, J. A. The natural history of rheumatoid arthritis over 20 years: clinical symptoms, radiological signs, treatment, mortality, and prognostic significance of early features. *Clin Rheumatol* 1987; **6** (Suppl. 2): 5–11.

82. Reilly, P. A., Cosh, J. A., Maddison, P. J., Rasker, J. J., and Silman, A. Mortality and survival in rheumatoid arthritis: a 24-year prospective study of 100 patients. *Ann Rheum Dis* 1990; **49**: 363–9.

83. Eberhardt, K., Larsson, B. -M., and Nived, K. Early rheumatoid arthritis: some social, economical, and psychological aspects. *Scand J Rheumatol* 1993; **22**: 119–23.

84. van der Heijde, D. M. F. M., van Leeuwen, M. A., van Riel, P. L. C. M. *et al.* Biannual radiographic assessment of hands and feet in a three-year prospective follow-up of patients with early rheumatoid arthritis. *Arthritis Rheum* 1992; **35**: 26–34.

85. Kaarela, K., Kauppi, M. J., and Lehtinen, K. E. S. The value of the ACR 1987 criteria in a very early rheumatoid arthritis. *Scand J Rheumatol* 1995; **24**: 279–81.

86. Fex, E., Jonsson, K., Johnson, U., and Eberhardt, K. Development of radiologic damage during the first 5–6 yr of rheumatoid arthritis: a prospective follow-up study of a Swedish cohort. *Br J Rheumatol* 1996; **35**: 1106–15.

87. Plant, M. J., Jones, P. W., Saklatvala, J., Ollier, W. E. R., and Dawes, P. T. Patterns of radiological progression in early rheumatoid arthritis: results of an 8 year prospective study. *J Rheumatol* 1998; **25**: 17–26.

88. Young, A., Jaraquemada, D., Awad, J., Festenstein, H., Corbett, M., Hay, F. C., and Roitt, I. Association of HLA-DR4/Dw4 and DR2/DW2 with radiologic changes in a prospective study of patients with rheumatoid arthritis: preferential relationship with HLA-Dw rather than HLA-DR specificities. *Arthritis Rheum* 1984; **27**: 20–5.

89. Kaarela, K., and Kautiainen, H. Continuous progression of radiological destruction in seropositive rheumatoid arthritis. *J Rheumatol* 1997; **24**: 1285–7.

90. Isomäki, H. Long-term outcome of rheumatoid arthritis. *Scand J Rheumatol* 1992; **21** (Suppl. 95): 3–8.

91. Larsen, A., Dale, K., and Eek, M. Radiographic evaluation of rheumatoid arthritis and related conditions by standard reference films. *Acta Radiol Diagn* 1977; **18**: 481–91.

92. Isomäki, H., Kautiainen, H., Kaarela, K., and Nieminen, M. Low 20-year mortality in RA patients with early hospitalisation. *Scand J Rheumatol* 1995; **24**: 189.

93. Weisman, M. H. Natural history and treatment decisions in rheumatoid arthritis revisited. *Arthritis Care Res* 1989; **2** (Suppl.): S75–S83.

94. Alarcón, G. S. Predictive factors in rheumatoid arthritis. *Amer J Med* 1997; **103** (Suppl. 6A): 19S–24S.

95. Lindqvist, E., Jonsson, K., Saxne, T., and Eberhardt, K. Course of radiographic damage over 10 years in a cohort with early rheumatoid arthritis. *Ann Rheum Dis* 2003; **62**: 611–16.

96. Möttönen, T., Paimela, L., Leirisalo-Repo, M., Kautiainen, H., Ilonen, J., and Hannonen, P. Only high disease activity and positive RF indicate poor prognosis in patients with early rheumatoid arthritis treated with 'sawtooth' strategy. *Ann Rheum Dis* 1998; **57**: 533–9.

97. Sherrer, Y. S., Bloch, D. A., Mitchell, D. M., Roth, S. H., Wolfe, F., and Fries, J. F. Disability in rheumatoid arthritis: comparison of prognostic factors across three populations. *J Rheumatol* 1987; **14**: 705–9.

98. Yelin, E., Meenan, R., Nevitt, M., and Epstein, W. Work disability in rheumatoid arthritis: effects of disease, social, and work factors. *Ann Int Med* 1980; **93**: 551–6.

99. Leigh, J. P., and Fries, J. F. Mortality predictors among 263 patients with rheumatoid arthritis. *J Rheumatol* 1991; **18**: 1307–12.

100. Ragan, C., and Farrington, E. The clinical features of rheumatoid arthritis. *JAMA* 1962; **181**: 663–7.

101. Erhardt, C. C., Mumford, P. A., Venables, P. J. W., and Maini, R. N. Factors predicting a poor life prognosis in rheumatoid arthritis: an eight year prospective study. *Ann Rheum Dis* 1989; **48**: 7–13.

102. van der Heijde, D. M. F. M., van Riel, P. L. C. M., van Rijswijk, M. H., and van de Putte, L. B. A. Influence of prognostic features on the final outcome in rheumatoid arthritis: review of the literature. *Semin Arthritis Rheum* 1988; **17**: 284–92.

103. Hassell, A. B., Davis, M. J., Fowler, P. D. *et al.* The relationship between serial measures of disease activity and outcome in rheumatoid arthritis. *Quart J Med* 1993; **86**: 601–7.

104. Combe, B., Eliaou, J. F., Daurès, J. P., Meyer, O., Clot, J., and Sany, J. Prognostic factors in rheumatoid arthritis: comparative study of two subsets of patients according to severity of articular damage. *Br J Rheumatol* 1995; **34**: 529–34.

105. Paimela, L., Palosuo, T., Leirisalo-Repo, M., Helve, T., and Aho, K. Prognostic value of quantitative measurement of rheumatoid factor in early rheumatoid arthritis. *Br J Rheumatol* 1995; **34**: 1146–50.

106. Meyer, O., Combe, B., Elias, A., Benali, K., Clot, J., Sany, J., and Elianou, J. F. Autoantibodies predicting the outcome of rheumatoid arthritis: evaluation in two subsets of patients according to severity of radiographic damage. *Ann Rheum Dis* 1997; **56**: 682–5.

107. Meyer, O., Labarre, C., Dougados, M. *et al.* Anticitrullinated protein/peptide antibody assays in early rheumatoid arthritis for predicting five year radiologic damage. *Ann Rheum Dis* 2003; **62**: 120–6.

108. Lindqvist, E., Eberhardt, K., Bendtzen, K., Heinegård, D., and Saxne, T. Prognostic laboratory markers of joint damage in rheumatoid arthritis. *Ann Rheum Dis* 2005; **64**: 196–201.

109. Paimela, L., Heiskanen, A., Kurki, P., Helve, T., and Leirisalo-Repo, M. Serum hyaluronate level as a predictor of radiologic progression in early rheumatoid arthritis. *Arthritis Rheum* 1991; **34**: 815–21.

110. Fex, E., Eberhardt, K., and Saxne, T. Tissue-derived macromolecules and markers of inflammation in serum in early rheumatoid arthritis: relationship to development of joint destruction in hands and feet. *Br J Rheumatol* 1997; **36**: 1161–5.

111. Forslind, K., Eberhardt, K., Jonsson, A., and Saxne, T. Increased serum concentrations of cartilage oligomeric matrix protein: a prognostic marker in early rheumatoid arthritis. *Br J Rheumatol* 1992; **31**: 593–8.

112. Kotaniemi, A., Isomäki, H., Hakala, M., Risteli, L., and Risteli, J. Increased type I. collagen degradation in early rheumatoid arthritis. *J Rheumatol* 1994; **21**: 1593–6.

113. Paimela, L., Leirisalo-Repo, M., Risteli, L., Hakala, M., Helve, T., and Risteli, J. Type I collagen degradation product in serum of patients with early rheumatoid arthritis: relationship to disease activity and radiological progression in a 3-year follow-up. *Br J Rheumatol* 1994; **33**: 1012–16.

114. Hakala, M., Åhman, S., Luukkainen, R., Risteli, H. L., Kauppi, M., Nieminen, P., and Risteli, J. Application of markers of collagen metabolism in serum and synovial fluid for assessment of disease process in patients with rheumatoid arthritis. *Ann Rheum Dis* 1995; 54: 886–90.

115. Emery, P., Salmon, M., Bradley, H., Wordsworth, P., Tunn, E., Bacon, P., and Waring, R. Genetically determined factors as predictors of radiological change in patients with early symmetrical arthritis. *Br Med J* 1992; 305: 1387–9.

116. Eberhardt, K., Fex, E., Johnson, U., and Wollheim, F. A. Associations of HLA-DRB and -DQB genes with two and five year outcome in rheumatoid arthritis. *Ann Rheum Dis* 1996; 55: 34–9.

117. van Zeben, D., Hazes, J. M. W., Zwinderman, A. H., Vandenbroucke, J. P., and Breedveld, F. C. Factors predicting outcome of rheumatoid arthritis: results of a follow-up study. *J Rheumatol* 1993; 20: 1288–96.

118. Iannuzzi, L., Dawson, N., Zein, N., Kushner, I. Does drug therapy slow radiographic deterioration in rheumatoid arthritis. *New Engl J Med* 1983; 309: 1023–8.

119. Pincus, T. Long-term outcomes in rheumatoid arthritis. *J Rheumatol* 1995; 34 (Suppl. 2): 59–73.

120. Luukkainen, R. Chrysotherapy in rheumatoid arthritis with particular emphasis on the effect of chrysotherapy on radiological changes and on the optimal time of initiation of therapy. *Scand J Rheumatol* **Suppl.** 1980; 34: 1–56.

121. Devlin, J., Gough, A., Huissoon, A. *et al.* The acute phase and function in early rheumatoid arthritis: C-reactive protein levels correlate with functional outcome. *J Rheumatol* 1997; 24: 9–13.

122. Egsmose, C., Lund, B., Borg, G. *et al.* Patients with rheumatoid arthritis benefit from early 2nd line therapy: 5 year follow-up of a prospective double blind placebo controlled study. *J Rheumatol* 1995; 22: 2208–13.

123. Munro, R., Hampson, R., McEntegard, A., Thomson, E. A., Madhok, R., and Capell, H. Improved functional outcome in patients with early rheumatoid arthritis treated with intramuscular gold: results of a five year prospective study. *Ann Rheum Dis* 1998; 57: 88–93.

124. Smolen, J., and Aletaha, D. Therapeutic strategies in early rheumatoid arthritis. *Best Practice Res Clin Rheumatol* 2005; 19: 163–77.

125. Möttönen, T., Hannonen, P., Leirisalo-Repo, M. *et al.* Comparison of combination therapy with single-drug therapy in early rheumatoid arthritis: a randomised trial. FIN-RACo trial group. *Lancet* 1999; 353: 1568–73.

126. Korpela, M., Laasonen, L., Hannonen, P. *et al.* Retardation of joint damage in patients with early rheumatoid arthritis by initial aggressive treatment with disease-modifying antirheumatic drugs: five-year experience from the FIN-RACo Trial Group. *Arthritis Rheum* 2004; 50: 2072–81.

127. O'Dell, J. R., Haire, C. E., Erikson, N. *et al.* Treatment of rheumatoid arthritis with methotrexate alone, sulfasalazine and hydroxychloroquine, or a combination of all three medications. *N Engl J Med* 1996; 334: 1287–91.

128. Möttönen, T., Hannonen, P., Korpela, M. *et al.* Delay of institution of therapy and induction of remission during single-drug or combination-disease-modifying antirheumatic drug therapy in early rheumatoid arthritis. *Arthritis Rheum* 2002; 46: 894–8.

129. Epstein, W. V., Henke, C. J., Yelin, E. H., and Katz, P. P. Effect of parenterally administered gold therapy on the course of adult rheumatoid arthritis. *Ann Int Med* 1991; 114: 437–44.

130. Lehtinen, K., and Isomäki, H. Intramuscular gold therapy is associated with long survival in patients with rheumatoid arthritis. *J Rheumatol* 1991; 18: 524–9.

131. Capell, H. A., Murphy, E. A., and Hunter, J. A. Rheumatoid arthritis: workload and outcome over 10 years. *Quart J Med* (new series) 1991; 290: 461–76.

132. Hakala, M., and Nieminen, P. Functional status assessment of physical impairment in a community based population with rheumatoid arthritis: severely incapacitated patients are rare. *J Rheumatol* 1996; 23: 617–23.

133. Fries, J. F., Williams, C. A., Morfeld, D., Singh, G., and Sibley, J. Reduction in long-term disability in patients with rheumatoid arthritis by disease-modified antirheumatic drug-based treatment strategies. *Arthritis Rheum* 1996; 39: 606–22.

134. Lindqvist, E., and Eberhardt, K. Mortality in rheumatoid arthritis patients with disease onset in the 1980s. *Ann Rheum Dis* 1999; 58: 11–14.

135. Peltomaa, R., Paimela, L., Kautiainen, H., and Leirisalo-Repo, M. Mortality in patients with rheumatoid arthritis treated actively from the time of diagnosis. *Ann Rheum Dis* 2002; 61: 889–94.

136. McDougall, R., Sibley, J., Haga, M., Russell, A. Outcome in patients with rheumatoid arthritis receiving prednisone compared to matched controls. *J Rheumatol* 1994; 21: 1207–13.

137. Saag, K. G. Low-dose corticosteroid therapy in rheumatoid arthritis: balancing the evidence. *Am J Med* 1997; 103 (Suppl. 4): 31S–39S.

138. Puolakka, K., Kautiainen, H., Möttönen, T. *et al.* Impact of initial aggressive drug treatment with a combination of disease-modifying antirheumatic drugs on the development of work disability in early rheumatoid arthritis. *Arthritis Rheum* 2004; 50: 55–62.

139. Puolakka, K., Kautiainen, H., Möttönen, T. *et al.* Early suppression of disease activity is essential for maintenance of work disability in patients with recent-onset rheumatoid arthritis. *Arthritis Rheum* 2005; 52: 36–41.

140. Grigor, C., Capell, H., Stirling, A. *et al.* Effect of treatment strategy of tight control for rheumatoid arthritis (the ICORA study): a single-blind randomised controlled trial. *Lancet* 2004; 364: 263–9.

141. Lehtimäki, M. Y., Kaarela, K., and Hämäläinen, M. Incidence of hip involvement and need for total hip replacement in rheumatoid arthritis: an eight-year follow-up study. *Scand J Rheumatol* 1986; 15: 387–91.

142. Palm, T. M., Kaarela, K., Hakala, M. S., Kautiainen, H., Kröger, H. P., and Belt, E. A. *Clin Exp Rheumatol* 2002; 20: 392–4.

143. Eberhardt, K., Fex, E., Johnsson, K., and Geborek, P. Hip involvement in early rheumatoid arthritis. *Ann Rheum Dis* 1995; 54: 45–8.

144. Wolfe, F., and Zwillich, S. H. The long-term outcomes of rheumatoid arthritis: a 23-year prospective, longitudinal study of total joint replacement and its predictors in 1,600 patients with rheumatoid arthritis. *Arthritis Rheum* 1998; 41: 1072–82.

21 | Biomarkers for cartilage and bone in rheumatoid arthritis

Tore Saxne, Bengt Månsson, and Dick Heinegård

Introduction

A biological marker (biomarker) can by consensus be defined as a characteristic that is objectively measured and evaluated as an indicator of normal biological processes, pathological processes, or responses to a therapeutic intervention[1]. This definition includes a variety of methods that relate to the presence and severity of a disease and could comprise both biochemical assays and imaging techniques. In a more restricted sense we consider biomarkers to be such that can be measured in patient samples, that is, blood, urine, synovial fluid, or tissue specimens. This type of marker is often developed following discoveries in basic biology, for example the identification and characterization of a matrix molecule in a certain tissue involved in the pathophysiology of a disease, such as a cartilage protein in rheumatoid arthritis (RA)[2].

In RA, which is characterized by progressive destruction of articular cartilage and bone, the release of matrix macromolecules or their fragments reflects processes in these tissues that can be detected at an early stage both quantitatively and qualitatively. The approach has promise for assessing the disease process and also for evaluating effects of therapy on these tissues. Such molecular markers reflect the activity of the process in the tissue at the time of sample retrieval. This contrasts to classical imaging techniques which provide a cumulative account of damage that has already occurred. Thus measurements of molecular markers of cartilage and bone in body fluids add information that is not accessible by other available tools. It needs to be emphasized that this information depicts parameters of the disease process quite different from those obtained by radiography (Fig. 21.1). Thus, marker levels will often not correlate to radiographic appearance of joints. For instance, increased concentrations of a certain marker, for example cartilage oligomeric matrix protein (COMP), may be found in serum in patients with early RA with normal radiographs of clinically affected joints[3]. This could be the very first sign of a pathological tissue process that eventually will result in tissue destruction. Consequently, markers provide a possibility for identifying processes which might be addressed by more active therapy before tissue destruction has become detectable by imaging.

In this chapter, we focus on biomarkers/molecular markers released from cartilage and bone, that is, intact or fragmented matrix molecules providing non-invasive means of monitoring processes in these tissues. The objective is to highlight some of the basic principles of the molecular marker approach to the study of the pathophysiology of tissue destruction in RA and also to point out the possible clinical applications. The potentials but also some of the limitations that currently exist will be discussed. Key results that illustrate principles will be given and a list of markers currently available will be provided.

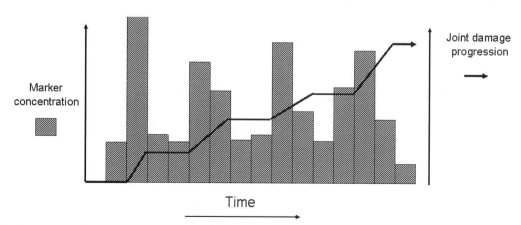

Fig. 21.1 Relation between joint damage progression as depicted by radiography and serum concentrations of a cartilage marker. Radiography provides a historic account of progressive joint destruction whereas a cartilage biomarker provides dynamic information on the current activity of the tissue process. Note that increased concentrations are seen prior to progression of radiographic changes. The correlation between marker concentrations at a given time point and radiographic score is therefore expected to be weak, whereas the correlation between marker concentrations and subsequent joint damage should be higher. Estimation of time-integrated marker levels in relation to progression of joint damage should be considered.

Cartilage and bone turnover

Both cartilage and bone are tissues that can be viewed as composite materials with an abundant extracellular matrix, which provides the tissue properties. In bone this organic matrix guides the deposits of mineral, essential for the tissue properties[4].

The only cell type in cartilage, the chondrocyte, is capable of both synthesizing and degrading all matrix components. Normally the cartilage matrix turnover is a highly controlled and finely tuned process. Newly synthesized molecules are secreted into the pericellular zone where some of them are deposited. The cells receive information from the matrix enabling them to maintain tissue homeostasis. It is reasonable to speculate that molecules responsible for matrix to cell signalling are enriched in the pericellular zone. Other molecules are transported further away to become incorporated in the territorial and interterritorial matrix, respectively, providing for the structural properties of the matrix.

A major feature of these tissues particularly apparent for bone is its continuous remodeling. It is particularly important since load causes fatigue and often altered requirements of the tissue architecture. Thus, there is a characteristic bone remodeling cycle that removes old less functional bone, which is replaced with new bone. This remodeling cycle has two phases. In the initial stage bone breakdown is executed by the osteoclasts, which adhere to the bone surface and create a function of a secondary lysosome having an acid pH to dissolve the hydroxyapatite mineral. This structure underneath the cells contains a variety of lysosomal enzymes with capacity to attack, degrade, and dissolve the organic matrix. The second, rebuilding phase depends on recruitment of osteoblasts that lay down an osteoid, which in a tightly regulated fashion becomes mineralized[4].

In RA, the normal balance of synthesis and degradation is disturbed and shifted towards degradation in established disease. This eventually leads to disruption of the structural and functional integrity of the joint. As a consequence of the disturbed matrix turnover, increased amounts of macromolecules or fragments thereof (molecular markers) are released into synovial fluid and may subsequently reach the bloodstream, and some fragments may also be found in the urine. The main difference between cartilage and bone in this respect is that for bone, markers show the level of turnover, where mechanisms are likely to be similar in both normal and pathological conditions, whereas in cartilage, markers can show a turnover in pathological states that is different from normal homeostasis. Thus lessons learnt from studies of bone markers in osteoporosis should not be extrapolated to cartilage in RA.

Cartilage and bone matrix

The cartilage matrix contains several matrix molecules specific for the tissue, but also many molecules with a ubiquitous distribution among connective tissues[2,4,5]. The major components are collagen type II and the large aggregating proteoglycan, aggrecan, both essentially cartilage specific. The collagen fibers with their other constituent molecules form a network in the tissue, with major functions of providing tensile stiffness and distributing load. The interactions between collagen fibrils, essential for the properties of the collagen network, as well as those between collagen fibers, largely rely on a number of other matrix proteins which often are proteoglycans, for example decorin and fibromodulin, but also on integral, minor collagens[2]. Furthermore, COMP, which has been extensively studied as a biomarker, has a role in stabilizing the collagen network[2,6,7]. These proteins apparently also have the potential to regulate collagen fibril formation and thus to modulate matrix assembly[2,8]. Figure 21.2 shows a schematic drawing of the cartilage matrix.

Cell appearance and matrix structure are not homogeneous throughout the articular cartilage. In the superficial layer the cells are relatively scarce, have a somewhat flattened shape, and are oriented in parallel to the surface. Deeper in the cartilage the cells are somewhat more abundant and have a rounded shape. The extracellular matrix also differs at different depths of the cartilage. Collagen type II fibers exemplify this. In the superficial layers collagen fibers run in parallel to the surface but deeper in the cartilage they run more perpendicular to the surface, which meets varying types of load. Also, aggrecan abundance varies between different parts of the cartilage, with lower concentration in the superficial than in the deep layers[2].

In each layer there is also a heterogeneity in the composition of the matrix depending on the distance from the cells (Fig. 21.2). Light and/or electron microscopy reveals thin, less dense collagen fibres around the cells and an abundance of metachromatically stained (negatively charged) material. This zone is called the territorial matrix. In the periphery of the territorial matrix the collagen fibers become more dense and form the so-called basket. The matrix localized outside the basket is called interterritorial matrix. The different distribution of matrix constituents may indicate different functional roles. This information must be considered when applying the molecular marker technology. Another consequence of the variable distribution is that molecules or fragments thereof detected in body fluids may be used to localize a disease process to a certain zone or compartment at a certain stage of, for example, RA.

The extracellular organic matrix of bone consists of predominantly type I collagen[2,4,5]. The triple helical structure of the molecule provides strength as well as flexibility to the tissue. Cross-links formed post-translationally stabilize the matrix. About 5% of the extracellular matrix of bone is made up of non-collagenous proteins[2,4,5]. These proteins have roles in regulating mineral homeostasis and in regulating bone turnover in an interplay with the osteoblasts and osteoclasts[2,4,5]. Some of these proteins are bone-specific, for example bone sialoprotein, osteocalcin, and osteoadherin. Others have a more ubiquitous distribution, for example osteopontin, osteonectin, fibromodulin, decorin, and biglycan. In osteoporosis, procollagen propeptides and telopeptides have proven useful as molecular markers for assessing therapy, but few results pertaining to their utility in RA are available as yet. Some evidence suggesting a role for bone sialoprotein and possibly osteocalcin as molecular markers in RA is available[9].

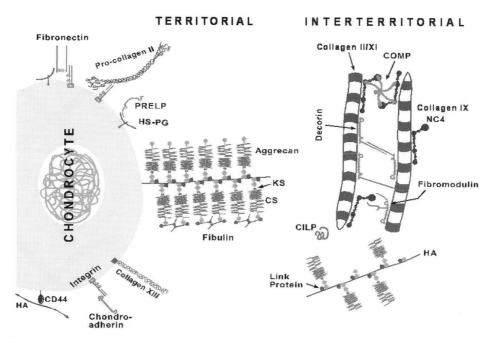

Fig. 21.2 Schematic illustration of the constituents of cartilage matrix. The spatial relationships of the various constituents to the chondrocyte, that is, their presence in the territorial (close to the cell) or interterritorial matrix (furthest away from the cell) are shown and the macromolecular organization of matrix molecules is indicated. CILP, cartilage intermediate layer protein; HA, hyaluronan; KS, keratan sulfate; CS, chondroitin sulfate; PRELP, proline arginine-rich end leucine-rich protein; HS-PG, heparan sulfate proteoglycan. See also colour plate section.

Progressive molecular events in cartilage and bone destruction

An important feature of the marker approach to the study of joint tissue pathology in RA and other joint diseases is the potential to detect early pathological tissue events. Also the use of a panel of markers makes it possible to depict a sequence of processes involving different parts of the matrix. This opens avenues for 'grading the tissue lesion at the molecular level'[10]. A suggested sequence of events in the progression of cartilage damage is shown in Fig. 21.3.

Structural disturbances close to the chondrocyte are probably easier to correct than those occurring in the interterritorial matrix, where the distance to the cell is larger and the assembly of the structural elements will be more complex to regulate. In a given compartment the organization of the matrix is finely regulated and the cells may be able to repair damaged structures. Aggrecan fragments may be lost and replaced without influencing the long-term function or structure, as demonstrated by the marked synovial fluid release of aggrecan in patients with reactive arthritis[11]. If more profound structural derangement occurs, including impaired function of the collagen network, irreversible joint damage is likely to follow. Thus, in early stages of disease one can expect one pattern of fragmentation of macromolecules whereas in later stages another pattern may emerge due to involvement of different compartments of the tissue. The challenge is to be able to detect the early reversible events occurring close to the cell in a reproducible and sensitive way in the individual patient in order to develop rational interventional strategies.

The concept of assessing the damage at the molecular level has been substantiated in both cross-sectional and longitudinal studies of patients with RA. In early stages high synovial fluid content of fragments of the core protein of aggrecan is found, even before any radiographic changes are apparent[12]. Subsequently, as the tissue damage increases the levels gradually decrease, most likely reflecting a reduction of cartilage mass. The G1 domain of aggrecan, bound to hyaluronan, is initially retained in the tissue but released later at a more advanced stage of the process[13]. Synovial fluid COMP levels also decrease with progressive cartilage destruction[14]. Increasing synovial fluid content of bone sialoprotein (BSP), a protein synthesized by the osteoblast, is first seen in advanced stages of arthritis, presumably reflecting the later involvement of the subchondral bone where this bone-specific protein is enriched[15]. Figure 21.4 illustrates the progressive molecular events in the degradation process by the synovial fluid content of some tissue markers at different stages of knee joint damage in patients with RA. These results corroborate the sequential molecular events suggested in Fig. 21.3.

In summary, the sequential nature of cartilage degradation in RA indicates that a specific marker may be more informative at a certain stage of the process, which underlines the fact that a panel of markers is needed to depict the state of the tissue process. Each marker may have 'a window' where increased release occurs, and defining this in relation to its tissue distribution and possibly its function will increase the utility of a particular marker.

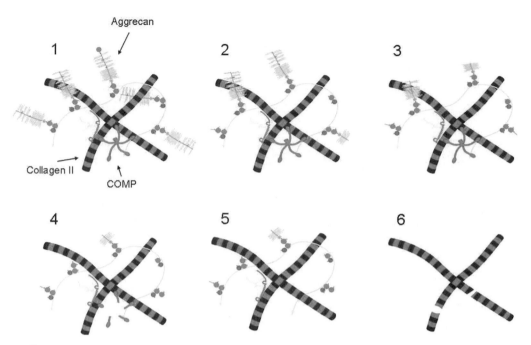

Fig. 21.3 Schematic illustration of a suggested sequence of events in the cartilage matrix during progressive cartilage damage resulting in sequential release of matrix macromolecules. Initially aggrecan molecules are degraded and released. This step is potentially reversible. Then other non-collagenous matrix macromolecules, for example COMP, are fragmented and released. This eventually leads to instability in the collagen network and a step of irreversibility when this network is disrupted and fragments of collagen are being released. At this stage molecules at the cartilage–bone interface, for example bone sialoprotein, may also be released. See also colour plate section.

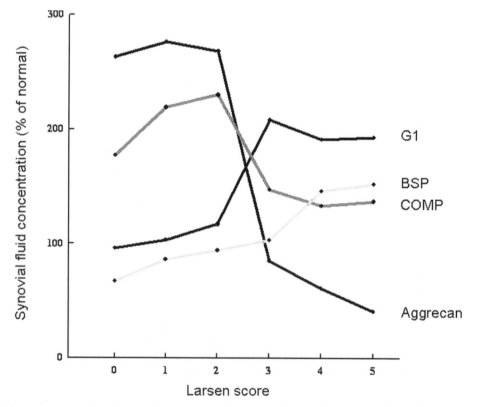

Fig. 21.4 Synovial fluid concentrations of cartilage and bone macromolecules in patients with RA with different degrees of radiographic knee joint damage. Values are expressed as a percentage of the mean concentration in synovial fluids from 10 healthy controls. Radiographic scoring was performed using the Larsen index, which takes into account both cartilage and bone changes. The score 0 denotes a normal appearing joint, and 5 the most advanced changes. Aggrecan, epitopes in the chondroitin–sulfate rich region of aggrecan; G1, the hyaluronan binding region of aggrecan; BSP, bone sialoprotein.

Markers of synthesis or degradation of matrix components

Both normal turnover and pathologic processes involve degradation as well as matrix repair. It is important to depict the balance between these processes when using the marker technology. This is, however, hampered by the often-observed release of newly synthesized molecules or fragments thereof not yet incorporated in the matrix. These fragments may be indistinguishable from those derived from resident structural molecules. It is therefore at present somewhat misleading to classify molecular markers as either reflecting matrix synthesis or degradation[9]. More work is needed in which marker release is related to other ways of depicting tissue events, as can be done by histopathological studies in experimental animals[16,17]. Another possible way to overcome this obstacle would be to characterize released fragments and discern patterns of fragments specifically related to synthesis or degradation. At present a certain marker still might reflect different processes in different diseases or different stages of a certain disease.

Currently available molecular markers for cartilage and bone

Table 21.1 summarizes knowledge about tissue distribution and clinical documentation of a number of the currently studied cartilage and bone markers. Key references describing the characteristics of each marker are cited.

Potential clinical applications of molecular markers for cartilage and bone in RA

In Table 21.2, examples of potential applications of molecular markers are listed. It is important to emphasize that the list includes both clinical and research applications. This underlines the notion that characterization and further development of this technology require collaborative efforts between clinical and basic science. Thus, a biologically sound hypothesis is the basis for optimal assessment, interpretation, and validation of results of molecular marker measurements in a clinical setting[2,50].

Diagnostic test

Ideally a diagnostic molecular marker would be released exclusively as a consequence of pathological tissue turnover. This could be a molecular fragment of a cartilage protein which would not be detectable during normal turnover but only appeared due to cleavage by an enzyme activated in a certain phase of disease, for example in early RA before any changes are detectable by imaging techniques. This would be similar to current cardiology practice, where assays for enzymes leaking from the cardiac muscle during a myocardial infarction have become key instruments for diagnosing this condition. These tests have a sensitivity that is far better than electrocardiography. Such tests are not yet available in rheumatology to measure tissue damage. In part this is due to disease heterogeneity. As expected, a number of studies show group average differences for serum levels between patients with different forms of arthritides and 'normal' individuals, but the overlap of individual specimens is pronounced[9,13,14,51]. At present the diagnostic utility of molecular markers lies in their ability to identify stages of tissue pathology with increased release of matrix macromolecular fragments. Thus assaying COMP in serum, for example, helps to identify RA patients with pathophysiological and prognostic features that differ. Measurement of COMP also offers the possibility of distinguishing between patients with or without ongoing cartilage pathology at their first consultation for musculoskeletal symptoms.

Monitor and predict progression of tissue damage

The underlying assumption is that changes in the content of tissue-derived molecules or their fragments in synovial fluid/blood/urine reflect the disease process in the tissue. Increased release of cartilage or bone fragment molecules accordingly should indicate an accelerated tissue turnover with an emphasis on degradation. If the dysregulated turnover persists in RA the result will be permanent joint damage. This suggested scenario forms the rationale for measurements of tissue markers to identify patients prone to rapid progression of joint damage and to distinguish them from those having a more favorable prognosis.

Information in support of this approach is accumulating. Initial studies suggested successful identification of patients with rapid progression of hip joint damage using serum COMP measurements[3]. These studies have been corroborated and extended to include a prognostic value regarding development of destruction of small joints and development of reduced physical function as measured by performance tests[29,52]. Also in osteoarthritis, serum COMP has been shown to identify patients with progressive joint damage[53,54]. Figure 21.5 illustrates the relation between serum COMP obtained at diagnosis of RA and the risk of progression of joint damage in hands and feet over five years in a cohort of conservatively treated patients monitored prospectively since the late 1980s[29]. Other cartilage and bone markers have also shown promise as prognostic indicators in RA, including aggrecan and collagen I and II epitopes[19,55,56]. It has been possible to identify rapid progressors whereas the identification of slow progressors has proven much more difficult for all markers tested. Prognostic markers have not yet reached the sensitivity which would make them useful in management of individual patients. Future assays, specific for fragments released only under pathologic conditions, will have much higher sensitivity and improve the ability to identify alterations in a given patient. At present it is quite clear that markedly high release of, for example, COMP is an unfavorable prognostic sign. However, a moderately increased serum level of COMP is less informative. For good reasons, patients are already currently treated aggressively at early stages of the disease, for example with tumor necrosis factor (TNF)-blockers, which

Table 21.1 Currently available cartilage and bone markers

	Tissue distribution	Remarks	Key references
Aggrecan: G1	Cartilage Trace in tendon and atherosclerotic lesions	Retained bound to HA in tissue after aggrecan is cleaved and the C-terminal part is released	13
Aggrecan: Chondroitin sulfate-region peptides	Cartilage	Fragments like these containing large number of charged groups are efficiently eliminated in the lymph nodes on passage from the joint via the lymphatics. Serum levels do not provide a good indicator of a joint process	12, 13, 18, 19
Aggrecan: Chondroitin sulfate epitopes (846, 7D4, 3B3)	Cartilage 846 appears in cartilage in early life and in osteoarthritis. Other tissues?	Number of epitopes of 846 per aggrecan very different in different disease groups and does not provide a measure of level of new synthesis, although its presence requires new synthesis	3, 20–22
Aggrecan: Keratan sulfate	Cartilage, cornea	Keratan sulfate-containing fragments are likely to be cleared in lymph nodes. Applications should be restricted to synovial fluid	20, 21, 23–26
Aggrecan: Aggrecanase cleavage neoepitopes	The enzyme is present widely but its substrate aggrecan is restricted	Aggrecanase cleaves at four sites along aggrecan. One site is present in the interglobular domain. Assay complicated by the necessity to remove a keratan sulfate chain	27, 28
Aggrecan: MMP (matrix metalloproteinase) cleavage neoepitopes	Several MMPs can accomplish cleavage. Wide tissue distribution		(27)
COMP (thrombospondin-5)	Particularly prominent in cartilage and most so in articular cartilage and the intervertebral disc	Produced by synovial cells, but presence in synovial capsule 1/100 of that in synovial fluid. Presence in tendon, particularly pressure-bearing parts. No detectable increase in blood in tendonitis	3, 14, 29–31
Matrilin-1	Only cartilage and not in articular cartilage. Particularly abundant in tracheal cartilage	May be used to depict contributions from processes in non-articular cartilage	32, 33
CILP (cartilage intermediate layer protein)	Restricted to cartilage and particularly in an intermediate zone	Protein synthesis and amount increased in early osteoarthritis	34
Collagen II: C-terminal propeptide	Cartilage	Apparently an indicator of new synthesis cleaved upon procollagen processing for fibrillogenesis	3, 22
Collagen II: cross-links	Cartilage	Cross-links are only formed after assembly of supramolecular structures. The cross-links thus represent a true degradation indicator Release particularly prominent in late stage disease	9, 35–38
Collagen II: collagenase cleavage neoepitope	Cartilage	Collagen cleavage appears to occur late in cartilage destruction. Cleavage products may result from cleavage of resident fibers as well as of newly synthesized collagen	39

Table 21.1　*(Continued)*

	Tissue distribution	Remarks	Key references
Osteocalcin	Bone and dentine, osteoblasts and odontoblasts	Conflicting data in RA	40–43
Bone sialoprotein	Bone, osteoblasts. Enriched in bone-cartilage interphase	Increased in RA. Relates to joint damage	15, 44, 45
Collagen I: N- and C-procollagen propeptides	Ubiquitous. Changes in body fluids mainly reflecting bone turnover	Few data in RA. Putative marker of synthesis	46, 47
Collagen I: N-and C-telopeptides	Ubiquitous. Changes in body fluids mainly reflecting bone turnover	Few data in RA. Putative marker of degradation	37, 43, 48, 49

Table 21.2　Examples of potential applications of molecular markers for cartilage or bone involvement in rheumatoid arthritis

1. Diagnostic test
2. Monitor and predict progression of tissue damage
3. Monitor response to therapy/provide proof of concept in experimental animals and clinical trials
4. Elucidate pathophysiological mechanisms for cartilage destruction
   - Define cleavage patterns of macromolecules which will reveal the enzymatic mechanisms for cleavage and thereby facilitate development of inhibitors
   - By monitoring effects of therapy molecular markers will aid in understanding how mediators, e.g. cytokines, drive the destructive process

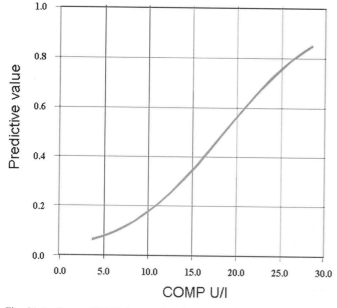

Fig. 21.5　Serum COMP in samples obtained at baseline in a prospective study of patients with early RA (disease duration median 11 months) in relation to development of joint damage as visualized radiographically in hands and feet after five years. The graph illustrates the predictive value for a certain COMP value for developing extensive joint damage, that is, to have a Larsen score >75th percentile of the cohort after five years. The calculations are based on values in 183 patients[29].

modify the disease progression and thereby reduce the possibility of evaluating prognostic markers[57]. Therefore data derived from old, carefully monitored cohorts of RA patients managed more conservatively may be a prerequisite for establishing the relevance of new assays[29].

Monitor response to therapy/provide proof of concept in experimental animals and clinical trials

The concept of assessing tissue-protective or damaging effects of therapeutic interventions by analyses of tissue-derived molecular markers is attractive. Ideally, it would provide a means of obtaining information on the influence on the tissue much earlier than is now possible by using imaging techniques. A first step to exploring this application is to study how a marker behaves in relation to biochemical markers of inflammation and to histopathological tissue changes in experimental arthritis. In a second step the influence of therapeutic intervention in animal models of arthritis should be performed. Finally, in the third step, its utility for assessing therapy potentially retarding damage in human disease should be examined. This gives information both on how the marker relates to the tissue process and on how a specific treatment affects the tissue and the marker release. To illustrate this approach we will examine how COMP has been characterized in this respect.

In studies of collagen II-induced arthritis in rats and mice and pristane-induced arthritis in rats, serial observations show that release of serum COMP increases during development of arthritis to reach a maximum coinciding with presence of cartilage changes, as confirmed by histopathologic observations[44,58]. The increase in serum fibrinogen or serum hyaluronan, markers of generalized and local inflammation, occurs considerably earlier during arthritis development than that of COMP and peaks at a time when the serum COMP levels are only slightly increased (Fig. 21.6)[59]. Furthermore, the levels of the inflammatory markers in most cases have returned to normal at a stage when the COMP levels are most markedly elevated.

Collagen II induced arthritis in rats

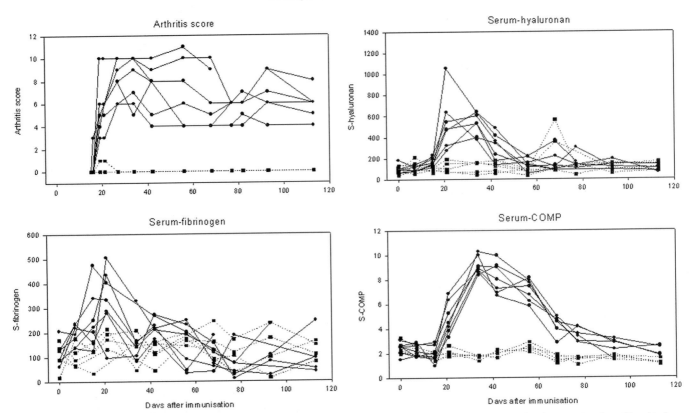

Fig. 21.6 Changes in arthritis score and serum concentrations of fibrinogen (marker of generalized inflammation), hyaluronan (marker of local inflammation) and COMP (marker of cartilage turnover) in experimental arthritis in male DA-rats induced by collagen II prepared from rat chondrosarcoma injected intradermally at the base of the tail. The unbroken lines denote the animals that exhibited signs of arthritis. The dotted lines denote the animals with no signs of arthritis after immunization. Note the different kinetics of the increase in concentrations of the markers of inflammation and cartilage involvement. The increase in serum concentrations of COMP occurs at a later stage, coinciding with marked histopathological changes in the cartilage. (Adapted from Ref. 59.)

Cytokine modulating treatment, which reduced cartilage pathology, also reduced serum COMP, whereas treatment which only reduced inflammation without influencing cartilage pathology did not influence the serum levels of COMP[16]. In recent experiments in which glucocorticoid treatment prevented cartilage damage in established collagen II arthritis in rats, the increased serum COMP at initiation of treatment was normalized, correlating with the tissue response to therapy[17]. Also, treatment with an experimental drug, CNI-1493, an inhibitor of the synthesis of pro-inflammatory cytokines, normalized serum COMP and prevented joint damage in this model[60]. Taken together, these observations show that changes in serum COMP are related to cartilage involvement in these models, but apparently not mechanistically directly linked to inflammation.

It has been shown that TNF-blockers retard the development of joint damage in RA[61,62]. We have monitored serum COMP during treatment of RA patients with infliximab or etanercept and shown that both drugs reduce circulating COMP regardless of clinical inflammatory response[63]. Thus serum COMP decreased both in patients in whom the signs of inflammation were reduced and in those where inflammation persisted, corroborating findings in the ATTRACT (Anti-Tumor Necrosis Factor Trial in Rheumatoid Arthritis with Concomitant Therapy)

study of infliximab, where joint damage retardation seemed to occur regardless of clinical response[62]. The dissociation between changes in serum COMP and variables of inflammation underlines that circulating COMP primarily reflects the cartilage process and supports that in RA there is a partial uncoupling of inflammation and tissue destruction[64].

Thus, COMP should be a suitable marker for monitoring cartilage response to therapy. The results demonstrate that a matrix macromolecule that is not completely tissue-specific may be useful for evaluating changes in a particular tissue. Importantly, the crucial experiments to establish the role of a marker for a particular tissue are such that relate changes in marker concentrations to events in the tissue depicted by other measures as has been illustrated here. Thus the fact that small amounts of COMP can be produced in the synovial membrane does not preclude its utility as a cartilage marker[65]. In support, we have shown that the concentration gradient of the tissue content for COMP between cartilage, synovial fluid, and synovial membrane is 100/10/1 (Månsson, Heinegård, and Saxne, unpublished). In other species an even greater synovial fluid/synovial membrane (100/1) gradient has been found[30].

In future experiments it will be possible to measure select fragments of COMP, which will provide new insight into the pathophysiological mechanisms operating in different stages or types of arthritides and in cytokine pathophysiology. The sequence of experiments described for evaluating COMP as a therapeutic marker serves as an example of how the initial evaluation of the biological rationale for using other markers in this application could be performed. By combining a set of markers with different specificity it should eventually be possible to monitor the arthritis process and the influence of therapy in all tissues in the joint.

Potential difficulties and factors to consider when interpreting results of cartilage and bone marker measurements

The molecular marker approach, although very promising, has some inherent difficulties that need to be sorted out for each marker and should be considered when interpreting results. As long as these factors are taken into account they do not preclude the exploration of molecular marker measurements as instruments for monitoring tissue involvement in disease. Some aspects of potentially confounding conditions regarding molecular marker measurements are reviewed below.

Formation and clearance of fragments in the joint

It is important to understand the generation and clearance of molecular fragments (Fig. 21.7)[66]. Macromolecules that are enzymatically cleaved in articular cartilage will be released into synovial fluid and/or taken up by the chondrocytes and degraded further. One fraction of the molecules may be phagocytosed and further degraded by cells in the synovial lining or in the joint fluid, but it appears that the bulk of fragments leave the joint cavity via lymphatic drainage. The half-life in synovial fluid of the fragments varies with the permeability of the synovial interstitium to different macromolecules. Thus, accelerated clearance has been observed in conditions with inflammation in the synovial lining cells[67]. Differences in marker concentrations between inflamed and non-inflamed joints may therefore underestimate the corresponding differences between release rates. As mentioned, the joint fluid content of cartilage-derived molecules may also be influenced by the amount of cartilage remaining in the joint[12]. This correlation outweighs the influence of synovial inflammation and has proved useful in monitoring the tissue damage. The concentration of a protein in synovial fluid is highly dependent on the amount of effusion present. Assessment of the synovial fluid volume can be done by magnetic resonance imaging or by a principle of dilution[68] but results are somewhat imprecise. We have found a surprisingly close correlation between concentration and total amount (concentration corrected for fluid volume) of individual fragments in most studied synovial fluid samples. The use of ratios of concentrations of two markers instead of absolute concentrations is an attractive way to make

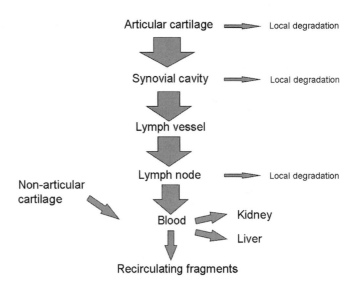

Fig. 21.7 Pathways for release and catabolism of joint cartilage or bone macromolecules. Macromolecules are fragmented by proteases and released into synovial fluid. Fragments are eliminated by lymphatic drainage to the blood and are then removed by hepatic degradation or renal clearance. Note influx of fragments from extra-articular cartilage or bone.

the results less influenced by volume alterations. This approach has proven most useful, particularly in longitudinal studies of patients and when lavage procedures are used to obtain fluid[18,69]. Another method for correcting for the unknown dilution of synovial fluid during lavage is to use a molecule that is neither synthesized nor metabolized by joint tissues to determine the dilution factor. One such molecule is urea, where one can assume that the concentrations are similar in synovial fluid and in serum[70].

Factors affecting the interpretation of serum analyses

A substantial portion of released fragments are entrapped and further degraded or eliminated in the regional lymph nodes (Fig. 21.7). The remainder reaches the bloodstream. Thus up to 80% of aggrecan core protein antigenic fragments are removed in the lymph node[71]. In contrast, the majority of antigenic fragments of COMP passes the lymph node, suggesting that serum COMP better represents events in the joint than serum aggrecan[71].

The macromolecules in the circulation are variably eliminated by uptake in the liver or by renal clearance (Fig. 21.7). The hepatic or renal elimination is dependent on the function of these organs, the function of which may be altered by disease processes or drug treatment. Clearly, the recirculating pool of any tissue marker represents only a fraction of all fragments released from the tissue. The clearance of fragments of COMP has been studied in RA and osteoarthritis (OA) patients and the half-life in the circulation appears to be around 7 h[72]. In these studies we also showed that there is a diurnal variation of serum levels of COMP, with the lowest levels at night during bed-rest, whereas the levels are stable during daytime, that is, during the period when serum sampling normally occurs[72]. Thus, although the contribution from single joints must be significant to become detectable against the background of normal turnover, it is possible to identify increased release due to joint pathology. Identification of fragments only released during pathological turnover of joint cartilage or bone would of course facilitate the development of the technology.

Another possible confounder when applying marker analyses in longitudinal studies of patients, for example in relation to therapy, is the influence of physical activity. It has recently been shown that serum COMP increases significantly during dynamic exercise and decreases slightly but significantly during rest. The increase may either be due to mobilization of COMP from the tissue during exercise or, more likely, be a consequence of increased transport from the joint cavity into the bloodstream. After 30 min levels had returned to baseline and it is therefore recommended that serum sampling is performed after at least 30 min of rest in a seated position[73,74]. Few data on other markers regarding this issue are available.

Other variables to consider regarding interpretation of serum analyses pertain to the influence of demographic factors such as gender, age, ethnicity, body mass index, etc. Some information on these variables is available, for example regarding COMP, hyaluronan, and collagen I and II biomarkers, mostly derived from studies of OA[75-79]. For example, serum COMP and serum hyaluronan are both higher in men than in women and serum COMP is higher in African-American women than in Caucasian women[75,76]. Also, levels of COMP and hyaluronan were associated with age[75,76]. However, when controlling for these factors a correlation between these markers and radiographic OA remains. Thus it seems important to control for such factors in studies of cohorts of patients but it may be less important in studies where individual patients are monitored over time.

Synovial fluid versus serum analysis

In studies of a joint tissue marker initial analyses should be performed on synovial fluid in order to establish what factors are influencing data outcome, provided the caveats discussed above are kept in mind. This will allow the correlating of alterations demonstrated by, for example, imaging technologies or histopathology to findings of altered marker levels or patterns. When a promising marker has been identified in synovial fluid, serum analyses may be explored. A joint fluid sample will obviously provide information on the condition of that particular joint while serum and urine samples will give an integrated measure of all tissues in the body containing a particular molecular marker, that is, in most cases for cartilage both articular and extra-articular cartilage. Thus it is anticipated that the serum level should not correlate to the synovial fluid level in a single joint in a polyarticular disease but could possibly do so in a monoarticular condition[11].

What is a normal value of a tissue marker measured in serum or synovial fluid?

The definition of the normal concentration range in serum for a marker is hampered by the confounding factors discussed above. It should be stressed that in a number of situations where

molecular marker analyses can be applied knowledge of normal values is not a confounding factor. This includes situations where individual patients are monitored, for example in relation to therapy, where changes of marker levels rather than absolute values are monitored, and also when markers are used for prognostic purposes. However, if one wants to use a marker for diagnostic purposes, that is, to detect whether a pathological turnover of, for example, cartilage is ongoing, reference guidelines are needed.

The problem encountered in identifying the normal serum range for a certain cartilage marker is illustrated by the age-dependent variations of serum concentrations of COMP. In children, common to many cartilage and bone markers, serum COMP shows high levels, which typically decrease to adult levels around 15 years of age (Månsson and Saxne, unpublished). This is most likely due to the higher tissue turnover during growth particularly in the growth plates, with release of both newly synthesized fragmented molecules not incorporated in the matrix and resident molecules being degraded. In blood donors, the serum concentrations of COMP do not vary with age in individuals between ages 20 and 50 years. However, in blood donors aged between 50 and 65 about 20% show serum concentrations above the upper normal range for the blood donors in the younger age group[80]. The higher levels in these apparently healthy individuals are most likely due to asymptomatic OA.

In summary, ideally normal values should be related to age and probably also to gender and ethnicity to be fully applicable[80,81]. One way to partially circumvent the problem is to define concentrations which, based on values in large cohorts of apparently healthy individuals, can identify pathological values, for example such that fall above the 95th percentile of values in healthy individuals. This will ensure that patients with pathological values will be identified; that is, the method will be specific but with fairly low sensitivity. This approach has been successfully used in a study of early RA using serum COMP[52]. Furthermore, this procedure is currently being applied in a clinical setting as recommended by the manufacturer of a commercial assay (AnaMar Medical, Sweden).

Validation of the role of molecular markers for tissue involvement in RA

The validation of molecular markers for investigations of the mechanisms of tissue damage in RA or for more clinically oriented applications depends on insights into biology, since tissue-derived markers represent a unique way of assessing tissue involvement in arthritis (Table 21.3). The molecular markers measure a feature of the disease process not contained in routinely used clinical or imaging procedures. Thus, there is no universal 'gold standard'. One issue is that changes in serum concentrations of a molecular marker may reflect a process in the tissue long before alterations are visible on radiographs or even by magnetic resonance imaging, since imaging techniques do not validate ongoing tissue pathology. However, imaging may be used as an end-point to examine whether early changes in marker

Table 21.3 Examples of factors to consider when validating the role of a molecular marker for tissue involvement in rheumatoid arthritis

1. Is there a biologic rationale for measuring the marker?
2. Do marker concentrations relate to processes in the tissue depicted by other techniques?
3. Is the technical performance of the assay adequate?
4. Is more than one assay available? Do results concur, i.e. do assays measure similar fragments?
5. Are marker levels influenced by demographic characteristics of patients?
6. Does physical activity influence marker levels?
7. Is there any diurnal variation of marker levels?
8. Do marker levels relate to measures of inflammation?
9. Are marker levels sensitive to spontaneous or drug-induced changes in the disease process?
10. Is the marker informative in all stages of the disease?

levels relate to subsequent joint damage, thus validating the prognostic potential of the process activity.

A primary requirement for a putative marker is that there is a biological rationale for its application. This means that a cartilage marker should be present in this tissue and convincing information should indicate that the marker is released during tissue turnover. Preferably, knowledge of its function or role in the tissue should be available since this will facilitate interpretation of the biological consequences of alterations. An example of a strategy for validation in this sense is given in the section where markers for monitoring of response to therapy are discussed. In accordance, results in initial experiments performed in animal models can subsequently be evaluated in studies in human subjects.

Furthermore, the technical performance of each assay needs careful validation. It is, however, beyond the scope of this review to detail the requirements of a reliable assay. It should be emphasized that if there are several assays for a certain marker it is essential to evaluate the performance of each assay. Different assays for a given protein may well show different results, since the antibodies used, polyclonal or monoclonal, may vary in specificity and recognize distinct fragments of the protein[14,29,82].

As discussed, it is important to define whether marker levels are influenced by demographic characteristics and physical activity. The need to examine presence of diurnal variation and to estimate turnover rate in the circulation for each marker have to be emphasized. To date information on these issues is scarce, with few exceptions.

Another issue to consider is whether changes in, for example, serum concentrations of a cartilage or bone marker are related to changes in the inflammatory process which can be measured by indicators of inflammation. If a close correlation is found between variables of inflammation, for example C-reactive protein and a cartilage marker, such a marker may not contribute significant new information. If, on the other hand, levels of a tissue marker vary independently compared to, for example, C-reactive protein, it is likely that this marker reflects a process which is not primarily driven by inflammation. Very little correlation exists between changes in COMP levels in serum and changes in C-reactive protein in all reported comparisons. A good example is the reduction in COMP levels seen during TNF-inhibition regardless of reduction of C-reactive protein[63].

Conclusion

We predict that developments in the area will make it possible to identify a set of cartilage and bone markers suitable for application in research and clinical practice. Each marker will have strengths and weaknesses, but by combining a number of well-characterized and validated markers, which need not be the same for use in research and clinical practice, the non-invasive biochemical monitoring of disease processes in joint tissues will be greatly facilitated, as shown by examples given in this chapter.

References

1. Biomarkers Definitions Working Group, and Bethesda M. Biomarkers and surrogate endpoints: preferred definitions and conceptual framework. *Clin Pharm Ther* 2001; **69**: 89–95.
2. Heinegård, D., Lorenzo, P., and Saxne, T. Matrix glycoproteins and proteoglycans in cartilage. In *Kelley's textbook of rheumatology* (Harris, E. D. Jr., Budd, R. C., Firestein, G. S., Genovese, M. C., Sergent, J. S., Ruddy, S. *et al.*, eds), pp. 48–62. Philadelphia: Elsevier Saunders; 2005.
3. Månsson, B., Carey, D., Alini, M. *et al.* Cartilage and bone metabolism in rheumatoid arthritis: differences between rapid and slow progression of disease identified by serum markers of cartilage metabolism. *J Clin Invest* 1995; **95**: 1071–7.
4. Heinegård, D., Saxne, T., and Lorenzo, P. Non-collagenous proteins: glycoproteins and related molecules. In *Dynamics of bone and cartilage metabolism* (Seibel, M. J., Robins, S. P., Bilezikian, J. P., eds), pp. 59–69. San Diego, Academic Press. 1999.
5. Eyre, D. R. Collagens and cartilage matrix homeostasis. *Clin Orthop Relat Res* 2004; **427 Suppl.**: S118–S122.
6. Hedbom, E., Antonsson, P., Hjerpe, A. *et al.* Cartilage matrix proteins: an acidic oligomeric protein (COMP) detected only in cartilage. *J Biol Chem* 1992; **267**: 6132–6.
7. Svensson, L., Oldberg, A., and Heinegård, **D**. Collagen binding proteins. *Osteoarthritis Cartilage* 2001; **9 Suppl A**: S23–S28.
8. Rosenberg, K., Olsson, H., Mörgelin, M., and Heinegård, D. Cartilage oligomeric matrix protein shows high affinity zinc-dependent interaction with triple helical collagen. *J Biol Chem* 1998; **273**: 20397–403.
9. Garnero, P., Rousseau, J. C., and Delmas, P. D. Molecular basis and clinical use of biochemical markers of bone, cartilage, and synovium in joint diseases. *Arthritis Rheum* 2000; **43**: 953–68.
10. Saxne, T., and Heinegård, D. Matrix proteins: potentials as body fluid markers of changes in the metabolism of cartilage and bone in arthritis. *J Rheumatol Suppl* 1995; **43**: 71–4.
11. Saxne, T., Glennås, A., Kvien, T. K., Melby, K., and Heinegård, D. Release of cartilage macromolecules into the synovial fluid in patients with acute and prolonged phases of reactive arthritis. *Arthritis Rheum* 1993; **36**: 20–5.
12. Saxne, T., Heinegård, D., Wollheim, F. A., and Pettersson, H. Difference in cartilage proteoglycan level in synovial fluid in early rheumatoid arthritis and reactive arthritis. *Lancet* 1985; **2**: 127–8.
13. Saxne, T., and Heinegård, D. Synovial fluid analysis of two groups of proteoglycan epitopes distinguishes early and late cartilage lesions. *Arthritis Rheum* 1992; **35**: 385–90.
14. Saxne, T., and Heinegård, D. Cartilage oligomeric matrix protein: a novel marker of cartilage turnover detectable in synovial fluid and blood. *Br J Rheumatol* 1992; **31**: 583–91.
15. Saxne, T., Zunino, L., and Heinegård, D. Increased release of bone sialoprotein into synovial fluid reflects tissue destruction in rheumatoid arthritis. *Arthritis Rheum* 1995; **38**: 82–90.
16. Joosten, L. A., Helsen, M. M., Saxne, T., van De Loo, F. A., Heinegård, D., and van den Berg, W. B. IL-1 alpha beta blockade

prevents cartilage and bone destruction in murine type II collagen-induced arthritis, whereas TNF-alpha blockade only ameliorates joint inflammation. *J Immunol* 1999; **163**: 5049–55.

17. Larsson, E., Erlandsson-Harris, L., Larsson, A., Månsson, B., Saxne, T., and Klareskog, L. Corticosteroid treatment of experimental arthritis retards cartilage destruction as determined by histology and serum COMP. *Rheumatology (Oxford)* 2004; **43**: 428–34.

18. Månsson, B., Geborek, P., and Saxne, T. Cartilage and bone macromolecules in knee joint synovial fluid in rheumatoid arthritis: relation to development of knee or hip joint destruction. *Ann Rheum Dis* 1997; **56**: 91–6.

19. Saxne, T., Wollheim, F. A., Pettersson, H., and Heinegård, D. Proteoglycan concentration in synovial fluid: predictor of future cartilage destruction in rheumatoid arthritis? *Br Med J (Clin Res Ed)* 1987; **295**: 1447–8.

20. Poole, A. R., Ionescu, M., Swan, A., and Dieppe, P. A. Changes in cartilage metabolism in arthritis are reflected by altered serum and synovial fluid levels of the cartilage proteoglycan aggrecan: implications for pathogenesis. *J Clin Invest* 1994; **94**: 25–33.

21. Belcher, C., Yaqub, R., Fawthrop, F., Bayliss, M., and Doherty, M. Synovial fluid chondroitin and keratan sulphate epitopes, glycosaminoglycans, and hyaluronan in arthritic and normal knees. *Ann Rheum Dis* 1997; **56**: 299–307.

22. Fraser, A., Fearon, U., Billinghurst, R. C. *et al.* Turnover of type II collagen and aggrecan in cartilage matrix at the onset of inflammatory arthritis in humans: relationship to mediators of systemic and local inflammation. *Arthritis Rheum* 2003; **48**: 3085–95.

23. Mehraban, F., Finegan, C. K., and Moskowitz, R. W. Serum keratan sulfate: quantitative and qualitative comparisons in inflammatory versus noninflammatory arthritides. *Arthritis Rheum* 1991; **34**: 383–92.

24. Sharif, M., Osborne, D. J., Meadows, K. *et al.* The relevance of chondroitin and keratan sulphate markers in normal and arthritic synovial fluid. *Br J Rheumatol* 1996; **35**: 951–7.

25. Spector, T. D., Woodward, L., Hall, G. M. *et al.* Keratan sulphate in rheumatoid arthritis, osteoarthritis, and inflammatory diseases. *Ann Rheum Dis* 1992; **51**: 1134–7.

26. Thonar, E. J., Lenz, M. E., Klintworth, G. K. *et al.* Quantification of keratan sulfate in blood as a marker of cartilage catabolism. *Arthritis Rheum* 1985; **28**: 1367–76.

27. Lark, M. W., Bayne, E. K., Flanagan, J. *et al.* Aggrecan degradation in human cartilage: evidence for both matrix metalloproteinase and aggrecanase activity in normal, osteoarthritic, and rheumatoid joints. *J Clin Invest* 1997; **100**: 93–106.

28. Tortorella, M. D., Pratta, M., Liu, R. Q. *et al.* Sites of aggrecan cleavage by recombinant human aggrecanase-1 (ADAMTS-4). *J Biol Chem* 2000; **275**: 18566–73.

29. Lindqvist, E., Eberhardt, K., Bendtzen, K., Heinegård, D., and Saxne, T. Prognostic laboratory markers of joint damage in rheumatoid arthritis. *Ann Rheum Dis* 2005; **64**: 196–201.

30. Skiöldebrand, E., Lorenzo, P., Zunino, L. *et al.* Concentration of collagen, aggrecan and cartilage oligomeric matrix protein (COMP) in synovial fluid from equine middle carpal joints. *Equine Vet J* 2001; **33**: 394–402.

31. Smith, R. K., and Heinegård, D. Cartilage oligomeric matrix protein (COMP) levels in digital sheath synovial fluid and serum with tendon injury. *Equine Vet J* 2000; **32**: 52–8.

32. Saxne, T., and Heinegård, D. Involvement of nonarticular cartilage, as demonstrated by release of a cartilage-specific protein, in rheumatoid arthritis. *Arthritis Rheum* 1989; **32**: 1080–6.

33. Saxne, T., and Heinegård, D. Serum concentrations of two cartilage matrix proteins reflecting different aspects of cartilage turnover in relapsing polychondritis. *Arthritis Rheum* 1995; **38**: 294–6.

34. Lorenzo, P., Bayliss, M. T., and Heinegård, D. Altered patterns and synthesis of extracellular matrix macromolecules in early osteoarthritis. *Matrix Biol* 2004; **23**: 381–91.

35. Christgau, S., Garnero, P., Fledelius, C. *et al.* Collagen type II C-telopeptide fragments as an index of cartilage degradation. *Bone* 2001; **29**: 209–15.

36. Lohmander, L. S., Atley, L. M., Pietka, T. A., and Eyre, D. R. The release of crosslinked peptides from type II collagen into human synovial fluid is increased soon after joint injury and in osteoarthritis. *Arthritis Rheum* 2003; **48**: 3130–9.

37. Garnero, P., Landewe, R., Boers, M. *et al.* Association of baseline levels of markers of bone and cartilage degradation with long-term progression of joint damage in patients with early rheumatoid arthritis: the COBRA study. *Arthritis Rheum* 2002; **46**: 2847–56.

38. Ishikawa, T., Nishigaki, F., Christgau, S. *et al.* Cartilage destruction in collagen induced arthritis assessed with a new biochemical marker for collagen type II C-telopeptide fragments. *J Rheumatol* 2004; **31**: 1174–9.

39. Poole, A. R., Ionescu, M., Fitzcharles, M. A., and Billinghurst, R. C. The assessment of cartilage degradation in vivo: development of an immunoassay for the measurement in body fluids of type II collagen cleaved by collagenases. *J Immunol Methods* 2004; **294**: 145–53.

40. Campion, G. V., Delmas, P. D., and Dieppe, P. A. Serum and synovial fluid osteocalcin (bone gla protein) levels in joint disease. *Br J Rheumatol* 1989; **28**: 393–8.

41. Gevers, G., Devos, P., De Roo, M., and Dequeker, J. (1986). Increased levels of osteocalcin (serum bone Gla-protein) in rheumatoid arthritis. *Br J Rheumatol* **25**: 260–2.

42. Sambrook, P. N., Ansell, B. M., Foster, S. *et al.* Bone turnover in early rheumatoid arthritis. 1. Biochemical and kinetic indexes. *Ann Rheum Dis* 1985; **44**: 575–9.

43. Garnero, P., Jouvenne, P., Buchs, N., Delmas, P. D., and Miossec, P. Uncoupling of bone metabolism in rheumatoid arthritis patients with or without joint destruction: assessment with serum type I collagen breakdown products. *Bone* 1999; **24**: 381–5.

44. Larsson, E., Müssener, A., Heinegård, D., Klareskog, L., and Saxne, T. Increased serum levels of cartilage oligomeric matrix protein and bone sialoprotein in rats with collagen arthritis. *Br J Rheumatol* 1997; **36**: 1258–61.

45. Hultenby, K., Reinholt, F. P., Norgård, M., Oldberg, Å, Wendel, M., and Heinegård, D. Distribution and synthesis of bone sialoprotein in metaphyseal bone of young rats show a distinctly different pattern from that of osteopontin. *Eur J Cell Biol* 1994; **63**: 230–9.

46. Hakala, M., Aman, S., Luukkainen, R. *et al.* Application of markers of collagen metabolism in serum and synovial fluid for assessment of disease process in patients with rheumatoid arthritis. *Ann Rheum Dis* 1995; **54**: 886–90.

47. Kroger, H., Risteli, J., Risteli, L., Penttila, I., and Alhava, E. Serum osteocalcin and carboxyterminal propeptide of type I procollagen in rheumatoid arthritis. *Ann Rheum Dis* 1993; **52**: 338–42.

48. Hakala, M., Risteli, L., Manelius, J., Nieminen, P., and Risteli, J. Increased type I collagen degradation correlates with disease severity in rheumatoid arthritis. *Ann Rheum Dis* 1993; **52**: 866–9.

49. Clemens, J. D., Herrick, M. V., Singer, F. R., and Eyre, D. R. Evidence that serum NTx (collagen-type I N-telopeptides) can act as an immunochemical marker of bone resorption. *Clin Chem* 1997; **43**: 2058–63.

50. Poole, A. R. Biochemical/immunochemical biomarkers of osteoarthritis: utility for prediction of incident or progressive osteoarthritis. *Rheum Dis Clin North Am* 2003; **29**: 803–18.

51. Garnero, P., Piperno, M., Gineyts, E., Christgau, S., Delmas, P. D., and Vignon, E. Cross sectional evaluation of biochemical markers of bone, cartilage, and synovial tissue metabolism in patients with knee osteoarthritis: relations with disease activity and joint damage. *Ann Rheum Dis* 2001; **60**: 619–26.

52. Svensson, B., and Saxne, T. Serum cartilage oligomeric matrix protein (COMP): a predictor of joint damage and physical function in early rheumatoid arthritis. *Arthritis Rheum* 2004; **50** (9 Suppl.): 158–9.

53. Conrozier, T., Saxne, T., Fan, C. S. *et al.* Serum concentrations of cartilage oligomeric matrix protein and bone sialoprotein in hip osteoarthritis: a one year prospective study. *Ann Rheum Dis* 1998; **57**: 527–32.

54. Sharif, M., Kirwan, J. R., Elson, C. J., Granell, R., and Clarke, S. Suggestion of nonlinear or phasic progression of knee osteoarthritis

based on measurements of serum cartilage oligomeric matrix protein levels over five years. *Arthritis Rheum* 2004; **50**: 2479–88.

55. Garnero, P., Geusens, P., and Landewe, R. Biochemical markers of joint tissue turnover in early rheumatoid arthritis. *Clin Exp Rheumatol* 2003; **21**: S54–S58.

56. Landewe, R., Geusens, P., Boers, M. *et al.* Markers for type II collagen breakdown predict the effect of disease-modifying treatment on long-term radiographic progression in patients with rheumatoid arthritis. *Arthritis Rheum* 2004; **50**: 1390–9.

57. Lard, L. R., Boers, M., Verhoeven, A. *et al.* Early and aggressive treatment of rheumatoid arthritis patients affects the association of HLA class II antigens with progression of joint damage. *Arthritis Rheum* 2002; **46**: 899–905.

58. Vingsbo-Lundberg, C., Saxne, T., Olsson, H., and Holmdahl, R. Increased serum levels of cartilage oligomeric matrix protein in chronic erosive arthritis in rats. *Arthritis Rheum* 1998; **41**: 544–50.

59. Larsson, E., Erlandsson-Harris, L., Lorentzen, J. C. *et al.* Serum concentrations of cartilage oligomeric matrix protein, fibrinogen and hyaluronan distinguish inflammation and cartilage destruction in experimental arthritis in rats. *Rheumatology (Oxford)* 2002; **41**: 996–1000.

60. Larsson, E., Erlandsson-Harris, L., Palmblad, K., Månsson, B., Saxne, T., and Klareskog, L. CNI-1493, an inhibitor of proinflammatory cytokines, retards cartilage destruction in rats with collagen induced arthritis. *Ann Rheum Dis* 2005; **64**: 494–6.

61. Bathon, J. M., Martin, R. W., Fleischmann, R. M. *et al.* A comparison of etanercept and methotrexate in patients with early rheumatoid arthritis. *N Engl J Med* 2000; **343**: 1586–93.

62. Lipsky, P. E., van der Heijde, D. M., St Clair, E. W. *et al.* Infliximab and methotrexate in the treatment of rheumatoid arthritis. Anti-Tumor Necrosis Factor Trial in Rheumatoid Arthritis with Concomitant Therapy Study Group. *N Engl J Med* 2000; **343**: 1594–602.

63. Crnkic, M., Månsson, B., Larsson, L., Geborek, P., Heinegård, D., and Saxne, T. Serum cartilage oligomeric matrix protein (COMP) decreases in rheumatoid arthritis patients treated with infliximab or etanercept. *Arthritis Res Ther* 2003; **5**: R181–R185.

64. Kirwan, J. R. The synovium in rheumatoid arthritis: evidence for (at least) two pathologies. *Arthritis Rheum* 2004; **50**: 1–4.

65. Recklies, A. D., Baillargeon, L., and White, C. Regulation of cartilage oligomeric matrix protein synthesis in human synovial cells and articular chondrocytes. *Arthritis Rheum* 1998; **41**: 997–1006.

66. Simkin, P. A., and Bassett, J. E. Cartilage matrix molecules in serum and synovial fluid. *Curr Opin Rheumatol* 1995; **7**: 346–51.

67. Myers, S. L., Brandt, K. D., and Eilam, O. Even low-grade synovitis significantly accelerates the clearance of protein from the canine knee: implications for measurement of synovial fluid 'markers' of osteoarthritis. *Arthritis Rheum* 1995; **38**: 1085–91.

68. Geborek, P., Saxne, T., Heinegård, D., and Wollheim, F. A. Measurement of synovial fluid volume using albumin dilution upon intraarticular saline injection. *J Rheumatol* 1988; **15**: 91–4.

69. Månsson, B., Gűlfe, A., Geborek, P., Heinegård, D., and Saxne, T. Release of cartilage and bone macromolecules into synovial fluid: differences between psoriatic arthritis and rheumatoid arthritis. *Ann Rheum Dis* 2001; **60**: 27–31.

70. Kraus, V. B., Huebner, J. L., Fink, C. *et al.* Urea as a passive transport marker for arthritis biomarker studies. *Arthritis Rheum* 2002; **46**: 420–7.

71. Saxne, T., Heinegård, D., and Wollheim, F. A. Cartilage macromolecules and the development of new methods for the assessment of joint disease. *Rheumatol Europe* 1997; **26**: 108–10.

72. Andersson, M., Jonsson, N., Petersson, I. F., Heinegård, D., and Saxne, T. Diurnal variation of serum-COMP in individuals with knee pain and osteoarthritis. *Ann Rheum Dis* 2002; **61** (Suppl. I): 47–8.

73. Mundermann, A., Dyrby, C. O., Andriacchi, T. P., and King, K. B. Serum concentration of cartilage oligomeric matrix protein (COMP) is sensitive to physiological cyclic loading in healthy adults. *Osteoarthritis Cartilage* 2005; **13**: 34–8.

74. Andersson, M., Thorstensson, C., Roos, E., Petersson, I., Heinegård, D., and Saxne, T. Serum-COMP levels increase during physical exercise in patients with knee osteoarthritis. *Arthritis Rheum* 2003; **48** (9 Suppl.): 292.

75. Elliott, A. L., Kraus, V. B., Luta, G. *et al.* Serum hyaluronan levels and radiographic knee and hip osteoarthritis in African Americans and Caucasians in the Johnston County Osteoarthritis Project. *Arthritis Rheum* 2005; **52**: 105–11.

76. Jordan, J. M., Luta, G., Stabler, T. *et al.* Ethnic and sex differences in serum levels of cartilage oligomeric matrix protein: the Johnston County Osteoarthritis Project. *Arthritis Rheum* 2003; **48**: 675–81.

77. Jordan, J., Kraus, V., Renner, J. *et al.* Ethnic and gender differences in serum biomarkers of types I and II collagen cleavage and aggrecan turnover in African Americans and Caucasians. *Arthritis Rheum* 2004; **50** (9 Suppl.): 481.

78. Mouritzen, U., Christgau, S., Lehmann, H. J., Tanko, L. B., and Christiansen, C. Cartilage turnover assessed with a newly developed assay measuring collagen type II degradation products: influence of age, sex, menopause, hormone replacement therapy, and body mass index. *Ann Rheum Dis* 2003; **62**: 332–6.

79. Qvist, P., Christgau, S., Pedersen, B. J., Schlemmer, A., and Christiansen, C. Circadian variation in the serum concentration of C-terminal telopeptide of type I collagen (serum CTx): effects of gender, age, menopausal status, posture, daylight, serum cortisol, and fasting. *Bone* 2002; **31**: 57–61.

80. Månsson, B., Heinegård, D., and Saxne, T. Diagnosis of osteoarthritis in relation to molecular processes in cartilage: comment on the article by Clark et al. *Arthritis Rheum* 2000; **43**: 1425–7.

81. Clark, A. G., Jordan, J. M., Vilim, V. *et al.* Serum cartilage oligomeric matrix protein reflects osteoarthritis presence and severity: the Johnston County Osteoarthritis Project. *Arthritis Rheum* 1999; **42**: 2356–64.

82. Vilim, V., Voburka, Z., Vytasek, R. *et al.* Monoclonal antibodies to human cartilage oligomeric matrix protein: epitope mapping and characterization of sandwich ELISA. *Clin Chim Acta* 2003; **328**: 59–69.

SECTION 4 | *Drug therapy*

22 | NSAIDs and analgesics

Richard O. Day, Lynette M. March, Garry G. Graham, Kieran F. Scott, and Kenneth M. Williams

Introduction

The non-steroidal anti-inflammatory drugs (NSAIDs) and related drugs can be divided into two major groups (reviewed in Refs 1 and 2).

1 Non-selective NSAIDs, such as aspirin, ibuprofen and indomethacin, which also produce gastrointestinal damage, inhibit the aggregation of platelets, decrease kidney function in some patients, and precipitate aspirin-induced asthma (Table 22.1). These drugs inhibit both cyclooxygenase-1 (COX-1) and COX-2 which are central enzymes involved in the synthesis of prostaglandins and related compounds.

2 COX-2 selective inhibitors (coxibs or COX-1 sparing agents), which have similar therapeutic activities to the non-selective NSAIDs. Their actions are due to the selective inhibition of COX-2. Because of their very weak effect on COX-1, the COX-2 selective inhibitors have much better gastrointestinal tolerance than the non-selective NSAIDs, little or no effect on platelets, and no tendency to produce asthma (Table 22.1).

In addition, there are two drugs, salicylate and paracetamol, with similar actions to the NSAIDs. Although salicylate is now little used as a NSAID in the treatment of rheumatoid arthritis (RA), salicylate is still of clinical interest because its prodrug, aspirin, is widely used as an antiplatelet agent, occasional analgesic, and antipyretic (see section on Pro-drugs). Salicylate is a weak inhibitor of isolated COX-1 and COX-2, findings that have often been cited as indicating that salicylate and, possibly, other NSAIDs, may have actions other than on prostaglandin synthesis. Recent work, however, indicates that salicylate may very well act by effects on COX-2-dependent pathways (see section on Mechanism of action of NSAIDs: prostaglandin synthesis).

Paracetamol (acetaminophen, see section on Paracetamol) is a unique drug which has similar activities to the COX-2 selective inhibitors but has weaker anti-inflammatory activity. It is, however, widely used as an adjunct analgesic in the treatment of RA and may also potentiate the anti-inflammatory effects of the non-selective NSAIDs and the COX-2 selective inhibitors. The opioids, such as codeine, are also used to treat the pain of RA but only have a minor role in the treatment of this disease.

NSAIDs

Both groups of NSAIDs are widely used to decrease the symptoms of RA. While RA is a relatively common disease, affecting about 1% of the adult population, the NSAIDs are more widely used as analgesics, particularly for the treatment of osteoarthritis. Osteoarthritis is not primarily an inflammatory disease although

Table 22.1 The comparative pharmacological effects of the NSAIDs, paracetamol, and salicylate[1,2]

Action on	Non-selective NSAIDs	COX-2 selective inhibitors	Paracetamol	Salicylate
Pain	Analgesic	Analgesic	Analgesic	Analgesic
Fever	Antipyretic	Antipyretic	Antipyretic	Antipyretic
Inflammation	Anti-inflammatory	Anti-inflammatory	Inactive in RA[a]	Anti-inflammatory
Platelets	Inhibition of aggregation	No effect	Weak effect	No effect
Aspirin-induced asthma	Precipitation of asthma	No effect	Weak effect	No effect
Gastrointestinal damage	Damage	Little or no effect	No effect	No effect
Renal excretion of Na	Decrease	Decrease	No effect	?

[a]Active anti-inflammatory agent in other conditions (see section on paracetamol below).

some patients have significant inflammation of affected joints. Both groups of NSAIDs are also used in the treatment of less common inflammatory rheumatic diseases, such as acute gout, ankylosing spondylitis, and psoriatic arthritis.

Despite their clinically useful anti-inflammatory activity, the NSAIDs have limitations in the treatment of RA. Firstly, their effects are only mild to moderate. By no means do they entirely suppress the pain and inflammation of RA. Furthermore, the non-selective NSAIDs have no clear-cut inhibitory effect on the progression of RA. Thus, joint damage still continues. It is presumed that the COX-2 selective inhibitors are also ineffective in suppressing the long-term progression of RA although recent experimental work, if confirmed, on the COX-2 selective inhibitors on cartilage may alter this view (see section on Cartilage below). The disease modifying anti-rheumatic drugs (DMARDs), which slow the progression of the diseases in many patients, are considered to be of greater benefit then the NSAIDs in RA. The actions of the DMARDs take weeks to months to develop whereas the analgesic and anti-inflammatory effects of the NSAIDs are produced within a few days at most[3]. The NSAIDs are therefore very useful, particularly in the early weeks of treatment of RA with the DMARDs.

Of great interest has been the expansion of indications for both groups of NSAIDs beyond the rheumatic diseases. Inflammatory states, such as eye inflammation and post-operative inflammation, are being treated with the non-selective NSAIDs. Analgesic indications have widened to include cancer pain and pain associated with biliary and renal colic. Aspirin, the index NSAID, is very widely used now for the prevention of thrombosis. All four groups of NSAIDs and related drugs have antipyretic activity (Table 22.1), but the COX-2 selective inhibitors are rarely used for this action because paracetamol and the non-selective NSAIDs, particularly aspirin and ibuprofen, are cheap and effective antipyretic drugs. The non-selective NSAIDs and the COX-2 selective inhibitors are also being used to prevent colon cancer and are being widely investigated for their actions on other cancers.

The non-selective NSAIDs are associated with important adverse effects, particularly on the gastrointestinal and cardiovascular systems. The COX-2 selective inhibitors produce less gastropathy but they increase the risk of coronary heart disease and stroke to an extent which has led to, at least, the temporary withdrawal of two selective inhibitors, rofecoxib and valdecoxib, while the use of other drugs in the same group is presently uncertain. Adverse reactions to NSAIDs may occur at any age. However, the peak age of onset of RA is about 44–50 and, consequently, many patients with RA are middle aged and elderly. Thus, they are at an age where cardiovascular diseases are increasing and they may be at considerable risk of the cardiovascular problems seen with both groups of NSAIDs. It should be noted that RA is a systemic disease and this disease, in addition to the patient's age, may increase the risk of adverse reactions to the NSAIDs.

Mechanism of action of NSAIDs: prostaglandin synthesis

Inhibition of the enzymes COX-1 and COX-2, and therefore the synthesis of prostaglandins, explains most of the therapeutic and

toxic actions of NSAIDs[4]. The COX-1 isoenzyme is constitutive and is involved in the synthesis of prostaglandins involved in normal physiological functions in platelets, the gastrointestinal tract, and the kidney. COX-2 is generally an inducible isoform of cyclooxygenase with greatly increased expression occurring in sites of inflammation, thereby providing substantial amounts of prostaglandins to contribute to the inflammatory process. COX-2 interestingly has a limited distribution otherwise, namely in brain, spinal cord, kidney, and testes and is also present in the stomach.

The genes for COX-1 (PTGS-1) and COX-2 (PTGS-2) reside on chromosomes 9 and 1, respectively, PTGS-1 being a 22.5 kb gene and PTGS-2 being much smaller with 8.3 kb[5-7]. The PTGS-2 gene is one of a number of 'primary response' or 'immediate early' genes which also include the gene for inducible nitric oxide synthase. These genes are heavily induced by inflammatory cytokines, including IL-1β, and tumor necrosis factor (TNF)[8,9]. In contrast, the PTGS-1 gene is constitutive in most cells and not responsive to cytokines[10]. There is about 60% homology of the amino acid sequences of the COX-1 and COX-2 proteins, although there are very few differences in the amino acid sequences in the active sites of the enzymes[11]. The tertiary structures of COX-1 and COX-2 have been determined, an important contrast being a side pocket that forms part of the binding site of the COX-2 selective inhibitors on the enzyme[12]. The Vmax and Km for arachidonic acid are similar for the two isoforms but, in cells, COX-1 and COX-2 are regulated independently. Thus, COX-1 requires a higher concentration of arachidonic acid and more hydroperoxide to be activated than does COX-2[13]. There is also a spatial separation in cells. COX-1 is found on the endoplasmic reticulum only, whereas COX-2 is found on the nuclear envelope as well as the endoplasmic reticulum.

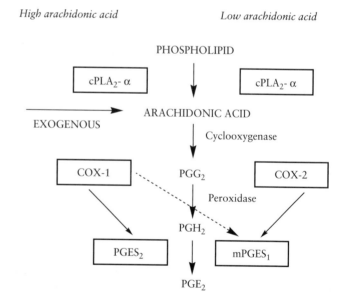

Fig 22.1 Scheme for synthesis of PGE$_2$ and the compartmentalization of enzymes involved in its synthesis. Both COX-1 and COX-2 have cyclooxygenase and peroxidase functions. Low concentrations of arachidonic acid are converted to PGE$_2$ mainly by COX-2 and prostaglandin E synthase-1 (mPGES$_1$) which is membrane associated. High concentrations of arachidonic acid are converted to PGE$_2$ by COX-1 and PGES$_2$ (a cytosolic enzyme), although mPGES$_1$ is also utilized.

Important aspects of the synthesis of prostaglandins by COX-1 and COX-2 are the compartmentalization of the enzymes and their dependence on the concentrations of arachidonic acid. In intact cells, low concentrations are metabolized to prostaglandin H_2 (PGH_2) and then to PGE_2 by COX-2 and membrane associated PGE synthase-1[13,14] (Fig. 22.1). Consistent with the association between COX-2 and the membrane associated PGE synthase-1, mice lacking this membrane associated PGE synthase have deficient and impaired inflammatory and pain responses[15].

Mechanism of action of NSAIDs in RA

The non-selective NSAIDs and the COX-2 selective inhibitors provide about equal symptomatic relief of RA, indicating that inhibition of COX-2 leads to the major desired effects of the non-selective NSAIDs in RA[16–18] (Table 22.1).

COX-2 inhibitors are also active in suppressing several animal models of arthritis. For example, the COX-2 selective inhibitors are active in several inflammatory tests in rat, such as paw edema[19]. Inhibition of COX-2 in the central nervous system may be an important aspect of the suppression of the pain associated with inflammation[20]. A selective COX-1 inhibitor is inactive in rat paw edema[19] but there are some experimental inflammatory processes, such as adjuvant-induced arthritis in the rat, which are decreased only by inhibition of both COX-1 and COX-2[19]. There are even some models of inflammation which are dependent upon COX-1[19].

The mechanism of the anti-inflammatory action of salicylate has been the subject of much argument. Although it is a weak inhibitor of isolated COX-1 and COX-2, it is a potent inhibitor of prostaglandin synthesis by intact cells, when the concentrations of the precursor, arachidonic acid, are low[1]. Under this condition, prostaglandins are synthesized primarily by a COX-2-dependent process[13] (Fig. 22.1). It is therefore not surprising that the effects of salicylate are similar to those of the COX-2 selective inhibitors (Table 22.1), although the molecular site of action of salicylate is still unclear. Salicylate also reduces the expression of COX-2 under some conditions[21] but the end result is still the same, that is, inhibition of COX-2 dependent processes. Aspirin, by contrast, inhibits both COX-1 and COX-2 although aspirin appears to have little or no effect in RA, with its metabolite, salicylate, being the major active species[22].

Selectivity of NSAIDs

Much has been made of the ratio of inhibitory concentrations against COX-1 and COX-2 of the NSAIDs. Most estimates of the potency ratio of NSAIDs as inhibitors of COX-1 and COX-2 have been derived from *in vitro* studies because these can be conducted quickly and reproducibly. However, there are many technical issues in establishing meaningful COX-2:COX-1 inhibitory potency ratios and there has been much criticism of the establishment and use of these ratios. The most reasonable ratios are those derived from *in vitro* assay systems in whole cells but the ratios vary depending on incubation times, whether exogenous or endogenous arachidonate substrate is used, the concentration of arachidonate employed, and the concentration of plasma proteins in the assay, amongst other variables. Despite the problems in the

determination of the ratios, there seems to be a very rough relationship between the COX-2:COX-1 inhibitory concentration ratio in intact cells and the relative risk for serious upper gastrointestinal bleeding or perforation[23]. Higher COX-2:COX-1 ratios are associated with greater gastrointestinal safety. These *in vitro* tests have therefore been important in the selection of COX-1 or COX-2 selective agents for further pharmacological examination and development.

The classification of the NSAIDs into non-selective NSAIDs and the COX-2 selective inhibitors can be regarded as the extremes of NSAIDs that are useful for the treatment of RA. Highly selective inhibitors of COX-1 have been prepared but, except for their activity in a couple of experimental systems, they are not effective anti-inflammatory agents[19]. Several older NSAIDs have considerable selectivity for COX-2-dependent synthesis of prostaglandins but may not be as selective as rofecoxib. Several were marketed before the identification of COX-2. These NSAIDs include etodolac, nimesulide, and meloxicam. Depending on the system, these three drugs are about as selective as celecoxib, although substantially less selective than the highly selective rofecoxib[23]. Of the remaining NSAIDs, the most selective in *in vitro* systems was diclofenac[23]. However, diclofenac appears much less selective in clinical practice because of the high incidence of adverse gastrointestinal effects during short-term treatment and its precipitation of aspirin-induced asthma.

Prostaglandin-independent effects of NSAIDs

NSAIDs have been reported to block a number of processes, other than prostaglandin synthesis. Several of these effects, such as inhibition of certain transcription factors, nuclear factor (NF)-κB and activator protein (AP)-1, could be important in suppressing the inflammatory response[24]. Several NSAIDs also inhibit the production of superoxide by neutrophils[25]. However, these effects have mainly been found in cellular systems *in vitro*, generally in media containing very little albumin, which is the major drug-binding protein in plasma. Under this condition, almost all the NSAID is not bound to albumin and, in general, the concentrations of NSAIDs in these *in vitro* studies are greater than the very low unbound concentration *in vivo*. This contrast makes it difficult to accept any causative relationship between these non-cyclooxygenase effects and the anti-inflammatory effects of NSAIDs[25]. Nevertheless, some parallel effects of NSAIDs in non-COX systems (inhibition of neutrophil aggregation, lysozyme release) are seen both *in vitro* and *ex vivo* in patients[26]. Furthermore, unlike S-flurbiprofen, R-flurbiprofen is a very weak inhibitor of prostaglandin synthesis but R-flurbiprofen is still anti-inflammatory in animal models[24] and, more importantly, it appears to be analgesic in humans[27]. Flurbiprofen is a phenyl-propionic acid but, unlike several other members of this group of NSAIDs, R-flurbiprofen is not inverted to S-flurbiprofen, which is an inhibitor of prostaglandin synthesis (see section on Pro-drugs below). Thus, effects of R-flurbiprofen cannot be due to its metabolic inversion to S-flurbiprofen.

Overall, many NSAIDs have pharmacological actions, independent of their actions on prostaglandin synthesis, but it is still not possible to make a definite conclusion about any non-prostaglandin action of NSAIDs in their suppression of the inflammation of RA.

Adverse reactions to NSAIDs

The drugs most commonly reported to adverse drug reaction reporting agencies are the non-selective NSAIDs. Up to 25% of all reports to these agencies relate to these drugs. Elderly patients are at greater risk than younger patients for adverse reactions in the gastrointestinal, renal, and central nervous systems. This difference is most likely due to a combination of reduced clearance of drug from the body and increased tissue sensitivity commonly observed in the elderly. As a result of greater risk in the elderly, a more cautious approach to the use of NSAIDs in this age group is warranted.

Gastrointestinal adverse reactions of the non-selective inhibitors

The non-selective NSAIDs are well known to produce adverse effects on the gastrointestinal tract. Erythema and ulceration are commonly seen on endoscopy and may progress to perforations, significant bleeding, and obstruction. From recent clinical trials, the cumulative annual incidence of serious gastrointestinal ulcer complications is about 1–2% of patients[16,17,28]. Gastric ulcers are located on the antral or prepyloric areas of the stomach. Duodenal injury is much less common than gastric injury but there is considerable loss of protein and blood across the mucosa and into the upper small intestine in patients taking non-selective NSAIDs[29].

The gastrointestinal symptoms from the NSAIDs include dyspepsia, epigastric pain, and, less commonly, nausea. Although lesions are found in many patients taking the non-selective NSAIDs, they are not necessarily associated with upper gastrointestinal symptoms, and the presence or absence of upper gastrointestinal symptoms is unsatisfactory as a predictor of serious bleeding from the upper gastrointestinal tract, especially in the elderly. However, upper gastrointestinal complaints, such as dyspepsia, are danger signals and it is of note that patients who know least about the risk of NSAIDs are more likely to continue therapy with the non-selective NSAIDs when upper gastrointestinal symptoms occur and are significantly more likely to bleed[30]. Patient education is therefore important in minimizing the gastrointestinal toxicity of the non-selective NSAIDs.

An individual's relative risk for serious complications of peptic ulcer disease as a result of taking the non-selective NSAIDs ranges from 2 to 6. The rate of severe adverse reactions requiring hospitalization in RA patients is high but has changed over the past 25 years. In a large survey in the USA, the rate increased from 0.6% in 1981 to 1.5% in 1992 but has declined and, in 2000, the rate was down to 0.5%[31]. An individual's absolute risk is still quite low but the total number of deaths attributable to these drugs is alarming due to the large number of the population that take them. Thus, deaths from the gastropathy caused by the non-selective NSAIDs are by no means uncommon. In the early 1990s, the annual deaths from the non-selective NSAIDs

were estimated to be ~7600 in the USA[32,33] and 1200 in the United Kingdom[34]. The majority of these deaths were probably in patients who were taking non-selective NSAIDs for pain, particularly for the pain of osteoarthritis, but it is unquestioned that deaths occurred in patients taking non-selective NSAIDs as part of the treatment of RA.

Patients at the highest risk of adverse gastrointestinal reactions from the non-selective NSAIDs are those with previous ulcers or gastrointestinal bleeding, cardiovascular disease, and those also taking anticoagulants, corticosteroids, or low dose aspirin[35–37]. The risk of gastropathy increases with increasing doses of non-selective NSAIDs. This places RA patients at an increased risk because high doses of NSAIDs are often required to decrease their inflammation. The optimal usage of NSAIDs in RA patients with gastrointestinal risk factors is still unclear although gastroprotective agents and COX-2 selective inhibitors (see below) are required for the many patients with risk factors for adverse reactions.

The short half-life NSAIDs, such as ibuprofen and diclofenac, are often ranked the safest while piroxicam, a long half-life NSAID, has been associated with a greater incidence of adverse gastrointestinal effects. However, the reason for the difference in risk between NSAIDs may be related largely to the relative potency of usual doses of individual NSAIDs. For example, low doses of ibuprofen are often used as occasional analgesics and produce a low incidence of gastropathy but, at full anti-inflammatory doses, the risk of gastrointestinal bleeding with ibuprofen is comparable to that produced by other non-selective NSAIDs[37].

The mechanism of the gastrointestinal damage induced by the NSAIDs is not as clear as is often assumed. It is generally claimed that the gastrointestinal damage is produced principally by inhibition of COX-1. However, it is more likely that the dual inhibition of COX-1 and COX-2 is required[38]. Experimentally, mice lacking COX-1 activity do not spontaneously develop damage to the gastrointestinal tract. Thus, selective inhibition of either COX-1 or COX-2 alone does not cause gastropathy[38].

The contribution of *Helicobacter pylori* to the risk of NSAID-induced gastrointestinal complications has been controversial but recent findings are that *H. pylori* can produce 'additive or synergistic gastric mucosal injury' with the NSAIDs[36]. It has been recommended that high-risk patients should be tested and treated for *H. pylori* prior to commencing NSAIDs if their long-term use is anticipated.

COX-2 selective inhibitors and drugs that reduce NSAID-induced gastropathy

The COX-2 selective inhibitors and the use of gastroprotective drugs are associated with a reduced risk of severe adverse gastrointestinal reactions. These treatments, along with reduced doses, are factors which have reduced the incidence of gastropathy from the NSAIDs in RA[31].

Three types of drugs decrease the risk of gastropathy: prostaglandin analogs (misoprostol), proton pump inhibitors (such as omeprazole and pantoprazole), and high doses of histamine-2 (H2) blockers[39,40]. Despite the general protective effect of these agents, the risk is not reduced to zero and may be particularly high in patients who have had previous ulcer bleeding, even if they are now *H. pylori* negative[41,42]. Proton pump inhibitors are well tolerated but the diarrhea and gastrointestinal discomfort that misoprostol often produces limits its acceptance by patients. This lack of tolerance of misoprostol may be a particular problem in elderly sick patients. High doses of several H2 blockers appear useful, but their effect may be limited to patients infected with *H. pylori*[37] or to patients with duodenal ulcer[39].

Histamine-2 antagonists, proton pump inhibitors, and misoprostol are effective in healing NSAID-induced mucosal damage. In the treatment of RA, the NSAIDs may have to be continued in patients, even though healing is then slower than if NSAIDs are discontinued[43]. Again, misoprostol is less advantageous than the proton pump inhibitors because of its tendency to produce diarrhea.

The availability of COX-2 selective inhibitors has led to their widespread use in the treatment of RA and for the pain of osteoarthritis. Initial endoscopic studies on substantial numbers of normal volunteers with rofecoxib and celecoxib, in repeated dose studies at the upper limit for clinical use or substantially higher, revealed gastrointestinal damage values indistinguishable from those seen with placebo and substantially less than ibuprofen and naproxen[44].

Large-scale controlled clinical trials have generally confirmed the gastrointestinal tolerability of the COX-2 selective inhibitors although there is still much debate about the results of the studies. Gastric and duodenal ulcers, and complications of ulcers such as bleeding, perforation, and obstruction, are all lower than during treatment with the non-selective NSAIDs[16,17,28,45] and, furthermore, the incidence of dyspepsia and related symptoms is reduced to the levels recorded with placebo[46]. The good gastrointestinal tolerability of the COX-2 selective inhibitors, however, appears to be totally lost in patients who are also taking low doses of aspirin for the prevention of thromboses[16,28] and therefore the prescription of the more expensive COX-2 selective inhibitors in these patients is questionable. Other antiplatelet agents, such as ticlopidine and clopidogrel, produce greater gastrointestinal bleeding than aspirin and, consequently, substitution of ticlopidine and clopidogrel for aspirin is not recommended in patients taking either non-selective NSAIDs or COX-2 selective inhibitors[37].

The relatively selective COX-2 inhibitors, meloxicam, etodolac, and nimesulide, are better tolerated than non-selective NSAIDs[47–51]. The incidence of ulcers and bleeding during treatment with etodolac is particularly low and much lower than that seen during treatment with equieffective doses of ibuprofen[49]. The incidence of perforations, ulcer, and bleeding during treatment with meloxicam was, however, not significantly lower than during treatment with diclofenac[47]. However, clinical comparisons with celecoxib are required. As is the case with the COX-2 selective inhibitors, the gastrointestinal tolerance of etodolac is negated by low-dose aspirin[52].

Cardiovascular adverse effects

Variable and sometimes very significant increases in blood pressure can occur in patients commenced on both groups of NSAIDs, particularly if they are elderly or marginally hypertensive, or treated with anti-hypertensives[53–55]. An increase in blood pressure has been observed particularly with indomethacin but can occur with any NSAID. Therefore, blood pressure should be more intensively monitored in hypertensive patients commencing NSAIDs and the increased blood pressure treated if continued treatment with a NSAID is considered necessary[55], as is often the case in RA patients.

The effect of the NSAIDs on blood pressure is, in part, due to their inhibition of the synthesis of vasodilatory prostaglandins in renal and vascular tissue. These important counter-regulatory hormones are secreted in response to treatment with diuretics and antihypertensive drugs. Removal of prostaglandins by NSAID inhibition of their synthesis then promotes an increase in blood pressure.

NSAIDs also worsen cardiac failure[56]. Of the COX-2 selective inhibitors, rofecoxib may have a greater tendency than celecoxib to contribute to cardiac failure[57,58], but at-risk patients taking any COX-2 selective inhibitor, or a non-selective NSAID, should be monitored carefully[55]. Elevation of systemic blood pressure during treatment with both the non-selective NSAIDs would be likely to increase the demands on the left ventricle but further work needs to be undertaken to determine the contribution of NSAIDs to cardiac failure.

Thrombosis and COX-2 selective inhibitors

For several years, there has been concern that the COX-2 selective inhibitors may cause thrombosis, resulting in infarction and stroke. The theoretical basis is that the prothrombotic thromboxane A_2 is synthesized by a COX-1-dependent pathway and is therefore not altered by the COX-2 selective inhibitors. This action could be accentuated by inhibition of the synthesis of prostacyclin, a vasodilator and antithrombotic mediator. Prostacyclin is produced largely by a COX-2-dependent pathway and therefore potentially inhibited by COX-2 selective inhibitors. Overall, it was suggested that the COX-2 selective inhibitors would increase the incidence of thrombosis. Such trends were found in several clinical studies on rofecoxib, celecoxib, and valdecoxib[16,59–61]. All these studies have provoked furious correspondence in medical journals and it is now recommended generally that the COX-2 selective inhibitors should be used only in the short term and at the lowest possible dose. Furthermore, the marketing of rofecoxib and, more recently, valdecoxib, have been suspended although these suspensions may be reconsidered.

While there is great concern that thrombosis is favored by selective COX-2 inhibition, the development of atherosclerosis or reactions following thrombosis in the heart may, in part, be inflammatory processes. Consequently, COX-2 inhibitors may usefully reduce this inflammation. Thus, the COX-2 selective inhibitors may be involved in a complex balance between thrombosis and protection against the progression of atherosclerosis.

The value, or the risks, of the COX-2 selective inhibitors is still not entirely clear but care must be taken in managing the many patients with both RA and atherosclerosis. RA patients taking low doses of aspirin as a prophylactic agent for thrombosis should continue taking the aspirin but, if treatment with a NSAID is indicated, a non-selective NSAID should be taken with low-dose aspirin and a gastroprotective drug.

Renal adverse effects

NSAIDs can affect the kidney in two ways: impairing kidney function and causing damage to kidney tissue[62]. The functional effects are more common than the tissue-damaging effects.

Renal prostaglandin synthesis is vital for the maintenance of renal function when renal perfusion is reduced in hypovolemic states (cirrhosis with ascites; nephrotic syndrome), ineffective circulatory volume (congestive heart failure), or primary renal disorders. In these conditions, vasoconstrictor hormones, such as noradrenaline and vasopressin, are secreted to maintain renal perfusion pressure. Compensatory secretion of prostaglandins by the kidney is essential to prevent unopposed vasoconstriction of renal blood vessels and thus damaging decreases in glomerular perfusion pressure. NSAIDs jeopardize this protective response by inhibiting the synthesis of the vasodilatory prostaglandins. This can lead to a decrease of glomerular filtration rate and renal blood flow that can progress to irreversible renal failure if prolonged. Concurrent diuretic therapy that leads to prostaglandin secretion in the kidney is another risk factor for NSAID impairment of renal function (see section on NSAID drug interactions, below). NSAID-induced renal functional impairment results in a rise in plasma creatinine within days of commencing the NSAID. Serum potassium also rises in more severe cases and weight gain is noted along with decreasing urine output. Cessation of the NSAID usually leads to rapid improvement. Careful monitoring of renal function is therefore important, especially in the elderly or renally impaired. Early recognition of functional impairment can prevent acute renal failure[63,64].

NSAID-induced sodium and water retention with dependent edema has been reported in up to 25% of patients given NSAIDs, with the greatest effect on patients in poor general health, with impaired renal function, and, particularly, in frail elderly patients[65]. Interestingly, at the start of treatment, both the non-selective NSAIDs and the COX-2 selective inhibitors reduce the output of sodium by about 15%, even in healthy subjects, but with continued dosage, the excretion recovers to baseline values within about three days[66]. It is suggested that recovery is less complete for patients with risk factors such as heart failure, treatment with diuretics, and cirrhosis with ascites.

Hyperkalemia can be marked but is uncommon. Risk factors identified are the patient's age, the presence of renal impairment, diabetes, and concurrent therapy with angiotensin-converting enzyme inhibitors, potassium-sparing diuretics, or cyclosporin.

Kidney tissue damage is uncommon with NSAIDs. Acute interstitial nephritis, with or without proteinuria in the nephrotic range, minimal change glomerulonephritis with nephrotic syndrome, papillary necrosis, acute tubular necrosis, and vasculitis are reported adverse reactions to NSAIDs. NSAID-induced interstitial nephritis is unusual but there are case reports linking this effect to most NSAIDs. Most commonly this adverse reaction occurs within 18 months of starting NSAIDs. Often proteinuria and renal failure occur but the abnormality recovers slowly over a year following the cessation of the NSAID. An important adverse renal effect of NSAIDs is associated with tiaprofenic acid. This drug is associated with intense interstitial cystitis in occasional patients. Unfortunately, quite a few patients have undergone investigation and multiple surgical interventions for this drug-induced problem[67]. Papillary necrosis was associated with the use of combination analgesics, particularly phenacetin, but the incidence has been declining since the removal of these analgesics.

Hematological adverse effects

Chronic therapy with the non-selective NSAIDs can be associated with anemia resulting from unsuspected blood loss from the gastrointestinal tract and, consequently, an occasional full blood count for any patient taking NSAIDs regularly is warranted. Anemia related to chronic inflammatory disease and vitamin and nutritional deficiencies may also contribute to anemia in patients with rheumatic disease. Serious NSAID-induced bone marrow toxicity is rare but was a significant problem with the old NSAID, phenylbutazone.

As discussed above, non-selective NSAIDs inhibit platelet COX-1 enzyme, thereby inhibiting platelet adhesiveness and prolonging the bleeding time. Low doses of aspirin irreversibly acetylate the COX-1 enzyme and bleeding time is prolonged significantly for up to 12 days, with the return to basal bleeding level being dependent upon the generation of new platelets. Other NSAIDs inhibit COX-1 reversibly so bleeding time decreases as the drugs are eliminated. For the majority of NSAIDs, bleeding time normalizes within 24 h of the last dose although platelet function may take longer to return to normal with NSAIDs with long half-lives, such as tenoxicam and piroxicam. Thus, it may be about three days after piroxicam is ceased before platelet function is normal. COX-2-specific inhibitors, such as celecoxib, do not inhibit platelet function or prolong bleeding time at clinically used or even supratherapeutic doses.

Thrombocytopenia is a rare, idiosyncratic adverse reaction that occurs with all non-selective NSAIDs but, because of the widespread use of NSAIDs, the total number of cases is substantial. The NSAID-induced thrombocytopenia is, however, usually mild and reversible but serious bleeding and death do occur and have been reported more often with phenylbutazone and indomethacin.

Neurological adverse effects

NSAID-induced central nervous system adverse effects are often overlooked in elderly patients. Confusion, cognitive dysfunction, somnolence, disturbances of behavior, and dizziness are some of the central nervous system adverse effects described[68]. In the absence of treatment with NSAIDs, these symptoms are not unusual in the elderly. Therefore, the link to NSAIDs is often unsuspected. Most reports implicate indomethacin, ibuprofen, and naproxen. Psychotic reactions have been reported with indomethacin and sulindac. Given that the antipyretic and at least a component of the analgesic effects of NSAIDs depend on central nervous system actions, it is to be expected that there will be other central nervous system effects. The effects of NSAIDs on the central nervous system may be related to COX-2-mediated conversion of the endocannabinoid, 2-arachidonylglycerol, to glyceryl prostaglandins[69], but further work is required.

Aseptic meningitis is an uncommon adverse reaction reported with ibuprofen and sulindac and occurs particularly in individuals with systemic lupus erythematosus or juvenile RA, while migraine type headaches are commonly noted in patients taking indomethacin, particularly if they are sufferers of migraine.

Hepatic adverse effects

NSAID-related hepatotoxicity leading to fibrosis or cirrhosis is quite rare and idiosyncratic when it does occur. Reversible liver function abnormalities are more common. Thus, anti-inflammatory doses of aspirin are associated with mild, usually asymptomatic elevations of hepatic enzymes in serum in 50% of patients, occurring within the first few weeks of therapy. Sulindac and diclofenac also appear to be associated with a higher incidence of reversible hepatotoxicity in comparison to other NSAIDs. Hepatotoxicity is more common in juvenile RA and in patients with systemic lupus erythematosus but there is no consistent liver function or histopathological abnormality in NSAID-induced hepatotoxicity. NSAID hepatotoxicity is a contraindication to further use in an affected patient. Hepatotoxicity from paracetamol is discussed below.

Rarely, severe liver toxicity occurs with aspirin even at low doses. Reye's syndrome, characterized by severe hepatic damage as well as encephalopathy, occurs mainly in children. Aspirin may contribute to the development of this syndrome although there is much argument about the association. However, Reye's syndrome is now very rare, possibly because aspirin is no longer recommended for use as an antipyretic in children less than 12 years of age[70].

Asthma

Asthma prescribers and patients need to be aware that aspirin and the non-selective NSAIDs can precipitate or exacerbate asthma. Aspirin or NSAID-induced bronchospasm is often acute and can be lethal. Those most at risk have a history of 'aspirin-allergy' and frequently have nasal polyps. Many tragedies from NSAID-bronchospasm occur when a new 'pain-relieving' drug is not known to be a NSAID by the prescriber or patient. It is commonly stated that about 4% of asthmatics have aspirin-induced asthma but recent provocative studies indicate that the respiratory function of about 20% of adult asthmatics is reduced by aspirin and the non-selective NSAIDs[71].

All the non-selective NSAIDs are contraindicated in this syndrome but the COX-2 selective inhibitors do not appear to produce this syndrome[72], although the current information sheets on celecoxib given to patients state that these drugs can precipitate asthma. A reduction in respiratory function can be produced by the relatively selective agents etodolac and meloxicam in a few patients, but the effect is small[73,74]. Paracetamol produces a similar small effect in small numbers of aspirin-sensitive asthmatics.

Dermatological adverse effects

Skin rashes are uncommon with NSAIDs although serious, idiosyncratic reactions such as erythema multiforme and blistering skin reactions are reported. Photosensitivity reactions are also well known although uncommon. Two COX-2 selective inhibitors, celecoxib and valdecoxib, are sulfonamides, but, although occasional rashes have been produced by these drugs, there does not appear to be any cross-reactivity with the antibacterial sulfonamides[75]. However, cross-reactivity with another closely related chemical group, the sulfonylurea antidiabetic drugs, is still possible. As with warnings for asthmatic patients,

however, the patient information on celecoxib is contrary to these research findings. The information sheet still states that patients who have had an allergic reaction with sulfonamides should not take celecoxib.

Cartilage and NSAIDs

It is widely considered that NSAIDs do not alter the course of RA. However, it has also been suggested that NSAID therapy may induce cartilage damage. *In vitro* studies indicate that NSAIDs might have a deleterious effect upon chondrocyte function but these have mostly been marred by employing supratherapeutic concentrations of the NSAIDs. In contrast, therapeutic concentrations of celecoxib decrease the cytokine-induced release of proteoglycans from cartilage[76] and celecoxib may cause less joint damage than non-selective NSAIDs in experimental inflammation in rats[77].

A clinical study in patients with osteoarthritis indicated that cartilage deterioration was more rapid in patients taking indomethacin, a potent prostaglandin synthetase inhibitor, than those taking azapropazone, a NSAID that is no longer used but may have been a weaker inhibitor of COX-1[78]. However, further clinical work is required on the favorable or unfavorable effects of NSAIDs on cartilage. No definite conclusions can be reached at this time.

NSAID chemistry

The non-selective NSAIDs, such as naproxen and ibuprofen, are mostly weak carboxylic acids with pKa values of about 4.5. The relatively selective agents, meloxicam and etodolac, and the COX-2 selective agent lumiracoxib, are also weak acids with similar pKa values. The percentage in the unionized forms in blood are therefore only about 0.1%. However, the high lipid solubility of the unionized forms and rapid equilibration of the unionized and ionized forms is considered to provide ready access to intracellular sites by passive diffusion. The passive diffusion in the unionized form is also thought to be the major mechanism of the oral absorption of these drugs and their rapid uptake into the central nervous system.

The atypical NSAIDs, aspirin and salicylate, are stronger acids than other non-selective NSAIDs. These two drugs have pKa values of 3.7 and 3, respectively. Consequently, in blood, the proportions in the unionized forms are even lower than those produced from other NSAIDs, but aspirin and salicylate are still considered to diffuse through cell membranes principally in the unionized forms.

Apart from lumiracoxib, the COX-2 selective inhibitors such as celecoxib, valdecoxib, etoricoxib, and rofecoxib are either totally or near totally unionized at physiological pH values. All these four COX-2 selective inhibitors are highly lipid soluble and, like the non-selective NSAIDs, should diffuse readily through cell membranes[79]. Celecoxib and valdecoxib are substituted sulfonamides and it has been of concern that patients with hypersensitivity reactions to the antimicrobial sulfonamides would also have similar reactions to celecoxib. However, as discussed above, there is no cross-reactivity[75].

A feature of the chemistry of several non-selective NSAIDs is that they contain a chiral center and are usually synthesized as the racemate, that is, a mixture containing equal amounts of the

Table 22.2 Dosage and approximate half-lives of elimination of NSAIDs. The dose forms of chiral compounds are indicated as racemate or individual S enantiomers. The dose of all NSAIDs should be decreased patients in renal and hepatic impairment and in the elderly

NSAID	Total daily dose range (mg); number of doses/day)	Half-life (h)	Notes
Non-selective			
Aspirin	4800; 2–3	0.25	Major activity in RA due to its metabolite, salicylate
Diclofenac	50–150; 1–3	1	
Diflunisal	500–1000; 2	11	
Fenbufen	900; 2	12 (active metabolite)	Racemate. Active metabolite biphenyl acetic acid
Fenoprofen	1200–2400; 2	3	Racemate. About 90% inversion of R to S enantiomer
Flurbiprofen	150–300; 2	3.5	Racemate No inversion of R to S in humans
Ibuprofen	1200–2400; 2–4	2	Racemate or active S. 60% of R inverted to S enantiomer
Indomethacin	25–150; 1–3	2.5	
Ketoprofen	100–300; 1 (sustained release) or 2 (rapid release)	2	Racemate or active S. enantiomer Commonly prescribed as slow release formulation
Ketorolac	60 (elderly)–90 (IM and IV); 30 (elderly)–40 (oral; 4–6 hourly for pain)	5	IM/IV and oral routes. Minor inversion of active S enantiomer to R enantiomer (6.5%)
Meclofenamate	200–400; 2	2.5	
Nabumetone	1000–2000; 1	23 (active metabolite)	Pro-drug Active metabolite 6-methoxy-2-naphthylacetic acid
Naproxen	500–1000; 2	14	S enantiomer only available
Oxaprozin	1200–1800; 1	55	
Piroxicam	10–20; 1	48	Decrease dose in liver disease
Salicylate	2000–4000; 3–4	2–15	Active metabolite of aspirin and salsalate. Half-life increases with increasing dose
Sulindac	200–600; 2	17 (sulfide)	Reduced to active sulfide metabolite. Enterohepatic cycling
Tenoxicam	10–20; 1	60	
Tiaprofenic acid	600; 2–3	3	
Tolmetin	1200–2000; 2–4	5	
COX-2 selective			
Celecoxib	100–200; 2	11	Sulfonamide 20–60% bioavailability
Valdecoxib	Up to 80; 2	7	Sulfonamide
Etodolac	400–600; 2	7	Racemate. No inversion of R to S in humans
Etoricoxib	60–90; 1	24	
Rofecoxib	25–50; 1	17	
Lumiracoxib	400; 1–2	5	

R and S enantiomers (Table 22.2, Fig. 22.2) The most important are the arylpropionic acids such as ibuprofen, fenoprofen, ketoprofen, naproxen, flurbiprofen, and tiaprofenic acid. Naproxen has only been available as the single S enantiomer and several pure S enantiomers of other arylpropionic acids are now available in some countries.

The clinical significance of the chiral structures of the arylpropionic acids is the different pharmacological activities of the two enantiomers. Only the S-configured enantiomers inhibit COX-1 and COX-2 and, therefore, prostaglandin production. However, some of the arylpropionic acids are metabolized in a very unusual fashion, namely that the inactive R enantiomers are inverted to the active S enantiomers (see section on Pro-drugs; Table 22.2,

Fig. 22.2). Etodolac is also a chiral compound but the inactive R enantiomer is not metabolized to the active S enantiomer.

Absorption of NSAIDs

Most non-selective NSAIDs are well absorbed after oral dosage. Their high oral bioavailabilities are due to:

1 high lipid solubilities of the unionized forms leading to passive diffusion from the gastrointestinal tract into blood.

2 Sufficient aqueous solubilities within the gastrointestinal tract. Some non-selective NSAIDs are administered as their sodium salts (e.g. naproxen sodium), which gives them high

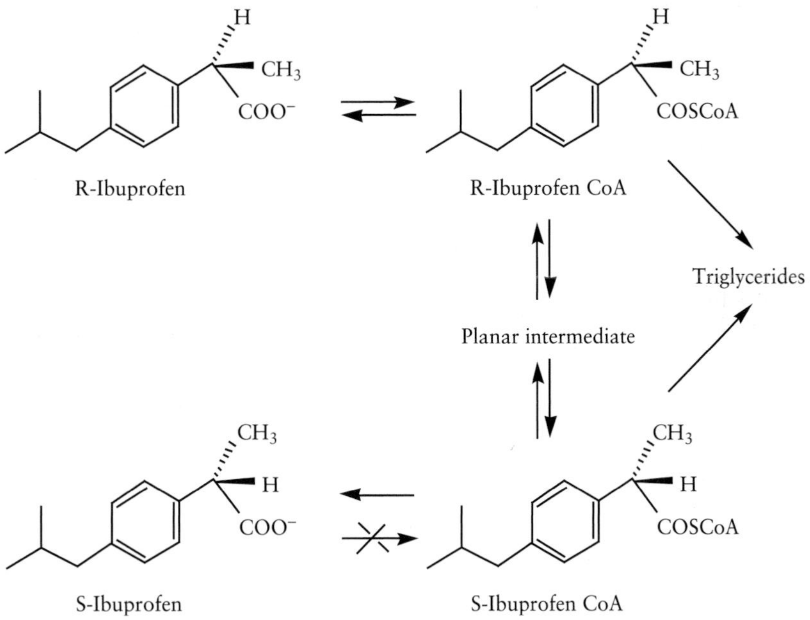

Fig. 22.2 Mechanism of inversion of ibuprofen and its uptake into 'hybrid' triglycerides through the intermediate formation of the coenzyme A thioesters. R ibuprofen is about 70% inverted to the therapeutically active S ibuprofen. The R enantiomers of fenoprofen and ketoprofen are inverted by the same mechanism.

aqueous solubilities but they are converted to their less soluble unionized forms in the acidic contents of the stomach. However, they still have sufficient aqueous solubility to be absorbed subsequently from the small intestine.

3 Resistance to hydrolytic enzymes.

4 Small hepatic clearance. Their hepatic clearances are generally small in relation to hepatic blood flow rates. Therefore, first pass metabolism in the liver is generally not significant.

Of the non-selective NSAIDs, only diclofenac and aspirin are exceptions. The bioavailability of diclofenac is about 50% and aspirin 50–70%. Their incomplete bioavailabilities are due to first pass metabolism. The incomplete absorption of aspirin is due to its first pass metabolism to an active metabolite, salicylate, but diclofenac is metabolized to inactive metabolites. The absorption of two COX-2 selective inhibitors is also incomplete; celecoxib (20–60%) and lumiracoxib (~74%)[79].

The absorption rate of NSAIDs is slowed when taken with food but the percentage absorbed is generally unaffected. Despite the effect on absorption rate, the non-selective NSAIDs should be taken with food to decrease the symptoms of gastric irritation. No decrement in the anti-inflammatory or analgesic efficacy in the treatment of RA is expected if the rate of absorption is slowed. Antacids taken with NSAIDs usually improve gastric tolerance but there is no reduction in the risk of serious upper gastrointestinal bleeding. Again, as with concurrent food intake, the bioavailability of NSAIDs is generally not affected by antacids.

The acidity of the stomach, together with the weakly acid nature and the high lipid solubility of the non-selective NSAIDs, leads to their concentration within the cells in the stomach wall; the build-up of these acidic drugs is most marked in the cells in

the parietal glands that secrete acid into the stomach[80]. These high cellular concentrations are considered to contribute to the gastropathy of the non-selective NSAIDs.

Several non-selective NSAIDs have been formulated as sustained release tablets and capsules in order to increase the duration of action of the drugs. No improvement in symptom control has been documented but administration can be less frequent. Thus, sustained release ketoprofen is given once daily as compared to two to three times daily for the conventional release formulation. Interestingly, studies with short half-life NSAIDs such as ibuprofen revealed that 8 or 12 hourly administration produced symptom control indistinguishable from a 6-hourly regimen of the same total daily dose. This result may be explained from the sustained concentrations in synovial fluid[81] (see section on Synovial fluid, below) or at other sites of action of the NSAIDs.

Pro-drugs

The metabolites of most NSAIDs are inactive, but several NSAIDs are administered as pro-drugs, that is, the parent drug is inactive and the activity resides in an active metabolite. Examples include nabumetone, sulindac, and fenbufen. Nabumetone is a widely used NSAID with relative safety for the upper gastrointestinal tract. It has no intrinsic activity until metabolized to 6-methoxy-2-naphthylacetic acid (6-MNA), which has an elimination half-life of about 24 h. Sulindac is metabolized by a reduction reaction to a sulfide metabolite, sulindac sulfide, by microflora in the large intestine[82]. This metabolite has a long half-life (16–18 h) and is responsible for the anti-inflammatory activity of sulindac. The conversion of sulindac to its sulfide is a reversible metabolic reaction and the sulfide is metabolized back to sulindac in the kidney. This conversion of the sulfide back to inactive sulindac in the kidney may explain the apparent diminished effect of sulindac on renal function compared to other NSAIDs, although the significance of this contrast with other NSAIDs is still uncertain[83]. Fenbufen, a non-selective NSAID, is activated by its metabolism to biphenylacetic acid. Parecoxib is a pro-drug, and is an injectable form which is hydrolyzed to the COX-2 selective agent valdecoxib.

Some of the arylpropionic acids are very unusual pro-drugs. These drugs are mostly administered as their racemates containing the inactive R enantiomers and the active S enantiomers. However, the inactive R enantiomers of some arylpropionic acids are metabolized to the active S enantiomers *in vivo* (Fig. 22.2). These R enantiomers can thus be considered pro-drugs for the active S enantiomers. Approximately 60% of the R-ibuprofen is converted to the active S enantiomer[84]. The inversion of R- to S-fenoprofen is also extensive but most other arylpropionates, such as flurbiprofen and tiaprofenic acid, undergo little or no inversion. Only about 10% of a dose of R-ketoprofen is converted to the active enantiomer, although the percentage conversion is increased in patients with very poor renal function[85] due to futile cycling of the glucuronide metabolite (see section on Renal clearance and futile cycling, below). Ketorolac differs from all other currently used arylpropionates in that a small amount of the S enantiomer (6.5%) is converted to the inactive R enantiomer[86].

The initial step in the R to S inversion of ibuprofen involves the stereoselective formation of a coenzyme A thioester which is then inverted and hydrolyzed (Fig. 22.2). The intermediate coenzyme A metabolites can also participate in fatty acid metabolism

such that the NSAID is incorporated into triglycerides. Interestingly, clofibrate increases the clearance of R-ibuprofen by both inversion and by non-inversion processes and may increase the incorporation of R-ibuprofen into triglycerides[87]. The biochemical reactions which result from the administration of R enantiomers of the inverted arylpropionic acids indicate potential toxicity but these drugs are still well tolerated. All that can be said at present is that the biochemical events which occur after the administration of the R enantiomers could be avoided by the use of other NSAIDs or by dosage with the pure S enantiomers. For those arylpropionates that undergo little or no inversion, the R enantiomer can be regarded as a 50% impurity.

Aspirin is both an active drug and a pro-drug (Fig. 22.3). It is an irreversible inhibitor of COX-1 and COX-2 through its acetylation of a serine residue in these enzymes. Currently, aspirin is used as an occasional analgesic, antipyretic, and, very commonly, in low dosage to prevent thrombosis. It is more gastrotoxic than most other non-selective NSAIDs.

Aspirin is also a pro-drug because it is hydrolyzed rapidly, yielding salicylate which is an active, analgesic, antipyretic, and anti-inflammatory agent, although it has no significant antiplatelet activity and does not precipitate aspirin-induced asthma (Table 22.1). Its half-life is longer than that of aspirin. Unusually, the half-life of elimination of salicylate increases with dose and ranges from about 2 to 15 h. Sodium and other salicylate salts were used widely in the treatment of RA but are rarely used for this indication in present medical practice. Salicylate is still, however, used as a reference anti-inflammatory drug in pharmacological and pharmacokinetic studies.

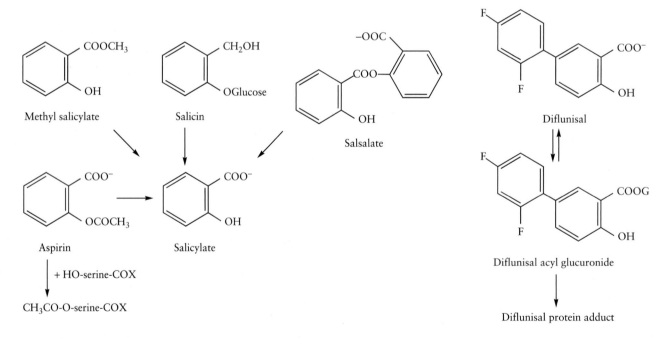

Fig 22.3 Structures and activation through metabolism of naturally occurring and synthetic salicylates. Methyl salicylate and salicin are naturally occurring while aspirin, diflunisal, salsalate, and salicylate are synthetic. Methyl salicylate is now synthesized and is used in liniments. Aspirin inhibits the COX isoenzymes by acetylation of an essential serine residue. One of the metabolites of diflunisal is an acyl glucuronide which is excreted in urine but is hydrolyzed back to the parent drug, diflunisal, to a greater extent if the excretion of the metabolite is reduced in patients with renal impairment or who are taking probenecid. G, glucuronide moiety.

The major problem with clinical use of salicylate is that good suppression of the inflammation of RA is produced only at high plasma concentrations of salicylate of 150–300 mg/L (1.1–2.2 mmol/L), concentrations that cause considerable tinnitus and deafness. The pharmacokinetics of salicylate also make its clinical use difficult. Salicylate is eliminated by saturable and self-inducible metabolism, which vary greatly between patients. Its renal excretion increases as urinary pH increases above about 6.5. All these unusual pharmacokinetic properties make it difficult to optimize the dosage of high dose aspirin or salicylate salts. Salicylate also displaces other drugs, most importantly phenytoin, from binding to plasma proteins. The unbound concentrations of phenytoin are not altered by salicylate and, consequently, salicylate should not potentiate the effects of phenytoin. Monitoring the plasma concentrations of phenytoin is, however, made more difficult by the increased unbound percentage of phenytoin in plasma because only the total plasma concentrations, not the unbound concentrations, are measured routinely. Salicylate also inhibits the renal excretion of cyclosporin.

Other pro-drugs of salicylate include salicin and salsalate. Salicin is the active principle in willow bark and is hydrolyzed and oxidized to salicylate while salsalate is a synthetic compound and a dimer of salicylate. Salsalate is well tolerated by the gastrointestinal tract but is hydrolyzed to salicylate and therefore has the disadvantage of producing tinnitus and deafness and the pharmacokinetic problems of salicylate (Fig. 22.3).

Half-lives of NSAIDs

The half-lives of elimination of the NSAIDs vary widely; from 1 h for diclofenac up to 2–3 days for tenoxicam and piroxicam (Table 22.2). The NSAIDs with short elimination half-lives are administered every 6–8 h and occasionally every 12 h. These intervals are substantially greater than their half-lives and, as expected, there are substantial fluctuations in plasma concentrations during therapy (Fig. 22.4). However, analgesic and anti-inflammatory activities are well maintained throughout the dosing interval. One possible reason for their long duration of effect may be their more sustained concentrations in synovial fluid (see section below on Synovial fluid). On the other hand, the NSAIDs with long half-lives are usually given once or twice daily. This is helpful for compliance and patient convenience, and the plasma concentrations of long half-life drugs do not fluctuate substantially during a dosing interval (Fig. 22.4).

A further difference between the two groups of NSAIDs is the time taken to accumulate to steady state. A general principle of pharmacokinetics is that drugs accumulate significantly for about 3–4 times the half-life of elimination. Thus, the plasma concentrations of NSAIDs with short half-lives achieve near steady state within 12 h, although tissue concentrations may take a longer time to achieve steady state. Loading doses of short half-life drugs are therefore not required. In clinical practice, the short half-life NSAIDs produce analgesia very quickly although their full anti-inflammatory effects may develop more slowly[3].

By contrast, NSAIDs with long half-lives accumulate significantly in plasma and for a considerable time after chronic dosing is commenced. For example, piroxicam, with a half-life of ~2 days, reaches 90% of its ultimate steady-state plasma concentration in

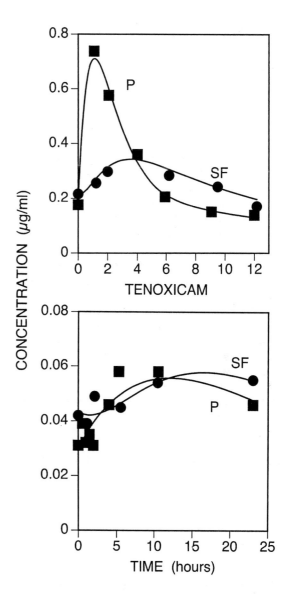

Fig. 22.4 Time courses of the concentrations of unbound naproxen and tenoxicam in plasma (P) and synovial fluid (SF) during long-term therapy in typical patients. Note the greater fluctuation in the plasma concentrations naproxen, the 'cross-over' in plasma, and synovial fluid concentrations for these drugs. (From Ref. 81, with permission.)

about 7 days. Naproxen has a shorter half-life of about 14 h (Table 22.2) and therefore accumulates for about two days following the onset of dosing. Loading doses may be employed to achieve steady-state concentrations of long half-life NSAIDs quickly, although this is uncommon in the treatment of patients with RA. However, it is recommended that naproxen 500–750 mg is given as a loading dose to be followed by 250 mg every 8 h in the treatment of acute gout[88].

Distribution and protein binding

The non-selective NSAIDs are extensively bound to plasma albumin and are weakly bound to tissues, thereby explaining the small volumes of distribution of these NSAIDs. Binding of NSAIDs to plasma albumin is a reversible reaction. An important equilibrium

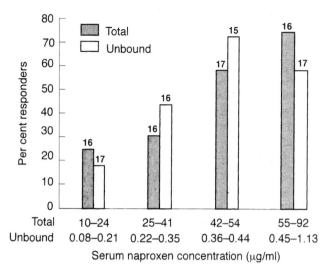

Fig. 22.5 Relationship between total and unbound plasma naproxen concentrations and the percentage of RA patients responding. The response to naproxen was determined using a 'summed' efficacy score. The numbers on the bars indicate the number of patients within each range of plasma concentrations. Note that not all patients respond, even at the highest plasma concentrations achieved. (From Ref. 91, with permission.)

between albumin bound NSAID, (bound drug), and unbound (free) NSAID in the plasma. The unbound drug is able to diffuse across cell membranes and bind to COX-1 and -2 intracellularly. The fraction of NSAID unbound is defined as the unbound drug/unbound plus bound drug. This ratio is altered by a number of factors such as the plasma albumin concentration, age, gender, renal and hepatic impairment, other albumin bound drugs, and pregnancy. The fraction unbound for NSAIDs increases when plasma albumin is low from any cause, in renal impairment and often in patients with active RA. It is important to remember that it is the unbound concentration which is critical to a change in performance of a drug, for example changes in efficacy or toxicity.

Free drug concentrations of naproxen are higher in the elderly and also in individuals whose RA activity has increased. These changes in free drug concentration are due to decreased clearance of free drug in the elderly and in patients with active RA[89]. As dosages of naproxen increase, the unbound naproxen concentrations increase linearly with dose but there is a less than proportional increment in total NSAID plasma concentrations (bound plus free concentrations). This phenomenon is due to the saturation of the available binding sites for NSAIDs on plasma albumin[90].

NSAIDs in synovial fluid

A major site of action of the NSAIDs is probably within the synovium of joints but there is little information on the distribution of the NSAIDs into this tissue. There is considerably more knowledge on the distribution in synovial fluid although practically all information has been obtained on the concentrations in synovial fluid of the knee because of the relatively easy access to this joint and the large volumes available for chemical analysis. Although there are substantial interpatient differences in the kinetics of transfer of NSAIDs between plasma and synovial fluid, it is evident that NSAIDs diffuse into and out of synovial fluid relatively slowly, with diffusion occurring mainly in the unbound forms. The result of the slow diffusion is that the pattern of distribution in synovial fluid depends on the plasma half-life of the NSAID[81].

NSAIDs with short and intermediate half-lives, such as ibuprofen and naproxen, show a crossover pattern during long-term dosage and the concentrations in synovial fluid are more sustained at a lower mean range than in plasma. Concentrations are lower in synovial fluid than in plasma for approximately the first 6 h post-dose, then higher than plasma concentrations subsequently (Fig. 22.4). Thus, the slow diffusion out of synovial fluid leads to more sustained levels of NSAIDs in synovial fluid than in plasma if the half-life of elimination of the NSAID is short or intermediate. By contrast, the crossover pattern is not seen with the long half-life NSAIDs, such as piroxicam and tenoxicam. For these NSAIDs, the concentrations of unbound drug are very similar in plasma and synovial fluid throughout the whole dosage interval (Fig. 22.4). Despite the different patterns in the time course of the concentrations in plasma and synovial fluid, the **mean** plasma concentrations over a dosage interval show a common pattern, irrespective of the half-life of elimination of the NSAIDs. Thus, the **mean total** concentrations (bound plus unbound) of NSAIDs in synovial fluid over a dosage interval are ~60% of the mean total concentration in plasma due to the lower levels of albumin and consequent lesser protein binding of NSAIDs in synovial fluid[81], whereas the **mean total unbound** concentrations are very similar.

Relationships between dose, plasma concentrations, and response

A feature of the pharmacokinetics of NSAIDs and many other groups of drugs is the interpatient differences in the plasma concentration during long-term dosage. Such interpatient differences would be expected to cause substantial differences in patient response. Relationships between the plasma concentrations of non-selective NSAIDs and anti-inflammatory response have been demonstrated in patients with RA although much variation in patient response remains unaccounted for (Fig. 22.5)[91]. The very variable absorption of celecoxib together with interpatient differences in its clearance may also lead to considerable interpatient differences in the response to this drug[79]. Overall, the data do not indicate that plasma NSAID concentration monitoring would substantially improve clinical outcomes although the variable plasma concentrations do support individualization of the dosage of NSAIDs.

Responders and non-responders to NSAIDs: relevance of pharmacokinetics

A proportion of patients with RA respond to some individual non-selective NSAIDs to a greater degree than to other non-selective NSAIDs; that is, they can be designated as responders or non-responders to individual NSAIDs[92,93]. Thus, a subset of RA patients sustain preferences for particular NSAIDs over considerable periods of time and in clinical trials involving blinded, re-exposure to drug. For example, some RA patients dosed with naproxen 1500 mg/day did not respond irrespective also of their plasma naproxen concentration, whereas the majority of subjects in this study had increasing anti-inflammatory effect with increasing dose of naproxen (Fig. 22.5)[91]. No pharmacokinetic contrasts for these non-selective NSAIDs, comparing responders to non-responders, have been discovered[93]. It is difficult to conceive that prostaglandin synthesis is not suppressed in all patients taking reasonable doses of NSAIDs. Mechanisms additional to inhibition of prostaglandin synthesis may be required for suppression of inflammation in some patients. An alternate NSAID may therefore work in some individuals because it has some mechanisms of action apart from inhibition of prostaglandin synthesis. Some RA patients who respond to particular NSAIDs contrast with non-responders in alterations in the plasma concentrations of markers of inflammation such as the acute phase reactants, effects not usually associated with NSAID action[94]. These effects on other components of the inflammatory response may hold the key to NSAID variability but much work remains to be done. The possible division of responders and non-responders of the COX-2 selective inhibitors has not been examined at this stage.

Saturable metabolism

The steady state concentrations of most NSAIDs increase in proportion to changes in dosage. Diflunisal, like salicylate, exhibits saturable metabolism and there is a disproportionate increase in the plasma concentrations with increasing dosage. The drug is a salicylate derivative but is not metabolized to salicylate (Fig. 22.3).

Hepatic clearance: liver failure

Both the non-selective NSAIDs and the COX-2 selective inhibitors are eliminated primarily by hepatic metabolism. The elimination of many NSAIDs has not been examined in patients with hepatic failure but the clearance of several, including ibuprofen[95], diclofenac, and salicylate is unaffected by liver failure. By contrast, the plasma concentrations of unbound naproxen are increased in patients with alcoholic liver disease and the concentrations of sulindac sulfide concentrations are increased about fourfold[95]. Substantial amounts of the parent inactive sulindac are normally excreted in bile and the consequent enterohepatic cycling tends to maintain the plasma concentrations of the active sulfide metabolite[96]. However, the biliary secretion of sulindac in patients with alcoholic liver disease is probably decreased well below normal levels and serves to maintain the plasma concentrations of the sulfide metabolite at higher than normal concentrations. NSAIDs other than naproxen and sulindac should be used in patients with liver diseases.

Renal clearance—renal failure

Only small proportions of the doses of most NSAIDs are excreted unchanged in urine, the only exception being salicylate which is excreted readily when urine is alkaline. The clearance of a number of NSAIDs, including ketoprofen, naproxen, diflunisal, fenoprofen, tolmetin, and indomethacin, decreases with renal impairment and during treatment with probenecid. This is surprising because of the small fraction excreted unchanged in urine. The reason is that acyl glucuronide metabolites of these drugs are retained to a greater extent than normal in renal failure and in patients taking probenecid. The retained acyl glucuronides are then hydrolyzed to their parent NSAIDs, thereby establishing a so-called 'futile cycle' and prolonging their presence in the body[97,98].

In the case of ketoprofen, the R and S acylglucuronides are retained in renal impairment. The retained glucuronide of R-ketoprofen is hydrolyzed to the R-ketoprofen, which is then inverted to the S enantiomer[85]. Thus, renal impairment produces a very considerable increase in the systemic exposure to the active S-ketoprofen and, therefore, increases the risk of further NSAID-induced renal failure which follows from inhibition of renal prostaglandin synthesis. All NSAIDs should be used with great care in the elderly and renally impaired. This applies particularly to NSAIDs which undergo futile cycling.

The acyl glucuronides of several acidic drugs, including some NSAIDs such as diflunisal and indomethacin, are also reactive, leading to the formation of adducts between proteins and the NSAID (Fig. 22.3)[97,98]. Surprisingly, these adducts are generally well tolerated but may be responsible for the uncommon hypersensitivity reactions to some NSAIDs and other acidic drugs.

Age and NSAID clearance

The clearance of naproxen and ketoprofen is reduced in the elderly while the clearance of piroxicam varies widely in elderly patients. As outlined above, the retention of the labile acyl glucuronide metabolites of several NSAIDs in renal impairment is a possible mechanism of the apparent reduced clearance. Toxicity has not been correlated directly with impaired NSAID clearance in individual elderly patients. However, the incidence of adverse reactions to all NSAIDs increases with dose, so it is sound practice to start with lower than usual doses of NSAIDs in elderly patients. Dosage can be increased if required and if side-effects are not problematic.

NSAID drug interactions

The NSAIDs interact with several other drug groups. Most of their interactions are considered to be due inhibition of the renal synthesis of prostaglandins.

Diuretics and antihypertensives NSAIDs, especially indomethacin, decrease the activity of diuretics and antihypertensives[99]. Although examined in greatest detail with the non-selective NSAIDs, it is probable that the same problems arise with the COX-2 selective inhibitors. Those most at risk are the elderly and patients with diabetes, or cardiovascular or renal diseases. Thus, these patient groups require increased surveillance particularly when treatment with NSAIDs is commenced. A particular problem occurs with the potassium-sparing diuretic triamterene, which can cause reversible renal failure with NSAIDs.

Lithium The clearance of lithium, which is largely renal, is reduced by the non-selective NSAIDs. Again, it is likely that the COX-2 selective inhibitors will have a similar effect. As plasma lithium concentrations need to be kept in a narrow therapeutic range, concentrations need to be monitored more frequently when NSAIDs are introduced or ceased. It is possible that sulindac may be less likely to cause this interaction because of lower exposure of kidney tissue to the active sulindac sulfide metabolite.

Digoxin The reduced renal function produced by the NSAIDs also decreases the clearance of digoxin. As a result, the dosage of digoxin should be monitored especially when treatment with NSAIDs is commenced or terminated.

Aminoglycosides Through their renal effects, the NSAIDs may increase the risk of nephrotoxicity with gentamicin and other aminoglycosides.

Warfarin A major interaction is the high chance of bleeding in patients taking the non-selective NSAIDs with warfarin. This interaction does not occur with the selective COX-2 inhibitors because of their insignificant effect on platelet COX-1.

Methotrexate An interaction between NSAIDs and methotrexate has been claimed but, although renal blood flow and renal function can be decreased by NSAIDs, prospective studies do not indicate any significant NSAID-induced decrease in the mean renal clearance of methotrexate, except during treatment with high doses of aspirin. However, the plasma concentrations of methotrexate may be increased by several NSAIDs in occasional patients. Although the data are limited, caution is still recommended when the dose of NSAIDs is changed in patients, particularly in the elderly and those with renal impairment[100].

Cholestyramine All acidic drugs, including the non-selective NSAIDs, the relatively selective inhibitors (meloxicam and etodolac), and the COX-2 selective agent lumiracoxib, are bound by cholestyramine. The result is decreased absorption of the NSAIDs, an interaction which can be very largely reduced by taking the NSAIDs and cholestyramine several hours apart. The chemical properties of paracetamol and the neutral COX-2 selective inhibitors, celecoxib, rofecoxib, valdecoxib, and etoricoxib, indicate that they should not interact with cholestyramine.

Hepatic metabolism The currently used NSAIDs do not interfere with the hepatic clearance of other drugs. The only exceptions include the now very rarely used NSAID phenylbutazone, which inhibited the metabolism of several drugs. Aspirin decreases the metabolism of valproate and an alternative NSAID is preferable unless the aspirin is used as an antiplatelet drug. With such a low dose of aspirin, a significant interaction is unlikely and, in any case, can be managed by monitoring the dose of valproate.

Management of NSAID dosage

The use of NSAIDs in RA is difficult because so many patients with RA have risk factors for actions on the gastrointestinal tract, and cardiovascular and renal systems, and NSAIDs may also interact with other drugs. Early, more aggressive treatment with combination DMARD therapy and corticosteroids is now recommended for RA, resulting in improved disease control. However, the non-selective NSAIDs and the COX-2 selective inhibitors provide considerable relief from the symptoms of RA and their use often cannot be avoided. Consequently, the use of NSAIDs must be managed. Ultimately, recommendations about the use of both groups of NSAIDs will depend upon the risk factors for gastrointestinal and cardiovascular toxicity in particular. Unfortunately, it is not possible to present firm recommendations about the use of NSAIDs, particularly because of the uncertain availability of the COX-2 selective inhibitors. To a large extent, the use of the COX-2 selective inhibitors will depend upon the perceived balance between the reduced gastrointestinal toxicity and the risk of thrombosis. Certainly, as the underlying risk of thrombosis increases, the non-selective NSAIDs will be used in preference to the COX-2 selective inhibitors. Conversely, the COX-2 selective inhibitors should be recommended if the patients are taking warfarin in order to prevent the combined inhibitory effect of a non-selective NSAID and warfarin on thrombosis.

Ibuprofen in its lowest effective dose is an appropriate first choice in patients with no gastrointestinal risk factors. In respect of dosing regimens, a once daily dosing with piroxicam, or slow release formulations of ketoprofen or naproxen, may be preferred to a twice or three times daily dosage with other NSAIDs such as ibuprofen and diclofenac. Many patients with inflammatory rheumatic diseases find that a NSAID suppository at night helps to control morning symptoms of pain and stiffness. However, indomethacin, the most widely used NSAID by rectal administration, is associated with a substantial incidence of headaches and other central nervous system effects.

The testing and eradication of *H. pylori* are important factors in patients starting NSAIDs but who have moderate to high risk factors for gastropathy[36,37]. Continuous therapy with a proton pump inhibitor is recommended after eradication of *H. pylori* in patients who have had bleeding, regardless of which kind of NSAID (non-selective or COX-2 selective) is being taken[101].

NSAID doses in RA ought to be the minimum to produce symptom relief. They should also be appropriate for the rheumatic condition and the age and general health of the patient. Thus, NSAID dose needs to be altered according to clinical response, the goal being to use the minimal effective dose, especially in the elderly who have an increased risk of serious adverse effects, and particularly in elderly patients with low body weight. Special care with dosing and monitoring is also needed for patients with hypertension or cardiac, renal, or liver impairment.

If NSAID dosage increases do not deliver a satisfactory response, then substitution with another NSAID is indicated. Why swapping one NSAID for another sometimes is successful is not understood. Concurrent paracetamol may also be helpful and may limit the gastrointestinal toxicity of the non-selective NSAIDs (Fig. 22.6)[102].

An important problem is that NSAIDs are too often prescribed indefinitely without careful, regular review. Any patient taking NSAIDs chronically requires evaluation as to ongoing need for the NSAID and with particular note of potential adverse reactions. Patients and their physician need to estimate the individual's baseline risk for serious gastrointestinal and cardiovascular adverse events and weigh these up against the benefits in quality of life achieved with the use of NSAIDs.

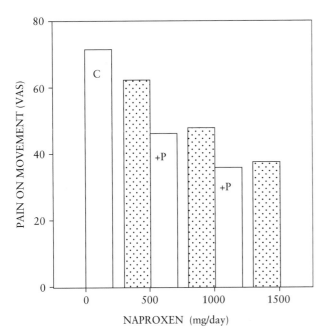

Fig. 22.6 Mean effects of naproxen (500, 1000, and 1500 mg/day). and paracetamol (4 g/day when dosed with naproxen). on pain in patients with rheumatoid arthritis. Histograms show the mean pain during treatment with placebo (C) or combinations of paracetamol (+P) with naproxen (500 and 1000 mg/day). Similar relative effects were observed with four of the other five measures of disease activity or responses to the drugs: pain at rest, joint index, global effect, and morning stiffness. (Redrawn from Ref. 102, with permission.)

Paracetamol (acetaminophen)

Therapeutic effects and adverse reactions of paracetamol

Paracetamol is an effective analgesic and antipyretic when given in appropriate doses. On average, it is slightly less efficacious than the NSAIDs as an analgesic in the treatment of osteoarthritis. However, it is often used as the first-line analgesic in osteoarthritis because of its efficacy in many patients and the excellent tolerance of therapeutic doses. Overall, the therapeutic and adverse reactions of paracetamol are very similar to those of the COX-2 selective inhibitors (Table 22.1). The important contrast with NSAIDs and the COX-2 selective inhibitors is that paracetamol has no significant anti-inflammatory action in RA[2], although paracetamol does show some therapeutic anti-inflammatory activity as demonstrated by its ability to reduce swelling after oral surgery[2]. Paracetamol also shows anti-inflammatory activity in animal models[2].

Although little studied, it appears that paracetamol potentiates the therapeutic effect of the non-selective NSAIDs in RA (Fig. 22.6)[102]. The result is that paracetamol can reduce the daily dose of NSAIDs in patients with RA. This does not lead to loss of overall analgesic efficacy but the risk for upper gastrointestinal toxicity may be reduced.

A major advantage for paracetamol in comparison with conventional NSAIDs is the absence of gastrointestinal toxicity, notably upper gastrointestinal ulceration, perforation, and bleeding. Serious hepatotoxicity occurs with paracetamol overdose and is the major problem with the drug. It has been claimed that hepatotoxicity can occur after therapeutic doses, particularly if taken with alcohol or taken by patients with liver failure. There are many published case histories in which it is claimed that hepatotoxicity has resulted from therapeutic doses but recent reviews of these histories indicate that the incidence of hepatotoxicity from therapeutic doses has been grossly overestimated[103]. Hepatotoxicity from therapeutic doses is an extremely rare event and paracetamol may be used in patients with liver disease at total doses up to 3 g daily[104].

Mechanism of action of paracetamol

Paracetamol is a weak inhibitor of isolated COX-1 and COX-2 but it is a potent inhibitor of prostaglandin synthesis in cellular systems when the concentrations of the precursor, arachidonic acid, are low[1,2]. Under this condition, there is marked inhibition of prostaglandin synthesis. These data suggest that paracetamol may suppress low-grade inflammation, such as may be associated with osteoarthritis, to a greater extent than in more inflammatory states such as RA. Animal studies indicate that paracetamol inhibits prostaglandin synthesis within the central nervous system and that its effects are due to activation of descending serotonergic pathways[105].

Pharmacokinetics and metabolism of paracetamol

Peak analgesic actions of paracetamol are observed about 2 h after an oral dose. The delay is due to the time taken for absorption and entry of paracetamol into the central nervous system. The plasma half-life is about 2 h. Dosing is usually six hourly, with a maximum daily dose of 4 g. This dose produces peak plasma concentrations of about 15 mg/L. Formulations that consist of fast and slow release components are now available. These formulations allow slightly less frequent dosing (e.g. eight hourly) and an improvement in the convenience associated with taking the drug.

The metabolism of paracetamol is of major importance in its toxic effects and, possibly, in its mechanism of action. Paracetamol is metabolized primarily to inactive glucuronide and sulfate conjugates but it is also metabolized oxidatively to a thiol reactive metabolite, N-acetylbenzoquinoneimine (NAPQI). At therapeutic doses of paracetamol, the metabolite reacts with glutathione and is inactivated but, at high doses, the reactive compound is not removed sufficiently and causes the well-known hepatotoxicity of paracetamol.

Paracetamol is also oxidized by the peroxidase functions of COX-1, and presumably also by COX-2, to NAPQI and to a free radical species (Fig. 22.7)[1,2]. Potentially, these reactive species could inhibit the COX isoenzymes but, at this stage, this suggested mechanism for inhibition is hypothetical. Paracetamol is also metabolized by the neutrophil enzyme, myeloperoxidase, the result being decreased production of the normal product, hypochlorous acid, by both intact neutrophils and isolated myeloperoxidase[106]. Recently it has been discovered that about 1–2% of a dose of paracetamol is deacetylated to *p*-aminophenol and then reacetylated to form paracetamol again[107]. The intermediate, *p*-aminophenol, is a renal toxin but it is not known

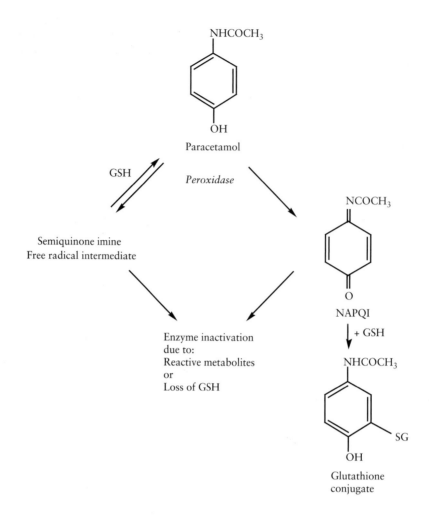

Fig. 22.7 Metabolism of paracetamol by myeloperoxidase, the peroxidase functions of COX-1 and COX-2, and cytochrome P450. It is proposed that the paracetamol inhibits the peroxidase functions of COX isoenzymes or other enzymes involved in prostaglandin synthesis either through direct inactivation by reactive paracetamol metabolites (free radical or NAPQI) or by depletion of the cofactor, reduced glutathione. NAPQI is the hepatotoxic metabolite of paracetamol. (From Ref. 2, with permission.)

where the process occurs or if toxic concentrations are achieved *in vivo*. The percentage of the dose undergoing this futile deacetylation pathway is low but, considering the high dose of paracetamol, up to 80 mg of *p*-aminophenol may be formed daily.

Drug interactions with paracetamol

The conversion of paracetamol to the glucuronide conjugate is inhibited by probenecid and, consequently, the half-life is increased from ~2 h to ~4 h. Consequently, the long-term dosage of paracetamol should be reduced during treatment with probenecid. Regular, high-dose paracetamol has been recorded as enhancing the anticoagulant effects of warfarin. However, the increase in prothrombin time reported is generally small and the strength of the evidence for a significant drug interaction is low[108].

Opioid analgesics

Opioids such as codeine, tramadol, and dextropropoxyphene are used extensively in the acute and chronic management of rheumatic disorders. However, the appropriate use of opioids in these disorders is contentious. There is little debate that short-term, oral use of opioids for problems such as acute mechanical back pain is appropriate. Once pain becomes chronic, as in RA, the use of opioids becomes problematic. Many of the patients with chronic rheumatic problems are elderly and the adverse effects of opioids become critically important. Constipation, cognitive impairment, drowsiness, increased risk of falls and fractures, and opioid dependence are well recognized problems with these drugs.

Codeine

Codeine is only an extremely weak ligand for opioid receptors but it is activated by its metabolism to morphine by the hepatic cytochrome P450 2D6 (CYP2D6). The activity of CYP2D6 shows very considerable interpatient variability due to genetic polymorphism and inhibition by some drugs. In particular, the metabolic activation and analgesic activity of codeine is very much decreased in 5–10% of Caucasians who have an abnormal CYP2D6. Also, the analgesic activity of codeine is reduced by inhibitors of cytochrome CYP2D6, such as quinidine and fluoxetine. Because of differences in the CYP2D6 phenotypes, codeine may be a weaker analgesic agent in Asians due to lower metabolism to morphine while the inhibitors of CYP2D6 have a lesser effect[109]. Morphine is metabolized further by glucuronidation to morphine 6-glucuronide and morphine 3-glucuronide. Morphine 6-glucuronide is also an agonist at the μ opioid receptor, producing analgesia and respiratory depression. It is retained in renal impairment and, therefore, if high doses of codeine are used in the management of rheumatic disorders, analgesic efficacy and careful monitoring for adverse effects are needed, especially in the elderly. Codeine has a half-life of elimination of approximately 3 h and its duration of action is therefore limited to 4–6 h.

Tramadol

Tramadol is a centrally acting analgesic with at least some opiate activity. It is a racemic mixture of (+)- and (−)-tramadol and has about 10% of the analgesic potency of morphine[109]. The (+) enantiomer of the parent drug and a demethylated metabolite are μ opioid agonists. Tramadol is converted to the active metabolite by CYP2D6 and, as is the case with codeine, the activation of tramadol shows marked interpatient variability. In particular, the analgesic activity of tramadol is reduced in patients who have an abnormal CYP2D6 or who take inhibitors of the cytochrome[110]. Tramadol also may have antidepressant-like activities; the (+)-enantiomer being an inhibitor of neuronal re-uptake of serotonin (like fluoxetine and other selective serotonin inhibitors) while the (−)-enantiomer inhibits the neuronal re-uptake of noradrenaline (like the tricyclic antidepressants). These activities are only weakly shown at therapeutic concentrations but may contribute to the analgesic activity of tramadol.

Tramadol is used as an analgesic in many clinical situations and, in rheumatic diseases, is mostly prescribed in combination with paracetamol in the treatment of osteoarthritis. In rheumatoid arthritis, its use should be limited to occasional analgesia. Tramadol is claimed to produce lesser respiratory depression than other opioids but, like the other opioids, it produces a considerable incidence of nausea and vomiting.

Dextropropoxyphene

Dextropropoxyphene is a controversial drug. It is a weak μ opioid agonist which has been used mainly in combination with paracetamol for the relief of the pain of osteoarthritis and other painful conditions. However, the combination does not appear to be superior to full doses of paracetamol and concerns about the efficacy of the combination, together with its toxicity, have led to its withdrawal in some countries. The drug has been associated with a number of sudden cardiac deaths, especially in overdose. There is some suspicion that elderly patients with coronary artery disease and renal impairment may be at greater risk for sudden cardiac death if taking dextropropoxyphene. The mechanism of increased cardiac risk is considered to be via the formation of nor-dextropropoxyphene, an oxidized metabolite, which is retained in renal failure. The risk of cardiotoxicity may be further increased by alcohol.

References

1. Graham, G. G., and Scott, K. F. Mechanisms of action of paracetamol and related analgesics. *Inflammopharmacology* 2003; **11**: 401–12.
2. Graham, G. G., Scott, K. F. Mechanism of action of paracetamol. *Am J Ther* 2005; **12**: 46–55.
3. Aarons, L., Grennan, D. M., and Rajapakse, C. *et al.* Anti-inflammatory (ibuprofen) drug therapy in rheumatoid arthritis: rate of response and lack of time dependency of plasma pharmacokinetics. *Br J Clin Pharmacol* 1983; **15**: 387–8.
4. Vane, J. R. Inhibition of prostaglandin synthesis as a mechanism of action for aspirin-like drugs. *Nature New Biol* 1971; **231**: 232–5.
5. Crofford, L. J. COX-1 and COX-2 tissue expression: implications and predictions. *J Rheumatol* 1997; **24** (Suppl. 49): 15–19.
6. Herschman, H. R. Prostaglandin synthase 2. *Biochim Biophys Acta* 1996; **1299**: 125–40.
7. Otto, J. C., and Smith, W. L. Prostaglandin endoperoxide synthases-1 and -2. *J Lipid Mediat Cell Signal* 1995; **12**: 139–56.
8. Smith, W. L., and DeWitt, D. L. Biochemistry of prostaglandin endoperoxide H. synthase-1 and synthase-2 and their differential susceptibility to nonsteroidal anti-inflammatory drugs. *Sem Nephrol* 1995; **15**: 179–94.
9. Appleby, S. B., Ristimaki, A., Neilson, K., Narko, K., and Hla, T. Structure of the human cyclo-oxogenase-2 gene. *Biochem J* 1994; **302**: 723–7.
10. Sirois, J., and Richards, J. S. Transcriptional regulation of the rat prostaglandin endoperoxide synthase 2 gene in granulosa cells: evidence for the role of a cis-acting C/EBP beta promoter element. *J Biol Chem* 1993; **268**: 21931–8.
11. Luong, C., Miller, A., Barnett, J., Chow, J., Ramesha, C., and Browner, M. F. Flexibility of the NSAID binding site in the structure of human cyclooxygenase-2. *Nature Struct Biol* 1996; **3**: 927–33.
12. Kurumbail, R. G., Stevens, A. M., and Gierse, J. K. *et al.* Structural basis for selective inhibition of cyclooxygenase-2 by anti-inflammatory agents *Nature* 1996; **38**: 644–8.
13. Murakami, M., and Kudo, I. Recent advances in molecular biology and physiology of the prostaglandin E2-biosynthetic pathway. *Progr Lipid Res* 2004; **43**: 3–35.
14. Scott, K. F., Bryant, K. J., and Bidgood, M. J. Functional coupling and differential regulation of the phospholipase A$_2$-cyclooxygenase pathways in inflammation. *J Leukoc Biol* 1999; **66**: 535–41.
15. Trebino, C. E., Stock, J. L., Gibbons, C. P. *et al.* Impaired inflammatory and pain responses in mice lacking an inducible prostaglandin E synthase. *Proc Natl Acad Sci U S A* 2003; **100**: 9044–9.
16. Silverstein, F. E., Faich, G., Goldstein, J. *et al.* Gastrointestinal toxicity with celecoxib vs nonsteroidal anti-inflammatory drugs for osteoarthritis and rheumatoid arthritis: the class study. A randomized trial. *JAMA* 2000; **284**: 1247–55.
17. Bombardier, C., Laine, L., Reicin, A. *et al.* Comparison of upper gastrointestinal toxicity of rofecoxib and naproxen in patients with rheumatoid arthritis. *N Engl J Med* 2000; **343**: 1520–8.
18. Simon, L. S., Weaver, A. L., Graham, D. Y. *et al.* Anti-inflammatory and upper gastrointestinal effects of celecoxib in rheumatoid arthritis: a randomized controlled trial. *JAMA* 1999; **282**: 1921–8.
19. Parente, L., and Perretti, M. Advances in the pathophysiology of constitutive and inducible cyclooxygenases: two enzymes in the spotlight. *Biochem Pharmacol* 2003; **65**: 153–9.
20. Warner, T. D., and Mitchell, J. A. Cycloxygenases: new forms, new inhibitors, and lessons from the clinic. *FASEB J* 2004; **18**: 790–804.

21. Cieslik, K. A., Zhu, Y., Shtivelband, M., and Wu, K. K. Inhibition of p90 ribosomal S6 kinase-mediated CCAAT/enhancer-binding protein β activation and COX-2 expression by salicylate. *J Biol Chem* 2005; **280**: 18411–7

22. The multicentre salsalate/aspirin comparison study group. Does the acetyl group of aspirin contribute to the antiinflammatory efficacy of salicylic acid in the treatment of rheumatoid arthritis? *J Rheumatol* 1989; **16**: 321–7.

23. Warner, T. D., Giuliano, F., Vojnovic, I., Bukasa, A., Mitchell, J. A., and Vane, J. R. Nonsteroid drug selectivities for cyclo-oxygenase-1 rather than cyclo-oxygenase-2 are associated with human gastrointestinal toxicity: a full in vitro analysis. *Proc Natl Acad Sci USA* 1999; **96**: 7563–8.

24. Tegeder, I., Pfeilschifter, J., and Geisslinger, G. Cyclooxygenase-independent actions of cyclooxygenase inhibitors. *FASEB J* 2001; **15**: 2057–72.

25. Friman, C., Johnston, C., Chew, C., and Davis, P. Effect of diclofenac sodium, tolfenamic acid and indomethacin on the production of superoxide induced by N-formyl-methionyl-leucyl-phenylaalanine in normal human polymorphonuclear leukocytes. *Scand J Rheumatol* 1986; **15**: 41–6.

26. Kaplan, H. B., Edelson, H. S., Korchak, H. M., Given, W. P., Abramson, S., and Weissmann, G. Effects of non-steroidal anti-inflammatory agents on human neutrophils functions in vitro and in vivo. *Biochem Pharmacol* 1984; **33**: 371–8.

27. Lötsch, J., Geisslinger, G., Mohammadian, P., Brune, K., and Kobal, G. Effects of flurbiprofen enantiomers on pain-related chemosomatosensory evoked potentials in human subjects. *Br J Clin Pharmacol* 1995; **40**: 339–46.

28. Schnitzer, T. J., Burmeister, G. R., Mysler, E. *et al.* Comparison of lumiracoxib with naproxen and ibuprofen in the Therapeutic Arthritis Research and Gastrointestinal Event Trial (TARGET), reduction in ulcer complications: randomised controlled trial. *Lancet* 2004; **364**: 665–74.

29. Bjarnason, I., Hayllar, J., MacPherson, A. J., and Russell, A. S. Side effects of nonsteroidal anti-inflammatory drugs on the small and large intestine in humans. *Gastroenterology* 1993; **10**: 1832–47.

30. Wynne, H. A., and Long, A. Patient awareness of the adverse effects of non-steroidal anti-inflammatory drugs (NSAIDs). *Br J Clin Pharmacol* 1996; **42**: 253–6.

31. Fries, J. F., Murtagh, K. N., Bennett, M., Zatarain, E., Lingala, B., and Bruce, B. The rise and decline of non-steroidal antiinflammatory drug-associated gastropathy in rheumatoid arthritis. *Arthritis Rheum* 2004; **50**: 2433–40.

32. Fries, J. F., Williams, C. A., Bloch, D. A., and Michel, B. A. Nonsteroidal anti-inflammatory drug-associated gastropathy: incidence and risk factor models. *Amer J Med* 1991; **91**: 213–22.

33. Fries, J. F., Williams, C. A., and Bloch, D. A. The relative toxicity of nonsteroidal antiinflammatory drugs. *Arthritis Rheum* 1991; **34**: 1353–60.

34. Griffin, M. R. Epidemiology of nonsteroidal anti-inflammatory drug-associated gastrointestinal injury. *Am J Med* 1998; **104**: 23S–29S.

35. Kimmey, M. B., and Lanas, A. Review article: appropriate use of proton pump inhibitors with traditional nonsteroidal anti-inflammatory drugs and COX-2 selective inhibitors. *Aliment Pharmacol Ther* 2004; **19**: (Suppl. 1), 60–5.

36. Peura, D. A. Prevention of nonsteroidal anti-inflammatory drug-associated gastrointestinal symptoms and ulcer complications. *Am J Med* 2004; **117**: (Suppl. 5A), 63S–73S.

37. Chan, F. K., and Graham, D. Y. Review article: prevention of nonsteroidal anti-inflammatory drug gastrointestinal complications—review and recommendations based on risk assessment. *Aliment Pharmacol Ther* 2004; **19**: 1051–61.

38. Hotz-Behofsits, C. M., Walley, M. J., Simpson, R., and Bjarnason, I. T. COX-1, COX-2 and the topical effect in NSAID-induced enteropathy. *Inflammopharmacology* 2003; **11**: 363–70.

39. Jacobsen, R. B., and Phillips, B. B. Reducing clinically significant gastrointestinal toxicity associated with nonsteroidal antiinflammatory drugs. *Ann Pharmacother* 2004; **38**: 1469–81.

40. La Corte, R., Caselli, M., Castellino, G., Bajocchi, G., and Trotta, F. Prophylaxis and treatment of NSAID-induced gastroduodenal disorders. *Drug Safety* 1999; **20**: 527–43.

41. Chan, F. K., Hung, L. C., Suen, B. Y. *et al.* Celecoxib versus diclofenac plus omeprazole in high-risk patients: results of a randomized double-blind clinical trial. *Gastroenterology* 2004; **127**: 1038–43.

42. Labenz, J., Blum, A. L., Bolten, W. W. *et al.* Primary prevention of diclofenac associated ulcers and dyspepsia by omeprazole or triple therapy in Helicobacter pylori positive patients: a randomised, double blind, placebo controlled, clinical trial. *Gut* 2004; **99**: 397–8.

43. Hawkey, C. J., Karrasch, J. A., Szczepanski, L. *et al.* Omeprazole compared with misoprostol for ulcers associated with nonsteroidal antiinflammatory drugs. Omeprazole versus Misoprostol for NSAID-induced Ulcer Management (OMNIUM) Study Group. *N Engl J Med* 1998; **338**: 727–34.

44. Simon, L. S., Lanza, F. L., Lipsky, P. E. *et al.* Preliminary study of the safety and efficacy of SC-58635, a novel cyclooxygenase 2 inhibitor: efficacy and safety in two placebo-controlled trials in osteoarthritis and rheumatoid arthritis, and studies of gastrointestinal and platelet effects. *Arthritis Rheum* 1998; **41**: 1591–602.

45. Deeks, J. J., Smith, L. A., and Bradley, M. D. Efficacy, tolerability, and upper gastrointestinal safety of celecoxib for treatment of osteoarthritis and rheumatoid arthritis: systematic review of randomised controlled trials. *BMJ* 2002; **325**: 619–26.

46. Bensen, W. G., Zhao, S. Z., Burke, T. A. *et al.* Upper gastrointestinal tolerability of celecoxib, a COX-2 specific inhibitor, compared to naproxen and placebo. *J Rheumatol* 2000; **27**: 1876–83.

47. Hawkey, C., Kahan, A., Steinbruck, K. *et al.* Gastrointestinal tolerability of meloxicam compared to diclofenac in osteoarthritis patients. International MELISSA Study Group. Meloxicam Large-scale International Study Safety Assessment. *Brit J Rheumatol* 1998; **37**: 937–45.

48. Dequeker, J., Hawkey, C., Kahan, A. *et al.* Improvement in gastrointestinal tolerability of the selective cyclooxygenase (COX)-2 inhibitor, meloxicam, compared with piroxicam: results of the Safety and Efficacy Large-scale Evaluation of COX-inhibiting Therapies (SELECT) trial in osteoarthritis. *Brit J Rheumatol* 1998; **37**: 946–51.

49. Jones, R. A. Etodolac (Lodine): profile of an established selective COX-2 inhibitor. *Inflammopharmacology* 2001; **9**: 63–70.

50. Degner, F., and Richardson, B. Review of gastrointestinal tolerability and safety of meloxicam. *Inflammopharmacology* 2001; **9**: 71–80.

51. Shah, A. A., Thjodleifsson, B., Murray, F. E. *et al.* Selective inhibition of COX-2 in humans is associated with less gastrointestinal injury: a comparison of nimesulide and naproxen. *Gut* 2001; **48**: 339–46.

52. Weideman, R. A., Kelly, K. C., Kazi, S. *et al.* Risks of clinically significant upper gastrointestinal events with etodolac and naproxen: a historical cohort analysis. *Gastroenterology* 2004; **127**: 1322–8.

53. Houston, M. C. Nonsteroidal anti-inflammatory drugs and antihypertensives. *Am J Med* 1991; **90** (5A): 42S–47S.

54. Johnson, A. G. NSAIDs and increased blood pressure: what is the clinical significance? *Drug Safety* 1997; **17**: 277–89.

55. LeLorier, J., Bombardier, C., Burgess, E. *et al.* Practical considerations for the use of nonsteroidal anti-inflammatory drugs and cyclo-oxygenase-2 inhibitors in hypertension and kidney disease. *Can J Cardiol* 2002; **18**: 1301–8.

56. Feenstra, J., Heerdink, E. R., Grobbee, D. E., and Stricker, B. H. Association of nonsteroidal anti-inflammatory drugs with first occurrence of heart failure and with relapsing heart failure. *Arch Int Med* 2002; **162**: 265–70.

57. Zhao, S. Z., Reynolds, M. W., Lejkowith, J., Whelton, A., and Arellano, F. M. A comparison of renal-related adverse drug reactions between rofecoxib and celecoxib, based on the World Health Organization/Uppsala Monitoring Centre safety database. *Clin Ther* 2001; **23**: 1478–91.

58. Mamdani, M., Juurlink, D. N., Lee, D. S. *et al.* Cyclo-oxygenase-2 inhibitors versus non-selective non-steroidal anti-inflammatory

drugs and congestive heart failure outcomes in elderly patients: a population-based cohort study. *Lancet* 2004; **363**: 1751–6.

59. Bresalier, R. S., Sandler, R. S., Quan, H. *et al*. Cardiovascular events associated with rofecoxib in a colorectal adenoma chemoprevention trial. *N Engl J Med* 2005; **352**: 1092–102.

60. Solomon, S. D., McMurray, J. J. V., Pfeffer, M. A. *et al*. Cardiovascular risk associated with celecoxib in a clinical trial for colorectal adenoma prevention. *New Engl J Med* 2005; **352**: 1071–80.

61. Nussmeier, N. A., Whelton, A. A., Brown, M. T. *et al*. Complications of the COX-2 inhibitors parecoxib and valdecoxib after cardiac surgery. *N Engl J Med* 2005; **352**: 1081–91.

62. Clive, D. M., and Stoff, J. S. Renal syndromes associated with non-steroidal antiinflammatory drugs. *N Engl J Med* 1984; **310**: 563–72.

63. Johnson, A. G., and Day, R. O. The problems and pitfalls of NSAID therapy in the elderly (Part I). *Drugs Aging* 1991; **1**: 130–43.

64. Johnson, A. G., and Day, R. O. The problems and pitfalls of NSAID therapy in the elderly (Part II). *Drugs Aging* 1991; **1**: 212–27.

65. Whelton, A., and Hamilton, C. W. Nonsteroidal anti-inflammatory drugs: effects on kidney function. *Journal of Clinical Pharmacology*, 1991; **31**: 588–98.

66. Catella-Lawson, F., McAdam, B., Morrison, B. W. *et al*. Effects of specific inhibition of cylooxygenase-2 on sodium balance, hemodynamics, and vasoactive eicosanoids. *J Pharmacol Exp Ther* 1991; **289**: 735–41.

67. O'Neill, G. F. Tiaprofenic acid as a cause of non-bacterial cystitis. *Med J Aust* 1994; **160**: 123–5.

68. Goodwin, J. S., and Regan, M. Cognitive dysfunction associated with naproxen and ibuprofen in the elderly. *Arthritis Rheum* 1982; **25**: 1013–15.

69. Kozak, K. R., Rowlinson, S. W., and Marnett, L. J. Oxygenation of the endocannabinoid, 2-arachidonylglycerol, to glyceryl prostaglandins by cyclooxygenase-2. *J Biol Chem* 2000; **275**: 33744–9.

70. Glasgow, J. F. T., and Hall, S. M. Reye's syndrome and aspirin. In *Aspirin and Related Drugs* (Rainsford K. D., ed.), pp. 555–85. New York: Taylor and Francis; 2004.

71. Jenkins, C., Costello, J., and Hodge, L. Systematic review of prevalence of aspirin induced asthma and its implications for clinical practice. *BMJ* 2004; **328**: 434–7.

72. West, P. M., and Fernandez, C. Safety of COX-2 inhibitors in asthma patients with aspirin hypersensitivity. *Ann Pharmacother* 2003; **37**: 1497–501.

73. Stevenson, D. D. Aspirin and NSAID sensitivity. *Immunol Allergy Clin North Am* 2004; **24**: 491–505.

74. DeBernardi, G., and Grassi, N. Tolerance of meloxicam in aspirin-sensitive asthmatics. *Am J Respir Crit Care Med* 1998; **157**: (Suppl.), A715.

75. Knowles, S., Shapiro, L., and Shear, N. H. Should celecoxib be contraindicated in patients who are allergic to sulfonamides? Revisiting the meaning of 'sulfa' allergy. *Drug Safety* 2001; **24**: 239–47.

76. Mastbergen, S. C., Lafeber, F. P., and Bijlsma, J. W. Selective COX-2 inhibition prevents proinflammatory cytokine-induced cartilage damage. *Rheumatology* 2002; **41**: 801–8.

77. Gilroy, D. W., Tomlinson, A., Greenslade, K., Seed, M. P, and Willoughby, D. A. The effects of cyclooxygenase 2 inhibitors on cartilage erosion and bone loss in a model of *mycobacterium tuberculosis*-induced monoarticular arthritis in the rat. *Inflammation* 1998; **22**: 509–19.

78. Rashad, S., Revell, P., Hemingway, A., Low, F., Rainsford, K., and Walker, F. Effect of non-steroidal anti-inflammatory drugs on the course of osteoarthritis. *Lancet* 1998; **2**: 519–22.

79. Brune, K., and Hinz, B. Selective cyclooxygenase-2 inhibitors: similarities and differences. *Scand J Rheumatol* 2004; **33**: 1–6.

80. Rainsford, K. D., and Brune, K. Role of the parietal cell in gastric damage induced by aspirin and related drugs: implications for safer therapy. *Med J Aust* 1976; **1**: 881–3.

81. Day, R. O., McLachlan, A. J., Graham, G. G., and Williams, K. M. Pharmacokinetics of non-steroidal anti-inflammatory drugs in synovial fluid. *Clin Pharmacokinet* 1999; **36**: 191–210.

82. Strong, H. A., Warner, N. J., Renwick, A. G., and George, C. F. Sulindac metabolism: the importance of an intact colon. *Clin Pharmacol Ther* 1985; **38**: 387–93.

83. Sedor, J. R., Williams, S. L., Chremos, A. N., Johnson, C. L., and Dunn, M. J. Effects of sulindac and indomethacin on renal prostaglandin synthesis. *Clin Pharmacol Ther* 1984; **36**: 85–91.

84. Lee, E. J, Williams, K., Day, R., Graham, G., and Champion, D. Stereoselective disposition of ibuprofen enantiomers in man. *Br J Clin Pharmacol* 1985; **19**: 669–74.

85. Grubb, N. G., Rudy, D. W., Brater, D. C., and Hall, S. D. Stereoselective pharmacokinetics of ketoprofen and ketoprofen glucuronide in end-stage renal disease: evidence for a 'futile cycle' of elimination. *Br J Clin Pharmacol* 1999; **48**: 4494–500.

86. Mroszczak, E., Combs, D., Chaplin, M. *et al*. Chiral kinetics and dynamics of ketorolac. *J Clin Pharmacol* 1996; **36**: 521–39.

87. Scheurer, S, Hall, S. D, Williams, K. M., and Geisslinger, G. Effect of clofibrate on the chiral inversion of ibuprofen in healthy volunteers. *Clin Pharmacol Ther* 1998; **64**: 168–76.

88. Sturge, R. A., Scott, J. T., Hamilton, E. B., Liyanage, S. P., Dixon, S. T., and Engler, C. Multi-centre trial of naproxen and phenylbutazone in acute gout. *Ad Exp Med Biol* 1977; **76B**: 290–6.

89. van den Ouweland, F. A., Franssen, M. J., van de Putte, L. B., Tan, Y., van Ginneken, C. A., and Gribnau, F. W. Naproxen pharmacokinetics in patients with rheumatoid arthritis during active polyarticular inflammation. *Br J Clin Pharmacol* 1987; **23**: 189–93.

90. Dunagan, F. M., McGill, P. E., Kelman, A. W., and Whiting, B. Naproxen dose and concentration: response relationship in rheumatoid arthritis. *Br J Rheumatol* 1988; **27**: 48–53.

91. Day, R. O., Furst, D. E., Dromgoole, S. H., Kamm, B., Roe, R., and Paulus, H. E. Relationship of serum naproxen concentration to efficacy in rheumatoid arthritis. *Clin Pharmacol Ther* 1982; **31**: 733–40.

92. Walker, J. S., Sheather-Reid, R. B., Carmody, J. J., Vial, J. H., and Day, R. O. Nonsteroidal antiinflammatory drugs in rheumatoid arthritis and osteoarthritis: support for the concept of 'responders' and nonresponders'. *Arthritis Rheum* 1997; **40**: 1944–54.

93. Baber, N., Halliday, L. D., van den Heuvel, W. J. *et al*. Indomethacin in rheumatoid arthritis: clinical effects, pharmacokinetics, and platelet studies in responders and non-responders. *Ann Rheum Dis* 1997; **38**: 128–36.

94. Cush, J. J., Lipsky, P. E., Postlethwaite, A. E., Schrohenloher, R. E., Saway, A., and Koopman, W. J. Correlation of serologic indicators of inflammation with effectiveness of nonsteroidal antiinflammatory drug therapy in rheumatoid arthritis. *Arthritis Rheum* 1990; **33**: 19–28.

95. Juhl, R. P., Van Thiel, D. H., Dittert, L. W., Albert, K. S., and Smith, R. B. Ibuprofen and sulindac kinetics in alcoholic liver disease. *Clin Pharmacol Ther* 1983; **34**: 104–9.

96. Dujovne, C. A., Pitterman, A., Vincek, W. C., Dobrinska, M. R., Davies, R. O., and Duggan, D. E. Enterohepatic circulation of sulindac and metabolites. *Clin Pharmacol Ther* 1983; **33**: 172–7.

97. Dickinson, R. G., and King, A. R. Studies on the reactivity of acyl glucuronides. II. Interaction of diflunisal acyl glucuronide and its isomers with human serum albumin in vitro. *Biochem Pharmacol* 1991; **42**: 2301–6.

98. McKinnon, G. E., and Dickinson, R. G. Covalent binding of diflunisal and probenecid to plasma protein in humans: persistence of the adducts in the circulation. *Res Comm Chem Pathol Pharmacol* 1990; **66**: 339–64.

99. Johnson, A. G., Seideman, P., and Day, R. O. Adverse drug interactions with nonsteroidal anti-inflammatory drugs (NSAIDs): recognition, management and avoidance. *Drug Safety* 1993; **8**: 99–127.

100. Bannwarth, B., Pehourcq, F., Schaeverbeke, T., and Dehais, J. Clinical pharmacokinetics of low-dose pulse methotrexate in rheumatoid arthritis. *Clin Pharmacokinet* 1996; **30**: 194–210.

101. Hunt, R. H., and Bazzoli, F. Review article: should NSAID/low-dose aspirin takers be tested routinely for H. pylori infection and treated if positive? Implications for primary risk of ulcer and ulcer relapse after initial healing. *Aliment Pharmacol Ther* 2004; **19** (Suppl. 1): 9–16.

102. Seideman, P. Additive effect of combined naproxen and paraceta-mol in rheumatoid arthritis. *Br J Rheumatol* 1993; **32**, 1077–82.

103. Graham, G. G., Scott, K. F., and Day, R. O. Tolerability of parac-etamol. *Drugs* 2003; **63** (Special Issue 2): 39–42.

104. McIntyre, N. Drugs and liver disease. In *Oxford textbook of clin-ical hepatology* (Bircher J, Benhamou J-P, McIntyre N, Rizzetto M., and Rodes J., eds), p. 1921. Oxford University Press; 1999.

105. Bonnefont, J., Courade, J. P., Alloui, A., Eschalier, A. Mechanism of the antinociceptive effect of paracetamol. *Drugs* 2003; **63** (Special Issue 2): 1–4.

106. Graham, G. G., Milligan, M. K., Day, R. O, Williams, K. M., and Ziegler, J. B. Therapeutic considerations from pharmacokinetics and metabolism: ibuprofen and paracetamol. In *Safety and Efficacy of Non-Prescription (Over-the-Counter). analgesics and NSAIDs* (Rainsford K. D., and Powanda M. C., eds), pp. 77–92. Dordrecht: Kluwer Press; 1997.

107. Nicholls, A. W., Farrant, R. D., Shockcor, J. P. *et al.* NMR and HPLC-NMR spectroscopic studies of futile deacetylation in paracetamol metabolites in rat and man. *J Pharm Biomed Anal* 1997; **15**: 901–10.

108. Bartle, W. R., and Blakely, J. A. Potentiation of warfarin anticoagu-lation by acetaminophen. *JAMA* 1991; **265**: 1260.

109. Caraco, Y., Sheller, J., and Wood, A. J. Impact of ethnic origin and quinidine coadministration on codeine's disposition and pharmacodynamic effects. *J Pharmacol Exp Ther* 1999; **290**: 413–22.

110. Grond, S., and Sablotzky, A. Clinical pharmacology of tramadol. *Clin Pharmacokinet* 2004; **43**: 879–923.

23 | Systemic and intra-articular glucocorticoids in rheumatoid arthritis

Johannes W. J. Bijlsma, Frank Buttgereit, and Johannes W. G. Jacobs

Introduction

Glucocorticoids (GCs) play a pivotal role in the management of rheumatoid arthritis (RA). The proportion of patients with RA that is treated with GCs by practicing rheumatologists on a daily basis is clearly in excess of the usually cautious recommendations in textbooks and review papers. Recent studies that demonstrate disease-modifying potential of low-dose GCs in RA have renewed the debate on the risk benefit ratio with this therapy[1]. GCs are still considered to be the most effective anti-inflammatory and immunosuppressive substances available[2], and our knowledge of the mechanisms of action has recently further increased. This knowledge may help us in the therapeutic use of GCs that are given orally, intra-articularly, and sometimes as intravenous pulse therapy[3]. The discussion on the use of GCs is often dominated by fear of a toxicity spectrum that is well engraved in international medical culture, but which is influenced highly by observations that are derived from the long-term usage of GCs at higher dosages. The evaluation of adverse events in relation to the dosage used, and especially in patients with RA, may help us

to better balance the advantages and disadvantages of GC treatment in RA[4]. Therefore, in this chapter emphasis is put on the balance between beneficial and unwanted effects of chronically administered low-dose GCs. Recent studies demonstrating the disease-modifying potential of low-dose GCs in RA have stimulated the interest of different pharmaceutical companies in developing a new generation of optimized GCs and GC receptor ligands; these developments will also be discussed.

Mechanisms of action

GCs have profound anti-inflammatory and immunosuppressive actions when used therapeutically. Different dosages and dosing regimens may have distinct therapeutically relevant effects mediated by different mechanisms.

Table 23.1 gives an overview of the relationship between clinical dosing and cellular actions of GCs[3,5]. In daily practice the rheumatologist increases the dosage with increasing clinical activity and severity of the disease. The mechanism behind this

Table 23.1 Relationship between clinical dosing and cellular actions of GCs

Terminology[a]	Clinical application in RA	Genomic actions (receptor saturation)[b]	Non-genomic actions[b]	
			Non-specific	cGCR-mediated
Low dose (≤7.5 mg/day)	Maintenance therapy	+ (< 50%)	−	?
Medium dose (>7.5 to ≤30 mg/day)	Treatment for minor extra-articular features	++ (> 50 to < 100%)	(+)	(+)
High dose (>30 to ≤100 mg/day)	Treatment for severe extra-articular features	++(+) (almost 100%)	+	+
Very high dose (>100 mg/day)	Initial treatment for acute and/or potentially life-threatening exacerbations of RA	+++ (almost 100%)	++	(+?)
Pulse therapy (≥250 mg for one or a few days)	For particularly severe and/or potentially life-threatening forms or to bridge the lag time of other treatments to exert effect	+++ (100%)	++(+)	+(++?)

[a] Values represent milligrams of prednisone equivalent per day. See Ref. 5 for further information.
[b] cGCR, cytosolic glucocorticoid receptor; ?, unknown; −, not relevant; (+), perhaps relevant, but of minor importance; +, relevant; ++, very relevant; +++, most relevant.

clinical decision is as follows. First, higher dosages increase the saturation of cytosolic glucocorticoid receptors (cGCRs) in a dose dependent manner, which intensifies the therapeutically relevant genomic actions that will be discussed below. Second, with increasing dosages, additional and qualitatively different non-specific (and perhaps also GC-mediated) non-genomic actions of GCs increasingly come into play.

Genomic actions

The anti-inflammatory and immunomodulatory effects of GCs are mediated predominantly by genomic mechanisms (Fig. 23.1). Binding to cGCR ultimately induces (transactivates) or inhibits (transrepresses) the synthesis of regulatory proteins[3]. These genomic actions are physiologically relevant and therapeutically effective at all dosages, even very small ones, but they are relatively slow. Significant changes in regulator protein concentrations are not seen within 30 min. The GC-induced synthesis of regulator proteins can be prevented by inhibition of transcription (such as by actinomycin D) or inhibition of translation (such as by cycloheximide).

GCs have a lipophilic structure and low molecular mass and thus may pass easily the cell membrane to bind the inactive cGCR (α-form). This is a 94 kD protein, in a complex bound with several heat shock proteins (chaperones). The complex interacts with immunophilins and several kinases of the mitogen-activated protein kinase (MAPK) signalling system, including Src, in order to bind and stabilize the proteins (Fig. 23.1). Rapid shedding of the chaperones follows binding of GCs to its receptor, enabling translocation into the cell nucleus, where the GCs/cGCR complex finally binds as a homodimer to specific DNA sites, the so-called GC response elements (GREs[6]). Within the cell nucleus, transcription is then either activated (transactivation) or inhibited (transrepression). Examples of outcome of the transactivation process are endocrine and metabolic effects of GCs; an example of transrepression is inhibition of pro-inflammatory cytokine synthesis.

Besides the interactions of GC/cGCR complexes with GREs, the interaction of activated cGCR monomers with transcription factors, such as activator protein-1 (AP-1), nuclear factor (NF)-κB, and nuclear factor of activated T cells (NF-AT), forms another important genomic mechanism of GCs. Inhibition of transcription factors also inhibits the expression of immunoregulatory and inflammatory cytokines. The above-described processes regulate a large number of genes. It has now become clear that adverse clinical effects are mostly based on transactivation mechanisms, while many important anti-inflammatory effects are mediated by transrepression mechanisms. This differential modulation has lead to drug discovery programs aiming at the development of so-called dissociating GCs (or selective glucocorticoids receptor agonists, SEGRAs; see section on Recent developments).

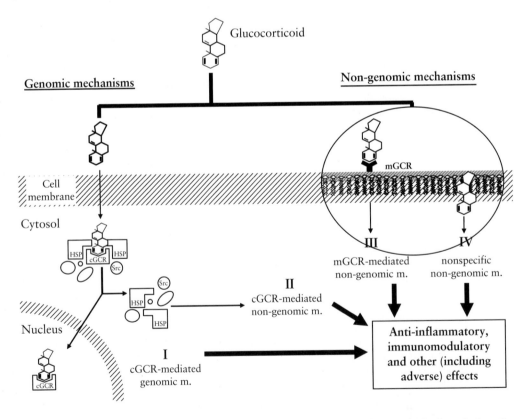

Fig. 23.1 Mechanisms of the cellular actions of GC. As lipophilic substances, GCs pass very easily through the cell membrane into the cell, where they bind to ubiquitously expressed cytosolic GC receptors (cGCRs). This is followed by either the classic cGCR-mediated genomic effects (I) or by cGCR-mediated non-genomic effects (II). Moreover, the GC is very likely to interact with cell membranes either specifically, via membrane-bound GC receptors (mGCRs) (III), or via non-specific interactions with cell membranes (IV). HSP, heat-shock protein; m., mechanism. (From Ref. 3, reproduced with permission.)

Non-genomic actions

Some regulating effects of GCs arise within a few seconds or minutes[7]. An example is the prevention of secondary damage in acute spinal or cerebral trauma by administration of ultrahigh methylprednisolone dosages; the preventive effect is virtually immediately present at the start of the infusion[8]. For these so-called non-genomic effects three mechanisms are relevant: (1) interaction with the cGCR; (2) non-specific interactions with cellular membranes and (3) (perhaps) specific interactions with membrane bound GCRs (mGCRs).

(Ad 1) After GC binding, the cGCR is released from the GC/cGCR, but there is also a rapid release of co-chaperones which may be responsible for producing effects such as the rapid inhibition of arachidonic acid release: non-transcriptional activation.

(Ad 2) Non-specific non-genomic actions in the form of physico-chemical interactions with biologic membranes occur. The resulting inhibition of calcium and sodium cycling across the plasma membrane of immune cells is thought to contribute to rapid immunosuppression and to a reduction of inflammatory processes[7]. These effects may (partially) explain the successful use of high dose GCs in various rheumatic diseases[9,10].

(Ad 3) GCs may also cause specific non-genomic actions that are mediated through mGCRs, see Fig. 23.1. It has been shown that in peripheral blood of patients with RA the number of mGCR-positive monocytes is increased and that this is positively correlated with disease activity[11]. It has been suggested that these mGCRs may play a role in the negative feedback regulation of RA.

Effects on the immune system

GCs reduce activation, proliferation, differentiation, and survival of a variety of inflammatory cells, including macrophages and T lymphocytes, and promote apoptosis, especially in immature and activated T cells. This is mainly mediated by changes in cytokine production and secretion. In contrast, B lymphocytes and neutrophils are less sensitive to GCs, and their survival may actually be increased by GC treatment. The main effect of GCs on neutrophils seems to be inhibition of adhesion to endothelial cells. GCs inhibit not only the expression of adhesion molecules, but also the secretion of complement pathway proteins and prostaglandins. At supraphysiological concentrations, GCs suppress fibroblast proliferation and interleukin (IL)-1 and tumor necrosis factor α (TNF-α)-induced metalloproteinase synthesis. By these effects, GCs may retard bone and cartilage destruction by inflammatory processes[12].

Leukocytes

Administration of GCs leads to a rise in the total leukocyte blood count due to an increase in neutrophils, though the number of other leukocytes in blood decreases. Table 23.2 summarizes the effects of GCs on specific leukocytes. The redistribution of lymphocytes, which is maximal 4–6 h after administration of a single high dose of prednisone and returns to normal within 24 h, has no clinical consequences; B cell function and immunoglobulin production are hardly affected. The effects of GCs on monocytes and macrophages might increase susceptibility to infection, however[13].

Table 23.2 Anti-inflammatory effects of GCs on immune modulatory cells

Cell type	Effects
Neutrophils	Increased blood count, decreasing trafficking, relatively unaltered functioning
Macrophages and monocytes	Decreased blood count, decreased trafficking, decreased phagocytosis and bacterial effects, inhibited antigen presentation, decreased cytokine and eicosanoid release
Lymphocytes	Decreased blood count, decreased trafficking, decreased proliferation and impaired activation, little effect on immunoglobulin synthesis
Eosinophils	Decreased blood count, increased apoptosis
Basophils	Decreased blood count, decreased release of their mediators of inflammation

Cytokines

The influence of GCs on the transcription and action of a large variety of cytokines with pivotal importance in the pathogenesis of RA represents one of the major mechanisms for GC action in RA. Most pro-inflammatory, T-lymphocyte helper (Th) 1-type cytokines are inhibited by GCs, including IL-1β, IL-2, IL-3, IL-6, TNF-α, interferon gamma, and granulocyte–macrophage colony-stimulating factor (GM-CSF). These cytokines are considered responsible for synovitis, cartilage degradation, and bone erosion in RA. Conversely, the production of Th2-type cytokines such as IL-4, IL-10, and IL-13 is either stimulated or not affected by GCs[14]. These cytokines have been related to the extra-articular features of erosive RA, associated with B cell over-activity, such as immune complex formation and vasculitis. Activation of Th2 cells can inhibit rheumatoid synovitis and joint destruction through the release of IL-4 and IL-10, which inhibit Th1 activity and down-regulate a number of monocyte and macrophage functions[15].

Adhesion molecules and permeability factors

Pharmacological doses of GCs dramatically inhibit exudation of plasma and migration of leukocytes into inflammatory sites. Adhesion molecules play a central role in chronic inflammatory diseases by controlling the trafficking of inflammatory cells into sites of inflammation. GCs reduce the expression of adhesion molecules, indirectly through the inhibition of pro-inflammatory cytokines and directly by inhibitory effects on the expression of adhesion molecules such as intercellular adhesion molecule-1 and E-selectin[16]. Chemotactic cytokines attracting immune cells to the inflammatory site, such as IL-8 and macrophage chemoattractant proteins, are also inhibited by GCs. Nitric oxide production in inflammatory sites is increased by pro-inflammatory cytokines and results in an increased blood flow, exudation, and probably amplification of the inflammatory response. The inducible (by cytokines) form of nitric oxide synthase is potently inhibited by GCs[17].

Inflammatory enzymes

An important part of the inflammatory cascade is the arachidonic acid metabolism, leading to the production of prostaglandins and leukotrienes, most of which are strongly pro-inflammatory. Through the induction of lipocortin (an inhibitor of phospholiphase A2), GCs inhibit the formation of arachidonic acid metabolites. GCs have also been shown to inhibit the production of cyclooxygenase (COX)-2 and phospholipase A2 induced by cytokines in monocytes and other inflammatory cells. In addition, GCs are potent inhibitors of the production of metalloproteinases *in vitro* and *in vivo*, especially collagenase and stromelysin, which are the main effectors of cartilage degradation induced by IL-1 and TNF-α[18].

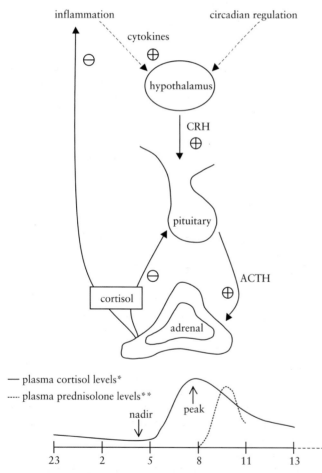

— plasma cortisol levels*
···· plasma prednisolone levels**

Fig. 23.2 Simplified scheme showing the HPA axis, plasma cortisol levels in RA, and plasma prednisolone levels after an oral dose at 8.00 a.m. Negative feedback loops of cortisol and exogenous GCs via pituitary (fast, major determinant serum half-life) and via inflammation (slow, major determinant biological half-life). *Scheme for control persons. Probably induced by cytokines, circadian rhythms are changed in RA, with a shift to an earlier cortisol peak (~1.5 h earlier). ** Oral administration of prednisolone at 8.00 a.m., peak plasma concentration in 1–3 h, plasma half-life in 2–3.5 h, biological half-life 6 h. (From pages 285–293, reproduced with permission.)

The hypothalamic–pituitary–adrenal axis

Pathophysiology

Pro-inflammatory cytokines, such as IL-1 and IL-6, as well as eicosanoids such as prostaglandin E2, and endotoxines, all activate corticotropin-releasing hormone (CRH) at the hypothalamic level. This in turn stimulates the secretion of adrenocorticotropic hormone (ACTH) by the pituitary gland, and thus of GCs by the adrenal glands. In otherwise healthy individuals in situations with severe infections or other major physical stress, cortisol production may increase to up to six times the normal amount[19]. However, in patients with active RA (and other chronic inflammatory diseases) the increase of cortisol driven by elevated cytokines might be inappropriately low[20], meaning that cortisol levels, although normal or elevated in the absolute sense, are insufficient to control the inflammatory response. This is the concept of relative **adrenal insufficiency**[19,21]. Both endogenous and exogenous GCs exert negative feedback control on the hypothalamic-pituitary-adrenal (HPA) axis, *directly* by suppressing secretion of pituitary ACTH and *indirectly* on the level of CRH, via suppression of release from inflammatory tissues of pro-inflammatory cytokines, see Fig. 23.2. This latter counter-regulation mechanism is possibly also less effective in RA than in healthy controls[22].

ACTH is secreted in brief episodic bursts, resulting in sharp rises in plasma concentrations of ACTH and cortisol, followed by slower declines in cortisol levels: the normal diurnal rhythm in cortisol secretion. The secretory ACTH episodic bursts increase in amplitude but not in frequency after 3–5 h of sleep, reach a maximum some hours before, and the hour after, awakening, decline throughout the morning, and are minimal in the evening. So cortisol levels are highest at about the time of awakening in the morning, are low in the late afternoon and evening, and reach their nadir an hour or so after falling asleep, see Fig. 23.2. GCs in the adrenal glands are not stored in sufficient amounts; therefore continuing synthesis and release are required to maintain basal secretion or to increase blood levels during stress. The total daily basal secretion of cortisol in humans has been estimated at 5.7 mg/m^2 [23].

Effects of glucocorticoids on the HPA axis

Chronic suppression of the HPA axis by pathologically increased endogenous GC secretion or administration of exogenous GCs leads to adrenal atrophy and loss of cortisol secretory capability. Patients have a failure of pituitary ACTH release as well as of adrenal responsiveness to ACTH; serum cortisol and ACTH levels are low. GC-induced secondary adrenal insufficiency is characterized by a selective ACTH deficit; other hypopituitary axes are normal. The time required to achieve suppression depends upon the dosage and the serum half-life of the GCs used, but also varies among patients, probably because of individual differences in rates of GC metabolism and sensitivity. This means that prediction with certainty of chronic suppression of the HPA axis and adrenal insufficiency is not possible. The duration of anti-inflammatory effect of one dose of a GC approximates the duration of HPA suppression. After a single oral dose, suppression for 1.25–1.5 days has been described after 250 mg hydrocortisone or cortisone, 50 mg prednisone or prednisolone, and 40 mg methylprednisolone. Duration of suppression after 40 mg triamcinolone and 5 mg dexamethasone was 2.25 and 2.75 days, respectively[6]. Following intramuscular administration of a single dose of 40–80 mg triamcinolone acetonide, duration of HPA suppression is 2–4 weeks and after 40–80 mg methylprednisolone, 4–8 days[24].

In case of chronic therapy: for patients who have had less than 10 mg of prednisone or its equivalent per day in one dose in the morning, the risk of clinical (symptomatic) adrenal insufficiency is not high but not absent. A recent review states that if the daily dose was 7.5 mg prednisolone (or equivalent) or more for at least three weeks, adrenal hypofunctioning should be anticipated, and that acute cessation of GCs in this situation could lead to problems[19]. Neither patients who have received GCs for less than three weeks nor those who have been treated with alternate-day prednisolone therapy have an absent risk of suppression of the HPA axis[25]. It seems prudent to consider these patients as having secondary adrenal insufficiency.

Mechanisms of glucocorticoid resistance

A small proportion of patients does not react favorably to GCs or even fails to respond to higher doses. Also, the susceptibility to adverse effects of GCs varies widely. Several different factors are involved in the variability of GC sensitivity in patients with RA, and understanding the mechanisms involved in sensitivity and especially resistance might eventually allow their modulation. GC resistance is a clinical problem in the treatment of RA. However, GC resistance in RA is not well defined; in daily practice waning of symptomatic relief is often considered to be a sign of resistance. According to this definition over 30% of patients with RA becomes resistant after 3–6 months. However, many relevant factors have not been taken into account for this definition, such as the prolonged beneficial effects of GCs on the progression of erosions or on the decrease in use of co-medication[26]. In Table 23.3 suggested mechanisms mediating GC resistance in RA are summarized[27], one of which is overexpression of GCRβ. GCRβ is an alternative splice variant of the GCR pre-mRNA that accounts for less than 1% of total GCR expression, but does not bind GCs. The suggestion that GCRβ plays a key role in mediating GC resistance is supported by the finding that overexpression of GCRβ reduces the GC effects. Furthermore, GCRβ is reported by some to be overexpressed by peripheral blood mononuclear cells from GC resistant RA patients[28].

mGCRs have been demonstrated on death cells in human leukemia and lymphoma cells. This led to the suggestion that mGCRs mediate cell lysis by inducing apoptosis. So reduced mCGR levels may also contribute to GC resistance. In a cohort of patients with RA a strong positive correlation between the number of mGCR positive monocytes and several parameters of disease activity was found. This may imply that mGCRs cause negative feedback regulation as follows. Immunostimulation (high disease activity) induces mGCR expression on immune cells such as monocytes. This leads to a significantly higher percentage of cells undergoing GC induced apoptosis, which decreases the activity of the immune system, that is, negative feedback regulation[11,27].

Table 23.3 Suggested mechanisms mediating GC resistance in patients with rheumatic diseases (selection)

Reduced number of GCRs and/or reduced affinity of the ligand
Polymorph changes and/or overexpression of chaperones/co-chaperones
Increased expression of inflammatory transcription factors
Changes in the phosphorylation status of the GCR
Overexpression of GCRβ
Multidrug resistance gene *MDR1*
Alteration in the expression of membrane-bound GCR

Therapeutic use

Many patients are using GCs: in a recent registration study for leflunomide, for instance, 54% of USA RA patients used concomitant GCs; a recent German survey indicated that 65% of RA patients treated by rheumatologists were using GCs[29,30].

GCs are used in various dosages in RA, depending on the indications for this therapy. For RA vasculitis, for instance, higher dosages are used than for control of joint inflammation. Based on pathophysiological and pharmacokinetic data, standardization has been proposed to minimize problems in interpretation of the generally used semiquantitative terms for dosages, like 'low', 'intermediate' or 'high', see Table 23.1[3].

Low dose maintenance therapy with GCs in RA

Signs and symptoms

In RA, GC therapy is often started and maintained low-dose, most often as additional therapy[31]. The rationale for this therapy is given in the previous paragraph. GCs are highly effective for relieving symptoms in patients with active RA in doses <10 mg; many patients are functionally dependent on this therapy and continue it long term[32]. A review of seven studies (in total 253 patients) evaluating the symptomatic effect of GCs in RA concluded that, when administered for a period of ~6 months, they are very effective[33]. Improvement has been documented in all clinical parameters, including pain scales, joint scores, morning stiffness, and fatigue, but also in parameters of the acute phase reaction, such as erythrocyte sedimentation rate (ESR) and C-reactive protein (CRP). After six months of therapy the beneficial effects of GCs in general seem to diminish[26,34,35]. However, if this therapy is then tapered off and stopped, patients often experience aggravation of symptoms for several months. In a randomized controlled trial, comparing 10 mg prednisolone with placebo in disease-modifying anti-rheumatic drug (DMARD)-naïve patients with early RA, a decreased need of 40% for intra-articular GC injections, of 49% for acetaminophen use, and of 55% for non-steroidal anti-inflammatory drug (NSAID) use was found in the prednisolone group, compared with the placebo group[26]. This might partially explain the finding in this, and perhaps other, studies that the effect of GCs on parameters of inflammation wanes after some months.

Radiological joint damage

Evaluation of disease-modifying properties of GCs in RA is particularly interesting. In 1995, joint-preserving effects of 7.5 mg prednisolone for two years in patients with RA of short and intermediate disease duration who also were treated with NSAIDs (95%) and DMARDs (71%) were described. The group of RA patients participating in this randomized placebo-controlled trial was heterogeneous, not only in respect to disease duration but also in stages of the disease and kind and dosages of DMARDs[35]. In another trial published in 1997, patients with early RA were randomized to either step-down therapy with two DMARDs (sulfasalazine and methotrexate) and prednisolone (start 60 mg/day, tapered in 6-weekly steps to 7.5 mg/day and stopped at 28 weeks), or sulfasalazine alone. In the combined drug strategy group, a statistically significant and clinically relevant effect in retarding joint damage was shown compared with the effect of sulfasalazine alone[36]. In an extension of this study, also long term (4–5 years), beneficial benefits were shown regarding radiological damage following the combination strategy[37]. A German study evaluated 200 patients with early RA, who were treated with methotrexate or intramuscular gold and randomized for additional treatment with 5 mg of prednisolone or placebo. After two years, progression of radiological damage proved to be less in the prednisolone-treated patients than in the patients treated with placebo-prednisolone[38]. In 2002 the results of a placebo-controlled trial on the effects of prednisolone in DMARD-naïve patients with early RA was published. Ten mg prednisolone daily in these patients (who only got DMARD therapy as rescue) clearly inhibited the progression of radiological joint damage, see Fig. 23.3[26]. Five-year follow-up of these patients confirmed a long-term beneficial effect of the early GC treatment[39].

There are also negative studies on the effect of GCs on radiological damage[34,40], but in *early* RA, evidence of joint sparing properties of GCs seems convincing. Nowadays GCs can be considered to have disease-modifying properties and may thus be called DMARDs[41]. The jury is still out, however, on whether or not GCs can also inhibit progression of erosions in *RA of longer duration*. It could well be that there is a so-called 'window of opportunity' in the treatment of RA[42]. If this window exists, effective treatment of early RA with GCs, as well as DMARDs, may result in an effect that lasts for a long period of time, whereas if effective treatment starts later, this opportunity may be lost and erosive progression may continue.

Some practical aspects

Dosing and timing

For symptomatic relief of the joint symptoms a dosage of 10 mg or less prednisone daily is usually sufficient. In some situations with extra-articular symptoms, such as pericarditis or pleuritis, dosages in the range of 20–30 mg prednisone are used[43]. In life-threatening situations high dosages or pulse therapy can be used (see next page).

There is a diurnal rhythm in the rheumatoid inflammatory process and symptoms: early in the morning patients experience the most extensive joint stiffness and other symptoms and signs. This is due to the long rest period during the night and the circadian rhythm of cortisol as described above[44]. In patients with

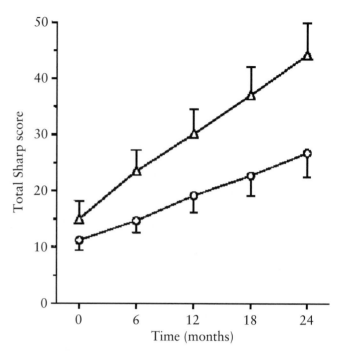

Fig. 23.3 Radiological joint damage according to the van der Heijde modification of the Sharp method. Means (standard errors) of hands and feet. Triangles, placebo group; circles, prednisolone group. From 12 months on, joint damage is significantly less among patients treated with prednisolone compared to patients taking placebo; $p = 0.04$ at 12 months and 0.02 at 24 months. (Based on Ref. 26, reproduced with permission.)

RA with low or moderate disease activity serum cortisol peak and nadir shift to earlier times of the day and night, whereas in patients with high disease activity, the circadian rhythm is markedly reduced or even lost[45]. So the timing of GC administration may be of importance for both efficacy and side-effects. However, data in literature are not unequivocal. In one study, administration of low doses of prednisolone at 2.00 am had more favorable effects on most clinical variables than administration of the same dosage at 7.30 am[46]. In another study, subjective and objective assessments showed no differences in effectiveness between three different times of administration of prednisolone.

Alternate-day regimens

Alternate-day regimens have been devised for oral long-term use of GC therapy, in an attempt to alleviate undesirable side-effects such as HPA axis suppression. These strategies consist of a single dose GC administered every other morning, usually in a dose equivalent to, or somewhat higher than twice the usual or pre-established daily dose. The rationale is that the body, including the HPA axis, is exposed to exogenous GCs only on alternate days. This only makes sense in cases where the patient has a responsive HPA axis. Unfortunately, alternate-day therapy is unsuccessful in most patients who require GCs; patients with RA often experience exacerbation of symptoms on the second day. This is in line with the clinical impression that a single dose of GC daily is less effective in RA than half that dose, given twice daily. In general, alternate-day regimens are used rarely in rheumatology today, except in patients with juvenile idiopathic arthritis, in whom alternate-day GC usage has the advantage of causing less inhibition of body growth[47].

Glucocorticoid withdrawal regimens

Because of potential side-effects, GCs generally are tapered off as soon as the disease is under control. This is probably only relevant for the symptomatic effects, but not for the disease-modifying effects of GCs. Tapering must be done carefully to avoid recurrent activity of the disease symptoms and to permit recovery of the adrenal function. There is no evidence-based scheme based on controlled, comparative studies for tapering GCs. It depends on the individual's disease, the disease activity and doses and duration of therapy and clinical response. Therefore only guidelines can be offered.

When patients are chronically treated with dosages of 10 mg prednisone or less, reduction by 2.5 mg every (second) month until a dosage of 5 mg daily is reached is often feasible. Thereafter, decreasing the dosage by 1 mg monthly is often possible.

If, because of extra-articular features, high dosages of prednisone are being used, in stable disease decrements of 5 mg every 1–2 weeks until a dosage of 20 mg/day is reached are advised, with 1–2.5 mg/day decrements every 2–3 weeks thereafter.

Immunomodulatory drugs, like methotrexate or azathioprine, can be added to therapy with GCs, to enable further reduction of the dose. These immunomodulatory drugs are then called GC-sparing agents.

Adaptations of glucocorticoid doses, stress regimens, and preoperative care

Patients on chronic low-dose GC medication have suppressed adrenal activity and should be advised to double their daily GC dose or to increase the dose to 15 mg prednisolone or equivalent a day in case of fever attributed to infection and to seek medical help. In case of major surgery, given the unreliable prediction of adrenal suppression on the basis of duration and dose of GC therapy, many physicians recommend 'stress doses' of GCs, also for patients with a low risk of adrenal suppression. The classic scheme of 100 mg hydrocortisone intravenously just before surgery, followed thereafter by 100 mg every 6 h for three days, is seldom necessary. A scheme with a lower dose, possibly reducing the risk of postoperative bacterial infectious complications, is to infuse 100 mg/24 h hydrocortisone intravenously the day of surgery, followed by 25–50 mg of hydrocortisone every 8 h for 2–3 days thereafter. An alternative is to administer on the day of surgery the usual dose of oral GCs orally or (the equivalent) parenterally, followed by 25–50 mg of hydrocortisone every 8 h for 2–3 days. In case of minor surgery, it is probably sufficient to double the oral dose or to increase the dose to 15 mg prednisolone or equivalent daily for 1–3 days. No comparative randomized studies on different peri-operative GC stress schemes have been published, however. Because in GC-induced loss of adrenal responsiveness aldosterone secretion is preserved by the intact rennin-angiotensin-aldosterone axis, in contrast to primary adrenal insufficiency, mineralocorticoid therapy is not necessary.

Drug interactions

Significant interactions between GCs and other drugs have been well documented. Drugs that *reduce* the systemic GC concentration may diminish clinical efficacy. They include large doses of aluminium/magnesium hydroxide, which decrease prednisone bioavailability by 30–40%[48], and most anticonvulsants (e.g. phenobarbital, phenytoin), which enhance the metabolism of GCs[49]. Rifampin accelerates the metabolism of synthetic steroids and may induce non-responsiveness to prednisone[50]. Drugs that *raise* the systemic GC concentration include some oral contraceptives[51] and antibiotics, for example erythromycin[52]. Antifungal agents, particularly ketoconazole, decrease GC-metabolizing enzymes[53]. Some data suggest that several NSAIDs, including indomethacin and naproxen, increase GC concentrations[54].

The other way round, GCs may affect serum concentration, efficacy, or toxicity of other drugs, such as warfarin and salicylates[55,56].

Glucocorticoid pulse therapy

In RA, GC pulse therapy is applied to treat some of the serious complications of the disease and to induce remission in active disease, often in the initiation phase of second-line anti-rheumatic treatment. In the latter patients, pulse therapy with schemes of 1000 mg methylprednisolone intravenously, 200 mg dexamethasone, or other equivalent doses, for one day or a few days, has been proven to be effective in most studies; the beneficial effect generally lasts for about six weeks, with a large variation in the duration of the effect[57]. Thus it does not seem sensible to apply pulse therapy in active RA unless a change is also made in the therapeutic strategy, for example with DMARD-treatment aimed to stabilize in the long term the remission induced by the pulse therapy. As described in the section Non-genomic actions, above, the mechanisms of action are not only genomic but also non-genomic, thus influencing the disease process differently than with oral lower dosage treatment[58]. The short-time effects of pulse therapy in patients with established, active RA on various dimensions of health status closely resemble the long-term effects of effective conventional DMARD therapy such as methotrexate in patients with early RA[10].

A mitigated form of pulse therapy is the parental use of 120 mg depot methylprednisolone acetate, quite popular in, amongst others, the UK.

Intra-articular glucocorticoid injections

Intra-articular injections with GCs are often used in RA. The effect depends on several factors, such as the treated joint (size, weight-bearing or non-weight-bearing), the activity of arthritis and volume of synovial fluid of the treated joint[59], application of arthrocentesis (synovial fluid aspiration) before injection, the choice and dose of the GC preparation, the injection technique, and application of rest to the injected joint. In a retrospective study the joints injected, especially knee joints, required at least one additional injection[60]. Arthrocentesis before injecting the GC preparation reduces the risk of relapse of arthritis[61].

Soluble GCs (e.g. phosphate salts) have a more rapid onset of action with probably less risk of subcutaneous tissue atrophy and depigmentation of the skin when given peri-articularly, but insoluble GCs are longer acting and might decrease soft tissue fibrosis more. So, insoluble GCs are given more safely into deep sites. Short-acting soluble GCs can be mixed with long-acting insoluble ones to combine rapid onset with long-acting effect. Triamcinolone hexacetonide, the least soluble preparation among the injectable GCs, shows the longest effect[62]. Co-administration of a local anesthetic with the GCs at intra-articular injection may provide immediate relief of pain.

Theoretically, rest of the injected joint minimizes leakage of the injected GC preparation to the systemic circulation (activity causes intra-articular pressure peaks), minimizes the risk of cartilage damage, and provides optimal conditions for repair of tissue damage. Advice and procedures for the post-injection period activity vary from none to the advice to take bed rest for three times 24 h following injection of a knee joint and splinting of injected joints. In a randomized controlled study, bed rest for 24 h following injection of a knee joint in patients with inflammatory arthritis such as RA prolonged duration of clinical response and reduced the need for additional injections, compared to the condition of injection in the outpatient setting, and no particular advice to rest the injected joint[63]. Favorable effects of resting the injected joints (e.g. by splinting in a cast or plaster) for three weeks in the case of a non-weight-bearing (upper extremity joint) and six weeks for a weight-bearing (lower extremity joint) have been described[60]. Based on literature, no definite evidence-based recommendation can be made, but it seems prudent to rest and certainly not to overuse the injected joint, even if pain is relieved.

It is recommended that intra-articular GC injections be repeated no more often than once every 3–4 weeks and be given no more frequently than 3–4 times a year in a weight-bearing joint to prevent GC-induced joint damage. This recommendation seems sensible, but there is no definite clinical evidence to support it. Accuracy of steroid placement influences the clinical outcome of GC injections; this is important as, for example, over half of shoulder injections are inaccurately placed[64].

The reported infection rate of joints following local injections with GCs is low and ranges from 1 case in 13 900—77 300 injections[65,66]. Putting it the other way around, how often is a proven bacterial arthritis due to a GC injection? In 214 documented cases of bacterial arthritis (including 58 joints with prosthesis or osteosynthetic material) in a prospective study in a population of over 1 000 000 persons over three years, only three joint infections were attributed to an intra-articular injection[67].

Other adverse effects of local GC injections are *systemic* adverse effects of the GCs, like disturbance of the menstrual pattern[68], hot flush-like symptoms the day of or the day after injection[69], and hyperglycemia in diabetes mellitus[70], and *local* complications, like subcutaneous fat tissue atrophy[71] especially after improper local injection, local depigmentation of the skin[72], tendon slip and tendon rupture[61], and lesions to local structures like nerves[73].

Adverse events of low-dose GC maintenance therapy

Studies of GC toxicity tend to be retrospective and observational. The lack of ability to differentiate bad outcomes that are attributable to GCs from those that occur as a result of the underlying disease or other comorbidities confounds the picture. In these studies a strong physician selection bias for GC use often exists, in other words, physicians are inclined to treat patients who have more severe disease with GCs. Less serious and near ubiquitous but eye-catching toxicities (such as Cushingoid appearance, skin thinning) may be of great concern to patients, whereas more debilitating but less conspicuous toxicity (such as osteoporosis, cataract, hypertension) initially may stay unrecognized or asymptomatic. The use of GCs at variable points in the disease, limited data to define the threshold dosage for particular adverse events, individual variability in sensitivity to adverse effects of GCs, the influence of the disease treated, and toxicity reports that cover a heterogeneous group of GCs, all confound the interpretation of toxicity data[4].

Compared with other anti-rheumatic agents, GCs have a low incidence of short-term symptomatic toxicity; it is uncommon for patients to discontinue therapy for these reasons[74,75]. Despite more than 50 years of use, robust data on long-term toxicity of GCs, such as from large prospective, randomized controlled trials (RCTs) with long-term follow-up are lacking. This present section is based on well-known data from literature and a survey of the reported toxicity data from four prospective RCTs of low-dose GCs in RA[4,26,35,38,76].

Endocrine and metabolic adverse effects

Glucose intolerance and diabetes

GCs increase serum glucose levels via an increase in hepatic glucose production and changes in insulin production and resistance[77]. In patients without pre-existing abnormalities of glucose tolerance, GCs will result in slightly increased fasting glucose levels and a more pronounced increase of postprandial values. It is uncommon for frank diabetes to develop *de novo* as a result of GC therapy[78].

GC-related hyperglycemia is dose-dependent. One case-control study suggested an increased risk (odds ratio 1.8) for initiation of anti-hyperglycemic drugs during therapy with 0.25–2.5 prednisone equivalent per day[79]. It is likely that subjects with risk factors for the development of diabetes mellitus (DM), such as a positive family history, increasing age, obesity, and previous gestational diabetes mellitus, are at increased risk of developing new-onset hyperglycemia during GC therapy[80]. This is usually rapidly reversed upon GC cessation, but some patients will go on to develop persistent DM[81]. Next to the average daily dose, the type of GC is of great importance. Dexamethasone is 30 times and prednisone 4 times as potent as hydrocortisone in the impairment of glucose metabolism[82].

Data from prospective RCT on low-dose GCs in RA are quite reassuring in this respect: no cases of new-onset DM were observed in either of these studies. The Utrecht trial, giving 10 mg prednisone for two years, found the least favorable results[26]: a significant increase in mean (SD) fasting glucose was seen in the prednisone group (from 5.1 (0.6) at baseline to 5.9 (1.9) mmol/L at two years, $p = 0.01$). However, even in this study, hyperglycemia, as defined by the World Health Organization, developed in only two patients in the prednisone group ($n = 40$) and one in the placebo group ($n = 41$).

There are no preventive measures apart from the use of lower doses of GCs and weight reduction. Alternate-day therapy is associated with alternate-day hyperglycemia[83].

There are no studies on the specific effects of low-dose GCs in diabetic patients, but a relevant and detailed discussion of glucose control under GC treatment has been published[84].

Fat redistribution and body weight

One of the most notable effects of chronic endogenous GC excess and of GC therapy is the redistribution of body fat. Centripetal fat accumulation with sparing and often even thinning of the extremities is a characteristic feature of patients exposed to long-term high-dose GCs. Potential mechanisms include hyperinsulinemia, changes in expression and activity of adipocyte-derived hormones and cytokines, such as leptin and TNF-α, increased food intake (GCs increase appetite), and muscle atrophy[85,86].

Review of toxicity data from prospective RCTs shows that low-dose prednisone in RA patients is associated with an increase of mean body weight over two years, in the range of 4–8%; this weight gain was significantly higher than in the placebo group[26,38].

Suppression of sex hormones secretion

GCs in high doses decrease gonadotropin-releasing hormone (GnRH) secretion from the hypothalamus, decrease basal and GnRH-stimulated luteinizing hormone (LH) secretion from the pituitary, and decrease the responsiveness of gonadal cells to LH, leading to lower levels of estrogens and testosterone[87]. In prospective RCTs on low-dose GCs in RA, decreased libido was not reported spontaneously.

Musculoskeletal adverse effects

Osteoporosis

Osteoporosis is a well-established side-effect and considered by some as the most potentially devastating complication of protracted GC therapy. GCs decrease calcium absorption, increase renal calcium loss, diminish sex hormone production, and inhibit osteoprotegerin; all of these lead to enhanced osteoclast-mediated bone resorption. However, a defect in bone formation may be the predominant pathway of importance[88]. GC-induced osteoporosis initially affects trabecular bone; however, with chronic GC use, cortical bone is also affected[89]. The deleterious effects of GCs on bone are already apparent at an early stage, with reported estimates of from 1.5 to even 20% losses of bone mineral density (BMD) in the first 6–12 months of use, followed by a slower rate of 1–3% loss per year thereafter[90,91].

The incidence of osteoporosis is time and dose dependent, but there is no 'safe' dose. Although some studies suggest that doses of 7.5 mg of prednisone per day or less are relatively safe, a longitudinal study observed an average loss of 9.5% from spinal trabecular bone over 20 weeks in patients exposed to 7.5 mg of prednisolone daily[92–94].

An exhaustive literature search for all prospective studies found 1200 patients in whom bone mass was studied prospectively while on GC treatment for any disease[95]. At a mean dose of almost 9 mg prednisone equivalent/day, the best estimate of bone loss overall in spine and hip (without bisphosphonate therapy) is 1.5% per year. Important predictive factors include height of starting dose and duration of chronic usage, and, in the spine, GC dose and lack of vitamin D supplementation.

Inflammatory disease activity has been shown to be an independent risk factor for osteoporosis, at least in RA. Disease activity leads to reduced physical activity (and thus less exposure to sunlight and, because of muscle atrophy, a propensity to falls) and elevated levels of inflammatory cytokines such as TNF-α, which stimulate differentiation of osteoclasts both directly and indirectly via receptor activator of NF-κB (RANK) ligand (osteoclast differentiation factor) and thus to bone loss. In a recent multicenter cross-sectional study, 205 patients with RA who were receiving GCs orally on a daily basis were compared with 205 matched RA patients who did not receive GCs. Vertebral deformities were found in 25% of patients on GCs versus in 13% of controls. The occurrence of vertebral deformities was dependent on daily dose[94].

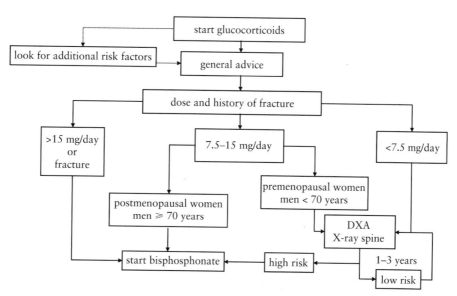

Fig. 23.4 Stream diagram for osteoporosis prevention during the use of GC; key message is that treatment with bisphosphonates should be started immediately in patients at high risk. General advice includes lifestyle, calcium and vitamin D suppletion. (Based on Ref. 98, reproduced with permission.)

It is, therefore, possible that GCs in RA, by decreasing disease activity and increasing physical activity, may cause less bone loss and fractures than they would have in the absence of inflammatory disease. On the other hand, it seems quite likely that, as some studies suggested, fractures occur at less decreased BMD levels in GC-treated patients than in patients not treated with GCs[90].

Data from prospective RCTs on *low-dose* GCs in RA show that BMD loss over two years induced by low-dose prednisone was not significantly different from that associated with placebo[26,76]. Osteoporosis is probably the most common adverse effect of chronic GC use, but fortunately it is preventable. Strategies for the prevention and treatment of GC-induced osteoporosis are well established and have been the object of recent extensive reviews, and authoritative guidelines[96–98]. A practical example is the stream diagram depicted in Fig. 23.4.

Osteonecrosis

Osteonecrosis (avascular necrosis of bone) has been considered an important consequence of high-dose GC use. Data on low-dose GC treatment is scarce and mostly anecdotal; one study reported osteonecrosis in 2.4% of patients receiving GC replacement therapy[99]. No case of avascular necrosis was observed in prospective RCTs on low-dose GCs in RA, nor in the COBRA trial[26,35,38,76]. In RA patients treated with low dosages of GCs, osteonecrosis is seldom noted.

Myopathy

Based on the scarce information available, myopathy is exceedingly rare with GC doses below 7.5 mg prednisolone equivalent daily. The clinical picture of chronic steroid myopathy can be difficult to distinguish from the effects of the underlying disease, especially in the case of musculoskeletal conditions such as RA[100]. When steroid myopathy is suspected, diagnosis can be ascertained by muscle biopsy, showing atrophy of type II fibers, and absence of inflammation[101].

Infectious diseases

The use of GCs is associated with increased susceptibility to various viral, bacterial, fungal, and parasitic infections. The mechanisms underlying this effect, such as the decrease in function of monocytes, subside rapidly with treatment interruption, an observation that may explain the relatively low infectious risk with the use of short-acting GCs and alternate-day therapy[102]. The risk of infection increases with dose and duration of treatment, but tends to remain low in patients exposed to low doses, even with high cumulative dosages[103]. In a meta-analysis of 71 trials involving over 2000 patients with different diseases and different dosages of GCs, a relative risk of infection was found of 2.0[104]. Five of these 71 trials involved patients with rheumatic diseases and showed no increased relative risk. In a study specifically on RA, the incidence of serious infections attributable to GCs was found to be similar or only slightly increased compared to that of placebo[105]. In prospective RCTs of low-dose GC therapy in RA, prednisone in doses of up to 10mg/day was not associated with increased incidence of any kind of infections over the two years of the trials[26,76].

In patients treated with GCs, physicians should anticipate the risk of infections with both usual and unusual microorganisms, realizing that GCs may blunt or mask the classic clinical features of infections and thus delay the diagnosis. Often missed diagnoses are diverticulitis (sometimes with perforation) and appendicitis.

Cardiovascular adverse effects

Dyslipidemia, atherosclerosis, and cardiovascular disease

GC treatment is considered to be a risk factor for dyslipidemia (increase in total plasma cholesterol, low-density lipoprotein cholesterol, and triglycerides, and decrease in high-density lipoprotein cholesterol) and atherosclerosis[106]. Beyond induction of dyslipidemia, the role of GCs in actual atherosclerosis is controversial. Increasing attention to accelerated atherosclerotic disease in RA and other inflammatory conditions has raised interesting questions about the role of chronic inflammation on the vascular endothelium[107,108]. Inflammation causes endothelial dysfunction, a risk factor for cardiovascular disease. This and the recognition of an association between elevated C-reactive protein (indicating inflammatory mechanisms) and accelerated coronary artery disease offer a theoretical basis for GC benefit on atherosclerotic disease in the context of inflammatory diseases[109]. Furthermore, recent data show that RA disease activity unfavorably alters the blood lipid profile, and treatment (including GC treatment) can improve this altered profile[110].

Recently, a record linkage database study on 68 781 GC users (of whom 1115 patients had RA) and 82 202 non-users was published[111]. The incidence of all cardiovascular diseases, including myocardial infarction, heart failure, and cerebrovascular disease was not increased in patients using <7.5 mg prednisolone on a chronic basis. However, it was increased in patients using dosages ≥7.5 mg daily: relative risk adjusted for all other known risk factors 2.6 (95% confidence interval (CI): 2.2–3).

In summary, research data do not support a significant role for low-dose GC treatment in the development of cardiovascular disease in RA, in contrast to higher dosages. In patients on low-dose GCs, the disease itself and, according to recent data, also medication with COX-2-selective NSAIDs, seem to be greater risk factors than GCs.

Water and electrolyte balance, edema, and renal and heart function

Hypernatremia, hypokalemia, and sodium and water retention are mineralocorticoid effects, produced by endogenous GCs at supraphysiologic concentrations. These effects may lead to edema and contribute to hypertension and heart failure in patients with Cushing's disease. Synthetic GCs (prednisone, prednisolone, methylprednisolone, dexamethasone) have little or no mineralocorticoid effects, and their administration increases glomerular filtration rate and induces kaliuresis and natriuresis without significant change in plasma volume[112]. A small number of trials has evaluated chronic GC administration in moderate to high doses in patients with heart failure. No significant detrimental effect on heart function emerged from these studies[113]. In the prospective RCTs on low-dose GC treatment in RA as well as in the COBRA trial, no cardiac insufficiency attributable to GCs occurred.

Hypertension

Despite increasing data that synthetic GCs do not cause significant fluid retention, induction of hypertension is a well-demonstrated adverse effect of GCs, observed in about 20% of patients exposed to exogenous GCs[114].

Toxicity data from prospective RCTs on low-dose GCs in RA are reassuring in respect to blood pressure: there were no significant effects of prednisone upon blood pressure in any of the trials. During the first phase of the COBRA trial, while intermediate to high doses of GCs were used, the mean blood pressure was at some points in time higher in the prednisone group than in the placebo group. It should be noted, however, that patients with severe or inadequately treated hypertension were excluded from most of these trials.

Data suggest that GC-induced hypertension is dose related and less likely with medium- or low-dose therapy. Individual variation in susceptibility, and factors such as the level of starting blood pressure, diet salt, renal function, associated diseases, and drug therapy (e.g. ciclosporine) may play a role in the development of GC-induced hypertension[114]

Other cardiac adverse effects

Arrhythmia and sudden death are very rare and mostly limited to patients receiving pulse GCs[115].

Gastrointestinal adverse effects

Peptic ulcer disease

The association between GC use and the risk of peptic ulcer disease has been the subject of extensive debate and contradictory trial results. The influence of the underlying disease on the risk of peptic ulceration is difficult to isolate from that of GCs. In a classical study 1415 patients admitted to the hospital for gastro-duodenal ulcer or hemorrhage were compared with 7063 randomly selected controls from Medicaid[116] The overall estimated relative risk for peptic ulcer disease amongst current GC users was 2.0 (95% CI: 1.3–3.0). However, this increased risk was nearly completely due to co-therapy with NSAIDs: the risk for patients co-medicated with NSAIDs was 4.4 (95% CI: 2.0–9.7), but for those receiving only GCs there was no significant increase in risk: 1.1 (95% CI: 0.5–2.1). In large-scale studies based on the UK General Practice Research Database, the relative risk of upper gastrointestinal (GI) complications was 1.8 (95% CI: 1.3–2.4) for users of GCs compared to non-users[117]. The risk tended to be greater for higher GCs doses but this trend was not statistically significant. Data from prospective RCTs with low-dose GCs and from the COBRA study show no increased incidence of upper GI ulcers and bleeds, but these events are relatively uncommon and may not be detected in a relatively low number of participating patients. In patients treated with GCs without concomitant use of NSAIDs, there thus seems to be no indication for gastro-protective agents if there are no (other) risk

factors for peptic complications. GCs are considered to be considerably less toxic to the upper GI tract than NSAIDs.

Pancreatitis

Although GCs are usually listed as one of the many potential causes of pancreatitis, evidence for such an association is weak and difficult to separate from the influence of the underlying disease, such as systemic lupus erythematosus (SLE) or vasculitis. In one postmortem study, acute pancreatitis or fat necrosis was observed in 29% of those treated with ACTH or GCs vs 4% in the controls[118]. However, none of these patients had been diagnosed with pancreatitis *premortem*, suggesting that clinically relevant pancreatitis due to GCs is rare.

Dermatological adverse effects

Even at low dosages, skin thinning and ecchymoses represent some of the most common adverse events of long-term GC therapy. Other clinically relevant adverse effects include easy bruisability, purpura, striae, impaired wound healing, steroid acne, thinning of scalp hair, and hypertrichosis[119]. Cushingoid phenotype is observed in over 5% of the patients exposed to ≥5 mg prednisone equivalent for ≥1 year[120]. Incidence of iatrogenic Cushing's syndrome is dose dependent and in general becomes evident after at least one month of GC therapy. Catabolic effects on the skin may appear during local and systemic GC therapy. Cutaneous atrophy mainly results from the effect of GCs on keratinocytes and fibroblasts. Decreased vascular structural integrity is probably a key determinant of purpura and easy bruisability in GC-treated patients. These effects were also reported to affect over 5% of those exposed to ≥5 mg prednisone equivalent for ≥1 year[121]. Wound healing impairment seems uncommon at low dose, but there are no exact data on prevalence. There are no data on incidence of steroid acne, striae, hirsutism, and thinning of scalp hair: they are more frequent with long-term treatment with moderate to high doses of GCs, but do occur at low doses such as are often used in RA. There is no strong evidence to support the claim that use of the lowest possible dose and alternate-day therapy may fully prevent these adverse effects.

Most of the cutaneous adverse effects of GCs are not serious for the doctor, but represent a very significant social problem for the patient.

Ophthalmologic adverse effects

Cataract

Long-term use of systemic GCs may induce formation of posterior sub-capsular cataract, characterized by disruption of the ordered maturation of the lens fibres, which then accumulate on the front surface of the posterior lens capsule. Cortical cataracts have also been attributed to GCs[122].

Reports on the frequency of cataract with long-term low-dose systemic GC therapy are scarce. In a group of RA patients treated with 5–15 mg/day of prednisone for six years, 15% was found to have cataracts, compared with 4.5% of matched RA controls not using prednisone[105]. Cataract formation is irreversible and there is no evidence regarding the possibility of halting progression with dose reduction or treatment interruption. More detailed prospective assessment of cataract formation among GC users is needed to definitively address this item. In prospective RCTs on low-dose GC treatment in RA, excess cataracts were not reported, but trial duration was probably too short for development of this complication and only two of the four extensively reviewed trials on low-dose GC treatment in RA included a regular routine ophthalmologic check in a significant number of patients.

Glaucoma

Systemic GC treatment increases the risk of glaucoma, which may result in visual field loss or even blindness. In the general population, 18–36% of those exposed to GCs experience an increase in intraocular pressure[123]. However, the occurrence and magnitude of elevation of intraocular pressure with GC administration is highly variable between individuals. High frequency of this adverse effect on GCs tends to occur in families, suggesting a genetic basis[124]. Patients with pre-existing glaucoma are especially sensitive: 46–92% of patients with open-angle and 65% of those with closed-angle glaucoma will have this condition aggravated upon exposure to GCs[123]. Open-angle glaucoma was found in 6 of 32 RA patients exposed to ≥7.5 mg of prednisone equivalent for more than a year (19%) and in 1 out of 38 treated with <7.5 mg of prednisone equivalent (2.6%—A Tryc, B Bartholome, F Buttgereit *et al.*, unpublished data). Patients with DM, high myopia, and relatives of those with open-angle glaucoma are reported to be more vulnerable to GC-induced glaucoma[123]. Elevation of intraocular pressure with exogenous GCs is generally reversible upon cessation, although it may take several weeks. Concomitant medication that lowers intraocular pressure may control even a significant pressure increase induced by GCs. As glaucoma is often asymptomatic and can lead to severe loss of sight, regular eye pressure checks seem thus recommendable for patients on high-dose long-term systemic GC treatment, especially for those with associated risk factors for glaucoma. For patients on low-dose GC therapy and no additional risk factors for glaucoma, it is generally accepted that routine checks are not indicated.

Neuropsychiatric disturbances

Psychosis

Estimates of the incidence of GC psychosis vary greatly in literature (0–60%), due to differences in study populations and methodology of assessing this adverse event. In the Boston Cooperative Drug Surveillance Program the incidence of psychosis in 718 prednisone-treated patients (with lupus nefritis) was 1.3% at <40 mg daily, 4–5% at 41–80 mg, and over 18% with higher doses[125]. In prospective RCTs on low-dose GC treatment in RA this adverse event was not reported. Overt psychosis attributable to GCs is extremely rare with the low- and medium-dose regimes usually employed in rheumatology[126].

Minor mood disturbances

GC treatment has been associated with a variety of low-grade disturbances such as depressed or elated mood (euphoria), irritability or emotional lability, anxiety and insomnia, memory and cognition impairments. The exact incidence of such symptoms in rheumatic patients exposed to GCs cannot be drawn from the literature. Most studies relate to doses of 80–160 mg of prednisone equivalent per day, far exceeding common regimes in rheumatology. Doses of less than 20–25 mg prednisone equivalent are associated with few or no significant disturbances[127]. However, individual susceptibility is highly variable and there are a few published cases in which a relationship between low-dose GCs, and even topical steroids and psychotic episodes seems hard to doubt.

Practical guidelines

The balance of risks and benefits of low-dose therapy clearly differs from that of medium- and high-dose therapy, in which the mechanisms of action of GCs may be different[5]. This may explain why GCs are used in practice in more patients than official recommendations suggest. Physicians, and probably patients, seem to value the benefit/risk ratio of low-dose GCs. There is surprisingly weak evidence to support clear recommendations to tackle or prevent toxicity of low-dose GCs. The literature, especially recent RCT results, suggests that *routine* toxicity monitoring for patients on low-dose GCs is currently not justifiable or cost effective. However, patients with additional risk factors (e.g. osteoporosis, obesity, hypertension, family history of diabetes or glaucoma) merit more careful observation. Apart from the preventive measures with regard to osteoporosis (see above) the following GC-related adverse effects may justify clinical checkup:

- Cushingoid symptoms
- Adrenal crisis on GC withdrawal
- Growth retardation in children
- New onset of DM in subjects at risk for developing DM
- Worsening of glycemic control in patients with DM
- Cataract and glaucoma
- Peptic ulcer (if associated with NSAIDs)
- Hypertension

Recent developments

Recent studies demonstrating the disease-modifying potential of low-dose GCs in RA have renewed the debate on the risk/benefit ratios associated with this therapy. In this section we will discuss recent developments that might positively influence these risk/benefit ratios, thus enabling us to optimize GC treatment. These developments regard improvements in drugs and their delivery, including designer GCs, with potential lower toxicity and increases in the effective dosage of GCs by time-release or targeted formulations[1,128,129].

Designer glucocorticoids

As discussed in the section Genomic actions above, GCs produce their cardiovascular, metabolic, and antigrowth adverse effects through molecular mechanisms distinct from those involved in immunomodulation. Transrepression is considered the key mechanism for the anti-inflammatory activity of GCs. In contrast, adverse effects are thought to be predominantly mediated via trans-activation. Ligands that preferentially induce the transrepression, and not transactivation function of the GCR, the selective gluco-corticoid receptor agonists (SEGRAs), theoretically should be as effective as conventional GCs, but with fewer adverse effects[1,130].

SEGRAs

A number of selective GC receptor agonists was described recently:

A276575 was described in 2002; it exhibits, similar to dexam-ethasone, high affinity for GCR and potently represses IL-1β-stimulated IL-6 production. However, in contrast to dexamethasone, A276575 causes smaller induction of aromatase activity[131].

AL-438, a ligand that exhibits a selective gene regulation profile, is able to repress and activate only a subset of the genes normally regulated by GCs. *In vivo* AL-438 has full anti-inflammatory effi-cacy and potency similar to GCs, but its negative effects on bone metabolism and glucose control are less[132].

ZK216348 is a non-steroidal SEGRA that shows similar anti-inflammatory activity to prednisolone in inflammation models of rats and mice regarding inhibition of edema and peroxidase activ-ity. In these models, the side-effects of ZK216348 with regard to increases in blood glucose, spleen involution, and skin atrophy were clearly less than that of prednisolone treatment[130]. This seems attributable to its low transactivation activity, which is about 60 times weaker than that of prednisolone.

Of course further *in vitro/vivo* investigations and clinical trials will have to define in more detail the safety-efficacy profile of this potentially new class of drugs.

Nitric oxide glucocorticoids

Coupling nitric oxide (NO) to GCs results in NO GCs, which have synergistic anti-inflammatory effects. NO GCs (nitrosteroids) also bind to the GCR, but they additionally slowly release low levels of NO. NO has several actions, including important anti-inflamma-tory effects, especially if slowly released. These include reduced leukocyte adhesion to the endothelium, diminished mast cell acti-vation, and inhibited synthesis of inflammatory mediators[1,133,134]. Apart from these additional anti-inflammatory properties, NO GCs have reduced side-effects, especially on bone (less osteoporo-sis), compared to conventional GCs. The prototype of these NO GCs is 21-NO-prednisolone, or NCX-1015. This NO GC is much more potent than prednisolone in models of acute and chronic inflammation, including collagen II-induced arthritis in mice. In addition, it has been shown that NCX-1015 did not activate osteo-clast activity in an *in vitro* assay of bone resorption, whereas pred-nisolone does[135]. Since the adverse effect of GCs on bone is considered a major drawback of GC treatment, this observation will stimulate clinical studies of this first available NO GC.

Alterations in glucocorticoid bioactivity: glycyrrhetinic acid

The cellular actions of GCs are largely mediated through binding to nuclear receptors that act as ligand-inducible transcription factors. In tissues, the two isozymes of 11β-hydroxysteroid dehy-drogenase (11β-HSD-1 and 11β-HSD-2) have a pivotal role in the regulation of GC hormone activity. 11β-HSD-1 catalyzes the conversion of the inactive 11-ketoforms (cortisone and 11-dehydrocorticosterone) into hormonally active, natural GCs (cortisol and corticosterone, respectively) and vice versa[136]. Although 11β-HSD-1 is thus bi-directional, *in vivo* it acts pre-dominantly as reductases generating the biologically active corti-sol. The human 11β-HSD-2 isozyme, however, is a unidirectional dehydrogenase that converts cortisol to the biologically inactive cortisone[137]. Alterations (decrements) in its activity have been implicated in several human diseases, including hypertension, intra-uterine growth retardation, and obesity. Peripheral tissues (eyes, adipose tissue, bone, and others) have been shown to be able to regulate corticosteroid concentrations through these 11β-HSD isozymes. *In vitro* studies showed that cortisol has a stimulatory effect on the differentiation of adipose stromal cells to mature adipocytes, while inhibition of 11β-HSD-1 by glycyrrhetinic acid prevented this cortisone-induced differentia-tion[138]. Modulation of 11β-HSD-1 activity could possibly influ-ence tissue GC concentrations, in order to circumvent the negative consequences of systemic GC excess.

Timing of glucocorticoid treatment

Clinical observations indicate that individual patients with RA differ in their subjective response to low-dose GC treatment administration times, some having better symptomatic relief from night time, or split morning and evening schedules. Timing of GC treatment at very early morning might be more effective and per-haps enable patients to use lower dosages[139]. Presently, different pharmaceutical companies are in the process of developing timed-release capsules or tablets to enable dosage of GCs very early in the morning.

Joint targeting by liposomes

When GCs are given intravenously, there is a rapid clearance and a large volume of distribution, which hamper clinical use. However, GCs can be incorporated in particulate carriers that show accumulation into inflammatory target sites. For RA, long-circulating liposomes seem to be the most interesting carriers for drug targeting. These liposomes are small lipid bilayer vesicles (100 nm in diameter) with an aqueous core that can be used to entrap water-soluble agents[1]. Water-soluble polymers like poly-ethylene glycol (PEG) can be attached to the surface of these lipo-somes to reduce adhesion of opsonic plasma proteins which would otherwise induce immune recognition and rapid removal from circulation by macrophages in the liver and spleen. PEG-coated, long-circulating liposomes can remain in the circulation with a half-life as long as 50 h. Studies with radiolabels entrapped in PEG liposomes have indicated that PEG liposomes can selec-tively extravasate to inflammatory tissues, by virtue of the increased permeability of the local vascular endothelium and the presence of activated macrophages. As a consequence, very high concentrations ($>10^{-5}$ M) are present at the site of inflammation for several hours, leading to a 100% genomic effect (mediated by the cGCR as described in the section Genomic actions, above), as well as to significant non-genomic effects (such as biophysical interactions with cellular membranes of immune cells)[3].

Rats with adjuvant-induced arthritis were treated intravenously with liposomal or free prednisolone phosphate a few days after the first signs of arthritis[140]. The effect on paw inflammation scores during the weeks after treatment was evaluated. Liposomal prednisolone proved to be highly effective: a single injection resulted in complete remission of the inflammatory response for almost a week. The same dosage of unencapsulated free prednisolone did not reduce inflammation. These experiments were successfully repeated in mice with collagen type II-induced arthritis[141]. A beneficial effect on cartilage destruction was also documented. These experiments suggest that it is possible to use long-circulating liposomes to target the synovial lining selectively in inflamed joints, and thus increase the local anti-inflammatory activity of GCs by using the location of actions more efficiently. It has been shown that this preferential GC delivery leads to (very) high GC concentration in the inflamed joint, but to low plasma concentrations, with perhaps a lower rate of side-effects.

The given examples of new GCs are incomplete, but indicate that with the increased evidence of the efficacy of GCs many efforts are now undertaken to decrease the toxicity of these drugs. This exciting development will without doubt show progress in the years to come.

References

1. Bijlsma, J. W. J., Saag, K. G., Buttgereit, F., and da Silva, J. A. P. Developments in glucocorticoid therapy. *Rheum Dis Clin N Am* 2005; **31**: 1–17.
2. Bijlsma, J. W., Straub, R. H., Masi, A. T., Lahita, R. G., and Cutolo, M. Neuroendocrine immune mechanisms in rheumatic diseases. *Trends Immunol* 2002; **23**: 59–61.
3. Buttgereit, F., Straub, R. H., Wehling, M., and Burmester, G.-R. Glucocorticoids in the treatment of rheumatic diseases. *Arthritis Rheum* 2004; **50**: 3408–17.
4. Da Silva, J. A. P., Jacobs, J. W. G., Kirwan, J. R. *et al*. Low-dose glucocorticoid therapy in rheumatoid arthritis. A review on safety: published evidence and prospective trial data. *Ann Rheum Dis*, 2006; **65**: 285–293.
5. Buttgereit, F., da Silva J. A., Boers, M. *et al*. Standardised nomenclature for glucocorticoid dosages and glucocorticoid treatment regimens: current questions and tentative answers in rheumatology. *Ann Rheum Dis* 2002; **61**: 718–22.
6. Almawi, W. Y. Molecular mechanisms of glucocorticoid effects. *Mod Asp Immunobiol* 2001; **2**: 78–82.
7. Buttgereit, F., and Scheffold, A. Rapid glucocorticoid effects on immune cells. *Steroids* 2002; **67**: 529–34.
8. Bracken, M. B., Shepard, J. M., Collens, W. F. *et al*. A randomized controlled trial of methylprednisolone or naloxane in the treatment of acute spinal cord injury. *N Engl J Med* 1990; **322**: 1405–11.
9. Badsha, H., and Edwards, C. J. Intravenous pulses of methyprednisolone for systemic lupus erythematosus. *Sem Arthritis Rheum* 2003; **32**: 370–7.
10. Jacobs, J. W., Geenen, R., Evers, A. W. *et al*. Short term effects of corticosteroid pulse treatment on disease activity and the wellbeing of patients with active rheumatoid arthritis. *Ann Rheum Dis* 2001; **60**: 61–4.
11. Bartholome, B., Spies, C. M., Gaber, T. *et al*. Membrane glucocorticoid receptors (mGCR) are expressed in normal peripheral blood mononuclear cells and upregulated following in vitro stimulation and in patients with rheumatoid arthritis. *FASEB J* 2004; **18**: 70–80.
12. Boumpas, D. T., Chrousos, G. P., Wilder, R. L., Cupps, T. R., and Balow, J. E. Glucocorticoid therapy for immune-mediated diseases: basic and clinical correlates. *Ann Intern Med* 1993; **119**: 1198–208.
13. Leonard, J. P., and Silverstein, R. L. Corticosteroids and the haematopoietic system. In *Principles of corticosteroid therapy* (Lin AN, and Paget SA, eds), pp. 144–9. New York: Arnold; 2002.
14. Verhoef, C. M., van Roon, J. A., Vianen, M. E., Lafeber, F. P., and Bijlsma, J. W. The immune suppressive effect of dexamethasone in rheumatoid arthritis is accompanied by upregulation of interleukin 10 and by differential changes in interferon gamma and interleukin 4 production. *Ann Rheum Dis* 1999; **58**: 49–54.
15. Morand, E. F., Jefferiss, C. M., Dixey, J., Mitra, D., and Goulding, N. J. Impaired glucocorticoid induction of mononuclear leukocyte lipocortin-1 in rheumatoid arthritis. *Arthritis Rheum* 1994; **37**: 207–11.
16. Cronstein, B. N., Kimmel, S. C., Levin, R. I., Martiniuk, F., and Weissmann, G. A mechanism for the antiinflammatory effects of corticosteroids: the glucocorticoid receptor regulates leukocyte adhesion to endothelial cells and expression of endothelial-leukocyte adhesion molecule 1 and intercellular adhesion molecule 1. *Proc Natl Acad Sci U S A* 1992; **89**: 9991–5.
17. Di Rosa, M., Radomski, M., Carnuccio, R., and Moncada, S. Glucocorticoids inhibit the induction of nitric oxide synthase in macrophages. *Biochem Biophys Res Commun* 1990; **172**: 246–52.
18. DiBattista, J. A., Martel-Pelletier, J., Wosu, L. O. *et al*. Glucocorticoid receptor mediated inhibition of interleukin-1 stimulated neutral metalloprotease synthesis in normal human chondrocytes. *J Clin Endocrinol Metab* 1991; **72**: 316–26.
19. Cooper, M. S., and Stewart, P. M. Corticosteroid insufficiency in acutely ill patients. *N Engl J Med* 2003; **348**: 727–34.
20. Neeck, G. Fifty years of experience with cortisone therapy in the study and treatment of rheumatoid arthritis. *Ann N Y Acad Sci* 2002; **966**: 28–38.
21. Gudbjornsson, B., Skogseid, B., Oberg, K., Wide, L., and Hallgren, R. Intact adrenocorticotropic hormone secretion but impaired cortisol response in patients with active rheumatoid arthritis: effect of glucocorticoids. *J Rheumatol* 1996; **23**: 596–602.
22. Bijlsma, J. W., Cutolo, M., Masi, A. T., and Chikanza, I. C. The neuroendocrine immune basis of rheumatic diseases. *Immunol Today* 1999; **20**: 298–301.
23. Esteban, N. V., Loughlin, T., Yergey, A. L. *et al*. Daily cortisol production rate in man determined by stable isotope dilution/mass spectrometry. *J Clin Endocrinol Metab* 1991; **72**: 39–45.
24. AHFS Drug Information. Bethesda, MD: American Society of Health-System Pharmacists, Inc.; 2001.
25. Schlaghecke, R., Kornely, E., Santen, R. T., and Ridderskamp, P. The effect of long-term glucocorticoid therapy on pituitary-adrenal responses to exogenous corticotropin-releasing hormone. *N Engl J Med* 1992; **326**: 226–30
26. Van Everdingen, A. A., Jacobs, J. W., Siewertsz Van Reesema, D. R., and Bijlsma, J. W. Low-dose prednisone therapy for patients with early active rheumatoid arthritis: clinical efficacy, disease-modifying properties, and side effects. A randomized, double-blind, placebo-controlled clinical trial. *Ann Intern Med* 2002; **136**: 1–12.
27. Buttgereit, F., Saag, K. G., Cutolo, M., da Sila, J. A. P., and Bijlsma, J. W. J. The molecular basis for the effectiveness, toxicity, and resistance to glucocorticoids: focus on the treatment of rheumatoid arthritis. *Scand J Rheumatol* 2005; **34**: 1–8.
28. Chikanza, I. C., and Kozaci, D. L. Corticosteroid resistance in rheumatoid arthritis molecular and cellular perspectives. *Rheumatology* 2004; **43**: 1337–45.
29. Weinblatt, M. E., Kremer, J. M., Coblyn, J. S. *et al*. Pharmacokinetics, safety, and efficacy of combination treatment with methotrexate and leflunomide in patients with active rheumatoid arthritis. *Arthritis Rheum* 1999; **42**, 1322–8.
30. Thiele, K., Buttgereit, F., Huscher, D. *et al*. Current use of glucocorticoids in patients with rheumatoid arthritis in Germany. *Arthritis Rheum*. [In press.], 2005.
31. Buchanan, W. W., Stephen, L. J., and Buchanan, H. M. Are 'homeopathic' doses of oral corticosteroids effective in rheumatoid arthritis? *Clin Exp Rheumatol* 1988; **6**: 281–4.
32. ACR Subcommittee on Rheumatoid Arthritis Guidelines. Guidelines for the management of rheumatoid arthritis: update. *Arthritis Rheum* 2002; **46**: 328–46.

33. Criswell, L. A., Saag, K. G., Sems, K. M. *et al*. Moderate-term, low-dose corticosteroids for rheumatoid arthritis. *Cochrane Database Syst Rev*; 2000; CD001158.

34. Hansen, M., Podenphant, J., Florescu, A. *et al*. A randomised trial of differentiated prednisolone treatment in active rheumatoid arthritis: clinical benefits and skeletal side effects. *Ann Rheum Dis* 1999; **58**: 713–18.

35. Kirwan, J. R. The effect of glucocorticoids on joint destruction in rheumatoid arthritis. The Arthritis and Rheumatism Council Low-Dose Glucocorticoid Study Group. *N Engl J Med* 1995; **333**: 142–6.

36. Boers, M., Verhoeven, A. C., Markusse, H. M. *et al*. Randomised comparison of combined step-down prednisolone, methotrexate and sulphasalazine with sulphasalazine alone in early rheumatoid arthritis. *Lancet* 1997; **350**: 309–18.

37. Landewe, R. B., Boers, M., Verhoeven, A. C. *et al*. COBRA combination therapy in patients with early rheumatoid arthritis: long-term structural benefits of a brief intervention. *Arthritis Rheum* 2002; **46**: 347–56.

38. Wassenberg, S., Rau, R., Steinfeld, P., and Zeidler, H. Very low dose prednisolone in early rheumatoid arthritis retards Radiographic progresssion over two years. A multicenter, double-blind placebo controlled study. *Arteritis Rheum* 2005; **52**, 3371–80.

39. Jacobs, J. W. G., van Everdingen, A. A., Verstappen, S. M. M., and Bijlsma, J. W. J. The beneficial effect of low dose glucocorticoids in early RA persists after a 2-year-trial of 10 mg prednisone therapy versus placebo. *Arthritis Rheum*. 2006; [In press.]

40. Paulus, H. E., Di Primeo, D., Sanda, M. *et al*. Progression of radiographic joint erosion during low dose corticosteroid treatment of rheumatoid arthritis. *J Rheumatol* 2000; **27**: 1632–7.

41. Khanna, D., and Paulus, H. E. Corticosteroids. In *Rheumatoid Arthritis* (St. Clair, E. W., Pisetsky, D. S., and Haynes, B. F., eds), pp 283–302. Philadelphia: Lippincott Wiliams & Wilkins; 2004.

42. O'Dell, J. R. Treating rheumatoid arthritis early: a window of opportunity? *Arthritis Rheum* 2002; **46**: 283–5.

43. Jacobs, J. W. G., and Bijlsma, J. W. J. Glucocorticoid therapy. In *Kelley's Textbook of Rheumatology* (Harris ED, Budd RC, Firestein GS *et al*. eds), pp. 859–76. Philadelphia: Elsevier Saunders; 2005.

44. Neeck, G., Federlin, K., Graef, V. *et al*. Adrenal secretion of cortisol in patients with rheumatoid arthritis. *J Rheumatol* 1990; **17**: 24–9.

45. Dekkers, J. C., Geenen, R., Godaert, G. L. R. *et al*. Diurnal rhythm of salivary cortisol in patients with rheumatoid arthritis of recent onset. *Arthritis Rheum* 2000; **43**: 465–6.

46. Arvidson, N. G., Gudbjornsson, B., Larsson, A., and Hallgren, R. The timing of glucocorticoid administration in rheumatoid arthritis. *Ann Rheum Dis* 1997; **56**: 27–31.

47. Kimura, Y., Fieldston, E., Devries-Vandervlugt, B., Li, S., and Imundo, L. High dose, alternate day corticosteroids for systemic onset juvenile rheumatoid arthritis. *J Rheumatol* 2000; **27**: 2018–24.

48. Tanner, A. R., Caffin, J. A., Halliday, J. W., and Powell, L. W. Concurrent administration of antacids and prednisone: effect on serum levels of prednisolone. *Br J Clin Pharmacol* 1979; **7**: 397–400.

49. Evans, P. J., Walker, R. F., Peters, J. R., Dyas, J., Riad-Fahmy, D., Thomas, J. P. *et al*. Anticonvulsant therapy and cortisol elimination. *Br J Clin Pharmacol* 1985; **20**: 129–32.

50. Kyriazopoulou, V., Parparousi, O., and Vagenakis, A. G. Rifampicin-induced adrenal crisis in addisonian patients receiving corticosteroid replacement therapy. *J Clin Endocrinol Metab* 1984; **59**: 1204–6.

51. Gustavson, L. E., Legler, U. F., and Benet, L. Z. Impairment of prednisolone disposition in women taking oral contraceptives or conjugated estrogens. *J Clin Endocrinol Metab* 1986; **62**: 234–7.

52. LaForce, C. F., Szefler, S. J., Miller, M. F., Ebling, W., and Brenner, M. Inhibition of methylprednisolone elimination in the presence of erythromycin therapy. *J Allergy Clin Immunol* 1983; **72**: 34–9.

53. Zurcher, R. M., Frey, B. M., and Frey, F. J. Impact of ketoconazole on the metabolism of prednisolone. *Clin Pharmacol Ther* 1989; **45**: 366–72.

54. Rae, S. A., Williams, I. A., English, J., and Baylis, E. M. Alteration of plasma prednisolone levels by indomethacin and naproxen. *Br J Clin Pharmacol* 1982; **14**: 459–61.

55. Kaufman, M. Treatment of multiple sclerosis with high-dose corticosteroids may prolong the prothrombin time to dangerous levels in patients taking warfarin. *Mult Scler* 1997; **3**: 248–9.

56. Klinenberg, J. R., and Miller, F. Effect of corticosteroids on blood salicylate concentration. *JAMA* 1965; **194**: 601–4.

57. Weusten, B. L., Jacobs, J. W., and Bijlsma, J. W. Corticosteroid pulse therapy in active rheumatoid arthritis. *Semin Arthritis Rheum* 1993; **23**: 183–92.

58. Buttgereit, F., Burmester, G. R., and Bijlsma, J. W. Which dose regimen for glucocorticoid pulse therapy in patients with severe refractory RA? *Ann Rheum Dis* 2005; **64**: 171–2.

59. Gaffney, K., Ledingham, J., Perry, J. D. Intra-articular triamcinolone hexacetonide in knee osteoarthritis: factors influencing the clinical response. *Ann Rheum Dis* 1995; **54**: 379–81.

60. McCarty, D. J., Harman, J. G., Grassanovich, J. L., and Qian, C. Treatment of rheumatoid joint inflammation with intrasynovial triamcinolone hexacetonide. *J Rheumatol* 1995; **22**: 1631–5.

61. Weitoft, T., and Uddenfeldt, P. Importance of synovial fluid aspiration when injecting intra-articular corticosteroids. *Ann Rheum Dis* 2000; **59**: 233–5.

62. Blyth, T., Hunter, J. A., and Stirling, A. Pain relief in the rheumatoid knee after steroid injection: a single-blind comparison of hydrocortisone succinate, and triamcinolone acetonide or hexacetonide. *Br J Rheumatol* 1994; **33**: 461–3.

63. Chakravarty, K., Pharoah, P. D., and Scott, D. G. A randomized controlled study of post-injection rest following intra-articular steroid therapy for knee synovitis. *Br J Rheumatol* 1994; **33**: 464–8.

64. Eustace, J. A., Brophy, D. P., Gibney, R. P., Bresnihan, B., and Fitzgerald, O. Comparison of the accuracy of steroid placement with clinical outcome in patients with shoulder symptoms. *Ann Rheum Dis* 1997; **56**: 59–63.

65. Gray, R. G., Tenenbaum, J., and Gottlieb, N. L. Local corticosteroid injection treatment in rheumatic disorders. *Sem Arthritis Rheum* 1981; **10**: 231–54.

66. Seror, P., Pluvinage, P., d'Andre, F. L., Benamou, P., and Attuil, G. Frequency of sepsis after local corticosteroid injection (an inquiry on 1160000 injections in rheumatological private practice in France). *Rheumatology (Oxford)* 1999; **38**: 1272–4.

67. Kaandorp, C. J., Krijnen, P., Moens, H. J., Habbema, J. D., and van Schaardenburg, D. The outcome of bacterial arthritis: a prospective community-based study. *Arthritis Rheum* 1997; **40**: 884–92.

68. Mens, J. M., Nico, d. W., Berkhout, B. J., and Stam, H. J. Disturbance of the menstrual pattern after local injection with triamcinolone acetonide. *Ann Rheum Dis* 1998; **57**: 700.

69. DeSio, J. M., Kahn, C. H., and Warfield, C. A. Facial flushing and/or generalized erythema after epidural steroid injection. *Anesth Analg* 1995; **80**: 617–19.

70. Black, D. M., and Filak, A. T. Hyperglycemia with non-insulin-dependent diabetes following intraarticular steroid injection. *J Fam Pract* 1989; **28**: 462–3.

71. DiStefano, V., and Nixon, J. E. Skin and fat atrophy complications of local steroid injection. *Pa Med* 1974; **77**: 38.

72. Stapczynski, J. S. Localized depigmentation after steroid injection of a ganglion cyst on the hand. *Ann Emerg Med* 1991; **20**: 807–9.

73. Linskey, M. E., and Segal, R. Median nerve injury from local steroid injection in carpal tunnel syndrome. *Neurosurgery* 1990; **26**: 512–15.

74. Pincus, T., Marcum, S. B., Callahan, L. F. *et al*. Longterm drug therapy for rheumatoid arthritis in seven rheumatology private practices. II. Second line drugs and prednisone. *J Rheumatol* 1992; **19**: 1885–94.

75. Fries, J. F., Williams, C. A., Ramey, D., and Bloch, D. A. The relative toxicity of disease-modifying antirheumatic drugs. *Arthritis Rheum* 1993; **36**: 297–306.

76. Capell, H. A., Madhok, R., Hunter, J. A., Porter, D., Morrison, E., Larkin, J. *et al*. Lack of radiological and clinical benefit over two years of low dose prednisolone for rheumatoid arthritis: results of a randomized controlled trial. *Ann Rheum Dis* 2004; **63**: 797–803.

77. Kautzky-Willer, A., Thomaseth, K., Clodi, M., Ludvik, B., Waldhausl, W., Prager, R. *et al*. Beta-cell activity and hepatic insulin extraction following dexamethasone administration in healthy subjects. *Metabolism* 1996; **45**: 486–91.

78. Olefsky, J. M., Kimmerling, G. Effects of glucocorticoids on carbohydrate metabolism. *Am J Med Sci* 1976: **271**, 202–10.

79. Gurwitz, J. H., Bohn, R. L., Glynn, R. J., Monane, M., Mogun, H., and Avorn, J. Glucocorticoids and the risk for initiation of hypoglycemic therapy. *Arch Intern Med* 1994; **154**: 97–101.

80. Hirsch, I. B., and Paauw, D. S. Diabetes management in special situations. *Endocrinol Metab Clin North Am* 1997; **26**: 631–45.

81. Hricik, D. E., Bartucci, M. R., Moir, E. J., Mayes, J. T., and Schulak, J. A. Effects of steroid withdrawal on posttransplant diabetes mellitus in cyclosporine-treated renal transplant recipients. *Transplantation* 1991; **51**: 374–7.

82. Liapi, C., and Chrousos, G. P. Glucocorticoids. In *Pediatric pharmacology* (Yaffe SJ, Arand JV, eds), pp. 466–75. Philadelphia, WB Saunders, 1992.

83. Greenstone, M. A., and Shaw, A. B. Alternate day corticosteroid causes alternate day hyperglycaemia. *Postgrad Med J* 1987; **63**: 761–4.

84. Hoogwerf, B., and Danese, R. D. Drug selection and the management of corticosteroid-related diabetes mellitus. *Rheum Dis Clin North Am* 1999; **25**: 489–505.

85. Stewart, P. M., and Tomlinson, J. W. Cortisol, 11 beta-hydroxysteroid dehydrogenase type 1 and central obesity. *Trends Endocrinol Metab* 2002; **13**: 94–6.

86. Tataranni, P. A., Larson, D. E., Snitker, S., Young, J. B., Flatt, J. P., and Ravussin, E. Effects of glucocorticoids on energy metabolism and food intake in humans. *Am J Physiol* 1996; **271**: E317–E325.

87. Hampson, G., Bhargava, N., Cheung, J., Vaja, S., Seed, P. T., and Fogelman, I. Low circulating estradiol and adrenal androgens concentrations in men on glucocorticoids: a potential contributory factor in steroid-induced osteoporosis. *Metabolism* 2002; **51**: 1458–62.

88. Manolagas, S. C., and Weinstein, R. S. New developments in the pathogenesis and treatment of steroid-induced osteoporosis. *J Bone Miner Res* 1999; **14**: 1061–6.

89. Nishimura, J., and Ikuyama, S. Glucocorticoid-induced osteoporosis: pathogenesis and management. *J Bone Miner Metab* 2000; **18**: 350–2.

90. Sambrook. P., and Lane, N. E., Corticosteroid osteoporosis. *Best Pract Res Clin Rheumatol* 2001; **15**: 401–13.

91. Bijlsma, J. W. J. Prevention of GC induced osteoporosis. *Ann Rheum Dis* 1997; **56**: 507–9.

92. Van Staa, T. P., Leufkens, H. G., and Cooper, C. The epidemiology of corticosteroid-induced osteoporosis: a meta-analysis. *Osteoporos Int* 2002; **13**: 777–87.

93. Laan, R. F., van Riel, P. L., van de Putte, L. B., van Erning, L. J., van't Hof, M. A., and Lemmens, J. A. Low-dose prednisone induces rapid reversible axial bone loss in patients with rheumatoid arthritis: a randomized, controlled study. *Ann Intern Med* 1993; **119**: 963–8.

94. De Nijs, R. N., Jacobs, J. W., Bijlsma, J. W., Lems, W. F., Laan, R. F., Houben, H. H. *et al.* Prevalence of vertebral deformities and symptomatic vertebral fractures in corticosteroid treated patients with rheumatoid arthritis. *Rheumatology (Oxford)* 2001; **40**: 1375–83.

95. Lodder, M. C., Lems, W. F., Kostense, P. J., Verhoeven, A. C., Dijkmans, B. A., and Boers, M. Bone loss due to glucocorticoids: update of a systematic review of prospective studies in rheumatoid arthritis and other diseases. *Ann Rheum Dis* 2003; **62**: 94.

96. Anonymous. Recommendations for the prevention and treatment of glucocorticoid-induced osteoporosis: 2001 update. American College of Rheumatology Ad Hoc Committee on Glucocorticoid-Induced Osteoporosis. *Arthritis Rheum* 2001; **44**: 1496–503.

97. The Royal College of Physicians, The Bone and Tooth Society of Great Britain, The National Osteoporosis Society. *Glucocorticoid-Induced Osteoporosis: Guidelines for Prevention and Treatment*. London, Royal College of Physicians. 2002.

98. Geusens, P. P., de Nijs, R. J., Lems, W. F. *et al.* Prevention of glucocorticoid osteoporosis: a consensus document of the Dutch Society of Rheumatology. *Ann Rheum Dis* 2004; **63**: 324–5.

99. Vreden, S. G., Hermus, A. R., van Liessum, P. A., Pieters, G. F., Smals, A. G., and Kloppenborg, P. W. Aseptic bone necrosis in patients on glucocorticoid replacement therapy. *Neth J Med* 1991; **39**, 153–7.

100. Danneskiold-Samsoe, B., and Grimby, G. The influence of prednisone on the muscle morphology and muscle enzymes in patients with rheumatoid arthritis. *Clin Sci (Lond)* 1986; **71**: 693–701.

101. Moxley, R. T. Metabolic and endocrine myopathies. In *Disorders of Voluntary Muscle* (Walton, J. N., Karpati, G., and Jones, D. H., eds), pp. 647–716. Edinburgh, Churchill Livingstone. 1994.

102. Dale, D. C., Fauci, A. S., and Wolff, S. M. Alternate-day prednisone: leukocyte kinetics and susceptibility to infections. *N Engl J Med* 1974; **291**: 1154–8.

103. Stracher, A. R., and Soave, R. Infectious complications of corticosteroid therapy. In *Principles of corticosteroid therapy* (Linn AN, and Paget SA, eds), pp. 419–30. London, Arnold. 2002.

104. Stuck, A. E., Minder, C. E., Frey, F. J. Risk of infectious complications in patients taking glucocorticosteroids. *Rev Infect Dis* 1989; **11**: 954–63.

105. Saag, K. G., Koehnke, R., Caldwell, J. R., Brasington, R., Burmeister, L. F., Zimmerman, B. *et al.* Low dose long-term corticosteroid therapy in rheumatoid arthritis: an analysis of serious adverse events. *Am J Med* 1994; **96**: 115–23.

106. Becker, D. M., Chamberlain, B., Swank, R., Hegewald, M. G., Girardet, R., Baughman, K. L. *et al.* Relationship between corticosteroid exposure and plasma lipid levels in heart transplant recipients. *Am J Med* 1998; **85**: 632–8.

107. Pasceri, V., and Yeh, E. T. H. A tale of two diseases: atherosclerosis and rheumatoid arthritis [editorial]. *Circulation* 1999; **100**: 2124–6.

108. Park, Y. B., Ahn, C. W., Choi, H. K., Lee, S. H., In, B. H., Lee, H. C. *et al.* Atherosclerosis in rheumatoid arthritis: morphologic evidence obtained by carotid ultrasound. *Arthritis Rheum* 2002; **46**: 1714–19.

109. Munford, R. S. Statins and the acute-phase response. *N Engl J Med* 2001; **344**: 2016–18.

110. Boers, M., Nurmohamed, M. T., Doelman, C. J., Lard, L. R., Verhoeven, A. C., Voskuyl, A. E. *et al.* Influence of glucocorticoids and disease activity on total and high density lipoprotein cholesterol in patients with rheumatoid arthritis. *Ann Rheum Dis* 2003; **62**: 842–5.

111. Wei, L., MacDonald, T. M., and Walker, B. R. Taking glucocorticoids by prescription is associated with subsequent cardiovascular disease. *Ann Intern Med* 2004; **141**: 764–70.

112. Whitworth, J. A., Gordon, D., Andrews, J., and Scoggins, B. A. The hypertensive effect of synthetic glucocorticoids in man: role of sodium and volume. *J Hypertens* 1989; **7**: 537–49.

113. Mason, J. W., O'Connell, J. B., Herskowitz, A., Rose, N. R., McManus, B. M., Billingham, M. E. *et al.* A clinical trial of immunosuppressive therapy for myocarditis. The Myocarditis Treatment Trial Investigators. *N Engl J Med* 1995; **333**: 269–75.

114. Whitworth, J. A. Mechanisms of glucocorticoid-induced hypertension. *Kidney Int* 1987; **31**: 1213–24.

115. Smith, R. S., and Warren, D. Effects of high-dose intravenous methylprednisolone on circulation in humans. *Transplantation* 1983; **35**: 349–51.

116. Piper, J. M., Ray, W. A., Daugherty, J. R., and Griffin, M. R. Corticosteroid use and peptic ulcer disease: role of nonsteroidal anti-inflammatory drugs. *Ann Intern Med* 1991; **114**: 735–40.

117. Garcia Rodriguez, L. A., and Hernandez-Diaz, S. The risk of upper gastrointestinal complications associated with nonsteroidal anti-inflammatory drugs, glucocorticoids, acetaminophen, and combinations of these agents. *Arthritis Res* 2001; **3**: 98–101.

118. Carone, F. A., and Liebow, A. A. Acute pancreatic lesions in patients treated with ACTH and adrenal corticoids. *N Engl J Med* 1957; **257**: 690–7.

119. Wolverton, S. E. Corticosteroids and the integument. In *Principles of corticosteroid therapy* (Lin AN, and Paget SA, eds), pp. 166–72. London; Arnold; 2002.

120. Covar, R. A., Leung, D. Y., McCormick, D., Steelman, J. Zeitler, P. and Spahn, J. D. Risk factors associated with glucocorticoid-induced adverse effects in children with severe asthma. *J Allergy Clin Immunol* 2000; **106**: 651–9.

121. Caldwell, J. R., and Furst, D. E. The efficacy and safety of low-dose corticosteroids for rheumatoid arthritis. *Semin Arthritis Rheum* 1991; **21**: 1–11.

122. Klein, R., Klein, B. E., Lee, K. E., Cruickshanks, K. J., and Chappell, R. J. Changes in visual acuity in a population over a 10-year period: The Beaver Dam Eye Study. *Ophthalmology* 2001; **108**: 1757–66.

123. Tripathi, R. C., Parapuram, S. K., Tripathi, B. J., Zhong, Y., and Chalam, K. V. Corticosteroids and glaucoma risk. *Drugs Aging* 1999; **15**: 439–50.

124. Stone, E. M., Fingert, J. H., Alward, W. L., Nguyen, T. D., Polansky, J. R., Sunden, S. L. *et al.* Identification of a gene that causes primary open angle glaucoma. *Science* 1997; **275**: 668–70.

125. Gourley, M. F., Austin, H. A., III, Scott, D., Yarboro, C. H., Vaughan, E. M., Muir, J. *et al.* Methylprednisolone and cyclophosphamide, alone or in combination, in patients with lupus nephritis: a randomized, controlled trial. *Ann Intern Med* 1996; **125** 549–57.

126. Patten, S. B., and Neutel, C. I. Corticosteroid-induced adverse psychiatric effects: incidence, diagnosis and management. *Drug Saf* 2000; **22**: 111–22.

127. Reckart, M. D., and Eisendrath, S. J. Exogenous corticosteroid effects on mood and cognition: case presentations. *Int J Psychosom* 1990; **37**: 57–61.

128. Song, I. H., Gold, R., Straub, R. H., Burmester, G. R., and Buttgereit, F. New glucocorticoids on the horizon. *J Rheumatology* 2005; **32**: 1199–207.

129. Buttgereit, F., Burmester, G. R., and Lipworth, B. J. Optimized glucocorticoid therapy: the sharpening of an old spear. *Lancet* 2005; **365**: 801–3.

130. Schäcke, H., Schottelius, A., Döcke, W. D. *et al.* Dissociation of transactivation from transrepression by a selective glucocorticoid receptor agonist leads to separation of therapeutic effects from side effects. *Proc Natl Acad Sci U S A* 2004; **101**: 227–32.

131. Lin, C. W., Nakane, M., Stashko, M. *et al.* Trans-Activation and repression properties of the novel nonsteroid glucocorticoid receptor ligand 2,5-dihydro-9-hydroxy-10-methoxy-2,2,4-trimethyl-5-(1-methylcyclohexen-3-y1)-1H-[1] benzopyrano [3,4-f] quinoline (A276575) and its four stereoisomers. *Mol Pharmacol* 2002; **62**: 297–303.

132. Coghlan, M. J., Jacobson, P. B., Lane, B. *et al.* A novel anti-inflammatory maintains glucocorticoid efficacy with reduced side effects. *Mol Endocrinol* 2003; **17**: 860–9.

133. Perretti, M., Paul-Clark, M. J., Mancini, L., and Flower, R. J. Generation of innovative anti-inflammatory and anti-arthritic glucocorticoid derivatives that release NO: the nitro-steroids. *Dig Liver Dis* 35 (Suppl. 2), 2003; 41–8.

134. Paul-Clark, M. J., Gilroy, D. W., Willis, D., Willoughby, D. A., and Tomlinson, A. Nitric oxide synthase inhibitors have opposite effects on acute inflammation depending on their route of administration. *J Immunol* 2001; **166**: 1169–77.

135. Paul-Clark, M. J., Mancini, L., Del Soldato, P. *et al.* Potent antiarthritic properties of a glucocorticoid derivative, NCX-1015, in an experimental model of arthritis. *Proc Natl Acad Sci U S A* 2002; **99**: 1677–82.

136. Walker, E. A., and Stewart, P. M. 11β-hydroxysteroid dehydrogenase: unexpected connections. *Trends Endocrinol Metab* 2003; **14**: 334–9.

137. Stewart, P. M., and Krozowski, Z. S. 11b-hydroxysteroid dehydrogenase. *Vitam Horm* 1999; **57**: 249–324.

138. Bujalska, I. J. Differentiation of adipose stromal cells: the role of glucocorticoids and 11β-hydroxysteroid dehydrogenase. *Endocrinology* 1999; **140**: 3188.

139. Cutolo, M., and Masi, A. T. Circadian rhythms. *Rheum Dis Clin N Am* 2005; **31**: 115–29.

140. Metselaar, J. M., Wauben, M. H. M., Wagenaar-Hilbers, J. P. A. *et al.* Complete remission of experimental arthritis by joint long-circulating liposomes. *Arthritis Rheum* 2003; **48**: 2059–66.

141. Metselaar, J. M., Van den Berg, W. B., Holthuysen, A. E. M. *et al.* Liposomal targeting of glucocorticoids to synovial lining cells strongly increases therapeutic benefit in collagen type II arthritis. *Ann Rheum Dis* 2004; **63**: 348–53.

24 | *The new frontiers in pathogenesis and treatment: methotrexate and leflunomide*

Rolf Rau

Methotrexate

Introduction

In 1947, aminopterin was synthesized as an antifolate for the treatment of tumors. Four years later, Gubner[1] reported the successful treatment of seven patients with rheumatoid arthritis (RA) with aminopterin. Methotrexate (MTX) (amethopterin), synthesized in 1948, proved to be less toxic than aminopterin and more feasible for longer term treatment. However, because of the dramatic effects of corticosteroids in the treatment of RA, few rheumatologists were interested in MTX. The first pilot studies only appeared in the early 1980s, encouraging a systematic evaluation of low-dose MTX treatment in RA.

The introduction of MTX is one of the major achievements in the pharmacotherapy of RA. MTX is very effective, has a relatively rapid onset of action, is well tolerated, and can be prescribed in a wide dose range, taking into account the needs of each individual patient. Today, MTX is the most widely used disease-modifying anti-rheumatic drug (DMARD) worldwide, and most DMARD combinations use MTX as one of their components. MTX also adds to the efficacy of tumor necrosis factor-α (TNF-α) blockers.

Pharmacokinetics

Bioavailability

Bioavailability of MTX decreases with increasing dose. With low doses it is ~70%. In the same individual, absorption remains constant with doses of 7.5 mg but decreases by 13.5% at the maintenance dose of 17 mg. Taking the drug after meals does not change the absorption rate significantly.

Plasma kinetics

After low oral dosage (7.5–15 mg/week) peak plasma concentrations ranged between 0.31 and 0.72 μM. Synovial fluid concentrations are comparable to plasma concentrations. Glomerular filtration eliminates 50–80% of the drug unchanged, with a half-life of 2–4 h[2]. The mean renal clearance is 110 mL/min/m²; 9–26% of MTX is eliminated through the bile. The terminal phase of MTX excretion refers to enterohepatic circulation and release from tissues. Total half-life ranges between 6 and 7 h.

Impaired renal function and older age may lead to decreased clearance and increased toxicity.

Metabolism

Less than 50% of MTX is bound to plasma proteins. Approximately 10% is oxidized to 7- Hydroxy-MTX, a less potent inhibitor of dihydrofolate reductase. Both enter the cells in polyglutamated forms (MTX-glu), maintaining constant concentrations over one week.

Drug interactions

Displacement of MTX from its binding to plasma proteins by aspirin and non-steroidal anti-inflammatory drugs (NSAIDs) has only minor impact since less than 50% of MTX is bound to plasma proteins. However, NSAIDs and aspirin may significantly reduce renal MTX clearance. This did not affect pharmacokinetic variables at weekly doses of 7.5 mg, but reduced the renal clearance of both MTX and creatinine by 20% at mean doses of 17 mg/week[3]. There are substantial inter-individual variations regarding drug interactions, and single cases with severe side-effects due to drug interactions have been reported. Long-term corticosteroid therapy reduced MTX clearance by ~20%, but short-term administration of 15 mg did not affect MTX pharmacokinetics[4]. Probenecid also decreases MTX clearance, leading to an increase of the 24 h plasma levels of up to 400%.

Mechanism of action

The mechanism of action of MTX in the treatment of RA is still incompletely understood. MTX is an antifolate with a chemical structure similar to that of folic acid and folinic acid (Fig. 24.1). MTX inhibits dihydrofolate reductase (DHFR), thereby preventing the reduction of folic acid to tetrahydrofolic acid, which is needed for the synthesis of pyrimidines and purines. The polyglutamyl derivatives of MTX are even stronger inhibitors of DHFR and several other important folate dependent enzymes in the purine biosynthesis pathway, that is, aminoimidazole–carboxamide–ributide–transformylase (AICAR-transformylase) and thymidilate-synthetase[5]. The role of adenosine as an important factor for the anti-inflammatory effects of MTX[6] has been questioned: in rat adjuvant arthritis there was no attenuation of anti-arthritic effects when adenosine antagonists were combined with MTX[7]. Moreover, 24 h urinary adenosine excretion was not elevated with MTX treatment, while AICA (substrate of AICAR-transformylase) excretion was elevated[8]. This may indicate some blockade in purine nucleotide biosynthesis. Folinic acid blocked the increase of AICA while folic acid in low dose did not, presumably because MTX blocks folate reduction by inhibiting DHFR[8]. The mechanism of action is illustrated in Fig. 24.2.

Immune system

Profound immunosuppressive effects have not been demonstrated with low-dose MTX treatment in RA. However, after antigen-stimulated proliferation of lymphocytes, proliferation of fibroblasts, the clonal growth of T and B cells, and IgM-RF production by mononuclear cells can be inhibited by adding MTX at therapeutic concentrations[9,10].

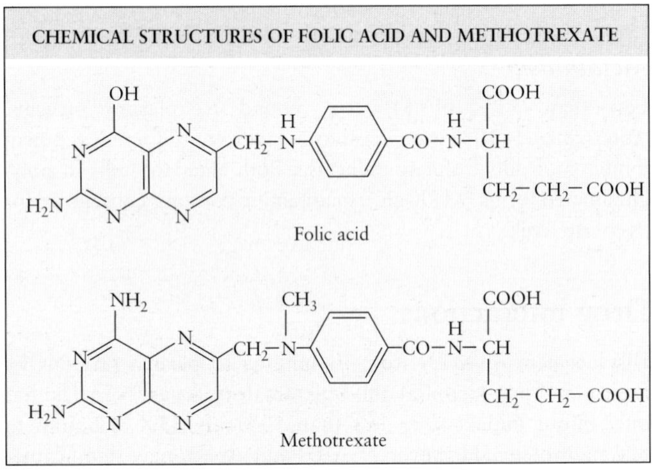

CHEMICAL STRUCTURES OF FOLIC ACID AND METHOTREXATE

Folic acid

Methotrexate

© www.rheumtext.com–Hochberg et al. (eds)

Fig. 24.1 Chemical structures of folic acid and methotrexate.

Cytokines

Several studies examined the influence of MTX on the production and activity of different cytokines. MTX significantly decreased the production of interleukin (IL)-1 in experimental arthritis. In RA patients, MTX sharply decreased IL-1 production by mononuclear cells *ex vivo* while IL-1 serum concentrations remained unchanged[11]. *In vitro* inhibition of IL-1 production by MTX can be abolished by folinic acid[12]. Liposome preparations of MTX dramatically inhibit TNF-α production *in vitro*. In adjuvant arthritis MTX decreased TNF-α concentrations in the synovial fluid, while in RA patients TNF-α concentrations remained unchanged[13]. Soluble IL-2 receptors (sIL2R) are elevated in active RA but decline with MTX treatment[14]. The production of the pro-inflammatory cytokines IL-6 and IL-8 are inhibited by MTX[15,16]. Enhanced *in vitro* production of IL-10 by peripheral blood mononuclear cells is associated with clinical response to MTX treatment[17]. Albumin-coupled MTX is significantly superior to MTX in suppressing collagen-induced arthritis. This confirms the prominent role of peripheral blood (PB) mononuclear cells (MCs) as a target of MTX since albumin is taken up by a high percentage of PBMCs in patients with RA[18].

The *in vitro* modulation of the cytokine network by MTX, increasing Th2 cytokines, and decreasing Th1 cytokines could explain its anti-inflammatory and immunoregulatory actions *in vivo*[19]. Synovial tissue metalloproteinase levels decrease after MTX therapy.

Anti-inflammatory effects

A rapid anti-inflammatory action is indicated by a significant decrease of C-reactive protein (CRP) and erythrocyte sedimentation rate (ESR) within days of a single MTX injection. Blood concentrations of hypoxanthine and uric acid even decrease within 2 h[20]. In different animal models of arthritis an inhibition of macrophage activation, granuloma formation, and lymphoid cell infiltration has been demonstrated. MTX decreases chemotaxis of polymorphonuclear

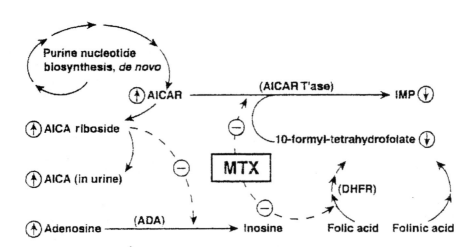

Fig. 24.2 Effect of MTX on folate and purine metabolism. AICAR, 5-aminoimidazole-4-carboxamide ribonucleotide; T'ase, transformylase; IIMP, inosine monophosphate; AICA, 5-aminoimidazole-4-carboxamide; ADA adenosine deaminase; DHFR = dihydrofolate reductase. Broken lines with encircled minus signs indicate inhibition of enzymes by MTX and AICA riboside. Encircled arrows indicate an increase (↑) or a decrease (↓) in metabolite levels when MTX inhibits DHFR or AICAR transformylase and when AICA riboside inhibits ADA. Note that folinic acid, but not folic acid, can bypass MTX inhibition of DHFR and replete pools of 10-formyl-tetrahydrofolate. (From Ref. 8, reproduced with permission).

Table 24.1 Long-term observational studies (selection)

Author	Year	n	Type of study	Disease duration (years)	Treatment duration in months (range)	Dose (mg/week)	Efficacy	Treatment continued (%)	After years
Kremer[29]	1992	29	Prospective	11.7	90 (79–107)	11.7	Good	62	71/2
Weinblatt[30]	1992	26	Prospective	8.9	84	10.2	Good	46	7
Sany[32]	1991	191	Prospective	8.5	19 (3–58)	10.2	Good	46	5
Hanrahan[33]	1989	128	Prospective	12	22 (1–60)	12.8	Moderate	50	5
Rau[37]	1997	271	Prospective	8.5	31.4 (1–108)	12.1	Good	60	5
Krause[34]	2000	271	Prospective	8.5	120 (12–198)	11.7	Good	60	10
Bologna[100]	1997	453	Retrospective	–	35 (3–106)	–	Good	73	5
Wluka[39]	2000	460	Retrospective	7.5	105 (40.4)	–	–	53 (17)[a]	–
Hoekstra[36]	2003	1022	Retrospective	4.0	–	9.2	–	50[b]	9

[a] If treatment discontinuation over three months was classified as termination the number was 38%; if patients starting a combination treatment were also excluded the number was 17%.
[b] Probability of being treated.

cells, activation and migration of neutrophils through capillary membranes, and leucotriene-B4 induced infiltration of psoriatic skin. MTX also reduces *in vitro* prostaglandin-E2 release and substantially inhibits neutrophil chemotaxis in RA. Cronstein has reviewed the molecular mechanisms of action of MTX[6,21].

Clinical efficacy

Placebo-controlled studies

In the early 1980s, 30 years after the first report by Gubner[1], open pilot studies indicated effectiveness of 7.5–15 mg MTX weekly in RA patients not responding to conventional DMARDs[22–24]. Between 1984 and 1989, four randomized, placebo-controlled trials over 6–26 weeks with weekly oral MTX doses of 7.5–25 mg demonstrated a significant improvement in the patients' clinical status[25]. A significant dose–response relationship of MTX was documented[26], and confirmed in terms of a rapid and excellent response to weekly intravenous (IV) doses of up to 50 mg[27]. Switching patients with incomplete response to 15–20 mg oral MTX weekly to 15 mg MTX intramuscular (IM) weekly improved the DAS28. However, further dose escalation up to 45 mg MTX IM did not seem to improve disease control further[28].

Long-term observational studies

Multiple, carefully monitored, long-term observational studies have documented lasting clinical effectiveness and good tolerability of MTX with low discontinuation rates[29–36] (Table 24.1). Most patients included in these studies suffered from long-lasting disease unresponsive to previous DMARD treatment. MTX improved all clinical and laboratory measures of disease activity significantly, with the peak effect reached after six months, usually sustained during the entire follow-up period. Marked improvement (>50%) in the number of swollen joints occurred in more than 50%[37] and 69%[31] of patients. Clinical remissions according to the American College of Rheumatology (ACR) criteria, however, were infrequent and are difficult to achieve in patients with severe destructive disease.

A long adherence to a treatment can serve as a surrogate for both good tolerability and effectiveness. 'Drug survival rates' of more than five years occurred in over 50% of patients. MTX treatment was continued substantially longer than treatment with other DMARDs in routine clinical care[38]. In community-based practice the probability of treatment continuation was found to be 64–75% after 5 and 6 years and ~50% after 9 and 12 years, respectively[36,39]. However, due to withdrawals for side-effects, two other studies showed no difference regarding continuation of treatment after four years between MTX and other DMARDs[40]. A selection of long-term observational studies is shown in Table 24.1.

One of the reasons for the long treatment continuation of MTX is the ability to adjust the dose in a wide range to the needs of the individual patient. The patient must be observed carefully and a reliable effective/highest-tolerated dose maintained; otherwise an initially improved disability index may deteriorate again and reach baseline values after ~8 years[35]. In patients older than 65 years, MTX was shown to be equally effective.

MTX has an eminent steroid-sparing effect since in all studies documenting the steroid dose it could be significantly reduced. Effective MTX treatment was also shown to increase life expectancy: after a mean observation period of 10 years in 271 patients with severe RA, the standardized mortality ratio (SMR) was 1.47 in patients who had improved by >50% after one year of treatment, 1.85 in those with a 20–50% improvement, and 4.11 in patients who had not improved[34]. In a cohort of 1240 patients from Wichita the 'mortality hazard ratio' for MTX use after adjustment for confounding factors was 0.4 when compared with RA patients with no MTX use set as 1.0[41]. Healing of erosive changes with MTX monotherapy has also been documented[42].

Effect on X-ray progression

The most important goal of treatment is to inhibit damage progression. Inhibition of progression as seen on radiographs is one of the most important criteria by which to judge the effectiveness of a DMARD. In most long-term studies documenting radiographic outcomes, most patients demonstrated ongoing progression under MTX treatment[29,30,37]. However, these patients still had clinically active disease, while patients who achieved a clinical remission displayed an arrest of progression[29,30,37]. When comparing a period of clinically insufficient pretreatment with the following period of effective MTX treatment in 18 RA patients, there was no difference in radiological progression[43]. In another study, the progression rate during MTX treatment was significantly reduced when compared to a pretreatment period[44]. In 31 patients who switched to MTX because of rapid radiographic progression, the mean progression was significantly reduced during 3.9 years of MTX treatment when compared with a mean observation period of 2.2 years while on treatment with other DMARDs[45]. In a three-year study comparing IM gold with IM MTX there was a significant flattening of the progression curve with time in both groups[46,47]. Further studies confirmed a reduction of progression with MTX treatment[48,49]. All these observations confirm that MTX delays radiological progression in patients that also respond clinically.

Comparison with other DMARDs

The relative efficacy and toxicity of MTX in comparison with other DMARDs has been investigated in several studies. MTX doses of 7.5–15 mg weekly were superior to 6–9 mg auranofin daily in improving disease activity, and caused fewer withdrawals, while in another study 7.5 mg MTX weekly and 6 mg auranofin/day were equally effective. A meta-analysis of clinical trials in 3957 patients found MTX to be more effective than auranofin and comparable to D-penicillamine and parenteral gold[56].

Three clinical trials found no significant difference in clinical improvement between parenteral gold and MTX, while MTX appeared to be slightly less toxic. In 174 patients with active early erosive RA parenteral MTX (15 mg weekly) and parenteral gold (50 mg weekly) improved all disease activity parameters significantly by >50% after one and three years without significant inter-group differences. Marked improvement (>50%) occurred in 68% of patients treated with MTX and 76% of patients treated with gold. Tolerability was significantly better with MTX[50,51]. In 141 patients all efficacy parameters improved significantly with parenteral gold or MTX treatment by 24 weeks without differences in efficacy; but gold caused significantly more withdrawals for toxicity[52].

Two trials have demonstrated more clinical benefit from treatment with MTX than with azathioprine[53,54]. A selection of comparative studies is shown on Table 24.2.

Leflunomide achieved higher ACR20/50/70 response rates than MTX supplemented with 1–2 mg folic acid per day in a large American one-year study[57]. The ACR response rates were maintained over 24 months[58]. In a European study, where only 10% of MTX-treated patients had folate supplementation, all efficacy parameters were significantly more improved with MTX than

with leflunomide. However, more patients on MTX were withdrawn due to liver enzyme elevations[59].

So far, there is only one study comparing MTX with one of the recently introduced TNF-inhibitors, etanercept. In patients with early RA, clinical response occurred earlier with etanercept, otherwise there were no important differences between the drugs. The later response with MTX may have resulted from a (too) low initial dose of 7.5 mg weekly (with folate supplementation) which could be increased after four and eight weeks to 15 and 20 mg, respectively, in case of insufficient response[49]. Only after 24 months was etanercept significantly better than MTX regarding ACR responses[60].

Results of different studies have to be compared with caution because of differences in patient selection, methodology, dosing, outcome parameters, etc. However, such comparisons have been made between different step-up combinations of MTX with TNF-α blockers[61]. In a similar comparison, conventional DMARDs including MTX compared favorably with the biologic agents based on outcome in composite scores (ACR, European league against rheumatism (EULAR)), ESR, CRP, swollen joint count, and radiographic progression[62].

Combination with other DMARDs

For a full treatment of MTX combination therapy see Chapter 26.

Effect on extra-articular manifestations of RA

In Felty's syndrome, treatment with MTX increased the number of neutrophils and reduced the ESR and the number of swollen joints, while the corticosteroid dose could be reduced[63]. MTX treatment may heal vasculitic ulcerations and digital infarctions but can also induce vasculitic lesions[64,65].

Toxicity of low-dose MTX

Its superior 'drug survival rate' may indicate a favorable effectiveness and limited toxicity of MTX in RA patients. Most adverse events are related to the antifolate activity of MTX and mimic symptoms of folate deficiency. Clinically relevant side-effects are fortunately rare. In prospective long-term studies with frequent visits[29,30,32,37], as well as in studies with IV application of higher MTX doses, 60–85% of patients reported adverse events and 10–30%

Table 24.2 Comparative studies with other DMARDs (selection)

Author	Year	Drugs	Centers	*n*	Disease duration	Treatment duration	MTX dose (mg)	MTX efficacy	MTX tolerability
Weinblatt[101]	1990	MTX/auran	Multi	281	6 years	36 weeks	7.5–15	Superior	Superior
Williams[55]	1992	MTX/auran	Multi	229	5 years	48 weeks	7.5–15	Equal	Superior
Suarez-Almasor[102]	1988	MTX/auran	1	40	6 years	26 weeks	10	Equal	Superior
Rau[50]	1997	MTX/auran	2	174	11 months	2 years	15	Equal	Superior
Hamdy[53]	1987	MTX/AZA	1	42	8.7 years	24 weeks	10	Equal/superior	Equal
Willkens[54]	1992	MTX/AZA	Multi	212	8.0 years	48 weeks	7.5–15	Superior	Superior
Jeurissen[48]	1991	MTX/AZA	1	64	10 years	48 weeks	7.5–15	Superior	superior

Aura, auranofin; AZA, azathioprine.

discontinued MTX due to toxicity. Elevated creatinine serum levels, advanced age, and low folic acid levels predispose to adverse events. Most side-effects are reversible when MTX is discontinued. Approximately 10% of patients suffer a post-dosing reaction characterized by arthralgias/myalgias or fatigue/malaise within hours after dosing.

Gastrointestinal tract

Nausea, malaise, abdominal pain, and vomiting were observed in 10–50% of patients in prospective studies. The symptoms start 1–8 h after administration and may last from a few hours to one week. Some patients are unable to work after dosing and take MTX only on weekends. Healing of peptic ulcers related to concomitant NSAID medication may be delayed.

Mucous and skin membranes

Stomatitis and painful ulcerations of the oral mucosa have been reported in long-term studies in up to 37% of patients and caused discontinuation in less than 10%. Mild rashes may occur early in treatment and represent allergic reactions to the drug. Urticaria, small vessel vasculitis[64], and granulomatous vasculitis are rare. Multiple small nodules with central necrosis, histologically indistinguishable from the 'usual' rheumatoid nodules, may develop at the hands and feet in ~8% of RA patients treated with MTX[65,66].

Hematopoetic system

MTX-related bone marrow suppression is a relatively rare but potentially fatal complication that has been observed in short-term studies in 2–3%, but in long-term studies in up to 24% of patients[67]. The most frequent abnormality is mild to moderate leucopenia[29]. Seventy patients with pancytopenia were published in the medical literature between 1980 and 1995; 12 of these patients (17%) died[68]. Important risk factors for haematologic complications are impaired renal function, multiple co-medication, interactions of MTX with NSAIDs, concurrent infections, particularly parvovirus B19, and, most important, folate deficiency[68]. The latter may be induced by concomitant treatment with other antifolates (i.e. trimetoprim-sulfametoxazol) and may cause severe bone marrow depression. Usually, mild to moderate abnormalities normalize within two weeks, but severe bone marrow suppression may require folinic acid supplementation: parenteral application of 10–20 mg leucovorin every 6 h until blood MTX levels are undetectable or until peripheral leukocyte and platelet counts show a return to normal[68]. This procedure can be combined with 100 mg hydrocortisone IV and granulocyte colony-stimulating factor (G-CSF)[69].

Respiratory system

MTX-induced lung disease is a rare but potentially life-threatening complication. The predominant symptoms of MTX pulmonitis are shortness of breath, dry non-productive cough, and fever, accompanied by headache, malaise, cyanosis, hypoxemia, and restrictive pulmonary function changes[70]. Rales can be present, and chest radiographs may demonstrate interstitial infiltrates.

Lung biopsy reveals hypersensitivity pneumonitis with massive interstitial and alveolar infiltration with inflammatory cells, predominantly lymphocytes, with granuloma formation and giant cells. Other causes of pulmonary disease, for example nosocomial infections, have to be excluded before a diagnosis of MTX-induced pneumonitis can be established.

In clinical studies, pulmonary adverse events were observed in 0–6.8% of patients[71]. In an overview of 95 patients a mortality rate of ~17.5% was documented[70]. Pre-existing lung disease does not predispose to MTX pulmonary complications. There is no evidence that lowdose MTX is associated with chronic interstitial lung disease[72].

Liver

Hepatotoxicity is a potentially serious problem in the long-term treatment with low-dose MTX. Among patients with psoriasis treated with daily dosing, liver fibrosis and cirrhosis developed with increasing cumulative dose in up to 24% of patients[73]. After introduction of weekly dosing and emphasis on alcohol abstinence, hepatotoxicity, fortunately, has been less of a problem than initially feared. Already proposals have been made to change the guidelines for monitoring liver function tests. However, transient slight elevations of liver enzymes in around 50% of patients have been observed in a recent study[74]. Frequent elevations of liver enzymes have been found to indicate structural liver abnormalities and could be correlated significantly with liver biopsy grades[75]. Usually, elevated liver function tests returned to normal after dose reduction of MTX, change in the concurrent NSAID therapy, folic acid supplementation, or even unchanged continuation of treatment[29,37].

Histologic changes in the liver originally attributed to MTX treatment may be related to the underlying disease[76]. Liver biopsy studies did not show differences between biopsies taken before and during MTX treatment in a number of histologic parameters, among them 'necrosis', 'inflammation', and 'fibrosis'[77]. Minor fibrosis was present in ~25% of patients before and during MTX treatment[77]. Only 5 of 25 liver biopsies demonstrated minor fibrosis in patients who received MTX for more than 10 years[78]. In contrast, Kremer observed an increase in fibrosis and in the Roenigk score over six years in 29 patients with sequential biopsies[79]. Over 3.5 years no progression of histological abnormalities and no correlation of liver enzyme elevations to concentrations of MTX or glutamated MTX in the liver could be demonstrated[80].

In an ACR overview of 16 600 RA patients treated with MTX the incidence of cirrhosis was estimated to be 1:1000[81]. Thus, liver biopsy is rarely indicated in RA patients on MTX treatment since the risk of complications may be greater than the risk of cirrhosis.

Infections and wound healing

Infections occur more often in patients treated with MTX than with other DMARDs[82], especially during the first years of treatment and in patients with severe RA[83]. The data may be confounded by a potentially higher rate of infections in patients with severe RA who tend to be treated more often with MTX than with other DMARDs. Opportunistic infections, serious fungal infections, more frequent herpes zoster, reactivation of hepatitis B, and tuberculosis have been reported. Some patients must discontinue MTX permanently because of recurrent infections, mostly affecting the small airways or the urinary tract.

It is still an open question as to whether perioperative infections or wound healing disturbances are increased with continuation of MTX since most studies are too small and inconclusive. In a recent study with 388 RA patients, the rate of infections in those who continued MTX was even smaller than those who interrupted therapy[84].

Kidneys

The excretion of MTX and its metabolites is delayed in patients with impaired renal function, leading to potentially increased toxicity. MTX treatment may also impair renal function, at least in elderly patients: two studies documented a reduction of the clearance of MTX and creatinine during weekly oral MTX treatment. These observations emphasize the need to monitor serum creatinine levels carefully during MTX treatment.

Reproductive system

Oligospermia, impotence, and gynecomastia have been reported with MTX treatment. Taken during pregnancy, the drug may cause fetal death, chromosomal abnormalities, and birth defects. Of 28 women treated with low-dose MTX during the first trimester of pregnancy, miscarriage occurred in 4 patients, 5 had elective termination of pregnancy, and among 19 life births only one child had minor anomalies[85]. In an other series of 10 pregnancies with MTX exposure during the first trimester no malformations were observed. A case with multiple congenital anomalies has been published.

Oncogenicity

Large studies of cancer and psoriasis treated with MTX did not establish an association between MTX and malignancies. In RA patients treated with MTX, lymphomas and leukemia have been reported. The majority suffered from non-Hodgkin lymphomas, most of which were associated with Epstein–Barr virus (EBV) infection[86]. Risk factors for RA patients to develop lymphoma while on MTX include severe disease, intense immunosuppression, genetic predisposition, and increased frequency of latent infections with pro-oncogenic viruses such as EBV[87]. Some lymphomas associated with EBV infection remit after the discontinuation of MTX[87,88]. In a study of 16 263 patients with RA, no increased rate of lymphomas was observed in patients taking MTX[89].

Central nervous system

Central nervous disturbances, including headache, dizziness, vertigo, light-headedness, and mood alterations, were reported in up to 36% in long-term studies[13]. Again, older age and elevated serum creatinine are predisposing factors[90]. In two of our patients with a history of epilepsy, seizures reappeared within six weeks of starting MTX treatment and disappeared only when MTX was discontinued.

Bone

Active RA is associated with osteoporosis, especially in patients taking corticosteroids. In rats treated with MTX a significant osteopenia developed through the suppression of osteoblast activity. In a three-year study in RA patients no difference in bone mineral density with or without MTX treatment was observed; however, the combination of prednisone ($\leq$5 mg/day) with MTX resulted in a significantly greater bone loss than the same prednisone dose without MTX[91].

Folate supplementation

Toxicity and efficacy of MTX is—at least in part—related to its anti-folate activity. Several randomized controlled trials have documented a reduction of MTX side-effects with folic acid or folinic acid supplementation. With the exception of one study[92], folate supplementation did not appear to interfere with MTX efficacy[93]. However, the number of patients in these studies was too small to reliably exclude a negative effect on the clinical efficacy of MTX. In a large 48-week, randomized study, 434 RA patients starting MTX treatment were supplemented with folic acid (1 mg/day), folinic acid (2.5 mg/week), or placebo. Supplementation with either folate regimen resulted in a reduction in the incidence of liver enzyme elevations but had no influence on the incidence, severity, or duration of other adverse events[74]. In that study, the weekly MTX dose to get an adequate clinical response was higher in patients with folate supplementation (18 vs. 14.5 mg, respectively). In a US trial, MTX with folate supplementation was less effective than leflunomide while in a corresponding European study without folate supplementation MTX was highly significantly superior to leflunomide[57,59]. These observations are compatible with the finding that best responders to MTX had significantly lower red blood cell folate levels than worst responders[94]. With folate supplementation, deficient blood folate levels and hyperhomocysteinemia can be prevented[95]. Increased homocysteine levels have been found to be a risk factor for cardiovascular mortality. However, several studies indicate that effective MTX treatment does not increase, but decreases mortality[34,41].

Recently it has been reported that hyperhomocysteinemia is not only related to folate deficiency but also to clinical disease activity and serum creatinine levels[96].

In vitro, several mechanisms of action of MTX can be blocked by folinic acid, but not by folic acid[8,97]. However, *in vivo*, folic acid is reduced to folinic acid. Furthermore, it could be shown that folic acid reduces the bioavailability of MTX in RA patients[98].

In conclusion, folate supplementation may improve MTX tolerability at the expense of reducing its efficacy. This may explain the steadily increasing weekly MTX doses reported from American long-term observational studies. The question of whether folic acid should be supplemented in all patients from the beginning of MTX treatment is still open[98].

Administration and drug monitoring

MTX is given once weekly and can be administered by the oral, intramuscular, intravenous, or subcutaneous route, with doses ranging from 7.5 to 30 mg. The dose may be influenced by disease activity, experience with efficacy and tolerability of previous treatments, renal function, concomitant disease, general health status, and body weight.

In our department, treatment usually was, and still is, started with a parenteral dose of 15 (−25) mg to exclude the individual differences in bioavailability of oral medication and to achieve a rapid response. After 6–12 weeks, we switch to oral medication and adjust the dose according to efficacy and tolerability. Most rheumatologists prefer to start with an oral dose of 7.5 mg and to increase the dose subsequently. Tolerability can often be improved by administering the drug in the evening or in divided doses over a 24 h period, by changing the route of administration (parenteral vs. oral), by reducing the dose, or by supplementation with folic acid. In case of nausea and vomiting medication of metoclopramide or dimenhydrinate *may mitigate the symptoms*. Possible interactions with NSAIDs should be taken into consideration. We add supplementation when side-effects occur in the presence of concomitant folate deficiency and stop it after normalization of folate levels. Most authors recommend permanent folic acid supplementation with 1 mg/day or 5 mg/week.

Relative or absolute contraindications to MTX treatment are listed in Table 24.3. If there is no alternative to MTX in a patient with renal impairment, we start with lower doses (i.e. 5 mg/week) and check the MTX serum level after 24 h to ensure that it is below 0.05 mM/L. Regular monitoring of serum creatinine is essential in all patients to avoid toxicity. Women with childbearing potential should practice adequate contraception. Women (and men) taking MTX should stop the drug three months before conception. Most rheumatologists will request alcohol abstinence or allow only one or two glasses of wine or beer per week while taking MTX.

During MTX treatment full blood counts, including differential and platelet count, serum creatinine, and aminotransferases should be monitored on a weekly basis during the first month, every two weeks during months 2 and 3, and monthly or bimonthly thereafter.

MTX should be discontinued temporarily under the following conditions: serum creatinine exceeding normal values; aminotransferases exceeding threefold the normal values; leucopenia or thrombocytopenia; stomatitis; acute infections; severe concurrent illness; concomitant treatment with trimethoprim-sulfamethoxazole; acute pulmonary symptoms.

Whether MTX should be discontinued before and after surgery should be decided in cooperation with the operating surgeon. *Most doctors do not routinely stop MTX during surgery. However, in case of wound-healing disturbances or infections MTX should tem-* *porarily be stopped*. Pre-treatment liver biopsies are recommended only in patients with a significant alcohol consumption or a history of liver disease. During MTX treatment liver biopsies should be performed only if over 50% of the ALT (alanine aminotransferase) level readings within one year are elevated or if the serum albumin concentration falls below normal. MTX should be permanently discontinued if biopsies reveal moderate to severe fibrosis or cirrhosis (Roenigk class IIIb or IV)[99].

Parameters of disease activity, radiographic progression, and functional capacity should be monitored regularly. In the case of unsatisfactory response the dose should be increased or MTX combined with another DMARD or a biologic agent.

Leflunomide

Introduction

Leflunomide (LEF) was developed in the 1980s as a compound capable of preventing mitogen-induced lymphocyte proliferation. It was found to have immunosuppressive and anti-inflammatory properties and was approved for the treatment of RA in the US in 1998 and in Europe in 1999.

Pharmacology and pharmacokinetics

LEF is an isoxazol derivative with no structural relationship with existing immunomodulatory drugs. It is a pro-drug which is rapidly converted into its active metabolite A77 1726, manolonitrilamide (Fig. 24.3). The conversion takes place in the submucosal wall of the intestinum and after its first passage in the liver.

LEF is completely absorbed. Due to its high protein binding (>99%) and its enterohepatic circulation A77 1726 has a long plasma half-life of ~15 days (range 5–40 days). Around 40% of the administered dose is excreted unchanged in the faeces and around 60% of A77 1726 is eliminated in the urine predominantly as glucoronide conjugates and oxanilic acid derivatives. Due to its enterohepatic circulation and its binding to cholestyramine, A77 1726 can be eliminated rapidly in case of toxicity by cholestyramine administration.

A77 1726 can increase the free fractions of diclophenac, ibuprofen, and tolbutamide, presumably by inhibiting cytochrome P450 which is responsible for the metabolizing of NSAIDs.

Mechanism of action

The active leflunomide metabolite A77 1726 inhibits the enzyme dihydroorotate dehydrogenase (DHODH) which is critical for the *de novo* synthesis of pyrimidines, thereby inhibiting RNA and DNA synthesis and decreasing the proliferation and differentiation of lymphocytes, particularly T cells[103]. This reaction can be blocked in a dose-dependent way by the addition of uridine. Other important mechanisms of action are the inhibition of the nuclear factor (NF)-κB, IL-1β expression, and matrix metalloproteinase (MMP)-1 production. It has also been shown to inhibit chemotaxis of peripheral blood neutrophils in RA patients[104].

Table 24.3 Contraindications for MTX treatment

1. Renal insufficiency (serum creatinine > upper limit)
2. Pregnancy or inadequate contraception
3. Active liver disease
4. Regular alcohol intake
5. Acute or chronic infection
6. Leucopenia or thrombocytopenia (exception: Felty's syndrome)
7. Serious underlying systemic disease
8. Non-compliance

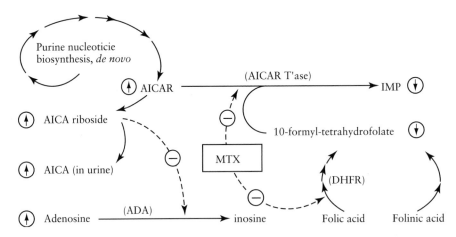

Fig. 24.3 Structure of leflunomide and its active metabolite.

Clinical efficacy

Safety and efficacy of LEF in RA was first investigated in the early 1990s in 350 patients treated with doses ranging from 5 to 25 mg/day, with 255 patients followed over 18 months[105].

Placebo-controlled studies

In a subsequent randomized, placebo-controlled dose finding study over 24 weeks involving 402 patients with a disease duration of 8.3 years, 25 mg/day performed somewhat better than 10 mg/day (ACR 20 in 60% and 52%, respectively), while 5 mg/day was no more effective than placebo[106].

A 12-month study performed in the United States (US 301) in 482 RA patients (mean disease duration seven years) compared LEF at a dose of 20 mg daily (after 100 mg loading doses on days 1–3) with MTX and placebo[57]. The initial MTX dose was only 7.5 mg weekly for nine weeks and could be increased to 15 mg weekly in case of inadequate therapeutic response (61% of the patients did so). Moreover, patients received 1–2 mg of folic acid per day. LEF was superior to MTX: 52% of patients treated with LEF achieved an ACR 20% response, compared to 46% of patients treated with MTX and 26% of patients on placebo. A statistically significant and clinically meaningful improvement in functional capacity measures and health-related quality of life was seen with LEF compared with placebo[107]. Both LEF and MTX inhibited radiographic progression significantly when compared with placebo. Of note, the potential of progression in these patients was low: the baseline value after seven years' disease duration was only 23 Sharp units, corresponding to ~5% of the maximum possible score. In a continuation study in those patients who completed 52 weeks the ACR 20 response rates (LEF 79% vs. MTX 67%; $p = 0.049$) were sustained in both active treatment groups[58]. The mean change in the total Sharp scores during the second year was 1.6 for LEF vs. 1.2 for MTX compared with 0.53 vs. 0.88 during the first year. The improvement in measures of function and quality of life were maintained in both active treatment groups. The Health Assessment Questionnaire (HAQ) disability index had improved significantly more with LEF than with MTX treatment.

In a multinational (predominantly European) study LEF ($n = 495$) was directly compared with MTX ($n = 489$) but without a placebo group in RA patients with a mean disease duration of 3.7 years[59]. Leflunomide was dosed as in the US 301 study; the initial MTX dose was 7.5 mg and could be increased to 15 mg after 4–12 weeks. In that study, the ACR response rate was significantly greater with MTX (65%) than with LEF (50.5%) after 12 months. Improvement was also significantly greater in the MTX group in tender and swollen joint counts, global assessments, and sedimentation rate. The reason for the better performance of MTX in this study compared to US 301 may be that only 10% of patients had folate supplementation. In those patients who continued treatment for a second year (LEF = 57%; MTX = 64%) the ACR 20 response rates were comparable with both drugs, but inhibition of radiographic progression was significantly greater with MTX[108].

In another double blind study in 358 patients the ACR 20 response rate with LEF 20 mg daily after six months was 55%; with sulfasalazine it was 56% compared with 29% with placebo. However, HAQ scores were significantly more improved in the LEF than in the sulfasalazine or placebo groups. Patients were given the option to continue treatment in a double blind fashion up to 12 and 24 months; patients in the placebo group were switched to sulfasalazine. While there was no difference between the treatment groups after 12 months, the ACR 20 response rate was significantly greater in the LEF than in the sulfasalazine group at 24 months[109]. The active treatment groups demonstrated less radiographic progression than the placebo group, but all together the progression was small[110]. Based on these studies it can be concluded that disease modification as measured radiographically is comparable with that of sulfasalazine and low to moderate doses of MTX[108].

Long-term observational studies

Patients completing the studies MN 301 and MN 302 were given the option to continue to be treated with LEF in an open label extension study. The extension study enrolled 22% of the patients of study MN301 and 37% of patients of study MN302. The study was terminated when LEF became commercially available. At that time 163 of 214 patients (76%) had received LEF for a mean treatment duration of 4.6 years. The ACR20, 50, and 70 response rates at year 4 or at study termination were 69%, 43%, and 20%, respectively, similar to the response rates after one, two, and three years. The CRP had decreased from ~4 to ~1.3 mg/dL (0–1.0), the HAQ scores had improved from ~1.0 to ~0.4 after two years, and deteriorated again to ~0.6 at study termination[111].

Combination of leflunomide with other DMARDs

DMARD combinations are especially advisable if the combined drugs have different mechanisms of action.

In 30 patients with incomplete response to a mean of 17 mg MTX/week, 10 mg LEF daily following a loading dose of 100 mg/day for two days was added, increased to 20 mg after three months in patients with persistently active disease. No significant pharmacokinetic interaction between both drugs was noted. An ACR 20 response was achieved by 20% of patients. However, liver enzyme elevations occurred in 63% of patients[112].

In a double-blind, randomized study in 263 patients with persistent disease activity in spite of MTX treatment for at least six months, the combination of MTX with LEF was compared with MTX + placebo. The LEF dosing was similar to that in the previous study. At 24 weeks, 46% of patients in the MTX + LEF group had a 20% ACR response compared to 19.5% in the MTX + placebo group ($p < 0.001$)[113].

In a six-month open label extension the patients in the combination group continued their treatment while patients previously on MTX alone received 10 mg/day LEF without a loading dose in addition to their MTX. At 48 weeks the ACR 20, ACR 50, and ACR 70 response rates were 58, 28, and 11.5%, respectively, indicating that the combination continued to be effective. Similar response rates were seen in the patients who had switched from the combination MTX + placebo to MTX + LEF during the extension period[114]. In the combination group liver enzymes were elevated in 28% of patients. In the original combination group treatment continued to be effective while patients switching from placebo to LEF experienced the same magnitude of response after six months.

Combination treatment is discussed in more detail in the Administration and drug monitoring section, below.

Toxicity of leflunomide in RA

The most frequently observed side-effects in the LEF groups in controlled clinical trials were diarrhea, nausea, abdominal pain, liver enzyme elevations, skin rashes, alopecia, and respiratory tract infections. This toxicity profile was in general similar to moderate doses of MTX and sulfasalazine, but due to the long half-life of the drug the side-effects persisted longer. Significant weight loss is a prominent feature of LEF toxicity and occurred in 7% of 70 patients starting LEF therapy[115].

The withdrawal rates for LEF due to adverse events were 22% in US 301 and 20% in MN 302 compared to 10% and 15% for MTX.

Skin

Rash, pruritus, and maculopapular reactions were seen in up to 24% of patients in clinical trials, occurred early, and resulted in discontinuation of therapy in only 1–2% of patients. Rare cases of Stevens Johnson syndrome and toxic epidermal necrolysis occurred in patients under combination treatment.

Infections

Due to its immunosuppressive effects, LEF treatment may be associated with an increased rate of infections. In clinical trials the rate of infections was similar to that seen with MTX, being only somewhat greater than in the respective placebo groups. LEF should not be started in patients with immunodeficiency, bone marrow impairment, and serious infections. If an infection occurs during combination therapy with another immunosuppressive agent, antibiotic therapy and discontinuation of combination is indicated. Patients with a history of tuberculosis should be carefully monitored for reactivation.

Nervous system

Side-effects of the nervous system include headache, dizziness, and paresthesia. These symptoms are usually mild to moderate and do not preclude continuation of treatment.

Hypertension

Hypertension developed in >10% of patients in US 301. In most cases this is an aggravation of an already existing hypertension.

Liver

In clinical trials with LEF monotherapy, 14–18% of patients had elevations of ALT up to twice the upper limit of normal, while elevations over three times normal were seen in less than 5%. Liver enzyme elevations were observed more frequently with MTX in MN 302 (without folate supplementation) and less frequently with MTX than with LEF in US 301 (with folate supplementation). The combination LEF/MTX caused substantially more enzyme elevations, up to 63[112] and 28%[115]. The European medicines evaluation agency (EMEA) reported 296 cases of hepatic abnormality in RA patients with a total drug exposure of 104 000 patient years[116]. The report included 129 cases of serious liver disease, 2 with cirrhosis, 15 with liver failure, and 15 deaths. Concomitant treatment with NSAIDs was a risk factor for hepatic abnormalities. In 2003, the Federal Drug Administration (FDA) reported 102 cases of serious hepatic events, observed from the approval of the drug until August 2002 in an estimated exposure time of 90 000–116 000 person years (Table 24.4). Liver failure can occur unpredictably at any time during LEF treatment.

Rare side-effects

While no hematologic adverse events were noted in US 301, mild leucopenia (2000–3000 cells/mm^3) occurred in 20 patients in MN 302, leading to withdrawal of 4 patients during the first year. During the second year eight additional cases occurred. Rare cases of pancytopenia have been observed in the post-marketing period, primarily in patients with known risk factors or combination treatment.

Cases of lymphoma have been observed in clinical studies. However, the frequency was in line with the expected rate of lymphoproliferative disorders in RA of 0.2%. Long-term follow-up

Table 24.4 Hepatic reactions in patients taking leflunomide reported by the EMEA and the FDA

Reporting agency variable	EMEA[a] (n)	FDA[b] (n)
All reactions	296	102
Serious reactions	129	54
Acute liver failure (ALF)	15	16
Fatal outcome		
ALF	9	8
Other causes	6	1
All causes	15	9
Possibly leflunomide related	10	5
Time to reaction (mean days; range)	Variable (3–1095)	135 (3–693)
Confounding factors (denominator)	129	54
Other hepatotoxic drugs (%)	78	74
Concomitant use of MTX and/or NASAIDS (%)	58	43
Comorbid conditions (%)	27	17

[a] European Medicines Evaluation Agency[116].
[b] US Food and Drug Administration[117].

is necessary to determine whether there is an increased risk for malignancy in patients treated with LEF.

Administration and drug monitoring

In clinical trials LEF treatment was usually started with a loading dose of 100 mg/day for three days, followed by 20 mg/day. However, due to toxicity concerns many rheumatologists start treatment with 20 mg/day and, if this is not well tolerated, reduce the daily dose to 10 mg. In combination with MTX and in patients with risk of toxicity the daily starting dose may be 10 mg, which can be increased to 20 mg after two months. In case of diarrhea with a 20 mg daily dose a good alternative is a 100 mg dose once a week.

At baseline, every two weeks for the first six months, and every eight weeks thereafter, a complete blood count, including differential white blood count and platelets, and liver function tests have to be performed.

In case of serious side-effects a washout with cholestyramine (8 g three times daily) for 11 days should be done.

LEF is contraindicated in patients with impaired liver function, severe renal impairment, severe hypoproteinemia, serious infections, known immunodeficiency, and bone marrow depression. LEF is also contraindicated in children since there is no experience in patients under 18 years of age.

LEF is absolutely contraindicated during pregnancy and in women who are breastfeeding. Women with childbearing potential must use a reliable contraception. In case of pregnancy a washout with cholestyramine should be performed as early as possible, and the plasma level of A77 1726 must be reduced below 0.02 mg/L.

References

1. Gubner, R., August, S., and Ginsberg, V. Therapeutic suppression of tissue reactivity. II. Effect of aminopterin in rheumatoid arthritis and psoriasis. *Am J Med Sci* 1951; **221**: 176–82.

2. Herman, R. A., van Pedersen, P., Hofman, J., and Furst, D. E. Pharmacokinetics of low dose methotrexate in rheumatoid arthritis patients. *J Pharm Sci* 1989; **78**: 165–71.
3. Kremer, J. M., and Hamilton, R. A. The effects of nonsteroidal anti-inflammatory drugs on methotrexate (MTX) pharmacokinetics: impairment of renal clearance of MTX at weekly maintenance doses but not at 7.5 mg. *J Rheumatol* 1995; **22**: 2072–7.
4. Lafforgue, P., Monjanel-Mouterde, S., Durand, A. *et al.* Is there an interaction between low doses of corticosteroids and methotrexate in patients with rheumatoid arthritis. *J Rheumatol* 1993; **20**: 263–7.
5. Baggott, J. E., Vaughn, W. H., and Hudson, B. B. Inhibition of 5-aminoimidazole-4-carboxamide ribotide transformylase, adenosine deaminase, and 5-adenylate deaminase by polyglutamates of methotrexate and oxidized folates and by 5'-aminoimidazole-4-carboxamide riboside and ribotide. *Biochem J* 1986; **236**: 193–200.
6. Cronstein, B. N. Molecular therapeutics: methotrexate and its mechanism of action. *Arthritis Rheum* 1996; **39**: 1951–60.
7. Andersson, S. E., Johansson, L. H., Lexmuller, K., and Ekstrom, G. M. Antiarthritic effect of methotrexate: is it really mediated by adenosine? *Eur J Pharm Sci* 2000; **9**: 333–43.
8. Morgan, S. L., Oster, R. A., Lee, J. Y., Alarcon, G. S., and Baggott, J. E. The effect of folic acid and folinic acid supplements on purine metabolism in methotrexate-treated rheumatoid arthritis. *Arthritis Rheum* 2004; **50**: 3104–11.
9. Olsen, N. J., and Murray, L. Antiproliferative effects of methotrexate on peripheral blood mononuclear cells. *Arthritis Rheum* 1989; **32**: 378–85.
10. Nakajiama, A., Hakoda, M., Yamanaka, H. *et al.* Divergent effects low methotrexate on the clonal growth of T and B lymphocytes and synovial adherent cells from patients with rheumatoid arthritis. *Ann Rheum Dis* 1996; **55**: 237–42.
11. Chang, D. M., Weinblatt, M. E., and Schur, P. H. The effects of methotrexate on interleukin 1 in patients with rheumatoid arthritis. *J Rheumatol* 1992; **19**: 1678–82.
12. Segal, R., Yaron, M., and Tartakovsky, B. Rescue of interleukin-1 activity by leucovorin following inhibition by methotrexate in a murine in vitro system. *Arthritis Rheum* 1990; **33**: 1745.
13. Seitz, M., Loetscher, P., Dewald, B. *et al.* Methotrexate action in rheumatoid arthritis: stimulation of cytokine inhibitor and inhibition of chemokine production by peripheral blood mononuclear cells. *Br J Rheumatol* 1995; **34**: 602–9.
14. Barrera, P., Boerbooms, A. M. T., Janssen, E. M. *et al.* Circulating soluble tumor necrosis factor receptors, interleukin-2 receptors, tumor necrosis factor α, and interleukin-6 levels in rheumatoid arthritis: longitudinal evaluation during methotrexate and azathioprine therapy. *Arthritis Rheum* 1993; **36**: 1070–9.
15. Segal, R., Mozes, E., Yaron, M., and Tartakovsky, B. The effects of methotrexate on the proliferation and activity of interleukin 1. *Arthritis Rheum* 1989; **32**: 370–7.
16. Seitz, M., Dewald, B., Ceska, M. *et al.* Interleukin-8 in inflammatory rheumatic diseases: synovial fluid levels, relation to rheumatoid factors, production by mononuclear cells, and effects of gold sodium thiomalate and methotrexate. *Rheumatol Int* 1992; **12**: 159–64.
17. Seitz, M., Zwicker, M., and Wider, B. Enhanced in vitro induced production of interleukin 10 by peripheral blood mononuclear cells in rheumatoid arthritis is associated with clinical response to methotrexate treatment. *J Rheumatol* 2001; **28**: 496–501.
18. Fiehn, C., Müller-Ladner, U., Gay, S., Krienke, S. *et al.* Albumin-coupled methotrexate (MTX-HAS) is a new anti-arthritic drug which acts synergistically to MTX. *Rheumatology* 2004; **43**: 1097–105.
19. Constantin, A., Loubet-Lescoulie, P., Lambert, N. *et al.* Antiinflammatory and immunoregulatory action of methotrexate in the treatment of rheumatoid arthritis. *Arthritis Rheum* 1998; **41**: 48.
20. Smolenska Z., Kaznowska, Z., Zarowny, D., Simmonds, H. A. *et al.* Effect of methotrexate on blood purine and pyrimidine levels in patients with rheumatoid arthritis. *Rheumatology* 1999; **38**: 997–1002.
21. Chan, E. S. L., and Cronstein, B. N. Molecular action of methotrexate in inflammatory diseases. *Arthritis Res* 2002; **4**: 266–73.
22. Willkens, R. F., Watson, M. A., and Paxson, C. S. Low-dose pulse methotrexate in rheumatoid arthritis. *J Rheumatol* 1980; **7**: 501–5.

23. Wilke, W. S., Calabrese, L. H., and Scherbel, A. L. Methotrexate in the treatment of rheumatoid arthritis: pilot study. Cleve Clin Q: 1980; **47**: 305–9.

24. Karger, T., and Rau, R. Treatment of rheumatoid arthritis with methotrexate. *Z Rheumatol* 1982; **41**: 164.

25. Weinblatt, M. E., Coblyn, J. S., Fox, D. A. *et al*. Efficacy of low-dose methotrexate in rheumatoid arthritis. *N Engl J Med* 1985; **312**: 818–22.

26. Furst, D. E., Koehnke, R., Burmeister, L. F. *et al*. Increasing methotrexate effect with increasing dose in the treatment of resistant rheumatoid arthritis. *J Rheumatol* 1989; **16**: 313–20.

27. Michaels, R. M., Nashel, D. J., Leonard, A., Sliwinski, J., and Derbes, S. J. Weekly intravenous methotrexate in the treatment of rheumatoid arthritis. *Arthritis Rheum* 1982; **25**: 339–41.

28. Lambert, C. M., Sandhu, S., Lochhead, A., Hurst, N. P., McRorie, E., and Dhillon, V. Dose escalation of parenteral methotrexate in active rheumatoid arthritis that has been unresponsive to conventional doses of methotrexate: a randomized, controlled trial. *Arthritis Rheum* 2004; **50**: 364–71.

29. Kremer, J. M., and Phelps, C. T. Long-term prospective study of the use of methotrexate in the treatment of rheumatoid arthritis. *Arthritis Rheum* 1992; **35**: 138–45.

30. Weinblatt, M. E., Weissman, B. N., Holdsworth, D. E. *et al*. Long-term prospective study of methotrexate in the treatment of rheumatoid arthritis: 84-month update. *Arthritis Rheum* 1992; **35**: 129–37.

31. Weinblatt, M. E., Kaplan, H., Germain, B. F. *et al*. Methotrexate in rheumatoid arthritis: a five-year prospective multicenter study. *Arthritis Rheum* 1994; **37**: 1492–8.

32. Sany, J., Anaya, J. M., Lussiez, V. *et al*. Treatment of rheumatoid arthritis with methotrexate: a prospective open longterm study of 191 cases. *J Rheumatol* 1991; **18**: 1323–7.

33. Hanrahan, P. S., Scrivens, G. A., and Russell, A. S. Prospective long term follow-up of methotrexate therapy in rheumatoid arthritis: toxicity, efficacy and radiological progression. *Brit J Rheum* 1989; **28**: 147–53.

34. Krause, D., Schleusser, B., Herborn, G., and Rau, R. Response to methotrexate treatment is associated with reduced mortality inpatients with severe rheumatoid arthritis. *Arthritis Rheum* 2000; **43**: 14–21.

35. Ortendahl, M., Holmes, T., Schettler, J. D., and Fries, J. F. The methotrexate therapeutic response in rheumatoid arthritis. *J Rheumatol* 2002; **29**: 2084–91.

36. Hoekstra, M., van de Laar, M. A. F. J., Bernelot Moens, H. J., Kruijsen, M. W. M., and Haagsma, C. J. Longterm observational study of methotrexate use in a Dutch cohort of 1022 patients with rheumatoid arthritis. *J Rheumatol* 2003; **30**: 2325–9.

37. Rau, R., Schleusser, B., Herborn, G., and Karger, T. Long-term treatment of destructive rheumatoid arthritis with methotrexate. *J Rheumatol* 1997; **24**: 1881–9.

38. Wolfe, F., Hawley, D. J., and Cathey, M. A. Termination of slow acting antirheumatic therapy in rheumatoid arthritis: a 14-year prospective evaluation of 1017 consecutive starts. *J Rheumatol* 1990; **17**: 994–1002.

39. Wluka, A., Buchbinder, R., Mylvaganam, A. *et al*. Longterm methotrexate use in rheumatoid arthritis: 12 year follow up of 460 patients treated in community practice. *J Rheumatol* 2000; **27**: 1864–71.

40. Furst, D. E. Proposition: methotrexate should not be the first second-line agent to be used in rheumatoid arthritis if NSAIDs fail. *Arthritis Rheum* 1990; **20**: 69–75.

41. Choi, H. K., Hernan, M. A., Seeger, J. D. *et al*. Methotrexate and mortality in patients with rheumatoid arthritis: a prospective study. *Lancet* 2002; **359**: 1173–7.

42. Wassenberg, S., and Rau, R. Radiographic healing with sustained clinical remission in a patient with rheumatoid arthritis receiving methotrexate monotherapy. *Arthritis Rheum* 2002; **46**: 2804–7.

43. Nordstrom, D. M., West, S. G., Andersen, P. A., and Sharp, J. T. Pulse methotrexate therapy in rheumatoid arthritis: a controlled prospective roentgenographic study. *Ann Intern Med* 1987; **107**: 797–801.

44. Reykdal, S., Steirisson, K., Sigurjonsson, K., and Brekkan, A. Methotrexate treatment of rheumatoid arthritis: effects on radiological progression. Scand *J Rheumatology* 1989; **18**: 221–6.

45. Rau, R., Herborn, G., Karger, T., and Werdier, D. Retardation of radiologic progression in rheumatoid arthritis with methotrexate therapy. *Arthritis Rheum* 1991; **10**: 1236–44.

46. Rau, R., Herborn, G., Menninger, H., and Sangha, O. Progression in early erosive rheumatoid arthritis: 12 month results from a randomised controlled trial comparing methotrexate and gold sodium thiomalate. *Brit J Rheumatol* 1998; **37**: 1220–6.

47. Rau, R., Herborn, G., Menninger, H., and Sangha, O. Radiographic outcome after three years of patients with early erosive rheumatoid arthritis treated with intramuscular methotrexate or parenteral gold: extension of a one-year double-blind study in 174 patients. *Rheumatology* 2002; **41**: 196–204.

48. Jeurissen, M. E. C., Boerbooms, A. M. T., van de Putte, L. B. A. *et al*. Methotrexate versus azathioprine in the treatment of rheumatoid arthritis: a forty-eight-week randomized, double blind trial. *Arthritis Rheum* 1991; **34**: 951–60.

49. Bathon, J. M., Martin, R. W., Fleischmann, R. M. *et al*. A comparison of etanercept and methotrexate in patients with early rheumatoid arthritis. *N Engl J Med* 2000; **343**: 1586–93.

50. Rau, R., Herborn, G., Menninger, H., and Blechschmidt, J. Comparison of intramuscular methotrexate and gold sodium thiomalate in the treatment of early erosive rheumatoid arthritis: 12 month data of a double-blind parallel study of 174 patients. *Brit J Rheum* 1997; **36**: 345–52.

51. Menninger, H., Herborn, G., Blechschmidt, J., and Rau, R. A 36-month comparative trial of methotrexate and gold sodium thiomalate in the treatment of early active and erosive rheumatoid arthritis. *Brit J Rheum* 1998; **37**: 1060–8.

52. Hamilton, J., McInnes, I. B., Thomon, E. S., Porter, D., Hunter, J. A. *et al*. Comparative study of intramuscular gold and methotrexate in a rheumatoid arthritis population from a socially deprived area. *Ann Rheum Dis* 2001; **60**: 566–72.

53. Hamdy, H., McKendry, R. J. R., Mierins, E., and Liver, J. A. Low-dose methotrexate compared with azathioprine in the treatment of rheumatoid arthritis. *Arthritis Rheum* 1987; **30**: 361–8.

54. Willkens, R. F., Urowitz, M. B., Stablein, D. M. *et al*. Comparison of azathioprine, methotrexate, and the combination of both in the treatment of rheumatoid arthritis: a controlled clinical trial. *Arthritis Rheum* 1992; **35**: 849–56.

55. Williams, H. J., Ward, J. R., Reading, J. C. *et al*. Comparison of auranofin, methotrexate and the combination of both in the treatment of rheumatoid arthritis. *Arthritis Rheum* 1992; **3**: 259–69.

56. Felson, D. T., Anderson, J. J., and Meenan, R. F. The comparative efficacy and toxicity of second-line drugs in rheumatoid arthritis. *Arthritis Rheum* 1990; **33**: 1449–60.

57. Strand, V., Cohen, S., Schiff, M. *et al*. Treatment of active rheumatoid arthritis with leflunomide compared with placebo and methotrexate. Leflunomide Rheumatoid Arthritis Investigators Group. *Arch Intern Med* 1999; **159**: 2542–50.

58. Cohen, S., Cannon, G. W., Schiff, M., Weaver, A., Fox, R. *et al*. Two year, blinded, randomized, controlled trial of treatment of active rheumatoid arthritis with leflunomide compared with methotrexate. *Arthritis Rheum* 2001; **44**: 1984–92.

59. Emery, P., Breedveld, F. C., Lemmel, E. M. *et al*. A comparison of the efficacy and safety of leflunomide and methotrexate for the treatment of rheumatoid arthritis. *Rheumatology* 2000; **39**: 655–65.

60. Genovese, M. C., Bathon, J. M., Martin, R. W., Fleischmann, R. M., Tesser, J. R. *et al*. Etanercept versus methotrexate in patients with early rheumatoid arthritis: two-year radiographic and clinical outcomes. *Arthritis Rheum* 2002; **45**: 1443–50.

61. Hochberg, M. C., Tracy, J. J. K., Hawkins-Holt, M., and Flores, R. H. Comparison of the efficacy of the tumour necrosis factor alpha blocking agents adalimumab, etanercept, and infliximab when added to methotrexate in patients with active rheumatoid arthritis. *Ann Rheum Dis* 2003; **62** (Suppl. 2): ii13–16.

62. Rau, R. Have traditional DMARDS had their day Clin Rheumatol. [First published online, 24 July.], 2004.

63. Wassenberg, S., Herborn, G., and Rau, R. Methotrexate treatment in Felty's syndrome. *Brit J Rheumatol* 1988; **37**: 908–11.

64. Marks, C. R., Willkens, R. F., Wilske, R., and Brown, P. B. Small vessel vasculitis and methotrexate. [Letter.] *Ann Intern Med* 1984; **100**: 916.

65. Segal, R., Caspi, D., Tishler, M. *et al*. Accelerated nodulosis and vasculitis during methotrexate therapy for rheumatoid arthritis. *Arthritis Rheum* 1988; **31**: 1182–5.

66. Kerstens, P. J. S. M., Boerbooms, A. M. T., Jeurissen, M. E. C. *et al*. Accelerated nodulosis during low dose methotrexate therapy for rheumatoid arthritis: an analysis of ten cases. *J Rheumatol* 1992; **19**: 867–71.

67. Alarcon, G. S., Tracy, I. C., and Blackburn, W. D. Jr. Methotrexate in rheumatoid arthritis: toxic effects as the major factor in limiting long-term treatment. *Arthritis Rheum* 1989; **32**: 671–6.

68. Gutierrez-Urena, S., Molina, J. F., Garcia, C. O., Cuellar, M., and Espinoza, L. R. Pancytopenia secondary to methotrexate therapy in rheumatoid arthritis. *Arthritis Rheum* 1996; **39**: 272–6.

69. Kam, H. Y., and Swee, C. N. Early onset methotrexate-induced pancytopenia and response to G-CSF: a report of two cases. *J Clin Rheumatol* 2001; **7**: 17–20.

70. Kremer, J. M., Alarcon, G. S., Weinblatt, M. E. *et al*. Clinical, laboratory, radiographic, and histopathologic features of methotrexate-associated lung injury in patients with rheumatoid arthritis: a multicenter study with literature review. *Arthritis Rheum* 1997; **40**: 1829–37.

71. Salaffi, F., Mangenelli, P., Carotti, M. *et al*. Methotrexate-induced pneumonitis in patients with rheumatoid arthritis and psoriatic arthritis: report of five cases and review of the literature. *Clin Rheumatol* 1997; **16**: 296–304.

72. Dawson, J. K., Graham, D. R., Desmond, J., Fewins, H. E., and Lynch, M. P. Investigation of the chronic pulmonary effects of low-dose oral methotrexate in patients with rheumatoid arthritis: a prospective study incorporating HRCT scanning and pulmonary function tests. *Rheumatology* 2002; **41**: 262–7.

73. Nyfors, A. Methotrexate hepatotoxicity in psoriasis and psoriatic arthritis: a review. In *Low Dose Methotrexate Therapy in Rheumatic Diseases* (Rau R, ed.). Basel: Karger; 1986.

74. van Ede, A. E., Laan, R. F., Rood, M. M. J. *et al*. Effect of folic or folinic acid supplementation on the toxicity and efficacy of methotrexate in rheumatoid arthritis: a forty-eight week, multicenter, randomized, double-blind, placebo-controlled study. *Arthritis Rheum* 2001; **44**: 1515–24.

75. Kremer, J. M., Furst, D. E., Weinblatt, M. E., and Blotner, S. D. Significant changes in serum AST across hepatic histological biopsy grades: prospective analysis of 3 cohorts receiving methotrexate therapy for rheumatoid arthritis. *J Rheumatol* 1996; **23**: 459–61.

76. Rau, R. *The Liver in Inflammatory Rheumatic Diseases* [German]. Darmstadt: Steinkopff; 1978.

77. Rau, R., Karger, T., Herborn, G., and Frenzel, H. Liver biopsy findings in patients with rheumatoid arthritis undergoing longterm treatment with methotrexate. *J Rheumatol* 1989; **16**: 489–93.

78. Aponte, J., and Petrelli, M. Histopathologic findings in the liver of rheumatoid arthritis patients treated with longterm bolus methotrexate. *Arthritis Rheum* 1988; **31**: 1457–64.

79. Kremer, J. M., Kaye, G. I., Kaye, N. W. *et al*. Light and electron microscopic analysis of sequential liver biopsy samples from rheumatoid arthritis patients receiving long-term methotrexate therapy: followup over long treatment intervals and correlation with clinical and laboratory variables. *Arthritis Rheum* 1995; **38**: 1194–203.

80. Fathi, N. H., Mitros, F., Hoffman, J., Straniero, N., Labreque, D. *et al*. Longitudinal measurement of methotrexate liver concentrations does not correlate with liver damage, clinical efficacy, or toxicity during a 3.5 year double blind study in rheumatoid arthritis. *J Rheumatol* 2002; **29**: 2092–8.

81. Walker, A. M., Funch, D., Dreyer, N. A. *et al*. Determinants of serious liver disease among patients receiving low-dose methotrexate for rheumatoid arthritis. *Arthritis Rheum* 1993; **36**: 329–35.

82. van der Veen, M. J., van der Heijde, A., Kruize, A. A., and Bijlsma J. W. Infection rate and use of antibiotics in patients with rheumatoid arthritis treated with methotrexate. *Ann Rheum Dis* 1994; **53**: 224–8.

83. Boerbooms, A. M., Kerstens, P. J., van Loenhout, J. W. *et al*. Infections during low-dose methotrexate treatment in rheumatoid arthritis. Semin *Arthritis Rheum* 1995; **24**: 411–21.

84. Grennan, D. M., Gray, J., Loudon, J. *et al*. Methotrexate and early postoperative complications in patients with rheumatoid arthritis undergoing elective orthopaedic surgery. *Ann Rheum Dis* 2001; **60**, 214–17.

85. Lewden, B., Vial, T., Elefant, E. *et al*. Low dose MTX in the first trimester of pregnancy: results of a French collaborative study. *J Rheumatol* 2004; **31**: 2360–5.

86. Dawson, T. M., Starkebaum, G., Wood, B. L., Willkens, R. F., Gown, A. M. *et al*. Epstein-Barr virus, methotrexate, and lymphoma in patients with rheumatoid arthritis and primary Sjogren's syndrome: case series. *J Rheumatol* 2001; **28**: 47–53.

87. Georgescu, L., Quinn, G. C., Schwartzman, S., and Paget, S. A. Lymphoma in patients with rheumatoid arthritis: association with the disease state or methotrexate treatment. *Semin Arthritis Rheum* 1997; **26**: 794–804.

88. Baird, R. D., van Zyl-Smit, R. N., Dilke, T., Scott, S. E., and Rassam, S. M. B. Spontaneous remission of low-grade B-cell non-Hodgkin's lymphoma following withdrawal of methotrexate in a patient with rheumatoid arthritis: case report and review of the literature. *Br J Haematol* 2002; **118**: 567–8.

89. Moder, K. G., Tefferi, A., Cohen, M. D. *et al*. Hematologic malignancies and the use of methotrexate in rheumatoid arthritis: a retrospective study. *Am J Med* 1995; **99**: 276–81.

90. Wernick, R., and Smith, D. L. Central nervous system toxicity associated with weekly low-dose methotrexate therapy. *Arthritis Rheum* 1989; **32**: 770–5.

91. Buckley, L. M., Leib, E. S., Cartularo, K. S. *et al*. Effects of low dose methotrexate on the bone mineral density of patients with rheumatoid arthritis. *J Rheumatol* 1997; **24**: 1489–94.

92. Morgan, S. L., Baggot, J. E., and Altz-Smith, M. Folate status of rheumatoid arthritis patients receiving long-term, low-dose methotrexate therapy. *Arthritis Rheum* 1987; **30**: 1348–56.

93. Whittle, S. L., and Hudges, R. A. Folate supplementation and methotrexate treatment in rheumatoid arthritis: a review. *Rheumatology* 2004; **43**: 267–71.

94. Kremer, J. M., Davey, B. T., Hall, M. J., and Lawrence, D. A. Significant differences in red blood cell folate levels between best and worst responders to methotrexate in patients with rheumatoid arthritis. *Arthritis Rheum* 1998; **41**: S158 [abstract].

95. van Ede, A. E., Laan, R. F., Blom, H. J., Boers, G. H., Haagsma, C. J. *et al*. Homocysteine and folate status in methotrexate-treated patients with rheumatoid arthritis. *Rheumatology* 2002; **41**: 658–65.

96. Jensen, O. K., Rasmussen, C., Mollerup, F., Christensen, P. B., Hansen, H. *et al*. Hyperhomocysteinemia in rheumatoid arthritis: influence of methotrexate treatment and folic acid supplementation. *J Rheumatol* 2002; **29**: 1615–18.

97. Genestier, L., Paillot, R., Quemeneur, L. *et al*. Mechanisms of action of methotrexate. *Immunopharmacology* 2000; **47**: 247–57.

98. Bressolle, F., Kinowski, J. M., Morel, J. *et al*. Folic acid alters methotrexate availability in patients with rheumatoid arthritis. *J Rheumatol* 2000; **27**: 2110–14.

99. Kremer, J. M., Alarcon, G. S., Lightfood, R. W. Jr. *et al*. Methotrexate for rheumatoid arthritis: suggested guidelines for monitoring liver toxicity. *Arthritis Rheum* 1994; **37**: 316–28.

100. Bologna, C., Viu, P., Picot, M. C. *et al*. Long-term follow-up in rheumatoid arthritis patients treated with methotrexate: a retrospective, observational study. *Br J Rheumatol* 1997; **36**: 535–40.

101. Weinblatt, M. E., Kaplan, H., and Germain, B. F. Low dose methotrexate compared with auranofin in adult rheumatoid arthritis. *Arthritis Rheum* 1990; **33**: 330–8.

102. Suarez-Almazor, M. E., Fitzgerald, A., Grace, M. *et al*. A randomised controlled trial of parenteral methotrexate compared with sodium aurothiomalate. *J Rheumatol* 1988; **15**: 753–6.

103. Fox, R. I., Hermann, M. L., Frangou, C. G. *et al*. Short analytical review: mechanism of action for leflunomide in rheumatoid arthritis. *Clin Immunol* 1999; **93**: 198–208.

104. Kraan, M. C., Reece, R. J., and Barg, E. C. Modulation of inflammatory and metalloproteinase expression in synovial tissue by

leflunomide and methotrexate in patients with active rheumatoid arthritis. *Arthritis Rheum* 2000; **43**: 1820–30.

105. Rozman, B., Domljan, Z., Popovic, M. *et al.* Long term administration of leflunomide to patients with rheumatoid arthritis. *Arthritis Rheum* 1994; **37** (Suppl.): 339.

106. Mladenovic, V., Domljan, Z., Rozman, B. *et al.* Safety and effectiveness of leflunomide in the treatment of patients with active rheumatoid arthritis: results of a randomized, placebo-controlled, phase II study. *Arthritis Rheum* 1995; **38**: 1595–603.

107. Strand, V., Tugwell, P., Bombardier, C. *et al.* Function and health-related quality of life: results from a randomized controlled trial of leflunomide versus methotrexate or placebo in patients with active rheumatoid arthritis. *Arthritis Rheum* 1999; **42**: 1870–8.

108. Sharp, J. T., Strand, V., Leung, H. *et al.* Treatment with leflunomide slows radiographic progression of rheumatoid arthritis. *Arthritis Rheum* 2000; **43**: 495–505.

109. Smolen, J. S., Kalden, J. R., Scott, D. L. *et al.* Efficacy and safety of leflunomide compared to placebo and sulfasalazine in active rheumatoid arthritis: a double blind randomized multicentre trial. *Lancet* 1999; **353**: 259–66.

110. Larsen, A., Kvien, T. K., Schattenkirchner, M., Rau, R. *et al.* Slowing of disease progression in rheumatoid arthritis patients during long-term treatment with leflunomide or sulfasalazine. *Scand J Rheumatol* 2001; **30**: 135–42.

111. Kalden, J. R., Schattenkirchner, M., Sörensen, H. *et al.* The efficacy and safety of leflunomide in patients with active rheumatoid arthritis. A five-year followup study. *Arthritis Rheum* 2003; **48**: 1513–20.

112. Weinblatt, M. E., Kremer, J. M., Coblyn, J. *et al.* Pharmocokinetics, safety and efficacy of combination treatment with methotrexate and leflunomide in patients with active rheumatoid arthritis. *Arthritis Rheum* 1999; **42**: 1322–8.

113. Kremer, J. M., Genovese, M. C., Cannon, G. W. *et al.* Concomitant leflunomide therapy in patients with active rheumatoid arthritis despite stable doses of methotrexate: a randomized, double-blind, placebo-controlled trial. *Ann Intern Med* 2002; **137**: 726–33.

114. Kremer, J. M., Genovese, M. C., Cannon, G. W. *et al.* Combination of leflunomide and methotrexate in patients with active rheumatoid arthritis failing MTX monotherapy: an open-label extension study. *Arthritis Rheum* 2001; **44**: S144.

115. Coblyn, J. S., Shadick, N., and Helfgott, S. Leflunomide-associated weight loss in rheumatoid arthritis. *Arthritis Rheum* 2001; **44**: 1048–51.

116. The European Agency for the Evaluation of Medical Products EMEA public statement of leflunomide (ARAVA): severe and serious hepatic reactions. EMEA March 12 (Doc. ref: EMEA/H/5611/01/en) 2001.

117. Arthritis Advisory Committee (2003). Briefing information regarding ARAVA (leflunomide). Food and Drug Administration, 5 March (www.fda.gov/ohrms/dockets/ac/03/briefing/3930b2.htm), 2003. Aventis Pharmaceutical.

25 | Gold, antimalarials, sulfasalazine, and other DMARDs

Piet L. C. M. van Riel and Eric-Jan J. A. Kroot

Introduction

Pharmacotherapy is still considered as the cornerstone in the management of rheumatoid arthritis (RA). Due to insights into the pathogenesis of RA and the availability of an increasing number of anti-rheumatic therapies, the strategy of the treatment of RA has changed dramatically in the past decade.

Changes in the pharmacotherapeutic management

Until half a century ago, only a few disease-modifying anti-rheumatic drugs (DMARDs) were available for the treatment of RA: antimalarials, sulfasalazine, d-penicillamine, and injectable gold salts. The management of RA at that time was mainly based on a 'wait and see' policy. This was on the assumption that prognosis was benign, the fear of adverse reactions, and on the lack of alternative treatments. It was common to treat the patient with active RA as long as possible with (bed)rest and salicylates; in the meantime the patient was reassured that the disease was not severe enough to 'dig up the gold'. From 1950 onwards, gradually more first- and second-line agents became available. Almost all the DMARDs were primarily developed for the treatment of other diseases and were found to be useful in the treatment of RA by coincidence. Only sulfasalazine was developed specifically for the treatment of RA and inflammatory bowel disease (IBD), on the assumption that both RA and IBD were caused by an infectious agent. As it was not directly clear in which order these drugs had to be used, the 'pyramid' treatment approach was followed. This strategy was mainly driven by the desire to avoid toxicity, which meant starting with the less toxic drug and keeping the more toxic drugs, which frequently appeared to be also the most effective, in reserve. In the 1980s the pyramid approach was abandoned, as it became clear that RA had a significant morbidity and mortality, with major consequences both for the individual and for society. In addition, it was shown that joint destruction started in the first years of disease and that it was possible to slow down this process both early and late in the disease course with DMARDs[1]. Moreover, results of several recent studies suggest that early treatment with two- and three-DMARD combinations produce superior benefits in comparison with DMARD monotherapy[2–7]. In addition, it was recently shown that a strategy of intensive monitoring and treatment of patients with RA with standard DMARDs aiming to achieve tight control of disease activity resulted in improved outcomes[8]. Due to the introduction of biological agents targeting the important mediators in the pathogenesis of RA such as tumor necrosis factor (TNF)-α, interleukin (IL)-1, or certain adhesion molecules (see Chapters 4 and 7), it is to be foreseen that in the coming years the early treatment strategies will be further adjusted (see Chapter 26). In addition, due to the new therapeutic possibilities that these innovative treatment strategies have created, several DMARDs discussed in this section will probably be removed from the anti-rheumatic therapeutic arsenal of RA in the near future.

Antimalarials

History

Hydroxychloroquine and chloroquine, two drugs used for the treatment and prophylaxis of malaria, have been widely used for the treatment of RA and systemic lupus erythematosus (SLE). In the early 1950s, Page first suggested remission of associated RA in his series of patients using antimalarials for other reasons[9]. Since that time, several double-blind, placebo-controlled trials have been conducted testing antimalarials in RA[9,10]. The efficacy has been proven to be somewhat weaker than that of most other DMARDs. However, one major advantage of antimalarials is their lack of life-threatening toxicity compared to other DMARDs. Therefore, antimalarials are frequently used in moderately active RA and in combination with other DMARDs for more severe disease[11,12].

Pharmacology

Both hydroxychloroquine and chloroquine are efficiently absorbed in the gastrointestinal tract and rapidly cleared from the plasma unchanged, after which their disposition is characterized by distribution in the tissues, including liver, spleen, kidney, and red and white blood cells[13]. Their extended half-lives of almost 40 days are caused by their unusually large volumes of distribution[11]. Thus steady state concentrations are only achieved after 3–4 months. This tissue accumulation can be explained by the avid intracellular uptake of antimalarials by acidic cytoplasmic vesicles, particularly by the lysosomes. This explains the high concentrations in the liver, which contains an abundance of lysosomes. Both drugs are metabolized by dealkylation. However, their excretion is different: chloroquine is predominantly excreted in the urine whereas hydroxychloroquine is predominantly excreted in the feces. Two studies have shown a correlation between a better clinical response and higher serum hydroxychloroquine levels[12,14]. However, there is a great inter-individual variability in serum levels of both drugs and evidence for a dose–response relationship needs further investigation[15].

Mechanism of action

The mechanism of action of chloroquine and hydroxychloroquine remains controversial. The most likely explanation is the inhibition of the antigen processing ability of macrophages and monocytes, leading to the inhibition of lymphocyte stimulation and proliferation, possibly leading to a down-regulation of autoimmune responses[16]. Antigen processing is inhibited by the reduction of lysosomal pH. Additional modes of action may include inhibition of chemotaxis, and IL-1 secretion by monocytes.

Therapeutic efficacy

Several double-blind, placebo-controlled clinical trials and randomized comparative studies in patients with RA have demonstrated efficacy[9,17,18]. Improved functional class, joint count, pain, grip strength, patient and observer's assessments, erythrocyte sedimentation rate (ESR), and hemoglobin have been reported. Studies comparing sulfasalazine and hydroxychloroquine showed no statistically significant differences in disease activity variables, including pain, general health, and number of tender and swollen joints. In one study, hydroxychloroquine had a slower onset of anti-rheumatic effect in comparison with sulfasalazine, but no difference was seen at 48 weeks[17]. However, sulfasalazine seemed to be effective in reducing radiological progression[1]. Improvements or slowing of joint destruction have not yet been demonstrated for antimalarials. A meta-analysis comparing the therapeutic efficacy of hydroxychloroquine and chloroquine, by using the generally accepted doses for both drugs (200–400 mg for hydroxychloroquine and 250 mg for chloroquine), showed that chloroquine was more effective than hydroxychloroquine, a finding that requires confirmation[19]. In a double-blind trial in which patients with juvenile RA were treated with hydroxychloroquine, no therapeutic effect was reported[20]. In conclusion, both hydroxychloroquine and chloroquine have been proven to be effective in the treatment of up to 60–80% of patients with RA or SLE. Maximum anti-rheumatic effect is usually achieved after 4–6 months of treatment.

Toxicity

The range of adverse effects is similar for hydroxychloroquine and chloroquine. However, hydroxychloroquine has been reported to have an incidence of adverse effects about half that of chloroquine in the usual doses. Both drugs have been shown to have the mildest toxicity profile in comparison with other DMARDs. Gastrointestinal side-effects are the most common and include epigastric discomfort and nausea. Headache and dermatological side-effects, such as urticaria, lichenoid changes, and

erythema multiforme, have also been reported in a number of studies[11,21]. The most serious side-effect reported so far is retinopathy. However, most case reports of retinopathy date from the 1960s when patients were prescribed higher doses than are now recommended. In these reports irreversible retinal damage (bull's eye retinopathy) involving blurred vision, accommodation problems, scotoma or night blindness, and loss of central vision have been reported. Retinal damage is not related to duration of therapy or to total cumulative dose, but rather to daily dose of the drug. Although severe toxicity is rare, baseline and six-monthly eye examination, including fundoscopy, colour vision testing, and visual field charting, are recommended[22,23].

Daily clinical practice

Dosage limits of 6 mg/kg/day for hydroxychloroquine and 4 mg/kg/day for chloroquine are recommended. These drugs should be used in patients with a normal liver function. Increases or decreases in dosing should be instituted when the body weight is outside the range of 60–70 kg[24]. Patients should be instructed to report any visual symptoms as soon as possible. Complete blood counts and urine analysis should be performed at the same intervals as the ophthalmological examinations. The drug should be used with caution in patients with renal disease or epilepsy. Use of antimalarials in pregnancy should be avoided[25].

Cyclosporin

History

Cyclosporin was first used in the management of rejection in solid organ transplantation. Borel discovered its immunosuppressive properties in 1972[26]. Shortly thereafter, cyclosporin was introduced for the treatment of several autoimmune diseases, including psoriasis, autoimmune eye disease, and inflammatory bowel disease[27]. In 1979, Hermann and Muller introduced cyclosporin for the treatment of RA[28]. Since then, several studies have confirmed the modest efficacy of cyclosporin in the treatment of RA[29–35].

Pharmacology

The cyclosporins, a family of nine distinct polypeptides (termed A to I), each composed of 11 amino acid residues, have been isolated from mycelia of two fungi, *Cyclocarpon leucidum* and *Trichoderma polysporum*. These fungi were found during the search for newer antimicrobial agents in Norway. Only cyclosporin A (cyclosporin) is immunologically active[27,36]. Cyclosporin, lipophilic by nature, is efficiently absorbed in the gastrointestinal tract and metabolized by the liver cytochrome P450-dependent mixed function oxidase system and eliminated in the bile. So the metabolism of cyclosporin may be affected by enzyme inhibitors and inducers. The elimination half-life is about 15 h in RA patients. Only 6% is eliminated through the urine[37]. Recently a microemulsion-based formulation of cyclosporin (neoral) has been developed, which possesses more predictable and improved absorption, with a consequent increased peak concentration and systemic bioavailability[38] with improved efficacy and better short-term safety profile.

Mechanism of action

Cyclosporin forms a complex with specific intracellular proteins known as cyclophilins. This cyclosporin/cyclophilin complex binds to calcineurin, thereby inhibiting its intracellular phosphatase activity[28]. As a result, there is inhibition of IL-2 production, which suppresses T cell activation. It also inhibits IL-1, IL-3, granulocyte-macrophage colony-stimulating factor, tumor and TNF-α secretion from macrophages[38,39]. The impaired production of these cytokines leads to inhibition of T cell activation and T cell-dependent immune responses. In addition, cyclosporin inhibits T cell initiation of humoral immunity, which means that immunoglobulin production is suppressed[38,39].

Therapeutic efficacy

Most studies investigating the efficacy of cyclosporin have been performed in RA patients refractory to other DMARDs. At the moment, only a small number of prospective, randomized, double-blind clinical trials on the efficacy of cyclosporin, at doses of 2.5–5 mg/kg per day, have been reported. Improvements in several clinical parameters and a 40% reduction in serum C-reactive protein (CRP) concentrations were noted compared with placebo[40]. Clinical benefit was evident after 3–6 months. No effect of cyclosporin on ESR has been reported in almost all studies evaluating the efficacy of cyclosporin. No long-term comparative trials have been performed to compare the efficacy of cyclosporin with that of methotrexate and azathioprine. In trials in which cyclosporin was compared with d-penicillamine (two years) and azathioprine (six months), comparable efficacy, but a higher number of adverse events for cyclosporin-treated patients was reported[41,42]. Retardation of radiological progression and clinical outcome in patients with active RA have been found in controlled clinical trials in which patients were treated with cyclosporin or placebo[40,43]. In another study no difference between cyclosporin and parenteral gold was found[44]. There have been two studies combining cyclosporin with another DMARD, methotrexate in particular. This combination appeared to be a promising option as clinical improvements without a substantial increase in adverse events were found[31,45]. But in neither of these two studies was the combination of cyclosporin and methotrexate able to induce clinical remission.

Toxicity

The most important side-effects leading to discontinuation of cyclosporin treatment include gastrointestinal intolerance and renal dysfunction. This renal toxicity is predictable and dose dependent. Measurement of 24 h urinary protein and plasma creatinine are recommended at the start of cyclosporin treatment. When, during treatment, the creatinine levels are persistently increased up to 30% of pretreatment levels, the dose should be reduced. It is possible that slowly progressive renal fibrosis, which

has been convincingly documented in patients with psoriasis[47], may also occur in RA patients. Cyclosporin treatment has been reported to be associated with an increased incidence of malignancies, lymphomas in particular[46]. Another common side-effect is hypertension, which is usually reversible by stopping the treatment or reducing the dose. Other frequently occurring side-effects include paresthesias, hypertrichosis, headaches, and gingival hyperplasia[46].

Daily clinical practice

The starting dosage for cyclosporin should be 2.5 mg/kg daily to 3.5 mg/kg daily as a twice-daily regimen, but in daily clinical practice the starting dose is often lower, 1–2 mg/kg daily. After 4–8 weeks the dose can be increased by increments of 0.5–1.0 mg/kg daily, up to a maximum of 5 mg/kg daily, at monthly or bimonthly intervals. Clinical response might be expected after 8–12 weeks. Cyclosporin should be stopped if no, or only partial, clinical response is achieved after three months, at maximal dosing of the drug. A complete blood count and liver function tests should be performed at baseline and periodically (once every two or three months) thereafter. When the dose is increased, monthly complete blood count and liver function tests, next to creatinine testing, are recommended for a period up to three months and periodically (once every two or three months) thereafter. The blood pressure and serum creatinine should be measured at baseline and biweekly for at least three months and monthly thereafter if a stable dose has been achieved. When creatinine increases to 30% above the baseline value, the dose has to be reduced. If the creatinine remains elevated the drug has to be discontinued. The drug has to be used with caution in patients with: age above 65 years, controlled hypertension, use of drugs with known cyclosporin interactions, use of NSAIDs, previous or concurrent use of alkylating agents, pre-malignant conditions, active infections, and pregnancy or breastfeeding. The drug is contraindicated in patients with known renal dysfunction, uncontrolled hypertension, current or past malignancy except for basal cell carcinoma, leucopoenia or thrombocytopenia, abnormal liver enzymes defined as twice the upper limit, or patients with an immunodeficiency disorder[48].

Gold salts

History

At the end of the last century the antimicrobial activity of gold salts *in vitro* was demonstrated[49]. Elsome showed that gold is highly active against the Gram-positive and some Gram-negative organisms and *Candida albicans in vitro*[49]. However, in patients with tuberculosis, treatment with intramuscular administered gold salts appeared not to be successful. As it was thought at that time that RA and tuberculosis had some similarities, being granulomatous diseases, gold salts were subsequently successfully tried in patients with RA by Forestier[50]. Most studies with gold salts have were performed in the 1970s and 1980s due to the introduction of an oral gold compound, auranofin, as at that time the intramuscular gold salts were viewed as the 'gold standard' disease-modifying agent. Although gold salts are no longer considered as the first choice in the treatment of RA, since the introduction of sulfasalazine and methotrexate, this oldest conventional DMARD is definitely not outdated, as modern DMARDs do not appear to be much better than it[51]. Therefore it is suggested that a sufficient trial of conventional DMARDs, including gold, should be considered preceding the introduction of treatment with the new and promising, but very expensive biologics[51]. However, it seems more likely to reflect clinical practice that gold salts are more likely to be used after failure of biological agents. The orally administered gold compound, auranofin, has a different efficacy and toxicity profile than the parenteral gold compounds and will be dealt with separately.

Parenteral gold compounds

Mechanism of action

Many effects of gold compounds on cellular and humoral immune responses have been demonstrated. However, the exact mechanism of action is still unknown. Worldwide, different gold compounds are used. The two most frequently used are sodium aurothiomalate and aurothioglucose. Both are water soluble and administered intramuscularly; sodium aurothiomalate is an aqueous solution while aurothioglucose is an oily suspension. Other parenteral preparations used include sodium aurothiopropanol sulfonate, aurothiopolypeptide, and sodium aurothiosulfate.

Therapeutic efficacy

The efficacy of the parenteral gold compounds has been clearly demonstrated in many controlled clinical trials. In addition to effects on clinical and laboratory features of RA, which are usually observed after a period of 8–12 weeks, it has been shown that treatment with parenteral gold compounds improves functional status and may slow down radiographic progression. Treatment with parenteral gold compounds resulted in similar efficacy percentages as treatment with sulfasalazine, d-penicillamine, azathioprine (2.5 mg/kg/day), cyclophosphamide (1.5 mg/kg/day), or methotrexate (15 mg/week). However, the withdrawal rate due to adverse reactions during gold treatment is significantly higher than during treatment with most other second-line agents[52]. Furthermore, a randomized 18-month open trial showed equivalence with cyclosporin A[44]. A recent study investigated whether the effect of intramuscular gold salts on functional status (Health Assessment Questionnaire, HAQ) was dependent on disease duration[53]. Significant reductions in disease activity variables were seen in all disease duration groups, although the HAQ only improved in the patient population with disease duration below two years. In another study, the efficacy and safety of intramuscular gold compounds was compared with methotrexate in 174 patients with a rather early (median disease duration of 11 months), erosive RA[54]. Patients were treated with weekly doses of either 50 mg aurothiomalate or 15 mg methotrexate. A significant response (more than 50% improvement in swollen and tender joints and ESR) was observed more frequently in the methotrexate-treated patients than in the gold-treated patients (76 versus 68%), while a complete remission was more frequently

observed in the gold-treated patients (24 versus 11%). As expected, significantly more gold-treated patients were withdrawn due to adverse reactions (6/87 versus 32/87). However, as has been observed earlier, those patients who were withdrawn due to adverse reactions on the gold compound experienced a marked improvement or even a clinical remission, which was sustained for months after stopping the treatment. This is never the case in methotrexate withdrawals. For many years it was not clear whether or not patients who were treated for the second time with a parenteral gold compound experienced the same response as during the first course. In a study in which the data from 45 patients who had received more than one gold course were reviewed it was shown that more than 95% of the patients who responded to the first course also responded to the second course[55]. The patients who had to discontinue the first course due to adverse reactions also developed an adverse reaction to the second course in 65% of the cases. Patients who did not respond to the first course also did not respond to the second one.

Toxicity

Sodium aurothiomalate is an aqueous gold salt that is rapidly absorbed from the injection site, in contrast to the lipid aurothioglucose, which is more slowly absorbed. The adverse reactions for both gold compounds are similar with one exception: 'nitritoid' cardiovascular reactions such as flushing, hypotension, tachycardia, and palpitations are unique to sodium aurothiomalate, probably due to the rapid absorption from the injection site. Treatment with gold salts is characterized by a high number of adverse reactions, the incidence varying from 25 to 40%. In particular, mucocutaneous reactions are frequently observed, followed by proteinuria and hematological adverse reactions such as leucopenia and thrombocytopenia; aplastic anemia is rarely observed. Some of the adverse reactions are at least partly dose dependent while others are fully idiosyncratic in nature. The dropout rate due to adverse reactions is 20–30%.

Daily clinical practice

Although several different dosing regimes are in use, most frequently one starts with a weekly dose of 50 mg for a period of 20 weeks. When a response occurs the dose can be gradually tapered by increasing the dosing interval. If no response is observed after 20 weeks, the dose can be increased up to 100 mg for a period of 6–8 weeks. Complete blood counts, urinalysis, renal and liver function tests, and chest radiograph should be performed before starting treatment. During the first eight weeks complete blood counts, liver function tests, and urinalysis should be performed every week, thereafter tests should be performed following every second injection. In the case of a mild adverse reaction it has to be decided whether to lower the dose or to temporarily withdraw the gold treatment until the adverse reaction has disappeared.

Oral gold

Mechanism of action

The orally absorbable gold compound, auranofin, is a lipid-soluble triethylphosphine monomeric gold compound. About 25% of auranofin is absorbed from the gastrointestinal tract; the blood levels of gold are one-quarter to one-sixth of those achieved with the parenteral administered gold compounds. Auranofin is more effective than the parenteral gold compounds in models of acute inflammation and is a potent inhibitor of lysosomal enzyme release and superoxide production. Like the parenteral gold compounds it affects cellular and humoral immune reactions.

Efficacy

Auranofin has a slow onset of response—first effects on inflammatory symptoms are seen after 4–6 months, the plateau being reached after six months. Auranofin is less effective than aurothioglucose and aurothiomalate but better tolerated. Auranofin has been found to be less effective than most of the other second-line agents but also less toxic, except for hydroxychloroquine[56]. However, early therapy with auranofin has been found to retard radiographic progression after two and five years[57]. A report with five years' follow-up data of a randomized study in which sulfasalazine was compared to auranofin showed that significantly more patients were still on sulfasalazine after five years follow-up[58]. Those patients who did not respond, or had adverse reactions, to previous parenteral gold treatment had the most unfavorable results: only 4% of those patients were still on auranofin after five years.

Toxicity

The nature of the adverse reactions with auranofin appears to be similar to, but generally less severe than that with parenteral gold compounds. Adverse reactions affecting the lower gastrointestinal tract (loose stools and diarrhea) are the most common complaints. Most adverse reactions occur during the first months of treatment, and are the reason to discontinue the treatment[59] in less than 10% of the patients.

Daily clinical practice

Auranofin is effective in doses of 6–9 mg daily; the usual starting dose is 6 mg, which in case of inefficacy can be increased up to 9 mg. Complete blood counts, urinalysis, and renal and liver function tests should be performed before starting treatment. During the first 12 weeks complete blood counts, liver function tests, and urinalysis should be performed biweekly, thereafter monthly. In the event of adverse reactions, the severity will determine whether one should only lower the dose or withdraw the treatment temporarily or permanently.

Immunosuppressive agents

The two most frequently used immunosuppressive agents at present, the 'anticancer' agents cyclophosphamide and azathioprine, were introduced for the treatment of RA in the 1960s. Their efficacy in the treatment of RA has been clearly demonstrated in many studies. However, especially for cyclophosphamide, the indications for its use in RA have become restricted due to the severe adverse reactions.

Cyclophosphamide

Cyclophosphamide, an alkylating agent, has long been thought to be the most effective anti-rheumatic drug in the treatment of RA. In a recent review cyclophosphamide appeared to have a clinically and statistically significant benefit on the disease activity of RA patients, similar to some other DMARDs such as antimalarials or sulfasalazine but lower than methotrexate[60]. Unfortunately it is also the most toxic agent, limiting its use given the low benefit–risk ratio compared to other anti-rheumatic agents. Potential severe adverse reactions include bone marrow suppression, infections, gonadal failure, hemorrhagic cystitis, alopecia, and the risk of developing malignancies, especially of the skin and bladder[61]. Cyclophosphamide and its metabolites are mainly excreted by the kidney. Hemorrhagic cystitis results from contact of the bladder with the metabolite and its occurrence can be reduced by ingestions of large amounts of fluid and administration of cyclophosphamide in a single morning dose. Cyclophosphamide is usually given as a daily oral dose (1.5 up to 2 mg/kg). It is not clear whether intermittent intravenous pulse treatment dose (5–10 mg/kg weekly or 500–1000 monthly) is of any benefit in RA. It is mostly indicated in patients with severe extra-articular vasculitic complications. In these patients the drug may be lifesaving, but meticulous monitoring and good clinical judgement are definitely required to use it effectively.

Azathioprine

Azathioprine, a purine analog, is used in the treatment of RA, in patients who are unable to tolerate or do not respond to other agents. It is regularly used in the management of other autoimmune diseases, SLE in particular, as a steroid-sparing agent. Azathioprine is usually given in an oral dose of 100–150 mg/day (1.25–3 mg/kg) although there are schemes in which 300 mg azathioprine given on alternative days might be useful as well[62,63]. It has been suggested that an intravenous loading dose of 40 mg/kg could speed up onset of clinical response, which is usually in excess of 8 weeks[64]. Azathioprine in a maximum dose of 150 mg appeared to be less effective in the treatment of RA than methotrexate in a maximum dose of 15 mg weekly, with respect to signs and symptoms as well as radiographic damage[62,63]. As with cyclophosphamide, dose-related bone marrow suppression is the most frequent adverse reaction to azathioprine. Next to this, gastrointestinal intolerance (nausea, vomiting, and diarrhea), susceptibility to infections, alopecia, and liver function test abnormalities can be observed. Second only to cyclophosphamide, treatment with azathioprine is associated with an increased risk of malignancies, particularly lymphomas[65].

D-penicillamine

History

Penicillamine has been used in the treatment of RA and systemic sclerosis for more than 30 years. During this period, a number of placebo-controlled studies have documented the clinical efficacy of penicillamine in the treatment of RA[66]. Whereas the mechanism of action of penicillamine is easily understood in the treatment of Wilson's disease, heavy-metal poisoning, and cystinuria, the mechanism of action of penicillamine as a DMARD in the treatment of RA remains unclear[67]. The beneficial effect has to be balanced against the serious side-effects that have been reported in several studies. Nevertheless penicillamine remains a therapeutic option in the treatment of RA.

Pharmacology

Penicillamine can be obtained by hydrolytic degradation of penicillin or can be chemically synthesized. Penicillamine exists as D and L enantiomers; the D enantiomer is clinically used because of the greater toxicity of the L enantiomer. The bioavailability is 50–70% after gastrointestinal absorption, but can be reduced by concurrent food, antacids, and oral iron preparations. Peak plasma concentrations of D-penicillamine (penicillamine) occur 1.5–4 h after oral dosage, and can be raised to 4–6 days in patients on long-term therapy. Penicillamine is rapidly cleared through oxidation to form disulfides with plasma proteins with reactive sulfhydryl groups, such as albumin, α_1-antitrypsin, IgA, L-cysteine, homocysteine, and with itself, resulting in penicillamine disulfide. The disulfides are mainly excreted in urine, and only partly in the feces[66,67]. Mixed disulfides with penicillamine, for example on cell surfaces, are probably involved in the biological effect in RA.

Mechanism of action

The mode of action remains, like that of most other DMARDs, unclear. It seems likely that the thiol group on penicillamine and oxidative reactions involved in the metabolism of penicillamine are responsible for the disease-modifying effect[66]. Also, the modulation of the immune system via sulfhydryl exchange reactions in various cells has been proposed as an important mode of action[67]. Penicillamine has a more inhibitory effect on T cell-mediated B cell expansion and activation than on direct action on B cells. Penicillamine is associated with limited suppression of the synthesis of immunoglobulins. This may be mediated by the effects of penicillamine/copper sulfate complexes on helper T cells. Penicillamine has also been reported to reduce tissue damage by inhibiting the granular enzyme myeloperoxidase[66].

Therapeutic efficacy

The therapeutic efficacy of penicillamine has been proven in a number of placebo-controlled trials, whereas there are only a few studies comparing penicillamine with other DMARDs[68]. Not only clinical improvements, but also reductions in ESRs, rheumatoid factors (RFs), immunoglobulins, hemoglobin, and circulating immune complexes have been reported in placebo-controlled trials[66]. However, it can take 3–6 months before full clinical response is apparent. No significant differences in efficacy between doses of 600 and 1200 mg/day were found. Lower doses have not been found to be effective. Comparative trials, with sulfasalazine, antimalarials, azathioprine, and intramuscular gold, have not reported better response rates for penicillamine[66,67].

There are few long-term efficacy data for penicillamine, but discontinuation of the drug due to lack of efficacy or side-effects has been frequently reported[69]. After five years, only 20% of the patients remained on penicillamine treatment, but intermittent treatment may sustain response in the longer term[66].

Toxicity

Discontinuation of penicillamine therapy due to drug toxicity is seen in up to 50% of patients. Most of these patients experience an adverse drug reaction during the first six months of treatment. One of the most important side-effects leading to discontinuation of penicillamine treatment is mucocutaneous reactions, including mouth ulcers, and urticarial and pruritic skin rashes[70]. Proteinuria due to immune complex-mediated glomerulonephritis in particular, is the most important renal complication, resolving in most patients after drug discontinuation. Adverse drug reactions occur significantly more often in human leukocyte antigen (HLA)-DR3 positive patients than among HLA-DR3 negative RA patients[71]. This link to HLA-DR3 has been the first example of immunopharmacogenetics[71]. Gastrointestinal side-effects include dysgeusia and nausea. Pancytopenia is the most common cause of death related to penicillamine. Other less serious hematological side-effects include thrombocytopenia and leucopenia. Despite the immunomodulatory effect of penicillamine, a number of autoimmune diseases such as myasthenia gravis, polymyositis, Goodpasture's syndrome, SLE, and pemphigus may occur[72]. These diseases resolve after discontinuation of penicillamine treatment. Another very rare side-effect is mammary hyperplasia, after which penicillamine treatment has to be stopped immediately.

Daily clinical practice

Penicillamine is administered in a non-enteric-coated form and should be taken without meals (1 h before), antacids, and iron tablets. Some advocate taking the penicillamine at bedtime. To avoid toxicity, the starting dose is 125 mg/day; thereafter dosing increments of 125 mg/day at 4–8-week intervals are added until response is satisfactory or a dose of 750 mg/day is achieved. Doses up to 1000–1500 mg/day have been reported, but the risk of toxicity is then substantially increased. It can take up to six months before full clinical response is apparent. Complete blood counts and urine analysis should be monitored biweekly until a stable dose is achieved. Thereafter monitoring can be reduced to every four weeks. Patients should be instructed to report symptoms that might indicate myelosuppression (edema, rash, bleeding, abnormal bruising, fever, and mouth ulceration), after which the drug has to be stopped immediately. The drug should be used with caution in patients with hepatic or renal failure. No special precautions are required in the elderly.

Sulfasalazine

History

Sulfasalazine was developed and used in the treatment of RA during the 1940s. At that time, RA was thought to have an infective etiology and therefore an anti-inflammatory agent

(5-aminosalicylic acid) and an antibiotic (sulfapyridine) were combined, which resulted in the development of sulfasalazine[73]. After encouraging results in the first decade, the drug fell out of favor due to conclusions based on a badly designed controlled study on the one hand and the spectacular results of corticosteroids on the other. In the late 1970s, after a period in which sulfasalazine was mainly used in the treatment of inflammatory bowel disease, the drug was rediscovered for the treatment of RA by McConkey *et al.*[74] In recent decades, the second-line effect has been established in several placebo-controlled trials and randomized controlled studies[19,56,75–80]. Today its use as monotherapy has frequently been replaced by the more effective use in combination therapies of two or three complementary drugs in active RA.

Pharmacology

Sulfasalazine consists of 5-aminosalicylic acid (5-ASA) and sulfapyridine linked by a diazo bond. As sulfasalazine is quite insoluble, the drug is poorly absorbed (10–20%). The drug is split into sulfapyridine and 5-aminosalicylic acid by bacterial azoreductases in the large intestine[73]. About 30% of 5-ASA is excreted in the urine following acetylation, whereas 50% is excreted unchanged in feces. Sulfapyridine blood levels appear 3–6 h post dosing. It undergoes acetylation in the liver to acetylsulfapyridine, hydroxylation to 5-hydroxysulfapyridine, and subsequent glucuronidation of these metabolites. Both acetylsulfapyridine and 5-hydroxysulfapyridine are excreted in the urine, either unchanged or after glucuronidation. As the rate of hepatic acetylation and oxidation is genetically determined, differences in rates of metabolism and plasma concentrations of sulfapyridine occur[74,81].

Mechanism of action

The mechanism of action of sulfasalazine is still unknown, but most evidence favors sulfapyridine rather than 5-ASA as the active moiety, both clinically and also in producing side-effects. A therapeutic action by the 30% of sulfasalazine that is absorbed unaltered cannot be excluded[81]. The sulfapyridine moiety seems to have immunomodulatory effects influencing prostaglandin synthesis, superoxide scavenging, lymphocyte function, polymorphonuclear leukocyte chemotaxis, inhibition of folate-dependent enzymes, and synovial neovascularization. In inflammatory bowel diseases, however, it has been shown that 5-amino salicylate acid is the active moiety[73,81]. It is of interest that sulfasalazine is an inhibitor of nuclear factor (NF)-κB[82]. Transcription factors of the NF-κB are critical for inducible expression of multiple genes involved in inflammatory responses. The specific inhibition of NF-κB activation by sulfasalazine is therefore an important target of sulfasalazine-mediated immunosuppression.

Therapeutic efficacy

Many randomized, placebo-controlled trials and non-comparative studies have demonstrated the efficacy of sulfasalazine in the treatment of RA[19]. Significant improvement in ESR, Ritchie articular index (RAI), number of swollen joints, grip strength, and duration of early morning stiffness has been reported in double-blind, placebo-controlled trails of sulfasalazine 2.0–3.0 g/day in patients with RA. In a comparative clinical trial, in which sulfasalazine was compared with hydroxychloroquine, significantly reduced radiological progression was observed within one year of treatment, and was still sustained after three years of follow-up[83]. A large meta-analysis of patients completing DMARD therapy in clinical trials demonstrated little difference in efficacy of sulfasalazine, methotrexate, parental or intramuscular gold, and D-penicillamine[19]. Only the rate of onset of action has been reported to be more rapid with sulfasalazine than with other DMARDs. Better drug survival rates have been found for sulfasalazine in comparison with aurothioglucose and hydroxychloroquine[84]. Clinical benefit was evident after 4–8 weeks of sulfasalazine treatment in some studies, before the comparator DMARD (respectively, hydrochloroquine and hydroxychloroquine) showed effect[17,18]. Combination therapy of methotrexate and sulfasalazine in patients who responded inadequately to sulfasalazine alone showed significant clinical improvements in a 24-week, randomized, non-blinded study[85]. Combination therapy of sulfasalazine with D-penicillamine, parental gold, or azathioprine has also been successful in several clinical studies, but was generally less well tolerated than monotherapy[86,87].

Toxicity

The adverse reaction profile of sulfasalazine is extensively known since it has been used in the treatment of inflammatory bowel diseases for more than 40 years. Gastrointestinal and central nervous system reactions are the most frequently reported adverse reactions[84]. Up to half of the patients may suffer from these reactions at some time. Nausea, vomiting, anorexia, dyspepsia, headache, and dizziness are the most common side-effects[88]. The gastrointestinal side-effects, particularly, seem to be dose related. The bulk of evidence favours sulfapyridine rather than 5-ASA as the therapeutic active moiety, as well as the main producer of these side-effects. Dose reduction with or without interruption of the medication for a couple of days is often effective in reducing these adverse effects[81]. The majority of these side-effects occur in the first 2–3 months of treatment and are less likely if dosage is increased gradually or when enteric-coated tablets are used[73]. Most of these effects disappear spontaneously after withdrawal of sulfasalazine. As most side-effects occur early in the treatment, biweekly monitoring of full blood counts and liver function tests during the first three months and once every 4–12 weeks thereafter have been recommended. Other less frequent adverse reactions include: skin rash, leucopenia and mild hemolysis, hepatitis, eosinophilic pneumonia, agranulocytosis, and hypogammaglobulinemia. The most severe hematological adverse reaction, agranulocytosis, is most likely to occur in the first six months of treatment. It is reversible in most cases after dose cessation or reduction[74]. No teratogenic effect or perinatal morbidity or mortality in the progeny of male or female patients taking sulfasalazine at conception or during pregnancy have been reported, but the use of this drug should be avoided in these circumstances, if possible. Also, fertility is often reduced in male patients treated with sulfasalazine due to a reversible effect on sperm motility and absolute sperm count[74]. Withdrawal rates for adverse reactions in sulfasalazine recipients varied from 10 to 36% in large comparative studies[19,56]. No differences in withdrawals due to adverse reactions have been reported between sulfasalazine, auranofin, and D-penicillamine[73]. Immunomodulation associated with sulfasalazine treatment has been reported to contribute to the development of lupus-related reactions in genetically predisposed individuals. The development of SLE-like symptoms and SLE-related autoantibody production (including increased levels of anti-DNA) were observed more commonly than expected in sulfasalazine-treated patients, with an increased risk in patients with SLE-related HLA haplotypes, increased serum IL-10 levels, and ANA in speckled patterns[89].

Daily clinical practice

Sulfasalazine is administered orally as enteric-coated tablets in the treatment of RA. Patients usually start with 0.5 g/day; thereafter the daily dose is increased by 0.5 g at four-day intervals. The usual maintenance dose is 2.0–3.0 g/day given in two divided doses. Complete blood counts and liver function tests should be performed before starting treatment and at least every four weeks during the first six months of treatment, and every three months thereafter. As there is always a possibility of serious hematological side-effects, patients should be instructed to learn to recognize warning clinical signs such as bruising, rash, fever, or significant malaise. As the drug is extensively metabolized by the liver and excreted by the kidney, it should be used with caution in patients with hepatic or renal disease. By incrementing the dose at four-day intervals, gastrointestinal side-effects are usually avoided. In patients with an ileostomy the drug is contraindicated[90].

Conclusion

In the last years of the previous decade and in the first years of the present decade an increasing number of anti-rheumatic agents have become available that have influenced the pharmacological therapy of RA. The old pyramid approach has been abandoned, replaced by a more aggressive treatment early in the disease course with effective, fast-acting DMARDs[91]. Due to new insights (change in dosages or route of administration, different ways of combining therapies, etc.) and the development of new therapies, the current drug therapy of RA is undergoing changes all the time. It is therefore not possible to present a fixed treatment outline. In general, one should try to suppress the disease activity rapidly and as completely as possible with the least toxic agent(s), singly or in combination, as it has been shown that this improves the clinical and radiological outcomes significantly[8].

References

1. Heijde van der, D. M., Riel van, P. L., Nuver-Zwart, H. H., Gribnau, F. W., and Putte van de, L. B. Effects of hydroxychloroquine and sulphasalazine on progression of joint damage in rheumatoid arthritis. *Lancet* 1989; I: 1036–38.
2. Geletka, R., and St Clair, E. W. Treatment of early rheumatoid arthritis. *Best Pract Res Clin Rheumatol* 2003; 17: 791–809.
3. Hurst, S., Kallan, M. J., Wolfe, F. J., Fries, J. F., and Albert, D. A. Methotrexate, hydroxychloroquine, and intramuscular gold in rheumatoid arthritis: relative area under the curve effectiveness and sequence effects. *J Rheumatol* 2002; 29: 1639–45.
4. O'Dell, J. R., Haire, C. E., Erikson, N., Drymalski, W., Palmer, W., Eckhoff, P. J. et al. Treatment of rheumatoid arthritis with methotrexate alone, sulphasalazine and hydroxychloroquine, or a combination of all three medications. *N Engl J Med* 1996; 334: 1287–91.
5. O'Dell, J. R., Leff, R., Paulsen, G., Haire, C., Mallek, J., Eckhoff, P. J. et al. Treatment of rheumatoid arthritis with methotrexate and hydroxychloroquine, methotrexate and sulphasalazine, or a combination of the three medications: results of a two-year, randomized, double-blind, placebo-controlled trial. *Arthritis Rheum* 2002; 46: 1164–70.
6. Mottonen, T., Hannonen, P., Leirisalo-Repo, M., Nissila, M., Kautiainen, H., Korpela, M. et al. Comparison of combination therapy with single-drug therapy in early rheumatoid arthritis: a randomised trial. FIN-RACo trial group. *Lancet* 1999; 353: 1568–73.
7. Ferraccioli, G. F., Gremese, E., Tomietto, P., Favret, G., Damato, R., and Di Poi, E. Analysis of improvements, full responses, remission and toxicity in rheumatoid patients treated with step-up combination therapy (methotrexate, cyclosporin A, sulphasalazine) or monotherapy for three years. *Rheumatology* 2002; 41: 892–8.
8. Grigor, C., Capell, H., Stirling, A., McMahon, A. D., Lock, P., Vallance, R. et al. Effect of a treatment strategy of tight control for rheumatoid arthritis (the TICORA study): a single-blind randomised controlled trial. *Lancet* 2004; 364: 263–9.
9. Clark, P., Casas, E., Tugwell, P., Medina, C., Gheno, C., Tenorio, G., and Orozco, J. A. Hydroxychloroquine compared with placebo in rheumatoid arthritis: a randomized controlled trial. *Ann Intern Med* 1993; 119: 1067–71.
10. A randomized trial of hydroxychloroquine in early rheumatoid arthritis: the HERA Study. *Am J Med* 1995; 98: 156–68.
11. Tett, S., Culter, D., and Day, R. Antimalarials in rheumatic diseases. *Baillieres Clin Rheumatol* 1990; 4: 467–89.
12. Tett, S. E., Day, R. O., and Cutler, D. J. Concentration-effect relationship of hydroxychloroquine in rheumatoid arthritis: a cross sectional study. *J Rheumatol* 1993; 20: 1874–9.
13. Cutler, D. J., MacIntyre, A. C., and Tett, S. E. Pharmacokinetics and cellular uptake of 4-aminoquinoline antimalarials. *Agents Actions Suppl* 1988; 24: 142–57.
14. Miller, D. R., Fiechtner, J. J., Carpenter, J. R., Brown, R. R., Stroshane, R. M., and Stecher, V. J. Plasma hydroxychloroquine concentrations and efficacy in rheumatoid arthritis. *Arthritis Rheum* 1987; 30: 567–71.
15. McLachlan, A. J., Tett, E., Cutler, D. J., and Day, R. O. Bioavailability of hydrochloroquine tablets in patients with rheumatoid arthritis. *Br J Rheumatol* 1994; 33: 235–9.
16. Fox, R. Mechanism of action of hydroxychloroquine as an antirheumatic drug. *Semin Arthritis Rheum* 1993; 23 (Suppl. 1): 82–91.
17. Nuver-Zwart, I. H., van-Riel, P. L., van-de-Putte, L. B., and Gribnau, F. W. A double blind comparative study of sulphasalazine and hydrochloroquine in rheumatoid arthritis: evidence of an earlier effect of sulphasalazine. *Ann Rheum Dis* 1989; 48: 389–95.
18. Faarvang, K. L., Egsmose, C., Kryger, P., Podenphant, J., Ingeman-Nielsen, M., and Hansen, T. M. Hydroxychloroquine and sulphasalazine alone and in combination in rheumatoid arthritis: a randomised double blind trial. *Ann Rheum Dis* 1993; 52: 711–15.
19. Felson, D. T., Anderson, J. J., and Meenan, R. F. The comparative efficacy and toxicity of second-line drugs in rheumatoid arthritis: results of two metaanalyses. *Arthritis Rheum* 1990; 33: 1449–61.
20. Brewer, E., Giannini, E., Kuzmina, N., and Alekseev, L. Penicillamine and hydroxychloroquine in the treatment of severe juvenile rheumatoid arthritis. *N Engl J Med* 1986; 314: 1269–76.
21. Rynes, R. I. Toxicity of antimalarial drugs in rheumatoid arthritis. *Agents Actions Suppl* 1993; 44: 151–7.
22. Bernstein, H. N. Ocular safety of hydroxychloroquine. *Ann Ophthalmol* 1991; 23: 292–6.
23. Easterbrook, M. The ocular safety of hydroxychloroquine. *Semin Arthritis Rheum*, 1993; 23 (2 Suppl. 1): 62–7.

24. Paulus, H. Antimalarial agents compared with or in combination with other disease modifying antirheumatic drugs. *Am J Med* 1988; **85**: 45–52.

25. American College of Rheumatology Ad Hoc Committee on Clinical Guidelines. Guidelines for monitoring drug therapy in rheumatoid arthritis. *Arthritis Rheum* 1996; **39**: 723–31.

26. Borel, J. F., Feurer, C., Gubler H. U., and Stahelin H. Biological effects of cyclosporin A: a new antilymphocytic agent. *Agents Actions* 1976; **6**: 468–75.

27. Yocum, D. Immunological actions of cyclosporin A in rheumatoid arthritis. *Br J Rheumatol* 1993; **32** (Suppl. 1): 38–41.

28. Chaudhuri, K., Torley, H., and Madhok, R. Disease-modifying antirheumatic drugs: cyclosporin. *British J Rheumatol* 1997; **36**: 1016–21.

29. Dougados, M., and Torley, H. Efficacy of cyclosporin A in rheumatoid arthritis: worldwide experience. *British J Rheumatol* 1993; **32** (Suppl. 1): 57–9.

30. Wells, G., and Tugwell, P. Cyclosporin A in rheumatoid arthritis: overview of efficacy. *Br J Rheumatol* 1993; **32** (Suppl. 1): 51–6.

31. Gerards, A. H., Landewe, R. B., Prins, A. P., Bruijn, G. A., Goei, The H. S., Laan, R. F., and Dijkmans, B. A. Cyclosporin A monotherapy versus cyclosporin A and methotrexate combination therapy in patients with early rheumatoid arthritis: a double blind randomised placebo controlled trial. *Ann Rheum Dis* 2003; **62**: 291–6.

32. Marchesoni, A., Battafarano, N., Arreghini, M., Panni, B., Gallazzi, M., and Tosi, S. Radiographic progression in early rheumatoid arthritis: a 12-month randomized controlled study comparing the combination of cyclosporin and methotrexate with methotrexate alone. *Rheumatology* 2003; **42**: 1545–9.

33. Marchesoni, A., Battafarano, N., Arreghini, M., Pellerito, R., Cagnoli, M., Prudente, P. *et al.* Step-down approach using either cyclosporin A or methotrexate as maintenance therapy in early rheumatoid arthritis. *Arthritis Rheum* 2002; **47**: 59–66.

34. Kim, W. U., Seo, Y. I., Park, S. H., Lee, W. K., Lee, S. K., Paek, S. I. *et al.* Treatment with cyclosporin switching to hydroxychloroquine in patients with rheumatoid arthritis. *Ann Rheum Dis* 2001; **60**: 514–17.

35. Sarzi-Puttini, P., D'Ingianna, E., Fumagalli, M., Scarpellini, M., Fiorini, T., Cherie-Ligniere, E. L. *et al.* An open, randomized comparison study of cyclosporine A, cyclosporine A + methotrexate and cyclosporine A + hydroxychloroquine in the treatment of early severe rheumatoid arthritis. *Rheumatol Int* 2005. [First published online, 7 Oct 2003.]

36. Rainsford, K. D. Disease-modifying antirheumatic and immunoregulatory agents. *Baillieres Clin Rheumatol* 1990; **4**: 405–32.

37. Faulds, D., Goa, K. L., and Benfield, P. Cyclosporin: a review of its pharmacodynamic and pharmacokinetic properties, and therapeutic use in immunoregulatory disorders. *Drugs* 1993; **45**: 953–1040.

38. Richardson, C., and Emery, P. Clinical use of cyclosporin in rheumatoid arthritis [published erratum appears in *Drugs* 1996 Apr; **51**: 570]. *Drugs*, 1995; **50** (Suppl. 1): 26–36.

39. Bentin, J. Mechanism of action of cyclosporin in rheumatoid arthritis. *Clin Rheumatol* 1995; **14** (Suppl. 2): 22–5.

40. Tugwell, P., Bombardier, C., Gent, M., Bennett, K. J., Bensen, W. G., Carette, S. *et al.* Low-dose cyclosporin versus placebo in patients with rheumatoid arthritis. *Lancet* 1990; **335**: 1051–5.

41. Tugwell, P., Bombadier, C., Gent, M. *et al.* Low dose cyclosporin in rheumatoid arthritis: a pilot study. *J Rheumatol* 1987; **14**: 1108–14.

42. Van Rijthoven, A. W., Dijkmans, B. A., Goeithe, H. S. *et al.* Comparison of cyclosporin and D-penicillamine for rheumatoid arthritis: a randomized, double blind, multicenter study. *J Rheumatol* 1991; **18**: 815–20.

43. Pasero, G., Priolo, F., Marubini, E., Fantini, F., Ferraccioli, G., Magaro, M. *et al.* Slow progression of joint damage in early rheumatoid arthritis treated with cyclosporin A. *Arthritis Rheum* 1996; **39**: 1006–15.

44. Zeidler, H., Kvien, T., Hannonen, P., Wollheim, F., Forre, O., Geidel, H. *et al.* Progression of joint damage in early active severe rheumatoid arthritis during 18 months of treatment: comparison of low-dose cyclosporin and parenteral gold. *British J Rheumatol* 1998; **37**: 874–82.

45. Tugwell, P., Pincus, T., Yocum, D., Stein, M. *et al.* Combination therapy with cyclosporin and methotrexate in severe rheumatoid arthritis. *N Engl J Med* 1995; **333**: 137–41.

46. Dijkmans, B. A. Safety aspects of cyclosporin in rheumatoid arthritis. *Drugs* 1995; **50** (Suppl. 1): 41–7.

47. Zachariae, H., Kragballe, K., Hansen, H., Marcussen, N., and Olsen, S. Renal biopsy findings in long-term cyclosporin treatment of psoriasis. *Br J Dermatol* 1997; **136**: 531–5.

48. Panayi, G. S., and Tugwell, P. The use of cyclosporin A in rheumatoid arthritis: conclusions of an international review. *Br J Rheumatol* 1994; **33**: 967–9.

49. Elsome, A. M., Hamilton-Miller, J. M., Brumfitt, W., and Noble, W. C. Antimicrobial activities in vitro and in vivo of transition element complexes containing gold(I) and osmium(VI). *J Antimicrob Chemother* 1996; **37**: 911–18.

50. Kean, W. F., Forestier, F., Kassam, Y., Buchanan, W. W., and Rooney, P. J. The history of gold therapy in rheumatoid disease. *Semin Arthritis Rheum* 1985; **14**: 180–6.

51. Rau, R. Have traditional DMARDs had their day? Effectiveness of parenteral gold compared to biologic agents. *Clin Rheumatol* 2005. [First published online, 24 July 2004.]

52. Gestel van, A. M., Haagsma, C. J., Furst, D. E., and Riel van, P. L. C. M. Treatment of early rheumatoid arthritis patients with slow-acting anti-rheumatic drugs (SAARDs). *Ballieres Clin Rheumatol* 1997; **11**: 65–82.

53. Munro, R., Hampson, R., McEntegart, A., Thomson, E. A., Madhok, R., and Capell, H. Improved functional outcome in patients with early rheumatoid arthritis treated with intramuscular gold: results of a five year prospective study. *Ann Rheum Dis* 1998; **57**: 88–93.

54. Rau, R., Herborn, G., Menninger, H., Blechschmidt, J. Comparison of intramuscular methotrexate and gold sodium thiomalate in the treatment of early erosive rheumatoid arthritis: 12 month data of a double-blind parallel study of 174 patients. *Br J Rheumatol* 1997; **36**: 345–52.

55. Klinkhoff, A. V., and Teufel, A. The second course of gold. *J Rheumatol* 1995; **22**: 1655–66.

56. Felson, D. T., Anderson, J. J., and Meenan, R. F. Use of short-term efficacy/toxicity tradeoffs to select second-line drugs in rheumatoid arthritis. A metaanalysis of published clinical trials. *Arthritis Rheum* 1992; **35**: 1117–25.

57. Egsmose, C., Lund, B., Borg, G., Petterson, H., Berg E., Brodin, U., and Trang, L. Patients with rheumatoid arthritis benefit from early 2nd line therapy: 5 year followup of a prospective double blind placebo controlled study. *J Rheumatol* 1995; **22**: 2208–13.

58. McEntegart, A., Porter, D., Capell, H. A., and Thomson, E. A. Sulphasalazine has a better efficacy/toxicity profile than auranofin: evidence from a 5 year prospective, randomized trial. *J Rheumatol* 1996; **23**: 1887–90.

59. van Riel, P. L., Gribnau, F. W., van de Putte, L. B., and Yap, S. H. Loose stools during auranofin treatment: clinical study and some pathogenetic possibilities. *J Rheumatol* 1983; **10**: 222–6.

60. Suarez-Almazor, M. E., Belseck, E., Shea, B., Wells, G., and Tugwell, P. Cyclophosphamide for rheumatoid arthritis. *Cochrane Database Syst Rev* 2000; **2**: CD001157.

61. Radis, C. D., Kahl, L. E., Baker, G. L., Morgan Wasko, M. C., Cash, J. M., Gallatin A. *et al.* Effects of cyclophosphamide on the development of malignancy and on long-term survival of patients with rheumatoid arthritis: a 20 year followup study. *Arthritis Rheum* 1995; **38**: 1120–7.

62. Jeurissen, M. E. C., and Boerbooms, A. M. Th., Putte van de, L. B. A., Doseburg, W. H., and Lemmens, A. M. Influence of methotrexate and azathioprine on radiologic progression in rheumatoid arthritis. *Ann Intern Med* 1991; **114**: 999–1004.

63. Jeurissen, M. E. C., Boerbooms, A. M. Th., Putte van de, L. B. A., Doesburg, W. H., Mulder, J., Rasker, J. J. *et al.* Methotrexate versus azathioprine in the treatment of rheumatoid arthritis: a forty-eight-week randomized, double-blind trial. *Arthritis Rheum* 1991; **34**: 961–72.

64. Durez, P., Desager, J. P., and Appelboom, T. Intravenous loading dose of azathioprine in active rheumatoid arthritis. *Arthritis Rheum* 1998; **41** (Suppl.): Abstract 726, S153.

65. Aguilar, H. I., Burgart, L. J., Geller, A., and Rakela, J. Azathioprine-induced lymphoma manifesting as fulminant hepatic failure. *Mayo Clin Proc* 1997; **72**: 643–5.

66. Munro, R., and Capell, H. A. Penicillamine. *Br J Rheumatol* 1997; **36**: 104–9.

67. Joyce, D. A. D-penicillamine. *Baillieres Clin Rheumatol* 1990; **4**: 553–74.

68. Eberhardt, K., Rydgren, L., Fex, E., Svensson, B., and Wollheim, F. A. D-penicillamine in early rheumatoid arthritis: experience from a 2-year double blind placebo controlled study. *Clin Exp Rheumatol* 1996; **14**: 625–31.

69. Joyce, D. A. Variability in response to D-penicillamine: pharmacokinetic insights. *Agents Actions Suppl* 1993; **44**: 203–7.

70. Situnayacke, R. D., Gurindulis, K. A., and McConkey, B. Longterm treatment of rheumatoid arthritis with sulphasalazine, gold or penicillamine: a comparison using life table methods. *Ann Rheum Dis* 1987; **46**: 177–83.

71. Dahlqvist, S. R., Strom, H., Bjelle, A., and Moller, E. HLA antigens and adverse drug reactions to sodium aurothiomalate and D-penicillamine in patients with rheumatoid arthritis. *Clin Rheumatol* 1985; **4**: 55–61.

72. Barrera, P., den Broeder, A., van der Hoogen, F., van Engelen, B. G., and van de Putte, L. B. Postural changes, dysphagia, and systemic sclerosis. *Ann Rheum Dis* 1998; **57**: 331–8.

73. Rains, C. P., Noble, S., and Faulds, D. Sulphasalazine: a review of its pharmacological properties and therapeutic efficacy in the treatment of rheumatoid arthritis. *Drugs* 1995; **50**: 137–56.

74. Porter, D. R., and Capell, H. A. The use of sulphasalazine as a disease modifying antirheumatic drug. *Baillieres Clin Rheumatol* 1990; **4**: 535–51.

75. Smolen, J. S., Kalden, J. R., Scott, D. L., Rozman, B., Kvien, T. K., Larsen, A. *et al.* and the European Leflunomide Study Group. Efficacy and safety of leflunomide compared with placebo and sulphasalazine in active rheumatoid arthritis: a double blind, randomised, multicentre trial. *Lancet* 1999; **353**: 259–66.

76. Scott, D. L., Smolen, J. S., Kalden, J. R., van de Putte, L. B., Larsen, A., Kvien T. K. *et al.* and the European Leflunomide Study Group. Treatment of active rheumatoid arthritis with leflunomide: two year follow up of a double blind, placebo controlled trial versus sulphasalazine. *Ann Rheum Dis* 2001; **60**: 913–23.

77. Kalden, J. R., Scott, D. L., Smolen, J. S., Schattenkirchner, M., Rozman, B., Williams, B. D. *et al*; European Leflunomide Study Group. Improved functional ability in patients with rheumatoid arthritis: longterm treatment with leflunomide versus sulphasalazine. European Leflunomide Study Group. *J Rheumatol* 2001; **28**: 1983–91.

78. Larsen, A., Kvien, T. K., Schattenkirchner, M., Rau, R., Scott, D. L., Smolen, J. S. *et al*; European Leflunomide Study Group. Slowing of disease progression in rheumatoid arthritis patients during long-term treatment with leflunomide or sulphasalazine. *Scand J Rheumatol* 2001; **30**: 135–42.

79. Choy, E. H., Scott, D. L., Kingsley, G. H., Williams, P., Wojtulewski, J., Papasavvas, G. *et al.* Treating rheumatoid arthritis early with disease modifying drugs reduces joint damage: a randomised double blind trial of sulphasalazine vs diclofenac sodium. *Clin Exp Rheumatol* 2002; **20**: 351–8.

80. Dougados, M., Emery, P., Lemmel, E., Zerbini, C., Brin, S., and Van Riel, P. Patients failing a DMARD: to switch to sulphasalazine or to add sulphasalazine to ongoing leflunomide. Results from the 12-month relief study. *Ann Rheum Dis* 2005. [First published online, 22 July 2004.]

81. Bird, H. A. Sulphasalazine, sulfapyridine or 5-aminosalicylic acid: which is the active moiety in rheumatoid arthritis? *Br J Rheumatol* 1995; **34** (Suppl. 2): 16–19.

82. Wahl, C., Liptay, S., Adler, G., and Schmid, R. Sulphasalazine: a potent and specific inhibitor of nuclear factor kappa B. *J Clin Invest* 1998; **101**: 1163–74.

83. van der Heijde, D. M., van Riel, P. L., Nuver-Zwart, I. H., and van de Putte, L. B. Sulphasalazine versus hydroxychloroquine in rheumatoid arthritis: 3-year follow-up. *Lancet* 1990; **335**: 539.

84. van Riel, P. L., van Gestel, A. M., and van de Putte, L. B. Longterm usage and side-effect profile of sulphasalazine in rheumatoid arthritis. *Br J Rheumatol* 1995; **34** (Suppl. 2): 40–2.

85. Haagsma, C. J., van Riel, P. L., de Rooij, D. J., Vree, T. B., Russel, F. J., van't Hof, M. A., and van de Putte, L. B. Combination of methotrexate and sulphasalazine vs methotrexate alone: a randomized open clinical trial in rheumatoid arthritis patients resistant to sulphasalazine therapy. *Br J Rheumatol* 1994; **33**: 1049–55.

86. Conaghan, P. G., and Brooks, P. Disease-modifying antirheumatic drugs, including methotrexate gold, antimalarials, and D-penicillamine. *Current Opin Rheumatol* 1995; **7**: 167–73.

87. McEntegart, A., Porter, D., Capell, H. A., and Thomson, E. A. Sulphasalazine has a better efficacy/toxicity profile than auranofin: evidence from a 5 year prospective, randomized trial. *J Rheumatol* 1996; **23**: 1887–90.

88. The Australian Multicentre Clinical Trial Group. Sulphasalazine in early rheumatoid arthritis. *J Rheumatol* 1992; **19**: 1672–7.

89. Gunnarsson, I., Nordmark, B., Hassan Bakri, A., Grondal, G., Larsson, P., Forslid, J. *et al.* Development of lupus-related side-effects in patients with early RA during sulphasalazine treatment: the role of IL-10 and HLA. *Rheumatology* 2000; **39**: 886–93.

90. Dougados, M. Sulphasalazine. In *Therapy of systemic rheumatic disorders* (Van de Putte, L. B., ed.), pp. 165–83. New York: Marcel Dekker; 1998.

91. van de Putte, L., van Gestel, A., and van Riel, P. Early treatment of rheumatoid arthritis: rationale, evidence, and implications. *Ann Rheum Dis* 1998; **57**: 511–12.

26 | Combination therapy with synthetic DMARDs in the treatment of rheumatoid arthritis

Antonios O. Aliprantis and Michael Weinblatt

Introduction

Treatment of rheumatoid arthritis (RA) with disease-modifying anti-rheumatic drugs (DMARDs) is the standard of care in rheumatology practices throughout the world. DMARDs include synthetic, low molecular weight compounds such as methotrexate (MTX), sulfasalazine (SSZ), and hydroxychloroquine (HCQ), and the more recently developed biologic response modifiers, etanercept, infliximab, adalimumab, and anakinra. Initiation of DMARD therapy early in the disease can profoundly impact functional and radiographic outcomes, strongly supporting an early, aggressive treatment approach[1,2]. Unfortunately, DMARDs rarely induce remission as monotherapy, including biologic agents[3–6]. As such, the majority of RA patients in clinical practice are on more than one drug[7,8].

In this chapter, a historical perspective on the use of combination therapy in RA will be presented. Then, the major clinical trials combining synthetic DMARDs will be discussed (see Table 26.1). Studies evaluating combination therapy with biologic agents are covered elsewhere in this book (see Chapter 27). The applicability of trial results to clinical practice will be our focus. Each section will address adverse events and, when known, pharmacokinetic interactions. The chapter will end with a discussion of the role of combination therapy with synthetic DMARDs within the landscape of the modern approach to the RA patient.

Historical perspective

The concept of combination therapy to treat RA was derived from the experience of oncologists and infectious disease specialists who used multiple drug regimens for years to combat a myriad of malignancies and infectious agents[9]. In 1963, Sievers and Hurri, working in Finland, were of the first to report on combination DMARD therapy for RA[10,11]. This unblinded, non-randomized trial compared a cohort of RA patients treated with either chloroquine (CHL) alone, or CHL plus intramuscular gold. Modest, non-significant beneficial effects were observed in the combination therapy arm.

The first report of effective combination therapy for RA came from McCarty and colleagues 20 years later[9]. The authors described the uncontrolled treatment of 17 patients with active, erosive RA with a combination of cyclophosphamide, azathioprine (AZA), and HCQ. Compared with baseline values, impressive positive effects on morning stiffness, joint swelling, and grip strength were found. Recortication and 'filling in' of erosions was enticingly reported. A high proportion of infectious complications tempered their positive results. The authors concluded, 'Until data from a controlled study are available . . . this genie should be kept in a bottle.' A follow-up study published four years later reported similar findings[12]. Although, 23 of the 31 patients achieved near or complete remission, four malignancies and three deaths were noted.

Three papers published between 1984 and 1987 examined combination therapies, including D-penicillamine (D-PCN). Combination with antimalarial compounds did not offer any advantage over D-PCN monotherapy[13,14]. The addition of SSZ to D-PCN did favor combination therapy in an open-label study, but the magnitude of the benefit was small[15]. Other contemporary studies were similarly disappointing. In 1989, a placebo-controlled, randomized trial of 101 RA patients treated with either gold alone or gold plus HCQ for one year favored combination therapy[16]. However, an intention to treat analysis was not performed and almost twice as many withdrawals due to adverse event occurred in the combination therapy arm. Another controlled study showed no benefit from the addition of HCQ to patients with a suboptimal response to gold[17]. The combination of MTX and auranofin (AUR) was evaluated in a large multicenter, randomized, placebo-controlled trial[18]. Other than an increase in the dropout rate due to lack of efficacy in the AUR arm, no clinical advantage to combination therapy was observed. However, the dose of MTX employed in this study was well below the optimal dose of 10 mg/m^2 [19].

It was upon this backdrop that Felson and colleagues published a comprehensive meta-analysis of combination therapy in 1994[20]. In this study, the authors pooled data from five controlled, randomized trials that had evaluated combinations of DMARDs at clinically effective doses. A statistically significant, but small, decrease in the tender joint count was found in the combination therapy arm. No differences were detected in any other clinical parameters. Moreover, the dropout rate due to side-effects was 9% higher among patients treated with combination therapies, though severe adverse events were rare. The authors concluded

Table 26.1   Combination therapy with synthetic DMARDs: a summary of the randomized trials performed to date

Author	Year	# patients	Early RA?	Treatment arms	Duration	Outcome	Ref.
Gibson	1987	72	No	CHL/D-PCN vs. CHL vs. D-PCN	12 months	No advantage to COMB	14
Bunch	1984	56	No	HCQ/D-PCN vs. HCQ vs. D-PCN	24 months	No advantage to COMB	13
Taggart	1987	30	No	SSZ/D-PCN vs. SSZ	6 months	Small benefit to COMB	15
Scott	1989	101	No	Gold/HCQ vs. gold	12 months	Small benefit to COMB	16
Porter	1992	142	No	Gold/HCQ vs. gold	6 months	No advantage to COMB	17
Williams	1992	335	No	AUR/MTX vs. AUR vs. MTX	48 weeks	No advantage to COMB	18
Trnavsky	1993	40	No	MTX/HCQ vs. HCQ	6 months	Clinical/radiographic variables favored COMB	26
Clegg	1997	141	No	HCQ/MTX then MTX vs. HCQ	60 weeks	All improved on COMB HCQ maintained benefit	27
Haagsma	1994	40	No	SSZ/MTX vs. MTX	24 weeks	Favored COMB	29
Haagsma	1997	105	Yes	SSZ/MTX vs. SSZ vs. MTX	52 weeks	No advantage to COMB	31
Dougados	1999	205	Yes	SSZ/MTX vs. SSZ vs. MTX	52 weeks	No advantage to COMB	32
Willkens	1992	209	No	MTX/AZA vs. MTX vs. AZA	24 weeks	No advantage of COMB	38
Tugwell	1995	148	No	MTX/CSA vs. MTX	6 months	Clinical variables favored COMB	47
Gerards	2003	120	Yes	MTX/CSA vs. CSA	48 weeks	Radiographic variables favored COMB	48
Ferracioli	2002	126	Yes	SSZ vs. MTX/CSA/SSZ	36 months	Favored 'step-up' therapy with MTX/CSA/SSZ	52
Marchesoni	2003	61	Yes	MTX/CSA vs. MTX	12 months	Slower radiographic progression with COMB	51
Kremer	2002	263	No	MTX/LFL vs. MTX	24 weeks	Clinical variables favored COMB	58
O'Dell	1996	102	No	MTX/SSZ/HCQ vs. SSZ/HCQ vs. MTX	24 months	Clinical variables favored triple therapy	62
O'Dell	2002	171	No	MTX/SSZ/HCQ vs. MTX/HCQ vs. MTX/SSZ	24 months	Clinical variables favored triple therapy	63
Boers	1997	155	Yes	MTX/SSZ/CCS vs. SSZ	56 weeks	Radiographic variable favored COMB	66
Mottonen	1999	199	Yes	MTX/SSZ/HCQ/CCS vs. monotherapy	24 months	Clinical/radiographic variables favored COMB	68
Grigor	2004	111	Yes	'Intensive' COMB vs. monotherapy	18 months	Clinical/radiographic variables favored COMB	73

COMB, combination therapy; LFL, leflunomide. See text for definition of other abbreviations.

that combination therapy did not offer patients a substantial increase in efficacy and was more toxic than single drug therapy. They recommended against its widespread use. In the past 11 years, the perspective on combination synthetic DMARD therapy for RA has undergone an exciting transformation. This is largely due to positive results from well-designed clinical trials combining therapeutic doses of MTX and other DMARDs.

Combination therapy regimens

MTX and antimalarials

The use of MTX with the antimalarial compound HCQ is an attractive clinical combination. MTX has a relatively prompt onset of action, but its therapeutic efficacy often reaches a plateau by six months[21]. HCQ exhibits a slower onset of action that frequently leads to withdrawal due to inefficacy[22]. The combination therefore might afford patients a rapid initial response, along with a more sustained and continued improvement from a regimen of two active DMARDs. In addition, the toxicities of these medications do not overlap[23]. Moreover, HCQ may protect patients from MTX-related acute liver injury. Levels of serum liver enzymes were evaluated in a cross-sectional cohort study of nearly 2600 patients with RA[24]. None of the 38 patients taking MTX and HCQ had elevations in their serum glutamic oxaloacetic transaminase level. The mechanism of this protective effect may be related

to a decrease in the maximal serum concentration of MTX when it is co-administered with HCQ[25]. Despite its allure, only two clinical trials have evaluated this combination. More clinically relevant is the combination of HCQ, MTX, and SSZ. This cocktail, often referred to as 'triple therapy,' is discussed below.

A six-month, randomized, placebo-controlled trial comparing HCQ versus HCQ plus MTX was performed on 40 patients with established RA (disease duration >2 years) at a single center in the Czech Republic[26]. The doses of HCQ and MTX were relatively low and fixed at 200 mg/day and 7.5 mg/week, respectively. Compared with patients in the placebo arm, those receiving combination therapy had a statistically significant reduction in painful and swollen joints, and scored better on a self-reported assessment of function and pain. The combination of MTX and HCQ was further evaluated in a multicenter trial reported in 1997[27]. In the initial, open-label, 24-week phase of this trial, 141 patients with active, established RA (disease duration >6 months) were treated with 400 mg of HCQ daily and 7.5–15 mg MTX weekly. Disease variables, including joint pain and swelling, and functional class, improved significantly from baseline values. In the second phase of the trial, patients randomly received maintenance therapy with either (a) HCQ with placebo for an arthritis flare, (b) HCQ with MTX for a flare or (c) placebo with MTX for a flare. The primary end-point, median time to first disease flare, was significantly delayed in patients receiving daily HCQ. No differences in adverse events were noted between the groups. These two trials helped establish combination therapy with MTX and HCQ as an effective and safe DMARD regimen. However, neither contained an

MTX-only arm. Therefore, whether this combination is better than MTX alone is unresolved.

MTX and SSZ

In 1989, marked clinical improvement was reported in four RA patients treated with MTX and SSZ[28], including three with history of a sub-optimal response to MTX. A randomized, open trial of 40 patients with SSZ-resistant RA published five years later had a similar conclusion[29]. A retrospective study found no difference in adverse events between 63 patients treated with MTX and 32 prescribed MTX and SSZ[30]. Despite these encouraging reports, the results of subsequent randomized, placebo-controlled trials have been disappointing.

A randomized, controlled, double blind study was performed at a single institution in the Netherlands to evaluate the combination of MTX and SSZ versus each of the individual drugs in 105 patients with early, active RA (disease duration <1 year)[31]. Despite provisions for dose escalation to meaningful doses, no significant difference was observed between the three arms in disease activity scores. A similarly designed trial was published two years later. In this double blind, placebo-controlled study, 205 patients with early, active RA were randomized to receive daily SSZ, weekly MTX, or both[32]. A statistically significant improvement at 52 weeks was reported in patients treated with combination therapy versus those who received only MTX. However, the magnitude of the benefit was small and no difference was found between combination therapy and SSZ alone. Moreover, the number of patients who fulfilled American College of Rheumatology (ACR) response criteria[33] or achieved a good European League Against Rheumatism (EULAR) response[34] was similar among the three treatment groups. A five-year follow-up study of this cohort showed that early intervention with the combination of MTX and SSZ had no effect on disease activity, structural changes, or disability compared to monotherapy[35].

The lack of an additive benefit between MTX and SSZ is not due to alterations in the serum levels of these drugs when they are combined[36]. A more likely explanation is that SSZ is a potent inhibitor of the reduced foliate carrier, the major cell membrane transporter for natural folates and MTX. In the presence of SSZ, the uptake and anti-proliferative effects of MTX are inhibited[37]. Regardless of the mechanism, unbiased clinical studies do not support the use of this combination of DMARDs.

MTX and AZA

Combination therapy with MTX and AZA has been evaluated in one multicenter, placebo-controlled trial, published in two parts[38,39]. In the initial report, 212 patients with established, active RA (disease duration > 6 months) were randomly assigned to receive 24 weeks of AZA, MTX, or combination therapy. The maximum doses of MTX and AZA were 15 mg/week and 150 mg/day in the monotherapy arms, and 7.5 mg/week and 100 mg/day in the combination therapy group. Unfortunately, 28 of the 73 patients randomized to receive AZA withdrew from the study. The most common reasons for withdrawal in this group were gastrointestinal symptoms (16 patients), lack of efficacy (6 patients), and elevations in liver function tests (3 patients). In contrast, 5 and 18 patients withdrew in the MTX and combination therapy arms, respectively. The 30% response rates were 41%, 57%, and 58% in the AZA, MTX, and combination therapy groups, respectively. The authors concluded that, in this short-term trial measuring disease activity, combination therapy offered no advantage over monotherapy with MTX. At 48 weeks the 30% response rates were 26%, 45%, and 38% in the AZA, MTX, and combination therapy groups, respectively[39]. The significantly worse response rates at this time point are accounted for by a large number of withdrawals and crossovers. A trend toward reduced radiographic progression on hand and wrist films was observed in the MTX arm versus AZA. In conclusion, this study does not support the combination of low-dose MTX and AZA for the treatment of RA. Whether using higher and more therapeutic doses of azathioprine and methotrexate together would have led to a better response is unknown.

MTX and cyclosporin A

The initial trials of oral cyclosporin A (CSA) in RA used relatively high doses (5–10 mg/kg/day) and uniformly showed efficacy, but with unacceptable levels of nephrotoxicity[40–42]. Although studies using lower doses (1–3.8 mg/kg/day) showed less impact on renal function, the magnitude of clinical benefit was also diminished[43,44]. In 1991, Brahn *et al.* showed that combination therapy with MTX and CSA was superior to either drug alone in suppressing inflammation and radiographic damage in a rat model of rheumatoid arthritis[45]. A pilot study in humans, published in 1994, examined the addition of CSA to the medication regimen of 20 RA patients with active disease despite treatment with MTX[46]. Significant improvements in all clinical parameters including painful and swollen joint counts were observed compared to baseline values. Though a statistically significant 20.8% rise in the mean serum creatinine was observed, the authors argued that this was similar to prior studies of CSA monotherapy. Moreover, no significant elevations in liver enzymes were reported.

The following year, a multicenter trial comparing MTX alone versus MTX plus CSA was reported[47]. In this trial 148 patients with established RA (mean disease duration 10.3 years) and active disease despite at least three months of MTX were randomized to receive low-dose CSA (initial dose 2.5 mg/kg/day) or placebo for 24 weeks. The CSA dose was increased to a maximum of 5 mg/kg/day if joints remained inflamed. Evidence of nephrotoxicity prompted a reduction in the dose. All patients continued MTX. A statistically significant decrease in the tender joint count was observed in the combination therapy arm versus placebo. In addition, 48% of patients in the CSA group met ACR criteria for improvement in RA[33] compared with only 16% in the placebo group. As expected, a small rise in the mean serum creatinine was observed in the CSA arm, but only one patient withdrew because of renal toxicity. In the 24-week open label extension of this trial, patients initially randomized to the CSA and MTX arm continued this treatment (group 1), while patients in the placebo arm had CSA added to their weekly MTX (group 2). At week 48, the clinical improvements observed during weeks 0–24 were maintained in patients in group 1. Accordingly, the majority of clinical scores in patients in group 2 approached those of group 1 by 48 weeks. However, by the end of the study, 36% and 16% of patients had greater than a 30% rise of their baseline serum creatinine in groups 1 and 2, respectively. CSA monotherapy was compared to combination therapy with MTX in 120 patients with active, early RA (disease duration <3 years) in a 48-week, double blind, randomized, placebo-controlled trial performed at multiple centers across the Netherlands[48]. The primary end-point of clinical remission[49] at week 48 was only achieved by four patients in the monotherapy and six in the combination groups. ACR50 response rates occurred more frequently and favored combination therapy (25% vs. 48%). Interestingly, median Larson scores[50], a measure of radiographic progression, increased 7.5 points in the CSA-only group, but only 2 points in the combination therapy arm. Hypertension and a rise in the serum creatinine were common. Marchesoni et al. addressed the question of whether the clinical benefit seen in these combination studies was solely due to MTX[51]. Sixty-one patients with early, active RA were randomized to receive either MTX alone or combination therapy with MTX and low-dose CSA. Mean damage scores increased 300% in the MTX group, but only 40% in the combination therapy arm. No significant differences were found in the ACR response rates between the two treatment arms. These findings suggest that CSA may uncouple joint inflammation and bone erosion.

Ferraccioli et al. reported a clinical trial in 2002 designed to better approximate clinical practice[52]. In this trial, 126 patients with early RA (mean disease duration 1–2 years) and active disease despite antimalarial drugs were randomized to one of three groups and started on MTX (Group 1), CSA (Group 2), or SSZ (Group 3), respectively. At six months, patients in groups 1 and 2 who did not fulfill the primary end-point, an ACR50 response, were given both MTX and CSA. SSZ was added if an ACR50 response was not attained at 12 months. Group 3 was maintained on SSZ regardless of disease course. By six months, 57% of patients taking MTX had reached an ACR50 improvement. In contrast only 31% and 33% of patients in groups 2 and 3, respectively, had a similar response. After the addition of MTX to CSA the percentage of patients in group 2 with an ACR50 improvement rose to 76% at 12 months. At 18 months, 90% and 88% of patients in groups 1 and 2, respectively, reached an ACR50 response. In contrast, only 24% of patients in group 3 had such a response. Only four cases of decreased GFR were noted. Many patients in group 3 withdrew due to lack of efficacy. Since the MTX arm was not extended beyond six months, these data do not exclude the possibility that MTX is as effective as combination therapy.

Taken together, data from trials of combination therapy with MTX and CSA suggest that this strategy is more effective than either drug alone at retarding radiographic progression. Though the mechanism of this interaction is not known, a pharmacokinetic analysis has shown that CSA increases serum levels of MTX and greatly diminishes the conversion to its major, inactive metabolite, 7-hydroxymethotrexate[53]. However, whether combination therapy is better than MTX monotherapy at controlling clinical disease activity, other than in patients who have had a sub-optimal response to MTX[46,47], is unresolved.

MTX and leflunomide

Leflunomide is a relatively new DMARD. Its active metabolite, A77 1726, inhibits dihydroorotate dehydrogenase, a key enzyme in the *de novo* synthesis of pyrimidines, a requisite step for T cell proliferation[54,55]. At the doses used for the treatment of RA, MTX has little effect on T cell proliferation but promotes the release of the anti-inflammatory molecule adenosine[56]. These potentially complementary mechanisms of action made MTX and leflunomide an intriguing DMARD regimen, though overlapping hepatic toxicity profiles were a consideration.

In a safety and pharmacokinetic study, leflunomide with a loading dose was added to the medical regimen of 30 patients with active RA despite therapeutic doses of MTX for at least six months[57]. The combination was generally well tolerated and no significant pharmacokinetic interactions were observed. However, 63% of the patients developed elevated levels of liver enzymes. In the majority of cases, the elevation resolved without adjusting the leflunomide dose. By 52 weeks, over half the patients achieved an ACR20 response. These results indicated that combination therapy with MTX and leflunomide had therapeutic potential, but raised the concern for synergistic liver toxicity.

In a multicenter trial, Kremer et al. randomly assigned 263 patients with active RA to receive leflunomide or placebo in addition to pre-existing MTX therapy[58]. As in the prior study, a loading dose of leflunomide was employed. At 24 weeks, 46.2% of patients in the leflunomide group achieved ACR20 criteria compared with only 19.5% in the placebo group. ACR50 and ACR70 response rates, as well as physical function scores, also favored leflunomide. The incidence of elevated liver enzyme levels was much higher in the combination therapy arm (31.5% vs. 6.8%). Again, the majority of elevations resolved without a change in dose. Following this study, patients were enrolled in a 24 week, open label extension, in which all patients were given leflunomide without a loading dose[59]. Three important findings were reported: (a) the clinical benefit achieved by patients originally randomized to the leflunomide arm was maintained; (b) ACR20 response rates were similar between the original placebo and leflunomide groups after all patients received leflunomide; and (c) the incidence of elevated transaminases was much lower when a loading dose of leflunomide was omitted from the dosing regimen. Although no cases of leukopenia, neutropenia, or serious liver disease occurred in either trial, a recent case series associated the combination of MTX and leflunomide with pancytopenia[60] and there is a case report of cirrhosis in a patient receiving this combination[61]. At this time, it is not known whether this combination is more effective than leflunomide alone or better than monotherapy in early RA. In addition, radiographic progression has not been evaluated and the long-term consequences of this combination on liver function is not known. Certainly, if leflunomide is added to pre-existing MTX therapy, a loading dose should be avoided and liver function tests monitored closely.

'Triple therapy': MTX, HCQ, and SSZ

The first randomized trial to explore more than two drugs for the treatment of RA appeared in 1996[62]. In this two-year, double blind study, 102 patients with established RA received either MTX alone (Group 1), HCQ plus SSZ (Group 2), or all three drugs (Group 3—triple therapy). The dose of MTX was increased over six months to 17.5 mg/week if a patient was not in remission. The doses of HCQ (400 mg/day) and SSZ (1000 mg/day) were held constant. Of the patients receiving triple therapy, 77%

achieved a 50% improvement at two years. In contrast, only 33% and 40% of patients in Groups 1 and 2, respectively, had a similar outcome. Toxic effects, including elevation in liver enzymes, were not observed more frequently in the triple therapy arm than in the other groups. A similar trial compared triple therapy to MTX plus HCQ and MTX plus SSZ in 171 patients with established RA (disease duration > 6 months)[63]. The ACR20 and ACR50 response rates for patients on triple therapy were 78% and 55%, respectively. These outcomes were substantially better than patients treated with MTX and SSZ (49% and 29%) and modestly higher than those who received MTX and HCQ (60% and 40%). Triple therapy was well tolerated and not associated with any specific toxicity. An open, but randomized, trial on 180 RA patients performed in Turkey also found improved efficacy of triple therapy over monotherapy, or combinations of two drugs[64]. Triple therapy is now being compared to anti-TNF (tumor necrosis factor) therapy in a randomized study in early RA.

Combination therapy trials that include corticosteroids as a controlled variable

Many of the trials discussed thus far in this chapter have permitted the use of oral corticosteroids (CCSs) by study participants. Though a cap on the total daily dose of steroids was usually included in the design of the trial, the decision to start or taper this medication was often discretionary and uncontrolled. In addition, the dose of steroids at baseline and total cumulative dose of steroids was rarely reported. However, even low-dose steroids suppress disease activity and slow radiographic progression[65]. Three trials have formally addressed this issue in the context of combination therapy: COBRA, FIN-RACo, and TICORA.

The COBRA investigators postulated that aggressive therapy in early RA could alter the course of the disease, well after the initial medications were discontinued[66]. In this multicenter, double blind trial, 155 patients with early RA (median disease duration <4 months) were randomized to receive either SSZ alone or combination therapy with SSZ, MTX, and high-dose prednisolone. The starting doses of prednisolone and MTX were 60 mg/day and 7.5 mg/week, respectively. The target dose of SSZ was 2000 mg/day. Initially, clinical scores of disease activity improved more in the combination therapy arm. The prednisolone was tapered and stopped by week 35. MTX was tapered off by week 46. Both groups were maintained on SSZ after week 46 until the end of the 56 week trial. At this time point, measures of joint inflammation converged. However, radiographic damage scores were substantially lower in the patients who had received early, aggressive combination therapy. A follow-up study of the COBRA cohort showed that this approach continued to affect the rate of radiographic progression five years later[67]. Withdrawal rates for adverse events and lack of efficacy were less in the combination therapy arm.

The FIN-RACo trial group has extensively evaluated the benefit of triple therapy plus steroids in early rheumatoid arthritis (disease duration <2 years). In their initial publication, they described 199 patients with early RA who were randomly assigned to receive single drug therapy or triple therapy plus low-dose prednisolone in an unblinded study[68]. To mimic practice situations, an intricate method for increasing or decreasing DMARD doses based on disease activity was outlined prior to the trial. Patients in the single drug arm were started on SSZ and, though other drugs could be substituted, they were not permitted to take more than one DMARD. Based on an intention to treat analysis, at two years 37% and 18% of patients in the triple and single therapy arms, respectively, were in remission. ACR50 response rates also favored combination therapy, but did not reach statistical significance. Adverse events did not occur more frequently in the combination therapy arm. At the end of the two-year trial, the restriction on the use of DMARDs was lifted and the patients were followed for an additional three years. The FIN-RACo investigators have recently published a series of longitudinal follow-up studies on this cohort. They found that patients in the combination therapy arm had lower Larsen scores[69], less risk of atlantoaxial subluxation[70], and a lower cumulative duration of work disability[71,72], despite similar scores on measures of disease activity. The data from FIN-RACo support the use of triple therapy plus prednisolone over monotherapy in early RA. Though no increase in serious adverse events were reported after five years of follow-up[69], the impact of daily CCSs on bone density and cardiovascular outcomes is a long-term concern with this strategy.

The TICORA study[73] attempted to unite the proven approach of aggressive, combination therapy in early RA with the preference of most rheumatologists to initiate therapy with one drug and 'step-up' to multidrug therapy in patients with recalcitrant disease[74]. To this end, the investigators randomly assigned 111 patients with relatively early RA (disease duration <5 years, median 19–20 months) to receive routine or intensive care. Only the assessors of disease activity were blinded to treatment allocation. Patients in the routine care group were followed in a rheumatology clinic every three months and no formal composite of disease activity was used to guide treatment decisions. DMARDs were started, stopped, and added at the discretion of the treating physicians. In the intensive therapy group, a single rheumatologist evaluated each patient once per month and escalated oral DMARD therapy if their disease activity score was greater than a pre-defined value. Oral therapy started with SSZ and progressed to triple therapy. Oral CCSs were added if there was an inadequate response to triple therapy. Finally, combination therapy with MTX and CSA or alternative DMARDs, like leflunomide, could be substituted. Intra-articular steroids were used liberally. At the end of the 18-month study, 82% of patients in the intensive therapy arm achieved the primary end-point of a 'good response' according to EULAR criteria[34]. In contrast, only 44% of patients who received routine care had a similar response. Remission rates were 65% and 16%, respectively, in the intensive and routine care groups. Assessments of functional status and radiographic progression also strongly favored intensive therapy. Interestingly, total costs were lower in the group that received intensive therapy, largely due to lower inpatient expenses. Adverse events and withdrawals due to lack of efficacy were not more common in the intensive therapy group. The impressive positive results of this trial need to be validated outside the structured and funded trial setting, where constraints on clinical practices may obstruct the frequency and intensity of monitoring and prescribing outlined in this trial.

Concluding remarks

Combination therapy with multiple synthetic DMARDs that include MTX as the anchor drug has been shown to be a safe and effective option for the treatment of RA. However, not all combinations are superior to MTX monotherapy (e.g. MTX/SSZ and MTX/AZA) or free of potential synergistic toxicity (e.g. MTX/LFL). Most promising is triple therapy with MTX, SSZ, and HCQ with or without the addition of CCSs[62,63,68,73]. Triple therapy is currently being evaluated against anti-TNF modalities in early RA and if as effective would no doubt be a more cost-effective first-line therapy. The COBRA[66], FIN-RACo[68], and TICORA[73] trials illustrate a key principle of the modern approach to the patient with early RA: aggressive therapy with combinations of DMARDs is effective at controlling both synovial inflammation and joint destruction and is not necessarily more toxic or costly. Moreover, long-term follow-up of the COBRA and FIN-RACo cohorts strongly suggests that early control of the disease can impact on the rate of radiographic and functional deterioration[67,69,71]. Certainly the liberal use of CCSs in these trials is a concern. As the rheumatology literature continues to advance from an era of case reports and single arm cohort studies to one of controlled, multicenter, randomized trials, our knowledge of the best initial and rescue combinations will evolve. Until then, rheumatologists will need to tailor combination DMARD regimens to individual patients with timely control of disease activity as a reasonable and attainable goal.

References

1. Lard, L. R., Visser, H., Speyer, I., vander Horst-Bruinsma, I. E., Zwinderman, A. H., Breedveld, F. C. et al. Early versus delayed treatment in patients with recent-onset rheumatoid arthritis: comparison of two cohorts who received different treatment strategies. Am J Med 2001; 111: 446–51.
2. Stenger, A. A., Van Leeuwen, M. A., Houtman, P. M., Bruyn, G. A., Speerstra, F., Barendsen, B. C. et al. Early effective suppression of inflammation in rheumatoid arthritis reduces radiographic progression. Br J Rheumatol 1998; 37: 1157–63.
3. Wolfe, F., and Hawley, D. J. Remission in rheumatoid arthritis. J Rheumatol 1985; 12: 245–52.
4. Redlich, K., Schett, G., and Steiner, G., Hayer, S., Wagner, E. F., Smolen, J. S. Rheumatoid arthritis therapy after tumor necrosis factor and interleukin-1 blockade. Arthritis Rheum 2003; 48: 3308–19.
5. Klareskog, L., van der Heijde, D., de Jager, J. P., Gough, A., Kalden, J., Malaise, M. et al. Therapeutic effect of the combination of etanercept and methotrexate compared with each treatment alone in patients with rheumatoid arthritis: double-blind randomised controlled trial. Lancet 2004; 363: 675–81.
6. Kathon, J. M., Martin, R. W, Fleischmann, R. M., Tesser, J. R., Schiff, M. H., Keystone, E. C. et al. A comparison of etanercept and methotrexate in patients with early rheumatoid arthritis. N Engl J Med 2000; 343: 1586–93.
7. Verhoeven, A. C., Boers, and, M., Tugwell, P. Combination therapy in rheumatoid arthritis: updated systematic review. Br J Rheumatol 1998; 37: 612–19.
8. Pincus, T., O'Dell, J. R., and Kremer, J. M. Combination therapy with multiple disease-modifying antirheumatic drugs in rheumatoid arthritis: a preventive strategy. Ann Intern Med 1999; 131: 768–74.
9. McCarty, D. J., and Carrera, G. F. Intractable rheumatoid arthritis: treatment with combined cyclophosphamide, azathioprine, and hydroxychloroquine. JAMA 1982; 248: 1718–23.
10. Sievers, K., and Hurri, L. Combined therapy of rheumatoid arthritis with gold and chloroquine. I. Evaluation of the therapeutic effect. Acta Rheumatol Scand 1963; 9: 48–55.
11. Sievers, K., Hurri, L., and Sievers, U. M. Combined therapy of rheumatoid arthritis with gold and chloroquine. II. Evaluation of the side effects. Acta Rheumatol Scand 1963; 9: 56–64.
12. Csuka, M., Carrera, G. F., and McCarty, D. J. Treatment of intractable rheumatoid arthritis with combined cyclophosphamide, azathioprine, and hydroxychloroquine: a follow-up study. JAMA 1986; 255: 2315–19.
13. Bunch, T. W., O'Duffy, J. D., Tompkins, R. B., and O'Fallon, W. M. Controlled trial of hydroxychloroquine and D-penicillamine singly and in combination in the treatment of rheumatoid arthritis. Arthritis Rheum 1984; 27: 267–76.
14. Gibson, T., Emery, P., Armstrong, R. D., Crisp, A. J., and Panayi, G. S. Combined D-penicillamine and chloroquine treatment of rheumatoid arthritis: a comparative study. Br J Rheumatol 1987; 26: 279–84.
15. Taggart, A. J., Hill, J., Astbury, C., Dixon, J. S., Bird, H. A., and Wright, V. Sulphasalazine alone or in combination with D-penicillamine in rheumatoid arthritis. Br J Rheumatol 1987; 26: 32–6.
16. Scott, D. L., Dawes, P. T., Tunn, E., Fowler, P. D., Shadforth, M. F., Fisher, J. et al. Combination therapy with gold and hydroxychloroquine in rheumatoid arthritis: a prospective, randomized, placebo-controlled study. Br J Rheumatol 1989; 28: 128–33.
17. Porter, D. R., Capell, H. A., and Hunter, J. Combination therapy in rheumatoid arthritis: no benefit of addition of hydroxychloroquine to patients with a suboptimal response to intramuscular gold therapy. J Rheumatol 1993; 20: 645–9.
18. Williams, H. J., Ward, J. R., Reading, J. C., Brooks, R. H., Clegg, D. O., Skosey, J. L. et al. Comparison of auranofin, methotrexate, and the combination of both in the treatment of rheumatoid arthritis: a controlled clinical trial. Arthritis Rheum 1992; 35: 259–69.
19. Furst, D. E., Koehnke, R., Burmeister, L. F., Kohler, J., and Cargill, I. Increasing methotrexate effect with increasing dose in the treatment of resistant rheumatoid arthritis. J Rheumatol 1989; 16: 313–20.
20. Felson, D. T., Anderson, J. J., and Meenan, R. F. The efficacy and toxicity of combination therapy in rheumatoid arthritis: a meta-analysis. Arthritis Rheum 1994; 37: 1487–91.
21. Weinblatt, M. E., Maier, A. L., Fraser, P. A., and Coblyn, J. S. Longterm prospective study of methotrexate in rheumatoid arthritis: conclusion after 132 months of therapy. J Rheumatol 1998; 25: 238–42.
22. Tett, S., Cutler, D., and Day, R. Antimalarials in rheumatic diseases. Baillieres Clin Rheumatol 1990; 4: 467–89.
23. Fries, J. F., Williams, C. A., Ramey, D., and Bloch, D. A. The relative toxicity of disease-modifying antirheumatic drugs. Arthritis Rheum 1993; 36: 297–306.
24. Fries, J. F., Singh, G., Lenert, L., and Furst, D. E. Aspirin, hydroxychloroquine, and hepatic enzyme abnormalities with methotrexate in rheumatoid arthritis. Arthritis Rheum 1990; 33: 1611–19.
25. Carmichael, S. J., Beal, J., Day, R. O., and Tett, S. E. Combination therapy with methotrexate and hydroxychloroquine for rheumatoid arthritis increases exposure to methotrexate. J Rheumatol 2002; 29: 2077–83.
26. Trnavsky, K., Gatterova, J., Linduskova, M., and Peliskova, Z. Combination therapy with hydroxychloroquine and methotrexate in rheumatoid arthritis. Z Rheumatol 1993; 52: 292–6.
27. Clegg, D. O., Dietz, F., Duffy, J, Willkens, R. F., Hurd, E., Germain, B. F. et al. Safety and efficacy of hydroxychloroquine as maintenance therapy for rheumatoid arthritis after combination therapy with methotrexate and hydroxychloroquine. J Rheumatol 1997; 24: 1896–902.
28. Shiroky, J. B., Watts, C. S., and Neville, C. Combination methotrexate and sulfasalazine in the management of rheumatoid arthritis: case observations. Arthritis Rheum 1989; 32: 1160–4.
29. Haagsma, C. J., van Riel, P. L., de Rooij, D, J., Vree, T. B., Russel, F. J., van't Hof, M. A. et al. Combination of methotrexate and sulphasalazine

vs methotrexate alone: a randomized open clinical trial in rheumatoid arthritis patients resistant to sulphasalazine therapy. *Br J Rheumatol* 1994; **33**: 1049–55.

30. Nisar, M., Carlisle, L., and Amos, R. S. Methotrexate and sulphasalazine as combination therapy in rheumatoid arthritis. *Br J Rheumatol* 1994; **33**: 651–4.

31. Haagsma, C. J., van Riel, P. L., de Jong, A. J., and van de Putte, L. B. Combination of sulphasalazine and methotrexate versus the single components in early rheumatoid arthritis: a randomized, controlled, double-blind, 52 week clinical trial. *Br J Rheumatol* 1997; **36**: 1082–8.

32. Dougados, M., Combe, B., Cantagrel, A., Goupille, P., Olive, P., Schattenkirchner, M. et al. Combination therapy in early rheumatoid arthritis: a randomised, controlled, double blind 52 week clinical trial of sulphasalazine and methotrexate compared with the single components. *Ann Rheum Dis* 1999; **58**: 220–5.

33. Felson, D. T., Anderson, J. J., Boers, M., Bombardier, C., Furst, D., Goldsmith, C. et al. American College of Rheumatology. Preliminary definition of improvement in rheumatoid arthritis. *Arthritis Rheum* 1995; **38**: 727–35.

34. van Gestel, A. M., Prevoo, M. L., van't Hof, M. A., van Rijswijk, M. H., van de Putte, L. B., and van Riel, P. L. Development and validation of the European League Against Rheumatism response criteria for rheumatoid arthritis: comparison with the preliminary American College of Rheumatology and the World Health Organization/International League Against Rheumatism Criteria. *Arthritis Rheum* 1996; **39**: 34–40.

35. Maillefert, J. F., Combe, B., Goupille, P., Cantagrel, A., and Dougados, M. Long term structural effects of combination therapy in patients with early rheumatoid arthritis: five year follow up of a prospective double blind controlled study. *Ann Rheum Dis* 2003; **62**: 764–6.

36. Haagsma, C. J., Russel, F. G., Vree, T. B., Van Riel, P. L., and Van de Putte, L. B. Combination of methotrexate and sulphasalazine in patients with rheumatoid arthritis: pharmacokinetic analysis and relationship to clinical response. *Br J Clin Pharmacol* 1996; **42**: 195–200.

37. Jansen, G., van der Heijden, J., Oerlemans, R., Lems, W. F., Ifergan, I., Scheper, R. J. et al. Sulfasalazine is a potent inhibitor of the reduced folate carrier: implications for combination therapies with methotrexate in rheumatoid arthritis. *Arthritis Rheum* 2004; **50**: 2130–9.

38. Willkens, R. F., Urowitz, M. B., Stablein, D. M., McKendry, R. J., Jr., Berger, R.G., Box, J. H. et al. Comparison of azathioprine, methotrexate, and the combination of both in the treatment of rheumatoid arthritis: a controlled clinical trial. *Arthritis Rheum* 1992; **35**: 849–56.

39. Willkens, R. F., Sharp, J. T., Stablein, D., Marks, C., and Wortmann, R. Comparison of azathioprine, methotrexate, and the combination of the two in the treatment of rheumatoid arthritis: a forty-eight-week controlled clinical trial with radiologic outcome assessment. *Arthritis Rheum* 1995; **38**: 1799–806.

40. van Rijthoven, A. W., Dijkmans, B. A., Goei The, H. S., Hermans, J., Montnor-Beckers, Z. L., Jacobs, P. C. et al. Cyclosporin treatment for rheumatoid arthritis: a placebo controlled, double blind, multicentre study. *Ann Rheum Dis* 1986; **45**: 726–31.

41. Dougados, M., and Torley, H. Efficacy of cyclosporin A in rheumatoid arthritis: worldwide experience. *Br J Rheumatol* 1993; **32** (Suppl. 1): 57–9.

42. Weinblatt, M. E., Coblyn, J. S., Fraser, P. A., Anderson, R. J., Spragg, J., Trentham, D. E. et al. Cyclosporin A treatment of refractory rheumatoid arthritis. *Arthritis Rheum* 1987; **30**: 11–17.

43. Tugwell, P., Bombardier, C., Gent, M., Bennett, K. J., Bensen, W. G., Carette, S. et al. Low-dose cyclosporin versus placebo in patients with rheumatoid arthritis. *Lancet* 1990; **335**: 1051–5.

44. Yocum, D. E., Klippel, J. H., Wilder, R. L., Gerber, N. L., Austin, H. A., 3rd, Wahl, S. M. et al. Cyclosporin A in severe, treatment-refractory rheumatoid arthritis: a randomized study. *Ann Intern Med* 1988; **109**: 863–9.

45. Brahn, E., Peacock, D. J., and Banquerigo, M. L. Suppression of collagen-induced arthritis by combination cyclosporin A and methotrexate therapy. *Arthritis Rheum* 1991; **34**: 1282–8.

46. Bensen, W., Tugwell, P., Roberts, R. M., Ludwin, D., Ross, H., Grace, E. et al. Combination therapy of cyclosporine with methotrexate and gold in rheumatoid arthritis (2 pilot studies). *J Rheumatol* 1994; **21**: 2034–8.

47. Tugwell, P., Pincus, T., Yocum, D., Stein, M., Gluck, O., Kraag, G. et al. Combination therapy with cyclosporine and methotrexate in severe rheumatoid arthritis. The Methotrexate-Cyclosporine Combination Study Group. *N Engl J Med* 1995; **333**: 137–41.

48. Gerards, A. H., Landewe, R. B., Prins, A. P., Bruyn, G. A., Goei The H. S., Laan, R. F. et al. Cyclosporin A monotherapy versus cyclosporin A and methotrexate combination therapy in patients with early rheumatoid arthritis: a double blind randomised placebo controlled trial. *Ann Rheum Dis* 2003; **62**: 291–6.

49. Pinals, R. S., Masi, A. T., and Larsen, R. A. Preliminary criteria for clinical remission in rheumatoid arthritis. *Arthritis Rheum* 1981; **24**: 1308–15.

50. Larsen, A. How to apply Larsen score in evaluating radiographs of rheumatoid arthritis in long-term studies. *J Rheumatol* 1995; **22**: 1974–5.

51. Marchesoni, A., Battafarano, N., Arreghini, M., Panni, B., Gallazzi, M., and Tosi, S. Radiographic progression in early rheumatoid arthritis: a 12-month randomized controlled study comparing the combination of cyclosporin and methotrexate with methotrexate alone. *Rheumatology (Oxford)* 2003; **42**: 1545–9.

52. Ferraccioli, G. F., Gremese, E., Tomietto, P., Favret, G., Damato, R., and Di Poi, E. Analysis of improvements, full responses, remission and toxicity in rheumatoid patients treated with step-up combination therapy (methotrexate, cyclosporin A, sulphasalazine) or monotherapy for three years. *Rheumatology (Oxford)* 2002; **41**: 892–8.

53. Fox, R. I., Morgan, S. L., Smith, H. T., Robbins, B. A., Choc, M. G., and Baggott, J. E. Combined oral cyclosporin and methotrexate therapy in patients with rheumatoid arthritis elevates methotrexate levels and reduces 7-hydroxymethotrexate levels when compared with methotrexate alone. *Rheumatology (Oxford)* 2003; **42**: 989–94.

54. Cherwinski, H. M., Cohn, R. G., Cheung, P., Webster, D. J., Xu, Y. Z., Caulfield, J. P. et al. The immunosuppressant leflunomide inhibits lymphocyte proliferation by inhibiting pyrimidine biosynthesis. *J Pharmacol Exp Ther* 1995; **275**: 1043–9.

55. Cherwinski, H. M., Byars, N., Ballaron, S. J., Nakano, G. M., Young J. M., and Ransom, J. T. Leflunomide interferes with pyrimidine nucleotide biosynthesis. *Inflamm Res* 1995; **44**: 317–22.

56. Cronstein, B. N., and Merrill, J. T. Mechanisms of the effects of methotrexate. *Bull Rheum Dis* 1996; **45**: 6–8.

57. Weinblatt, M. E., Kremer, J. M., Coblyn, J. S., Maier, A. L., Helfgott, S. M., Morrell, M. et al. Pharmacokinetics, safety, and efficacy of combination treatment with methotrexate and leflunomide in patients with active rheumatoid arthritis. *Arthritis Rheum* 1999; **42**: 1322–8.

58. Kremer, J. M., Genovese, M. C., Cannon, G. W., Caldwell, J. R., Cush, J. J., Furst, D. E. et al. Concomitant leflunomide therapy in patients with active rheumatoid arthritis despite stable doses of methotrexate: a randomized, double-blind, placebo-controlled trial. *Ann Intern Med* 2002; **137**: 726–33.

59. Kremer, J., Genovese, M., Cannon, G. W., Caldwell, J., Cush, J. Furst, D. E. et al. Combination leflunomide and methotrexate (MTX) therapy for patients with active rheumatoid arthritis failing MTX monotherapy: open-label extension of a randomized, double-blind, placebo controlled trial. *J Rheumatol* 2004; **31**: 1521–31.

60. Chan, J., Sanders, D. C., Du, L., and Pillans, P. I. Leflunomide-associated pancytopenia with or without methotrexate. *Ann Pharmacother* 2004; **38**: 1206–11.

61. Weinblatt, M. E., Dixon, J. A., and Falchuk, K. R. Serious liver disease in a patient receiving methotrexate and leflunomide. *Arthritis Rheum* 2000; **43**: 2609–11.

62. O'Dell, J. R., Haire, C. E., Erikson, N., Drymalski, W., Palmer, W., Eckhoff, P. J. et al. Treatment of rheumatoid arthritis with methotrexate alone, sulfasalazine and hydroxychloroquine, or a combination of all three medications. *N Engl J Med* 1996; **334**: 1287–91.

63. O'Dell, J. R., Leff, R., Paulsen, G., Haire, C., Mallek, J., Eckhoff, P. J. et al. Treatment of rheumatoid arthritis with methotrexate and hydroxychloroquine, methotrexate and sulfasalazine, or a combination of the three medications: results of a two-year, randomized, double-blind, placebo-controlled trial. *Arthritis Rheum* 2002; **46**: 1164–70.

64. Calguneri, M., Pay, S., Caliskaner, Z., Apras, S., Kiraz, S., Ertenli, I. et al. Combination therapy versus monotherapy for the treatment of patients with rheumatoid arthritis. *Clin Exp Rheumatol* 1999; **17**: 699–704.

65. Pincus, T., Ferraccioli, G., Sokka, T., Larsen, A., Rau, R., Kushner, I. *et al.* Evidence from clinical trials and long-term observational studies that disease-modifying anti-rheumatic drugs slow radiographic progression in rheumatoid arthritis: updating a 1983 review. *Rheumatology (Oxford)* 2002; **41**: 1346–56.

66. Boers, M., Verhoeven, A. C., Markusse, H. M., van de Laar, M. A., Westhovens, R., van Denderen, J. C. *et al.* Randomised comparison of combined step-down prednisolone, methotrexate and sulphasalazine with sulphasalazine alone in early rheumatoid arthritis. *Lancet* 1997; **350**: 309–18.

67. Landewe, R. B., Boers, M., Verhoeven, A. C., Westhovens, R., van de Laar, M. A., Markusse, H. M. *et al.* COBRA combination therapy in patients with early rheumatoid arthritis: long-term structural benefits of a brief intervention. *Arthritis Rheum* 2002; **46**: 347–56.

68. Mottonen, T., Hannonen, P., Leirisalo-Repo, M., Nissila, M., Kautiainen, H., Korpela, M. *et al.* Comparison of combination therapy with single-drug therapy in early rheumatoid arthritis: a randomised trial. FIN-RACo trial group. *Lancet* 1999; **353**: 1568–73.

69. Korpela, M., Laasonen, L., Hannonen, P., Kautiainen, H., Leirisalo-Repo, M., Hakala, M. *et al.* Retardation of joint damage in patients with early rheumatoid arthritis by initial aggressive treatment with disease-modifying antirheumatic drugs: five-year experience from the FIN-RACo study. *Arthritis Rheum* 2004; **50**: 2072–81.

70. Neva, M. H., Kauppi, M, J., Kautiainen, H., Luukkainen, R., Hannonen, P., Leirisalo-Repo, M. *et al.* Combination drug therapy retards the development of rheumatoid atlantoaxial subluxations. *Arthritis Rheum* 2000; **43**: 2397–401.

71. Puolakka, K., Kautiainen, H., Mottonen, T., Hannonen, P., Hakala, M., Korpela, M. *et al.* Predictors of productivity loss in early rheumatoid arthritis: a 5 year follow up study. *Ann Rheum Dis* 2005; **64**: 130–3.

72. Puolakka, K., Kautiainen, H., Mottonen, T., Hannonen, P., Korpela, M., Julkunen, H. *et al.* Impact of initial aggressive drug treatment with a combination of disease-modifying antirheumatic drugs on the development of work disability in early rheumatoid arthritis: a five-year randomized followup trial. *Arthritis Rheum* 2004; **50**: 55–62.

73. Grigor, C., Capell, H., Stirling, A., McMahon, A. D., Lock, P., Vallance, R. *et al.* Effect of a treatment strategy of tight control for rheumatoid arthritis (the TICORA study): a single-blind randomised controlled trial. *Lancet* 2004; **364**: 263–9.

74. O'Dell, J. R. Treating rheumatoid arthritis early: a window of opportunity? *Arthritis Rheum* 2002; **46**: 283–5.

27 | Biologics in the treatment of rheumatoid arthritis

Zuhre Tutuncu and Arthur Kavanaugh

Introduction

The treatment of rheumatoid arthritis (RA) has evolved rapidly during the last couple of decades. With the improved understanding of pathophysiologic mechanisms involved in the development and the progression of RA, and the progress in biotechnology, further targets are coming to light, and newer drugs are continually becoming available. While the effects of certain biologic agents on RA were recognized several decades ago, the development of biologics for the treatment of RA is still an area of intense activity and rapid progress. The cause of immunologically driven inflammation in RA is not completely understood. Nevertheless, it is well recognized that multiple exogenous and endogenous antigenic triggers result in series of autoimmune responses. These responses are sustained by cell–cell interactions, including cell types such as T cells, endothelial cells, macrophages, monocytes, dendritic cells, B cells, and mast cells. These complex interactions result in the production of cytokines, prostaglandins, and many other mediators. Biologics that specifically target individual pro-inflammatory cytokines, chemokines, adhesion molecules, costimulatory molecules, proteolytic enzymes, and angiogenic factors are now believed to represent a viable therapeutic strategy for arresting disease progression. Tumor necrosis factor alpha (TNF-α) and interleukin-1 (IL-1) are considered the major pro-inflammatory cytokines involved in the pathogenesis of many immune-mediated disorders[1]. While many of the targets are being investigated in clinical trials, TNF-α and IL-1 blocking therapy have already been approved for use and their efficacy and clinical applications have been validated in clinical practice. The success with TNF blocking agents in a significant proportion of patients with RA and other inflammatory conditions has stimulated interest in defining alternative strategies to control disease progression.

TNF-α blocking therapy

By modulating the growth, differentiation, and trafficking of cells, TNF-α has a central role in the pathogenesis of RA and other inflammatory disorders. TNF-α is produced primarily by monocytes and macrophages, but also by B cells, T cells, mast cells, and fibroblasts. Two different forms of TNF-α are responsible for its biologic activities. TNF-α is synthesized and expressed as a transmembrane protein on monocytes, macrophages, lymphocytes, and natural killer cells. Transmembrane (mTNF-α) levels increase upon cell activation and they can stimulate other cells via their TNF receptors. Soluble TNF-α (sTNF-α) is produced by proteolytic cleavage of membrane bound TNF-α by a specific metalloproteinase (TNF-α converting enzyme (TACE)). sTNF-α is thought to be the form responsible for most pathogenic effects of TNF-α in RA. The actions of TNF-α are mediated through two structurally distinct cell-associated receptors: TNF-RI (55kD; CD120a), and TNF-RII (75kD; CD120b). The two receptors differ in their binding abilities, and signaling properties; these differences also reflect the differences in their primary functions[2]. The biologic activity of TNF-α can be attenuated by soluble forms of TNF-α receptors. The binding of TNF-α to its receptor can initiate several signaling pathways. Signaling cascades include activation of transcription factors (e.g. nuclear factor-kappa B (NF-κB)), protein kinases (intracellular enzymes that mediate cellular responses to inflammatory stimuli: e.g. c-Jun N-terminal kinase (JNK), p38 MAP (mitogen-activated protein) kinase) and proteases (enzymes that cleave peptide bonds: e.g. caspases)[3]. TNF-α may contribute to the pathogenesis of RA by induction of pro-inflammatory cytokines such as IL-1 and IL-6, enhancement of leukocyte migration by increasing endothelial layer permeability and expression of adhesion molecules by endothelial cells and leukocytes, activation of neutrophils and eosinophils, induction of the synthesis of acute phase reactants, other liver proteins, and tissue-degrading enzymes (matrix metalloproteinase enzymes) produced by synoviocytes and/or chondrocytes. Elevated levels of TNF-α are found in involved tissues of patients with RA, psoriatic arthritis (PsA), and ankylosing spondylitis (AS). The role of TNF-α in mediating diverse inflammatory activities provided the initial rationale for blocking this cytokine[4]. Scientific and clinical evidence demonstrate that blocking TNF-α provides dramatic improvements in disease activity and quality of life, and attenuating radiographic progression in RA. Recently, three biological agents that inhibit TNF-α have been approved for use in RA and some other autoimmune disorders: a soluble p75 TNF-receptor IgG1-Fc fusion construct (etanercept), a chimeric anti-TNF-α IgG1 monoclonal antibody (mAb) (infliximab), and a human IgG1anti-TNF-α mAb (adalimumab).

Infliximab, etanercept, adalimumab

Mechanism of action

Analysis of samples from treated RA patients, shows that blockade of TNF-α activity may lead to clinical benefit in patients with RA by various mechanisms, including down-regulation of local and systemic pro-inflammatory cytokine production, reduction of lymphocyte migration into the joint, and reduction of angiogenesis in the joints[2,3]. The relevance of these has been demonstrated with post-treatment synovial biopsies that showed reduced cellular infiltrates, with fewer numbers of T cells and macrophages present[5]. Also, changes in soluble E-selectin, soluble intercellular adhesion molecule (ICAM)-1, vascular endothelial growth factor (VEGF), and circulating lymphocytes with anti-TNF-α therapy correlated with clinical outcome[6].

Although all three agents are TNF inhibitors, there are differences among them. The mAb infliximab and adalimumab are specific for TNF-α; etanercept binds TNF-α as well as LT-α. Both adalimumab and infliximab are IgG1 antibodies, and etanercept contains an IgG1 portion, but different antibody variable regions can confer different binding properties, and functional differences. In addition to sharing the ability to inhibit TNF, all three agents bind to TNF with high affinity, and all three agents are virtually the same in their ability to neutralize soluble and transmembrane TNF[7-9]. Effector functions, such as induction of cell lysis, were demonstrated by *in vitro* studies with infliximab and adalimumab, and apoptosis was demonstrated by both *in vitro* and *in vivo* studies for all three agents[10], although this is an area where conflicting data have been observed.

Clinical pharmacology and dosing

Clinical pharmacology studies demonstrate that infliximab has a dose-dependent PK profile following infusions of 3–20 mg/kg. In combination therapy with methotrexate (MTX) (7.5 mg once a week), serum infliximab concentrations tended to be slightly higher than when administered alone[8]. It has been estimated that the half-life of infliximab is around 8–9.5 days at the 3 mg/kg dose, although longer values have been reported for higher doses[11]. The volume distribution (Vd) of infliximab at steady state is independent of dose, suggesting predominantly intravascular distribution[9,12]. Median Vd ranges from 3 to 5 L. The clearance of infliximab is ~0.01L/h. The initial recommended dose of infliximab is 3 mg/kg given as an intravenous (IV) infusion followed by doses at two and six weeks after the first infusion, then every eight weeks thereafter. Infliximab is approved for use in combination with MTX, although patients have received infliximab with other disease-modifying anti-rheumatic drugs (DMARDs) or as monotherapy. At the recommended initial dose, about 25% of patients will have trough concentrations below 1 mg/mL; this is associated with lesser clinical response[9]. In that case higher doses and/or shorter intervals may be used.

Etanercept is given by self-administered subcutaneous injection at 25 mg twice weekly, or 50 mg once a week. Etanercept is approved for use either alone or in conjunction with methotrexate. When administered subcutaneously, etanercept is absorbed slowly, reaching a mean peak concentration at ~50 h after a single 25 mg dose. The immunoglobulin structure affords a half-life of 3–4.8 days. Serum concentration profiles at steady state were comparable among patients with RA treated with 50 mg once weekly and 25 mg twice weekly. Vd suggests predominantly intravascular distribution[13]. The route of clearance from the circulation is unclear, although it is presumed that it is mediated through Fc binding by the reticuloendothelial system. The clearance of etanercept is

0.16 L/h. Methotrexate has no effect on the pharmacokinetics of etanercept.

The peak serum adalimumab concentration and area under the curve increase linearly with dose over the range of 0.5–10 mg/kg. Adalimumab appears to have a low clearance and distributes mainly in the vascular compartment. Its elimination half-life is 10–13.6 days. Adalimumab has been studied with different doses at different intervals. The recommended dose is 40 mg every other week administered subcutaneously, with the possibility of changing dose frequency to weekly. After a single 40 mg subcutaneous dose, the maximum serum concentration is achieved within 131 h. Distribution of adalimumab is largely confined to the vascular department. Adalimumab is recommended to be used alone and in combination with methotrexate. Methotrexate has been shown to reduce the adalimumab clearance after single and multiple dosing by 29% and 44%, respectively[14].

Given intravenously, infliximab has a high peak concentration followed by steady state elimination, whereas etanercept and adalimumab, because they are given subcutaneously, have more 'flat' pharmacokinetic profiles. These peak plasma concentrations of TNF antagonists may influence their tissue penetration and their local impact on cell trafficking, function, and survival. However, half-life differences among TNF antagonists do not account for clinical differences during continuous anti-TNF treatment. Interestingly, the failure of a patient to respond to a single TNF antagonist should not be taken to mean that the patient is refractory to all TNF blockers. Studies have shown success with infliximab in patients who have failed to respond to etanercept therapy, and vice versa[15].

Efficacy

In recent years, true disease modification has become a realistic goal in the clinical care of patients with RA. With early and aggressive treatment involving new drugs and drug combinations, it may be possible to substantially ameliorate the physical, social, and economic consequences of RA. Anti-TNF-α agents are very effective, as demonstrated by a number needed to treat (NNT) of 2 to produce a 20% improvement. For all agents, the NNT for American College of Rheumatology (ACR)50 is 4 and for ACR70 it is 8[16]. The clinical benefits of TNF-α blockers are associated with an improvement in various serological parameters, including as C-reactive protein, serum amyloid-A, erythrocyte sedimentation rate (ESR), matrix metalloproteinase (MMP)-1 and MMP-3 levels[17]. Double blind, placebo-controlled, randomized clinical trials (DBPCRCTs) have demonstrated clinical benefit associated with significant improvement in patients with severe disease, often when conventional treatments are unsuccessful. Initial clinical studies based on the use of anti-TNF therapy have suggested a potential beneficial effect in inducing reduction of inflammatory parameters in patients with long-standing active RA. In the earliest controlled trials, the efficacy and tolerability of the TNF-α blockers in refractory RA patients were demonstrated[18-20]. This, along with the growing safety of experience gained with therapy, provided the rationale for studies with longer duration of therapy.

Multicenter DBPCRCTs with infliximab have evaluated the effects of multiple doses over longer time periods. In the

ATTRACT trial, addition of infliximab (3 mg/kg or 10 mg/kg every four or eight weeks) to patients with active RA despite concurrent methotrexate was significantly superior to treatment with methotrexate alone defined by ACR response criteria. The initial promising results from six months of treatment have been shown to be sustained through 54 weeks of follow-up[11,21]. In addition to achieving substantial efficacy as measured by ACR20 clinical response criteria, the use of infliximab was associated with significant improvement in functional status and quality of life[21]. The radiographic progression of joint damage was measured by modified Sharp score. The progression of radiographic damage was significantly less for all the infliximab-treated groups in comparison with methotrexate alone. Patients receiving infliximab had an arrest of the progression of joint damage as assessed by X-ray change scores[9,21]. The ASPIRE trial compared the effects of infliximab plus methotrexate and methotrexate alone in patients with early RA (i.e. <3 years duration). At 54 weeks the percentage of patients achieving an ACR20 response was significantly higher in the infliximab group. In addition, a significant increase in radiological destruction was observed in patients treated only with methotrexate, whereas a reduction in the progression of disease by ~90% was observed in infliximab plus methotrexate groups[22]. In the START trial, a large group of patients with active RA on usual background DMARD therapy were treated with either 3 mg/kg or 10 mg/kg of infliximab for 46 weeks[23]. Patients were allowed to dose escalate for lack of response. ACR responses were similar to the ATTRACT and ASPIRE trials. However, there was a statistically significant increase in serious infectious events in the 10 mg/kg group.

Initial studies have demonstrated the efficacy and tolerability of etanercept in both early and refractory disease and also established the optimal dose of 25 mg twice weekly[19,20]. In a six-month DBPCRCT with etanercept (10 or 25 mg twice weekly), patients with active and long-standing RA, etanercept was shown to be effective in rapidly reducing disease activity[24]. The efficacy and safety of etanercept together with methotrexate was demonstrated in another trial, where addition of etanercept resulted in rapid and sustained improvement[25]. In the open-label extension part of this study, the patients were able to sustain the improvement and the majority of them were able to decrease their use of methotrexate and/or corticosteroid dose. In one trial two doses of etanercept (10 or 25 mg twice weekly) were compared with an accelerated dosing of methotrexate in methotrexate naïve RA patients with less than three years of disease[26]. Radiographic assessments at 0, 6, and 12, 24 months showed that the rate of X-ray progression appeared to be slowed by both agents; the effect of 25 mg of etanercept being greater than that of methotrexate. The TEMPO study compared the effects of etanercept only, methotrexate only, and etanercept plus methotrexate on patients with established disease. Results showed that the combination of etanercept and methotrexate maintained significant, consistent efficacy advantage over monotherapy groups over two years. The mean total Sharp score decreased by 0.5 units with etanercept plus methotrexate, which was significantly better than the increase of 0.5 units observed in patients treated with etanercept alone and the increase of 2.8 units in those treated with methotrexate alone[27].

In a DBPCRCT phase II trial, 284 patients were treated with placebo or one of three doses of adalimumab (20, 40, or 80 mg) by weekly subcutaneous injection for 12 weeks[28]. Clinical results demonstrated the efficacy of adalimumab in comparison to placebo. In a subsequent DBPCRCT, the ARMADA trial, adalimumab was given to patients with active RA despite long-term methotrexate therapy at doses of 20, 40, and 80 mg every other week. Adalimumab at all doses provided significant, rapid, and sustained improvement in disease activity over 24 weeks compared with methotrexate alone[29]. The ARMADA trial also demonstrated sustained improvements in ACR criteria, Health Assessment Questionnaire (HAQ) scores after three years of combined treatment with adalimumab and methotrexate[30]. In a multicenter DBPCRCT, 619 patients with active RA with inadequate response to methotrexate were randomized to receive adalimumab 40 mg every other week, adalimumab 20 mg weekly, or placebo[31]. Both adalimumab regimens were found to be significantly more effective at reducing signs and symptoms measured with ACR20 response, and also improving physical function in comparison to placebo. In addition, modified total Sharp scores showed significantly smaller changes in patients treated with adalimumab, and significantly fewer patients had new erosions compared with those taking placebo. A study evaluating the health related quality of life (HRQoL) in two DBPCTs demonstrated that adalimumab plus methotrexate provides statistically significant improvements in HRQoL[32]. Long-term treatment efficacy with adalimumab was evaluated in patients with long-standing RA and adalimumab was found to be efficacious and safe for up to six years[33].

TNF inhibitors in inflammatory disorders other than RA

Psoriatic arthritis

Biopsy specimens of skin lesions and synovial tissue from patients with PsA have shown increased expression of TNF-α. The safety and efficacy of etanercept was assessed in a DBPCRT in 205 patients with PsA. Compared to placebo, treatment with etanercept resulted in significant improvements in measures of disease activity defined by ACR response criteria. Psoriatic skin lesions measured by psoriasis area and severity index (PASI) improved modestly with etanercept treatment compared to placebo[34]. The results of infliximab multinational psoriatic arthritis controlled trial (IMPACT) had also shown that rapid improvements in disease activity measures by ACR response criteria and psoriatic skin lesions by PASI with infliximab treatment at week 16 were sustained through week 50 with a good safety profile[35]. Adalimumab's effect on PsA has also been investigated in a double blind phase III study[36]. Substantial improvements in arthritis and skin disease were noted compared to placebo.

Ankylosing spondylitis

TNF-α was found to be abundantly expressed in the sacroiliac joints of AS patients. In addition, inflammatory arthritis resembling AS developed in a transgenic mouse engineered to overexpress murine TNF-α. Following initial pilot studies with etanercept and infliximab the safety and efficacy of etanercept were assessed in a DBPCRT in 277 patients with AS; 20, 50, and

70% improvements in assessment in ankylosing spondylitis (ASAS) response criteria were statistically significant compared to placebo at weeks 12 and 24. Sustained efficacy and safety of etanercept were reported up to 18 months in 99 patients[37]. Infliximab's safety and efficacy were assessed in a DBPCRT. Rapid and significant improvement in disease activity measured by Bath ankylosing spondylitis disease activity index (BASDAI) was maintained through week 54[38]. Trials are underway to show the efficacy of adalimumab on patients with AS.

Juvenile idiopathic arthritis (JIA)

Based on the promising results of a clinical trial in 69 children with active JIA who had inadequate response to methotrexate therapy, etanercept has been approved for the therapy of JIA, and further safety was demonstrated in a long-term trial[39,40]. Infliximab and adalimumab are being studied in JIA.

Crohn's disease

The number of TNF-α-secreting cells is increased in the mucosa of inflamed intestine and TNF-α has been shown to exert deleterious effects in the pathophysiology of Crohn's disease. Clinical trials and clinical experience with currently available TNF inhibitors have yielded non-parallel results. The efficacy of infliximab on active fistulas and long-term maintenance of Crohn's disease has been proven in several clinical trials[41,42]. However, etanercept at a dose of 25 mg twice weekly was found to be ineffective for the treatment of patients with moderate to severe Crohn's disease[43]. Adalimumab has been studied and has also shown efficacy in Crohn's disease.

Safety

Clinical trials, post-marketing experience, and pharmacovigilance programs have begun to yield a large safety profile for TNF blocking agents[44]. Although generally TNF blockers have been shown to have a good safety profile, there are issues of safety that should be taken into consideration. DBPCRT and long-term safety data from an open label extension trial with the three TNF blockers demonstrated that these agents can be safe and well tolerated for up to seven years and rates of adverse events were consistent with those seen in controlled trials[11,16,24–26,33]. Since their introduction, the three TNF inhibitors have been used by more than one million patients worldwide.

Infusion reactions/injection site reactions

Clinical trial data have shown that about 20% of infliximab-treated patients have experienced an infusion reaction. However, less than 1% of infliximab-treated patients develop serious infusion-related reactions, and only 2.5% of these reactions result in discontinuation of therapy. Headache (20%) and nausea (15%) are the most common infusion reactions. These are usually transient, rarely severe, and can typically be controlled by slowing the rate of infusion or by treatment with acetaminophen or antihistamines[11,24].

With etanercept and adalimumab, cutaneous reactions at injection sites represent the most frequent side-effect, although they rarely cause discontinuation of therapy[24,25,31]. Injection site reactions, which occur in ~34–37% of patients treated with etanercept and 20–23% of those treated with adalimumab, typically consist of erythematous or urticarial lesions[31,44]. Although they can arise at sites of previous injections, these reactions seem to be limited to the skin and are not associated with other features of immediate hypersensitivity. Reactions typically occur close to initiation of treatment and abate over time, even with continued dosing.

Infection

Infections occur more frequently and are important contributors to the accelerated morbidity of RA patients compared to the general population. Comorbidities, such as diabetes mellitus, heart disease, disability, and concurrent immunosuppressive medication (e.g. steroid, cytotoxic) all contribute to the risk of infection[45]. In RA trials with anti-TNF therapies, the number of reports of infections tended to be somewhat higher among patients receiving TNF-α inhibitors; however, there were not usually significant sequelae occurring as a consequence of these infectious episodes. In all studies the most frequent infection was upper respiratory infection. Other frequent infections included sinusitis, urinary tract infection, bronchitis, and pharyngitis.

Experimental data demonstrate that anti-TNF therapy interferes with the ability to mount an inflammatory response against intracellular organisms. Some concerns were aroused with the emergence of opportunistic infections, including tuberculosis (TB) in patients treated with TNF antagonists, in the period following approval of these agents. The incidence of serious infections (infections requiring hospitalization or parenteral antibiotics) in patients with RA before the anti-TNF era ranged from ~0.02 to 0.12 per patient year[46,47]. The incidence of severe infections in the patients treated with TNF antagonists in clinical trials has been comparable to that seen in the placebo groups. The incidence of serious infection rates per patient year according to clinical trials were 0.04 in both etanercept and placebo groups; 0.03 in both infliximab and placebo groups; 0.04 and 0.02 in adalimumab and placebo groups, respectively[48]. Post-marketing data indicate an incidence of 0.007 serious infections per patient year in etanercept-treated patients, although under-reporting can not be ruled out. Post-marketing surveillance has not detected any change in the incidence of serious infections in patients treated with infliximab. Data from post-marketing indicate that an apparently higher number of cases of certain opportunistic infections with infliximab than etanercept (26 *Pneumocystis carinii* and 18 histoplasma infections per 271 000 infliximab-treated patients) (4 *Pneumocystis carinii* and 1 histoplasmosis per 121 000 etanercept treated patients)[49]. Although these results are reassuring, precautions should be taken to prevent or minimize serious infections that might occur while a patient is receiving TNF antagonists. Anti-TNF agents should not be administered to patients with acute infection.

TNF antagonist therapy can interfere with organisms' ability to fight against TB. TNF plays an important role in the formation and maintenance of granulomas. TB cases have been seen in patients treated with any of the available anti-TNF agents, but most cases occur within a few months of initiating treatment, therefore they are thought to represent reactivation of existing disease. Of note, more patients treated with TNF inhibitors have extrapulmonary and disseminated TB[50]. Additionally, the rates of TB associated with the use of TNF antagonists have been shown to be higher in geographic regions where TB is more prevalent in the general population[51]. Although no cases of TB occurred in etanercept-treated patients during clinical trials, there have been 38 confirmed cases of etanercept-associated TB worldwide in 150000 patients treated through December 2002. For infliximab, 441 cases of TB among 492 874 infliximab-treated patients were reported, while only six cases of infliximab-related TB cases were reported in clinical trials. Ninety-seven percent of the infliximab-related cases occurred within seven months, with a median time of onset of 12 weeks. The incidence of TB in clinical trials with adalimumab was higher in earlier clinical trials when the dose of adalimumab was higher. The incidence dropped to 1% after adalimumab was reduced to its current dose, and after screening for latent TB infection was instituted prior to therapy (21 cases in 2400 patients). To date, a greater number of cases have been seen among patients receiving infliximab than the other TNF inhibitors, but this may in part relate to issues such as the particular patient population exposed, screening procedures, and other factors. The increased risk and unusual presentations of TB in anti-TNF-treated patients compared with the overall population deserves clinical suspicion and close follow-up. The risk of developing TB with TNF antagonists is significantly reduced with screening and appropriate clinical monitoring. Current US guidelines recommend purified protein derivative (PPD) skin testing and chest X-ray prior to TNF antagonist therapy. If the PPD test is positive without evidence of active infection, then treatment for latent TB should commence before or with anti-TNF therapy.

Malignancy

The overall rate of malignancy in patients with RA is the same as in the normal population; however, the risk of lymphoma is increased in patients with RA. Although the actual reason is not known, the severity and the duration of the disease, and the use of immunomodulatory agents, such as methotrexate, seem to play a role. Overall standardized incidence ratios (SIRs) of lymphoma in the RA population are reported to be 2.0–8.0. Anti-TNF drugs can theoretically affect the host defense against malignancy. To date, the occurrence of lymphoma seen in clinical trials and long-term follow-up of patients from clinical trials of the various TNF inhibitors in RA patients does not appear to exceed the rate that would be expected in this population, namely, RA patients with severe active disease. The SIR for etanercept was 3.5, for infliximab 6.4, and for adalimumab 4.35 in the RA patients treated in clinical trials. According to a prospective analysis of 18 572 patients with RA, the overall SIR among RA patients was 1.9; it was 1.7 for methotrexate, 2.9 for biologic use, 2.6 for etanercept, and 3.8 for infliximab[52]. However, these differences in SIRs are generally viewed as slight and the candidates for anti-TNF therapy are severe cases of RA, who already have a higher risk of lymphoma. Longer-term follow-up of larger numbers of patients treated with TNF inhibitors will provide clinicians with a better view about the safety of these agents as regards any risk for lymphoma.

Autoimmune responses

As is true for any therapeutic agent, especially large protein molecules, some of which contain foreign sequences, antibodies to anti-TNF agents can develop. Although their clinical relevance

is presently unclear, these antibodies can diminish the half-life of the therapeutic agent and consequently decrease its efficacy. They might also lead to adverse effects, including immune-complex formation or hypersensitivity reactions. Approximately 3% of the etanercept-treated patients developed antibodies to etanercept[53]. In one study antibodies to infliximab developed in 53, 21, and 7% of patients who were receiving 10, 3, and 1 mg/kg of infliximab, respectively[54]. RA trials of infliximab with or without concomitant methotrexate treatment revealed that immunogenicity was decreased by concomitant MTX, due perhaps in part to the increase in the half-life of infliximab associated with MTX use[8]. A multi-center trial of infliximab therapy in Crohn's disease revealed that the induction of these anti-infliximab antibodies might have contributed to hypersensitivity reaction in some patients who had been treated with this drug. Antibodies to adalimumab developed in about 12% of patients; the rate was reduced to 1% with concurrent methotrexate treatment[54]. Although it is believed that there is a trend towards higher clearance of infliximab and adalimumab in the presence of anti-adalimumab and anti-infliximab antibodies, routine testing for antibodies to TNF inhibitors is not currently recommended.

Although a substantial minority of RA patients has serum anti-nuclear antibodies (ANA), the prevalence of ANA has been reported to be increased with anti-TNF agents. The mechanism and the significance of the development of antibodies are uncertain[44,55]. Antibodies to double-stranded DNA (ds-DNA) have also been reported to develop in about 5–10% of RA patients treated with all anti-TNF therapies[54]. However, few (0.2–0.4%) treated patients developed symptoms consistent with drug-induced lupus, and among these who did, the manifestations eventually ceased after the treatments were stopped[11,25,55]. A few patients have been also reported to develop anti-cardiolipin antibodies, mostly asymptomatic.

Demyelinating syndromes

A full epidemiology of demyelinating disorders in RA has not been determined. Clinical data suggest that TNF antagonists may exacerbate existing demyelinating disease[56]. Post-marketing surveillance data reveal cases of demyelinating disorders with all available TNF inhibitors. Although there is supporting evidence that the incidence of multiple sclerosis (MS) may be increased in patients with RA, it is recommended that clinicians should exercise caution when considering a TNF antagonist for a patient with a pre-existing or recent onset central nervous system demyelination disorder.

Congestive heart failure (CHF)

TNF-α levels are found to be consistently elevated in patients with CHF, and patients with RA are known to have an elevated risk of CHF. Pre-clinical and early clinical studies suggested that anti-cytokine therapy could prove beneficial in the treatment of patients with heart failure. However, clinical trials with high-dose infliximab (10 mg/kg) in patients with CHF were discontinued early, because of an increase in deaths and worsening of CHF in patients with class III–IV CHF. Etanercept trials with CHF were also stopped early due to lack of efficacy. On the contrary, in RA clinical trials TNF antagonists were not associated with new onset CHF and they might actually reduce risk[57]. Nevertheless, increased caution is recommended when using anti-TNF agents in patients with CHF, especially with Classes III and IV.

Other adverse events

Rare reports of pancytopenia, including aplastic anemia, have been reported in patients treated with anti-TNF agents. Several cases of elevations in aminotransferases, and autoimmune hepatitis have been reported with anti-TNF usage. While many reports have described increased susceptibility to intracellular pathogens in patients with chronic viral infections in preliminary studies, TNF-α inhibitors have displayed a reasonable safety profile in the setting of some chronic viral infections, including hepatitis C, hepatitis B, and HIV, and in certain circumstances have demonstrated adjunctive activity in the treatment of these infections[58,59]. However, additional studies are needed to assess the risks and benefits of anti-TNF therapy in chronic viral infections.

Pregnancy and lactation

There are cases reported where patients became pregnant when they were being treated with TNF inhibitors. The rates of normal births were similar to the published rates from the general population. There are insufficient data to advise continuation or starting of anti-TNF therapy if a patient becomes pregnant[60]. It is not known if TNF blocking agents are secreted in human milk. The safety of these agents during lactation has not been established.

Monitoring

Everyone who is under consideration for anti-TNF treatment should be carefully evaluated for the presence of infection, malignancy, demyelinating disorders, or any other chronic condition which may predispose to infections. In addition, potential adverse effects of TNF-α inhibition must be weighed against the potential clinical benefits before initiating the therapy with these agents. Physicians are recommended to exercise caution when patients develop a new infection while undergoing treatment with anti-TNF agents. Prophylactic antituberculous treatment should be started if latent tuberculosis is discovered. PPD is recommended before starting treatment with a TNF inhibitor. In addition, chest X-ray is recommended if PPD skin test is positive. Although no specific laboratory monitoring is required by regulatory agencies, it is highly recommended that physicians obtain complete blood count and liver function tests regularly on patients treated with anti-TNF agents. Assiduous monitoring of patients for any sign and symptom of infection, demyelinizing disease, and malignancy is requisite during treatment with TNF inhibitors.

While currently available TNF blockers have undoubtedly constituted a considerable advance in the management of RA and other inflammatory conditions, there are future challenges. For example, further basic research and clinical trials could help identify factors that would predict clinical response or toxicity to these agents.

Other TNF blockers under investigation

Despite the success with the currently available TNF antagonists, there is still room for additional TNF-directed therapies in treating RA and other inflammatory disorders. A variety of other strategies are being tested with the ultimate goal of inhibiting the function of TNF. Some of these are macromolecules, including the PEGylated human anti-TNF-α mAb Fab fragment CDP870 (humanized Fab anti-TNF fragment), and PEGylated soluble p55 TNF receptor construct. Polyethylene glycol (PEG) is a construct with high molecular weight which has been shown to increase the half-life of compounds it is bound to. Subcutaneous injection of ascending doses of chimeric PEGylated CDP870 was well tolerated among patients with active RA and the results showed rapid improvement in ACR responses[61]. Further studies are ongoing. A PEGylated recombinant soluble inhibitor of p55 receptors was reportedly effective in several hundred patients in a Phase II trial[62]. TACE is a transmembrane protein that cleaves cell surface-bound TNF-α to release soluble, mature TNF-α. Inhibition of TACE is shown to inhibit TNF-α secretion by human synovium tissue explants of RA patients[63]. Antisense oligonucleotides have nucleotide sequences complementary to the mRNA sequences encoding the targeted protein. When they bind to mRNA, they block the production of the targeted protein. Human TNF antisense oligonucleotides are currently being investigated. The impact of these new approaches remains to be seen.

IL-1 blocking therapy

Members of the IL-1 family include IL-1α, IL-1β, and the IL-1 receptor antagonist (IL-1Ra). Specific cellular proteases process IL-1α and IL-β to their 17 kDa mature forms. Pro IL-1α precursor (proIL-1α) is active intracellularly. However, proIL-1β is not active before cleavage with IL-1β-converting enzyme (ICE). After cleavage it is secreted and is fully functional. IL-1Ra is a naturally occurring antagonist protein with amino acid sequence homology to IL-1α and IL-1β. Multiple forms of this protein exist. One is secreted, and functions as a competitive inhibitor of IL-1α and IL-1β, binding to the same counter-receptor but transducing no signal. Other forms of IL-1Ra are intracellular; although they may serve inhibitory functions, their roles have not been fully defined. The IL-1 polypeptides bind to two cell-surface receptors: type 1(IL-1R1) and type 2 (IL-1R-II). IL-1RI is found on most cell types, while IL1-RII occurs mainly on the surface of neutrophils, monocytes, B cells, and bone marrow progenitor cells. When IL-1 binds to IL-1RI, the signal transduction is mediated through association of a second receptor unit, IL-R accessory protein (IL-1R-AcP). Binding of IL-1 to IL1-RII does not lead to signal transduction. IL-1RII acts like a decoy receptor and competitive inhibitor. Soluble forms of IL-1RII inhibit IL-1 activity by competing with IL-1RI for IL-1 binding.

Like TNF-α, IL-1 is one of the key mediators of inflammatory response. Although IL-1 can be synthesized by many different cell types, it is produced at inflammatory sites primarily by macrophages. IL-1 exhibits both local and systemic biologic effects. Systemic effects of IL-1 include fever, muscle breakdown, and induction of acute phase proteins in the liver. IL-1 induces the production of other cytokines, including TNF-α, IL-6, and IL-8. IL-1 enhances the expression of adhesion molecules on endothelial cells and induces chemotaxis of neutrophils, monocytes, and lymphocytes. IL-1 has both angiogenic and angiostatic activities[64].

Anakinra

Structure and mechanism of action

Anakinra (designated IL-1ra) is a recombinant non-glycosylated homolog of IL-1Ra that differs from native human IL-1Ra by the addition of a single methionine residue at its amino terminus. Anakinra blocks the activity of IL-1 by competitively inhibiting IL-1 binding to the IL-1RI receptor. Levels of the naturally occurring IL-1Ra, which are elevated in the synovium and synovial fluid from RA patients, appear to be insufficient for the excess amount of locally produced IL-1.

Clinical pharmacology

In subjects with RA, maximum plasma concentrations of anakinra occurred 3–7 h after subcutaneous administration of anakinra at clinically relevant doses (1–2 mg/kg). The terminal half-life ranged from 4 to 6 h. In RA patients, no unexpected accumulation of anakinra was observed after daily subcutaneous doses for up to 24 weeks. The estimated anakinra clearance increased with increasing creatinine clearance and body weight. Humans with renal disfunction have markedly decreased clearance of anakinra, therefore dose adjustment is required. The recommended dose of anakinra for the treatment of patients with moderate to severely active RA is 100 mg/day administered daily by subcutaneous injection.

Efficacy

The clinical efficacy of IL-Ira as a monotherapy in patients with active RA was demonstrated in 472 patients in a placebo-controlled study[66]. Three different doses of anakinra (30, 75, and 150 mg) resulted in improvement in ACR criteria in comparison to placebo group, with better response rates with higher doses. However, the overall magnitude of reductions in clinical symptoms and signs (20–30%) was relatively modest when compared to those reported in TNF-α blocking agents. In the open label extension study, ACR20 was achieved in 71% of the patients who received the highest dose of anakinra (150 mg/day). Additionally, each dose of IL-1ra was associated with a reduction in radiographic progression relative to placebo[66].

The efficacy of anakinra plus methotrexate was evaluated in a 24-week DBPCT on patients with active RA despite methotrexate therapy. Patients were treated with 0, 0.04, 0.1, 1.0, or 2.0 mg/kg anakinra per day. The optimal dose of anakinra was 1.0 mg/kg. The combination therapy with methotrexate was also significantly more effective than methotrexate alone[67].

Importantly, an increased incidence of serious infections, and no additional clinical benefit, were reported when anakinra was used in combination with etanercept in a trial of 244 RA patients[68]. Therefore, despite promising results in animal models of RA, combination therapy with inhibitors of TNF and IL-1 is not recommended. The safety of anakinra alone was also evaluated in a trial with 1414 patients which allowed a wide variety of comorbid conditions and concomitant DMARDs[79]. The results showed that anakinra is a generally well-tolerated treatment for RA in patient populations representative of those seen in normal clinic settings.

Safety

The most common adverse event is dose-dependent injection site reaction (ISR), occurring in 50–80% of patients in trials[65]. These reactions were generally mild and transient, and resolved rapidly.

Infections were uncommon and occurred at a similar rate to placebo group. Infections that required antibiotic therapy were 12% of the placebo-treated group, and 15–17% of the treatment group. The infections consisted primarily of bacterial events such as cellulites, pneumonia, and bone and joint infections. Serious infections occurred in 2.1% of patients treated with anakinra, as compared to 0.4% of those receiving placebo. The incidence of pulmonary infections may be higher among patients with underlying asthma. In placebo-controlled studies up to 8% of patients receiving anakinra showed reductions in their neutrophil count compared to 2% of the placebo patients. Other reported adverse events were headache, nausea, diarrhea, sinusitis, influenza-like syndrome, and abdominal pain. The development of TB or other opportunistic infections, malignancy rate, and incidences were similar to those expected for the populations studied[70].

Clinical use and monitoring

Anakinra may be useful in patients who have no response, or who are unable, to tolerate TNF blocking agents. Anakinra can be used alone or in combination with MTX. Because of the potential for increase in rate of infections, it is not recommended for use in conjunction with TNF inhibitors. Patients should be closely monitored for signs and symptoms of infection. Anakinra treatment needs to be discontinued if a patient develops serious infection. Neutrophil count should be assessed prior to initiating anakinra treatment and, while receiving anakinra therapy, monthly for three months, and then every four months up to one year. There are case reports of adult onset Still's disease, familial Mediterranean fever, JIA, and familial cold anti-inflammatory disease who showed improvement in disease activities with anakinra treatment[71].

Pregnancy and lactation

Reproductive studies have only been performed on rats and rabbits and they have not revealed any evidence of harm to the fetus. Because there are no well-controlled studies in pregnant women, anakinra should only be used in a pregnant mother if clearly needed. It is not known if anakinra is secreted in human milk.

Other IL-1 blockers under investigation

There are several other IL-1-inhibiting strategies that are in development for the treatment of rheumatic diseases. IL-1 first binds to IL-1R type I and then recruits the cell surface IL-1R accessory protein (IL-1RAcP). IL-1 Trap is a high affinity inhibitor of IL-1 consisting of the Fc portion of human IgG1 and extracellular domains of IL-1R type I and IL-1RAcP. Efficacy of IL-1 Trap was evaluated in 201 patients with active RA, who were allowed to take stable doses of DMARD treatment. Patients received 25, 50, 100 mg IL-1 Trap, or placebo subcutaneously. There was no difference between groups in terms of ACR responses at the end of a 12-week treatment. However, the 100 mg group showed good to moderate improvement in DAS28 responses[72]. An inhibitor of IL-1 converting enzyme (ICE, also called caspase-1), a metalloproteinase that facilitates the secretion of IL-1β and IL-18, is orally active agent that targets IL-1[73].

IL-6 blocking therapy

IL-6 is a pleiotropic cytokine that regulates the immune response, inflammation, hematopoiesis, and bone metabolism. IL-6 acts by binding to a specific receptor (IL-6R) which binds to another protein responsible for signal transduction. Elevated IL-6 levels both in the serum and synovial fluid in patients with RA were shown to correlate with the disease activity and radiographic joint damage[74]. Administration of a mouse monoclonal IL-6 antibody to five patients with RA resulted in amelioration of disease activity[75]. A humanized anti-human IL-6 receptor monoclonal antibody (MRA) that inhibits binding of IL-6 to IL-6R was later developed. MRA is composed of human IgG1 and murine complementarity determining regions (CDRs).

In a DBPCT, 164 patients with refractory RA were randomly assigned to an intravenous placebo, 4 mg/kg, or 8 mg/kg of MRA every four weeks. At the end of three months, 78% of patients in the 8 mg/kg group, 57% in the 4 mg/kg group, and 11% in the placebo group achieved at least ACR20, and 40% in the 8 mg/kg group achieved ACR50[76]. Although generally well tolerated, significant increases in cholesterol and triglyceride levels, as well as liver function test levels, were observed with both MRA groups in comparison to the placebo group. Long-term trials are underway to evaluate the further efficacy and safety of this drug.

Blockade of costimulatory pathways

Autoreactive T cells stimulated by one or more unidentified autoantigens presumably play a central role in triggering RA. Activation of T cells requires both antigen presentation and costimulation by the antigen-presenting cells (APCs) (Fig. 27.1). The first signal is generated when an antigen/MHC class II complex binds to the specific T cell receptor. Although essential for initiating T cell activation, this signal is not sufficient to induce a productive immune response. A second, costimulatory signal occurs when cell-surface molecules on the APC (CD80 or CD86) interact with a heterodimeric cell-surface protein receptor (CD28) on the T cell surface. Cytotoxic T lymphocyte-associated antigen 4 (CTLA-4), which is an important negative regulator of CD80/CD86–CD28, is a molecule that is transiently expressed at the surface of the T cells. CTLA-4 is expressed by T cells early after activation, but not on resting T cells, and transduces an inhibitory signal. As CTLA-4 binds to CD80/CD86 on the APC with a greater avidity than CD28, it also competes with CD28 binding to CD80/CD86, thereby leading to incomplete T cell activation.

Abatacept

These observations led to the development of abatacept, CTLA-4-immunoglobulin (CTLA-4Ig), a soluble receptor construct composed of the extracellular domain of CTLA-4 and an IgG1

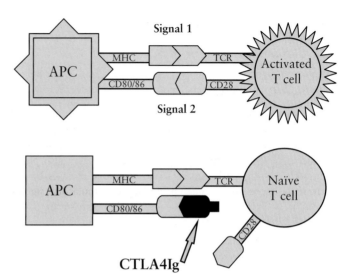

Fig. 27.1 Activation of T cells requires two signals. The first signal is generated when the MHC class II/antigen complex binds a T cell receptor. The second signal is generated by costimulation of CD28 on T cells by CD80 or CD86 molecules on APCs. CTLA-4Ig binding prevents this activation. TCR, T cell receptor.

Fc piece. Pre-clinical studies with CTLA-4Ig fusion proteins have shown a inhibition of T cell-mediated immune responses. The first evidence that CTLA-4Ig was clinically effective came from a small open label trial in patients with psoriasis[77]. In another pilot study, abatacept was evaluated in patients with RA for safety and dose-finding[78]. Recently, abatacept's safety and efficacy were evaluated in a DBPCT with 339 patients with active RA despite methotrexate therapy[79]. Patients were randomized to receive 2 mg/kg, 10 mg/kg of abatacept, or placebo intravenously on days 1, 15, and 30, and then monthly thereafter for a total of six months. The percentage of patients who achieved ACR20 was significantly higher in the 10 mg/kg CTLA-4Ig group compared to placebo. One-year analysis of this study also revealed that abatacept treatment was associated with rapid and a sustained increase in remission rates as defined by DAS28[80]. The rates of adverse effect were similar in both abatacept plus methotrexate and methotrexate only groups, while rates of serious adverse events were less common in the abatacept group[79].

Abatacept was also evaluated in patients with inadequate response to etanercept, who were randomized to receive either CTLA-4Ig or placebo in addition to etanercept[81]. Combination therapy with etanercept and abatacept resulted in statistically significant improvement in ACR response criteria in comparison to placebo group. The combination therapy with abatacept and etanercept was well tolerated, with a safety profile comparable to etanercept alone. Further studies are in progress that will provide more information on the long-term safety, effectiveness, and tolerance of abatacept.

A number of anti-CD80/86 monoclonal antibodies are in development. The anti-CD80 molecule IDEC-114 blocks costimulatory signaling by binding directly to CD80. Clinical data for this drug are just beginning to emerge. In addition, inducible costimulator (ICOS), another member of the CD28/CTLA-4 family, is an important costimulatory receptor expressed on activated T cells. ICOS may be of particular relevance to the activation of memory T cells. In collagen-induced arthritis, ICOS regulates *in vivo* and *in vitro* expression of IL-17, a pro-inflammatory cytokine implicated in RA.

Targeting B cells

Until recently the T cell was believed to be the main immune cell involved in the abnormal self-antigen recognition that characterizes autoimmune diseases. Over the last few years, however, considerable evidence has emerged that B cells may also play a central role in the pathogenesis of autoimmune diseases by presenting antigens to T cells, providing costimulatory signals, secreting cytokines, and also by producing autoantibodies. B cells' critical role in T cell activation has justified the trial of several therapeutic agents.

Rituximab

CD20 is a surface antigen that is expressed only on mature B cells. Rituximab is a genetically engineered chimeric monoclonal antibody to anti-CD20 IgG1, which has been approved for the treatment of B cell lymphoma since 1997. Rituximab causes selective and rapid transient depletion of the CD20+ B cell population. B cell depletion by rituximab may be mediated by various mechanisms, including antibody-dependent cellular cytotoxicity, complement-mediated B cell lysis, and induction of apoptosis.

The first evidence of efficacy of rituximab came from an open label trial in 5 patients, which was subsequently extended to 22 patients[82,83]. In both studies, however, rituximab was given in conjunction with high-dose glucocorticoids and cyclophosphamide, raising doubts about effects related to rituximab itself. The first DBRPCT compared rituximab to placebo in 161 patients with methotrexate-resistant RA[84]. Patients were given two intravenous infusions of 1000 mg rituximab two weeks apart. Patients were randomly assigned to receive one of four treatments: methotrexate only, rituximab only, rituximab + cyclophosphamide, and rituximab + methotrexate. All patients received glucocorticoid therapy for two weeks, with a total dose of 930 mg. At the end of six months, the rituximab + methotrexate and rituximab + cyclophosphamide groups had significantly greater ACR50 rates compared to the methotrexate alone group. In all groups treated with rituximab a significantly higher proportion of patients reached ACR20. This dramatic clinical efficacy after two rituximab infusions was maintained after 48 weeks in the group that received rituximab + methotrexate and continued to receive methotrexate (ACR20 65%, and ACR50 35%). Rituximab therapy induced profound peripheral blood B cell depletion for six months or more, and the therapy was also associated with a decrease in rheumatoid factor (RF) levels that was maintained after 24 weeks. Levels of other immunoglobulins decreased only slightly and remained within normal ranges. Of note, in this one-year study, infections were not more common with rituximab than with methotrexate alone. Infusion-related events, including transient hypotension, cough, pruritus, and rash were the most common side-effects during the first rituximab infusion.

For instance, Rituximab may be effective in other autoimmune diseases. The drug was effective and safe in small open label trials

Table 27.1 Future Potential therapentic agents

Tareting inflammatory cytokines	• IL-15
	• IL-17
	• IL-18
Targeting anti-inflammatory cytokines	• IL-4
	• IL-10
	• IL-11
Targeting adhesion molecules	• IL-8
	• CCRI
Targeting adhesion molecules	• ICAM-1
	• VCAM-1
	• CD11a/CD18
	• E-selectin
Targeting angiogenesis	• VEGF
	• EGF
	• α V/β III
Targeting T cells	• IL-2
	• CD4
	• LFA3/CD2
	• CD25
Targeting B cells	• BAFF-R/BlyS
Targeting innate immunity	• Complements (e.g. C5a)
	• TLR
Targeting intracellular signals	• NFκB
	• MAPK

of systemic lupus erythematosus[85]. Modest benefit was reported in patients with other inflammatory conditions, including primary Sjogren's syndrome, JIA, and vasculitis[86]. Additional trials are underway that should answer questions regarding dosing, treatment intervals, safety, and tolerability.

Future directions

In the near future biotechnological advances will allow improved treatment of those who do not respond to current therapies and possibly will lead to new strategies for treating systemic inflammatory disease. Several other promising biologic agents directed at a variety of targets are now being investigated (Table 27.1).

High concentrations of several pro-inflammatory cytokines have been shown to be present at elevated concentrations in the synovial fluid and synovial membranes of affected joints. A fully human mAb to IL-5 has been investigated in a phase II trial in patients with RA. The results were very promising, with dose-dependent clinical efficacy and a good safety profile reported[87]. Pre-clinical studies in arthritis models suggest that other pro-inflammatory cytokines, including IL-17 and IL-18, may also be possible targets.

Chemokines and chemokine receptors control the recruitment of leukocytes to the sites of inflammation. IL-8 is a chemotactic cytokine that affects lymphocyte and neutrophil migration through interaction with IL-8 receptors. Several chemokine antagonists, including CXCL-8/IL-8 antibody and CCR1 antagonist, are under development for the treatment of rheumatic diseases. ABX-IL8 is a fully human monoclonal antibody that binds free IL-8. Preliminary studies of this agent have been conducted in RA, with promising results.

Modulation of anti-inflammatory cytokines, inhibition of adhesion molecules, inhibition of angiogenesis, T cell-directed therapies, inhibition of complements (e.g. antiC5a), inhibition of

Toll-like receptors, and inhibition of intracellular signaling molecules are among other potential future therapeutic candidates. Although there are many questions to be answered, these biological agents will serve as a new hope in the management of refractory inflammatory conditions.

References

1. Koch, A. E., Kunkel, S. L., and Strieter, R. M. Cytokines in rheumatoid arthritis. *J Investig Med* 1995; **43**: 28–38.
2. Bazzoni, F., and Beutler, B. The tumor necrosis factor ligand and receptor families. *N Engl J Med* 1996; **334**: 1717–25.
3. Beg, A., and Baltimore, D. An essential role for NF-κB in preventing TNF-α-induced cell death. *Science* 1996; **274**: 782–4.
4. Feldman, M., Elliott, M. J., Woody, J. N., and Maini R. N. Anti-tumor necrosis factor-α therapy of rheumatoid arthritis. *Adv Immunol* 1997; **64**: 283–350.
5. Tak, P. P., Taylor, P. C., Breedveld, F. C., Smeets, T. J. M., Daha, M. R. *et al.* Decrease in cellularity and expression of adhesion molecules by anti-tumor necrosis factor α monoclonal antibody treatment in patients with rheumatoid arthritis. *Arthritis Rheum* 1996; **39**: 1077–81.
6. Paleolog. E., Young, S., McCloskey, R. V. *et al.* Angiogenesis as a therapeutic target in rheumatoid arthritis: serum vascular endothelial growth factor is decreased by anti-TNFα therapy. *Clin Exp Rheumatol* 1998; **16**: 232.
7. Lee, H., Kimko, H. C., Rogge, M., Wang, D., Nestorov. I., and Peck, C. C. Population pharmacokinetic and pharmacodynamic modeling of etanercept using logistic regression analysis. *Clin Pharmacol Ther* 2003; **73**: 348–65.
8. Maini, R. N., Breedveld, F. C., Kalden, J. R. *et al.* Therapeutic efficacy of multiple intravenous infusions of anti-tumour necrosis factor-alpha monoclonal antibody combined with low-dose weekly methotrexate in rheumatoid arthritis. *Arthritis Rheum* 1998; **41**: 1552–63.
9. St Clair, E., Wagner, C., Fasanmade, A., Wang, B., Schaible, T., Kavanaugh, A., and Keystone, E. Relationship of serum infliximab concentrations to clinical improvement in rheumatoid arthritis. *Arthritis Rheum* 2002; **46**: 1451–9.
10. Scallon, B. J., Moore, M. A., Trinh, H. *et al.* Chimeric anti TNFα monoclonal antibody cA2 binds recombinant transmembrane TNFα and activates immune effector functions. *Cytokine* 1995; **7**: 251–9.
11. Maini, R., St Clair, E. W., Breedweld. F. *et al.* Infliximab (chimeric anti-tumour necrosis factor α monoclonal antibody) versus placebo in rheumatoid arthritis patients receiving concomitant methotrexate: a randomized phase III trial. *Lancet* 1999; **354**: 1932–9.
12. Kavanaugh, A., St Clair, E. W., McCune, W. J. *et al.* Chimeric anti-tumour necrosis factor α monoclonal antibody treatment of patients with rheumatoid arthritis receiving methotrexate therapy. *J Rheumatol* 2000; **27**: 841–50.
13. Korth-Bradley, J. M., Abbe, S. R., Roberta, K. H. *et al.* The pharmacokinetics of etanercept in healthy volunteers. *Ann Pharmacother* 2000; **34**: 161–4.
14. Abbott Laboratories. Humira: package insert. Abbott Park, IL; 2000.
15. Yocum, D. Effective use of TNF antagonists. *Arthritis Res Ther* 2004; **6** (Suppl. 12): S24–S30.
16. Jobanputra, P., Barton, P., Bryan, S., and Burls, A. The effectiveness of infliximab and etanercept for the treatment of rheumatoid arthritis: a systemic review and economic evaluation. *Health Technol Assess* 2002; **6**: 1–110.
17. Brennan, A., Browne, K. A., Green, P. A., Jaspar, J. M., Maini, R. N., and Feldman, M. Reduction of serum matrix metalloproteinase 1 and matrix metalloproteinase 3 in rheumatoid arthritis patients following anti-tumour factor-alpha (cA2) therapy. *Br J Rheumatol*; **36**: 643–50.
18. Elliott, M. J., Maini, R. N., and Feldman, M. Randomized double-blind comparison of chimeric monoclonal antibody to tumor necrosis factor alpha (cA2) versus placebo in rheumatoid arthritis. *Lancet* 1994; **344**: 1105–10.
19. Moreland, L. W., Margolies, G., Heck, L. W. *et al.* Recombinant soluble tumor necrosis factor receptor (p80) fusion protein: toxicity and dose finding trial in refractory rheumatoid arthritis. *J Rheumatol* 1996; **23**: 1849–55.
20. Moreland, L. W., Baumgartner, S. W., Schiff, M. H. *et al.* Treatment of rheumatoid arthritis with a recombinant human tumour necrosis factor receptor (p75)-Fc fusion protein. *N Engl J Med* 1997; **337**: 141–7.
21. Lipsky, P. E., Desiree, M. F. M., van der Heijde. *et al.* Infliximab and methotrexate in the treatment of rheumatoid arthritis. *N Engl J Med* 2000; **343**: 1594–602.
22. St Clair, E. W., van der Heijde, D. M., Smolen, J. S., Maini, R. N. *et al.* Combination of infliximab and methotrexate therapy for early rheumatoid arthritis: a randomized, controlled trial. *Arthritis Rheum* 2004; **50**: 3432–43.
23. Westhovens, R., Wolfe, F., Rahman, M. U., Han, J., and Yocum, D. Infliximab dose escalation in patients with rheumatoid arthritis: results from the SRART trial. *Arthritis Rheum* 2004; **50** (Suppl.): S185.
24. Moreland, L. W., Schiff, M. H., Baumgartner, S. W. *et al.* Etanercept therapy in rheumatoid arthritis: a randomized, controlled trial. *Ann Intern Med* 1999; **130**: 478–86.
25. Weinblatt, M. E., Kremer, K. M., Bankhurst, A. D. *et al.* A trial of etanercept, a recombinant tumor necrosis factor receptor: Fc fusion protein in patients with rheumatoid arthritis receiving methotrexate. *N Engl J Med* 1999; **340**: 253–9.
26. Genovese, M. C., Bathon, J. M., Martin, R., Fleischmann, R. *et al.* Etanercept versus methotrexate in patients with early rheumatoid arthritis: two year radiographic and clinical outcomes. *Arthritis Rheum* 2002; **46**: 1443–50.
27. Klareskog, L., van der Heijde, D., de Jager. *et al.* Therapeutic effect of the combination of etanercept and methotrexate compared with each treatment alone in patients with rheumatoid arthritis: double-blind randomized controlled trial. *Lancet* 2004; **363**: 675–81.
28. Van de Putte, L. B. A., Rau, R., Breedveld, F. C., Kalden, J. R. *et al.* Efficacy and safety of the fully human anti-TNF-alpha monoclonal antibody adalimumab (D2E7) in DMARD refractory patients with rheumatoid arthritis: a 12 week, phase II study. *Ann Rheum Dis* 2003; **62**: 1168–77.
29. Weinblatt, M., Keystone, E., Furst, D., Moreland, L. W. *et al.* Adalimumab, a fully human anti-tumor necrosis factor α monoclonal antibody, for the treatment of rheumatoid arthritis in patients taking concomitant methotrexate. *Arthritis Rheum* 2003; **48**: 35–45.
30. Schiff, M. H., Weisman, M., Furst, D. E. *et al.* Adalimumab (Humira) plus methotrexate in patients with rheumatoid arthritis: continued efficacy up to 4 years in open label trials. *Ann Rheum Dis* 2004; **63** (Suppl. 1): 269.
31. Keystone, E., Kavanaugh, A., Sharp, J., Tannenbaum, H. *et al.* Adalimumab (D2E7), a fully human anti-TNFα monoclonal antibody, inhibits the progression of structural damage in patients with active rheumatoid arthritis despite concomitant methotrexate therapy. *Arthritis Rheum.* 2002; **46** (Suppl. 9): S205. Abstract 468.
32. Torrance, G. W., Tugwell, P., Amorosi, S., Chartash, E., and Sengupta, N. Improvement in health utility among patients with rheumatoid arthritis treated with adalimumab plus methotrexate. *Rheumatology* 2004; **43**: 712–18.
33. Breedweld, F. C. *et al.* Adalimumab is efficacious and safe: persistent remission observed in patients with rheumatoid arthritis treated for up to 6 years. *Arthritis Rheum* 2004; **50** (Suppl.): S188.
34. Mease, P. J., Kivitz, A. J., Burch, F. X., Siegel, E. L., Cohen, S. B. *et al.* Etanercept treatment of psoriatic arthritis: safety, efficacy, and effect on disease. *Arthritis Rheum* 2004; **50**: 2264–72.
35. Antoni, C., Kavanaugh, A., Kirkham, B., Tutuncu, Z., Burmester, G., Manger, B. *et al.* The infliximab multinational psoriatic arthritis controlled trial (IMPACT). Arthritis Rheum. [In press.]
36. Mease, P., Gladman, D., Ritclin, C. *et al.* Adalimumab therapy in patients with psoriatic arthritis: 24 week results of a phase III study. *Arthritis Rheum* 2004; **50**: 4097.
37. Davis, J. C. Jr., Van Der Heijde, D., Braun, J., Dougados, M., Cush, J., Clegg, D. O. *et al.* Recombinant human tumor necro-

factor receptor (etanercept) for treating ankylosing spondylitis: a randomized, controlled trial. *Arthritis Rheum* 2003; **48**: 3230–6.

38. Braun, J., Brandt, J., Listing, J., Zink, A., Alten, R., Burmester. G. *et al.* Long-term efficacy and safety of infliximab in the treatment of ankylosing spondylitis: an open, observational, extension study of a three-month, randomized, placebo-controlled trial. *Arthritis Rheum* 2003; **48**: 2224–33.

39. Lovell, D. J., Giannini, E. H., Reiff, A. *et al.* Etanercept in children with polyarticular juvenile rheumatoid arthritis. *N Engl J Med* 2000; **342**: 763–9.

40. Lovell, D. J., Giannini, E. H., Reiff, A. *et al.* Long-term efficacy and safety of etanercept in children with polyarticular-course juvenile rheumatoid arthritis: interim results from an ongoing multicenter, open-label, extended-treatment trial. *Arthritis Rheum* 2003; **48**: 218–26.

41. Breese, E. J., Michie, C. A., Nicholls, S. W., Murch, S. H., Williams, C. B. *et al.* Tumor necrosis factor alpha-producing cells in the intestinal mucosa of children with inflammatory bowel disease. *Gastroenterology* 1994; **106**: 1455–66.

42. Present, D. H., Rutgeerts, P., Targan, S., Hanauer, S. B., Mayer, L. *et al.* Infliximab for the treatment of fistulas in patients with Crohn's disease. *N Engl J Med* 1999; **340**: 1398–405.

43. Sandborn, W. J., Hanauer, S. B., Katz, S., Safdi, M., Wolf, D. G., Baerg, R. D. *et al.* Etanercept for active Crohn's disease: a randomized, double-blind, placebo-controlled trial. *Gastroenterology* 2001; **121**: 1088–94.

44. Fleischman, R., and Yocum, D. Does safety make a difference in selecting the right TNF antagonist? *Arthritis Res Ther* 2004; **6** (Suppl. 2): S12–S18.

45. Wolfe, F., Mitchell, D., and Sibley, J. The mortality of rheumatoid arthritis. *Arthritis Rheum* 1994; **37**: 481–94.

46. Doran, M. F., Crowsan, C. S., Pond, G. R., O'Fallon, W. M., and Gabriel, S. E. Predictors of infection in rheumatoid arthritis. *Arthritis Rheum* 2002; **46**: 2294–300.

47. Jeurissan, M. E., Boerbooms, A. M., van de Putte, L. B., Doesburg, W. H. *et al.* Methotrexate versus azathioprine in the treatment of rheumatoid arthritis: a forty week randomized, double blind trial. *Arthritis Rheum* 1991; **34**: 961–72.

48. Kavanaugh, A., and Keystone, E. The safety of biologic agents in early rheumatoid arthritis. *Clin Exp Rheumatol* 2003; **21**: S203–S208.

49. Lee, J. H., Slifman, N. R., Gershon, S. K., Edwards, E. T., Schwieterman, W. D. *et al.* Life threatening histaplasmosis complicating immunotherapy with tumor necrosis factor alpha antagonists infliximab and etanercept. *Arthritis Rheum* 2002; **46**: 2565–70.

50. Keane, J., Gerson, S., Wise, R. P., Mirabile-Levens, E., Kasznica, J. *et al.* Tuberculosis associated with infliximab, a tumor necrosis factor α-neutralizing agent. *N Engl J Med* 2001; **345**: 1098–104.

51. Wolfe, F., Michaud, K., Anderson, J., and Urbansky, K. Tuberculosis infection in patients with rheumatoid arthritis and the effect of infliximab therapy. *Arthritis Rheum* 2004; **50**: 372–9.

52. Wolfe, F., and Michaud, K. Lymphoma in rheumatoid arthritis. *Arthritis Rheum* 2004; **50**: 1740–51.

53. Bathon, J. M., Martin, R. W., Fleischmann, R. M. *et al.* A comparison of etanercept and methotrexate in patients with early rheumatoid arthritis. *N Engl J Med* 2003; **343**: 1586–93.

54. Olsen, N. J., and Stein, C. M. New drugs for rheumatoid arthritis. *N Engl J Med* 2004; **350**: 2167–79.

55. Charles, P. J., Smeenk, R. J. T., De Jong, J., Feldmann, M., and Maini, R. N. Assessment of antibodies to DsDNA induced in rheumatoid arthritis (RA) patients following treatment with infliximab, a monoclonal antibody to TNF alpha. *Arthritis Rheum* 2000; **43**: 2383–90.

56. Mohan, N., Edwards, E. T., Cupps, T. R. *et al.* Demyelination occurring during anti-tumor necrosis factor alpha therapy for inflammatory arthritides. *Arthritis Rheum* 2001; **44**: 2862–9.

57. Wolfe, F., and Michaud, K. Heart failure in rheumatoid arthritis: rates, predictors, and the effect of anti-TNF therapy. *Am J Med* 2004; **116**: 305–11.

58. Calabrese, L. H., Zein, N., Vassilopoulos, D. Safety of antitumor necrosis factor (anti-TNF) therapy in patients with chronic viral infections: hepatitis C, hepatitis B, and HIV infection. *Ann Rheum Dis* 2004; **63** (Suppl. II): ii18–ii24.

59. Parke, F. A., and Reveille, J. D. Anti-tumor necrosis factor agents for rheumatoid arthritis in the setting of chronic hepatitis c infection. *Arthritis Care Res* 2004; **51**: 800–4.

60. Furst, D. E., Breedveld, F. C., Kalden, J. R., Smolen, J. S. *et al.* Updated consensus statement on biological agents, specifically tumor necrosis factor α (TNF α) blocking agents and interleukin 1 antagonist (IL-1ra) for the treatment of rheumatic diseases, 2004. *Ann Rheum Dis* 2004; **63** (Suppl. II): ii2–ii12.

61. Hazleman, B., Smith, M., Moss, K. *et al.* Efficacy of a novel PEGylated humanized anti-TNF fragment (CDP870) in patients with rheumatoid arthritis: a phase II double-blind, randomized, dose escalating trial. *Rheumatology* 2002; **41**: 1133–7.

62. Schiff, M., Furst, D., and Cohen, S. The long term safety of pegylated recombinant methionyl human soluble tumor necrosis factor type I (PEG STRF-RI): an extension study for rheumatoid arthritis patients completing previous PEG STNF clinical studies. *Arthritis Rheum* 2001; **44**: S79.

63. Zhang, Y., Xu, J., Levin, J., Hegen, M. *et al.* Identification and characterization of 4-((4-(2-butynyloxy)phenyl)sulfonyl)-N-hydroxy-2, 2-dimethyl-(3S)thiomorpholinecarboxamide (TMI-1), a novel dual tumor necrosis factor-alpha-converting enzyme/matrix metalloprotease inhibitor for the treatment of rheumatoid arthritis. *J Pharmacol Exp Ther* 2004; **309**: 348–55.

64. Arend, W. P., Malyak, M., Smith, M. F. Jr. *et al.* Binding of IL-1a, IL-1b, and IL-1 receptor antagonist by soluble IL-1 receptors and levels of soluble IL-1 receptors in synovial fluids. *J Immunol* 1994; **153**: 4766–74.

65. Bresnihan, B., Alvaro-Garcia, J. M., Cobby, M. *et al.* Treatment of rheumatoid arthritis with recombinant human interleukin-1 receptor antagonist. *Arthritis Rheum* 1998; **41**: 2196–204.

66. Jiang, Y., Genant, H. K., Watt, I., Cobby, M. *et al.* A multicenter, double-blind, dose raging, randomized and placebo controlled study of recombinant human interleukin-1 receptor antagonist in patients with rheumatoid arthritis: radiologic progression and correlation of Genant and Larsen scoring methods. *Arthritis Rheum* 2000; **43**: 1001–9.

67. Cohen, S., Hurd, E., Cush, J. J. *et al.* Treatment of rheumatoid arthritis with anakinra, a recombinant human interleukin-1 receptor antagonist, in combination with methotrexate: results of a twenty-four-week, multicenter, randomized, double-blind, placebo-controlled trial. *Arthritis Rheum* 2002; **46**: 614–24.

68. Genovese, M. C., Cohen, S., Moreland, L., Lium, D., Robbins, S., Newmark, R., Bekker, P. *et al.* Combination therapy with etanercept and anakinra in the treatment of patients with rheumatoid arthritis who have been treated unsuccessfully with methotrexate. *Arthritis Rheum* 2004; **50**: 1412–19.

69. Fleischmann, R. M., Schechtman, J., Bennett, R. *et al.* Anakinra, a recombinant interleukin-1 receptor antagonist (r-metHuIL-1ra), in patients with rheumatoid arthritis: a large, multinational, multicenter, placebo-controlled trial. *Arthritis Rheum* 2003; **48**: 927–34.

70. Fleischmann, R. M. Safety of anakinra, a recombinant interleukin-1 receptor antagonist (r-metHuIL-1ra), in patients with rheumatoid arthritis and comparison to anti-TNF-alpha agents. *Clin Exp Rheum* 2002; **20** (5 Suppl.): S35–S41.

71. Hoffman, H. M., Rosengren, S., Boyle, D. L., Cho, J. Y., Nayar, J. *et al.* Prevention of cold-associated acute inflammation in familial cold autoinflammatory syndrome by interleukin-1 receptor antagonist. *Lancet* 2004; **364**: 1779–85.

72. Bingham, C. O., III, Genovese, M. C., Moreland, L. W., Grimes, I. *et al.* Results: of a phase II study of IL-1 Trap in moderate to severe rheumatoid arthritis. *Arthritis Rheum* 2004; **50** (Suppl.): s237.

73. Gabay, C. IL-1 trap: Regeneron/Novartis. *Curr Opin Investig Drugs* 2003; **4**: 593–7.

74. Dasgupta, K. E., Corkill, M., Kirham, B., Gibson, T., and Panayi, G. Serial estimation of interleukin 6 as a measure of systemic disease in rheumatoid arthritis. *J Rheumatol* 1992; **19**: 22–5.

75. Wendling, D., Racadot, E., and Wijdenes, J. Treatment of severe rheumatoid arthritis by interleukin 6 monoclonal antibody. *J Rheumatol* 1993; **20**: 259–62.

76. Nishimoto, N., Yoshizaki, K., Miyasaka, N., Yamamoto, K., Kawai, S., Tekeuchi, T. *et al.* Treatment of rheumatoid arthritis with

humanized anti-interleukin-6 receptor antibody. *Arthritis Rheum* 2004; **50**: 1761–9.

77. Abrams, J. R., Lebwohl, M. G., Guzzo, C. A., Jegasothy, B. V., Goldfarb, M. T., Goffe, B. S. *et al*. CTLA4-Ig-mediated blockade of T-cell costimulation in patients with psoriasis vulgaris. *J Clin Invest* 1999; **103**: 1243–52.

78. Moreland, L. W., Alten, R., Van den Bosch, F. *et al*. Costimulatory blockade in patients with rheumatoid arthritis: a pilot, dose finding, double-blind, placebo controlled clinical trial evaluating CTLA-4Ig and LEA29Y eighty-five days after the first infusion. *Arthritis Rheum* 2002; **46**: 1470–9.

79. Kremer, J. M., Westhovens, R., Leon, M., Di Georgio, E., Alten, R., Steinfel, S. *et al*. Treatment of rheumatoid arthritis by selective inhibition of T-cell activation with fusion protein CTLA4Ig. *N Engl J Med* 2003; **20**: 1907–15.

80. Emery, P., Combe, B., Nuamah, I. *et al*. Patients with rheumatoid arthritis treated with abatacept (CTLA4Ig; BMS-188667) report rapid improvements in pain, disease activity and physical function. *Ann Rheum Dis* 2004; **63** (Suppl. 1): 525.

81. Windblast, M., Schiff, M., Goldman, M. *et al*. A pilot, multicenter, randomized, double-blind, placebo controlled trial of a co-stimulatory blocker (CTLA-4Ig) (2 mg/kg) given monthly in combination with etanercept in active rheumatoid arthritis. *Arthritis Rheum* 2002; **46** (Suppl): S204.

82. Edwards, J. C. W., and Cambridge, G. Sustained improvement in rheumatoid arthritis following a protocol designed to deplete B lymphocytes. *Rheumatology* 2001; **40**: 205–11.

83. Leonardo, M. J., Edwards, J. C. W., and Cambridge, G. Clinical outcome in 22 patients with rheumatoid arthritis treated with B lymphocyte depletion. *Ann Rheum Dis* 2002; **61**: 883–8.

84. Edwards, J. C. W., Szczepanski, L., Szechinski, J., Filipowicz-Sosnowska, A., Emery, P. *et al*. efficacy of B-cell-targeted therapy with rituximab in patients with rheumatoid arthritis. *N Engl J Med* 2004; **350**: 2572–81.

85. Cambridge, G., Leandro, M. J., Isenberg, D. A. *et al*. B cell depletion therapy in systemic lupus erythematosus: effect of autoantibody and anti-microbial antibody profile. *Arthritis Rheum* 2004; **50** (Suppl.): s227.

86. Pijpe, J., Bootsma, H., van Imhoff, G. *et al*. Rituximab (anti-CD20) for the treatment of primary Sjogren's syndrome. *Arthritis Rheum* 2004; **50** (Suppl.): S575

87. McInnes, I. B., and Gracie, J. A. Targeting cytokines beyond tumor necrosis factor-alpha and interleukin-1 in rheumatoid arthritis. *Curr Rheumatol Rep* 2004; **6**: 336–42.

Non-drug therapy

Introduction

Decline of function over time is found in most patients with rheumatoid arthritis (RA). About 50% of patients show evidence of articular damage with radiographic joint space narrowing and/or erosions within the first two years of disease[1]. Early retirement, within three years, has been found in 37% of early cases of rheumatoid arthritis[2]. The main functional limitations pertain to pain, decreased joint motion, muscle weakness, reduced endurance, and limitations in aerobic capacity. The unpredictable course of the disease often causes anxiety and depression, and reduces self-efficacy.

Physiotherapy is an essential part of comprehensive management for patients with rheumatoid arthritis, and there is a growing body of knowledge concerning the efficacy of physiotherapeutic interventions[3,4]. Most recent research on physiotherapy has focused on exercise therapy. The aim of physiotherapy is to prevent or reduce functional consequences of the disease. The basis of intervention are needs experienced by the patient and relevant findings of manifest or imminent functional impairment. In addition, cognitive and behavioral factors have to be taken into account[4,5].

Exercise therapy

Range of motion (ROM) exercises

Decreased range of passive motion may be due to capsular swelling and increased intra-articular fluid volume. In more advanced stages, contracture and articular structural changes contribute. Adhesions sometimes add to the restriction. The increased frictional force, due to cartilage destruction, on ROM becomes apparent when the joint is loaded. In the unloaded joint, cartilage destruction and joint space narrowing appear to play a minor role among factors contributing to stiffness. Elastic, as well as viscous, joint stiffness are more closely related to local, active inflammatory changes such as capsular swelling[6]. External restrictions of flexibility are pain-induced muscle tension or increased stiffness of muscle tissue. Inflammatory changes in flexor and extensor tendons cause increased viscous stiffness of, for example, finger joints[6]. Destruction of stabilizing tissues impairs mobility because of incongruency of the joint.

There are three types of ROM exercises: passive, assisted, and active. In order to increase extensibility, terminal stretching is applied. It is a general rule that the stretch should be held at the maximally achieved range for 5–20 s, with at least three repetitions. However, the implications of different tissue changes limiting joint motion have not been tested. ROM exercises are usually combined with strength training. Muscle function is necessary to preserve mobility.

Only a few randomized controlled studies have tested the effect of joint-specific ROM exercise programs in RA patients. A home training program for patients with arthritic shoulder dysfunction has been evaluated by Mannerkorpi and Bjelle[7]. Twenty-eight consecutive female outpatients with shoulder pain, functional classes I and II, were randomly assigned to two groups. One group (*n* = 14) received instructions for shoulder training to be performed three times a week, comprising (1) warming up and relaxation exercises, (2) retraction exercises of the shoulder blades, (3) pulley-assisted movements in flexion and abduction, (4) light stretching of shoulder muscles (6–10 s), and (5) endurance training of the outward rotator muscles with an elastic rubber band. The number of repetitions was individually adapted depending on pain, limitation of ROM, and endurance. No instructions were given to the control group. After eight weeks, the training group reported decreased pain on active motion. Abduction of the left arm and hand-to-neck mobility of the right arm were improved compared with the controls. Muscle endurance in both arms was increased. There was a trend towards improvement of the arm activities of daily living (ADL) index in the training group; however, the difference was not significant. The long-term effect was not studied. No adverse effects were observed.

The role of exercise with particular reference to the RA hand has been highly controversial[8]. It has been suspected that resistive exercises accelerate the development of hand deformities. The effect of daily, simple hand exercises has been tested in a randomized, controlled, 48-month trial in 44 female patients with seropositive, active RA for at least one year and erosions in the metacarpophalangeal (MCP) and/or proximal interphalangeal (PIP) joints[8]. All patients were classified as functional class I. None had severe deformities. The exercise program comprised warm-up exercises, stretching, dexterity training, grip strengthening exercises, and flexion and extension training of the MCP and PIP joints, with 5–10 repetitions each. The patients were strongly encouraged to perform the exercises on a regular basis. The control group was given no exercise instructions. Parameters recorded were grip strength, pincer grip strength, and flexion and extension ROM of individual MCP and PIP joints. The examiner was blinded. About 80% of the patients completed the study. At the end of the 48 months, grip strength and pincer grip strength were significantly improved in the training group, while there was a significant deterioration in the control group. There was a significant loss of MCP joint extension in both groups, somewhat less in the training group. Flexion in the MCP joints deteriorated in the control group but this did not reach statistical significance; nor was the improvement of flexion in the training group significant. Changes in the flexion and extension of the PIP joints did not reach statistical significance. It can be concluded that this type of simple exercise regimen improves muscle strength but is less efficacious with regard to joint motion. No adverse effects were observed.

The effect of 12 weeks of home hand exercises performed for 10–20 min twice a day has been studied in 44 patients, functional classes II and III[9]. The patients were randomly assigned to one of three exercise groups or a control group. The exercise groups were ROM exercises, resistive (RES), and RES + ROM exercises. Immediate and short-term effects at three months follow-up were studied. The exercises were well tolerated and only caused transient, mild to moderate discomfort. Examinations were performed by a blinded observer. There were no significant changes in range of motion of the PIP and MCP joints over the study period, with the exception of increased left PIP extension in the RES group. There were no significant changes in deformities, ulnar deviation, or joint circumference. Compared with the control group, there was a significant decrease in right hand joint count in the ROM group and an increase in left hand dexterity in the RES + ROM group. The combined intervention groups gained significant strength in the left hand after three months of exercise (RES 22%, ROM 6%). Follow-up evaluation three months after the exercise period revealed no statistically significant changes in any of the intervention groups.

The effect of active exercises and warm wax bath treatment was evaluated in 52 rheumatoid arthritis patients, functional classes I and II, with a mean age of 53 years and an average duration of the disease of 7.6 years[10]. The patients were randomized into four groups: (1) both exercise and wax bath, (2) exercise only, (3) wax bath only, and (4) controls. Treatment was given three times a week for four weeks. Twenty minutes of wax bath treatment was followed by hand exercises, including eight different movements with slight resistance (soft exercise dough) for 20 min. Active exercise was found to significantly reduce pain with non-resistant motion, stiffness, and flexion deficits. Total grip function and pinch test improved significantly in group 1 compared to all other groups. No significant effect was observed with wax bath except that pain relief was registered immediately after treatment in groups 1 and 3. Stiffness was reduced in all treatment groups immediately after treatment.

Dynamic exercise programs intended to improve muscle function and aerobic capacity may have a short-term effect on joint mobility. During a 12-week, high-intensity exercise program joint flexibility improved significantly in the high-intensity group only, and in particular in the joints of the lower extremities[11]. Range of motion was not changed significantly in the control groups which had programs including ROM exercises. There was no significant difference between the groups at 24 weeks follow-up, except knee extension with high-intensity training.

A long-term (two-year) program comprising different training modalities was not found to prevent deterioration of joint function measured as the functional score of 26 joints[12]. The decrease in joint function was not associated with any increase in pain experience or disease activity. Radiographic examination revealed progression of joint destruction in both the experimental and the control group.

There is a lack of controlled clinical trials concerning the effect of passive ROM exercises. During the recent four decades a special manual therapy has been introduced to improve joint mobility by passive accessory joint movements, muscle stretching, and soft tissue mobilization. At present no evidence-based clinical practice guidelines exist on manual therapy for RA conditions[3].

To summarize, capsular and muscular stiffness are temporarily reduced by regular motion exercises. However, in the long run, reduced mobility associated with progressive joint destruction cannot be significantly prevented by ROM exercises.

Training of muscle strength, endurance, and aerobic capacity

Changes in muscle strength have been found to be closely correlated with changes in systemic disease activity[6]. The inflammatory process and physical inactivity have a catabolic effect on muscle[13]. Pain or inhibition caused by pressure-induced joint capsular distension can result in muscular weakness[14]. Except for intrinsic muscles of the hand, electromyographic signs of myopathy or neuropathy are an unusual finding in patients with RA[15]. Rheumatoid arthritis patients also experience impaired control of balance, and an increased body-sway in standing position has been found[16]. This might partly be due to proprioceptive dysfunction of joints and muscles[17].

Training of muscle strength introduces a considerable load on the joint on which the muscles act. Compressive forces in the knee joint in the extended position are about 10 times higher than the load applied at the ankle during training of the quadriceps muscle. During maximal contraction of the knee extensor muscles, an increased intra-articular hydrostatic pressure varying between 15 and >380 mmHg has been observed in RA patients, depending on the volume of joint effusion and capsular stiffness[14]. An increase in the intra-articular pressure of as little as 20 mmHg decreases synovial blood flow significantly, inducing a risk of anoxic joint destruction. Because of possible risks induced by intensive muscle training, articular rest and static training with low loads have been recommended[18]. Rest is therefore indicated in patients with acute and very active arthritis[19], but the majority of patients need physical activity to preserve joint and muscle function and to overcome the effect of inactivation. During the last three decades it has become apparent that short-term, high-intensity static or dynamic training of patients with non-acute RA can improve strength, aerobic capacity, and physical performance without increasing disease activity or accelerating joint destruction[3,4,20]. However, previous reviews include, to a varying extent, trials that were not randomized; also, outcome evaluations confined to subgroups have low power and introduce a risk of bias[21].

The following review is based on randomized, controlled trials comparing high-intensity with low-intensity training. As a rule, the studies include only patients with stable medication and low to moderate disease activity, except in one of the trials testing the effect of intensive exercise on patients with active arthritis[22]. The disability level was usually low to moderate (Table 28.1). The compliance in the different intervention studies was satisfactory: around 85%[70–91] completed the program. A considerable variety in study design, with regard to types of training, intensity, frequency, and duration, was found, which, in part, was due to the different aims of the studies.

Out-come measures were according to the following methods. Muscle strength, mostly of the lower extremities, was tested

Table 28.1 Randomized controlled trials of exercise interventions in RA

Study	Patients (*n*)	Functional class	Age	Duration (years)	Inclusion criteria	Exclusion criteria
Harkcom (28)	20	II	52	9	NR	NR
Minor (23)	40	NR	54	11	Symptomatic weight-bearing joints	Not on stable medication
					Age > 20 years	Currently exercising
Ekdahl (24)	67	II	53	11	Functional class II	Other disease states that might
					Age: 20–65 years	influence the results
Hansen (12)	75	I–II	52	7	Age: 20–60 years	Training 3 times per week
					Functional classes I–II	Comorbidity
Lyngberg (29)	24	I–III	67	9	Corticosteroid treatment >6 months	Heart disease
						Unable to train
Hakkinen (25, 35)	43	NR	44	1	Recent-onset arthritis	NR
Stenström (30, 36)	54	I–II	54	14	Functional classes I and II	NR
					Age: <65 years	
Van den Ende (11)	100	NR	52	10	Age: 20–70 years	Arthroplastics of weight-bearing
					Able to bicycle	joints, comorbidity
Komatireddy (27)	49	II–III	61	11	NR	Chest pain, abnormal ECG
						Pulmonary function
						abnormalities
Van den Ende (22)	64	NR	60	8	Active disease	Arthroplasties
					ARA criteria	
					Ability to walk	
Hakkinen (26)	62	NR	49	0.75	ARA criteria	NR
Bearne (17)	93	NR	60	11	Duration: > 2 years	Acute exacerbation
					Definite RA	Hypertension, diabetes, steroids
					Lower limb involvement	Wheelchair-bound

NR, not reported.

isometrically, isokinetically, or with a dynamometer for isotonic contraction. Evaluation of muscle training in one study was based on an index of muscle function, including endurance, and balance/coordination. Aerobic capacity was measured with a cycle ergometer or treadmill test. Goniometer and/or flexibility scores were used to assess joint mobility. Assessment of physical capacity included a stair-climbing test, walk test, grip test, step test, and/or sit-to-stand time. Conventional methods were used to assess disease activity, such as the Ritchie index, tenderness, number of swollen joints, morning stiffness, and pain rating. Evaluations were performed by examiners who were blinded to the experimental condition, in all but three studies.

The results confirm previous non-randomized trials[31–33]. Dynamic training with moderate to high intensity improves muscle strength and physical capacity significantly. Measurement of the cross-sectional area of the femoral quadriceps muscle by means of computerized tomography in one of the experimental groups with high-intensity training revealed a significant increase (5.5%) after six months[25]. Low-intensity static training, however, did not improve strength significantly. In a group of elderly subjects, dynamic training did not improve muscle strength[29]. On the other hand, muscle strength decreased more than 20% in the control group during the same time. The effect of exercise therapy on impairment of balance was tested in one study only[24]. No significant differences in standing balance were found during the training period of 18 weeks despite intensive, dynamic training of the lower extremities. It has also been shown that successful muscular rehabilitation does not improve proprioceptive acuity when joint position sense is tested[17].

Weight-bearing exercises were used in several studies. This type of closed chain-training instead of open chain-training (isokinetic training or quadriceps table) has become popular in sports medicine rehabilitation. During this type of strength training, the extremity is loaded as a functional unit with activation of all stabilizing muscles of the extremity. If load tolerance is reduced in one of the joints of the extremity, open-chain training may be used. Isokinetic training has been shown to be safe and effective[34], but the equipment is expensive. Isometric training is equally effective and strength training can be performed with the joint in a pain-free position.

High-intensity training three times a week increased aerobic capacity significantly. No improvement was found in groups with aerobic training once a week only[12], or with repetitive resistive exercises with moderate exertion[27].

Follow-up studies

Increases in muscle strength in patients with early RA were lost to a great extent during the follow-up period of three years, during which the patients had resumed their habitual physical activities[35]. If training activities are continued, improvements in muscle strength and endurance can be maintained. This has been shown for a follow-up time of three months after six weeks of supervised high-intensity training[24], and for three years after two years' supervised, home-based training[26]. Similar results have been reported by Minor[23]. Re-examination nine months after physical conditioning showed persistent improvement of aerobic capacity, 50-foot walking time, and grip strength. The patients had been encouraged to continue exercising but the compliance was not studied. Aerobic capacity and joint mobility appear to be more sensitive to detraining than muscle strength and physical capacity[11].

In order to maintain the improved physical fitness, continued exercise is required. The outcome depends on the compliance of the patient. Compliance with a one-year home exercise program was found to be predicted by habitual, regular ROM exercises before the intervention and by high self-efficacy for exercises[36]. Interestingly, health status, initial disease activity, or treatment priorities had no influence.

The impact on functional ability and well-being

Different performance tests such as walking test and stair-climbing test showed significant improvement in the majority of the studies reviewed, confirming previous reports (reviewed in Ref. 3). To assess functional capacity for activities of daily living the Health Assessment Questionnaire (HAQ)[37] was used in eight of the studies. This instrument showed that the majority of patients were mildly to moderately disabled before training; the median HAQ score varied between 0.53 and 1.83. A significant improvement in the score of the experimental groups was reported in five of the studies[17,22,25–27]. The HAQ score seems insensitive to measuring outcome in short-term exercise trials, at least in patients with a low degree of disability.

Significant improvement in Arthritis Impact Measurement Scale (AIMS) scores of physical activity and depression[39] was reported after 12 weeks of physical conditioning exercises[23]. However, the effect on depression was not maintained at the follow-up three months later. Another exercise trial with high or low-intensity training during 12 weeks did not change the AIMS score of depression[11]. The Nottingham Health Profile was used in one of the studies[30]. Strength and mobility training as a home exercise resulted in only minor physical improvements and had no effect on the total score or the subscores. Progressive relaxation training of the control group was found to reduce lack of energy. Cognitive and behavioral effects of exercise therapy have been described in previous studies (reviewed in Ref. 4).

The heterogeneity of outcome measures makes it difficult to compare the different studies. It is apparent that more long-term studies are needed to clarify the effect of physiotherapeutic interventions on activities of daily living and well-being.

Adverse effects

The dynamic training did not increase the progression of joint destruction. However, no protective effect, as described by Nordemar and coworkers[32], was found. No negative effect on the experience of pain or disease activity was observed except in studies on patients with active arthritis[22]. The exercise load of the resistance exercises had to be reduced in 65% of the patients in 50% of the exercise sessions.

Reduced signs of activity and discomfort were found at follow-up. It has been suggested that an increase of circulating neuropeptides after exercise training might reduce pain caused by physical loading of inflamed joints[3]. A study of neuropeptide levels in RA patients and in healthy subjects after high-intensity training for six weeks showed a significant increase in the corticotropin-releasing hormone levels in RA patients but not in the healthy training group. In addition, significantly higher levels of β-endorphin were found in arthritis patients compared to healthy controls after high-intensity training and after low-intensity

training for another six months[40]. This interesting observation needs to be confirmed and its molecular mechanism should be analyzed.

Aerobic training has been shown to have an effect on immune parameters in healthy subjects with increase in natural killer cytotoxicity, monocyte concentration, and interleukin (IL)-1 levels in plasma[41]. Eight weeks of bicycle training increased aerobic capacity significantly in patients with RA but did not induce changes in blood mononuclear cell sub-populations, proliferative response, or natural killer cell activity[41]. Furthermore, there was no change in plasma concentrations of IL-1β and IL-6. Exercise sessions with repeated (25 times) maximal voluntary quadriceps contractions did not increase plasma concentrations of TNF-α, IL-1β, or IL-6 in rheumatoid arthritis patients[17].

As a rule, the patients were instructed to reduce the training load and/or the number of repetitions for some days if the training caused pain lasting for more than 2 h. To influence pain behavior in other chronic musculoskeletal disorders, the training intensity has been based on goal-setting and not on pain attention. This approach has been found to be effective in, for example, chronic low back pain. A comparative study has therefore been performed, with RA patients in a home training program, to investigate whether additional cognitive training with goal setting and reinterpretation of pain versus a recommendation to avoid overload and increased pain, would influence the exercise results[42]. After 12 weeks no significant difference was noted between the groups with regard to functional capacity or joint mobility. However, the goal-setting group had a significantly larger decrease in the Ritchie's index and pain rating during one of the lifting tasks. In addition, self-efficacy for mood and fatigue had increased.

Hydrotherapy

Pool exercise

Exercises in heated swimming pools have a long tradition. The weight-relieving effect of water immersion allows easier movement with less pain. Increased water resistance during rapid movements can be used to train muscle strength[43] and aerobic capacity[23].

Despite its popularity, the efficacy of this therapy has not been adequately evaluated in the treatment of RA[44]. In a randomized, controlled trial comprising 130 patients with RA involving at least six joints, exercise hydrotherapy was compared with seated immersion in a pool with a water temperature of about 36°C, land exercise, or progressive relaxation[44]. All interventions were limited to two sessions per week for four consecutive weeks. The outcome was evaluated immediately after the intervention and three months later. The overall effect was a significant reduction in joint tenderness after intervention, but between groups the difference was significant for the hydrotherapy only. At follow-up the reduction was no longer significant. Grip strength, range of motion, and duration of morning stiffness did not change significantly. There was no significant reduction in pain or improvement of health status (AIMS 2) for individual groups.

However, hydrotherapy patients had a significantly better emotional and psychological state than the other groups at follow-up.

The effect of four years intensive dynamic training in water once a week as a complement to traditional physiotherapy was studied in 30 arthritis patients in functional class II. A matched control group of another 30 patients had ROM exercises, static muscle strength training, and passive treatment only[45]. The hydrotherapy group showed a significantly higher physical activity level after the intervention and at follow-up two years later. For the control group there were significantly more admissions for acute hospital care during the training period. Significantly better grip strength was measured in the hydrotherapy group. No significant differences between the two groups were noted with regard to work capacity, functional ability, pain rating, Ritchie's index, or radiographic changes.

Studies are needed to evaluate the effect of hydrotherapy in patients with more advanced disabilities and restriction of mobility.

Balneotherapy

Balneotherapy (spa therapy) is a popular form of treatment with traditions from ancient times. In many places in Europe it has been claimed to constitute a special form of physiotherapy. The term is used for bathing in thermal or mineral water, for example sodium chloride baths, Dead Sea salt baths, sulfur baths, or mud baths. A review comprising six studies, representing 355 patients with definite or classical rheumatoid arthritis, shows that most studies report positive findings (the absolute improvement in measured outcomes ranged from 0 to 44%) but they all have methodological flaws[46]. For example, only two of the randomized clinical trials included comparison of effects between groups. *Therefore, the studies do not permit reliable conclusions concerning possible effectiveness of balneotherapy in RA.* Most methodological flaws could be avoided in future research.

Pain treatment

Pain experience, and its impact on function and quality of life in RA, is one of the most important reasons for seeking medical care. Therefore, one of the aims of physiotherapeutic interventions in RA is to reduce pain and the consequences of pain for physical function and capacity. Pain in RA is caused not only by the inflammatory process but also by periarticular tissue changes with reduced extensibility and muscle spasm. Altered biomechanical conditions reduce load tolerance. As in other chronic pain conditions, peripheral and central nociceptive sensitization may increase the intensity of perceived pain. Among different physical treatment modalities, heat and cold are those used most frequently. Other types of treatment are transcutaneous electrical nerve stimulation (TENS), low-energy laser therapy, and acupuncture.

Heat treatment

Heating elevates pain threshold, decreases muscle tension, and increases extensibility of connective tissue[47,48]. Therefore, heat treatment is usually combined with exercise therapy. Infrared light, liquid paraffin, and hot packs heat superficial tissue layers, while short-wave diathermy (SWD), microwave diathermy (MWD), and ultrasound (US) deliver deep heat.

Physiological effect

Superficial heating reduces synovial blood flow by shunting blood from periarticular tissue to superficial layers. Radiant heat, for example infrared light, decreases synovial blood flow by more than 20% in active arthritis[48]. Similar effects are caused by heat delivered by conduction, for example hot packs or paraffin. It has been suggested that the decrease in synovial blood flow might decrease the inflammatory process associated with RA[48], but no experimental studies have tested this hypothesis. External heat application causes only a minor increase in the intra-articular temperature (IAT), but this depends on the distance between the superficial heat source and the joint. Swelling and hypertrophy in arthritic joints reduce penetration of heat.

Deep heating (SWD, MWD, US) increases the IAT to a varying extent depending on the degree of inflammatory activity. An increase of nearly 6°C has been described in knee joints of healthy subjects as compared to less than 3°C in RA patients with active arthritis[48]. Similar increases are caused by continuous US. It has been suspected that an increase in the IAT might accelerate degradation of cartilage collagen. *In vitro* studies have shown that synovial collagenase was four times more active at 36°C than at 30°C[48]. Therefore, the use of deep heating may be hazardous in the treatment of joints with ongoing arthritis.

Superficial and deep heating cause a temporary elevation of the pain threshold[47]. However, there is no convincing clinical evidence that these treatment modalities cause a more longstanding reduction of tenderness of inflamed joints.

As mentioned, heating of connective tissue increases the extensibility, as demonstrated in animal experiments. The effect on connective tissue changes in RA has not been studied so far.

Clinical effects

Superficial heat is soothing in painful conditions, and it improves the outcome of ROM exercises[10,49]. However, superficial heat without exercise produces no persisting therapeutic benefit. During the past 50 years, numerous papers on the mode of action and clinical effects of deep heating have been published and reviewed by the so-called Ottawa Panel[49]. Regarding ultrasound treatment only one study was accepted. Continuous ultrasound (0.5 W/cm^2) applied in water to the dorsal and palmar aspect of the hand (10 min on alternate days, 3 weeks) had a significant effect on tender joints when compared to placebo at 10 weeks.

Adverse effects

Local heat treatment may be hazardous and cause burns when arterial circulation and cutaneous sensation are impaired.

Cold

Cold treatment is used especially in acute painful conditions. It is delivered by means of packs, ice water, vapocoolant sprays, and baths.

Physiological effects

Cold increases the pain threshold and causes vasoconstriction followed by vasodilatation. Prolonged cooling of joints for more than 10 min reduces the IAT by 2–3°C. Vapocoolant sprays are most effective. Experimental studies show no histological evidence suggesting an effect on progression of inflammatory joint disease[48]. Twenty-four subjects with knee synovitis were treated with ice bags for 20 min, three times a day for four weeks. The synovial fluid demonstrated no change of joint fluid pH, white cell count, T and B lymphocytes, protein levels, or immune complexes after the course of treatment.

Clinical effects

Several studies indicate a beneficial effect of cold treatment on pain and pain-induced stiffness[48], but there is a lack of randomized, controlled clinical trials.

Adverse effects

Patients with vasomotor instability have a reduced tolerance for cold. Increased tendency to develop vasospasm is often found in smokers.

Transcutaneous electrical nerve stimulation

TENS has been used for many years in the treatment of acute and chronic pain conditions. Besides its effect on pain transmission, experimental studies indicate a direct effect on the inflammatory process. Stimulation with high frequencies (70 Hz) appears to be more effective than low frequencies (3 Hz)[50]. There have been only two randomized, controlled trials of TENS treatment in RA[51,52] plus a non-randomized exploration of TENS placebo effects[53]. These studies have been confined to treatment of wrist pain in RA. In one of the studies, there was no difference with regard to pain, joint tenderness, or grip strength when high-frequency TENS was compared to 'acupuncture-like' TENS or placebo TENS[52]. The other two studies indicate a better effect of active TENS than placebo with regard to pain, muscle strength[51], and load tolerance[53]. TENS stimulation at a distance from the pain source has less effect than stimulation over the painful joint[53]. A duration of pain relief after cessation of stimulation for up to 18 h has been reported[50].

Additional randomized, controlled trials, also including other painful conditions in RA, are needed before definite conclusions can be drawn regarding the therapeutic value of TENS in inflammatory joint diseases.

Low-level laser therapy (LLLT)

Laser (light amplification by stimulated emission of radiation) can be delivered as continuous or pulsed irradiation, and different wavelengths can be chosen. The energy output of low-energy laser is below 0.5 W. The laser types most frequently used in the treatment of painful musculoskeletal disorders are the gallium arsenid (GaAs) and gallium-arsenid-aluminium midlaser, with a wave length of 904 nm and 830 nm, respectively[54]. Laser light has been shown to have an effect on cells in tissue cultures, an effect of both stimulation and inhibition depending on the intensity of irradiation. However, reflection and absorption of the laser light in the skin reduces the energy input considerably in deeper layers of the tissue. Less than 20% of the GaAs-irradiation penetrates the skin.

LLLT applied to the foot, knee, or hand versus placebo had a significant effect on pain at three months, but no benefit regarding function, tender joints, muscle force, or ROM[49]. The effect of low-energy laser on finger synovitis in RA patients has been tested in four randomized, controlled trials. It was found that this type of laser had a significant effect on joint pain in only one study[56], but no effect on tenderness, or range of motion[54–57].

Acupuncture

Acupuncture has for a long time been used to treat painful musculoskeletal disorders. Sensory stimulation by means of acupuncture has also been suggested to have an anti-inflammatory effect. Therefore, acupuncture might be expected to be of interest in the treatment of patients with rheumatoid arthritis. In a review, 12 studies were examined with regard to scientific quality and efficacy of acupuncture in RA[58]. Most of these studies failed to meet quality standards. Thus, there exists no convincing evidence at present that acupuncture is efficacious in RA.

Acupuncture has no effect on erythrocyte sedimentation rate (ESR), C-reactive protein (CRP), pain, number of swollen and/or tender joints, or the patient's global assessment[59], indicating that acupuncture has no anti-inflammatory effect in rheumatoid arthritis.

Conclusion

Most RA patients in clinical settings have evidence of a progressive disease that has deleterious consequences with regard to their functional capacity. The traditional treatment approach, with passive treatment modalities and low-load exercises, has been replaced by a more active attitude stressing an active role for the patient in the rehabilitation process. High-intensity training of muscle function and aerobic capacity has been found to be highly efficacious in patients with low to moderate disease activity, but continued exercise is needed to maintain improved physical fitness. In order to achieve this goal, the patient needs support and advice by a physiotherapist. More long-term studies are needed to clarify the effect of physiotherapeutic interventions on outcome with regard to activities of daily living and well being. The need for cognitive and behavioral training in this context should be observed. Cognitive behavior therapy, when it is the only intervention in RA, has been found to be ineffective in changing patients' physical, psychological, or social health status[60]. Therefore it is important to combine the different approaches.

References

1. Pincus, T., and Callahan, L. F. What is the natural history of rheumatoid arthritis? *Rheum Dis Clin North Am* 1993; 13: 123–51.
2. Eberhardt, K., Larsson, B. M., and Nived, K. Early rheumatoid arthritis: some social, economical and psychological aspects. *Scand J Rheumatol* 1993; 22: 119–23.
3. Ottawa Panel. Ottawa Panel evidence-based clinical practice guidelines for therapeutic exercises in the management of rheumatoid arthritis in adults *Phys Ther* 2004; 84: 934–72.
4. Stenström, C. H. Therapeutic exercise in rheumatoid arthritis. *Arthritis Care Res* 1994; 7: 190–7.
5. Keefe, F. J., and Van Horn Y. Cognitive-behavioral treatment of rheumatoid arthritis pain. *Arthritis Care Res*, 1993; 6: 213–22.
6. Tiselius, P. Studies on joint temperature, joint stiffness and muscle weakness in rheumatoid arthritis. *Acta Rheumatol Scand*, 1969; 14: (Suppl.): 7–106.
7. Mannerkorpi, K., and Bjelle, A. Evaluation of instruction for home training of shoulder dysfunction in rheumatoid arthritis patients. *Physiother Theory Pract* 1994; 10: 69–76.
8. Brighton, S. W., Lubbe J. W., and Van der Merve C. A. The effect of a long-term exercise programme on the rheumatoid hand. *Br J Rheumatol* 1993; 32: 392–5.
9. Hoening, H., Groff, G., Pratt, K., Goodberg, E., and Franck, W. A randomized controlled trial of home exercise on the rheumatoid hand. *J Rheumatol* 1993; 20: 785–9.
10. Dellhag, B., Wollersjö, I., Bjelle, A. Effect of active hand exercise and wax bath treatment in rheumatoid arthritis. *Arthritis Care Res* 1992; 5: 87–92.
11. Van den Ende, C. H. M., Hazes, J. M. W., le Cessie, S. et al. Comparison of high and low intensity training in well controlled rheumatoid arthritis: results of a randomized clinical trial. *Ann Rheum Dis* 1996; 55: 798–805.
12. Hansen, T. M., Hansen, G. F., Langgaard, A. M., and Rasmusson, J. O. Longterm physical training in rheumatoid arthritis: a randomized trial with different training programs and blinded observers. *Scand J Rheumatol* 1993; 22: 107–12.
13. Roubenoff, R. Exercise and inflammatory disease. *Arthritis Rheum* 2003; 49: 263–6.
14. Geborek, P., Moritz, U., and Wollheim, F. A. Joint capsular stiffness in knee arthritis: relationship to intraarticular volume, hydrostatic pressure, and extensor muscle function. *J Rheumatol*, 1989; 16: 1351–8.
15. Moritz, U. Electromyographic studies in adult rheumatoid arthritis. *Acta Rheum Scand Suppl* 1963; 6: 1–123.
16. Ekdahl, C., and Andersson, S. I. Standing balance in rheumatoid arthritis: a comparative study with healthy subjects. *Scand J Rheumatol* 1989; 18: 33–42.
17. Bearne, L. M., Scott, D. L., and Hurley, M. V. Exercise can reverse quadriceps sensorimotor dysfunction that is associated with rheumatoid arthritis without exacerbating disease activity. *Rheumatology* 2002; 41: 157–66.
18. Kottke, T. K., Caspersen, C. J., and Hill, C. S. Exercise in the management and rehabilitation of selected chronic diseases. *Preventive Med* 1984; 13: 47–65.
19. Alexander, G. J. M., Hortas, C., and Bacon, P. A. Bed rest, activity and the inflammation of rheumatoid arthritis. *Br J Rheumatol* 1983; 22: 134–40.
20. Hazes, J. M. W., and Van den Ende, C. H. M. How vigorously should we exercise our rheumatoid arthritis patients? *Ann Rheum Dis* 1996; 55: 861–2.
21. Van den Ende, C. H. M., Vliet Vlieland, T. P. M., Munneke, M., and Hazes, J. M. W. Dynamic exercise therapy in rheumatoid arthritis: a systematic review. *Br J Rheumatol* 1998; 37: 677–87.
22. Van den Ende, C. H. M., Breedveld, F. C., le Cessie, S. et al. Effect of intensive exercise on patients with active rheumatoid arthritis: a randomized clinical trial. *Ann Rheum* 2000; 59: 615–21.
23. Minor, M. A., Hewett, J. E., Webel, R. R. et al. Efficacy of physical conditioning exercise in patients with rheumatoid arthritis and osteoarthritis. *Arthritis Rheum* 1989; 32: 1396–405.
24. Ekdahl, C., Andersson, S. I., Moritz, U., and Svensson, B. Dynamic versus static training in patients with rheumatoid arthritis. *Scand J Rheumatol* 1990; 19: 17–26.
25. Hakkinen, A., Hakkinen, K., and Hannonen, P. Effects of strength training on neuromuscular function in patients with recent-onset inflammatory arthritis. *Scand J Rheumatol* 1994; 25: 237–42.
26. Hakkinen, A., Sokka, T., and Hannonen, P. A home-based two-year strength training period in early rheumatoid arthritis led to good long-term compliance: a five-year followup. *Arthritis Rheum* 2004; 51: 56–62.
27. Komatireddy, G. R., Leitch, R. W., Cella, K. et al. Efficacy of low load resistive muscle training in patients with rheumatoid arthritis class II and III. *J Rheumatol* 1997; 24: 1531–9.
28. Harkcom, T. M., Lampman, R. M., Banwell, B. F., and Castor, C. W. Therapeutic value of graded aerobic exercise training in rheumatoid arthritis. *Arthritis Rheum* 1985; 28: 329.
29. Lyngberg, K. K., Harrby, M., Bentzen, H. et al. Elderly rheumatoid arthritis patients on steroid treatment tolerate physical training without increase in disease activity. *Arch Phys Med Rehabil* 1994; 75: 1189–95.
30. Stenström, C. H., Arge, B., and Sundbom, A. Dynamic training versus relaxation training as home exercise for patients with inflammatory rheumatic diseases: a randomized controlled trial. *Scand J Rheumatol* 1996; 25: 28–33.
31. Ekblom, B., Lovgren, O., Alderin, M. et al. Effect of short term physical training on patients with rheumatoid arthritis. *Scand J Rheumatol* 1975; 4: 80–6.
32. Nordemar, R., Edström, L., and Ekblom, B. Changes in muscle fibre size and physical performance in patients with rheumatoid arthritis after short-term physical training. *Scand J Rheumatol* 1976; 5: 70–6.
33. Nordemar, R., Ekblom, B., Zachrisson, L., and Lundqvist, K. Physical training in rheumatoid arthritis: a controlled long-term study I. *Scand J Rheumatol* 1981; 10: 17–23.
34. Lyngberg, K. K., Ramsing, B. U., Nawrocki, A. et al. Safe and effective isokinetic knee extension training in rheumatoid arthritis. *Arthritis Rheum* 1994; 37: 623–8.
35. Hakkinen, A., Malkia, E., Hakkinen, K. et al. Effects of detraining subsequent to strength training on neuromuscular function in patients with inflammatory arthritis. *Br J Rheumatol* 1997; 36: 1075–81.
36. Stenström, C. H., Arge, B., and Sundbom, A. Home exercise and compliance in inflammatory rheumatic diseases: a prospective clinical trial. *J Rheumatol* 1997; 24: 470–6.
37. Fries, J. F., Spitz, P. W., Kraines, R. G., and Holman, H. R. Measurement of patient outcome in arthritis. *Arthritis Rheum* 1980; 23: 137–45.
38. Van den Ende, C. H. M., Breedveld, F. C., Dijkmans, B. A. C., and Hazes, J. M. W. The limited value of the health assessment questionnaire as an outcome measure in short term exercise trials. *J Rheumatol* 1997; 24: 1972–7.
39. Meenan, R. F., Gertman, P. M., Mason, J. H., and Dunaif, R. The Arthritis Impact Measurement Scales: further investigations of a health status measure. *Arthritis Rheum* 1982; 25: 1048–53.
40. Ekdahl, C., Ekman, R., Petersson, I., and Svensson, B. Dynamic training and circulating neuropeptides in patients with rheumatoid arthritis: a comparative study with healthy subjects. *Int J Clin Pharm Res* 1994; 14: 65–74.
41. Baslund, B., Öyngberg, K., and Andersen, V. Effect of 8 wk of bicycle training on the immune system of patients with rheumatoid arthritis. *J Appl Phys* 1993; 75: 1691–5.
42. Stenström, C. H. Home exercise in rheumatoid arthritis functional class II: goal setting versus pain attention. *J Rheumatol* 1994; 21: 627–34.
43. Danneskiold-Samsoe, B., Lyngberg, K., Risum, T., Telling, M. The effect of water-exercise given to patients with rheumatoid arthritis. *Scand J Rehab Med* 1987; 19: 31–5.
44. Hall, J., Skevington, S. M., Maddison, P. J., and Chapman, K. A randomized and controlled trial of hydrotherapy in rheumatoid arthritis. *Arthritis Care Res* 1996; 9: 206–15.

45. Stenström, C. H., Lindell, B., Swanberg, E. *et al.* Intensive dynamic training in water for rheumatoid arthritis functional class II: a long-term study of effects. *Scand J Rheumatol* 1991; 20: 358–65.

46. Verhagen, A. P., Bierma-Zeinstra, S. M., Cardoso, J. R. *et al.* Balneotherapy for rheumatoid arthritis. *Cochrane Database Syst Rev* 2000; 4: CD000518.

47. Minor, M. A., and Sanford, M. K. Physical intervention in the management of pain in arthritis: an overview for research and practice. *Arthritis Care Res* 1993; 6: 197–206.

48. Hayes, K. W. Heat and cold in the management of rheumatoid arthritis. *Arthritis Care Res* 1993; 6: 156–66.

49. Ottawa Panel. Ottawa Panel evidence-based clinical guidelines for electrotherapy and thermotherapy interventions in the management of rheumatoid arthritis in adults. *Phys Ther* 2004; 84: 1016–43.

50. Mannheimer, C., and Carlsson, C. A. The analgesic effect of transcutaneous electrical nerve stimulation (TNS) in patients with rheumatoid arthritis: a comparative study of different pulse patterns. *Pain* 1979; 6: 329–34.

51. Abelson, K., Langley, G. B., Sheppeard, H. *et al.* Transcutaneous electrical nerve stimulation in rheumatoid arthritis. *N Z Med J* 1983; 96: 156–8.

52. Langley, G. B., Sheppeard, H., Johnson, M., and Wigley, R. D. The analgesic effects of transcutaneous electrical nerve stimulation and placebo in chronic pain patients: a double-blind non-crossover comparison. *Rheumatol Int* 1984; 4: 119–23.

53. Kumar, V. N., and Redford, J. B. Transcutaneous nerve stimulation in rheumatoid arthritis. *Arch Phys Med Rehabil* 1982; 63: 595–6.

54. de Bie, R. A., Verhagen, A. P., Lenssen, A. F. *et al.* Efficacy of 904 nm laser therapy in the management of musculoskeletal disorders: a systematic review. *Phys Ther Rev* 1998; 3: 59–72.

55. Nyholm Gam, A., Thorsen, H., and Lonnberg, F. The effect of low-level laser therapy on musculoskeletal pain: a meta-analysis. *Pain* 1993; 52: 63–6.

56. Johannsen, F., Hauschildt, B., Remvig, L. *et al.* Low energy laser therapy in rheumatoid arthritis. *Scand J Rheumatol* 1994; 23: 145–7.

57. Hall, J., Clarke, A. K., Elvins, D. M., and Ring, E. F. J. Low level laser therapy is ineffective in the management of rheumatoid arthritis finger joints. *Br J Rheumatol* 1994; 33: 142–7.

58. Lautenschlager, J. Akupunktur bei der Behandlung entzundlich-rheumatischer Erkrankungen. *Z Rheumatol* 1997; 56: 8–20.

59. Casimiro, L, Brosseau, L, Milne, S. *et al.* Acupuncture and electroacupuncture for the treatment of RA. *Cochrane Database Syst Rev* 2002; 3: CD003788.

60. Kraaimaat, F. W., Brons, M. R., Geenen, R., and Bijlsma, W. J. The effect of cognitive behavior therapy in patients with rheumatoid arthritis. *Behav Res Ther* 1995; 33: 487–95.

29 | Patient education

Ylva Lindroth

Introduction

Patient education has been defined as 'a planned learning experience using a combination of methods such as teaching, counseling, and behavior modification techniques which influence patients' knowledge and health behavior . . .[and which] involves an interactive process which assists patients to participate actively in their health care, and provides them with information about available health service and their use'[1]. It should be distinguished from primary prevention strategies such as health education and health promotion programs. The latter may be of importance for some forms of arthritis, for example osteoarthritis (weight reduction in obesity) or osteoporosis (increase in calcium intake and physical activity). For patients with chronic disease, the goal of patient education is to minimize the consequences of the disease and maximize the capacity of the individual to enjoy a high quality of life[2]. Even as recently as 1976, the importance of educating arthritis patients was neither acknowledged in medical textbooks, nor mentioned in printed matter on arthritis written expressly for patients[3]. In 1982, a meta-analysis of patient education programs identified 63 as having been experimental studies with control groups, of which 30 involved chronic disease; none, however, included arthritis as a target subject[4]. The number of patient education programs and the topics with which they dealt have increased during the past several years. From 1990–98, Medline cites 4324 studies on patient education. These address a great variety of conditions, including infections, diabetes, asthma, hypertension, cardiac disorders, cancer, multiple sclerosis, dental care, schizophrenia, and arthritis. In a recent systemic review of Rheumatoid Arthritis Patient Education[5], 1423 publications were found eligible for inclusion as patient education intervention. However, when literature research was restricted to randomized control trials in rheumatoid arthritis (RA) using outcome measures agreed upon by Outcome Measures in Rheumatology Clinical Trials (OMERACT)[6], only 31 studies could be included.

Rationale for arthritis patient education

It has been established that patients desire greater medical knowledge about their disease. They believe that the more they know about RA, the better they can cope with it[7–9]. However, patients often have long-standing misconceptions about arthritis. As shown in interviews, patients with RA thought it could have been caused by injury or cold, damp weather. More than half of the patients interviewed had no idea why they needed to have blood tests so frequently. They could not distinguish between anti-inflammatory and disease-modifying drugs[10]. Other patients with RA believed that diet or infection was the culprit. Their main sources of information were television, books, and magazines[8]. Furthermore, patients have certain lay beliefs about their disease which they base on their own experience[11]. New information must filter through the patient's own preconceived notions before being accepted. Education is not simply transferring knowledge from educators to patients, that is, from active group leaders to passive participants; it is an interactive, two-way process. Patients assess the pain, stiffness, and severity of their disease by what they can or cannot do, rather than in terms of biochemical or pathological processes. They can adopt scientific ideas only if these fit their own conception of their disease. Patients with arthritis develop their own way of coping by using common sense or feedback from their environment. Compliance with any type of regime suggested at a consultation or discussed in education groups is dependent on how such information accords with the lay beliefs of patients. It has, therefore, been suggested that one explores such beliefs and then provides the individual patient with information based on such understanding[11].

Needs assessment

Before planning a patient education program, it is essential to assess the needs and problems of those being served. Surveys have indicated disagreement as to the foremost complaints of arthritis patients. Some patients report dealing with pain as their main problem[12]. Others are concerned more with the origin of their disease and with diagnostic procedures. They find their greatest problems alleviated in learning to communicate with their physician, understanding medication, dealing with the impact of arthritis on work, and confronting their worries about the future[7]. When patients were asked to state spontaneously what troubled them the most, they cited functional disability, feeling dependent on others, and pain. Psychological factors, family, and marital problems were seldom mentioned. However, when the same patients were given a preformatted list, they did reveal psychological problems, the most prevalent one being uncertainty regarding the future course of their disease[13]. Disruption of leisure activities was often singled out as a distressing aspect of living with chronic arthritis[14–16].

Language barriers and cultural background may need to be addressed by other strategies. For example, individuals who come as refugees from other countries or who live in remote areas may find it hard to sit down and discuss their problems in a group with other patients. In Java, leather puppets in 'Wayang Kulit,' a local cultural event, have been used as a basis for teaching villagers[17].

Table 29.1 Different methods of arthritis patient education

Type of education	First author	Publication year	Reference number
Groups led by health professionals	Althoff B	1977	19
	Cohen JL	1986	21
	Lindroth Y	1989	15
	Taal E	1993	13
	Hammond A	1994	37
Groups led by lay leaders	Lorig K	1985	22
	Goeppinger J	1989	20
	Cohen JL	1986	21
Home study	Goeppinger J	1989	20
Cognitive—behavioral	Keefe FJ	1996	40
Groups	Calfas KJ	1992	45
Support groups	Potts M	1985	46
	Radojevic V	1992	47
Individual strategy	Lorish CD	1985	48
	Hammond A	1994	37
Telephone information service	Weinberger M	1989	25
Pamphlets, books	Vignos PJ	1976	3
Computer-based programs	Wetstone SC	1985	26
'Wayang kulit', leather puppets	Darmawan J	1992	17
Part of day care	Jacobsson L	1998	49

Approaches to arthritis patient education

The best way to deliver patient education has yet to be determined. Local traditions and available resources play an important part in the choice of method. In some countries, group programs for the education of arthritis patients are administered by the overall healthcare system. Shared care is a part of rheumatology units and involves a professional team with rheumatologists, nurses, physiotherapists, occupational therapists, social workers, and sometime psychologists, dietitians and podiatrists as well[18,19]. Patient education can also be organized and led by lay leaders in the community as self-management courses[20–22]. Inexpensive methods of education such as pamphlets and booklets have been shown to be effective in increasing patient knowledge about arthritis[3,23]. However, instruction from a health professional resulted in greater comprehension than distributing a booklet alone. Furthermore, increased knowledge alone had no effect on alleviating disability or improving quality of life[24]. Other low-cost methods of providing information to arthritis patients have been employed, such as telephone contacts, audio-visual tapes, and computer-based education[25,26].

Outline of arthritis patient education

The patient's knowledge of arthritis

Understanding the nature of the disease, the theoretical background of different symptoms, and the rationale for treatment options are fundamental to all arthritis education programs (see Table 29.2). Nevertheless, knowledge by itself is not sufficient to change behavior and thereby affect the outcome of the disease[27]. In order to take an active part in rehabilitation programs and communicate better with health professionals, patients need, and in fact want, to know more about arthritis[7–9].

Behavior modification

Most arthritis education programs aim to develop patients' skills and change their behavior. This has been proven to be more effective than cognitive change alone[4]. These modifications in a patient's lifestyle involve exercise, rest, joint protection, and adherence to medication. Participatory sessions teach exercises to be performed daily, demonstrate technical aids, instruct in work simplification methods, and train the group in relaxation techniques.

Psychosocial aspects

For many patients, the mere fact of living with arthritis presents them with the difficult task of tolerating the uncertainties of a chronic disease. These individuals need to develop strategies to balance their fear of progressive worsening and the threat of dependency against their hopes for relief and remission[28]. To address these issues, many programs include sessions about self-awareness, communication skills, and stress management[13,15,22]. Self-efficacy has been defined as people's judgements of their capabilities to organize and execute courses of action required to attain designated types of performance. It is concerned not with the skills one has, but with the judgement of what one can do with whatever skills one possesses[29]. Goal setting and feedback about performance have been shown to be effective in strengthening patients' self-efficacy and skill acquisition[13,30].

Effects of arthritis patient education

Change in patient knowledge

In a review of 76 patient education studies, 34 measured patients' knowledge; of these, 94% found an increase[31]. In a later review of 25 studies, 8 of them studied change in knowledge and 7 of the 8 found an increase[32]. During the last few years, a trend away from studies measuring cognitive change has emerged, with the focus shifting toward studies that include three or more disease-outcome categories[33].

Change in behavior

The changes in behavior most frequently prescribed in arthritis patient education programs were the increased compliance with medication[33], practice of exercise, and relaxation techniques[34,35]. Also recommended were joint protection, and work simplification[36,37]. In long-term follow-up old habits of neglect with regard to exercise prevailed after 12 months. In contrast, the practice of joint protection and work simplification and remained unchanged after five years, in both the short and long-term[38,39].

Change in health status

Does patient education have an impact on the outcome of rheumatic disease? There are as yet no studies regarding the effect of patient education programs on mortality, and only limited information is available on whether they can reduce the side-effects of drugs, or favorably alter the economic consequences of arthritis[40]. The impact of patient education with regard to pain is a matter of controversy. Some studies have reported a reduction in pain[20,22,41], whereas others show either no effect[13,15] or suggest increased pain[42]. Patients reported knowing how to deal with pain better after going through an education program[9]. In a review of 14 studies measuring pain, 50% showed pain was reduced significantly after patient education[34]. A meta-analysis compared trials of patient education and non-steroidal anti-inflammatory drug (NSAID) treatments. Patient education accounted for a diminution in pain approaching 20–30% of that achieved by NSAID treatment[43].

Evaluating the success of patient education intervention on psychosocial status should be done with caution. Assessments have been difficult to quantify, and questions have therefore been raised about statistical reliability[31]. As psychosocial variables are often closely related to such things as disease activity, the progression of pain, and disability, it may prove difficult to determine if alterations in these variables are the result of an intervention, or represent natural changes in the disease process. Meta-analysis of psycho-educational interventions shows a modest effect size of 0.28 for depression[33].

In summary the effect of patient education is modest when outcome measures similar to studies on pharmacological treatment are used. However, it must be remembered that the effect of patient education is an added resource to standard medical care and in that sense a complement which may provide important improvements to the quality of life for patients with RA[44].

The future of patient education

Patient education has undergone fundamental changes during the last 30 years, going from hand-out materials and lecture programs to cognitive, behavioral, and interactive educational-behavioral self-management courses. If a similar development continues, we can expect to see the emergence of better methods based on research from other fields such as education, sociology, and psychology. New approaches involving computer-based Internet technology may supplement personal interactive meetings. Problem-based programs have now appeared and the further development of these strategies may better meet the needs of individual patients, as well as increase their motivation to learn. Economic analyses may look closer at the cost-effectiveness of patient education in the totality of the healthcare system: does it reduce or add to the total cost? Traditional evaluation methods may not be optimal for finding the true effect of patient education; new methods may develop to better acknowledge beneficial effect for the patients. Comparisons between different types of programs will be necessary; that is, telephone contact versus visiting a physician, community support groups as opposed to a multisession program of structured education, community-based self-management courses instead of multidisciplinary education. International and national standards using similar methods of evaluation will make it easier to compare the effectiveness of different programs. New methods also need to be developed for individuals with other ethnic backgrounds, as well as for those who cannot read, or who live in remote areas. It is to be hoped that patient education will be offered increasingly to a wider spectrum of patients suffering from rheumatic diseases and that such programs, designed to meet specific patient needs, will achieve acceptance as part of the total management of chronic illness.

References

1. Bartlett, E. E. Forum: patient education. Eight principles from patient education research. *Prev Med* 1985; **14**, 667–9.
2. Bauman, A., Lindroth, Y., and Daltroy, L. H. Health promotion and patient education for people with arthritis. In *Rheumatology* (Klippel JH and Dieppe PA, eds), London: Mosby; 1998.
3. Vignos, P. J., Parker, W. T., and Thompson, H. M. Evaluation of a clinic education program for patients with rheumatoid arthritis. *J Rheumatol* 1976; **3**: 155–65.
4. Mazzuca, S. A. Does patient education in chronic disease have a therapeutic value? *J Chron Dis* 1982; **35**: 521–9.
5. Riemsma, R. P, Taal, E., Kirwan, J. R., and Rasker, J. J. , Systematic review of rheumatoid arthritis patient education. *Arthritis Rheum* 2004; **51**: 1045–59.
6. Brooks, P., and Hochberg, M. Outcome measures and classification criteria for the rheumatic diseases: a compilation of data from OMERACT (Outcome Measures for Arthritis Clinical Trials), ILAR (International League of Associations for Rheumatology), regional leagues and other groups. *Rheumatology* 2001; **40**: 896–906.
7. Silvers, I. J., Melbourne, F. H., Weisman, M. H., and Mueller, M. R., Assessing physician/patient perceptions in rheumatoid arthritis: a vital component in patient education. *Arthritis Rheum* 1985; **28**: 300–7.
8. Kay, E. A, and Punchak, S. S. Patient understanding of the causes and medical treatment of rheumatoid arthritis. *Br J Rheumatol* 1998; **27**: 396–8.

9. Lindroth, Y., Brattström, M., Bellman, I. *et al.* A problem-based education program for patients with rheumatoid arthritis: evaluation after three and twelve months. *Arthritis Care Res* 1997; **10**: 325–32.

10. Hill, J., Bird, A., Hopkins, R., Lawton, C., and Wright, V. The development and use of a patient knowledge questionnaire in rheumatoid arthritis. *Br J Rheumatol* 1991; **30**: 45–9.

11. Donovan, J. L., Blake, D. R., and Fleming, W. G. The patient is not a blank sheet: lay beliefs and their relevance to patient education. *Br J Rheumatol* 1989; **28**: 58–61.

12. Lorig, K., Cox, T., Cuevas, Y., Kraines, R. G., and Britton, M. C. Converging and diverging beliefs about arthritis: Caucasian patients, Spanish-speaking, and physicians. *J Rheumatol* 1984; **11**: 76–9.

13. Taal, E., Riemsma, R. P., Brus, H. L., Seydel, E. R., Rasker, J. J., and Wiegman, O. Group education for patients with rheumatoid arthritis. *Patient Educ Couns* 1993; **20**: 177–87.

14. Eberhardt, K., Larsson, B. M., and Nived, K. Early rheumatoid arthritis: some social, economic and psychological aspects. *Scand J Rheumatol* 1993; **22**: 119–23.

15. Lindroth, Y., Bauman, A., Barnes, C., McCredie, M., and Brooks, P. M. A controlled evaluation of arthritis education. *Br J Rheumatol* 1989; **28**: 7–12.

16. Fex, E., Larsson, B. M., Nived, K., and Eberhardt, K. Effect of rheumatoid arthritis on work status and social and leisure time activities in patients followed 8 years from onset. *J Rheumatol* 1989; **25**: 44–50.

17. Darmawan, J., Muriden, K. D., Wigley, R. D., and Valkenburg, H. A. Arthritis community education by leather puppet (wayang kulit) shadow play in rural Indonesia (Java). *Rheumatol Int* 1992; **12**: 97–101.

18. Brattström, M. *Ledskydd och rehabilitering*. Lund: Studentlitteratur; 1970.

19. Althoff, B., Nordenskiöld, U., and Hansen, A. M. Ledskydd: ett skonsamt levnadssätt. *Riksförbundet Mot Reumatism*, Stockholm: 1977.

20. Goeppinger, J., Arthur, M. W., Baglioni, A. J., Brunk, S. E., and Brunner, C. M. A re-examination of the effectiveness of self-care education for persons with arthritis. *Arthritis Rheum* 1989; **32**: 706–16.

21. Cohen, J. L., Sauter, S. H., De Vellis, R. F., and De Vellis, B. M. Evaluation of arthritis self-management courses led by laypersons and by professionals. *Arthritis Rheum* 1986; **29**: 388–93.

22. Lorig, K., Lubeck, D., Kraines, R. G., Seleznick, M., and Holman, H. R. Outcomes of self-help education for patients with arthritis. *Arthritis Rheum* 1985; **28**: 680–5.

23. Moll, J. M. H., and Wright, V. Evaluation of the arthritis and rheumatism council handbook on gout. *J Chron Dis* 1972; **31**: 405–11.

24. Maggs, F. M., Jubb, R. W., and Kemm, J. R. Single-blind randomized controlled trial of an educational booklet for patients with chronic arthritis. *Br J Rheumatol* 1996; **35**: 775–7.

25. Weinberger, M., Tierny, W. M., Booher, P., and Katz, B. P. Can the provision of information to patients with osteoarthritis improve functional status? *Arthritis Rheum* 1989; **32**: 1577–83.

26. Wetstone, S. C., Sheehann, T. J., Votaw, R. G., Peterson, M. G., and Rothfield, N. Evaluation of a computer based education lesson for patients with rheumatoid arthritis. *J Rheumatol* 1985; **2**: 907–3.

27. Lorig, K., Seleznick, M., Lubeck, D., Ung, E., Chastain, R. L., and Holman, H. R. The beneficial outcomes of the arthritis self-management course are not adequately explained by behavior change. *Arthritis Rheum* 1989; **32**: 91–5.

28. Wiener, C. L. The burden of rheumatoid arthritis: tolerating the uncertainty. *Soc Scien Med* 1975; **9**: 97–104.

29. Bandura, A. Self-efficacy: toward a unifying theory of behavior change. *Psychol Rev* 1977; **84**: 191–215.

30. Lorig, K., Chastain, R. L., Ung, E., Shoor, S., and Holman, H. R. Development and evaluation of a scale to measure perceived self-efficacy in people with arthritis. *Arthritis Rheum* 1989; **32**: 37–44.

31. Lorig, K., Konkol, L., and Gonzales, V. Arthritis patient education: a review of the literature. *Patient Educ Couns* 1987; **10**: 207–52.

32. Hawley, D. J. Psycho-educational interventions in the treatment of arthritis. *Baillieres Clin Rheumatol* 1995; **9**: 803–23.

33. Hill, J., Bird, H., and Johnson, S. Effect of patient education on adherence to drug treatment for rheumatoid arthritis: a randomized controlled trial. *Ann Rheum Dis* 2001; **60**: 869–75.

34. Hirano, P. C., Laurent, D. D., and Lorig, K. Arthritis patient education studies, 1987–1991: a review of the literature. *Patient Educ Couns* 1994; **24**: 9–54.

35. Stenström, C. H., Arge, B., and Sundbom, A. Dynamic training versus relaxation training as home exercise for patients with inflammatory rheumatic diseases. *Scand J Rheumatol* 1996; **25**: 28–33.

36. Nordenskiöld, U. Evaluation of assistive devices after a course in joint protection. *Int J Technol Assess Health Care* 1994; **10**: 293–304.

37. Hammond, A. Joint protection behavior in patients with rheumatoid arthritis following an education program. *Arthritis Care Res* 1994; **7**: 5–9.

38. Lindroth, Y., Bauman, A., Brooks, P. M., and Priestley, D. A 5-year follow-up of a controlled trial of an arthritis education program. *Br J Rheumatol* 1995; **34**: 647–52.

39. Hammond, A., and Freeman, K. The long-term outcomes from a randomized controlled trial of an educational-behavioural joint protection programme for people with rheumatoid arthritis. *Clin Rehabil* 2004; **18**: 520–8.

40. Lorig, K., and Holman, H. R. Arthritis self-management studies: a twelve-year review. *Health Educ Q* 1993; **20**: 17–28.

41. Keefe, F. J., Caldwell, D. S., Baucom, D. *et al.* Spouse-assisted coping skills training in the management of osteoarthritic knee pain. *Arthritis Care Res* 1996; **9**: 279–91.

42. Parker, J. C., Singsen, B. H., Hewett, J. E. *et al.* Educating patients with rheumatoid arthritis: a prospective analysis. *Arch Phys Med Rehab* 1984; **65**: 771–4.

43. Superio-Cabuslay, E., Ward, M. M., and Lorig, K. Patient education intervention in osteoarthritis and rheumatoid arthritis: a meta-analytic comparison with non steroid antiinflammatory drug treatment. *Patient Educ Couns* 1996; **9**: 292–301.

44. Riemsma, R. P., Taal, E., Kirwan, J. R., and Rasker, J. J. Patient education programmes for adults with rheumatoid arthritis. *BMJ* 2002; **325**: 558–9.

45. Calfas, K. J., Kaplan, R. M., and Ingram, R. I. One-year evaluation of cognitive-behavioral intervention in osteoarthritis. *Arthritis Care Res* 1992; **5**: 202–9.

46. Potts, M., and Brandt, K. D. Analysis of education-support groups for patients with rheumatoid arthritis. *Patient Couns Health Educ* 1985; **4**: 161–6.

47. Radojevic, V., Nicassio, P. M., and Weisman, M. H. Behavioral intervention with and without family support for rheumatoid arthritis. *Behavior Therapy* 1992; **23**: 13–30.

48. Lorish, C. D., Parker, J., and Brown, S. Effective patient education: a quasi-experiment comparing an individualized strategy with a routinized strategy. *Arthritis Rheum* 1985; **28**: 1289–97.

49. Jacobsson, L., Fritiof, M., Olofsson, Y., Runesson, I., Strömbeck, B., and Wikström, I. Evaluation of a structured multidisciplinary day care program in rheumatoid arthritis. *Scand J Rheumatol* 1998; **27**: 117–24.

30 | Occupational therapy and assistive products and technology

Ulla Nordenskiöld

Introduction

The main goal of occupational therapy is to improve individual patient's health and well-being by adjusting their environment, supplying assistive devices, and by teaching strategies[1]. Promoting activity is a central concept in occupational therapy and includes all aspects of an individual's physical and mental life. The importance of activity to health is central. The World Health Organization (WHO) is committed to promoting the empowerment of persons with disabilities so that they will not be disentitled or discriminated against[2].

Health, according to Pörn[3], consists of three basic components in the dynamics of the individual: the repertoire, the environment, and the goals of the subject. Repertoire is defined as the individual's skills. New skills can be acquired and skills deteriorate when they are not used. Occupational therapy, based on a holistic view, teaches that individuals must be actively involved in, for example, personal care, living conditions, work, leisure, and relationships with other people. Occupational therapy seeks to prevent disability while re-establishing and maintaining abilities. Individuals with rheumatoid arthritis (RA) have problems conducting their daily lives because of pain, muscle weakness, and fatigue. They are often unable to perform daily activities in a normal manner. Pincus et al.[4] also noted that difficulties in daily activities were among the predictors of a higher mortality rate in RA patients.

The ICF: a model for functioning, disability, and health

The International Classification of Functioning, Disability, and Health (ICF)[2], developed by the WHO, is a model that focuses on function instead of impairment. The overall aim of the classification is to establish a common language for describing health and health-related conditions in order to improve communication between health professionals, researchers, and the public, including people with disabilities. The ICF has two parts, each with two components. Part 1 covers Functioning and Disability and includes the components body functions and body structures, and activities and participation. Part 2 covers contextual factors and includes the components environmental factors and personal factors Each component can be expressed in both positive and negative terms.

When analysing the situation of patients with RA, the occupational therapist finds the classification helpful with the different perspectives of health: biological, individual, and social. As well, the classification can be used as a clinical tool in needs assessment, matching treatment and outcome evaluation. However, the way in which a person reacts to difficulties and hardship depends not only on disabilities but also, to a great extent, on the individual's personality and social situation[5]. Some patients feel threatened or guilty, while others may see a challenge in learning to cope with their life situation and 'take charge'[6].

You must fight and not just now but for your whole life.

Disability: body functions and structures

Impairments are problems in body functions or structures. For example in RA this applies to joint function, pain, stiffness, fatigue, reduced grip force, and deformities. Pain contributes to fatigue and pain management is a major component in clinical care. The hand has a very complex structure and, when inflamed, the possibilities for reduced mobility and muscle function, as well as instability, are manifold. Pain reducing the strength of the wrist and fingers often occurs early in the disease, and has a strong impact on the person's daily activity. The functional and structural changes in RA resulting in deformity and functional impairment are detailed in Chapter 35. Smith et al.[7] maintain that the internal force required in the metacarpophalangeal (MCP) joints to carry out the pinch grip is six times as much as is required for the pinch grip itself. The more the MCP joint is flexed, the greater the component on the volar side. When the ligamentous structures become insufficient, in RA, the proximal phalanges will be pulled in the volar direction, resulting in volar subluxation. Chao et al.[8] have confirmed Smith's estimates concerning the volar and radial forces on the MCP joints.

This is the theory of protecting the MCP joints, on which the use of assistive devices with enlarged handles is based.

Patient-experienced needs: occupational therapy interventions

Stability without pain is required for good hand function and normal hand force. Instability and dislocation of carpal joints result in a weak grip. The general purpose of an elastic wrist orthosis (orthosis = to make straight) in connection with RA is

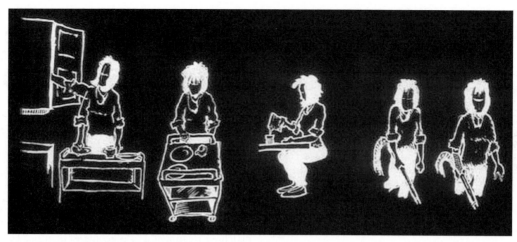

Fig. 30.1 Pain decreased significantly when an elastic wrist orthosis was used in three ADL situations: setting a breakfast table, pouring out of a milk carton, and vacuum cleaning, compared to not using the orthosis.

stabilization of the inflamed joints, immobilization to control the inflammation and pain, protection of the ligaments, prevention of deformities, and relief of pain. A wrist orthosis allows full mobility of the MCP, proximal interphalangeal (PIP), and distal interphalangeal (DIP) joints, and the carpometacarpal (CMC) joint of the thumb. The volar support in the palm should not be extended beyond the distal palmar crease, the so-called lifeline. Studies[9–11] have demonstrated that when a patient used a prefabricated elastic wrist orthosis the grip force was significantly increased. Pain also decreased significantly when the subject used the orthosis in three activities of daily living (ADL) situations: setting a breakfast table, pouring out of a milk carton, and vacuum cleaning, compared to performing the same tasks without the orthosis (Fig. 30.1). In one study[10] focused on possible negative long-term effects, no increased muscle weakness was detected after six months. A hand exercise program including training of 'the gliding surfaces' combined with analgetic paraffin bath treatment has also been developed[12], tested, and shown to have a positive effect on the flexion and extension in the finger joints and to reduce pain[13].

Dynamic orthoses are often used in *pre-and postoperative* treatment, as discussed in Chapter 35. They are applied preoperatively to increase force and correct the tendency to subluxation of the tendons. In the postoperative period it is extremely important that the gliding surfaces be made to function correctly. The orthoses are individually designed according to the type of operation.

To decrease or eliminate the reduced joint function and pain,*ergonomically designed assistive devices* such as an upright-handled bread knife and cheese slicer are used. Using assistive devices such as a spring-assisted scissors, a cheese slicer, a broad-handled potato peeler, and a designed bread knife, resulted in significant pain reduction compared with using ordinary household tools[9] (Fig. 30.2). The hand and finger joints were positioned in an ergonomically more comfortable grip, since the handles are designed with a wider gripping area[12].

An electronic grip force measuring instrument, Grippit® (Fig. 30.3)[14], has been developed to measure both the peak grip force and the mean grip force over a set period of time (10 s) in newtons (N). The grip device and an arm-support are mounted on a transportable base and standard arm and grip positioning is ensured. As early as 2 years after onset of disease, grip force is on average reduced by 50%, and after 7 and 14 years of disease the loss is 68% and 79%, respectively [14–16].

To what extent patients' ADL problems can be explained by reduced grip force has been analyzed in one daily task—vacuuming[17]. Vacuuming was avoided by 8 of the 41 women; the mean grip force in these women was 42 N (confidence interval (CI): 25–58). The women who were still doing the vacuuming had a mean grip force value of 80 N (CI: 63–100) (Fig. 30.4). Thus the threshold value of grip force for performing vacuum-cleaning would be 60 N. Studies[18,19] have suggested that a grip force level below 88 N was the threshold level for performing daily activities, and that the level for lifting a frying pan weight (1250 g) was below 76 N. Such information could be used for designing technical adaptations, since the results showed the relationship between grip force, pain, and difficulty in daily activities.

Disability: activities and participation

Activity limitations and participation restriction are difficulties an individual has in activities and in involvement in life situations. Verbrygge and Jette[20] distinguish between intrinsic disability (without personal assistance or equipment assistance) and actual disability (with such assistance) and stress the scientific importance of measuring both levels of disability. There is no general concept of ADL. The term is used both in a narrow way and a wide sense, classified as personal care, home maintenance, work/school, and leisure/recreation.

Patient-experienced needs: occupational therapy interventions

ADL assessments are used by the occupational therapist to describe patients' problems and needs, identify suitable intervention measures, establish goals, follow changes in ADL, evaluate treatment, and predict outcome. The ADL instruments can also be used to measure what forms a difficulty for performing an activity, or whether

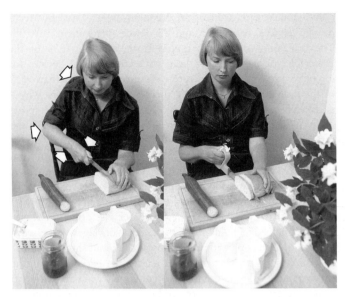

Fig. 30.2 The ergonomically designed breadknife has a handle with a wider gripping area and is specially designed for people with reduced grip force. It can be used as a general-purpose knife ('products for all').

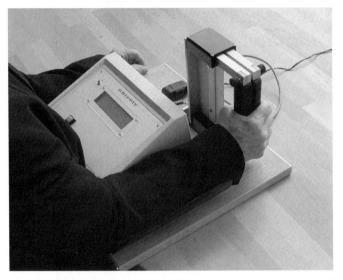

Fig. 30.3 The Grippit®: an electronic grip force instrument developed to measure peak grip force and mean grip force over a set period of time in newtons. Reference values and standard positions are documented.

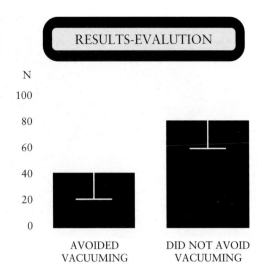

RESULTS-EVALUTION

Fig. 30.4 The grip force was significantly ($p < 0.036$) lower in the 8 women who avoided vacumming than the 3.3 women who did not avoid. The threshold value of grip force for performing vacuum-cleaning would be 60 N.

the individual can perform the activity in a way that is satisfactory to the individual with assistance, or after special interventions. One of the instruments, the self-reported diagnosis-specific Evaluation of Daily Activities Questionnaire, EDAQ[16,21], describes assistive devices as specific interventions and identifies the individual's own techniques for solving problems. The instrument also analyses ergonomics as interventions with both hands, and indicates in detail the activities for which new solutions have to be developed. EDAQ consists of 102 daily activities divided into 11 dimensions, as eating/drinking, dressing, toileting, transferring, bathing/showering, cooking, washing/clothes care, cleaning, and mobility indoors/outdoors, and can be used to evaluate both the intrinsic and actual disability. If the Health Assessment Questionnaire (HAQ)[22] has been

used for this purpose the result will be a higher HAQ score (decreased function), since the scale steps '2' in the HAQ rank the use of assistive devices in the same category as 'with much difficulty'. The problem with the widely used HAQ model is therefore that it mixes two different aspects of disability, that is, perceived difficulty and dependence on devices or another person's help[17,23,24].

A self-administered checklist with defined assistive devices is included in the EDAQ instrument, listing their number, use, and the individual's opinion[17].

A significant reduction was noted in patients' difficulties when they use *assistive devices and altered working methods*[16,21]. The number of items affected by assistive devices varies between the dimensions. In the dimension Eating/Drinking, for example, all items except 'opening can' and 'opening bottle' showed decreased difficulty in most patients with devices such as the special breadknife, cheese slicer, springy scissors and tongs, elongated handles on knife and fork, and two-hand grip. The items 'raising from toilet' and 'washing hands' in the dimension Toileting and 'managing faucet' in the dimension Bathing showed increased ability in all subjects with difficulties who used the raised toilet seat, the lengthened faucet, and the elongated lever, respectively.

As an example of *changed working methods*, in the dimension Cooking most patients described difficulty in 'lifting frying pan with one hand' or 'taking down sugar', but with a two-hand grip the majority could do it with no or little difficulty. In the dimension Washing/Clothes care, there were several items with few changes in difficulty, as in the items 'opening/folding ironing board', 'ironing', 'washing in machine', 'washing up in washbowl', 'hanging out wash', and 'putting in and out of plug'. In the dimension Cleaning, most did not gain anything from using tools when 'wringing out cloth', and 'sweeping floor'.

By using the Rasch mode1[25] to transform ordinal scores from an instrument to one-dimensional linear measures, one can analyse whether items change from hard to easy and monitor changes in the subject's performance. In a report[21] using the Rasch analysis to transform the patients' ratings on the ordinal scale to a linear measure, it was possible to construct a

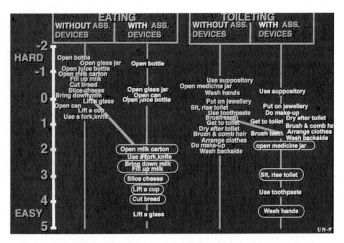

Fig. 30.5 The dimensions Eating (12 items) and Toileting (13 items) in the instrument EDAQ are analysed with the Rasch analysis. The items have been marked on the scale, which ranges from 'hard' to 'easy' both without assistive devices/altered working methods and with devices/altered methods.

hierarchical model ranging from difficult items to easy ones and with the patients' overall difficulties ranging from less able to more able. Changes in difficulty were clearly identified and it was possible to demonstrate a positive effect of assistive devices in most women (Fig. 30.5). The use of devices or altered methods led to a reduction in perceived difficulty in 42% of the ratings. As expected, Thyberg et al.[15] demonstrated that the use of assistive devices was related to subgroups with severe disease and more disability in both women and men with early RA and that the use of devices significantly reduced difficulties. This clearly shows the importance of providing assistive devices for patients with RA.

Environmental factors: ergonomically designed assistive devices

Barriers and hindrances are the negative aspect of environmental factors. It is recognized that any product or technology can be assistive. For the purpose of the ICF of environmental factors, assistive products are defined as any product, instrument, equipment, or technology adapted or specially designed for improving the functioning of a disabled person.

Assistive technology is used by people with disabilities, with the intention of decreasing their difficulties and maximizing the quality of activities[2]. Technology for the patients has a wide meaning, and includes both equipment and the procedures used to select and evaluate the equipment. The policy regarding assistive technology is based on integration and normalization. Sweden has a well-developed provision system for assistive devices, which is integrated with the healthcare system. The development of devices with good function and appealing design has become an area of increasing interest in Sweden. The term 'universal design'[26] is used to emphasize the combination of applied ergonomics research and product development. It can lead to better products for general use as well, '*products for all*'.

Individuals with arthritis are frequent users of assistive technology devices, between 5 and 23 devices per person[9,15,16,27,28]. The utilization of devices ranges from 95% to 75% of the prescribed devices. After a joint protection course devices for kitchen work and personal care were used by no less than 95% of the individuals[9,10]. However, there are several reasons why it is difficult to draw firm conclusions. Caveats regarding reports on usage of assistive devices include influences of social and economic factors, the method used for providing devices, and the stage of the disease. The prescription, provision, cost[9,17], utilization, and feelings about assistive devices, including orthoses, have demonstrated how individual perspectives vary; for example, they: opened the patients' world for activities (some now dare go out, sure that they will be able to unlock the door), increased function, helped in maintaining a role as a working woman (when driving, able to cope with job as postal clerk and shop assistant), in leisure (support when knitting, gardening, biking, picking up children, and sailing), 'otherwise I would behave in an odd way', 'using the devices at work-not afraid to show my pain', 'both the office chair and the adapted keyboard are big help when I'm working at the computer'.

Patient education: health education

Patient education is activity designed to improve the way patients manage their health behaviour[29,30] and is approached in the previous chapter.

Joint protection: a pedagogical model

Joint protection—for active living,[12] a written educational model, is a syllabus for patient education that has been developed to facilitate the treatment of the consequences of a disease and, hopefully, to allow patients to better maintain an active lifestyle with fewer difficulties; it has played an important role in rehabilitation in the last few decades. The principles were first presented in the United States by the occupational therapist J. Cordery[31,32], following the biomechanical analyses of Smith et al. The focus has been on minimizing the biomechanical forces acting upon joints as much as possible in order to reduce the risk of joint damage, that is, to strive for the best possible function with the least possible pain. However, it has not been shown whether it is possible to halt or delay structural damage of the joints by these measures.

Joint protection for active living was built up as an equilateral triangle, where the triangle illustrates how *knowledge, emotion (inspiration),* and *action* support each other (*the cognitive triad*), and the value of meeting others through group education (Fig. 30.6), with the patient's own activity being in focus. By focusing on the patient's needs in daily activities and own experience of the disease (patient-orientated), one avoids the introduction of information that may be incompatible with the patient's views or emotional state. The course includes 13 lesson hours

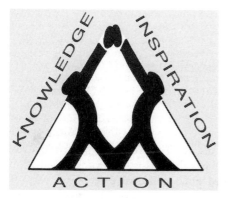

Fig. 30.6 An educational model for patient education where the triangle illustrates how knowledge, emotion (inspiration), and action support each other (the cognitive triad) and the value of meeting others through group education.

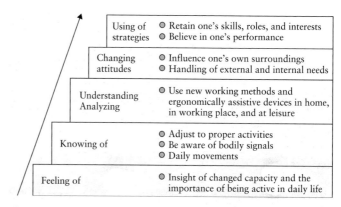

Fig. 30.7 The 'educational staircase' illustrates the process for achieving the establishment of an active lifestyle and adaptation to the new situation. Having alternative working methods and attitudes, and using new strategies requires more engagement than just 'knowing about' something.

over a period of three weeks, and is led by a team consisting of an occupational therapist, a physician and/or nurse, a physiotherapist, and a social worker.

One afternoon group session with information for *relatives* is also included in the model.

The fundamental principles are: a written course booklet for the patients and a guide for the counsellors, small groups of about five participants, alternating theory and practice with repetition, *dialogue communication*-with mutual esteem between individuals, practical homework as a '*contract*' following each meeting, and the ultimate goal of stimulating the participants to find their own solutions. By sharing experiences, difficulties, and solutions, patients realize that they are by no means alone. Studies[9,33,34] have found that programs based on learning theories, such as changing methods when doing daily tasks and daring to discuss the problems with family and co-workers, had a positive effect on patients' behaviour in the workplace, as well as changing leisure activities: 'I have had to stop bowling, I teach others instead'; 'I practice running instead of playing golf'.

Hammond *et al.*[33] have suggested that there was pain relief and an increase in functional ability in a follow-up study four years after joint protection instruction.

The 'educational staircase' illustrates the process of change: insight leads to changes in attitudes, and then to changes in behaviours and strategies, maintaining established goals/needs and an individual adaptation to the new life situation (Fig. 30.7).

Cost-effectiveness/utility analysis

Economy in healthcare implies using the resources in the most effective way. Consequently, occupational therapists should describe their aims, measurements, and treatments and establish the effects on the patients of the interventions. The 'direct' cost could comprise costs for the selection process, the devices, and the domestic services. The 'indirect' costs reflect resource use in other areas not directly concerned with the provision of services[35]. The method for economic evaluation (Fig. 30.8) is an attempt to illustrate the costs for the personnel and devices as well as the effects from the patients' perspective. When analyzing and describing effectiveness (utility) in the healthcare system

one must identify the effect on the subject, otherwise the system can only be described as showing the productivity. The cost of patient education, in the form of the joint protection course, including provision of assistive devices, *could be judged to be low in relation to its effectiveness—the utility to the patient*[9].

Outcome measurements

Occupational therapists, like other health professionals, will feel obliged to use more *evidence-based methods*. Instruments which are specifically developed for people with arthritis must include the patients' own experiences as well as the sensitivity of the instruments for describing important changes within an individual. In order to understand why a person is more, or less, able to do the activities and satisfied with the treatment, it is important to consider both the person's physical capacity and the person's mental ability to perform in relevant situations. Other types of evaluation, such as the quality of life and well-being[36], may help to understand the patient's total situation and avoid the label 'someone with a chronic disease'. The Canadian Occupational Performance Measure, COPM, is designed to identify problems within different areas and to investigate the individuals' satisfaction with the performance of the occupations[37]. When developing new instruments it is of value to use the terms in ICF as well as the 'core sets' for RA[38].*Focus groups* with discussions about questions relating to outcomes from, and satisfaction/dissatisfaction with, RA treatment can highlight shortcomings and effects of the interventions[6,39]. It is always the prerogative of the subject to determine whether the interventions affected the quality of his/her activity.

Combined early assessment and treatment of impaired grip force, pain, and impaired hand function[40,41] should be given priority, and the patient's perspective on needs and limitations in activities and restrictions in participation of performing daily tasks need to be incorporated. Patient education, with two-way communication, introducing assistive devices, alternative methods and strategies, or modifying work place and leisure activities[42] are others. Both the benefit of assistive technology in relation to the individual's goals/needs and their own solutions should be identified, since no single measure can account for all aspects. By means of the ICF, interventions such as hand movements, hand

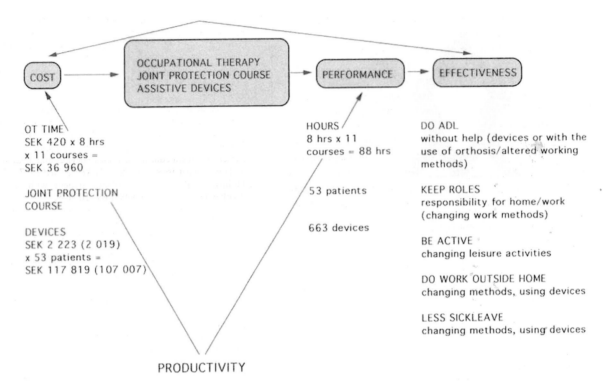

Fig. 30.8 A cost-effectiveness analysis of the joint protection course, the assistive devices, and the utility to the patient. SEK = Swedish Crown; OT time = occupational therapist's time.

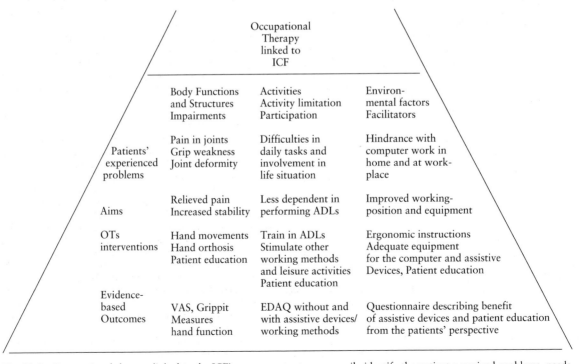

Fig. 30.9 Occupational therapy linked to the ICF's components, to more easily identify the patient-perceived problems, needs, and goals as well as occupational therapy's interventions and outcome measures. VAS = Visual analogue scale.

orthoses, ADL training, ergonomic devices, and patient education can be appropriately targeted and their effects on levels of body function, activity/participation, and environmental factors monitored, measured, and evaluated–occupational therapy should be used holistically (Fig. 30.9).

The role of an occupational therapist entails great responsibility for developing the ability to switch between the role of an 'efficient professional' and that of a caring fellow human being, with the ability to see the person/patient with RA as both healthy and sick. The most important goal is to build a basis for the individual's creative thinking that will enable them to find their own solutions to their problems and an insight into their own possibilities. After a joint protection course women with RA may deliver comments such as:

I'm not alone with my problems, I can–I have important experiences and knowledge.

I want and know how to influence around me.

It shows that society wants us. It does not feel so shameful to have the disease.

References

1. Yerxa, E. In search of good ideas for occupational therapy. *Scand J Occup Ther* 1994; **1**: 7–15.
2. World Health Organization *International Classification of Functioning, Disabilities and Health, ICF.* Geneva: World Health Organization; 2001.
3. Pörn, I. Health and adaptedness. *Theor Med* 1993; **14**: 295–303.
4. Pincus, T., Callahan, L. F., and Vaughn, W. K. Questionnaire, walking time and button test measures of functional capacity as predictive markers for mortality in rheumatoid arthritis. *J Rheumatol* 1987; **14**: 240–51.
5. Berglund, K., Persson, L. O., and Brattström, M. Effects of group counselling for rheumatoid arthritis patients on measures of psychological adjustment to illness. In *Rheumatology State of the Art* (Balint, G., ed.), pp. 432–5. Amsterdam: Elsevier Science; 1992.
6. Ahlmen, M., Nordenskiöld, U., Archenholtz, B., Thyberg, I., Rönnquist, R. M., Linden, L. *et al.* Rheumatology outcomes; the patient's perspective: a multicentre focus group interview study of Swedish rheumatoid arthritis patients. *Rheumatology* 2005; **44**: 105–10.
7. Smith, E., Juvinal, R., Bender, L., and Pearson, R. Role of the finger flexors in rheumatoid deformities of the metacarpophalangeal joints. *Arthritis Rheum* 1964; **7**: 467–80.
8. Chao, E. Y., Opgrande, J. D., and Axmear, F. E. Three dimensional force analysis of finger joints in selected isometric hand functions. *J Biomechanics* 1976; **9**: 387–96.
9. Nordenskiöld, U. Evaluation of assistive devices after a course in joint protection. *Int J Technol Assess Health Care* 1994; **10**: 294–304.
10. Kjeken, I., Möller, G., and Kvien, T. Use of commercially produced elastic wrist orthoses in chronic arthritis: a controlled study. *Arthritis Care Res* 1995; **8**: 108–13.
11. Steultjens, E., Dekker, J., Bouter, L., van Schaardenburg, D., van Kuyk, M-A., and van den Ende, C. Occupational therapy for rheumatoid arthritis: a systematic review. *Arthritis Care Res* 2002; **47**: 672–85.
12. Althoff, B., and Nordenskiöld, U. *Joint Protection: for Active Living.* Course booklet. Nordenskiöld, U., Althoff, B., and Hansen, A. M. *Joint Protection for Active Living.* Guide. Stockholm: Swedish Rheumatism Association; 1994.
13. Dellhag, B., Wollersjö, I., and Bjelle, A. Effect of active hand exercise and waxbath treatment in rheumatoid arthritis patients. *Arthritis Care Res* 1992; **5**: 287–92.
14. Nordenskiöld, U., and Grimby, G. Grip force in patients with rheumatoid arthritis and fibromyalgia and in healthy subjects: a study with the Grippit instrument. *Scand J Rheumatol* 1993; **22**: 14–19.
15. Thyberg, I., Hass, U., Nordenskiöld, U., and Skogh, T. Survey of the use and effect of assistive devices in patients with early rheumatoid arthritis: a two year followup of women and men. *Arthritis Care Res* 2004; **4**: 413–28.
16. Nordenskiöld, U., Grimby, G., and Dahlin-Ivanoff, S. Questionnaire to evaluate the effects of assistive devices and altered working methods in women with rheumatoid arthritis. *Clin Rheumatol* 1998; **17**: 6–16.
17. Nordenskiöld, U. Daily activities in women with rheumatoid arthritis: aspects of patient education, assistive devices and methods for disability and impairment assessment. *Scand J Rehab Med* 1997; **37** (Suppl.):1–72.
18. Philips, C. Rehabilitation of the patient with rheumatoid hand involvement. *Phys Ther* 1989; **69**: 1091–9.
19. Turner, D. Relation between handgrip strength, upper limb disability and handicap among elderly women. *Clin Rehabil* 1992; **6**: 117–23.
20. Verbrugge, L. M., and Jette, A. M. The disablement process. *Soc Sci Med* 1994; **38**: 1–14.
21. Nordenskiöld, U., Grimby, G., Hedberg, M., Wright, B., and Linacre, J. M. The structure of an instrument for assessing the effect of assistive devices and altered working methods in women with rheumatoid arthritis. *Arthritis Care Res* 1996; **9**: 21–30.
22. Fries, J. F., Spitz, P., Krainer, G., and Holman, H. Measurement of patient outcome in arthritis. *Arthritis Rheum* 1980; **23**: 137–45.
23. Tennant, A., Hillman, M., Fear, J., Pickering, A., and Chamberlain, M. A. Are we making the most of Stanford Health Assessment Questionnaire? *Br J Rheumatol* 1996; **35**: 574–8.
24. Stucki, G. Understanding disability. *Ann Rheum Dis* 2003; **62**: 289–90.
25. Wright, B. D., and Masters G. *Rating Scale Analysis: Rasch Measurement.* Chicago: MESA; 1982.
26. Benktzon, M. Designing for our future selves: the Swedish experience. *Appl Ergon* 1993; **24**: 19–27.
27. Rogers, J. C., and Holm, M. B. Trajectory of assistive device usage and user and no-user characteristics: long handled bath sponge. *Arthritis Rheum* 2002; **15**: 645–50.
28. Mann, M. Assistive technology for persons with arthritis. In *Rheumatologic rehabilitation* (Melvin J., and Jensen G., eds), pp. 369–92. Bethesda, MD: American Occupational Therapy Association; 1998.
29. Hoffmann, T., and Worrall, L. Designing effective written health education materials: considerations for health professionals *Disabil Rehabil* 2004; **26**: 1166–73.
30. Lindroth, Y., Nilsson, J. Å., and Wollheim, F. A. Demographic variables and knowledge, behaviour and health outcome among patients with rheumatoid arthritis: correlation before and seven years after a patient education program. In Lindroth, Y., Development and evaluation of patient education in rheumatoid arthritis. Thesis. Lund, 1997, pp. 109–28.
31. Cordery, J. Joint protection: a responsibility of the occupational therapist. *Am J Occup Ther* 1965; **19**: 285–94.
32. Cordery, J., and Rocchi, M. Joint protection and fatigue management. In *Rheumatologic Rehabilitation* (Melvin, J., and Jensen, G., eds), pp. 279–322. Bethesda, MD: American Occupational Therapy Association; 1998.
33. Hammond, A., Young, A., and Kidao, R. A randomized controlled trial of occupational therapy for people with early rheumatoid arthritis. *Ann Rheum Dis* 2004; **63**: 23–30.
34. Stamm, T., Machold, K., Smolen, J., Fisher, S., Redlish, K., Graninger, W., Ebner, W., and Erlasher, L. Joint protection and home hand exercises improve hand function in patients with hand osteoarthritis: a randomized controlled trial. *Arthritis Care Res* 2002; **47**: 44–9.
35. Andrich, R., Ferrario, M., and Moi, M. A model of cost-outcome analysis for assistive technology. *Disabil Rehabil* 1998; **20**: 1–24.
36. Sandqvist, G., Åkesson, A., and Eklund, M. Daily occupations and wellbeing in women with limited systemic sclerosis. *Am J Occup Ther* 2005; **59**: 390–7.
37. Law, M., Baptiste, S., and Carswell, A. *et al. Canadian Occupational Performance Measure.* Manual. Toronto: Canadian Association of Occupational Therapists; 1994.

38. Stucki, G., Cieza, A., Geyh, S. *et al.* ICF Core Sets for rheumatoid arthritis. *J Rehabil Med* 2004; **44** Suppl.: 87–93.

39. Carr, J., Hewlett, S., Hughes, R. *et al.* Rheumatology outcomes: the patient's perspective. *J Rheumatol* 2003; **30**: 880–3.

40. Dellhag, B., and Bjelle, A. A grip ability test use in rheumatology practice. *J Rheumatol* 1995; **22**: 1559–65.

41. Fitinghoff, H., Söderback, I., and Nordemar, R. An activity analysis of hand grips used in housework by female rheumatoid arthritics. *Work* 1994; **4**: 128–36.

42. Wikström, I., Isaksson, Å., and Jakobsson, L. Leisure activities in rheumatoid arthritis: change after disease onset and associated factors. *Br J Occup Ther* 2001; **64**: 87–92.

31 | Psychological and social aspects

Tore Kristian Kvien and Liv Marit Smedstad

Introduction

Rheumatoid arthritis (RA) is a chronic and potentially disabling disease with pervasive negative impacts on the functional, social, and mental status of affected individuals. Long-term disease outcome varies from minimal loss of function to a mortality and morbidity approaching that of a malignant disease[1]. Substantial variation in function is readily observed among persons with RA. Much of the variation that is observed is the result of a multifactorial, complex interaction between the disease process and personal and social factors[2,3]. In spite of a growing body of studies addressing associations between the above variables in RA, their inter-relationships are still insufficiently explored, and remain issues of controversy.

In the traditional biomedical model, disease is conceptualized as an accurate pathological condition due to a well-defined cause and requiring definitive treatment. This single cause, single effect model of disease was challenged by Engel in 1977[4], who argued that the medical model was no longer adequate for the scientific tasks and social responsibilities of medicine. An alternative biopsychosocial model was proposed, in which illness and illness outcome were conceptualized as determined by biological, psychological, and social variables. During the 1980s, the multidimensional paradigm of illness offered by the biopsychosocial model gradually gained general acceptance in medicine. The model was assumed to imply that emotional, behavioral, and social processes are implicated in the development, course, and outcome of most illness[5].

Most chronic rheumatic disorders do not fit easily into the traditional biomedical model. Rheumatic diseases in general and RA in particular can be described with considerable accuracy in diagnostic and pathological terms, yet their cause is unknown, their course is unpredictable, and their treatment regimens are only partly effective[6]. Thus, paralleling the shift of paradigm in medicine in general over the past two decades, rheumatology moved from a strict biomedical model of disease towards a biopsychosocial model distinguished by a multicause, multieffect relationship[7]. Likewise, the importance of behavioral variables in the pathogenesis, morbidity, and mortality of rheumatic diseases was emphasized[8]. Thus, rheumatology is in the forefront of the medical specialities that conceptualize and assess disease outcome within a multidimensional framework. This chapter reviews the literature on psychosocial aspects in RA.

Chronic diseases and their inter-relationship with psychosocial aspects

Most chronic diseases will have an impact on the psychological as well as the social functioning of the individual. Life with a chronic disease, regardless of whether it is pulmonary, cardiovascular, or musculoskeletal, will lead to loss of physical function, changes in the ability to perform valued activities, and have impact on psychosocial variables. This has also been supported by clinical research. For example Wells et al.[9] examined psychiatric disorders and eight chronic medical conditions in a community sample of 2554 persons. They found that arthritis, cancer, lung disease, neurological disorder, heart disease, and physical handicap were strongly associated with psychiatric disorders. The prevalence of psychiatric disorders was higher among persons with one or more medical conditions compared to persons without any medical condition. Persons with chronic medical conditions were more likely to have recent affective and anxiety disorders.

A great body of literature deals with the relationships and possible causal directions of psychological dysfunction and chronic pain. Chronic musculoskeletal pain in the general population is associated with higher depression scores than in the normal population and also with higher numbers of depressive cases[10,11]. This relationship between anxiety, depression, and pain, is a challenge for the clinician facing individuals without any biomedical condition that fully explains the pain reported by the patient. Pain in RA is a major component of the disease, and is explained partly by the inflammatory process, partly by destructive changes of the joints. However, pain in a patient with RA may be associated with depression, which in its turn exaggerates the patient's perception of pain.

How to measure psychological and social health status

A variety of measures and instruments are available to assess the psychological and social aspects of RA. However, the understanding of certain concepts is required to use the various instruments correctly. Therefore, the terminology most commonly used when measuring psychosocial health in clinical research will be briefly reviewed.

Process and outcome measures

Process measures in RA are temporary variables reflecting the fluctuating process of disease; that is, the pathology preceding the level of impairment. Measures of the biomedical process have an intrinsic importance to the extent that they serve as proxies for outcome measures[12]. While most process measures are unidimensional, arthritis outcome measures have been designed to reflect several dimensions of arthritis[13]. Furthermore, process and outcome measures differ in another principal way—while the disease process is usually measured by an external rater or by a technical procedure, most non-fatal disease outcomes are measured by patients' self-reports. Self-report measures are designed to capture the subjective nature of disease impact and, as such, their subjectivity is not a bias but rather a deliberate integral component. On the other hand, objective process measures provide information complementary to the subjective outcome measures. Thus, subjective and objective measures represent separate, though related, disease dimensions. Measures of psychosocial function can be considered both as outcome measures and as possible predictors or covariates important for longitudinal observational studies[14].

Impairment, disability, and handicap

Whereas impairment represents disturbances at the organ level caused by a pathological process, disability reflects the consequences of impairment in terms of functional performance[2,15]. Subsequently, handicap is the social disadvantage which results from an interaction between impairment and/or disability and a range of factors external to the disease process[16]. The relationship between impairment, disability, and handicap may appear hierarchical, inasmuch as the greater the impairment, for example the joint damage, the more disabled and socially handicapped the individual will be. However, this is not necessarily the case. As pointed out by Carr and Thompson[17], rheumatologists will be familiar with patients with mild RA who seem inappropriately crippled by their disease and, conversely, of patients functioning normally despite severe joint deformities. Thus, since individuals perceive, assess, and defend themselves against the loss of health in a highly subjective manner[5], factors other than the disease process may be important in determining the level of handicap in the individual patient with arthritis. Consequently, the identification of factors external to the disease process, heralding adverse disease outcomes, is a major challenge in rheumatological research. However, the measurement of handicap in chronic diseases is in its infancy, as recently pointed out by Carr *et al.*[18]. The London Health Impact Questionnaire is a generic instrument measuring the handicap state of an individual by comparison with the normal activities/lifestyle of someone of a similar age, sex, and background who does not have health problems[19]. A disease-specific measure of patient-perceived handicap in RA, the Disease Repercussion Profile, has also been developed and validated[17]. This tool provides an individualized measure of patient-perceived handicap in RA.

In recent years, the new International Classification of Functioning, Disability, and Health (ICF) created by the World Health Organization has provided both a framework and a

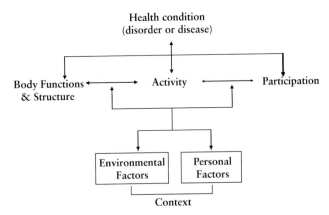

Fig. 31.1 The International Classification of Functioning, Disability and Health (ICF).

classification that comprehensively represents the experience of patients with RA (Fig. 31.1). This classification system also provides a universal language understood by health professionals, researchers, policy makers, and patients alike. A brief and a comprehensive set of core measures in RA have been developed[20]. The ICF provides a means of mapping different factors that describe the process of functioning and disability. Three components constitute the ICF: body functioning and structure, activities and participation, and environmental factors. Unlike the preceding ICIDH 1, the ICF has been approved by the World Health Assembly, and all of the member states have been asked to implement the classification system. In conclusion, the ICF represents the currently most promising classification tool which offers a framework for assessing the multidimensional impacts of RA[21].

Health status and health-related quality of life

It is widely accepted that quality of life measures should be included in all clinical studies. However, controversies still exist regarding definitions and concepts. Muldoon and coworkers[22] have suggested a simple framework for description of the core elements of quality of life related to health status. They propose a division into functional status and subjective well-being and, further, to divide health into physical and mental domains. As shown in Fig. 31.2, assessment of physical functioning (top left) involves measuring the ability to perform specific tasks (e.g. activities of daily living or climbing stairs) as well as less easily-defined concepts related to role performance (e.g. the ability to continue employment as a carpenter). Thus, the measurement of physical functioning is in many respects similar to the assessment of physical disability. Mental functioning (Fig. 31.2, bottom left) is reflected in the patient's ability to meet cognitive and social challenges ranging from specific tasks to complex social interactions. The complementary perspective on quality of life assigns central importance to individuals' subjective appraisal of their state of health. This definition implies that quality of life is a reflection of the way that the patients perceive and react to their health status and to other non-medical aspects of their lives. Physical well-being (Fig. 31.2, top right) concerns the sense of discomfort arising from a particular symptom and extends to vitality or

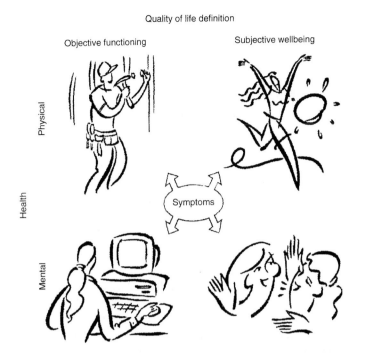

Quality of life definition

Objective functioning   Subjective wellbeing

Physical

Health

Mental

Symptoms

Fig. 31.2 A classification scheme of quality of life measures (daily function and sense of well-being) related to health (mental and physical). (From Ref. 22, reproduced with permission.)

general satisfaction with physical health. A patient's appraisal of his or her mental well-being is usually interpreted as the absence of psychological distress and can also include emotional ties and social support. Thus, a main issue is to distinguish objective functioning from subjective well-being[22].

Depression versus psychological distress

As pointed out by DeVellis[23], there are three different systems for classifying psychiatric disorders and at least twice as many interview schedules that correspond to these classification systems. These schedules have standardized criteria for diagnosing depressive disorders and other types of psychiatric illness. However, diagnostic interviews to classify patients into diagnostic categories take 60–90 min to administer, even with trained personnel[23].

Another and more commonly used approach, in both practice and research, is to examine depressive symptoms and anxiety symptoms by using self-administered instruments. It has been practice to assign cut-off points to self-report symptom scores, resulting in the respondents being classified as above or below some criteria level of depressive symptoms. However, such cut-off points of symptom scores have been insufficiently validated against the gold standard, that is, the interview approach to classify patients into psychiatric disorders.

During the past two decades, self-report questionnaires have gained widespread acceptance as useful tools in rheumatological research[24]. Some instruments have been developed to capture specifically depressive symptoms; others represent disease-specific or generic health status measures where psychological symptoms constitute one out of several dimensions of health that are being measured[25].

Several of the depression scales contain items that are influenced by aspects of the disease process, for example pain and

fatigue, and thus are not necessarily indicative of depression among persons with arthritis. For example The Center for Epidemiological Studies Depression Scale (CES-D) has been shown to include some somatic items that are likely to yield an overestimate of the association between disability and depression[26]. Patients with RA also generally had elevated scores on The Minnesota Multiphasic Personality Inventory (MMPI) scales for hypochondriasis, depression, and hysteria. Largely, five disease-related MMPI statements explained these elevated scale scores where patients with RA and normal subjects differed significantly in their responses[27].

Thus, questionnaires which include items tapping somatic symptoms may easily inflate estimates of the prevalence and severity of depressive symptoms among patients with RA[27,28], a phenomenon which is often called criterion contamination[28,29]. Suggested remedies to these problems include either to eliminate somatically related items from an instrument, or to increase the threshold for labeling symptoms of distress as suggestive of significant mental problems[28].

Measures of psychological health status

Several instruments are available to measure psychological health status (for review see Refs 25, 30–32). It has been agreed that health status represents one of five core domains that should be included in every longitudinal observational study of patients with rheumatic diseases. Within the domain of health status are listed subdomains such as quality of life/health status instruments, recording of symptoms, physical function, and measurement of psychosocial function[14].

Several instruments have been developed to measure psychological well-being and psychological symptoms. Important examples are the CES-D[26], the MMPI scales[27], and the General Health Questionnaire (GHQ)[33].

The multidimensional health status measures are most commonly used in RA patients, both in clinical practice and for research purposes. Examples of such measures are the generic instruments Short Form-36 Health Survey (SF-36), the Sickness Impact Profile (SIP) and the Nottingham Health Profile (NHP), and the disease-specific Arthritis Impact Measurement Scales (AIMS). All these measures contain scales capturing psychological symptoms.

The SF-36 measures eight of the most commonly used dimensions in health surveys. It contains 36 items, and is scored as eight multi-item scales plus one item measuring a self-evaluated change in health status. The SF-36 is a generic measure, meaning that its concepts are not specific to any age, disease, or treatment group. This allows for comparisons of the relative burdens of different diseases, and benefits of different treatments. It is suitable for self-administration. The eight multi-item scales are as follows: physical functioning (10 items), role limitations due to physical health (4 items), bodily pain (2 items), general health (5 items), vitality/energy/fatigue (4 items), social functioning (2 items), role limitations due to emotional problems (3 items), and mental health (5 items), plus the one item measure on reported health transition. Each scale has a score span of 0–100, where 100 represents the best health[34,35]. It performs similarly to disease specific measures in RA[36].

The SIP comprises 136 statements in 12 categories[37]. It consists of statements such 'I have difficulty reasoning and solving problems' and 'I laugh and cry suddenly'. The different items describe behaviors related to the following categories: sleep and rest, eating, work, home management, recreation and pastimes, ambulation, mobility, body care and movement, social interaction, alertness behavior, emotional behavior, and communication. It has been widely used in rheumatic diseases[38], but is rather time consuming. Therefore, a modified Shorter Sickness Impact Profile has also been validated in RA[39].

Part I of the NHP contains 38 items grouped in six subscales: physical abilities, sleep, social isolation, emotional reactions, pain, and energy[40]. Each item has a yes/no response to statements about health problems, for example 'I'm tired all the time', 'I feel as if I'm losing control', and 'I feel that life is not worth living'. Part II provides a brief indicator of handicap and contains seven items that record effect of health problems on occupations, jobs around the house, personal relationships, social life, sex life, hobbies, and holidays. The NHP is frequently used in different diseases and settings, but has a relatively complicated scoring, based on a weighting system.

The AIMS is a self-administered, multidimensional health status measure developed for use in arthritis patients. The psychometric properties of the instrument have been extensively examined[41,42]. The original AIMS questionnaire contained 45 items grouped into scales covering nine different areas. These scales could be combined to produce an overall score of health status with three or five components. Among the scales were one for assessing anxiety (six items) and one for symptoms of depression (six items). The item scores are added, and the sum is transformed to a 0–10 scale, with higher scores indicating more severe distress. With respect to the AIMS depression subscale, threshold values indicating possible and probable depression have been established in United States patients with RA[43].

A revised AIMS2[44] contains a total of 78 questions, of which the first 57 items are combined into 12 scales: mobility (five items), walking and bending (five items), hand and finger function (five items), arm function (five items), self-care tasks (four items), household tasks (four items), social activity (five items), support from family and friends (five items), arthritis pain (five items), work (four items), level of tension (five items), and mood (five items). One additional item estimates the overall impact of arthritis, and three items explore comorbidity. The scales may be combined into a five-component model reflecting the physical dimension (mobility level, walking and bending, hand and finger function, arm function, self-care tasks, household tasks), affect (level of tension, mood), symptoms (pain), social interaction (social activity, support from family and friends), and role (work). A short form of AIMS2 (SF-AIMS2) has been validated in both French and Norwegian patient populations and seems to perform well[45,46].

An instrument to detect psychological and psychosocial severity in RA and osteoarthritis was developed by Wolfe and Skevington[47]. The instrument is called the Rheumatology Distress Index (RDI), and is a self-report questionnaire made up of five variables, anxiety, depression, global severity, fatigue, and sleep disturbance. The instrument aims at offering a simple and easy to administer questionnaire that can be used to classify patients according to their level of distress. Pincus _et al._ have also developed a multidimensional health assessment questionnaire (MDHAQ) that includes items on demanding physical activities, but also on pain, fatigue, anxiety, and depression[48].

Measures of social health status

The term social health status has no universal definition. It seems appropriate to differentiate between two dimensions: one dimension is related to the _social functioning_ of the patient, that is, his/her relations to other individuals. The other is related to the patient's _ability to work_, and to the _monetary consequences_ of the disease, that is, to the economic burden for the patient and his/her family due to work disability, loss of income, and extra costs.

The social functioning may be measured by several of the multidimensional health status measures, both generic and disease specific, reviewed above. The scales measuring social functioning reflect the patients' social relationships rather than occupational aspects. For instance, the AIMS2 score for social interaction is an aggregate score for the components of support from family and social activity. The social functioning score in SF-36 is computed from the scores of two items that are related to health problems interfering with social activities and contact with family and friends.

The work status as well as the direct and indirect costs may be measured through questionnaires or interview. These variables are highly influenced by the social welfare, the availability of health service, and differences in socioeconomic systems across countries[14].

Psychological health status in rheumatoid arthritis

Anxiety and depression are prevalent problems in patients with RA[49,50]. Different studies present various prevalences of anxiety and depression in RA, which is not surprising since different instruments have been used. Creed[51] reviewed several studies and found that the reported prevalence of depression in RA patients varied from 0 to 53.5%; the majority having prevalences around 20–30%. Eberhardt _et al._[52] examined the psychological distress and several other outcomes in 84 early RA patients followed prospectively for two years. They found that the scores on the Symptom Check List (SCL-90) generally were not very pronounced, and fairly stable over time[52]. VanDyke _et al._[53] examined the level of anxiety experienced by individuals with RA and found significantly higher levels of both state and trait anxiety than a normative group of age-equivalent adults. Furthermore, high correlations between anxiety and both depression and stress were found, whereas no relation was found to disease duration. In a study by Dickens _et al._[54], 39% of the sample of 74 patients with RA were classified as being depressed using standardized research interviews. Furthermore, depressed patients had more marked social difficulties that were partly related to their disease, and partly not.

Prevalences of depression and other psychological dysfunction have mainly been studied in clinical samples identified through rheumatology practices or hospital settings. This approach has limitations as the results do not necessarily reflect the situation

Table 31.1 Mean (SD) scores of health status obtained in 2001 from 962 patients with RA from the RA county register in Oslo, Norway

Scales	Total (*n* = 962)	< 40 years (*n* = 60)	40–49 years (*n* = 120)	50–59 years (*n* = 170)	60–69 years (*n* = 204)	70–79 years (*n* = 276)	> 80 Years (*n* = 132)
SF-36 (0–100, 0 worst health)							
Physical	50.1	73.0	63.0	56.2	49.7	42.7	35.6
functioning	(26.6)	(20.3)	(23.9)	(23.5)	(24.8)	(25.6)	(25.9)
Role physical	28.4	53.4	47.8	30.5	30.0	17.6	15.6
	(36.9)	(42.3)	(41.3)	(36.8)	(35.8)	(30.6)	(29.0)
Bodily pain	42.9	52.1	48.8	43.4	43.7	39.3	38.6
	(22.3)	(23.8)	(23.1)	(22.3)	(19.8)	(21.8)	(23.1)
General health	45.2	51.2	49.6	45.8	46.0	40.4	45.9
	(22.1)	(24.2)	(23.3)	(22.5)	(22.7)	(19.2)	(22.2)
Vitality	41.8	47.5	44.9	41.5	44.3	38.5	39.9
	(22.1)	(19.9)	(22.5)	(22.8)	(21.3)	(22.6)	(20.8)
Social functioning	65.7	74.4	75.0	66.2	69.2	60.0	58.6
	(28.3)	(28.5)	(25.2)	(28.0)	(26.4)	(28.6)	(29.8)
Role emotional	53.6	73.0	70.0	60.2	56.5	42.8	36.8
	(42.3)	(37.7)	(40.8)	(42.0)	(41.2)	(40.4)	(40.4)
Mental health	70.1	73.1	74.9	71.0	72.6	66.5	66.9
	(20.1)	(17.9)	(18.5)	(19.5)	(19.7)	(20.6)	(21.6)
MHAQ (1–4, 4 worst health)	1.61	1.32	1.41	1.57	1.60	1.71	1.78
	(0.54)	(0.43)	(0.40)	(0.48)	(0.48)	(0.61)	(0.62)
AIMS 2 (0–10, 10 worst health)							
Physical	2.43	1.31	1.66	2.00	2.22	2.88	3.65
	(1.88)	(1.27)	(1.38)	(1.44)	(1.68)	(2.03)	(2.15)
Affect	3.32	3.03	3.05	3.32	3.07	3.63	3.48
	(1.76)	(1.58)	(1.77)	(1.59)	(1.74)	(1.81)	(1.91)
Symptom (pain)	4.97	4.08	4.41	4.92	4.87	5.51	4.99
	(2.61)	(2.70)	(2.52)	(2.55)	(2.53)	(2.57)	(2.75)
Social interaction	4.07	3.63	3.94	4.20	3.97	4.18	4.14
	(1.62)	(1.50)	(1.47)	(1.53)	(1.53)	(1.74)	(1.81)
VAS (0–100, 100 worst health)							
Pain	36.5	25.4	30.0	34.5	37.8	40.3	41.3
	(24.8)	(23.0)	(22.8)	(23.4)	(24.5)	(24.9)	(26.7)
Fatigue	47.3	39.1	44.9 (27.7)	46.2	47.7	49.6	49.6
	(29.3)	(30.6)	(27.7)	(29.3)	(29.1)	(28.9)	(30.8)

VAS, visual analog scale.

for the population sample of patients with RA. Data collected in 2001 from the patient population in the Oslo RA register are presented in Table 31.1. This register has been validated for its completeness[55]. The patients have self-reported their health status on visual analogue scales, and on generic (SF-36) and disease-specific (AIMS2) health status measures. The health status scores from this representative sample of RA patients demonstrate how self-reported levels of physical disability, but also mental distress, increase with increasing age (Table 31.1). Data from this register have indicated that the overall health of patients with RA has improved from 1994 to 2001. Scores for psychological distress were only numerically improved whereas statistically significant improvement was observed for physical functioning and pain[56].

Rather few studies have compared the magnitude of psychological problems between patients and healthy controls. Katz and Yelin[57] assessed depressive symptoms in RA with the Geriatric Depression Scale (GDS). Data were collected annually from 1986 through 1990. Sample sizes declined by about 7% each year of the study reflecting subject attrition due to death, refusal, and loss to follow-up. A cut-off point of 7 or greater on the GDS was used to define the presence of depressive symptoms; 15–17% of persons reported depressive symptoms each year, 4% every year, and over 29% equaled or exceeded the cut-off point in at least one year. To put these findings in perspective, Katz provided data on a comparison group of people without RA that were given the GDS between 1989 and 1991. The proportion of these people who exceeded the cut-off point of 7 between 1989 and 1991 ranged from 3 to 5%[23].

A Norwegian group of 238 RA patients aged up to 70 years and with disease duration of maximum four years was examined for psychological distress and compared with 116 healthy controls matched with respect to sex, age, and geographical area[58]. Psychological distress was measured by a generic self-report instrument, namely the GHQ. The patients reported significantly more severe mental distress than the controls. This was so for the GHQ sum score reflecting global mental distress as well as for each of the four subscales measuring symptoms of anxiety and depression, somatization, and social dysfunction, respectively. Twenty per cent of the patients had GHQ sum score values indicating possible psychiatric caseness compared to 6% of the controls. The percentage of *possible* depressive cases among patients was 22 when the AIMS depressive subscale was used as an indicator of possible caseness, whereas 11% were classified as *probable* psychiatric cases[58]. In another study, Gilboe *et al.*[59] found that RA and systemic lupus erythematosus (SLE) patients had consistently worse SF-36 health status scores compared with healthy individuals.

Psychological problems do not seem to be greater in RA than in other chronic rheumatic diseases. Hawley and Wolfe used 19 122 AIMS depression scores to compare depressive symptoms and scores between various rheumatic diseases. Depressive symptoms and depression scores in RA did not differ from other clinical patients taken as a whole and were less pronounced than in patients with fibromyalgia[43]. Matched RA and SLE patients had similar SF-36 scores within the dimension of mental health and role limitations due to emotional problems[59].

Social health status in RA

Some of the multidimensional generic and disease-specific health status measures also capture the social functioning, which reflects the patients' social relationships rather than occupational aspects. SF-36 and AIMS2 scores obtained by postal surveys to a community-based RA sample in Oslo are shown in Table 31.1. In a comparative study, Gilboe *et al*[59] have shown that the SF-36 social functioning score is similar between RA and SLE patients and lower (worse health) compared to matched, healthy controls.

Several studies have shown that RA with time is associated with a considerable work disability and decreased earnings[52,60,61]. Wolfe[13] reviewed four studies of work disability in a total of more than 2000 RA patients. These studies showed that approximately half of the patients were work disabled after about 10 years of disease. Pincus[62] has discussed the underestimated long-term medical and economic consequences of RA and documented that more than 50% of patients with RA less than 65 years, and who were working at onset of disease, received work disability payments.

In a study addressing work disability in relation to psychiatric comorbidity among patients with inflammatory rheumatic diseases, Lowe *et al.*[63] found that work disability was significantly affected by psychiatric comorbidity. Depression accordingly constitutes an independent risk factor of work disability in patients with inflammatory rheumatic disease.

Indirect costs account for activities that are foregone as a result of the disease. These activities may include paid or unpaid labor and tasks such as shopping, gardening, etc.[64]. Indirect costs in clinical samples of RA exceed direct costs and most of the indirect costs are related to wage losses[65]. Population studies have shown major earning gaps between individuals with symmetric polyarthritis and those in the general population[62].

How are psychological variables related to disease factors?

Relationships between psychological variables and disease factors have traditionally been examined as one-way directional effects, either by studying the disease impact in terms of psychological outcome, or by studying the impacts on clinical status by psychological variables. However, one-way directional effects between physical and psychological variables in RA are too simplistic. Even prospective, longitudinal studies with multiple time points will have difficulties testing causal models which allow for reciprocal (two-way) causation and feedback loops. This is probably the main reason why studies exploring causal relationships between psychosocial and physical variables in RA are relatively scarce. Nevertheless, the question of directionality is a key issue as evidence of causality may have considerable impact on clinical practice. If, for example, depression is a factor that enhances the pain level and not vice versa, then drug management of depression would be a therapeutic option to improve pain. If, on the other hand, pain is a primary phenomenon and depression secondary, pain treatment would be the major challenge, and successful treatment of pain could be expected to lead to lower levels of depression. Studies exploring these relationships can be divided into cross-sectional and longitudinal. The cross-sectional design has limitations because only relations between variables can be explored, whereas causal relationships can only be examined in studies using a longitudinal design.

Several cross-sectional studies have examined the relationships between pain and psychological distress and between disease activity variables and psychological measures. As expected, most of these studies have found significant correlations between anxiety and depression on one side, and pain and disability on the other. Weaker, but significant correlation has been found between joint counts acute phase reactants and depression/anxiety[66-68]. Multivariate analyses have also been used in these cross-sectional studies to identify primary versus secondary phenomena. Several studies have indicated that, for example, chronic pain adversely impacts on mood, and not supported the opposing hypothesis that negative mood is a predisposing factor in the development of chronic pain[67].

Different designs have been used for the longitudinal studies. Krotty *et al.*[69] examined 75 young women (median age 43 years) with early RA on frequent occasions, with a wide range of disease activity and disability measures (HAQ), and psychosocial variables. Psychosocial variables were as important as disease and pain in determining function. The result suggests that interventions based on the importance of maintaining social relationships could have impact on function. This study also demonstrates that complicated statistical approaches are required to show directional relationships in longitudinal studies.

Hawley and Wolfe[70] studied psychological and clinical factors in 400 patients with RA examined at six-month intervals over a mean of three years using the AIMS psychological scales. Development of depression was associated with socioeconomic but not clinical factors, and disease activity appeared to have a limited effect on psychological status. Initial psychological scores were associated with subsequent pain levels and number of physician visits. The same group later analyzed data from 713 patients with RA attending at two subsequent clinic visits[71]. Six demographic and seven clinical variables were assessed, including the AIMS depression score. They found that clinical changes explained about 20% of depressive changes between visits, while 34% of current depression scores were explained by demographic and clinical variables. Thus, changes in pain and disability score predicted changes in depression.

In a study by Affleck *et al.*[72], patients who described themselves as more depressed on a depression scale also reported more intense pain across the recording period, independent of the level of disease activity and disability.

Smedstad *et al.*[73] examined 216 RA patients annually for two years for symptoms of anxiety and depression measured by the Arthritis Impact Measurement Scales, tender joint counts, erythrocyte sedimentation rate (ESR), self-reported pain, measured by visual analogue scales, and disability measured by the Health Assessment Questionnaire. Strong cross-sectional relationships were found between symptoms of anxiety and depression, respectively, and the other clinical variables. Using a multivariate approach, pain and disability consistently were the two variables most strongly related to symptoms of anxiety and depression, whereas tender joint counts and ESR did not contribute significantly

to the explained variance in mental distress. High levels of disability predicted an increase in depressive symptoms over the next year. Otherwise, changes in psychological distress could not be predicted by the disease-related variables. However, the current level of mental distress significantly predicted the level of mental distress one year ahead, a finding which demonstrates the stability of mental distress over time. Exploring directional models between the one-year change in mental distress, and pain and disability, respectively, the only statistically significant finding was that a high level of disability at baseline significantly predicted an increase in depressive symptoms over the next year. Otherwise, the attempts at causal modeling failed to yield consistent results (Figs 31.3 and 31.4)[73].

Another methodological approach was used in a study showing that psychological distress was higher in 238 RA patients than in sex- and age-matched healthy controls[58]. When disease factors were introduced as covariates the group difference disappeared.

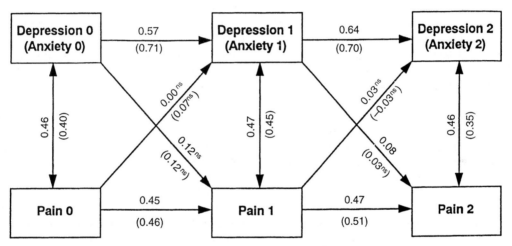

Fig. 31.3 Cross-lagged relationships between depression (anxiety) and pain at baseline (0), after one and two years' follow-up. Double-headed arrows show Pearson's correlation coefficients (r). Single-headed arrows show standard regression coefficients (beta values). ns, not significant at the 5% level. Other coefficients significant at the 5% level. (From Ref. 73, reproduced with permission.)

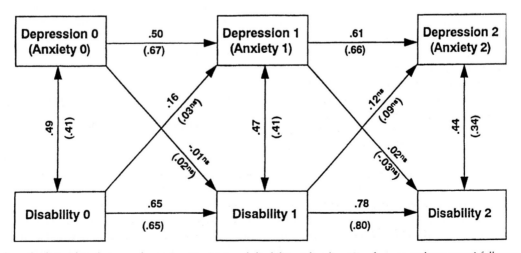

Fig. 31.4 Cross-lagged relationships between depression (anxiety) and disability at baseline (0), after one and two years' follow-up. Double-headed arrows show Pearson's correlation coefficients (r). Single-headed arrows show standard regression coefficients (beta value). ns, not significant at the 5% level. Other coefficients significant at the 5% level. (From Ref. 73, reproduced with permission.)

Thus cardinal features of RA, disability, pain, and fatigue, were separately able to explain the difference in psychological distress between patients and controls. This finding indicates that these three variables may act as mediators between the underlying disease process and mental distress[58]. The same cohort of patients have been followed longitudinally and the level of psychological distress was stable over time[74].

Katz and Yelin[75] have examined the role of function and functional changes in the development of depressive symptoms among women with RA. They found that loss of valued activities was a significant risk factor for developing depressive symptoms, whereas overall functional decline was not a significant risk factor. Thus, their study highlights that disability measures do not predict psychological symptoms, in contrast to measures that capture concepts that are valued by the patients[75]. In a study by Evers et al.[76] examining long-term predictors of anxiety and depressed mood in early RA, a worse clinical status, more neuroticism, and a lower educational level at the time of diagnoses were all significantly related to increased psychological distress three and five years later. The authors conclude that patient characteristics may predict the long-term susceptibility to distress in patients with early RA. Sharpe and colleagues[77] found that a set of five factors consistently predicted depression at recent onset RA at the following assessment. These were initial level of depression, disability, pain, beliefs about the consequences of arthritis, and coping strategies.

In summary, it appears that psychological variables are strongly correlated to disease variables, especially pain and disability, but consistent causal relationships have not been identified. However, most data indicate that psychological distress more frequently is a secondary consequence of the disease rather than vice versa.

The role of life events, coping, social support, and other intervening variables

Possible directional relationships between disease variables and psychological variables become even more complex if some potentially mediating factors are also considered, including life events, coping, and social support. Conway et al.[78] found, in a study of 60 consecutive outpatients with RA, a non-significant trend for an excess of life events before onset of disease compared with after. Other investigations indicate that negative life events may worsen the disease, and positive events may lead to improvement[79,80].

Several authors have suggested that social support is a powerful modulating factor. Fyrand et al. found that patients with RA had a smaller network than healthy controls[81], that disease duration correlated inversely with daily emotional support, and that high physical disability was associated with less social companionship[82]. In a randomized study the network intervention group reported an increase in network size[83]. However, more research is required to explore the independent role of social support

and social network on the perceived health status of patients with RA[84–86].

Coping factors gain importance from the observation that coping attitudes and behavior can be modified by interventions. Thus, understanding coping may explain some discrepancies between individual disease severity factors and health impact of the disease. A typical definition of coping is 'the cognitive, behavioral and emotional efforts individuals exert to manage specific external and/or internal demands'[87]. Examples of helpful coping strategies comprise information seeking, reorganization of routines, denial, wish fulfillment, distraction, seeking social support, expressing emotions, and seeking spiritual support[87]. Passive and active coping strategies have to be distinguished.

Self-efficacy in rheumatic diseases has been examined in an attempt to explain variations in pain and health status over time. In an observational study by Brekke et al.[88], 306 patients with RA were followed over five years, assessing changes in self-efficacy and health status. The authors found that the baseline level of self-efficacy seemed to influence future level of perceived pain, whereas baseline mental health status seemed to influence future self-efficacy[88]. In another study Brekke and coworkers[89] found differences in levels of self-efficacy as well as in patient-reported health between patients living in an affluent and non-affluent area of Oslo. Thus, even in a welfare society with universal access to healthcare, the disease impact seemed to be closely linked to the patient's socioeconomic situation[89].

With time, patients may improve their psychological adaptation as the patients learn to adjust to the disease and perhaps alter expectations. Time since diagnosis is associated with improved psychological well-being, controlling statistically for changes in disability[66]. Seeking information about the disease has also been found to be associated with improved outcome. Cognitive restructuring, which involves attempting to alter the patient's views or thoughts about the disease to be more positive, also leads to improved psychological well-being[87]. Newman et al.[90] divided a large sample of patients attending an outpatient rheumatology clinic into four distinct groups who attempted to cope with their disease in different ways. The four groups were almost indistinguishable on arthritis measures, but the patient group applying active coping strategies was found to report lower levels of pain and stiffness in addition to disability. They also had significantly higher levels of psychological well-being[90]. Identification of coping strategies also has implications for health education practice[91].

How are social variables related to disease factors?

Several studies have shown that work disability is associated with job characteristics, but also with the disease severity[13,52]. In a sample of 421 RA patients working at the time of the first clinic visit, six variables were independently associated with future work disability: VAS pain, rheumatoid factor, completion of high school, depression, body mass index, and joint count. Thus, work disability is explained by RA disease factors and psychosocial factors, as well as by job characteristics and setting[13]. In a

Swedish study, early retirement was predicted by physically demanding work and a high initial disability score[52]. In a more recent study Mau *et al.*[92] examined the occurrence of permanent work disability in prognostic groups of patients with RA. They examined 73 gainfully employed consecutive outpatients who were re-examined after a mean follow-up of six years. Permanent work disability occurred in 27 out of the 73 patients (37%). Age, disease activity, functional class, and strenuous job-related physical requirements appeared to be determinants of the permanent work disability. No case of permanent work disability occurred in 21 individuals aged less than 50 years, with a joint count less than 15, and less physically demanding jobs.

Therapeutic implications

Patients with RA frequently experience psychological and social problems. This calls for a biopsychosocial approach in the understanding and management of the patients. One major issue of therapeutic importance is the question of causal relationships between psychosocial health status on the one hand and traditional disease factors on the other. Several studies have demonstrated relationships between levels of psychological distress, pain, and disease activity, but consistent causal relationships have not been found[73].

A reasonable approach for patients with active disease, excess pain problems, and depressive symptoms, would therefore be to target the therapy against each of these disease manifestations. It will usually not be appropriate to refer a patient for therapy of the depressive symptoms without simultaneously considering adequate anti-inflammatory and or anti-rheumatic medication and relief of pain. Despite the lack of consistent causal relationships between psychological and traditional disease variables, there is more evidence suggesting that, for example, psychological distress appears as a phenomenon secondary to disease factors than as a factor aggravating arthritis activity[71,73]. However, it seems that all of these factors interact in complex reciprocal patterns that, so far, are poorly understood. As some of these variables represent opportunities for therapeutic interventions, it seems reasonable to have a wide therapeutic approach to hopefully counteract negative feedback loops leading to excess dysfunction and suffering.

Coping behavior may influence psychological and social functioning[93]. Cognitive behavioral patient education programs may improve health status[94-96]. In a blinded, randomized controlled trial by Sharpe *et al.*[97], half of the sample of patients with recent onset RA were allocated to receive a cognitive behavioral treatment of eight weeks' duration in addition to routine medical management. The group receiving adjunctive psychological intervention showed a reduction in depressive symptoms at both post-treatment and at six-month follow-up. Furthermore, the intervention group showed significant improvement in joint involvement at six month follow-up. This improvement was maintained over the ensuing 18 months, although similar improvements were seen in the group receiving routine clinical care[98]. The authors conclude that cognitive behavioral treatment offered as an adjunct to standard clinical management early in the course of RA is efficacious in producing improvements in both psychological and physical indices. However, in a study by Parker *et al.*[99] examining the effectiveness of a cognitive behavioral approach and pharmacologic treatment of depression in RA, cognitive behavioral approaches to the management of depression were not found to be additive to antidepressant medication alone. With respect to the effects of patient education programs in RA, this issue was reviewed in a meta-analysis by Riemsma *et al.*[100,101]. The authors included 31 studies in their review. Substantial evidence of the long-term effects of patient education programs in rheumatology seems limited, although several studies indicate a short-term improvement in health status. Lorig *et al.*[95,102] found that improvement in health status subsequent to the arthritis self-management program was probably mediated through improved self-efficacy.

Many studies have documented that various rehabilitation interventions are effective[103,104]. Furthermore, a biopsychosocial therapeutic approach also means a multidisciplinary approach. Hill *et al.*[105] compared the effect on disease course of a follow-up system with either a rheumatology nurse practitioner or a consultant rheumatologist. In the patients managed by the nurse practitioner pain, morning stiffness, psychological status, patient knowledge, and satisfaction had all improved significantly. One explanation might be that the patient managed by the nurse practitioner received more efficient information and educational material. More attention was probably also given to psychological factors as well as coping strategies.

In summary, these studies suggest that the organization of the healthcare system may be important and that the teamwork between nurse, rheumatologist, and other health professionals may lead to a more successful outcome when more time and attention is given to the psychosocial well-being of the patient. Psychosocial variables represent important outcome variables as well as predictors of an unfavorable outcome. As a consequence, the therapy has to target both biological and psychosocial aspects of the disease.

References

1. Pincus, T., and Callahan, L. F. Reassessment of twelve traditional paradigms concerning the diagnosis, prevalence, morbidity and mortality of rheumatoid arthritis. *Scand J Rheumatol* 1989; **18** (Suppl. 79): 67–96.
2. Liang, M. H., and Katz, J. N. Measurement of outcome in rheumatoid arthritis. *Baillieres Clin Rheumatol* 1992; **6**: 23–37.
3. Newman, S., and Mulligan, K. The psychology of rheumatic diseases. *Baillieres Best Pract Res Clin Rheumatol* 2000; **14**: 773–86.
4. Engel, G. L. The need for a new medical model: a challenge for biomedicine. *Science* 1977; **196**: 129–36.
5. Green, S. A. Supportive psychologic care of the medically ill: a synthesis of the biopsychosocial approach in medical care. In *Human Behavior: An Introduction for Medical Students* (Stoudemire, A., ed.), pp. 323–38. Philadelphia: J. B. Lippincott; 1990.
6. Shipley, M., and Newman, S. P. Psychological aspects of rheumatic diseases. *Baillieres Clin Rheumatol* 1993; **7**: 215–19.
7. Wegener, S. T. Psychosocial aspects of rheumatic disease: the developing biopsychosocial framework. *Curr Opin Rheumatol* 1991; **3**: 300–4.

8. Pincus, T. Formal educational level: a marker for the importance of behavioral variables in the pathogenesis, morbidity, and mortality of most diseases? *J Rheumatol* 1988; **15**: 1457–60.

9. Wells, K. B., Golding, J. M., and Burnam, M. A. Psychiatric disorder in a sample of the general population with and without chronic medical conditions. *Am J Psychiatry* 1988; **145**: 976–81.

10. Magni, G., Marchetti, M., Moreschi, C., Merskey, H., and Luchini, S. R. Chronic musculoskeletal pain and depressive symptoms in the National Health and Nutrition Examination. I. Epidemiologic follow-up study. *Pain* 1993; **53**: 163–8.

11. Magni, G., Caldieron, C., Rigatti-Luchini, S., and Merskey, H. Chronic musculoskeletal pain and depressive symptoms in the general population: an analysis of the 1st National Health and Nutrition Examination Survey data. *Pain* 1990; **43**: 299–307.

12. Fries, J. F., Spitz, P., Kraines, R. G., and Holman, H. R. Measurement of patient outcome in arthritis. *Arthritis Rheum* 1980; **23**: 137–45.

13. Wolfe, F. The natural history of rheumatoid arthritis. *J Rheumatol* 1996; **23** (Suppl. 44): 13–22.

14. Wolfe, F., Lassere, M., van der Heijde, D., Stucki, G., Suarez-Almazor, M., Pincus, T. *et al.* Preliminary core set of domains and reporting requirements for longitudinal observational studies in rheumatology. *J Rheumatol* 1999; **26**: 484–9.

15. Badley, E. M. The genesis of handicap: definition, models of disablement, and role of external factors. *Disabil Rehabil* 1995; **17**: 53–62.

16. Fitzpatrick, F., and Badley, E. M. An overview of disability. *Br J Rheumatol* 1996; **35**: 184–7.

17. Carr, A. J., and Thompson, P. W. Towards a measure of patient-perceived handicap in rheumatoid arthritis. *Br J Rheumatol* 1994; **33**: 378–82.

18. Carr, A. J., Thompson, P. W., and Kirwan, J. R. Quality of life measures. *Br J Rheumatol* 1996; **35**: 275–81.

19. Harwood, R. H., Gompertz, P., and Ebrahim, S. Handicap one year after a stroke: validity of a new scale. *J Neurol Neurosurg Psychiatry* 1994; **57**: 825–9.

20. Stucki, G., Cieza, A., Geyh, S., Battistella, L., Lloyd, J., Symmons, D. *et al.* ICF Core Sets for rheumatoid arthritis. *J Rehabil Med* 2004; **44**: 87–93.

21. Stucki, G., and Cieza, A. The International Classification of Functioning, Disability and Health (ICF) Core Sets for rheumatoid arthritis: a way to specify functioning. *Ann Rheum Dis* 2004; **63**: ii40–ii45.

22. Muldoon, M. F., Barger, S. D., Flory, J. D., and Manuck, S. B. What are quality of life measurements measuring? *BMJ* 1998; **316**: 542–5.

23. DeVellis, B. M. The psychological impact of arthritis: prevalence of depression. *Arthritis Care Res* 1995; **8**: 284–9.

24. Pincus, T., Callahan, L. F., Brooks, R. H., Fuchs, H. A., Olsen, N. J., and Kaye, J. J. Self-report questionnaire scores in rheumatoid arthritis compared with traditional physical, radiographic, and laboratory measures. *Ann Intern Med* 1989; **110**: 259–66.

25. Wolfe, F. Practical issues in psychosocial measures. *J Rheumatol* 1997; **24**: 990–3.

26. Blalock, S. J., DeVellis, R. F., Brown, G. K., and Wallston, K. A. Validity of the Center for Epidemiological Studies Depression Scale in arthritis populations. *Arthritis Rheum* 1989; **32**: 991–7.

27. Pincus, T., Callahan, L. F., Bradley, L. A., Vaughn, W. K., and Wolfe, F. Elevated MMPI scores for hypochondriasis, depression, and hysteria in patients with rheumatoid arthritis reflect disease rather than psychological status. *Arthritis Rheum* 1986; **29**: 1456–66.

28. DeVellis, B. M. Depression in rheumatological diseases. *Baillieres Clin Rheumatol* 1993; **7**: 241–57.

29. Pincus, T., and Callahan, L. F. Depression scales in rheumatoid arthritis: criterion contamination in interpretation of patient responses. *Patient Educ Couns* 1993; **20**: 133–43.

30. McDowell, I., and Newell, C. *Measuring Health*, 2nd edn. New York: Oxford University Press; 1996.

31. Bellamy, N. *Musculoskeletal Clinical Metrology*. Dordrecht: Kluwer Academic; 1993.

32. Brooks, P., McFarlane, A. C., Newman, S., and Rasker, J. J. Psychosocial measures. *J Rheumatol* 1997; **24**: 1008–11.

33. Goldberg, D., and Williams, P. *A User's Guide to the General Health Questionnaire*. Windsor: NFER-Nelson; 1988.

34. Ware, J. E., Jr., and Sherbourne, C. D. The MOS 36-item short-form health survey (SF-36). I. Conceptual framework and item selection. *Med Care* 1992; **30**: 473–83.

35. McHorney, C. A., Ware, J. E., Jr., Lu, J. F., and Sherbourne, C. D. The MOS 36-item Short-Form Health Survey (SF-36): III. Tests of data quality, scaling assumptions, and reliability across diverse patient groups. *Med Care* 1994; **32**: 40–66.

36. Kvien, T. K., Kaasa, S., and Smedstad, L. M. Performance of the Norwegian SF-36 Health Survey in patients with rheumatoid arthritis. II. A comparison of the SF-36 with disease-specific measures. *J Clin Epidemiol* 1998; **51**: 1077–86.

37. Bergner, M., Bobbitt, R. A., Kressel, S., Pollard, W. E., Gilson, B. S., and Morris, J. R. The Sickness Impact Profile: conceptual formulation and methodology for the development of a health status measure. *Int J Health Serv* 1976; **6**: 393–415.

38. Sullivan, M., Ahlmen, M., and Bjelle, A. Health status assessment in rheumatoid arthritis. I. Further work on the validity of the sickness impact profile. *J Rheumatol* 1990; **17**: 439–47.

39. Sullivan, M., Ahlmen, M., Bjelle, A., and Karlsson, J. Health status assessment in rheumatoid arthritis. II. Evaluation of a modified Shorter Sickness Impact Profile. *J Rheumatol* 1993; **20**: 1500–7.

40. Hunt, S. M., McEwen, J., and McKenna, S. P. Measuring health status: a new tool for clinicians and epidemiologists. *J R Coll Gen Pract* 1985; **35**: 185–8.

41. Meenan, R. F., Gertman, P. M., and Mason, J. H. Measuring health status in arthritis: the Arthritis Impact Measurement Scales. *Arthritis Rheum* 1980; **23**: 146–52.

42. Meenan, R. F., Gertman, P. M., Mason, J. H., and Dunaif, R. The arthritis impact measurement scales: further investigations of a health status measure. *Arthritis Rheum* 1982; **25**: 1048–53.

43. Hawley, D. J., and Wolfe, F. Depression is not more common in rheumatoid arthritis: a 10-year longitudinal study of 6,153 patients with rheumatic disease. *J Rheumatol* 1993; **20**: 2025–31.

44. Meenan, R. F., Mason, J. H., Anderson, J. J., Guccione, A. A., and Kazis, L. E. AIMS2: the content and properties of a revised and expanded Arthritis Impact Measurement Scales Health Status Questionnaire. *Arthritis Rheum* 1992; **35**: 1–10.

45. Guillemin, F., Coste, J., Pouchot, J., Ghezail, M., Bregeon, C., and Sany, J. The AIMS2-SF: a short form of the Arthritis Impact Measurement Scales 2. French Quality of Life in Rheumatology Group. *Arthritis Rheum* 1997; **40**: 1267–74.

46. Haavardsholm, E. A., Kvien, T. K., Uhlig, T., Smedstad, L., and Guillemin, F. A comparison of agreement and sensitivity to change between AIMS2 and short form of AIMS2 (AIMS-SF) in more than 1000 rheumatoid arthritis patients. *J Rheumatol* 2000; **27**: 2810–16.

47. Wolfe, F., and Skevington, S. M. Measuring the epidemiology of distress: the rheumatology distress index. *J Rheumatol* 2000; **27**: 2000–9.

48. Pincus, T., Swearingen, C., and Wolfe, F. Toward a multidimensional Health Assessment Questionnaire (MDHAQ): assessment of advanced activities of daily living and psychological status in the patient-friendly health assessment questionnaire format. *Arthritis Rheum* 1999; **42**: 2220–30.

49. Dickens, C., McGowan, L., Clark-Carter, D., and Creed, F. Depression in rheumatoid arthritis: a systematic review of the literature with meta-analysis. *Psychosom Med* 2002; **64**: 52–60.

50. Soderlin, M. K., Hakala, M., and Nieminen, P. Anxiety and depression in a community-based rheumatoid arthritis population. *Scand J Rheumatol* 2000; **29**: 177–83.

51. Creed, F. Psychological disorders in rheumatoid arthritis: a growing consensus? *Ann Rheum Dis* 1990; **49**: 808–12.

52. Eberhardt, K., Larsson, B. M., and Nived, K. Early rheumatoid arthritis: some social, economical, and psychological aspects. *Scand J Rheumatol* 1993; **22**: 119–23.

53. VanDyke, M. M., Parker, J. C., Smarr, K. L., Hewett, J. E., Johnson, G. E., Slaughter, J. R. *et al.* Anxiety in rheumatoid arthritis. *Arthritis Rheum* 2004; **51**: 408–12.

54. Dickens, C., Jackson, J., Tomenson, B., Hay, E., and Creed, F. Association of depression and rheumatoid arthritis. Psychosomatics 2003; 44: 209–15.

55. Kvien, T. K., Glennås, A., Knudsrød, O. G., Smedstad, L. M., and Førre, Ø. The prevalence and severity of rheumatoid arthritis in Oslo: results from a county register and a population survey. *Scand J Rheumatol* 1997; 26: 412–18.

56. Heiberg, T., Finset, A., Uhlig, T., and Kvien, T. K. Seven year changes in health status and priorities for improvement of health in patients with rheumatoid arthritis. *Ann Rheum Dis* 2005; 64: 191–5.

57. Katz, P. P., and Yelin, E. H. Prevalence and correlates of depressive symptoms among persons with rheumatoid arthritis. *J Rheumatol* 1993; 20: 790–6.

58. Smedstad, L. M., Moum, T., Vaglum, P., and Kvien, T. K. The impact of early rheumatoid arthritis (RA) on subjective well-being and mental distress: a comparison between 238 patients with RA and 116 matched controls. *Scand J Rheumatol* 1996; 25: 377–82.

59. Gilboe, I-M., Kvien, T. K., and Husby, G. Health status in systemic lupus erythematosus compared to rheumatoid arthritis and healthy controls. *J Rheumatol* 1999; 26: 1694–700.

60. Kochevar, R. J., Kaplan, R. M., and Weisman, M. Financial and career losses due to rheumatoid arthritis: a pilot study. *J Rheumatol* 1997; 24: 1527–30.

61. van Jaarsveld, C. H. M., Jacobs, J. W. G., Schrijvers, A. J. P., van Albada-Kuipers, G. A., Hoffman, D. M., and Bijlsma, J. W. J. Effects of rheumatoid arthritis on employment and social participation during the first years of disease in the Netherlands. *Br J Rheumatol* 1998; 37: 848–53.

62. Pincus, T. The underestimated long term medical and economic consequences of rheumatoid arthritis. *Drugs* 1995; 50 (Suppl. 1): 1–14.

63. Lowe, B., Willand, L., Eich, W., Zipfel, S., Ho, A. D., Herzog, W. et al. Psychiatric comorbidity and work disability in patients with inflammatory rheumatic diseases. Psychosom Med 2004; 66: 395–402.

64. Maetzel, A. Costs of illness and the burden of disease. *J Rheumatol* 1997; 24: 3–5.

65. Yelin, E. The costs of rheumatoid arthritis: absolute, incremental, and marginal estimates. *J Rheumatol* 1996; 44 (Suppl.): 47–51.

66. Newman, S. P., Fitzpatrick, R., Lamb, R., and Shipley, M. The origins of depressed mood in rheumatoid arthritis. *J Rheumatol* 1989; 16: 740–4.

67. Smedstad, L. M., Vaglum, P., Kvien, T. K., and Moum, T. The relationship between self-reported pain and sociodemographic variables, anxiety, and depressive symptoms in rheumatoid arthritis. *J Rheumatol* 1995; 22: 514–20.

68. Bendtsen, P., and Hornquist, J. O. Severity of rheumatoid arthritis, function and quality of life: sub-group comparisons. *Clin Exp Rheumatol* 1993; 11: 495–502.

69. Crotty, M., McFarlane, A. C., Brooks, P. M., Hopper, J. L., Bieri, D., and Taylor, S. J. The psychosocial and clinical status of younger women with early rheumatoid arthritis: a longitudinal study with frequent measures. *Br J Rheumatol* 1994; 33: 754–60.

70. Hawley, D. J., and Wolfe, F. Anxiety and depression in patients with rheumatoid arthritis: a prospective study of 400 patients. *J Rheumatol* 1988; 15: 932–41.

71. Wolfe, F., and Hawley, D. J. The relationship between clinical activity and depression in rheumatoid arthritis. *J Rheumatol* 1993; 20: 2032–7.

72. Affleck, G., Tennen, H., Urrows, S., and Higgins, P. Individual differences in the day-to-day experience of chronic pain: a prospective daily study of rheumatoid arthritis patients. *Health Psychol* 1991; 10: 419–26.

73. Smedstad, L. M., Vaglum, P., Moum, T., and Kvien, T. K. The relationship between psychological distress and disease activity: a 2 year old prospective study of 216 patients with early rheumatoid arthritis. *Br J Rheumatol* 1997; 36: 1–8.

74. Uhlig, T., Smedstad, L. M., Vaglum, P., Moum, T., Gerard, N., and Kvien, T. K. The course of rheumatoid arthritis and predictors of psychological, physical and radiographic outcome after 5 years of follow-up. *Rheumatology (Oxford)* 2000; 39: 732–41.

75. Katz, P. P., and Yelin, E. H. The development of depressive symptoms among women with rheumatoid arthritis: the role of function. *Arthritis Rheum* 1995; 38: 49–56.

76. Evers, A. W., Kraaimaat, F. W., Geenen, R., Jacobs, J. W., and Bijlsma, J. W. Longterm predictors of anxiety and depressed mood in early rheumatoid arthritis: a 3 and 5 year followup. *J Rheumatol* 2002; 29: 2327–36.

77. Sharpe, L., Sensky, T., and Allard, S. The course of depression in recent onset rheumatoid arthritis: the predictive role of disability, illness perceptions, pain and coping. *J Psychosom Res* 2001; 51: 713–19.

78. Conway, S. C., Creed, F. H., and Symmons, D. P. M. Life events and the onset of rheumatoid arthritis. *J Psychosom Res* 1994; 38: 837–47.

79. Klages, U. Life events and irrational attitudes in patients with rheumatoid arthritis: relations to pain, disability and general health condition. *Int J Psychosomatics* 1991; 38: 21–6.

80. Smedstad, L. M., Kvien, T. K., Moum, T., and Vaglum, P. Life events, psychosocial factors and demographic variables in early rheumatoid arthritis: relations to one-year changes in functional disability. *J Rheumatol* 1995; 22: 2218–25.

81. Fyrand, L., Moum, T., Wichstrom, L., Finset, A., and Glennas, A. Social network size of female patients with rheumatoid arthritis compared to healthy controls. *Scand J Rheumatol* 2000; 29: 38–43.

82. Fyrand, L., Moum, T., Finset, A., and Glennas, A. The impact of disability and disease duration on social support of women with rheumatoid arthritis. *J Behav Med* 2002; 25: 251–68.

83. Fyrand, L., Moum, T., Finset, A., and Glennas, A. The effect of social network intervention for women with rheumatoid arthritis. *Fam Process* 2003; 42: 71–89.

84. Revenson, T. A. The role of social support with rheumatic disease. *Baillieres Clin Rheumatol* 1993; 7: 377–96.

85. Krol, B., Sanderman, R., and Suurmeijer, T. P. Social support, rheumatoid arthritis and quality of life: concepts, measurement and research. *Patient Educ Couns* 1993; 20: 101–20.

86. Suurmeijer, T. P, Doeglas, D. M., Briancon, S., Krijnen, W. P., Krol, B., Sanderman, R. et al. The measurement of social support in the European research on incapacitating diseases and social support: the development of the social support questionnaire of transactions (SSQT). *Soc Sci Med* 1995; 40: 1221–9.

87. Newman, S. Coping with rheumatoid arthritis. *Ann Rheum Dis* 1993; 52: 553–4.

88. Brekke, M., Hjortdahl, P., and Kvien, T. K. Changes in self-efficacy and health status over 5 years: a longitudinal observational study of 306 patients with rheumatoid arthritis. *Arthritis Rheum* 2003; 49: 342–8.

89. Brekke, M., Hjortdahl, P., Thelle, D. S., and Kvien, T. K. Disease activity and severity in patients with rheumatoid arthritis: relations to socioeconomic inequality. *Soc Sci Med* 1999; 48: 1743–50.

90. Newman, S., Fitzpatrick, R., Lamb, R., and Shipley, M. Patterns of coping in rheumatoid arthritis. *Health Psychol* 1990; 4: 187–200.

91. Blalock, S. J., DeVellis, B. M., Holt, K., and Hahn, P. M. Coping with rheumatoid arthritis: is one problem the same as another? *Health Educ Q* 1993; 20: 119–32.

92. Mau, W., Bornmann, M., Weber, H., Weidemann, H. F., Hecker, H., and Raspe, H. H. Prediction of permanent work disability in a follow-up study of early rheumatoid arthritis: results of a tree structured analysis using RECPAM. *Br J Rheumatol* 1996; 35: 652–9.

93. Newman, S. P., and Revenson, T. A. Coping with rheumatoid arthritis. *Baillieres Clin Rheumatol* 1993; 7: 259–80.

94. Parker, J. C., Smarr, K. L., Buckelew, S. P., Stucky-Ropp, R. C., Hewett, J. E., Johnson, J. C. et al. Effects of stress management on clinical outcomes in rheumatoid arthritis. *Arthritis Rheum* 1995; 38: 1807–18.

95. Lorig, K., and Holman, H. Arthritis self-management studies: a twelve-year review. *Health Educ Q* 1993; 20: 17–28.

96. Parker, J. C., Bradley, L. A., DeVellis, R. M., Gerber, L. H., Holman, H. R., Keefe, F. J. et al. Biopsychosocial contributions to the management of arthritis disability: blueprints from an NIDRR-sponsored conference. *Arthritis Rheum* 1993; 36: 885–9.

97. Sharpe, L., Sensky, T., Timberlake, N., Ryan, B., Brewin, C. R., and Allard, S. A blind, randomized, controlled trial of cognitive-behavioural intervention for patients with recent onset rheumatoid arthritis: preventing psychological and physical morbidity. *Pain* 2001; **1989**: 275–83.

98. Sharpe, L., Sensky, T., Timberlake, N., Ryan, B., and Allard, S. Long-term efficacy of a cognitive behavioural treatment from a randomized controlled trial for patients recently diagnosed with rheumatoid arthritis. *Rheumatology (Oxford)* 2003; **42**; 435–41.

99. Parker, J. C., Smarr, K. L., Slaughter, J. R., Johnston, S. K., Priesmeyer, M. L., Hanson, K. D. *et al*. Management of depression in rheumatoid arthritis: a combined pharmacologic and cognitive-behavioral approach. *Arthritis Rheum* 2003; **49**: 766–77.

100. Riemsma, R. P., Kirwan, J. R., Taal, E., and Rasker, J. J. Patient education for adults with rheumatoid arthritis. *Cochrane Database Syst Rev* 2003; CD003688.

101. Riemsma, R. P., Taal, E., Kirwan, J. R., and Rasker, J. J. Systematic review of rheumatoid arthritis patient education. *Arthritis Rheum* 2004; **51**; 1045–59.

102. Lorig, K., Seleznick, M., Lubeck, D., Ung, E., Chastain, R. L., and Holman, H. R. The beneficial outcomes of the arthritis self-management course are not adequately explained by behavior change. *Arthritis Rheum* 1989; **32**: 91–5.

103. Stucki, G., and Liang, M. H. Efficacy of rehabilitation interventions in rheumatic conditions. *Curr Opin Rheumatol* 1994; **6**: 153–8.

104. Uhlig, T., Finset, A., and Kvien, T. K. Effectiveness and cost-effectiveness of comprehensive rehabilitation programs. *Curr Opin Rheumatol* 2003; **15**: 134–40.

105. Hill, J., Bird, H. A., Harmer, R., Wright, V., and Lawton, C. An evaluation of the effectiveness, safety and acceptability of a nurse practitioner in a rheumatology outpatient clinic. *Br J Rheumatol* 1994; **33**: 283–8.

32 | *Non-drug management of chronic pain*

Wolfgang Hamann

Introduction

Pain is a sensation following tissue damage or a sensory experience expressed in terms of tissue damage (International Association for the Study of Pain). In neurophysiological terms, pain is experienced when selected areas in the limbic system, particularly neurones in the cingulate gyrus and related areas of the somatosensory cortex are excited at the same time[1]. Physiologically, this condition arises when nociceptors in peripheral tissues are stimulated, as is the case following trauma in acute pain or in inflammatory pain (**nociceptive pain**). However, it is not uncommon that excitation of limbic and related somatosensory cortical neurones originate from abnormal, usually damaged, peripheral or central nervous tissue (**neuropathic pain**) or as the consequence of psychological mechanisms (**psychogenic pain**). For the individual it does not matter how the typical state of limbic and somatosensory cortex excitation comes about, because the end result is just as unpleasant. In order to control chronic pain successfully, it is important to establish first which combination of the above mechanisms one is dealing with in the individual patient. The final treatment plan needs to be multidisciplinary, taking account of all aspects of a particular pain condition[2].

It is a feature of the pain pathway that at each synaptic relay there are mechanisms for amplification as well as inhibition. Pain control in clinical practice is targeted either at the nociceptors themselves or at the extensive variety of inhibitory mechanisms, which may be segmental, descending from higher centers, or within the brain itself. Before concentrating on specific techniques or methods of pain control, it is helpful to follow the pain pathway from the periphery to the brain, looking out for the target points of known methods of pain relief.

Pain pathway

A schematic outline of the pain pathway is given in Fig. 32.1. The major functional compartments are (a) the somatosensory receptors; (b) the primary afferent fibers, including dorsal root ganglia; (c) the dorsal horn/trigeminal nuclei; (d) the ascending tracts, for example spino-thalamic tract; (e) the descending inhibitory or facilitatory tracts; (f) the brain stem; (g) the thalamus; (h) the limbic system, in particular the cingulate gyrus; and (i) the somatosensory cortex. Pain relieving techniques have targeted almost all of these structures.

Peripheral sensory receptors

Nociceptors (pain receptors) are the source of nociceptive pain. Their sensitivity is increased by the action of inflammatory substances. They are the main target of anti-inflammatory analgesia in rheumatoid arthritis (see Chapter 22). It is worth noting that some of these sensory receptors cannot be excited in the absence of inflammation (silent nociceptors).

Tactile and temperature receptors are the targets for some physical therapies in pain control. In the dorsal horn, inhibition is exerted by primary afferents from these receptors at post- and presynaptic terminals of nociceptor afferents. These inhibitory mechanisms may be activated by treatment with warmth, cold, or massage.

Primary afferent fibers

These may be the source of pain following nerve damage or following transection of peripheral nerves. In their search for peripheral sections of a severed peripheral nerve, sprouting nerve fibers may form neuromata. The increased number of Na^+ channels in the tips of sprouts are probably the reason for the increased nervous discharge that may originate from neuromata. More than 50% of individuals with large peripheral nerves severed in limb amputation will develop neuropathic pain in the form of phantom limb pain[4]. Sodium channel antagonists such as carbamazepine or mexilitine may be helpful in this condition. For temporary analgesia peripheral nerves can be blocked by infiltration with local anesthetics.

Terminal parts of primary afferent nerve fibers are also the target of two types of often very effective types of physical treatments, transcutaneous electrical nerve stimulation (TENS) and acupuncture. In TENS low threshold afferent nerve fibers are stimulated electrically. Nervous activity in these fibers will activate segmental inhibition as well as long inhibitory loops reaching up to the brainstem, both targeting nervous transmission through the pain pathway.

Dorsal root ganglia

Dorsal root ganglia have gained much more prominence recently, because they are not only the nutritive cell bodies for primary afferent fibers, but also the place of manufacture of many chemical mediators released either centrally or peripherally. Here it is substance P that is of particular interest. The majority of this substance is released peripherally. Centrally, it serves as an excitatory modulator substance in the dorsal horn. Topical application of

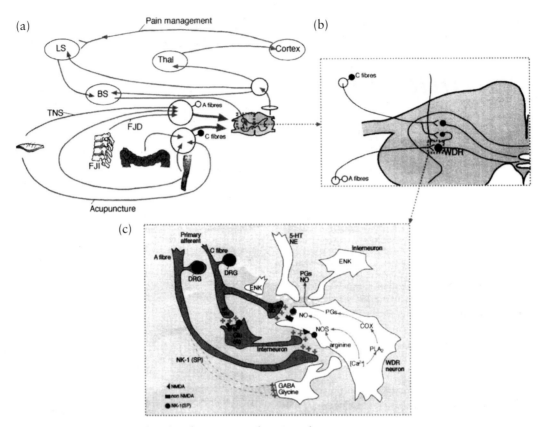

Fig. 32.1 Overview depicting access points of modes of treatment to the pain pathway.
(a)   Primary afferent fibers from skin, muscle, bone and other soft tissue and viscera. The term C-fiber includes small myelinated fibers. A-fibers are large myelinated fibers. Ascending pathways connect to the brainstem (BS), thalamus Thal, cortex, and limbic system (LS). Transcutaneous electrical nerve stimulation (TNS), facetjoint injection (FJI), facetjoint denervation (FJD).
(b)   Postsynaptic projections of primary afferent fibers in the dorsal horn. WDR wide dynamic range neurons.
(c)   Excitatory and injibitory synaptic connections to WDR-cell (white), excitatory neurones (blue), inhibitory neurons (yellow). Abbreviations DRG = dorsal root ganglion; ENK = enkephalin; NO = nitric oxide; NOS nitric oxide synthetase; PG = prostaglandin; COX = cyclo-oxygenase; NK-1 = neurokine 1; SP = substance P. (Modified from Yak S. (4).).

capsaicin to the skin can deplete primary afferents of substance P. This phenomenon is used in the topical use of capsaicin in a variety of neuropathic pain conditions.

Dorsal horn

The principal synaptic connections of nociceptor afferents in the dorsal horn can be summarized into reflex and ascending (pain pathway). Pre- and postsynaptically they are under the control of powerful segmental and descending inhibitory systems as described in the gate theory[4]. Nervous activity in large diameter afferent nerve fibers (touch and proprioception) has a strongly inhibitory effect on input from the population of small afferent fibers which contains the nociceptor (pain) fibers. The main excitatory transmitter substance is glutamate, together with an ever-increasing number of other substances, for example substance P. Two types of excitatory terminals are known:

(1) the nociception-specific small neurones in lamina I of the dorsal horn in the spinal cord;

(2) the so-called wide dynamic range neurones (WDR) in lamina V of the dorsal horn, which can be excited by tactile thermal proprioceptive and noxious stimuli. The WDR neurones have been widely investigated and much of the present knowledge about processing of nociceptive information comes from studies on these cells.

It is a significant feature of WDR cells that nervous impulses from non-myelinated nociceptor fibers result in depolarization and increased excitability outlasting the afferent activity by many seconds. This so-called wind-up phenomenon is mediated through glutamate released on to N-methyl-D-aspartate (NMDA) receptors on the WDR cells. Wind-up is an important functional mechanism of the gate theory[4], which states that increased nervous activity in small afferent nerve fibers opens the gate to the pain pathway, and conversely increased nervous activity in large diameter (tactile) nerve fibers has the opposite effect. Large afferent nerve fibers are the target of TENS (see below).

The number of chemical mediators affecting transmission through the pain pathway is considerable. Here we can only mention the substances that are directly implicated in current methods of pain control. Seventy-five per cent of opioidergic inhibition at the level of the dorsal horn is presynaptic. Mu receptor agonists are clinically the most significant analgesic drugs. Morphine and morphine-like drugs are, however, often not effective in neuropathic pain conditions, because cholecystokinine is up-regulated and counteracts the effect of mu-receptor agonists. Opioidergic inhibitory mechanisms are utilized in acupuncture. The insertion and manipulation of acupuncture needles is a mildly nociceptive stimulus activating small nociceptor afferents. Either directly, or through the descending non-specific inhibitory complex (DNIC)[5], endorphinergic inhibition is produced. The role of endorphins in acupuncture is underlined by the fact that pain relief through acupuncture is frequently accompanied by nausea. Gaba (gamma-amino-butyric acid)-ergic inhibition is activated by benzodiazepines.

Adrenergic and 5-hydroxy-tryptaminergic mechanisms are amplified by tricyclic antidepressants. NMDA effects of glutamate may be antagonized by, for example, ketamine.

Descending inhibitory mechanisms are often effectively activated by spinal cord stimulation. This technique is most effective in neuropathic pain conditions. It therefore has no role in the control of rheumatoid arthritis (RA) pain.

Brainstem and brain

The brainstem is the origin of powerful descending inhibition originating in particular from the periaquaeductal grey matter. Strong binding sites for mu-receptor agonists can be found in the brainstem and in the thalamus. Anxiolytics may be useful in curtailing the limbic aspects of pain perception. Finally, pain management, a combination of cognitive behavioral techniques and physical therapy, addresses at the same time limbic and cortical mechanisms in combination with improvement of physical parameters and peripheral sensory perception.

Stimulation analgesia

Stimulation analgesia targets either segmental inhibitory mechanisms activated by A-beta afferent fibers (TENS, peripheral nerve stimulation, and vibration), small afferent fibers to cause release of endorphins (acupuncture, acupuncture-like TENS), or descending inhibitory systems (spinal cord stimulation). Spinal cord stimulation will not be discussed any further, because its main indications are (non-inflammatory) neuropathic and ischemic pain conditions.

TENS

TENS is a commonly used form of stimulation analgesia. It has also proved itself as a pain control method in RA. For a more detailed review of this method of pain control the reader is referred to the excellent chapter by Thompson and Wolf in the *Textbook of pain*[6].

The technique

Transcutaneous electrical nerve stimulation is a form of pain control that mobilizes the body's own analgesic mechanisms. When it is used successfully there are few side-effects and almost no complications. It should therefore be used as an initial treatment in the management plan for the control of chronic pain. In order to achieve maximum effectiveness, qualified staff need to explain in layman's terms firstly what this technique is concerned with and, secondly, describe in detail how to test for efficacy and how to manage TENS on a daily basis. Wynn Perry[7] feels that it is often necessary to admit a patient for assessment purposes, although this is a minority view. There are no reliable criteria predicting that TENS will control a particular pain condition[8]. A detailed guide has been published by Thompson and Filshie[9] on how to establish whether TENS is effective and how to start treatment.

Equipment

The equipment consists of a set of electrodes connected through a set of highly flexible leads to a battery driven electrical stimulator. Modern transistorized stimulators can be quite small, even to the point that patients with hand deformities may not be able to operate them. It is important to select a model of appropriate dimensions for the individual. The price of transcutaneous nerve stimulators has come down dramatically over the years, so that all the equipment needed costs less than one consultant outpatient appointment.

TENS machines are designed as one or two channel devices with independent controls.

The device used must at least offer the following stimulation options: (1) regular repetitive, (2) burst mode, and (3) random stimulation. Stimulation frequencies available should cover the range 3–30 Hz (low frequency) and 31–120 Hz (high frequency as well as stimulus durations between 0.1 and 1 ms. The device should also be equipped with rechargeable batteries. The choice of electrodes is essentially between carbonized silicone rubber and adhesive electrodes. Silicone rubber electrodes have the advantage that they can be re-used many times. They have to be kept in position with micropore tape and sometimes do not stay as securely fixed as necessary. They may be dislodged, particularly during physical activity. It is important that proper saline gel is used. Without a proper contact gel there may be unreliable electrical contact and current sinks and surges may develop, resulting in irritation of the skin. An occasionally encountered complication is skin reaction. This can be minimized by the use of purpose-designed TENS gel, which is based on normal saline. Hypertonic gels, like ECG gel, should not be used. Occasionally, it may also be necessary to use a low allergy gel to overcome sensitivity problems.

Parameters of stimulation

There is no way of predicting which particular pattern of stimulation a patient will find most effective[6]. Several studies concentrating on this point have been unsuccessful in predicting whether continuous, burst, or random stimulation is most effective in certain situations. Physiologically, it is known that different patterns of afferent nervous discharge may result in the release of different transmitter substances. Empirically, it is important that any pattern tried needs to be used for at least one hour three times a day[9]. In terms of frequencies preferred, this is best left to the patient to decide. Usually, frequencies between 30 and 70 Hz are chosen. The strength of stimulation should be as high as can be tolerated comfortably. Ordinary TENS should not be painful, and there should be no muscle twitching. Other parameters offered on some devices are ramped or high frequency stimulation. Ramped stimuli may be experienced as more pleasant. They are functionally not different from the above types. High frequency stimulation is known to block nervous conduction in the fibers stimulated. Practically this can be seen to apply only to large afferent nerve fibers, because the strength of stimulation needed to excite C-fibers would have to be high and quite unpleasant. In the absence of nerve damage it is not helpful to block conduction in large sensory nerve fibers, because it is these fibers that mediate segmental inhibition of the pain pathway. Theoretically high frequency fiber block may be useful in situations where pain is mediated through large fibers, as is the case in some forms of allodynia. More research is needed on this topic.

Positioning of electrodes

The aim is to position the electrodes in the inhibitory cutaneous receptive field. Segmental inhibitory mechanisms are very powerful. The electrodes must therefore be placed in the same nervous segment[9]. This may be quite distant from the site of pain. Electrodes must never be placed on skin that is not intact.

Effectiveness of TENS

A 2005 Cochrane review on the effectiveness of TENS and acupuncture-like TENS in osteoarthritis of the knee found both forms of treatment superior to placebo[10]. The median methodological quality of the seven eligible trials was 3 out of 5.

A meta-analysis by Moore and McQuay[11] found that the use of TENS to control chronic pain 'may well be justified but it cannot be proved' with the clinical trial data available. Experimentally it is very difficult to design placebo TENS, which would be required for a double blind controlled study. There are two components in pain control with TENS, the segmental inhibition and the placebo effect. The placebo effect is significant during the first month of use. Research using placebo TENS has shown that after this time interval pain relief relies solely on segmental inhibition[6]. There is also a significant decline over time in the number of individuals who respond to TENS. Whilst at the beginning 60–80% of all individuals tested respond positively to TENS, this declines to 20–30% after one year[6].

It is important to appreciate that TENS is pain control and not cure. Pain relief is most commonly experienced when the stimulator is switched on. In some patients pain relief outlasts use of the stimulator by 10–30 min or even longer. In others two or more sessions are needed before significant pain relief is experienced. Except for patients with purely psychogenic pain, who tend not to respond to TENS, there are no distinct groups of chronic pain sufferers who do or do not respond[8]. Responsiveness to TENS needs to be established through a trial. It may of course still be necessary to supplement it with other forms of pain control.

Acupuncture-like TENS

This form of TENS is different from the above techniques, because stronger stimuli are employed so as to excite small nociceptor afferent nerve fibers, with the aim of effecting spinal release of endogenous opioids similar to the use of acupuncture. The electrodes are placed over known acupuncture points. This form of acupuncture may be mildly painful and there may also be some local contraction of muscle[6].

Acupuncture

Acupuncture is a form of stimulation analgesia targeting the small primary afferent fibers from nociceptors. Stimulation of this fiber group causes long-term inhibition lasting for several hours[12], as well as release of endogenous opioids through activation of the DNIC[5] in the central nervous system. Increased levels of the inhibitory transmitter substances enkephaline, 5-hydroxytryptamine, and

catecholamines have been found in the cerebrospinal fluid following acupuncture. The significance of this finding in relation to the direct analgesic action of acupuncture is, however, reduced by the observation that the placebo response is also mediated through an opioidergic link[13]. The use of placebo as part of an inherently active treatment is common in pain management and ethically acceptable. Although there is a sizeable literature on the use of acupuncture in musculoskeletal pain, reports of its use in rheumatoid arthritis are not common. Traditional Chinese acupuncture is the form used, in which specific points have been identified for specific effects. Probably for mnemonic convenience, a system of meridians has been introduced for the description of the location of individual points[14].

In Western acupuncture needles are positioned in the dermatome where the pain is localized. The needles are either manipulated in the traditional fashion between thumb and index finger or are connected to a low current source of repetitive electricity.

Acupuncture is now widely used for pain control. Initially, 49% of patients with nociceptive pain experienced pain relief in the study by Carlson and Sjolund[15] decreasing to under 17% after six months. Two meta-analyses[16,17] and a clinical update[18] produced equivocal results. In a third meta-analysis Ezzo et al.[19] came to the conclusion that there is limited evidence that acupuncture is more effective than no treatment, and inconclusive evidence that acupuncture is more effective than placebo. The absence of support or ambivalence in meta-analyses can be explained partly by the difficulty of designing a placebo acupuncture technique. Needling in apparently non-effective points will still induce a small tissue injury and activate the DNIC system.

Pain management

The experience of pain is based on simultaneous excitation of neurones in the somatosensory cortex and the limbic system. So far we have discussed pain control mechanisms targeting primary afferent fibers, the dorsal horn, and descending inhibitory systems. Pain management targets the cortex and the limbic system. The techniques employed are psychological, and the cognitive behavioral approach appears to be the most successful method[20].

The adaptation to chronic pain may be studied using the model of stress and coping. Chronic pain represents the stressor to which individuals respond with widely diverse adaptations, ranging from almost normal function to catastrophizing (e.g. expectation that the condition will lead to life in a wheelchair) and complete disability. Rheumatoid arthritis is a good test condition for this model, because the disease level can be quantified relatively well. In RA it has been found that adjustment to pain and functional impairment correlates more strongly with psychosocial factors such as depression and anxiety than with disease activity[21], which can be altered using techniques of cognitive evaluation and coping strategies. It has also been shown that pain coping strategies predict perceived control of pain[22]. Severe pain is unfortunately not easily controlled with cognitive evaluation and coping strategies. Keefe et al.[23] showed that higher levels of pain are related to lower levels of self-efficacy. However, after eliminating pain intensity as a component, pain coping strategies were found to explain 8–15% of self-efficacy. A great variety of topics are taught, including an educational overview of rheumatoid arthritis, a simplified version of the gate theory, information about acute versus chronic pain, information about medical management of pain, specific coping strategies like problem solving, relaxation, awareness of pain behaviour, strategies for attention diversion, and training in family dynamics and communication. Programs are either residential or outpatient based, and for patients with musculoskeletal impairment they are frequently run in combination with physiotherapists, who assist in realistically increasing goal setting and regaining of mobility. The setting up of a pain management program is a specialist task, but achievable even in the setting of a district general hospital[24]. For how long do the benefits last following a course? Lorig and Holman[25] looked at the long-term outcomes of an arthritis self-management study. They found the beneficial effects of the program sustained after 20 months. There were no differences between test groups with or without exposure to reinforcement.

Nerve blocks and radiofrequency procedures

Nerve blocks may be indicated in situations of entrapment, for example carpal tunnel syndrome or radiculopathy. In entrapment it is often useful to add steroid to the local anesthetic, because of the reduction of inflammatory swelling. Detailed descriptions of techniques can be found in Cousins and Bridenbaugh[26] and Wedley and Gauci[27].

Surgical transection of large sensory nerves or nerve roots for pain relief is a questionable technique in individuals with normal life expectancy, because it may result in neuropathic pain. More than 50% of limb amputees experience phantom limb pain[4].

Using radiofrequency (RF) or cryo-lesioning, nerves retain their physical continuity. Nerve fibers can regenerate and nerve pains in the form of anesthesia dolorosa are less likely to occur. Radiofrequency lesioning is the technique that permits the greatest degree of precision in targeting. It is also the least invasive technique. It is used for a variety of indications, of which facet joint denervation is the most relevant to rheumatoid arthritis.

Pulsed radiofrequency treatment (PRF, see below) is a modification of the continuous RF technique, where the mean temperature produced increases only slightly. Gauci[28] has published level V evidence (Table 32.1) that PRF applied to dorsal root ganglia may be used for the control of arthritic pain.

Pain originating from the zygo-apophyseal (facet) joints

Rheumatoid arthritis can affect any joint in the body. However, joints rarely involved are the distal interphalangeal, sacroiliac, and lumbar facet joints. Among the facet joints, the atlanto-occipital joints are a well recognized site giving rise to sometimes severe problems in the form of atlanto-occipital and atlanto-axial instability. The bulk of the literature about facet joints in rheumatoid arthritis is concerned with this problem, for which the reader is

Table 32.1

Levels of evidence	Type of evidence
I	Meta-analysis of several quality, randomized controlled trials (RCT)
II	One high-quality or several lower-quality RCTs
III	Well designed, but non-RCT studies
IV	Quality non-experimental studies
V	Case reports

After European Society for Medical Oncology minimum clinical recommendations; http://www.esmo.org

referred to the chapter about surgery. Like any other joint, facet joints may give rise to pain. Kaplan *et al.*[29] were able to show that distension of the capsule of facet joints causes pain and that this pain can be abolished reversibly by conduction block of the nerve supplying the facet joint with local anesthetic.

Dolan *et al.*[30] showed a good correlation between pain relief caused by injection of facet joints with local anesthetic which exhibited an increased uptake of technetium in single photon emission computerized tomography (SPECT). Pain relief was less likely to occur in apparently painful joints which did not show up on SPECT scanning. The physiological parameter measured with SPECT is an increase in localized blood flow, as is present in inflammation. Facet joint injections, nerve blocks and denervations have been performed for many years. The effectiveness of facet joint denervation for pain control has been established at evidence level II[31–33].

Clinical diagnosis of facet joint arthropathy

Within the term mechanical low back pain no pathognomonic clinical parameters have been identified for the diagnosis of the facet joint syndrome[34]. However, the following signs are commonly taken as indicative for this diagnosis. Facet joint pain may be episodic or continuous. It usually has a local component that may be sharp or aching and often a referred component that must not be of a radicular distribution. Movements that increase the pressure on the joint tend to aggravate the pain. At the same time, not to have any movement in a joint affected is often very unpleasant, resulting in the typical phenomenon that individuals with facet joint pain find it uncomfortable to be in a fixed position for any length of time. Patients with cervical facet joint pain present with a stiff and painful neck, possibly even torticollis. The pain may radiate into the head and shoulder in a non-radicular fashion[35]. The pain is exacerbated particularly by extension, rotation, and lateral flexion. There should be no neurological abnormalities. Radiographs, computerized tomography (CT) scans or magnetic resonance imaging (MRI) scans often show degeneration or appositional bone growth producing lipping of joints and various forms of misalignment of the joint surfaces. However, none of the structural radiological signs are sufficiently pathognomonic, because all these observations may be present without pain. As shown above, a positive SPECT scan strengthens the diagnosis[30]. Clinically it is not always possible to differentiate facet joint pain from discogenic, osteoporotic, or soft tissue pain. It is the absence of more clearly defined diagnostic criteria that make it essential to rely on procedural diagnostic measures before embarking on destructive forms of treatment.

Procedure-based diagnosis of facet joint pain

Two techniques with slightly different aims are used.

Medial branch block

The medial branch block[29,35] aims to identify facet joints suitable for denervation. The medial branches of the dorsal rami of spinal roots innervate the segmental facet joints and adjacent small portions of multifidus muscle. Under fluoroscopic control 0.5 mL of either lignocaine or bupivacaine are injected at the junction between pedicle and transverse process relating to the facet joint likely to be the source of pain, and the subject is asked to observe whether or not there is short-lasting pain relief for the duration of the effectiveness of the local anesthetic. There is no treatment value in itself in this procedure.

Facet joint injection

Facet joint injection[36] aims to identify facet joints suitable for denervation as well as to provide pain relief for more than a few hours. The fluoroscopic beam is moved into the plane of the facet joint and the needle is advanced into the joint employing tunnel vision. Two procedural questions have attracted attention in the literature, namely the volume of substrate to be injected and whether contrast should be used or not. Firstly, the volume of the extended joint capsule of a facet joint is probably less than 1 mL. Any volume injected in excess of the capsular capacity will result in periarticular deposit of the injectate, either with or without rupture of the joint capsule. More often than not, so-called facet joint injections are really combined intra-articular plus posterior compartment injections. Secondly, contrast used to verify intra-articular positioning of the needle will itself fill up capsular space and needs to be added to the total volume injected.

Aims and outcome of facet joint injections

Facet joint injections are performed either with the aim of curbing an episode of facet joint pain or as a diagnostic procedure to decide on a denervation of the joint in question. Nelemans et al.[37] could neither endorse nor reject injection treatment for pain control, including facet joint injection treatment of back pain in their meta-analysis on this topic.

In most studies the diagnosis of facet joint pain is based on clinical criteria or on the exclusion of other more clearly defined conditions. Lilius et al.[38] performed a randomized controlled study on 109 subjects with three types of injections: (1) cortisone and local anesthetic into facet joints; (2) the same mixture as a periarticular injection; and (3) physiological saline injected into two joints. A significant but treatment-independent improvement was noted in pain and disability scores but not in movements of the lumbar spine. Carette et al.[39] performed a double blind controlled study comparing injection with methyl prednisolone with saline in patients diagnosed as suffering from facet joint arthropathy by successful facet joint injection with lignocaine. No difference was found between the two groups that could be related to the use of methyl prednisolone. In this study the correct needle position in the joint to be injected was checked by injecting 0.5 mL of Omnipaque® contrast before injection of the test substance, so that the joint was largely filled with contrast medium before the test substance could be injected (see below). Roy et al.[40] did observe good but temporary pain relief following intra- or periarticular facet joint injection. Using a small volume of 1.5 mL local anesthetic, Moran et al.[36] observed pain relief only in 16.7% of their total sample of 143 facet joints in 54 patients. A recent, well designed trial appears to provide level II-type evidence that facet joint injection with local anesthetic and steroid may provide pain relief for several months[41]. Facet joint pain was diagnosed by reproduction of the typical pain through distension of the joint capsule whilst contrast medium was injected.

Denervation of cervical facet joints

The technique of RF denervation of facet joints was first described by Shealey[42]. RF-denervation does frequently provide long-lasting pain relief[32], although it is followed by nerve regeneration which can be quite rapid[43]. For cervical facet joint denervation, the patient is positioned in a supine position on a radiotranslucent table. The procedure is carried out under local anesthesia and sedation as required. Under fluoroscopic control the facet joint in question is displayed with the fluoroscope in an oblique position. Under local anesthesia with or without sedation the tip of a needle insulated except for the last 5 mm of the tip (Sluiter Mehta needle) is positioned on the facet joint 1–2 mm dorsal of the foramen. The target is the medial branch of the dorsal ramus of the spinal root where it runs around the superior margin of the transverse process. Following anatomical positioning of the needle tip, the proper positioning is ascertained functionally by electrical stimulation through the tip of the needle. A local change in sensation, for example a feeling of heaviness or tingling, should be felt during stimulation with not more than 0.5 V at a rate of 50/s. The rate of stimulation is then reduced to 2/s. The perception threshold at this rate of stimulation should exceed the 50/s value by 50% or more and no stimulation-synchronous distant muscle twitching should occur. The purpose of the low frequency stimulation is to make sure that no motor nerve is within reach of the tip of the needle. Recently, sensory stimulation has been questioned as a valid test for medial branch identification. Instead, localized multifidus muscle contraction has been taken as an indication that the RF electrode is near the medial branch[44]. Following the identification process, 1 mL of 2% lignocaine is injected and after 2 min a radiofrequency current is passed through the needle, raising the temperature to 80°C.

Future developments

Pulsed radiofrequency

Sluijter[45] developed a new form of applying RF in the form of short 20 msec pulses at 2 Hz following the observation by Slappendael[46] that continuous RF at 40°C applied to the dorsal root ganglia was as effective as RF at 67°C in controlling brachialgia pain.

Experimentally, it has been shown that PRF causes up-regulation of the early immediate genes C-fos postsynaptically in the dorsal horn[47,48] and Activating Transmission Factor 3 in the small neurones of dorsal root ganglia[49]. Level IV evidence for the clinical efficacy of this technique exists largely for neuropathic pain conditions[50]. Gauci[28] has used it successfully for the control of osteoarthritic pain. Further trials are needed.

Subcutaneous and peripheral nerve stimulation

Spinal cord stimulation and TENS rely on the activation of inhibitory pathways activated by primary afferent A alpha fibers. Certainly TENS has an analgesic effect almost exclusively when it is switched on. Acupuncture stimulates small diameter afferent delta fibers which activate long lasting inhibitory systems[12]. Subcutaneous and peripheral nerve stimulation is even more effective at recruiting delta fibers. Peripheral nerve stimulation has been used successfully for several years, whereas subcutaneous stimulation is at an experimental stage. Anecdotally it has been quite successful in controlling chronic inflammatory pain (Goroszeniuk *et al.*, in preparation).

Conclusions

This chapter has concentrated on non-drug forms of pain management in conventional medical practice. Alternative methods have not been included. This would have required a chapter in its own right. The techniques described have the advantage of avoiding drug side-effects. The levels of evidence for many of these techniques have improved during the last 10 years. However, more randomized, controlled trials are still needed.

References

1. Derbyshire, S. W., and Jones, A. K. Cerebral responses to a continual tonic pain stimulus measured using positron emission tomography. *Pain* 1998; **76**: 127–35.
2. Flor, H., Fydrich, T., and Turk, D. C. Efficacy of multidisciplinary pain treatment centers: a meta-analytic view. *Pain* 1992; **49**: 221–30.
3. Wartan, S. W., Hamann, W., Wedley, J. R., and McColl, I. Phantom pain and sensation among British veteran amputees. *British J Anaesth* 1997; **78**: 652–9.
4. Melzack, R., and Wall, P. D. Pain transmission: a new theory. *Science* 1965; **150**: 971–9.
5. Le Bars, D., Dickenson, A. H., Besson, J. M., and Villanueva, L. Aspects of sensory processing through convergent neurons. In *Spinal afferent processing* (Yaksh TL, ed.), pp. 467–504. New York: Plenum; 1986.
6. Woolf, C. J., and Thompson, J. W. Stimulation-induced analgesia: transcutaneous electrical nerve stimulation (TENS) and vibration. In *Textbook of Pain* (Wall, P. D., Melzack, R. eds), pp. 1191–208. Edinburgh: Churchill Livingstone; 1994.
7. Wynn, P. Pain in avulsion lesions of the brachial plexus. *Pain* 1980; **9**: 41–53.
8. Bates, J. A. V., and Nathan, P. W. Transcutaneous electrical nerve stimulation in chronic pain. *Anaesthesia* 1980; **35**: 817–22.
9. Thompson, J. W., and Filshie, J. Transcutaneous electrical nerve stimulation (TENS) and acupuncture. In *Oxford Textbook of Palliative Medicine* (Doyle D, Hanks G, and McDonald N, eds), pp. 229–44. Oxford University Press: 1993.
10. Osiri, M., Brosseau, L., McGowan, J., Robinson, V. A., Shea, B. J., Tugwell, P., and Wells, G. G. W. Transcutaneous electrical nerve stimulation for knee osteoarthritis. *Cochrane Database of Systematic Reviews.* 2005; Vol. 1.
11. McQuay, H. J., and Moore, R. A. Transcutaneous electrical nerve stimulation. In *An Evidence-Based Resource for Pain Relief* (McQuay, H. J., and Moore, R. A., eds), pp. 207–11. Oxford University Press: 1998.
12. Sandkuhler, J., Chen, J. G., Cheng, G., and Randic, M. Low-frequency stimulation of afferent A delta-fibers induces long-term depression at primary afferent synapses with substantia gelatinosa neurons in the rat. *J Neurosci* 1997; **10**: 6483–91.
13. ter Riet, G., de Craen, A. J. M., de Boer, A., and Kessels, A. G. H. Is placebo analgesia mediated by endogenous opioids? A systematic review. *Pain* 1998; **76**: 273–5.
14. Lim, J. Understanding acupuncture. PhD thesis. Cambridge, 1989.
15. Carlsson, C. P., Sjolund, B. H. Acupuncture and subtypes of chronic pain: assessment of long-term results. *Clin J Pain* 1994; **10**: 290–5.
16. Ernst, E., and White, A. R. Acupuncture for back pain: a meta analysis of randomized controlled trials. *Arch Intern Med* 1998; **158**: 2235–41.
17. ter Riet, G., Kleijnen, J., and Knipschild, P. Acupuncture and chronic pain: a criteria based meta analysis. *J Clin Epidemiol* 1990; **43**: 1191–9.
18. Thomas, M., and Lundeberg, T. Does acupuncture work? *Pain Clinical Updates* 1996; Vol. IV, Issue 3, pp. 1–4.
19. Ezzo, J., Berman, B., Hadhazy, V. A., Jadad, A. R., Lao, L., and Singh, B. B. Is acupuncture effective for the treatment of chronic pain? A systematic review. *Pain* 2000; **86**: 217–25.
20. Parker, J. C., Frank, R. G., Beck, N. C., Smarr, K. L., Buescher, K. L., Phillips, L. R. *et al.* Pain management in rheumatoid arthritis patients: a cognitive-behavioral approach. *Arthritis Rheum* 1988; **31**: 593–601.
21. Hagglund, K. J., Roth, D. L., Haley, W. E., and Alarcon, G. S. Discriminant and convergent validity of self-reported measures of affective distress in patients with rheumatoid arthritis. *J Rheumatol* 1989; **16**: 1428–32.
22. Haythornthwaite, J. A., Menefee, L. A., Heinberg, L. J., and Clark, M. R. Pain coping strategies predict perceived control over pain. *Pain* 1998; **77**: 33–9.
23. Keefe, F. J., Affleck, G., Lefebvre, J. C., Starr, K., Caldwell, D. S., and Tennen, H. Pain coping strategies and coping efficacy in rheumatoid arthritis: a daily process analysis. *Pain* 1997; **69**: 35–42.
24. Luscombe, F. E., Wallace, L., Williams, J., and Griffiths, D. P. G. A district general hospital pain management programme: first year experiences and outcomes. *Anaesthesia* 1995; **50**: 114–17.
25. Lorig, K., and Holman, H. R. Long-term outcomes of an arthritis self-management study: effects of reinforcement efforts. *Soc Sci Med* 1989; **29**: 221–4.
26. Cousins, M. J., and Bridenbaugh, P. O. *Neural Blockade in Clinical Anaesthesia and Pain Management.* Philadelpia: JB Lippincott; 1980.
27. Wedley, J. R., and Gauci, C. A. *Handbook of Clinical Techniques in the Management of Chronic Pain.* Chur: Harwood Academic; 1994.
28. Gauci, C. *Proceedings of World Wide Pain Conference*, San Francisco, July 2000.
29. Kaplan, M., Dreyfuss, P., Halbrook, B., and Bogduk, N. The ability of lumbar medial branch blocks to anaesthetize the zygoapophysial joint: a physiologic challenge. *Spine* 1998; **23**: 1847–52.
30. Dolan, A. L., Ryan, P. J., Arden, N. K., Stratton, R., Wedley, J. R., Hamann, W., Fogelman, I. and Gibson, T. The value of SPECT scans in identifying back pain likely to benefit from facet joint injection. *Br J Rheumatol* 1996; **35**: 1269–73.
31. Gallagher, J., Pettricioni di Vadi, P. L., Wedley, J. R., Hamann, W., Ryan, P., Chikanza, B. *et al.* Radiofrequency facet joint denervation in the treatment of low back pain: a prospective controlled double-blind study to assess its efficacy. *Pain Clinic* 1994; **7**: 193–8.

32. Lord, S. M., Barnsley, L., Wallis, B. J., McDonald, G. J., and Bogduk, N. Percutaneous radio-frequency neurotomy for chronic cervical zygapophyseal-joint pain. *New Eng J Med* 1996; **335**: 1721–6.

33. Dreyfuss, P., Halbrook, B., Pauza, K., Joshi, A., McLarty, J., and Bogduk, N. Efficacy and validity of radiofrequency neurotomy for chronic lumbar zygoapophysial joint pain. *Spine* 2000; **25**: 1270–7.

34. Schwarzer, A. C., Wang, S., Bogduk, N., McNaught, P. J., and Laurent, R. Prevalence and clinical features of lumbar zygapophysial joint pain: a study in an Australian population with chronic back pain. *Ann Rheum Dis* 1995; **58**: 100–6.

35. Dreyfuss, P., Schwarzer, A.C., Lau, P., and Bogduk, N. Specificity of lumbar medial branch and L5 dorsal ramus blocks: a computed tomography study. *Spine* 1997; **22**: 895–902.

36. Moran, R., O'Connel, D., and Walsh, M. G. The diagnostic value of facet joint injections. *Spine* 1998; **13**: 1407–10.

37. Nelemans, P. J., de Bie, R. A., deVet, H. C., and Sturmans, F. Injection therapy for subacute and chronic benign low back pain. *Spine* 2001; **26**: 501–15.

38. Lilius, G., Laasonen, E. M., and Myllynen, P. Chronic unilateral low-back pain: predictors of outcome of facet joint injections. *Spine* 1990; **15**: 780–2.

39. Carette, S., Marcoux, S., Truchon, R., Grondin, C., Gagnon, J., Allard, Y., and Latulippe, M. A controlled trial of corticosteroids into facet joints for chronic low back pain. *New Eng J Med* 1991; **325**: 1002–7.

40. Roy, D. F., Fleury, J., Fontaine, S. B., and Dussault, R. G. Clinical investigation of cervical facet joint infiltration. *Can Assoc Radiol J* 1988; **39**: 118–20.

41. Shih, C., Lin, G. Y., Yueh, K. C., and Lin, J. J. Lumbar zygapophyseal joint injections in patients with chronic lower back pain. *J Chin Med Assoc* 2005, **68**: 51–2.

42. Shealy, C. N. Percutaneous radiofrequency denervation of spinal facets: treatment of chronic back pain and sciatica. *J Neurosurg* 1975; **43**: 448–51.

43. Hamann, W., and Hall, S. Acute effect and recovery of primary afferent nerve fibres after graded radiofrequency lesions in anaesthetised rats. *Br J Anaesth* 1992; **68**: 443.

44. Van Kleef, M., Barendse, G. A. M., Kessels, A., Voets, H. M., Weber, W. E. J., and de Lange, S. Randomized trial of radiofrequency lumbar facet denervation for chronic low back pain. *Spine* 1999; **24**: 1937–42.

45. Sluijter, M. Non-thermal radiofrequency procedures in the treatment of spinal pain. Pain in Europe; 2nd Annual Congress of the European Federation of IASP Chapters, Barcelona, p. 326: 1997.

46. Slappendael, R., Crul, B. J. P., Braak, G. J. J., Geurts, J. W. M., Booij, L. H. D. J., Voerman, V. F., and Boo, T. D. The efficacy of radiofrequency lesioning of the cervical dorsal root ganglion in a double-blind randomized study: no difference between 40 and 67°C treatments. *Pain* 1997; **73**: 159–63.

47. Higuchi, Y., Nashold, Blaine, S. Jr., Sluijter, M., Cosman, E., and Pearlstein, R. D. Exposure of the dorsal root ganglion in rats to pulsed radiofrequency currents activates dorsal horn lamina I and II neurons. *Neurosurgery* 2002; **50**: 850–6.

48. Van Zundert, J., de Louw, A. J., Joosten, E. A., Kessels, A. G., Honig, W., Dederen, P. J. *et al.* Pulsed and continuous radiofrequency current adjacent to the cervical dorsal root ganglion of the rat induces late cellular activity in the dorsal horn. *Anaesthesiology* 2005; **102**: 1–3.

49. Hamann, W., Sherief, A. S., Thompson, T., and Standring, S. Pulsed radiofrequency applied to dorsal root ganglia causes a selective increase in ATF3 in small neurons. *European J Pain* 2006; **10**: 171–6.

50. Munglani, R. The long term effect of pulsed radiofrequency for neuropathic pain. *Pain* 1998; **90**: 437–9.

33 | *Health economics*

Leigh F. Callahan

Introduction

Arthritis and other rheumatic conditions are highly prevalent, a leading cause of disability, and contribute to substantial economic consequences[1–19]. These conditions as a whole impose less of an impact in terms of mortality compared to other chronic conditions, but a considerable burden in terms of morbidity and costs.[16] Rheumatoid arthritis (RA), the second most prevalent form of arthritis, is a progressive, systemic, chronic disease affecting 0.5–1% of the population[1,20–22]. RA results in significant morbidity and mortality[14,23]. Morbidity includes functional loss, pain and fatigue, substantial psychological and social effects, work disability, and time loss[24]. There are also significant economic consequences associated with RA for individual patients, their families, and society[12,18,19,25–51]. The costs of RA have been estimated at up to $14 billion dollars per year in the US[52], with estimates of $285 million in Sweden[53] and $990 million in the UK[19]. Yet, despite the documentation of the enormous impact of RA, the consequences and 'side-effects' of the disease have often been underestimated.

The changes in the healthcare environment demand the concomitant evaluation and measurement of the costs and benefits of interventions for RA[33,54–58]. Healthcare providers, hospitals, and systems of delivery need to demonstrate that they achieve appropriate patient outcomes in a cost-effective manner[56,58]. Cost of illness studies are generally used to estimate the different types of costs associated with a specific disease (Table 33.1) and economic evaluations are used to study the relationship between the effectiveness of interventions and their costs[33,57,59–61]. These studies and evaluations continue to receive increased attention as healthcare budgets are limited and decision makers in reimbursement agencies are forced to regulate the allocation of healthcare resources[62].

Cost of illness studies are generally divided into three categories (Table 33.1), direct costs, indirect costs, and intangible costs[16,50,63–67]. Direct costs are the costs that accrue when people receive medical care, such as physician visits, hospitalizations, medications, and diagnostic tests. Direct costs also include expenditures for other items such as adaptations to the home environment and transportation costs to visit healthcare providers, but it is often difficult to accurately estimate these other expenditures.

Indirect costs are costs for resources that are lost, but for which there is no direct payment actually made. They are usually calculated as the costs due to lost wages from a reduction in, or cessation of work. Indirect costs can be classified into two groups, morbidity and mortality costs[50,66]. Morbidity costs are mainly productivity losses borne by the individual, the individual's family, their employer, and society due to their illness. Mortality costs are the present value of lost production due to premature death caused by illness.

Intangible costs are the costs of individuals foregoing the activities they and society value. Intangible costs include the costs associated with a decline in functional capacity, increased pain, reduced quality of life, and increased mortality. These costs are difficult to quantify and are often not included in economic studies.

The purpose of an economic analysis is to identify, measure, value, and compare the costs and consequences of interventions. Three methods are commonly used for economic analyses: cost–benefit, cost–effectiveness, or cost–utility studies[33,59–61]. Cost-benefit analyses value the consequences or benefits in monetary terms. With cost-benefit analysis, outcomes or benefits are assigned a monetary value. Due to the reluctance of many clinicians to value human life in dollars, cost-benefit analyses are rarely done in rheumatology[59]. Cost-effectiveness analyses relate all costs to a single, common effect. These analyses highlight the aggregate benefits conferred in non-economic terms, such as dollars per life saved or dollars per year of life gained[59,60]. These are

Table 33.1 Categories of cost of illness studies

Category	Definition	Examples
Direct costs	Expenditures for medical care and related items	Hospitalizations Physician visits Nursing home stays Diagnostic tests Aids and divices Transportation
Indirect costs	Costs due to lost wages	Productivity loss by patients Productivity loss by caregivers Reduced family income
Intangible costs	Costs of an individual foregoing the activities they and society value	Pain Reduced quality of life Mortality

the types of economic analyses most commonly performed in the health arena. Cost-utility analyses are a type of cost-effectiveness analysis in which benefits are expressed as values or utilities assigned to a given status, such as quality-adjusted life years[59,60].

Currently, the economic evaluations in rheumatology employ a variety of methodologies, resulting in potential threats to validity, usability, and comparability of studies[58]. A set of minimum criteria for standardization of methods for economic evaluations in rheumatology has been proposed by the OMERACT (Outcomes Measures in Rheumatology) Economics Working Group[58]. The 13 proposed recommendations are: (1) model horizon; (2) duration of treatment; (3) extrapolation beyond trial duration; (4) modeling beyond trial duration; (5) synthesis of comparisons where clinical trials do not exist; (6) outcome measures; (7) mortality; (8) valuation of health; (9) resource use; (10) classification and reporting of adverse events; (11) discontinuation of treatment; (12) therapeutic strategies; and (13) population risk stratification[58].

This chapter focuses on the economic consequences of RA, reviewing the estimates of the direct, indirect, and intangible costs of the disease. In addition, the predictors of cost in economic evaluations of RA and studies examining cost-effectiveness of new drugs will be reviewed.

Direct costs

The economic costs of RA are high, approximately those of coronary heart disease[25,26,28–32,51,68,69]. The economic burden of RA significantly exceeds that related to osteoarthritis and high blood pressure[48]. The direct costs of RA have been estimated to be three times the costs of medical care for persons of the same age and gender who do not have RA in the US[30,71] and 2.5 times the costs of age- and gender-matched individuals in Sweden[72]. The projected annual US direct costs are US$ 3.6 billion for treating RA[70].

The majority of studies examining costs of RA have been conducted in clinical populations. The studies cannot be compared directly due to different costing methods, but some trends and similarities can be seen among the studies. A summary of studies conducted in the late 1970s to late 1990s is presented in Table 33.2[71]. The cost estimates from the original studies were updated to 1996 dollars by using the Consumer Price Index[68]. The direct costs ranged from US$2299/person/year in a study from Canada[73,74] to US$13 549 in a study from the US that focused only on patients who had been hospitalized[74]. All of the studies until 2000 report the costs of RA before the introduction and increasing use of biologic therapy.

In studies prior to the widespread introduction of biologics, hospitalizations accounted for more than 40% of the direct costs and surgery was responsible for the majority of inpatient costs (Table 33.2)[25,28,29,31,34,52,68,70,71,73–76]. Of the three categories of outpatient costs, healthcare visits, medications, and diagnostic tests, the largest category was medications (Table 33.2). The one study conducted prior to widespread biologic therapy introduction where inpatient costs were considerably lower than outpatient costs involved a cohort of patients with recent onset RA[77]. And, a more recent study of RA costs during the first year of disease from Sweden also reported lower inpatient costs (12%) compared to ambulatory healthcare (76%) and medications (9%)[41]. A study from the Netherlands also noted that the majority of costs in the first two years of disease were from consultations with healthcare workers[45], in contrast to devices and adaptations being the main contributors to total direct costs in individuals with more than 10 years of disease.

A comparative study of the societal economic burden of RA, osteoarthritis (OA), and hypertension was conducted in Ontario, Canada in early 2000 (Table 33.3)[48]. Costs were converted to 2000 US dollars. Total costs (direct and indirect) were substantially greater in the RA patients compared to the OA and hypertension patients (Table 33.3). The total direct costs for RA were US$2575, compared to US$1976 for OA, US$1536 for hypertension, and $US 2024 for individuals with both OA and hypertension. Direct costs accounted for a higher %age of total costs for patients with OA and patients with hypertension, compared to patients with RA. Unlike the majority of studies in the 1990s, direct costs were higher than indirect costs in RA patients and total drug costs accounted for the highest portion of the direct costs rather than hospitalization (Table 33.3).

The total direct medical costs in 7527 persons with RA were estimated in a three-year study in 2001 US dollars using the

Table 33.2   Summary of studies demonstrating the average direct costs per individual for patients with RA (1996 US dollars) [a]

Reference	Outpatient costs				Inpatient costs[c]	Other costs	Total direct costs
	Healthcare visits	Medications[b]	Diagnostic tests	Total			
73	108	396	155	731	1564	NA	2298
75	264	1342	86	1806	378	126	2310
28	525	1221	917	3006	3051	910	6967
25	564	504	582	1650	4610	385	6645
77	667	686	889	2242	298	NA	2540
70	423	486	NA	933	2867	400	4200
74	NA	NA	NA	NA	13549	NA	13549
31	1532	728	NA	2280	4522	1249	8051
76	733	1544	277	2554	5250	395	8500

Source: Lubeck DP, *Pharmacoeconomics* 2001; **19**: 811–18. Reproduced with permission.
NA, not applicable.
[a] Some totals include other categories, such as devices. Therefore, rows do not always sum to the total.
[b] NSAIDs (non-steroidal anti-inflammatory drugs) and DMARDs (disease-modifying anti-rheumatic drugs) for RA.
[c] Other costs include outpatient surgeries, rehabilitation care, and emergency department visits not otherwise classified

Table 33.3 Cost of Illness estimates for six months for patients with RA, OA, and high blood pressure (2000 US dollars)

	RA (*n* = 253)		OA and HBP (*n* = 191)		OA (*n* = 140)		HBP (*n* = 142)	
	$	%	$	%	$	%	$	%
Total costs	4674		2456		2856		1963	
Direct costs: total	2575	55.1	2024	82.4	1976	69.2	1536	78.3
Drugs total	1237		974		768		786	
Health professionals total	554		339		384		316	
Separately ordered total	278		110		119		100	
Hospitalizations total	264		393		439		313	
Community services	186		203		219		19	
Aids and devices	57		6		47		3	
Indirect costs: total	2098	44.9	432	17.6	880	30.8	427	21.7
Lost time doing chores, including paid help	1729	82.4	418	96.8	845	96.0	262	61.4
Time lost from work	326	15.5	14	3.2	33	3.8	164	38.3
Support person time lost from work	44	2.1	0	0.0	2	0.2	1	0.3

Source: Maetzel A, *et al. Ann Rheum Dis* 2004; **63**: 395–401. Reproduced with permission.
HBP, high blood pressure (hypertension).

Table 33.4 Direct annual medical costs for 7527 RA patients, by cost type (2001 US dollars)[a]

Cost type	Cost, $ (95% CI)	% (95% CI)
Outpatient costs: total	**1541 (1501–81)**	**16.2 (15.4–17.0)**
Physician and health professional	674 (662–686)	7.1 (6.8–7.4)
Radiographs	329 (311–347)	3.5 (3.2–3.7)
MRI, CT scans	199 (185–212)	2.1 (1.9–2.3)
Endoscopies	93 (86–99)	1.0 (0.9–1.1)
Other tests[b]	130 (126–134)	1.4 (1.3–1.4)
Outpatient surgery	114 (106–123)	1.2 (1.1–1.3)
Drug costs: total	**6324 (6172–6477)**	**66.4 (63.4–69.6)**
DMARDs	643 (619–667)	6.8 (6.4–7.2)
Biologic agents	3307 (3164–3451)	34.7 (32.5–37.1)
NSAIDs	591 (573–610)	6.2 (5.9–6.6)
GI medications and analgesics	518 (496–540)	5.4 (5.1–5.8)
Non-RA medications	1247 (1224–1270)	13.1 (12.6–13.7)
Hospitalization costs: total	**1573 (1450–1697)**	**16.5 (14.9–18.2)**
Total costs	**9519 (9301–9737)**	**100**

Source: Michaud *et al.*, *Arthritis Rheum* 2003; **48**: 10; 2750–62. Reproduced with permission.
CI, confidence interval; CT, computed tomography; GI, gastrointestinal; MRI, magnetic resonance imaging.
[a] Adjusted for age, sex, and calendar half-year.
[b] Includes laboratory tests, Doppler examinations, treadmill tests, mammograms, bone density tests, and other examinations.

Consumer Price Index[38]. This study provides the most comprehensive estimates to date of direct costs since the introduction of biologic agents into the treatment of RA. In 2001, the mean total annual direct medical care cost for a patient with RA was US$9519 (Table 33.4)[38]. Drug expenses were US$6324, representing 66% of total direct costs (Table 33.4). Hospitalization costs were US$1573 and outpatient costs were US$1541, 17% and 16% of total direct costs, respectively.

The largest component of the drug expenses was the cost of biologic therapy, US$3307 (Table 33.4), representing more than 50% of the total drug costs. Non-RA medications represented the second largest component, US$1247, followed by DMARDs, US$643, NSAIDs, US$591, and gastrointestinal medications US$518 (Table 33.4)[38]. Almost a quarter of the patients had received biologic therapy at some time during the study period,

and 26.1% were receiving biologic therapy during the last six months of 2001[38]. The total annual direct costs for patients receiving biologic therapy was US$19 016 compared to US$6164 for patients who did not receive biologic agents[38].

Indirect costs

Estimates of the indirect costs of RA, primarily lost income from work measured by the human capital approach, were three to four times higher than the direct costs of RA in studies conducted through the 1990s[25,28,30,52,68]. Indirect costs in clinical studies ranged from US$10 000 to US$50 000 in 1990 dollars[68]. Work disability has been reported after five years in 60–70% of patients with RA younger than 65 years who had been working at disease onset[78]. Of the individuals who stopped working, 10% indicated they had tried changes such as reducing their hours before stopping work[78].

A pilot study using job histories to estimate potential based on the US Department of Labor job analysis was conducted to examine financial and career loses due to RA. Results found that estimated earnings decreased from US$18 409 to US$13 000 per year[79]. Also, the number of jobs patients could perform was estimated to drop from 11.5 million to 2.6 million.

When the absolute and incremental indirect costs of RA were estimated in a national community-based sample in the United States, the absolute indirect costs were estimated to be $3.98 billion[31]. The incremental indirect costs that were due to RA were estimated to be $2.45 billion, more than 60% of the total wage loss costs of this condition[31]. Eighty per cent of the increment of the costs of RA was due to wage losses.

In England in 1992, the indirect costs resulting from production loss were estimated to be £651.5 million, 52% of the total costs[80]. Lost production among males and females was £177.2 million and £474.3 million, respectively[80]. The higher loss among the female population is a result of the higher prevalence of RA among females.

The effect of RA on working capabilities and social participation during the first six years of disease was studied in the Netherlands. The employment rate was low in the RA population compared to the Dutch population[81]. In the male 45–64-year-old group, 63% of RA patients were not employed compared to 32% of the Dutch population. Of the employed patients, 59% reported that RA affected their working capabilities. And, of the patients without a paying job, 41% believed that this was partly due to RA[81]. In addition, fewer RA patients had non-paying jobs and they performed fewer household activities compared to the Dutch population.

Patients with RA were significantly more likely to have lost their job or to have retired early due to their illness in a clinical study in Minnesota of the indirect and non-medical costs among people with RA and OA compared to non-arthritic controls[35]. They were also more likely to have reduced their work hours or stopped working entirely due to their illness, and they were three times more likely to have had a reduction in household family income than either individuals with OA or those without arthritis[35]. Fifteen per cent of the individuals with RA were unable to get a job because of their illness. In addition to the costs associated with labor force participation, the individuals with RA incurred significantly more expenditures for home or childcare compared to individuals without arthritis[35].

High indirect annual costs were observed in a study of early RA in Germany. The mean annual indirect costs were US$11 750[82]. During the first three years of disease, indirect costs were made up primarily from sick leave at the beginning and then from work disability as time progressed. These costs are higher than the indirect costs estimated in a Swedish study of early RA, US$5610[53]. These differences probably reflect variations in costing methods. The Swedish study did not take into account costs related to short-term sick leave.

In the Canadian study comparing the six-month economic burden of RA, OA, and hypertension, the total indirect costs were higher for the patients with RA compared to the patients with OA, hypertension, or OA and hypertension (Table 33.3)[48]. The total indirect costs for RA were US$2098. The largest portion of the indirect costs were attributed to lost time doing chores, including paid help, US$1729 (Table 33.3). This was followed by time lost from work, US$326, and support person time lost from work, US$44[48].

Although the indirect cost estimates of RA are substantial, they are most likely an underestimate of the true indirect costs of the condition. The human capital approach to estimating indirect costs tends to underestimate the work loss or disability days of older individuals and females. Homemaker costs are estimated using the wages of house cleaners and day care workers, not teachers or counselors. Also, older women have lower labor force participation rates, resulting in lower estimates of the economic impact.

Intangible costs

The costs of RA extend far beyond the medical care costs, work loss, and changes in economic status. The intangible costs of RA include pain, depression, anxiety, changes in family structure, limitations in instrumental and nurturant activities, and changes in appearance resulting from deformity[12,30,37,83–95]. The amount of time individuals spend engaging in activities such as shopping, and visiting the bank and supermarket, as well as the amount of time spent actively participating in hobbies, is significantly reduced in individuals with RA. Studies show that women with RA report limitations in numerous aspects of homemaking[96]. Household work disability is most substantial in women with moderate-to-severe RA[96]. In families in which the wife and/or mother has moderate to severe disease, the other family members spend seven more hours per week on household activity.

Limitations in instrumental activities, such as cleaning, laundry, shopping, cooking, and organizing finances are reported to range from 16 to 73%[97]. The range of reported limitations in nurturant activities, including listening, making arrangements, maintaining ties, care for the sick, and teaching, is 16–42%. It is very difficult to put a monetary price on these limitations, yet they have a significant impact on quality of life.

The impact of RA on psychological status has been measured in terms of depression, coping strategies, anxiety, cognitive changes, self-efficacy, and learned helplessness[90,91,98–103]. Most studies indicate higher levels of psychological distress in individuals with RA than in the general population. This higher level of distress is comparable with levels found among clinical samples of individuals with other chronic conditions[89].

Studies evaluating the rates of divorce in individuals with RA have yielded equivocal findings[104,105]: some studies have found that divorce rates are higher in individuals with RA compared with the general population, whereas others show no significant difference[104]. Hawley and colleagues did note a significant reduction in the rate of remarriage after divorce in individuals with RA[105]. Moreover, the studies in the literature have consistently shown that RA creates stress on marriages and on the healthy spouses[104].

There are no national data studies summarizing the psychological and social impacts of RA. Perhaps this is because it is difficult to quantify these consequences in a traditional population-based survey format, let alone price them in economic terms. The difficulty of data collection notwithstanding, information is needed to increase awareness of the many intangible costs of RA.

Table 33.5 Predictors costs in patients with RA

Predictors	Total direct costs	Same component of direct costs	Indirect costs
Increased disability (HAQ)	A, B, C, D, F, G, I, J		D, F
Poorer functional status (SF-36)	B, E		
Decreased global well-being VAS	A, G		
Increased comorbidity	B. H		
Female sex	E	A	
Higher education		A, B	
Higher income		B	
Younger age		A, B	
Shorter disease duration	H	A	
Majority ethnic status		B	
Private health insurance	E	B	
Pain VAS	A		
Pension	E		
Receiving assistance from others	E		
Poor hand function	C		
Igm RF	C		

A, Ref. 106; B, Ref. 38; C, Ref. 41; D, Ref. 42; E, Ref. 107; F, Ref. 47; G, Ref. 28; H, Ref. 77; I, Ref. 45; J, Ref. 76.

Predictors of cost

Several economic analyses have examined predictors of costs in patients with RA[28,38,41,42,45,47,76,77,106,107]. All of the studies including information about predictors of economic cost analyzed associations of the variables with total direct costs; some also analyzed associations with some of the components of direct costs[38,106], and a few also analyzed associations of predictor variables with indirect costs[42,107]. A summary of the predictor variables studied in economic analyses is depicted in Table 33.5 with reference to the studies. The Health Assessment Questionnaire (HAQ) disability scale was the predictor variable examined in the most studies (Table 33.5). Higher levels of disability were associated with higher total direct and indirect costs. Poorer functional status scores according to the Short Form-36 Health Survey (SF-36) and global well-being visual analog scale (VAS) were also associated with higher total direct costs. Other predictors of either total direct costs or subcomponents of direct costs include increased comorbidity, female sex, higher education and income, younger age, shorter disease duration, majority ethnic status, private health insurance, pain, pension, receiving assistance from others, poor hand function, and IgM rheumatoid factor (Table 33.5)

Conclusion

The direct, indirect, and intangible costs associated with RA are enormous. The long-term economic consequences include medical costs, lost wages due to frequent work disability and reductions in work capacity, psychological distress, and social dislocation. The indirect costs of RA are probably underestimated substantially with current costing methods, but even with underestimations they are significantly higher than the direct costs of RA. The majority of direct medical costs were due to hospitalizations and long-term care in the past. With the introduction of biological therapy, the majority of direct medical costs appear to be due to medication expenses. Poorer functional status appears to be the best predictor of higher direct and indirect costs. The intangible costs of RA are considerable, but difficult to quantify and price. Therapies and treatment of RA should be evaluated in terms of the many consequences of the disease.

References

1. Lawrence, R. C., Helmick, C. G., Arnett, F. C., Deyo, R. A., Felson, D. T., Giannini, E. H. *et al.* Estimates of the prevalence of arthritis and selected musculoskeletal disorders in the United States. *Arthritis Rheum* 1998; **41**: 778–99.
2. Helmick, C. G., Lawrence, R. C., Pollard, R. A., Lloyd, J. C., and Heyse, S. P. Arthritis and other rheumatic conditions: who is affected now, who will be affected later? *Arthritis Care Res* 1995; **8**: 203–11.
3. Reynolds, D., Chambers, L., Badley, E., Bennett, K., Goldsmith, C., Jamieson, E. *et al.* Physical disability among Canadians reporting musculoskeletal diseases. *J Rheumatol* 1992; **19**: 1020–30.
4. Reynolds, D., Torrance, G., Badley, E., Bennett, K., Chambers, L., Goldsmith, C. *et al.* Modelling the population health impact of musculoskeletal diseases: arthritis. *J Rheumatol* 1993; **20**: 1037–47.
5. Badley, E. M., Rasooly, I., and Webster, G. K. Relative importance of musculoskeletal disorders as a cause of chronic health problems, disability, and health care utilization: findings from the 1990 Ontario Health Survey. *J Rheumatol* 1994; **21**: 505–14.
6. Badley, E. M., and Tennant, A. Impact of disablement due to rheumatic disorders in a British population: estimates of severity and prevalence from the Calderdale Rheumatic Disablement Survey. *Ann Rheum Dis* 1993; **52**: 6–13.
7. Badley, E. M. The impact of disabling arthritis. *Arthritis Care Res* 1995; **8**: 221–8.
8. Verbrugge, L. M., Lepkowski, J. M., and Konkol, L. L. Levels of disability among U.S. adults with arthritis. *J Gerontol A Biol Sci Med Sci* 1991; **46**: S71–S83.
9. Verbrugge, L. M., Gates, D. M., and Ike, R. W. Risk factors for disability among U.S. adults with arthritis. *J Clin Epidemiol* 1991; **44**: 167–82.

10. Verbrugge, L., and Patrick, D. Seven chronic conditions: their impact on US adults' activity levels and use of medical services. *Am J Public Health* 1994; **85**: 173–82.

11. Coyte, P. C., Asche, C. V., Croxford, R., and Chan, B. The economic cost of musculoskeletal disorders in Canada. *Arthritis Care Res* 1998; **11**: 315–25.

12. Yelin, E., and Callahan, L. F. The economic cost and social and psychological impact of musculoskeletal conditions. *Arthritis Rheum* 1995; **38**: 1351–62.

13. Badley, E. M. The economic burden of musculoskeletal disorders in Canada is similar to that for cancer, and may be higher. *J Rheumatol* 1995; **22**: 204–6.

14. Callahan, L. F., and Yelin, E. H. *The social and economic consequences of rheumatic disease. The Arthritis Foundation Primer on Rheumatic Disease*, Atlanta, GA: Arthritis Foundation; 2001; 1–4.

15. Health Canada. *Arthritis in Canada: An Ongoing Challenge.* Ottawa: Health Canada; 2003.

16. Rice, D. P., Hodgson, T. A., and Kopstein, A. N. The economic costs of illness: a replication and update. *Health Care Financ Rev* 1985; 7: 61–80.

17. Hootman, J. M., Sniezek, J. E., and Helmick, C. G. Women and arthritis: burden, impact and prevention programs. *J Womens Health Gend Based Med* 2002; **11**: 407–16.

18. Reginster, J. Y. The prevalence and burden of arthritis. *Rheumatology (Oxford)* 2002; **41** (Suppl. 1): 3–6.

19. Jonsson, D., and Husberg, M. Socioeconomic costs of rheumatic diseases: implications for technology assessment. *Int J Technol Assess Health Care* 2000; **16**: 1193–200.

20. Silman, A. J., and Hochberg, M. C. *Epidemiology of rheumatic diseases.* Oxford University Press; 1993.

21. Abdel-Nasser, A. M., Rasker, J. J., and Valkenburg, H. A. Epidemiological and clinical aspects relating to the variability of rheumatoid arthritis. *Semin Arthritis Rheum* 1997; **27**: 123–40.

22. Kvien, T. K., Glennas, A., Knudsred, O. G., Smedstad, L. M., Mowinckel, P., and Forre, O. The prevalence and severity of rheumatoid arthritis in Oslo. *Scand J Rheumatol* 1997; **26**: 412–18.

23. Goronzy, J. J., and Weyand, C. M. Rheumatoid arthritis: epidemiology, pathology, and pathogenesis. In *Arthritis Foundation Primer on the Rheumatic Diseases* (Klippel JH, ed.), pp. 209–17. Atlanta, GA: Arthritis Foundation; 2001.

24. March, L., and Lapsley, H. What are the costs to society and the potential benefits from the effective management of early rheumatoid arthritis? *Best Pract Res Clin Rheumatol* 2001; **15**: 171–85.

25. Meenan, R. F., Yelin, E. H., Henke, C. J., Curtis, D. L, and Epstein, W. V. The costs of rheumatoid arthritis: a patient-oriented study of chronic disease costs. *Arthritis Rheum* 1978; **21**: 827–33.

26. Liang, M. H., Larson, M., Thompson, M., Eaton, H., McNamara, E., Katz, R. *et al.* Costs and outcomes in rheumatoid arthritis and osteoarthritis. *Arthritis Rheum* 1984; **27**: 522–9.

27. Stone, C. E. The lifetime economic costs of rheumatoid arthritis. *J Rheumatol* 1984; **11**: 819–27.

28. Lubeck, D. P., Spitz, P. W., Fries, J. F., Wolfe, F., Mitchell, D. M., and Roth, S. H. A multicenter study of annual health service utilization and costs in rheumatoid arthritis. *Arthritis Rheum* 1986; **29**: 488–93.

29. acobs, J., Keyserling, J. A., Britton, M., Morgan, G. J., Jr., Wilkenfeld, J., and Hutchings, H. C. The total cost of care and the use of pharmaceuticals in the management of rheumatoid arthritis: the Medi-Cal program. *J Clin Epidemiol* 1988; **41**: 215–23.

30. Allaire, S. H., Prashker, M. J., and Meenan, R. F. The costs of rheumatoid arthritis. *Pharmacoeconomics* 1994; **6**: 513–22.

31. Yelin, E. The costs of rheumatoid arthritis: absolute, incremental, and marginal estimates. *J Rheumatol* 1996; **23** (Suppl. 44): 47–51.

32. Pincus, T. The underestimated long term medical and economic consequences of rheumatoid arthritis. *Drugs* 1995; **50**: 1–14.

33. Lambert, C. M., and Hurst, N. P. Health economics as an aspect of health outcome: basic principles and application in rheumatoid arthritis. *Br J Rheumatol* 1995; **34**: 774–80.

34. Meenan, R. F., Yelin, E. H., Nevitt, M., and Epstein, W. V. The impact of chronic disease: a sociomedical profile of rheumatoid arthritis. *Arthritis Rheum* 1981; **24**: 544–9.

35. Gabriel, S.E., Crowson, C. S., Campion, M. E., and O'Fallon, W. M. Indirect and nonmedical costs among people with rheumatoid arthritis and osteoarthritis compared with nonarthritic controls. *J Rheumatol* 1997; **24**: 43–8.

36. Mitchell, J. M., Burkhauser, R. V., and Pincus, T. The importance of age, education, and comorbidity in the substantial earnings losses of individuals with symmetric polyarthritis. *Arthritis Rheum* 1988; **31**: 348–57.

37. Eberhardt, K., Larson, B. M., and Nived, K. Early rheumatoid arthritis: some social, economical, and psychological aspects. *Scand J Rheumatol* 1993; **22**: 119–23.

38. Michaud, K., Messer, J., Choi, H., K., and Wolfe, F. Direct medical costs and their predictors in patients with rheumatoid arthritis: a three-year study of 7,527 patients. *Arthritis Rheum* 2003; **48**: 2750–62.

39. Soderlin, M. K., Kautiainen, H., Jonsson, D., Skogh, T., and Leirisalo-Repo, M. The costs of early inflammatory joint disease: a population-based study in southern Sweden. *Scand J Rheumatol* 2003; **32**: 216–24.

40. Haglund, U., and Svarvar, P. The Swedish ACCES model: predicting the health economic impact of celecoxib in patients with osteoarthritis or rheumatoid arthritis. *Rheumatology (Oxford)* 2000; **39** (Suppl. 2): 51–6.

41. Hallert, E., Husberg, M., Jonsson, D., and Skogh, T. Rheumatoid arthritis is already expensive during the first year of the disease (the Swedish TIRA project). *Rheumatology (Oxford)* 2004; **43**: 1374–82.

42. Kobelt, G., Jonsson, L., Lindgren, P., Young, A., and Eberhardt, K. Modeling the progression of rheumatoid arthritis: a two-country model to estimate costs and consequences of rheumatoid arthritis. *Arthritis Rheum* 2002; **46**: 2310–19.

43. Ruof, J., Hulsemann, J. L., Mittendorf, T., Handelmann, S., der Schulenburg, J. M., Zeidler, H. *et al.* Costs of rheumatoid arthritis in Germany: a micro-costing approach based on healthcare payer's data sources. *Ann Rheum Dis* 2003; **62**: 544–9.

44. van den Hout, W. B., Tijhuis, G. J., Hazes, J. M., Breedveld, F. C., and Vliet Vlieland, T. P. Cost effectiveness and cost utility analysis of multidisciplinary care in patients with rheumatoid arthritis: a randomised comparison of clinical nurse specialist care, inpatient team care, and day patient team care. *Ann Rheum Dis* 2003; **62**: 308–15.

45. Verstappen, S. M., Verkleij, H., Bijlsma, J. W., Buskens, E., Kruize, A. A., Heurkens, A. H. *et al.* Determinants of direct costs in Dutch rheumatoid arthritis patients. *Ann Rheum Dis* 2004; **63**: 817–24.

46. Birnbaum, H. G., Barton, M., Greenberg, P. E., Sisitsky, T., Auerbach, R., Wanke, L. A. *et al.* Direct and indirect costs of rheumatoid arthritis to an employer. *J Occup Environ Med* 2000; **42**: 588–96.

47. Lajas, C., Abasolo, L., Bellajdel, B., Hernandez-Garcia, C., Carmona, L., Vargas, E. *et al.* Costs and predictors of costs in rheumatoid arthritis: a prevalence-based study. *Arthritis Rheum* 2003; **49**: 64–70.

48. Maetzel, A., Li, L. C., Pencharz, J., Tomlinson, G., and Bombardier, C. The economic burden associated with osteoarthritis, rheumatoid arthritis, and hypertension: a comparative study. *Ann Rheum Dis* 2004; **63**: 395–401.

49. Brouwer, W. B., van Exel, N. J., van de, B. B., Dinant, H. J., Koopmanschap, M. A., and van den Bos, G. A. Burden of caregiving: evidence of objective burden, subjective burden, and quality of life impacts on informal caregivers of patients with rheumatoid arthritis. *Arthritis Rheum* 2004; **51**: 570–7.

50. Cooper, N. J. Economic burden of rheumatoid arthritis: a systematic review. Rheumatology (Oxford) 2000; **39**: 28–33.

51. Gabriel, S. E., Crowson. C. S., Campion, M. E., and O'Fallon, W. M. Direct medical costs unique to people with arthritis. *J Rheumatol* 1997; **24**: 719–25.

52. Lubeck, D. P., The economic impact of rheumatoid arthritis. In *Rheumatoid arthritis: pathogenesis, assessment, outcome, and treatment* (Wolfe F, and Pincus T, eds), pp. 247–59. New York, Marcel Dekker; 1664.

53. Kobelt, G., Eberhardt, K., and Jonsson, L., Jonsson, B. Economic consequences of the progression of rheumatoid arthritis in Sweden. *Arthritis Rheum* 1999; **42**: 347–56.

54. Katz, J. N., and Sangha, O. Assessment of the quality of care. *Arthritis Care Res* 1997; **10**: 359–69.

55. Katz, P. P., and Showstack, J. A. Choosing quality and outcomes measures for rheumatic diseases. *Arthritis Care Res* 1997; **10**: 370–80.

56. Mason, J. H. Outcomes measurement in today's health care environment. *Arthritis Care Res* 1997; **10**: 355–8.

57. Ferraz, M. B., Maetzel, A., and Bombardier, C. A. summary of economic evaluations published in the field of rheumatology and related disciplines. *Arthritis Rheum* 1997; **40**: 1587–93.

58. Gabriel, S. E., Tugwell, P., and Drummond, M. Progress towards an OMERACT-ILAR guideline for economic evaluations in rheumatology. *Ann Rheum Dis* 2002; **61**: 370–3.

59. Ruchlin, H. S., Elkin, E. B., and Paget, S. A. Assessing cost-effectiveness analyses in rheumatoid arthritis and osteoarthritis. *Arthritis Care Res* 1997; **10**: 413–21.

60. Haddix, A. C., Teutsch, S. M., Shaffer, P. A., and Dunet, D. O. *Prevention Effectiveness: A Guide to Decision Analysis and Economic Evaluation*. New York, Oxford University Press; 1996.

61. Gold, M. R., Siegel, J. E., Russell, L. B., Weinstein, M. C. *Cost-Effectiveness in Health and Medicine*. New York: Oxford University Press; 1996.

62. Maztzel, A. Costs of illness and the burden of disease. *J Rheumatol* 1997; **24**: 3–5.

63. Hall, J., and Mooney, G. What every doctor should know about economics. Part I. The benefits of costing. *Med J Aust* 1990; **152**: 29–31.

64. Savage, R. L., Moller, P. W., Ballantyne, C. L., and Wells, J. E. Variation in the risk of peptic ulcer complications with nonsteroidal antiinflammatory drug therapy. *Arthritis Rheum* 1993; **36**: 84–90.

65. Hodgson, T. A., and Meiners, M. R. Cost-of-illness methodology: a guide to current practices and procedures. *Milbank Mem Fund Q Health Soc* 1982; **60**: 429–62.

66. Hodgson, T. A. The state of the art of cost-of-illness estimates. *Adv Health Econ Health Serv Res* 1983; **4**: 129–64.

67. Rice, D. P. Estimating the cost of illness. *Am J Public Health* 1967; **57**: 424–39.

68. Lubeck, D. P. The economic impact of arthritis. *Arthritis Care Res* 1995; **8**: 304–10.

69. van Jaarsveld, C. H. M., Jacobs, J. W. G., Schrijvers, H. J. P., Heurkens, A. H. M., Haanen, H. C. M., and Bijlsma, J. W. J. Direct cost of rheumatoid arthritis during the first six years: a cost-of-illness study. *Br J Rheumatol* 1998; **37**: 837–47.

70. Ward, M. M., Javtiz, H. S., and Yelin, E. H. The direct cost of rheumatoid arthritis. *Value in Health* 2000; **3**: 243–52.

71. Lubeck, D. P. A. review of the direct costs of rheumatoid arthritis: managed care versus fee-for-service settings. *Pharmacoeconomics* 2001; **19**: 811–18.

72. Jonsson, B., Rehnberg, C., Borgquist, L., and Larsson, S. E. Locomotion status and costs in destructive rheumatoid arthritis: a comprehensive study of 82 patients from a population of 13,000. *Acta Orthop Scand* 1992; **63**: 207–12.

73. Clarke, A. E., Zowall, H., Levinton, C., Assimakopoulos, H., Sibley, J. T., Haga, M. *et al*. Direct and indirect medical costs incurred by Canadian patients with rheumatoid arthritis: a 12 year study. *J Rheumatol* 1997; **24**: 1051–60.

74. Wolfe, F., Kleinheksel, S. M., Spitz, P. W., Lubeck, D. P., Fries, J. F., Young, D. Y. *et al*. A multicenter study of hospitalization in rheumatoid arthritis: effect of health care system, severity, and regional difference. *J Rheumatol* 1986; **13**: 277–84.

75. Lanes, S. F., Lanza, L. L., Radensky, P. W., Yood, R. A., Meenan, R. F., Walker, A. M. *et al*. Resource utilization and cost of care for rheumatoid arthritis and osteoarthritis in a managed care setting. *Arthritis Rheum* 1997; **40**: 1475–81.

76. Yelin, E., and Wanke, L. A. An assessment of the annual and long-term direct costs of rheumatoid arthritis. *Arthritis Rheum* 1999; **42**: 1209–18.

77. Newhall-Perry, K., Law, N. J., Ramos, B., Sterz, M., Wong, W. K., Bulpitt, K. J. *et al*. Direct and indirect costs associated with the onset of seropositive rheumatoid arthritis. *J Rheumatol* 2000; **27**: 1156–63.

78. Yelin, E., Meenan, R., Nevitt, M., and Epstein, W. Work disability in rheumatoid arthritis: effects of disease, social, and work factors. *Ann Intern Med* 1980; **93**: 551–6.

79. Kochevar, R. J., Kaplan, R. M., and Weisman, M. Financial and career losses due to rheumatoid arthritis: a pilot study. *J Rheumatol* 1997; **24**: 1527–30.

80. McIntosh, E. The cost of rheumatoid arthritis. *Br J Rheumatol* 1996; **35**: 781–90.

81. van Jaarsveld, C. H. M., Jacobs, J. W. G., Schrijvers, A. J. P., van Albada-Kuipers, G. A., Hofman, D. M., and Bijlsma, J. W. J. Effects of rheumatoid arthritis on employment and social participation during the first years of disease in the Netherlands. *Br J Rheumatol* 1998; **37**: 848–53.

82. Merkesdal, S., Ruof, J., Schoffski, O., Bernitt, K., Zeidler, H., and Mau, W. Indirect medical costs in early rheumatoid arthritis: composition of and changes in indirect costs within the first three years of disease. *Arthritis Rheum* 2001; **44**: 528–34.

83. Bradley, L. A. Psychological aspects of arthritis. Bull Rheum Dis 1985; **35**: 1–12.

84. Ehrlich, G. E. Social, economic, psychologic, and sexual outcomes in rheumatoid arthritis. *Am J Med* 1983; **75**: 27–34.

85. Spitz, P. W. The medical, personal, and social costs of rheumatoid arthritis. *Nurs Clin North Am* 1984; **19**: 575–82.

86. Skevington, S. M. Psychological aspects of pain in rheumatoid arthritis: a review. *Soc Sci Med* 1986; **23**: 567–75.

87. Fitzpatrick, R., Newman, S., Archer, R., and Shipley, M. Social support, disability and depression: a longitudinal study of rheumatoid arthritis. *Soc Sci Med* 1991; **33**: 605–11.

88. Parker, J. C., and Wright, G. E. The implications of depression for pain and disability in rheumatoid arthritis. *Arthritis Care Res* 1995; **8**: 279–83.

89. DeVellis, B. M. Depression in rheumatological diseases. *Baillieres Clin Rheum* 1993; 7: 241–57.

90. Zautra, A., and Manne, S. Coping with rheumatoid arthritis: review of a decade of research. Ann Behav Med 1992; **14**: 31–9.

91. Blalock, S. J., DeVellis, B. M., DeVellis, R. F., Giorgino, K. B., van, H., Sauter, S., Jordan, J. M. *et al*. Psychological well-being among people with recently diagnosed rheumatoid arthritis: do self-perceptions of abilities make a difference? *Arthritis Rheum* 1992; **35**: 1267–72.

92. Katz, P. P., and Yelin, E. H. Prevalence and correlates of depressive symptoms among persons with rheumatoid arthritis. *J Rheumatol* 1993; **20**: 790–6.

93. Smith, T. W., Peck, J. R., Milano, R. A., and Ward, J. R. Cognitive distortion in rheumatoid arthritis: relation to depression and disability. *J Consult Clin Psychol* 1988; **56**: 412–16.

94. Revenson, T. A., and Felton, B. J. Disability and coping as predictors of psychological adjustment to rheumatoid arthritis. *J Consult Clin Psychol* 1989; **57**: 344–8.

95. Zautra, A. J., Burleson, M. H., Matt, K. S., Roth, S., and Burrows, L. Interpersonal stress, depression, and disease activity in rheumatoid arthritis and osteoarthritis patients. *Health Psychol* 1994; **13**: 139–48.

96. Allaire, S. H., Meenan, R. F., and Anderson, J. J. The impact of rheumatoid arthritis on the household work performance of women. *Arthritis Rheum* 1991; **34**: 669–78.

97. Reisine, S. T., Goodenow, C., and Grady, K. E. The impact of rheumatoid arthritis on the homemaker. *Soc Sci Med* 1987; **25**: 89–95.

98. Manne, S. L., and Zautra, A. J. Coping with arthritis: current status and critique. *Arthritis Rheum* 1992; **35**: 1273–9.

99. Blalock, S. J., DeVellis, B. M., Holt, K., and Hahn, P. M. Coping with rheumatoid arthritis: is one problem the same as another? *Health Educ Q* 1993; **20**: 119–32.

100. Blalock, S. J., Afifi, R. A., DeVellis, B. M., Holt, K., and DeVellis, R. F. Adjustment to rheumatoid arthritis: the role of social comparison processes. *Health Educ Res* 1990; **5**: 361–70.

101. Lorig, K., Chastain, R. L., Ung, E., Shoor, S., and Holman, H. R. Development and evaluation of a scale to measure perceived self-efficacy in people with arthritis. *Arthritis Rheum* 1989; **32**: 37–44.

102. Nicassio, P. M., Wallston, K. A., Callahan, L. F., Herbert, M., and Pincus, T. The measurement of helplessness in rheumatoid arthritis: the development of the arthritis helplessness index. *J Rheumatol* 1985; **12**: 462–7.

103. Callahan, L. F., Brooks, R. H., and Pincus, T. Further analysis of learned helplessness in rheumatoid arthritis using a 'Rheumatology Attitudes Index'. *J Rheumatol* 1988; **15**: 418–26.

104. Revenson, T. A. The role of social support with rheumatic disease. *Baillieres Clin Rheum* 1993; 7: 377–96.

105. Hawley, D. J., Wolfe, F., Cathey, M. A., and Roberts, F. K. Marital status in rheumatoid arthritis and other rheumatic disorders: a study of 7,293 patients. *J Rheumatol* 1991; **18**: 654–60.

106. Clarke, A. E., Levinton, C., Joseph, L., Penrod, J., Zowall, H., Sibley, J. T. *et al*. Predicting the short term direct medical costs incurred by patients with rheumatoid arthritis. *J Rheumatol* 1999; **26**: 1068–75.

107. Lapsley, H. M., March, L. M., Tribe, K. L., Cross, M. J., Courtenay, B. G., and Brooks, P. M. Living with rheumatoid arthritis: expenditures, health status, and social impact on patients. *Ann Rheum Dis* 2002; **61**: 818–21.

SECTION
6

Surgical therapy

34 | Large joints and feet

Urban Rydholm

Introduction

Joint surgery in rheumatoid arthritis (RA) is an essential component of rheumatological rehabilitation, in particular large joint replacement procedures. Surgical synovectomy, however, has largely been replaced by local or systemic non-surgical measures (see Section 4). An increasing variety of joint prostheses are now in use. Immediate results are often dramatic but long-term, controlled trials are scarce.

The outcome of surgical procedures in the large joints and feet differ between patients with RA and osteoarthritis (OA), due to the systemic and progressive character of RA.

The number of RA patients undergoing orthopedic intervention is influenced by availability of resources for combined clinics where qualified orthopedic surgeons can cooperate with rheumatologists. More than 10% of RA patients treated medically for five years had undergone large- or small-joint surgery in a study by James et al.[1]. Rheumatoid factor (RF) positive women with rheumatoid nodules are at higher risk for surgery, and in order to reduce the eventual need for surgery, a therapeutic target in the first year of RA is the suppression of disease activity.

The need for surgery will probably diminish with time, as more patients will be offered early and more aggressive medical treatment. Many RA joints are, however, replaced due to 'secondary osteoarthritis' and it should be remembered that even joints with modest signs of inflammation may, with time, develop sever structural damage and require joint replacement. It is also possible that effective analgesic therapy may increase the risk of OA due to overuse of joints.

Indications and contraindications

Indications

Indications for surgical intervention are mainly as follows:

- *pain relief* when conservative measures have failed;
- *prevention* of nerve compression, tendon rupture, or further functional joint deterioration;
- *reconstruction* of damaged joints with the aim of improving function.

Relieving pain is the dominant overall indication.

The decision to perform surgery must always be based on a careful analysis of the origin of the pain, which may be caused by synovial inflammation in an intact joint, by destructive changes, or by a combination of inflammation and destruction. The radiographic appearance of the painful joint is of interest, since it is less likely that advanced radiographic changes will be reversible with non-surgical treatments. Surgical procedures involving removal of synovial tissue from tendon sheaths may prevent tendon rupture. Even if no preventive effect of synovectomy has ever been proven, it should be remembered that synovectomy temporarily reduces factors that are involved in the destruction of cartilage[2].

Correction of deformity and fusion of ankle and small joints in the foot may also prevent unfavorable loading conditions in proximal joints. Isolated correction of deformities is, however, often superfluous, since neighboring joints have commonly adapted to surrounding deformities. Reconstructive surgery can consist of replacement of destroyed joint surfaces with artificial materials, endoprostheses, or autologous tissue. Arthrodesis is also still useful, for example in the hindfoot where it may improve loading conditions for the knee and foot. Often a combination of indications is present.

Contraindications and risk factors

There are some risk factors related to rheumatoid disease that always should be taken into consideration in the planning of surgery (Table 34.1). Certain drugs may increase the risks associated with surgery, but perioperative guidelines have never been well established for a majority of the traditional anti-rheumatic drugs. Perioperative use of Cox inhibitors remains controversial, although they may be beneficial in preventing heterotopic bone formation[4] and decreasing the risk of postoperative stiffness and thromboembolism. Bleeding complications may be minimized by meticulous surgical technique and use of tranexamic acid[3]. Use of non-steroidal anti-inflammatory drugs (NSAIDs), steroids, methotrexate, hydroxychloroquine, or gold have not been shown to cause impaired healing or infectious complications[5]. While recommendations for the perioperative use of NSAIDs and glucocorticoids remain controversial most data support their use, and also methotrexate[6], in connection with joint surgery[7–9].

Immune suppressive therapy is increasingly used in the treatment of RA and may or may not affect wound healing[10,11]. Recently published data suggest that in patients with rheumatoid arthritis undergoing elective foot and ankle surgery, the use of tumor necrosis factor (TNF)-α inhibition agents is probably safe in the perioperative period[12]. Available data, however, so far do not support evidence-based recommendations. Severe and active disease, lack of motivation, and unrealistic patient expectations are relative contraindications.

Table 34.1 Risk factors related to rheumatoid arthritis

Increased disease or therapy-related risk of infection
Nutritional difficulties (temporomandibular arthritis, dysphagia secondary to cervical spine involvement)
Cardiovascular problems (vasculitis, valvular heart disease)
Renal insufficiency (e.g. amyloidosis)
Impaired bone quality (osteopenia)
Anesthesiological risks related to the cervical spine and temporomandibular joints

Strategic considerations

In order to optimize surgery in patients with several potential options for joint surgery during decades of disease, it is essential to assess the indications and priorities in combined clinics involving rheumatologists, orthopedic surgeons, hand surgeons, and health professionals. The experienced team will be aware of the many paradoxical effects that may result from individual joint procedures in patients with RA. Total knee replacement in a patient with valgus deformities of the knee may result in pain relief not only in the knee but also in the ankle and foot, due to improved loading position. On the other hand, replacement of the knee joints in a previously wheelchair-restricted patient may give rise to increased pain in adjacent joints caused by resumed physical activity, and thus require further surgery. Another example is the amelioration of elbow pain in patients dependent on assistive walking devices, by improving lower extremity function and eliminating the need for such devices.

The first in a series of planned operations should, if possible, be a small procedure, such as forefoot surgery or arthrodesis of a thumb. This will allow an appreciation of the patient's capacity to participate in postoperative rehabilitation after more complex procedures.

General anesthesia in patients with instability of the cervical spine and/or limited mouth opening due to temporomandibular arthritis needs special equipment and careful management. In such patients the possibility of multiple joint surgery in a single session should be considered in order to minimize the total need for anesthesia. Bilateral total hip or knee replacement and ipsilateral shoulder and elbow replacement can be performed without increased peri- or postoperative morbidity[13].

Non-cemented joint implants and conventional osteosynthetic devices may be impossible to use in RA patients with severe osteopenia. The risk of permanent deformities and osteopenia also contraindicates prolonged postoperative bed rest or joint immobilization in these patients. Postoperative exercises are possibly an important component for a good outcome.

Surgery of the shoulder

Among hospitalized rheumatic patients or patients with more than 15 years of illness, 80–90% have radiographic changes and more or less severe symptoms from the shoulder[14]. Arthritis is common in both the glenohumeral (GH) and acromioclavicular (AC) joints. Radiographic deterioration of the GH joint progresses as mobility is lost. Disease in the AC joint is an often overlooked cause of shoulder pain. Clinical signs of AC joint arthritis have been reported in 34%, and radiographic changes in 85%, in one report[14].

Indications and surgical methods

Painful AC joint arthritis can be treated by lateral clavicle resection, possibly in combination with anterior acromioplasty, a procedure which can provide good pain relief in patients with massive rotator cuff rupture. Lateral clavicle resection should probably be considered more often than is currently the case. The procedure is relatively minor and may possibly replace prosthetic surgery in some patients where the shape of the head of the humerus is retained and the articular cartilage of the glenohumeral joint is somewhat preserved[15].

Synovectomy

Synovectomy in the GH joint is seldom warranted, because when non-remitting shoulder problems develop, pronounced joint destruction is usually present. A patient with pain at rest, somewhat well-preserved joint surfaces, and a proliferative synovitis, could be a candidate for synovectomy, but there is no good published evidence for this. Arthroscopic synovectomy is a possibility.

Resection interposition arthroplasty

Resection interposition arthroplasty involves trimming the joint surfaces and interposing a membrane (Lyodura®, silicone, fascia) between the head of the humerus and the glenoid. The postoperative course is often long and troublesome and there is a risk of instability[16]. A prosthesis is most likely the superior material for interposition.

Shoulder replacement

Arthroplasty by endoprosthesis, in the form of either a hemiprosthesis or as a total joint prosthesis with a glenoid component (Fig. 34.1), has become an increasingly common procedure on the indication of painful motion of the shoulder with deterioration in the glenohumeral joint. The functional outcome of prosthetic surgery is determined by the quality of the soft tissue parts, not least the rotator cuff, in addition to the correct positioning of the prosthesis. Recent trends have favored modular humeral prostheses of various styles, with a conical connection between the humerus component's shaft and the articular head, making it possible to vary the humeral head size while keeping the same prosthetic humeral shaft. Hemiprostheses, rather than total joint

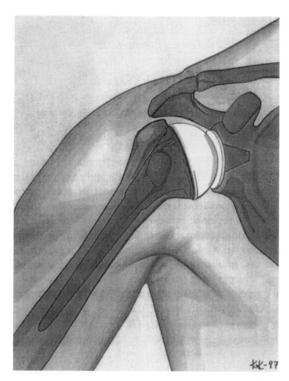

Fig. 34.1 The typical shoulder prosthesis is a design with a cemented or non-cemented stem, a modular head, and an optional glenoid component. As in the normal shoulder, the joint is stable through the tension of the joint capsule and muscles. (Reprinted with permission from Knutson K. (1998). Arthroplasty and its complications. In *Osteoarthritis* (ed. K. D. Brandt, M. Doherty, and L. S. Lohmander), pp. 388–402. Oxford University Press.)

Table 34.2 Average clinical results and radiographic findings in 558 replaced shoulders

Pain relief	89 (78–100)%
Pre- or postoperative complications	10 (0–24)%
Loosening of humeral component	6 (0–25)%
Loosening of glenoid component	8 (0–25)%

replacement, are still widely used, due to the lack of good methods for the fixation of a glenoid component.

There is agreement that arthroplasty with a prosthesis usually provides reliable pain relief and functional gain. The need to replace the glenoid is, however, controversial[17–19]. A disadvantage with hemiarthroplasty is that pain relief may be less reliable than after total shoulder replacement and that bone loss in the glenoid accelerates, which may make revision difficult. However, the bone quality of RA patients is often such that safe fixation of a glenoid component may be nearly impossible. This is reflected by the rather high frequency of development of radiolucent zones, probably a prostage to loosening, in many studies. Preservation of the original glenoid also excludes the possibility that plastic wear products will cause or accelerate prosthetic loosening.

Shoulder prostheses of various styles have now been used to treat rheumatic patients for several decades. Nevertheless, long-term follow-up is lacking. It is difficult to extract reliable data from the literature since different authors mix both diagnoses and prosthetic types in their studies. The majority of such mixed studies have average follow-up periods of 3–4 years. Since it is difficult to measure isolated mobility of the GH joint, usually total shoulder mobility is reported. Pain relief is good, and an ~90% outcome of 'good–excellent' is standard. Table 34.2 shows achieved average pain relief and radiographic findings in 558 procedures from 14 studies with a follow-up period exceeding three years[20]. None of the studies used randomized controlled protocols.

Radiographic loosening of the components is common, but causes only insignificant symptoms. An association between loosening of the glenoid component and concurrent occurrence of rotator cuff injury has been proven[21]. Proximal migration of the humerus is common, and may change the kinetics of the shoulder and increase the risk of prosthetic loosening. There is, however, no relationship between the clinical outcome and the degree of progressive proximal migration of the humerus[22].

Postoperative fracture occurs in less than 2% and nerve damage in less than 1%, with infection in ~0.5% of cases[23]. Use of a glenoid component may, however, increase the risk of complications.

Modular prostheses consisting of separate components provide better possibilities for achieving an optimal tension in soft tissues and restoring the center of mobility, but they also involve a risk for dislocations between the components, and corrosion between the components. There are no long-term results yet. Non-cemented glenoid components have shown promising short-term results, but have the disadvantage of potentially causing plastic wear[24]. Bipolar prostheses, with a small head articulating with polythene inside a larger metallic shell articulating against the glenoid, have also been introduced[25].

There is also the possibility of surface replacement on the same indications as for the conventional stemmed prostheses, and this procedure has the advantage of bone preservation as well as avoidance of the potential complications associated with a long humeral stem in rheumatoid bone. The procedure is not suitable for severely damaged joints in which the humeral head is insufficient or too soft[26].

The results of prosthetic surgery in the shoulder can be evaluated in terms of pain relief, improved mobility, functional improvement of the upper extremity, radiographic results, and complication frequency. It appears most relevant to evaluate the outcome based on function (Table 34.3)[27–30].

Arthrodesis

Arthrodesis is an option in younger patients with severe bone destruction, which precludes secure prosthetic fixation, or, rarely, when severe pain is present despite very limited range of motion. Long-term postoperative immobilization is required, with the risks involved of stiffening of the other joints in the upper extremity.

The elbow

Instability of the elbow is unusual and generally a sign of severe bone loss. The ulnar nerve passes close to the articular capsule, and nerve compression is not uncommon. Approximately half of all hospitalized patients experience elbow problems, often early

Table 34.3 Upper limb function following shoulder arthroplasty in patients with RA

Author(s)	No. of shoulders	Can manage personal hygiene		Can use a comb	
		Preop (%)	Follow-up (%)	Preop (%)	Follow-up (%)
Kelly (1987)	41	41	83	12	54
Barrett *et al.* (1989)	134	46	84	28	66
Rydholm and Sjögren (1993)	71	30	78	6	56
van Cappelle and Visser (1994)	41	39	71	29	61

in the disease[30]. Slow radiographic progression is the rule[31]. Although pain and limited range of motion are common, surgery rarely will be indicated until there is significant loss of cartilage.

Indications and surgical methods

Patients with instability may be helped by stabilizing orthoses that allow full motion. A sensible method for alleviating elbow symptoms in patients dependent on walking devices is to try to make the patient independent of these devices by improving leg function.

Synovectomy

The stable, somewhat movable, but painful elbow is well suited for synovectomy with concurrent removal of the radial head. Synovectomy may be performed both early and late in the course, and provides good pain relief with only minor effects on mobility. Removal of the radial head has been considered a condition for radical synovectomy, and is likely to contribute to the pain relief by disconnecting the radiohumeral and proximal radioulnar joints. Since the stability of the elbow is largely dependent on the congruence of the humeroulnar joint, instability problems after extirpation of the radial head are uncommon. Synovectomy can, however, also be performed radically with preservation of the radial head, whereby one avoids the risk for a potential sense of weakness in the forearm. It should always be remembered that synovectomy in a severely destroyed elbow can result in instability, and thus one problem is replaced by a new one.

Compression of the ulnar nerve at the elbow may, at times, also be an indication for synovectomy of the elbow, with or without concurrent neurolysis and nerve transposition. There are few long-term follow-up studies of elbow synovectomy in patients with RA[33], indicating long-term pain relief and minor improvement in flexion in approximately two-thirds of the patients. Late synovectomy yields only temporary pain relief with a high rate of elbow arthroplasties[34].

Synovectomy is not followed by progressive bone loss, and hence any subsequent prosthetic surgery is not rendered more difficult. Surprisingly the results are not appreciably affected by the degree of preoperative destruction.

Synovectomy may be superior to prosthesis, since it is simpler, less expensive, and has fewer complications, but still gives results comparable to those of prostheses[35,36]. The results concerning pain relief are, however, inferior to those achieved by prosthetic surgery.

Resection interposition arthroplasty

Resection interposition arthroplasty has been used to treat patients with an elbow which is painful and limited in mobility, but reasonably stable and radiographically intact. The affected joint surfaces are trimmed and covered with a material to prevent adhesion. A number of interposition materials have been used over the years. Usually, Lyodura®, abdominal skin, or muscle fascia from the thigh is used. The disadvantage of the method is the risk of progressive loss of bone with subsequent instability. Pain relief has generally been reported as good. Mobility and stability are, however, not improved[35,36], and ulnar nerve damage and fractures are relatively common. Loss of bone may, in the long run, be such that reoperation by prosthesis is rendered impossible. In the light of the improved results with prosthetic surgery, the method has slowly lost ground.

Elbow replacement

For elbows with severe pain on motion, limited range of motion, and pronounced loss of cartilage and bone, joint replacement is a well-established alternative. Development has been from hinged prostheses to prostheses with a sloppy hinge permitting some rotation and valgus–varus laxity, in order to decrease the forces on the bone–cement and cement–prosthesis interfaces. Most commonly used today are sloppy hinged implants and unlinked stemmed surface replacement prostheses of the same basic type as knee prostheses (Fig. 34.2). More than 90% of the patients are completely free from pain after surgery[37]. Flexion and rotation are usually improved postoperatively. Correct positioning of the prosthesis and careful handling of the soft tissues is critical for the outcome. The surgical technique is difficult, and the procedure is associated with a relatively high frequency of complications. Transient impairment of ulnar nerve function is common, but permanent ulnar nerve injury is uncommon[38].

Results of 1495 procedures reported in 18 studies are shown in Table 34.4[20].

Although the average gain in flexion was only 15° (8–25°), this may represent a substantial functional gain, allowing the patient to reach the mouth with the hand. The gain in extension of 8° (−2° to 21°) usually has little impact on function, in contrast to improved rotation of the forearm. For an elbow to be useful during daily activities, freedom from pain, mobility, and stability are required. It has been reported[39] that 43/50 surface-replaced elbows after three years showed negligible pain, a range of motion exceeding 100°, and instability of less than 10°.

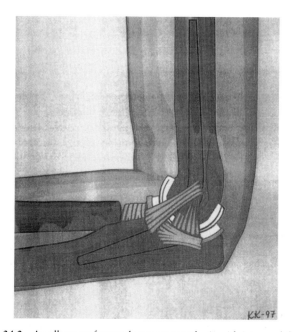

Fig. 34.2 An elbow surface replacement prosthesis with intramedullary humeral and ulnar stems. Some constrainment is achieved by the anatomy of the prosthetic joint surfaces. The ulnar component has an articulating surface from polyethylene. Joint stability is achieved by tension in ligaments and muscles. (Reprinted with permission from Knutson K. (1998). Arthroplasty and its complications. In *Osteoarthritis* (ed. K. D. Brandt, M. Doherty, and L. S. Lohmander), pp. 388–402. Oxford University Press.)

Table 34.4 Average clinical results of prosthetic surgery in the elbow

Pain relief	89 (70–100)%
Gain of flexion	15 (8–25) °
Gain of extension	8 (−2–21) °
Gain of supination	16 (4–28) °
Gain of pronation	14 (8–25) °

in flexion contracture, outward rotation, and adduction, and functional shortening of the limb, valgus stress in the knee joint, and malpositioning of the foot. Early in the course, radiographs may appear normal. Radiographic changes occur with time, but do not correlate closely with symptoms. RA of the hip may progress in an explosive way, when combined with infarction of the femoral head. Bone loss in the acetabulum results in protrusion of the head of the femur into the pelvis. This may not cause symptoms but, with progress, follows loss of mobility. Protrusion is observed in up to 40% of patients with RA[42]. Progression is usually slow, but may be explosive in some cases. Shortening of a limb can be accentuated by protrusion. Patients with protrusion should undergo regular radiographic check-ups so that bone loss does not reach a stage where prosthetic implantation becomes difficult or impossible.

Indications for surgery include severe pain on weight bearing or at rest. Limited range of motion and/or advanced protrusion occasionally indicate need for surgery.

Hip replacement

Total hip replacement (THR) was made practical by Sir John Charnley, and its astounding success has made other surgical alternatives most uncommon. In the absence of long-term follow-up studies of uncemented prostheses, prosthetic anchorage using bone cement (Fig. 34.3) is still considered to be the gold standard. Osteopenia and subchondral cyst formation reduce the chances for successful prosthetic anchorage, especially on the acetabular side. Even if the long-term loosening rate of cemented cups has been reduced with the most modern cementation technique[43], a trend has developed toward using non-cemented cups aiming at osseointegration through press–fit fixation to bone. Some evidence now also supports the use of uncemented femoral components.

Surgery in patients having a pronounced protrusion involves transplantation of donor bone and/or bone from the patient's femoral head or iliac crest to the acetabular roof. Such transplanted bone heals predictably and safely[44].

Mobilization following THR is usually unproblematic but may be more difficult in patients with poorly functioning upper extremities who have difficulty using walking devices. Patients with active polyarthritis may also find it difficult to avoid placing weight on the leg after extensive reconstructive surgery that involves bone transplantation.

Beneficial results of THR in hip RA are well established[43,45,46]. THR in patients with RA has a very low perioperative mortality, and the mortality during the three years following the procedure in patients older than 65 years does not differ from that in patients with OA[47]. Survival, when matched for age and gender,

The predominant complication is ulnar nerve damage, which, as a rule, is reversible and which may possibly be minimized by modification of the surgical technique. It is characteristic of surface replacement prostheses that early complication risks are frequent (ulnar nerve injury, dislocation, and infection) while long-term risks are few. For the linked prostheses, on the contrary, the long-term results are jeopardized by both wear of the coupling mechanism and mechanical prosthetic loosening. Due to the superficial location of the elbow, impaired wound healing is a significant risk for deep infection. The average risk of deep infection is 3%[38], which is in the same range as the risk after a knee prosthesis, but significantly higher than the risk for infection after hip or shoulder prostheses. The probability for survival of the prosthesis after synovectomy and vigorous antibiotic treatment is low. It is generally considered too risky to attempt a reimplantation after deep infection. These patients are submitted to a resection arthroplasty, and end up with significant loss of function. The results after revision performed due to aseptic prosthetic loosening, instability, material defects, or fracture are significantly better.

Surgery of the hip

The true rate of involvement of the hip in patients with RA is uncertain, since ultrasound screening shows that asymptomatic synovitis is as common as symptomatic[40]. Manifest hip problems occur in 20–40% of all patients with RA[41], and will often result

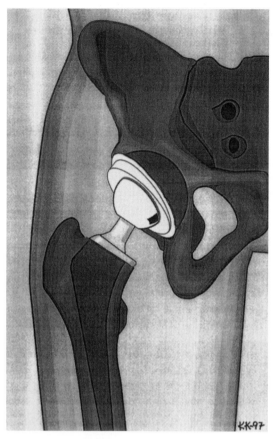

Fig. 34.3 Conventional hip prostheses have a cobalt–chromium stem fixed with bone cement to the femoral shaft. The head may be modular and made from cobalt–chromium alloy or ceramics. It is fixed to the neck with a taper lock. The polyethylene acetabular cup is fixed with bone cement. (Reprinted with permission from Knutson K. (1998). Arthroplasty and its complications. In *Osteoarthritis* (ed. K. D. Brandt, M. Doherty, and L. S. Lohmander), pp. 388–402. Oxford University Press.)

has even been found to be better than that in the non-operated population. The Swedish Hip Arthroplasty Register provides prosthetic survival data and is easily accessible on the Internet[48].

Complications from THR can be divided into early, general, local, and late. An early complication involves problems in wound healing, which appears to be more common in RA than in OA. Dislocation of the prosthetic joint usually occurs early, before the articular capsule has healed, or later when the plastic cup has worn and lost its hemispheric shape. The frequency has been reported to be about 2–3%.

Deep infection is a serious but rare (<1%) complication of THR and may occur early after preoperative contamination of the joint, or later in secondary surgery, or by hematological spreading. Infection can usually be treated by exchanging the prosthesis in one or two stages, using local and systemic antibiotic treatment in the interim.

Aseptic loosening of a prosthesis is the most common reason for revision. The risk is shown in Table 34.5. The problem is often solved by exchange of the loose prosthetic components for new cemented or sometimes non-cemented implants. However, some cases may require both bone transplantation and specific implants aimed at strengthening the hip bone weakened by disease and

prosthetic loosening. New methods, for example the use of morselized cancellous bank bone for reconstruction of bone deficiencies in the proximal femur or in the acetabulum (bone packing), are being developed to improve prosthetic anchorage associated with revision[51].

Radiostereometric analysis (RSA) is a high-precision research method, showing that some implanted components are imperfectly fixed and move at the implant–center or bone–cement interfaces[52,53]. This may stimulate resorption of the adjacent bone, revealed as a visible zone on radiography, which widens until a shift in the position of the prosthesis can be detected. Other mechanisms are also given as causes of zone changes, for example injury to the bone close to the prosthesis in surgical preparation, toxic effects of monomers leaking from bone cement, and heat damage from the exothermic cement hardening process. Loosening is difficult to evaluate in non-cemented prostheses, since these may shift, that is, migrate somewhat, before normal healing occurs.

Microscopic plastic particles break away because of wear of the cup, and are thought to contribute further toward loosening of the prosthesis when they penetrate into the thin zone between the prosthesis or cement and the bone bed. Here they promote an inflammatory process, causing more rapid bone resorption or cyst-like defects in the bone bed, accelerating the loosening process[54].

Surgery of the knee

The knee joints are involved in some 80% of patients with RA, and surgery is still frequently indicated when medical therapy has failed.

Indications and surgical methods

Synovectomy

Preventive effects of synovectomy have never been documented although the removal of large masses of tissue in the joint may have temporary biomechanical advantages. Transient pain relief can also be achieved. In recent years arthroscopic synovectomy has provided shorter rehabilitation times, and equally favorable clinical results[55].

It appears that damage to the cartilage is not affected by synovectomy, but continues or begins following synovectomy, and eventually leads to need for total knee replacement (TKR)[56]. Synovectomy is associated with minor risks, most notably loss of joint mobility due to scar formation in the capsule.

Arthrodesis osteotomy, and capsulotomy

Prior to the prosthetic knee era, various procedures were tested to reduce the effects of arthritis-induced joint damage and to restore joint function. Most of these procedures are now obsolete, for example primary arthrodesis due to poor acceptance of an immobile knee, and double osteotomy due to poor results.

Posterior capsulotomy can be performed to release a knee contracture in patients without cartilage damage. However, even pronounced flexion contracture and valgus malalignment can be successfully corrected by prosthetic surgery.

Table 34.5 Kaplan-Meier survivorship analysis of prosthetic loosening or revision after THR in patients with RA

Author(s)	No of joints	Age (years)	End-point	Risk at:				
				5 years (%)	7 years (%)	10 years (%)	12 years (%)	20 years (%)
Severt et al. (1991)	75	50	Loosening		7	23		
Joshi et al. (1993)[a]	74	<40	Revision					4
			Cup revision					1
			Femoral revision					4
Partio et al. (1994)[b]	84		Revision	3		9		
Önsten et al. (1994)[c]	201	64	Revision			7		
			Acetabular loosening			21		
			Operated <1981					
			Acetabular loosening	13				
			Femoral loosening	20				
			Operated >1981					
			Acetabular loosening	4				
			Femoral loosening	4				
Malchau et al. (1993)	1905	74–65 (f)	Revision	3	6			
	1434	64–55 (f)	Revision	5	11			
	1118	<55 (f)	Revision	7	18			
	558	74–65 (m)	Revision	7				
	503	64–55 (m)	Revision	10				
	669	<55 (m)	Revision	8	10			

f, females; m, males.
[a] Risk factors: men.
[b] Risk factor: age.
[c] Risk factor: young men and first generation cementation technique (<1981).

Corrective osteotomy may, in rare cases, be tried in order to achieve reposition of the knee joint without using TKR. These procedures may involve the correction of varus and valgus angles or improvement of extension defects. The latter, however, makes later prosthetic intervention substantially more difficult.

Knee replacement

The main indication for TKR is pain resulting from cartilage and bone damage, but other indications may include prevention related mainly to valgus deformity, resulting in imbalance with stress on the ankle and foot. Recent advances have generated prostheses that directly replace the joint surfaces in the three joint compartments of the knee, so-called tricompartmental prostheses (Fig. 34.4). Such prostheses can be used with or without a plastic component on the joint surface of the patella. Some tricompartmental prostheses have interconnecting parts to enhance the stability of the prosthesis, partly to replace the function of the posterior crucial ligament, partly to replace the collateral ligaments. Prostheses are affixed to the bone with bone cement or directly to bone, so called biological anchorage.

TKR is a safe method to correct malalignment, restore strength and stability, and to give the patient pain-free mobility of the knee. Good results require correct surgical management of soft tissues, restoration of a correct line of balance through the joint, restoration of the level and position of the patella, and correct

cementation. The aim is to give the patient a flexion capacity of at least 105°, as required to rise from a chair without help of the upper extremities.

Inpatient postoperative training is rarely required for more than 10 days after open synovectomy or knee arthroplasty. Treatment with mechanical devices providing passive movement helps to attain the final range of motion somewhat faster, but does not improve final outcome[57].

The aims of TKR are to correct malalignment, restore strength, mobility, and stability, relieve pain, and improve swelling. A substantial number of patients are relieved from pain, and most patients gain in mobility, but the most mobile may lose somewhat. Postoperative mobility is not affected by age, late mobilization, cementing, ligament release, or patellar component, but rather by previous synovectomy[58].

Prosthetic complications are more difficult to master surgically in the knee than in the hip. Prosthetic exchange can be performed in one or two stages, as in the hip joint, but the functional results after revision are seldom comparable to the results after primary surgery[59]. When exchange for a new prosthesis is no longer possible due to bone defects, it is usually still possible to perform an arthrodesis[60].

Fractures close to the prosthesis, supracondylar fractures of the femur in particular, present a problem with osteopenic bone. The consequences, in most cases, involve limb shortening, malalignment, pain, and impaired walking ability. Furthermore, there is an increased risk for prosthetic loosening and pseudarthrosis. The

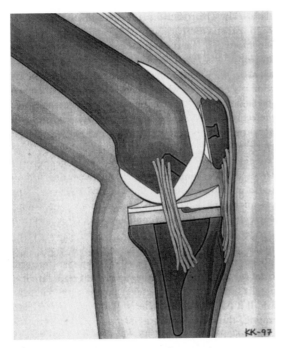

Fig. 34.4 A tricompartmental knee prosthesis. The femoral component is fixed with or without bone cement. The tibial component is a metal tray with an intramedullary stem fixed with bone cement. A polyethylene inlay of appropriate thickness is fitted in the tray. The joint becomes stable through the action of ligaments and muscles. A polyethylene button may be used to resurface the patella. (Reprinted with permission from Knutson K. (1998). Arthroplasty and its complications. In *Osteoarthritis* (ed. K. D. Brandt, M. Doherty, and L. S. Lohmander), pp. 388–402. Oxford University Press.)

Table 34.6 Survival analysis showing the cumulative risk of revision for a knee prosthesis in patients with RA

Author(s)	No.	Revised (%) 5 years	7 years	10 years
Knutson *et al.* (1986)	270	15	–	–
	1962	9	–	–
	296	10	–	–
	170	16	–	–
Ranawat *et al.* (1989)	73	–	–	0
Scuderi *et al.* (1989)	193	0	5	11
	193	3	3	3
	193	0	0	–
Laskin (1990)	80	6	10	19
Moran *et al.* (1991)	73	17	–	–
Rand and Ilstrup (1991)	2876	7	–	18
	779	2	–	–
Aglietti *et al.* (1995)	65	1	–	4
Elke *et al.* (1995)	61	9	–	19
Kolstad *et al.* (1996)	55	8	27	–
Robertsson *et al.* (1996)	1776	4	–	5
	1976	2	–	–
	189	16	–	–

treatment principles involve observing the risk for prosthetic complications from persistent malalignment.

Deep infection presents a serious complication since there is a risk of jeopardizing the knee joint. The infection risk has been estimated to be two to three times higher than in OA. The risk of infection is greater when using large prostheses with intramedullary stems[61]. Furthermore, RA patients may acquire deep infections more than three years after the surgery, probably via blood-borne infection, in particular when leg ulcers are present[42,59,62].

Loosening is less frequent when tricompartmental prostheses are used[50]. Component designs and cementing techniques have also improved results[51]. The claimed advantages of biological anchoring have not been confirmed concerning the attachment of the tibial component, which is most often affected by loosening[62].

Patellar problems have become more dominant as other complications decrease[61]. If a patellar component is not used, the risks for continued patellofemoral joint pain, attrition of the patella, and subsequent patellar instability or subluxation remain. If a patellar component is used, yet another particle-generating, thin plastic part is introduced, which may wear and loosen. Furthermore, the osteopenic patella may be weakened by surgical preparation, hence increasing the risk for fracture[63]. Opinions on the use of the patellar component are divergent and attempts to predict postoperative patellar pain for selective use of patellar components have been made[64].

In conclusion good results regarding pain relief, stability, and mobility can be expected after TKR with currently used tricompartmental prostheses, and the risk for revision within 10 years should be less than 10% (Table 34.6). The survival rate of prostheses with revision as the end-point was estimated to be 93.7% at 15 years[65].

In the Swedish Knee Arthroplasty Registry[66] the cumulative revision rate is about 5% at 10 years and the number of satisfied or very satisfied patients about 85%.

The problem of persistent patellar pain, however, remains to be solved.

Surgery of the ankle

Arthritis of the ankle seldom occurs in isolation, but follows arthritis of the hindfoot and middle foot. It may be severely debilitating and is perhaps the most common cause of more significant gait difficulties among rheumatics[75,76]. After 10 years of disease, nearly all patients show clinical signs of arthritis in one or more joints of the feet.

The ankle is affected by malalignment of the hind- and forefoot to a high degree, and it is usually appropriate to manage these (see below) before considering surgery of the ankle. It should also be remembered that pain from the hind- and middlefoot joints may cause symptoms which are perceived as originating from the ankle joint. A non-corrected malposition of the ankle or hindfoot may jeopardize gait improvement after a hip and knee arthroplasty.

Indications and surgical methods

Synovectomy

Synovectomy of the ankle is rarely performed. The opportunity for radical treatment is small, and joint destruction has usually

Table 34.7 Clinical and radiographic results of ankle arthrodesis in patients with RA

Author	No.	Mobility of foot (°)	Pain free (%)	Radiographically fused (%)
Sowa and Krackow (1989)	6	18 (0–30)	100	
Smith and Wood (1990)	11	4 (0–20)	91	82
Moran *et al.* (1991)	30	12	96	60
Cracchiolo *et al.* (1992)	32		71	78
Turan *et al.* (1995)	10		100	100

progressed too far when the patient's symptoms begin. Tenosynovectomy around the medial tendons is likely to be valuable in preventing rupture of the tibialis posterior tendon[77]. Such rupture is, however, uncommon and not the genesis of rheumatic valgus foot, but may cause an acute and further accentuated valgus deformity of the hindfoot.

Arthrodesis

Arthrodesis is the most established treatment for rheumatic destruction of ankle joints. The choice of surgical method is probably of lesser significance for healing, but may influence the degree and type of complications. Special consideration should be given to inferior bone quality and possible malalignment in adjacent joints in rheumatic patients. A malaligned heel can be corrected and fixed in the same session as the ankle arthrodesis by driving the fixation screws down through the talus and into the calcaneus. Mechanical studies have shown that good fixation is achieved by two or three crossed screws, and is fully comparable to that achieved with external fixation[78]. A recent method involves arthroscopic cleansing of the joint followed by percutaneous screwing, aiming to minimize the risk of disrupting healing in the skin and bone[79]. Arthroscopic methods aim at decreasing surgical trauma and hence postoperative complications in cases where there is minor malalignment, and percutaneous screw fixation, per se, may offer the same advantages[80].

Arthrodesis of the ankle usually relieves pain (Table 34.7) and is a good alternative in patients with somewhat well-maintained hind- and middle foot, with the possibility for these joints to take over some of the lost flexion and extension capacity of the ankle. Through these movements of the middle foot, the patient retains a good walking ability on flat ground. However, a long-term risk with ankle arthrodesis is progression of pathological changes in the middle foot due to such compensatory mobility. If middle foot movement is lacking due to earlier arthrodesis or spontaneous ankylosis, walking following ankle arthrodesis may still be possible with the help of adapted shoes. Arthrodesis remains a safer surgical option than arthroplasty, since late complications are seldom observed in a primarily successful arthrodesis.

Ankle replacement

Arthroplasty using endoprosthesis of the ankle is an appealing alternative since postoperative rehabilitation is short and retaining mobility of the ankle is functionally beneficial. A stiff ankle involves a risk for compensatory hypermobility of the joints in the middle foot with the risk for secondary osteoarthritis, a risk which may be avoided by using a prosthesis. However, implantation of a prosthesis involves a risk for deep infection after disturbed wound healing, prosthetic loosening, migration, and wear. Ankle prostheses have traditionally yielded poor outcome results[20]. Prosthetic survival after 10 years has been estimated at 60% in a mixed ankle study, where patients below the age of 57 years had only 42% prosthetic survival[85]. A prosthetic survival at five years of 78% has been reported for RA patients[86]. More recent reports[86] show more promise and the cumulative survival rate at five years was 92.7% in a mixed-case study[87].

Total ankle replacement may be a realistic alternative to arthrodesis, provided that the components are correctly positioned and are of the correct size. However, the risks of loosening and failure remain higher than after total hip or total knee replacement. The currently available literature has not yet shown that total ankle arthroplasty gives proven cost-effective results[88].

The ankle is more prone to wound healing problems than other joints, and the frequency of infection is high regardless of which type of implant is used. Late infection via blood-borne contamination occurs also in the ankle. In the event of loosening, the only remaining treatment is arthrodesis, involving extensive bone transplantation and prolonged fixation time[89]. Revision surgery is thus technically difficult and often hard on the patient. Non-healed arthrodesis on the other hand can, in some cases, be relatively pain free and may be managed by use of an orthosis or firmly supported shoes.

Surgery of the foot

The percentage of RA patients with foot pain is very high and increased with duration of the disease. Many of the foot problems can be dealt with by adapted shoes with or without different kinds of insoles. Some patients with ankle and hindfoot pain manage well with a stiff ankle joint cap.

Indications and surgical methods

The most important indication for surgery is pain on weight-bearing, which impedes walking. However, there is also a preventive indication, partly to avoid progressive malalignment and partly to avoid wound formation. Pressure from ill-fitting shoes can cause ulcerations and infections, which may cause late, hematogenous prosthetic infections, mainly in knee joints. Hence, it is always wise to try to provide rheumatic patients with a foot free from infection and weight-bearing pain, prior to proceeding to prosthetic surgery in the knee or hip. Furthermore, forefoot problems need to be taken care of prior to or concurrently with the ankle joint.

Surgery of the hindfoot

Since arthritis in the talonavicular joint is a common and early finding in RA, arthrodesis in this joint can be used to prevent development of pes planovalgus. An isolated talonavicular arthrodesis has been shown to limit mobility even in the remaining two hindfoot joints[91]. Joint destruction, with a reduction in joint space, is easy to detect radiographically in the talonavicular and calcaneocuboid joints, but much more difficult in the talocalcanear joint.

If the heel is already in a valgus position or if pain originates mainly in the talocalcanear joint, a complete triple arthrodesis should be considered, involving the joints between talus and the heel bone, between the talus and the navicular bone, and between the heel bone and the cuboid bone. In patients having major malalignment, corrective talocalcanear arthrodesis must be performed by removing a wedge of bone during the procedure. Arthrodeses of the hindfoot are often performed with transplantation of iliac crest bone.

The effect of arthrodesis on hindfoot pain is satisfactory (Table 34.8), regardless of whether or not radiographs show healing of the arthrodesis, indicating that fibrous healing is sufficient for relieving pain. Consequently, need for reoperation is unusual. Bone transplantation can be performed by simply using the dowel technique involving the use of an autologous bone cylinder for joint fusion. The fixation method per se (staple, screw, or pin) is of less importance. Progression of ankle pain does occur, and correlates with persistent valgus malalignment of the hindfoot[96].

Panarthrodesis (combined ankle and hindfoot arthrodesis) is sometimes required in patients with major deformities. A successful technique is the use of retrograde intramedullary nailing through calcaneus, talus, and tibia[98].

Surgery of the forefoot

Surgical treatment of forefoot problems includes everything from bursectomy, chiseling of exostoses, hallux valgus procedures, arthrodeses, joint resections, and osteotomies, to forefoot amputation. The two main types of surgical methods are joint preserving metatarsal osteotomies, and joint resections, possibly in combination with arthrodesis of the great toe.

Joint resections can be performed completely or partially involving the metatarsal articular heads or the toe bases, and the joints can be reached via dorsal or plantar incisions. These procedures can be completed with volar plate arthroplasty, flexor tendon centralization, and medial capsulorrhaphy. Several corrective hallux valgus procedures have been described, but the methods mainly used in RA include resection of the proximal first phalanx with or without capsuloplasty, metatarsal head resection, arthrodesis, metatarsal osteotomy, or implantation of silicone prostheses.

Forefoot surgery is among the most common rheumatic surgical procedures and the results are rather satisfactory[99–104]. The foot may, however, become shorter, and the toes functionally detached, which in turn affects walking ability. There is also a risk of relapse of hallux valgus due to poor lateral support from the other toes, which may be an argument for arthrodesis in the metatarsophalangeal (MTP) joint of the great toe.

When the MTP joints of the toes are relatively well preserved, osteotomy of the metatarsal bones may be a good alternative. Most surgical methods, however, involve resection of the MTP joints. These procedures yield clinical improvement in ~80–90% of cases. Walking distance improves and it is easier to fit shoes[101,104]. The initial gains in function and pain relief decline with time[105]. Isolated resection of the MTP joints of the small toes creates a risk for later problems in the first MTP joint, due to poor lateral support, even if the great toe appears to be unaffected at the time of surgery.

A study[106] comparing arthroplasty and non-surgical management shows a high frequency of relapse of metatarsalgia after forefoot arthroplasty, and results no better than those obtained by conservative treatment. Randomized prospective studies comparing different surgical methods and longer follow-up studies after forefoot surgery need to be performed.

There is no recognized optimal method for treating rheumatic hallux valgus. A retrospective study[102] shows similar results with and without arthrodesis of the great toe. Resection of the first MTP joint offers pain relief, but poor function of the great toe, decreased ability to bear weight on the medial forefoot, poorer balance, and a significant risk of hallux valgus relapse with the risk for lateralization of the small toes. In this respect, arthrodesis seems preferable. A disadvantage of arthrodesis is the increased risk for interphalangeal joint degeneration, either by

Table 34.8 Outcome of hind- and middle foot arthrodeses

Author	No. of feet	Results (%)	Fusion (%)	Complications (%)
Talonavicular arthrodesis				
Elboar *et al.* (1976)	26	85 better	?	19 (preoperative)
Ruff and Turner (1984)	10	70 good	70	0
Ljung *et al.* (1992)	19	89 good	63	0
Talocalcanear arthrodesis				
Russoti *et al.* (1988)	45	90 satisfied	98	2 (infection)
Triple arthrodesis				
Ruff and Turner (1984)	8	88 good	88	0
Figgie *et al.* (1989)	49	86 good	96	12 (wound problems)
Cracchiolo *et al.* (1990)	24	88 satisfied	100	21 (wound problems)

perioperative trauma of axial pins or later by increased load as the foot concludes the stepping motion. Results after great toe arthrodesis are poorest in fibrous healing of the arthrodesis.

Good results have been reported with silicone prostheses[107]. However, some silicone implants fracture, and prosthetic surgery of the great toe does not work well in conjunction with concurrent small toe resection, due to a loss of lateral support for the great toe.

Problems with overall outcome assessment of surgery in RA

Reports on the results of joint surgery are difficult to interpret since they are often based on heterogeneous clinical material with differing natural courses. Results of joint surgery are probably less dramatic in patients with RA than OA due to the systemic and more progressive type of disease.

Although validated assessment instruments have been devised for functional outcome in RA, the outcome of surgery is often reported as an improvement in some kind of in-house score, and most reports are retrospective and short term. Long-term follow-up studies in RA are furthermore complicated by heterogeneity in disease course.

The future of total joint replacement

Alternatives to bone cement fixation of prosthetic components have continuously been introduced to solve the problem of long-term implant fixation. Different surface finishes allow bone ingrowth, but retrieval studies have so far been able to show only partial success. Such microstructured or porous ingrowth prostheses require good bone quality and precise prosthetic fit, which may be an unrealistic ideal. Titanium alloys were introduced because of good biocompatibility, and the possibility of so-called osseointegration. The weight-bearing surface of a titanium implant must, however, be prepared to allow for articulation with polyethylene or it must involve a modular implant with a cobalt–chromium or ceramic bearing. A cemented titanium implant also means a risk of release of high concentrations of local and systemic metallic particles upon micromotion of the prosthesis inside the cement mantle[108].

Hydroxyapatite (HA) and tricalcium phosphate can be coated to an implant to enhance fixation to bone[109]. HA is bioactive, allowing bone ingrowth. Gaps of less than 2 mm can be bridged. HA coating also reduces the metallic contact surface to bone. HA will undergo dissolution, and the effects of the amount or rate of dissolution on prosthetic fixation is not yet known. There is also a risk of loose HA particles creating 'third' body wear in the articulation.

Bone morphogenic proteins and transforming growth factor-β may find use in enhancing the attachment of prostheses to bone[110].

Metal-against-metal articulations for the hip were already available in the 1950s. However, their use was abandoned due to the unsolved problem of fixation, and manufacturing problems with regard to the congruity between the ball and socket. The idea has been taken up again in recent years with implants of very

high quality. The metal release remains a concern, however, and the CoCr–CoCr articulation is hardly the final solution to the wear problem in total hip arthroplasty[111].

Ceramics (alumina, zirconium oxide) have been used for several decades as materials for bearing surfaces in THR. Their use has been limited chiefly due to the risk for fracture of the material. Alumina–polyethylene articulation, however, results in low wear rates and ceramic–ceramic couplings show almost no wear, that is, no particle production. Metal-backed ceramic acetabular cups, as well as polyethylene cups with a ceramic bearing surface, provide the possibility of ceramic–ceramic articulation. Improved quality control will perhaps result in an increased use of ceramics as prosthetic material in the future[112].

High-density polyethylene has been used for decades as the plastic material in all kinds of total joint prostheses, but modifications to improve its performance have been introduced. Wear characteristics may be improved by irradiation or by using cross-linking agents. Heat and high pressure during the manufacturing may help to give the material a more resistant structure[113].

References

1. James, D., Young, A., Kulinskaya, E., Knight, E., Thompson, W., Ollier, W., and Dixey, J. Early Rheumatoid Arthritis Study Group (ERAS), UK. Orthopaedic intervention in early rheumatoid arthritis: occurrence and predictive factors in an inception cohort of 1064 patients followed for 5 years. *Rheumatology (Oxford)* 2004; **43**: 369–76.
2. Kanbe, K., Takemura, T., Takeuchi, K., Chen, Q., Takagishi, K., and Inou, K. Synovectomy reduces stromal-cell-derived factor-1 (SDF-1) which is involved in the destruction of cartilage in osteoarthritis and rheumatoid arthritis. *J Bone Joint Surg Br* 2004; **86**: 296–300.
3. Benoni, G., and Fredin, H. Fibrinolytic inhibition with tranexamic acid reduces blood loss and blood transfusion after knee arthroplasty: a prospective, randomized double-blind study of 86 patients. *J Bone Joint Surg Br* 1996; **78**: 434–40.
4. Dorn, U., Grethen, C., Effenberger, H., Berka, H., Ramsauer, T., and Drekonja, T. Indomethacin for prevention of heterotopic ossification after hip arthroplasty: a randomized comparison between 4 and 8 days of treatment. *Acta Orthop Scand* 1998; **69**: 107–10.
5. Bibbo, C., Anderson, R. B., Davis, W. H., and Norton, J. The influence of rheumatoid chemotherapy, age, and presence of rheumatoid nodules on postoperative complications in rheumatoid foot and ankle surgery: analysis of 725 procedures in 104 patients [corrected]. *Foot Ankle Int* 2003; **24**: 40–4. Erratum in: *Foot Ankle Int* 2003; **24**: 118.
6. Rosandich, P. A., Kelley, J. T. 3rd., and Conn, D. L. Perioperative management of patients with rheumatoid arthritis in the era of biologic response modifiers. *Curr Opin Rheumatol* 2004; **16**: 192–8.
7. Grennan, D. M., Gray, J., Loudon, J., and Fear, S. Methotrexate and early postoperative complications in patients with rheumatoid arthritis undergoing elective orthopaedic surgery. *Ann Rheum Dis* 2001; **60**: 214–17.
8. Jain, A., Witbreuk, M., Ball, C., and Nanchahal, J. Influence of steroids and methotrexate on wound complications after elective rheumatoid hand and wrist surgery. *J Hand Surg [Am]* 2002; **27**: 449–55.
9. Sany, J., Anaya, J. M., Canovas, F., Combe, B., Jorgensen, C., Saker, S. *et al.* Influence of methotrexate on the frequency of postoperative infectious complications in patients with rheumatoid arthritis. *J Rheumatol* 1993; **20**: 1129–32.
10. Kasdan, M. L., and June, L. Postoperative results of rheumatoid arthritis patients on methotrexate at the time of reconstructive surgery of the hand. *Orthopaedics* 1993; **16**: 1233–5.

11. Perhala, R. S., Wilke, W. S., Clough, J. D., and Segal, A. M. Local infectious complications following large joint replacement in rheumatoid arthritis patients treated with methotrexate versus those not treated with methotrexate. *Arthritis Rheum* 1991; **34**: 146–52.

12. Bibbo, C., and Goldberg, J. W. Infectious and healing complications after elective orthopaedic foot and ankle surgery during tumor necrosis factor-alpha inhibition therapy. *Foot Ankle Int* 2004; **25**: 331–5.

13. Worland, R. L., Jessup, D. E., and Clelland, C. Simultaneous bilateral total knee replacement versus unilateral replacement. *Am J Orthop* 1996; **25**: 292–5.

14. Petersson, C. J. Painful shoulders in patients with rheumatoid arthritis. *Scand J Rheumatol* 1986; **15**: 275–9.

15. Kelly, I. G. The source of shoulder pain in rheumatoid arthritis: usefulness of local anaesthetic injections. *J Shoulder Elbow Surg* 1994; **3**: 62–5.

16. Milbrink, J., and Wigren, A. Resection arthroplasty of the shoulder in rheumatoid arthritis: a follow-up study. *J Orthop Rheumatol* 1990; **19**: 432–6.

17. Kechele, P., Bamania, C., Wirth, M. A., Seltzer, D. G., and Rockwood, C. A. Rheumatoid shoulder: hemiarthroplasty *vs* total shoulder arthroplasty. *J Shoulder Elbow Surg* 1995; **4**: 13.

18. Pollock, R. G., Deliz, E. D., McIlveen, S. J., Flatow, E. L., and Bigliani, L. U. Prosthetic replacement in rotator cuff-deficient shoulders. *J Shoulder Elbow Surg* 1992; **1**: 173–86.

19. Rodosky, M. W., and Bigliani, U. Indications for glenoid resurfacing in shoulder arthroplasty. *J Shoulder Elbow Surg* 1996; **5**: 231–48.

20. [No authors listed]. Rheumatic diseases: surgical treatment. A systematic literature review by SBU—the Swedish Council on Technology Assessment in Health Care. *Acta Orthop Scand Suppl* 2000; **294**: 1–88.

21. Franklin, J. L., Barret, W. P., Jackins, S. E., and Matsen, F. A. III. Glenoid loosening in total shoulder arthroplasty. *J Arthroplasty* 1988; **1**: 39–46.

22. Rydholm, U., and Sjögren, J. Resurfacing of the humeral head in rheumatoid arthritis. *J Shoulder Elbow Surg* 1993; **2**: 286–95.

23. Wirth, M. A., and Rockwood, C. A. Complications of total shouder-replacement arthroplasty. *J Bone Joint Surg Am* 1966; **78**: 603–16.

24. Cofield, R. H. Uncemented total shoulder arthroplasty: a review. *Clin Orthop* 1994; **307**: 86–93.

25. Lee, D. H., and Niemann, K. M. W. Bipolar shoulder arthroplasty. *Clin Orthop* 1994; **304**: 97–107.

26. Levy, O., Funk, L., Sforza, G., and Copeland, S. A. Copeland surface replacement arthroplasty of the shoulder in rheumatoid arthritis. *J Bone Joint Surg Am* 2004; **86-A**: 512–18.

27. Barret, W. P., Thornhill, T. S., Thomas, W. H., Gebhart, E. M., and Sledge, C. B. Nonconstrained total shoulder arthroplasty in patients with polyarticular rheumatoid arthritis. *J Arthroplasty* 1989; **4**: 91–6.

28. Kelly, I. G. Unconstrained shoulder arthroplasty in rheumatoid arthritis. *Clin Orthop* 1994; **307**: 94–102.

29. van Cappelle, H. G. J. and Visser J. D. Hemiarthroplasty of the shoulder in rheumatoid arthritis. *J Orthop Rheumatol* 1994; **7**: 43–7.

30. Amis, A. A., Hughes, S. J., Miller, J. H., and Wright, W. A functional study of the rheumatoid elbow. *Rheumatol Rehabil* 1982; **21**: 151–7.

31. Ljung, P., Jonsson, K., Rydgren, L., and Rydholm, U. The natural course of rheumatoid elbow arthritis: a radiographic and clinical 5-year follow-up. *J Orthop Rheumatol* 1995; **8**: 32–6.

32. Herold, N., and Schrøder, H. A. Synovectomy and radial head excision in rheumatoid arthritis. *Acta Orthop Scand* 1995; **66**: 252–4.

33. Wanivenhaus, A., and Bretschneider, W. Late synovectomy of the elbow joint. In *The Elbow: Endoprosthetic Replacement and Non-Endoprosthetic Procedures* (W. Rüther ed.), pp. 48–56. Berlin: Springer Verlag; 1995.

34. Maenpaa, H. M., Kuusela, P. P., Kaarela, K., Kautiainen., H. J., Lehtinen, J. T., and Belt, E. A. Reoperation rate after elbow synovectomy in rheumatoid arthritis. *J Shoulder Elbow Surg* 2003; **12**: 480–3.

35. Ljung, P., Jonsson, K., Larsson, K., and Rydholm, U. Interposition arthroplasty of the rheumatoid elbow. *J Shoulder and Elbow Surg* 1996; **5**: 81–5.

36. Milbrink, J. and Wigren, A. Resection interposition arthroplasty of the elbow in rheumatoid arthritis. *J Orthop Rheumatol*, 1990; **3**: 95–106.

37. Ewald, F. C., Simmons, E. D., Sullivan, J. A., Thomas, W. H., Scott, R. D., Poss, R. *et al.* Capitellocondylar total elbow replacement in rheumatoid arthritis: long-term results. *J Bone Joint Surg Am* 1993; **75**: 498–507.

38. Ljung, P. Arthroplasty of the rheumatoid elbow: with special reference to non-constrained replacement and its complications. Thesis, University of Lund, Sweden, 1995.

39. Ljung, P., Jonsson, K., and Rydholm, U. Short-term complications of the lateral approach for non-constrained elbow replacement. *J Bone Joint Surg Br* 1995; **77**: 937–42.

40. Eberhardt, K., Fex, E., Johnsson, K., and Geborek, P. Hip involvement in early rheumatoid arthritis. *Ann Rheum Dis* 1995; **54**: 45–8.

41. Lehtimäki, M. Y., Kaarela, K., and Hämäläinen, M. M. J. Incidence of hip involvement and need for total hip replacement in rheumatoid arthritis: an eight-year follow-up study. *Scand J Rheumatol* 1986; **15**: 387–91.

42. Poss, R., Maloney, J. P., Ewald, F. C., Thomas, W. H., Batte, N. J., Hartness, C., and Sledge, C. 6 to 11 years results of total hip arthroplasty in rheumatoid arthritis. *Clin Orthop* 1984; **182**: 109–16.

43. Önsten, I., Besjakov, J., and Carlsson, Å. S. Improved radiographic survival of the Charnley prosthesis in rheumatoid arthritis and osteoarthritis: results of new versus old operative techniques in 402 hips. *J Arthroplasty* 1994; **9**: 3–8.

44. Kinzinger, P. J. M., Karthaus, R. P., and Sloof, T. J. H. Bone grafting for acetabular protrusion in hip arthroplasty: 27 cases of rheumatoid arthritis followed for 2–8 years. *Acta Orthop Scand* 1991; **62**: 110–12.

45. Severt, R., Wood, R., Cracchiolo, A., and Amstutz, H. C. Long-term follow-up of cemented total hip arthroplasty in rheumatoid arthritis. *Clin Orthop* 1991; **265**: 137–45.

46. Malchau, H., Herberts, P., and Ahnfelt, L. Prognosis of total hip replacement in Sweden: follow-up of 92 675 operations performed in 1978–1990. *Acta Orthop Scand* 1993; **64**: 497–506.

47. Whittle, J., Steinberg, E. P., Anderson, G. F., Herbert, R., and Hochberg, M. C. Mortality after elective total hip arthroplasty in elderly Americans: age, gender, and indication for surgery predict survival. *Clin Orthop* 1993; **295**: 119–26.

48. www.jru.orthop.gu.se

49. Joshi, A. B., Porter, M. L., Trail, I. A., Hunt, L. P., Murphy, J. C. M., and Hardinge, K. Long-term results of Charnley low-friction arthroplasty in young patients. *J Bone Joint Surg Br* 1993; **75**: 616–23.

50. Partio, E., Von Bonsdorff, H., Wirta, J., and Avikainen, V. Survival of the Lubinus prosthesis. *Clin Orthop* 1994; **303**: 140–6.

51. Gie, G. A., Linder, L., Ling, R. S. M., Simon, J. P., Slooff, T. J., and Timperley, A. J. Impacted cancellous allografts and cement for revision total hip arthroplasty. *J Bone Joint Surg Br* 1993; **75**: 14.

52. Önsten, I., Bengnér, U., and Besjakov, J. Socket migration after Charnley arthroplasty in rheumatoid arthritis and osteoarthritis: roentgen stereophotogrammetric study. *J Bone Joint Surg Br* 1993; **75**: 677–80.

53. Önsten, I., Åkesson, K., Besjakov, J., and Obrant, K. J. Migration of the Charnley stem in rheumatoid arthritis and osteoarthritis: a roentgen stereophotogrammetric study. *J Bone Joint Surg Br* 1995; **77**: 18–22.

54. Schmalzried, T. P., Jasty, M., and Harris, W. H. Periprosthetic bone loss in total hip arthroplasty: polyethylene wear debris and the concept of the effective joint space. *J Bone Joint Surg Am* 1992; **74**: 849–63.

55. Ogilvie-Harris, D. J., and Basinski, A. Arthroscopic synovectomy of the knee for rheumatoid arthritis. *Arthroscopy* 1991; **7**: 91–7.

56. Doets, H. C., Bierman, B. T., and Von Soesbergen R. M. Synovectomy of the rheumatoid knee does not prevent deterioration: 7-year follow-up of 83 cases. *Acta Orthop Scan* 1989; **60**: 523–5.

57. Johnson, D. P. The effect of continuous passive motion on wound healing and joint mobility after knee arthroplasty. *J Bone Joint Surg Am* 1990; **72**: 421–6.

58. Harvey I. A., Barry, K., Kirby, S. P., Johnson, R., and Elloy, M. A. Factors affecting the range of movement of total knee arthroplasty. *J Bone Joint Surg Br* 1993; **75**: 950–5.

59. Wilson, M. G., Kelley, K., and Thornhill, T. S. Infection as a complication of total knee-replacement arthroplasty: risk factors and treatment in sixty-seven cases. *J Bone Joint Surg Am* 1990; **72**: 878–83.

60. Vlasak, R., Gearen, P. F., and Petty, W. Knee arthrodesis in the treatment of failed total knee replacement. *Clin Orthop* 1998; **321**: 138–44.

61. Knutson, K., Lindstrand, A., and Lidgren, L. Survival of knee arthroplasties: a nation-wide multicentre investigation of 8000 cases. *J Bone Joint Surg Br* 1986; **68**: 795–803.

62. Robertsson, O., Knutson, K., Lewold, S., Goodman, S., and Lidgren, L. (1996). Knee arthroplasty in rheumatoid arthritis: a report from the Swedish Knee Arthroplasty Register on 4,381 primary operations 1985–1995. *Acta Orthop Scand* 1997; **68**: 545–53.

63. Grace, J. N. and Sim, F. H. Fracture of the patella after total knee arthroplasty. *Clin Orthop* 1988; **230**: 168–75.

64. Fern, E. D., Winson, I. G., and Getty, C. J. Anterior knee pain in rheumatoid patients after total knee replacement: possible selection criteria for patellar resurfacing. *J Bone Joint Surg Br* 1992; **74**: 745–8.

65. Ito., J, Koshino, T., Okamoto, R., and Saito, T. 15-year follow-up study of total knee arthroplasty in patients with rheumatoid arthritis. *J Arthroplasty* 2003; **18**: 984–92.

66. www.ort.lu.se/knee

67. Ranawat, C. S., Padgett, D. E., and Ohashi, Y. Total knee arthroplasty for patients younger than 55 years. *Clin Orthop* 1989; **248**: 28–33.

68. Scuderi, G. R., Insall, J. N., Windsor, R. E., and Moran, M. C. Survivorship of cemented knee replacements. *J Bone Joint Surg Br* 1989; **71**: 798–803.

69. Laskin, R. S. Total condylar knee replacement in patients who have rheumatoid arthritis: a ten-year follow-up study. *J Bone Joint Surg Am* 1990; **72**: 529–35.

70. Moran, C. G., Pinder, I. M., Lees, T. A., and Midwinter, M. J. Survivorship analysis of the uncemented porous-coated anatomic knee replacement. *J Bone Joint Surg Am* 1991; **73**: 848–57.

71. Rand, J. A., and Ilstrup D. M. Survivorship analysis of total knee arthroplasty. *J Bone Joint Surg Am* 1991; **73**: 397–409.

72. Aglietti, P., Buzzi, R., Segoni, F., and Zaccherotti, G. Insall-Brustein posterior-stabilized knee prosthesis in rheumatoid arthritis. *J Arthroplasty* 1995; **10**: 217–12.

73. Elke, R., Meier, G., Warnke, K., and Morscher, E. Outcome analysis of total knee-replacements in patients with rheumatoid arthritis versus osteoarthrosis. *Arch Orthop Trauma Surg* 1995; **114**: 330–4.

74. Kolstad, K., Sahlstedt, B., and Bergström, B. Marmor modular knee plateau positioning and prosthesis survival in 55 knees with rheumatoid arthritis. *Arch Orthop Traumac Surg* 1996; **115**: 17–21.

75. Kerry, R. M., Holt, G. M., and Stockley, I. The foot in chronic rheumatoid arthritis: a continuing problem. *Foot* 1994; **4**: 201–3.

76. Michelson, J., Easley, M., Wigley, F. M., and Hellmann, D. Foot and ankle problems in rheumatoid arthritis. *Foot Ankle Int* 1994; **15**: 608–13.

77. Johnson, K. A., and Strom, D. E. Tibialis posterior tendon dysfunction. *Clin Orthop* 1989; **239**: 196–206.

78. Thordarson, B. D., Markolf, K. L., and Cracchiole III, A. Arthrodesis of the ankle with cancellous-bone screws and fibular strut graft: biomechanical analysis. *J Bone Joint Surg Am* 1990; **72**: 1359–63.

79. Turan, I., Wredmark, T., and Felländer-Tsai, L. Arthroscopic ankle arthrodesis in rheumatoid arthritis. *Clin Orthop* 1995; **320**: 110–14.

80. Lauge-Pedersen, H., Velasques, A., Rydholm, U., and Knutson, K. Percutaneous arthrodesis in the rheumatoid ankle. *Tech Orthop* 2003; **18**: 279–85.

81. Sowa, D. T., and Krackow, K. A. Ankle fusion: a new technique of internal fixation using a compression blade plate. *Foot Ankle* 1989; **9**: 222–40.

82. Smith, E. J., and Wood, P. L. Ankle arthrodesis in the rheumatoid patient. *Foot Ankle* 1990; **10**: 252–6.

83. Moran, C. G., Pindler, I. M., and Smith, S. R. Ankle arthrodesis in rheumatic arthritis: 30 cases followed for 5 years. *Acta Orthop Scand* 1991; **62**: 538–43.

84. Cracchiolo III, A., Cimino, W. R., and Lian, G. Arthrodesis of the ankle in patients who have rheumatoid arthritis. *J Bone Joint Surg Am* 1992; **74**: 903–9.

85. Kitaoka, H. B., Patzer, G. L., Ilstrup, D. M., and Wallrichs, S. L. Survivorship analysis of the Mayo total ankle arthroplasty. *J Bone Joint Surg Am* 1994; **76**: 974–9.

86. Anderson, T., Montgomery, F., and Carlsson, A. Uncemented STAR total ankle prostheses. *J Bone Joint Surg Am* 2004; **86** (Suppl. 1, Pt 2): 103–11.

87. Wood, P. L., and Deakin, S. Total ankle replacement: the results in 200 ankles. *J Bone Joint Sur Br* 2003; **85**: 334–41.

88. SooHoo, N. F., and Kominski, G. Cost-effectiveness analysis of total ankle arthroplasty. *J Bone Joint Surg Am* 2004; **86**: 2446–55.

89. Carlsson, A. S., Montgomery, F., and Besjakov, J. Arthrodesis of the ankle secondary to replacement. *Foot Ankle Int* 1998; **19**: 240–5.

90. Van Der Heijde, D. M. F. M., Van Leeuwen, M. A., Van Riel, P. L. C. M., Koster, A. M., Van't Hof, M., Van Rijswijk, M. H. *et al.* Biannual radiographic assessment of hands and feet in a three-year prospective follow-up of patients with early rheumatoid arthritis. *Arthritis Rheum* 1992; **35**: 26–34.

91. Carlsson. Å. S., Önsten, I., Besjakov, J., and Sturesson, B. Isolated talonavicular arthrodesis performed for non-inflammatory conditions block motion in healthy adjacent joints: a radiostereometric analysis of 3 cases. *Foot* 1995; **5**: 80–3.

92. Elboar, J. E., Thomas, W. H., Weinfeld, M. S. *et al.* Talonavicular arthrodesis for rheumatoid arthritis of the hindfoot. *Orthop Clin N Am* 1976; **7**: 821–6.

93. Ruff, M. E. and Turner, R. H. Selective hindfoot arthrodesis in rheumatoid arthritis. *Orthopaedics* 1984; **7**: 49–54.

94. Ljung, P., Kaij, J., Knutson, K., Pettersson, H., Rydholm, U. Talonavicular arthrodesis in the rheumatoid foot. *Foot Ankle*, 1992; **13**: 313–16.

95. Russotti, G. M., Cass, J. R., and Johnson, K. A. Isolated talocalcaneal arthrodesis: a technique using moldable bone graft. *J Bone Joint Surg Am* 1988; **70**: 1472–8.

96. Figgie, M. P., O'Malley, M. J., Ranawat, C., Inglis, A. E., and Sculco, T. P. Triple arthrodesis in rheumatoid arthritis. *Clin Orthop* 1993; **292**: 250–4.

97. Cracchiolo, III. A., Pearson, S., Kitaoka, H., and Grace, D. Hindfoot arthrodesis in adults utilizing a dowel graft technique. *Clin Orthop*, 1990; **257**: 193–203.

98. Rydholm, U. Surgical correction of severe deformities of the rheumatoid hindfoot. *Tech Orthop* 2003; **18**: 297–302.

99. Helal, B., and Greiss, B. Telescoping osteotomy for pressure metatarsalgia. *J Bone Joint Surg Br* 1984; **66**: 213–17.

100. Åström, M., and Cedell, C-A. Metatarsal osteotomy in rheumatoid arthritis. *Acta Orthop Scand* 1987; **58**: 398–400.

101. Stockley, I., Betts, R. P., Getty, C. J. M., Rowley, D. I., and Duckworth, T. A prospective study of forefoot arthroplasty. *Clin Orthop* 1989; **248**: 213–18.

102. Hughes, J., Grace, D., Clark, P., and Klenerman, L. Metatarsal head excision for rheumatoid arthritis. *Acta Orthop Scand* 1991; **62**: 63–6.

103. Van Der Heijden, K. W. A. P., Rasker, J. J., Jakobs, J. W. G., and Dey, K. Kates forefoot arthroplasty in rheumatoid arthritis: a 5-year followup study. *J Rheumatol* 1992; **19**: 1545–50.

104. Mann, R. A., and Schakel, M. E. Surgical correction of rheumatoid forefoot deformities. *Foot Ankle* 1995; **16**: 1–6.

105. Patsalis, T., Georgousis, H., and Göpfert, S. Long-term results of forefoot arthroplasty in patients with rheumatoid arthritis. *Orthopaedics* 1996; **19**: 439–47.

106. Craxford, A. D., Stevens, J., and Park, C. Management of the deformed rheumatoid forefoot: a comparison of conservative and surgical methods. *Clin Orthop* 1981; **166**: 121–6.

107. Cracchioleo, A., III, Weltmer, J. B. Jr., Lian, G., Dalseth, T., and Dorey, F. Arthroplasty of the first metatarsophalangeal joint with a double-stem silicone implant: results in patients who have degenerative joint disease, failure of previous operations or rheumatoid arthritis. *J Bone Joint Surg Am* 1992; **74**: 552–63.

108. Kärrholm, J., Frech, W., Nivbrant, B., Malchau, H., Snorrason, F., and Herberts, P. Fixation and metal release from the Tifit femoral stem prosthesis: 5-year follow-up of 64 cases. *Acta Orthop Scand* 1998; **69**: 369–78.

109. Önsten, I., Nordqvist, A., Carlsson, Å. S., Besjakov, J., and Shott, S. Hydroxyapatite augmentation of the porous coating improves fixation of tibial components: a randomized RSA study in 116 patients. *J Bone Joint Surg Br* 1998; **80**: 417–25.

110. Sumner, D. R., Turner, T. M., Purchio, A. F., Gombotz, W. R., Urban, R. M., and Galante, J. O. Enhancement of bone ingrowth by transforming growth factor-β. *J Bone Joint Surg Am,* 1995; **77**: 1135–47.

111. Saikko, V., Nevalainen, J., Revitzer, H., and Ylinen, P. Metal release from total hip articulations in vitro. *Acta Orthop Scand,* 1998; **69**: 449–54.

112. Saikko, V. and Pfaff, H. G. Low wear and friction in alumina/alumina total hip joints. *Acta Orthop Scand* 1988; **69**: 443–8.

113. Jazrawi, L. M., Kummer, F. J., and DiCesare, P. E. Alternative bearing surfaces for total joint arthroplasty. *J Am Acad Orthop Surg* 1998; **6**: 198–203.

Introduction

The human hand is mainly a prehensile organ most important for both occupational capacity and performing activities of daily living. The hand and its function, however, are also a part of the body language affecting social life and interpersonal relations to a very significant degree. A painful, swollen hand with deformities is therefore not only a prehensile disaster but might also lead to a most disabling, psychosocial handicap.

Hand function is based upon certain properties of the hand, which can be characterized as:

- freedom from pain;
- perceptual skin sensibility;
- optimal joint stability;
- functional range of motion;
- muscle strength.

These properties are listed in order of significance, freedom from pain and tactile sensibility being more important than range of motion and strength. This fact forms the basis for many of the surgical procedures used in rheumatoid arthritis (RA), for example when arthrodesis of a joint improves hand function through transforming a painful and unstable joint into a pain-free and stable fusion. The loss of joint motion after such a procedure is for certain joints, that is, the wrist joint and the metacarpophalangeal joint of the thumb, of minor importance compared to the improvement due to stability and pain relief.

Being unable to perform activities of daily living because of impaired hand function is often the main reason why institutional care is needed for a rheumatoid patient. Hand surgery might in such cases be of importance—even simple surgical procedures might significantly improve hand function and contribute to the patient's independence. The most common indication for surgery in rheumatoid arthritis is uncontrolled pain, which the patients consider the main reason for treatment. The timing, order, and type of surgical procedures must be discussed with the patient in detail. Patients are often well aware of the expected postoperative result, but not seldom are mainly informed by their neighbor patients. Rheumatoid patients often have strong feelings about the advantages and disadvantages of various procedures, and they must be allowed to have a main influence on the decision. Such a discussion is preferably performed in a team consisting of hand surgeon, rheumatologist, physical therapist, and occupational therapist.

Surgical procedures

The surgical options in RA include tenosynovectomy, that is, excision of synovitis from a tendon sheath, tendon transfer or tendon repair, soft tissue stabilizing procedures, excision of painful nodules, peripheral nerve release, arthrosynovectomy (implying removal of synovitis from a joint), arthrodesis, and arthroplasty, consisting of excision of a joint with or without endoprosthetic replacement. The main goals of hand surgery in RA patients are to obtain:

- pain relief;
- improved hand function;
- correction of deformities;
- prophylactic effects.

A combination of these goals is often achieved; endoprosthetic replacement of destroyed metacarpophalangeal (MCP) joints results, for example, in pain relief, improved function, and correction of deformity.

The indication for surgery is based mainly on symptoms and clinical findings rather than the radiographic appearance. The radiographs are, however, essential for the choice between different surgical alternatives. All patients in whom hand surgery is being considered therefore have to be radiographically examined. Rheumatoid joint destruction is commonly classified according to Larsen–Dale–Eek[1] in stages 1–6, with stage 1 corresponding to a normal radiographic appearance, stage 6 to a totally destroyed joint. Surgical treatment in RA has a long tradition, but many of commonly used procedures are based on empirical data and not controlled data. In a recent meta-analysis by the Swedish Council on Technology Assessment in Health Care[2], the main conclusion was that better documentation of both new and established surgical procedures is needed.

Tenosynovectomy and tendon repair

Tenosynovitis is common around the extensor tendons at the wrist, the flexor tendons in the carpal canal, and in the flexor tendon sheaths of the fingers. Tenosynovitis impairs the range of motion, but gives rise to pain mainly when peripheral nerves are involved, such as in the carpal canal. Tenosynovitis may take the form of inflammatory tissue on the tendon surface and of intra-tendinous rheumatoid nodules. Such nodules may impair the strength of the tendon; ruptures seem to increase in RA[3]. Tendon ruptures may also be a consequence of wear against sharp bony edges, so called attrition ruptures. These are seen around the ulnar head (caput ulna syndrome), in the carpal canal against the carpal bones, and volar to the MCP joints when the proximal phalanx is subluxated.

Surgical excision of the synovial sheath and intra-tendinous nodules (i.e. tenosynovectomy) improves the range of motion and probably minimizes the risk of rupture[4]. The technique should take great care of important structures, not severing tendons or the fibrous parts of the tendon sheath, the pulleys. Postoperatively, immediate exercises are performed under supervision of a physical or occupational therapist.

Tenosynovectomy results in improved range of motion, improved strength, and possibly less risk of rupture, though this has not been proven[4-6]. Tendon ruptures result in sudden loss of active motion. Ruptures of the finger extensors in the wrist region cause impaired active extension of the MCP joints, while ruptures of flexor tendons in the carpal canal cause impaired active flexion of one or more finger joints, depending on how many tendons that are involved. In cases of isolated rupture of the deep flexor tendons or the long thumb flexor, active flexion of the distal interphalangeal (DIP) and/or interphalangeal (IP) joints is lost. Fusion of the involved joints is a simple method of restoring stability and strength, since active motion in a single DIP joint is not important for a functional hand grip. However, if multiple tendons are ruptured, a tendon is required. Reconstruction of ruptured tendons with the help of tendon grafts implies an intact proximal muscle and a time-consuming and sometimes complicated postoperative rehabilitation. Most rheumatoid patients are better served with a transfer of one or more intact tendons to compensate for the loss of motion. Such tendon transfers give an improved range of motion, although it is not normalized[7].

Soft tissue procedures

A variety of surgical procedures, including reefing of ligaments, shortening or changing direction of tendons, and releasing contracted joint capsules, may be used to correct deformities and achieve improved hand function. In early stages of the disease, soft tissue stabilization may help to achieve joint stability when combined with synovectomies or other procedures. Excision of painful subcutaneous nodules is popular among patients because of beneficial effects on tenderness and pain, but the recurrence rate is high. Most subcutaneous nodules are, however, not tender.

Peripheral nerve surgery

Synovitis in joints and tendon sheaths may affect neighboring peripheral nerves. Raised tissue pressure may impair nerve function—compression neuropathy. The symptoms are paresthesis and pain, and later, loss of sensibility and/or motor function. Compression neuropathies are common in RA; however, the symptoms of pain and tingling are often masked by other kinds of chronic pain, and one has to ask specifically about paresthesis during the night, the main signals distinguishing nerve compression symptoms from joint pain. Compression of peripheral nerves may be caused by synovitis in nearby joints or tendon sheaths. The most common localization is in the carpal tunnel,

where the median nerve is prone to be compressed by tenosynovitis of the flexor tendons, resulting in paresthesias in the radial two-thirds of the hand. The prevalence of this condition is reported to be 10–69%[8]. A carpal tunnel release with a careful tenosynovectomy is a reliable procedure which will restore nerve function and finger flexor capacity.

Synovitis of the elbow joint may involve the ulnar nerve, causing paresthesis in the ulnar part of the lower arm and hand[9]. Release of the nerve from the sulcus cubiti may relieve symptoms, but preferably a nerve transposition should be performed. This will prevent recurrence of the nerve compression. Elbow synovitis may also influence the function of the median nerve in the elbow region (anterior interosseous syndrome)[10] or the posterior branch from the radial nerve[11].

Joint synovectomy

Surgical synovectomy may be performed to achieve pain relief and to reduce swelling and tenderness. The feasibility of complete surgical removal of synovial tissue between joints varies. In multi-chamber joints such as the hand, complete synovectomy is difficult or impossible.

Synovectomy should be performed in early stages, when radiographic changes are minimal (Larsen stages 1–3) and the result is influenced by the radicality of the removal, the degree of radiographic destruction, and the general development of the disease. Postoperatively the joint is immobilized for a few days, followed by a period of active physiotherapy. Satisfactory pain relief has been reported[12] but relapses do occur and long-term studies have not shown any retarding effect on radiographic progression[13,14]. Consequently, synovectomy is rarely performed as an isolated surgical procedure.

Arthrodesis (fusion)

Arthrodesis implies removal of all cartilage and subchondral bone from a joint, necessary to achieve bony healing between joint surfaces. The joint has to be immobilized internally with wires, pins, screws, or plates during the healing period. The osteosynthesis material can be removed after healing if local tenderness occurs. The surgical procedure should aim at achieving maximum stability with internal fixation in order to minimize the need of plaster or external splints. In some joints (i.e. the MCP and proximal interphalangeal (PIP) joints of the fingers) fusion impairs function to a significant degree, even if pain relief is achieved, and is thus rarely performed. In other joints, however (i.e. the wrist, the MCP joint of the thumb, the DIP joints of the fingers), fusion is an effective way of improving hand function because stability in these joints is more important for function than range of motion.

Arthroplasty

Destroyed joints with deformity, impaired range of motion, and pain can be resected and replaced by soft tissues (interposition arthroplasty) or with implants (endoprostheses). Interposition arthroplasty may be performed in joints without too much loading. Tendons, fascia or fibro-cartilage material can be interposed between the resected joint surfaces in order to obtain a joint-like function. The advantages with these procedures are low cost and low incidence of foreign body reactions. Arthroplasty with endo-prostheses is, however, a more common procedure, although development of implants for hand surgery has been slow compared with devices for larger joints. The problems in arthroplastic surgery are to achieve implant fixation to surrounding bone and to find a joint mechanism which combines optimal range of motion with stability. All joint prostheses are prone to tear and wear, particularly in joints exposed to load.

A detailed description of the various procedures and their reported results in the different joints is given below.

The wrist joint

The wrist is the fundament of the hand and any wrist disability will significantly affect the function of the hand.

It has a complex anatomy involving several joints, allowing motion between radius, ulna, and the eight carpal bones. The wrist consists of three different parts:

1. The **radiocarpal joint** is the main wrist joint between the distal surface of the radius and the proximal surfaces of the proximal row of carpal bones. About half of the flexion–extension capacity depends on this joint.

2. The intercarpal joints articulate the eight carpal bones. About half of the range of motion in flexion–extension depends on motion between the carpal bones, as does radial and ulnar mobility.

3. The **distal radioulnar (DRU)** joint is part of the rotating joints of the lower arm enabling pronation and supination of the hand.

In RA of the wrist the stabilizing structures (ligaments, tendons, and joint capsule) often become weakened by the synovitis. Instability and subsequent deformity follow.

Volar subluxation (Fig. 35.1) and reduced range of motion are typical for RA[15,16]. The intercarpal joints may develop either ankylosis or instability. In the DRU joint synovitis causes destruction of stabilizing structures, leading to displacement between the ulnar head and radius. Such a displacement impairs pronation–supination and may interfere with the surrounding tendons, especially the ulnarly located finger extensor tendons, which may rupture. The caput ulna syndrome[17] is characterized by weakness in the hand and wrist joint, pain and limited prosupination, and a dorsal protrusion of the ulnar head with crepitations and clicking. About 30% of patients with rheumatoid arthritis may become affected by a caput ulna syndrome[18].

The radiocarpal and intercarpal joints

Simmen[19] has defined three types of natural courses for the wrist joint in rheumatoid arthritis, which affect the indication for surgery and choice of surgical alternatives:

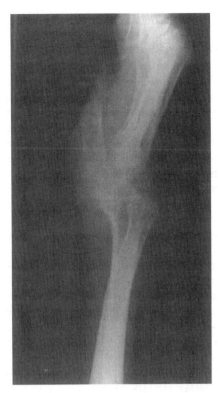

Fig. 35.1   Radiographic lateral view of a wrist joint with volar subluxation.

Type I Progressive destruction with moderate pain at loading leading to subsequent ankylosis without pain. This is a favorable development, since stability in the wrist is more important than range of motion. Surgery is rarely indicated. In type I disease, fusion of the intercarpal joints occurs spontaneously. Treatment aims at achieving a functional position for the ankylosis and splints are useful to prevent flexion or ulnar deformity. After spontaneous ankylosis the wrist becomes stable and pain free.

Type II Progressive erosive destruction; severe pain and ankylosis will not occur spontaneously. A progressive destruction with severe pain at loading may necessitate surgical arthrodesis, which is the method of choice in this type of disease. Range of motion after arthroplasty or partial wrist fusion is often limited.

Type III Progressive destruction with severe instability and/or deformity. The patient often experiences inflammatory symptoms and without treatment the end result is a grossly deformed wrist joint with major impairment of hand function. Surgery is strongly indicated to prevent disabling deformity with impaired range of motion. The aims of surgical intervention are to achieve pain relief and stability, and to prevent secondary tendon ruptures. Synovectomy, often combined with ulnar head resection or a ligament stabilizing procedure, total or partial fusion, and arthroplasty are the surgical alternatives of choice.

The distal radioulnar joint

Synovitis in the DRU joint often causes destruction of ligaments and joint surfaces of both ulna and radius, resulting in displacement and joint destruction. If the joint surfaces are intact, a synovectomy combined with ligament reconstruction around the ulnar head may restore function, but in most cases a resection of the ulnar head, (Darrach procedure) is needed. The Darrach procedure is effective in relieving pain, improving prosupination and preventing tendon ruptures, but should not be performed in wrists with ulnar translocation, in which severe ulnar deviation may develop. Ulnar head resection is often combined with soft tissue stabilization in order to avoid instability of the distal end of the ulna; fascia, capsular structures, or tendons (extensor carpi ulnaris or flexor carpi ulnaris) can be utilized for this purpose[20].

Although ulnar head resection helps to improve wrist function, complications do occur. Instability of the ulnar end is, in spite of stabilizing procedures, frequent, but rarely disabling. In wrist joints with ulnar translocation of the carpus, the ulnar head plays an important role as a support for the carpal bones; ulnar head resection in such individuals may result in severe ulnar deviation of the wrist. An alternative to ulnar head resection is the Sauvée–Kapandji procedure, which comprises of a fusion between the ulnar head and the radius in order to preserve the ulnar support for the carpus; prosupination is achieved through an osteotomy of the ulna proximal to the fusion. The Sauvée–Kapandji procedure was originally designed for post-traumatic problems of the DRU joint, but good results in RA have also been reported[21].

Synovectomy of the wrist

In early stages of rheumatic arthritis (Larsen stages 1–3) synovectomy can be an effective treatment to achieve pain relief in the wrist joint. Synovectomy is performed through a dorsal approach and should always include tenosynovectomy of the extensor tendons, and arthrosynovectomy of the radiocarpal, intercarpal, and distal radioulnar joints. This implies a broad surgical exposure of the wrist joint with expanded healing time and postsurgical loss of motion as a consequence. Arthroscopic synovectomy has been introduced to minimize the surgical trauma[22], but this technique is still not accepted as a routine procedure because it is time and resource consuming.

The initial result of wrist synovectomy is pain relief, but the range of motion in terms of flexion–extension capacity is always impaired; the prosupination is, however, often improved, especially if ulnar head resection is performed. Long-term studies have shown pain relief, but no preventive effect on progressive destruction[12]. Since the preventive effect of wrist synovectomy is doubtful, this procedure is rarely performed. Wrist tenosynovectomy has, however, proven effective in preventing tendon ruptures[23] and should therefore be considered in cases of wrist tenosynovitis.

Proximal carpectomy

In later stages of RA (Larsen 3–6) resection of the proximal carpal row might be an alternative to fusion in order to preserve some range of motion in the wrist joint. After bone resection, soft tissue interposition is sometimes performed to achieve stability and mobility[24].

Arthrodesis of the wrist

Fusion is a reliable procedure to achieve pain relief and stability, together with correction of any deformity of the wrist joint[25–27].

Various fusion techniques are described, using Steinmann pins, screws and plates, or bone grafts to achieve internal stability. It avoids prolonged external fixation, which can constitute considerable problems for patients with RA. The clinical results of wrist fusions are very satisfying, since, even when bilateral wrist fusions are performed, the pain-free and stable wrist always improves hand function[28]. Complications comprise failed healing, persisting pain, or median nerve compression, a complication seen especially when severe volar subluxation of the wrist joint is reduced by the fusion.

Limited wrist fusion

When only limited parts of the wrist are destroyed, a partial fusion of the wrist may be considered as an alternative to total wrist fusion in order to preserve some range of motion. Partial wrist fusion can be performed in the radiocarpal joint, with preservation of the intercarpal joints, or in the intercarpal joints, with preservation of the radiocarpal joint[29]. Fusion between os lunatum and radius is advocated in ulnar head resection to prevent deviation of the wrist joint in cases of ulnar translocation of the carpus[30,31].

Arthroplasty of the wrist

Replacement of the wrist joint with an endoprosthesis is still a controversial procedure, mainly because fusion is the gold standard for reconstruction of an unstable and painful wrist joint. However, when surgical intervention of both the right and left wrist joints is indicated, arthroplasty might be an alternative for one of the joints, taking into account that some range of wrist motion is useful when performing activities of daily living[32]. There are three problems with endoprosthetic replacement of the wrist: defining the center of rotation in the wrist, achieving implant fixation to bone, and balancing the forces acting on the wrist joint[33]. Both constrained hinge joints and non-constrained ball-in-socket joints have been advocated, but non-constrained designs are nowadays used to a very limited degree.

Constrained wrist implants

Silicone implants of Swanson's design have been in use for 20 years. Early results were encouraging, with immediate pain relief and a functional range of motion[34–39]. This implant is merely a spacer with silicone stems introduced into the marrow channels of the third metacarpal bone and the radius. Increasing reports of bone resorption and subsidence (70–100% in some studies), frequent fractures of the silicone implant, and development of foreign body reactions, 'silicone synovitis', have tempered the initial enthusiasm with this implant[40,41]. Titanium shields (grommets) have been introduced in order to improve the results, but their effect is unproven.

Silicone implants for replacement of the wrist joint have now been almost abandoned.

Non-constrained wrist implants

Various designs of ball-in-socket implants in the wrist joint have been suggested, the Volz and Meuli prostheses being the most

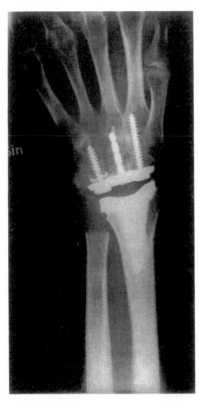

Fig. 35.2 Radiographic anteroposterior view of the Universal Total Wrist Implant (KMI®).

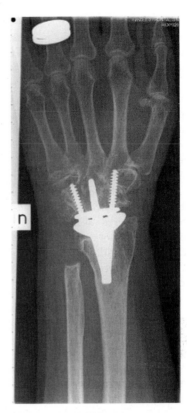

Fig. 35.3 Radiographic anteroposterior view of Avanta Total Wrist Implant (Avanta®).

used non-constrained implants. Both implants have spherical metal balls, articulating against sockets of polyethylene, with titanium stems enabling bone fixation with or without cement. Pain relief and 60–70° of flexion-extension are often achieved[42,43]. Loosening of the components, especially the distal stem is, however, a problem. Frequently the implant's center of rotation is malplaced in the wrist joint leading to ulnar deviation and/or flexion deformity of the wrist. Complications occurred in 44% of the procedures, with a total revision rate of 33% due to loosening, dislocation, or imbalance[44]. Beckenbaugh and Menon have presented an alternative non-constrained implant with ellipsoid balls (Fig. 35.2), aiming to improve the balance of the arthroplasty[45]. These implants can be used with or without cement fixation. Good short-term results have been reported[46], but long-term studies are still missing. Newer and improved implant designs are introduced to avoid reported early complications such as dislocation or loosening. Modular designs with a built-in rotational capacity are now available on the market.

The MCP joint and ulnar drift

The MCP joints of the fingers are ball-in-socket joints allowing some 90° of extension–flexion and 25° of ulnar-radial deviation. The range of motion of the MCP joints is important, both for opening the hand and for the grasping of objects. Lateral stability is needed, especially in the index finger when used in the lateral pinch.

Isolated synovectomy of the MCP joints was a frequent procedure in the past, but is now usually performed only as an adjunct to soft tissue stabilizing procedures.

The hands are, together with the face, the only parts of the body that are not covered by clothes. Hand deformities are therefore not only a cause of functional handicap, but may also impact on the patient psychologically. In most cases ulnar drift causes impaired prehensile function, the destroyed MCP joints loosing their extension capacity, with inability to open the hand to grasp a glass or to shake hands as a result. In some cases the pinch grip between the thumb and the fingertips is lost, leaving the lateral pinch between the thumb and the radial side of the index finger as the only remaining grip for manipulation[47]. Even if the prehensile function of the hand is not impaired, patients often experience ulnar drift as cosmetically disturbing and strongly urge a surgical correction.

Ulnar drift has a complex pathogenesis including:

* radial deviation of the wrist joint leading to hand scoliosis, with secondary ulnar deviation of the fingers;
* tenosynovitis of the flexor tendon sheath leading to weakening of annular ligaments with subsequent ulnarly directed forces of the flexor tendons onto the index and middle fingers;
* synovitis of MCP joints leading to weakening of the transverse ligaments of the extensor tendon 'hood' with subsequent ulnar luxation of the extensor tendons;
* common use of lateral pinch in which the thumb creates ulnarly directed forces to the radial side of the index finger.

These different forces produce not only ulnar deviation of the fingers but also volar subluxation of the proximal phalanx from the metacarpal heads, which is a mandatory part of the deformity and the main cause of extension loss of the MCP joints.

Three stages of ulnar drift can be distinguished[48]. **Fearnley 1:** where active reduction is possible; that is, there is a minor deformity which might be corrected by the muscle activity of the hand itself. Treatment by dynamic splinting with rubber bands, counteracting both the ulnar deviation and the volar subluxation of the fingers, is feasible. **Fearnley 2:** passive reduction is still possible but there is more severe deformity which, however, can be corrected with splints or with the help of the contralateral hand. The MCP joints are radiographically normal and soft tissue surgical procedures can be used to correct the ulnar deviation. **Fearnley 3:** there is fixed deformity combined with subluxation and/or radiographic destruction of the MCP joints. Soft tissue procedures are no longer successful and arthroplasty of the MCP joints is the recommended surgical procedure.

Soft tissue procedures in ulnar drift

The ulnar drift deformity often includes luxation of the extensor tendons ulnarly to the metacarpal heads due to synovitis of the MCP joint, which causes destruction of the tendon's stabilizing structures. Extension movements of the MCP joints will then cause ulnar deviation of the fingers due to the ulnarly luxated tendons. Early surgical correction of the tendon displacement may prevent ulnar drift in these cases[49]. Such a procedure, called centralization of the extensor tendons, can be done in Fearnley stages 1 or 2 and is performed with a release of the ulnar transverse ligament and a duplication of the radial transverse ligament of each of the MCP joints.

Correction of ulnar drift in Fearnley stage 2 can also be performed through transfer of the interosseous tendons from one proximal finger phalanx to its ulnarly situated neighbor, so-called crossed intrinsic transfer or Straub[50]. The interosseous muscles, which act on the lateral bands, produce ab- and adduction movements of the fingers and transfer of the ulnar lateral band (i.e. the intrinsic tendon) from each of the index, middle, and fourth fingers to the radial side of the middle, fourth, and fifth fingers, respectively; radial correction of ulnarly deviating fingers can be achieved.

After both procedures, postoperative early controlled motion is performed with the help of a dynamic splint which prevents the ulnar deviation of the fingers. Dynamic splinting is used for six weeks and a static splint worn at night is then used for three months or longer. About 80% good or excellent early results are reported with centralization when used in Fearnley stages 1 or 2[49]. However, long-term results are not known.

Arthrodesis of the MCP joints

A functional hand grip depends on proper range of motion in the MCP joints of the fingers, both for opening of the hand and for grasping. The adaptation of the fingers to different shapes of objects also depends on the ulnar–radial deviation of the fingers. Fusion of the MCP joints II–V is therefore not recommended,

at least not for the three ulnar fingers. In the thumb, however, fusion of the MCP joint of the thumb is useful. Fusion of the MCP joint of the index finger is sometimes performed in conjunction with arthroplasty of the remaining fingers, in order to achieve radial stability in the lateral pinch.

Arthroplasty of the MCP joints

In Fearnley stage 3 surgical procedures of the MCP joint itself are needed to improve joint function and to correct the ulnar drift. Since fusion is not a useful procedure for the MCP joints, except the thumb and perhaps the index finger, surgical alternatives are arthroplasties with or without endoprostheses.

Interposition arthroplasty

Various concepts of arthroplasties using different kinds of soft tissues for interposition and stabilization of the MCP joints have been described, commonly using the extensor tendon[51] or the volar plate[52] as the interposed structure. A disadvantage is that the range of motion is often limited and tends to deteriorate with time. Published data with these procedures are sparse.

Arthroplasty with endoprostheses

The first reported surgical procedure using an endoprosthesis for replacement of the MCP joints was performed in the beginning of 1950 and since then a variety of endoprostheses have been presented[53]. The joint mechanism might be constrained using a polymere (silicone) as the flexible hinge, or non-constrained using a ball-in-socket concept. The stem of the endoprosthesis might be fixed into the bone marrow channels, with or without cement, or might be encapsulated by soft tissues as the main fixation. A new principle of non-cemented fixation is the osseointegration concept, in which titanium fixtures anchored to the surrounding bone tissue are used for implant fixation.

Silicone implants

Swanson's arthroplasty using silicone implants has for more than 20 years been the gold standard for endoprosthetic replacement of the MCP joints[54–57]. The concept is based on a flexible silicone spacer with proximally and distally directed stems (Fig. 35.4), which after resection of the metacarpal head are introduced into the marrow channels of the metacarpal bone and the proximal phalanx, respectively. The spacer is subsequently 'encapsulated' into surrounding soft tissues for implant fixation. The radial collateral ligaments, at least for the index finger, are reinserted to bone before implantation of the spacers. With the Swanson arthroplasty immediate pain relief, proper correction of deformity, and adequate range of motion are often obtained. With time, however, bone reactions tend to occur around the implants, both as new bone formation and as bone resorption due to movements between implant and bone as described as early as 1975[58]. The range of motion deteriorates due to subsidence of the implants into the surrounding bone. Silicone particle-induced synovitis has mainly been described around silicone implants in larger joints, but it can occasionally occur in MCP joints as

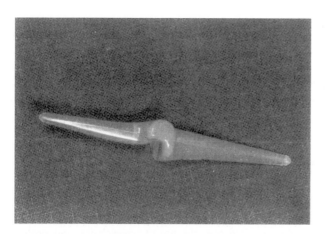

Fig. 35.4   Silicone MCP implant of Swanson type.

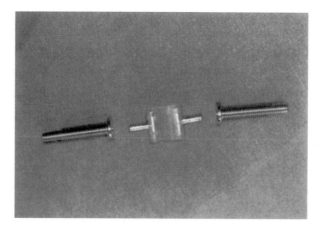

Fig. 35.6   Silicone MCP implant with titanium fixtures a.m. Brånemark.

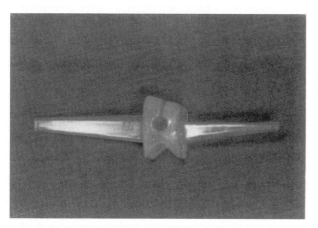

Fig. 35.5   Silicone MCP implant of Sutter (Avanta) type.

Osseointegrated implants

The osseointegration concept was introduced by Brånemark and has been used extensively for fixation of artificial teeth[66]. Preliminary experience from silicone implants with titanium stems anchored to titanium screw-shaped fixtures in the marrow channels of the surrounding bone (Fig. 35.6) were encouraging. In published series 90–100% osseointegration (measured from X-ray examinations) and excellent clinical results have been reported[67,68]. High fracture rates of the silicone were, however, a problem, with 6% silicone fractures occurring after 2.5 years[69]. An alternative implant design with better durability has been presented as a prototype.

The PIP joint

The PIP joint is a hinge joint with about 100° of flexion–extension and with no lateral motion. Synovectomy is sometimes performed, sometimes in addition to reefing the central tendon in order to treat button hole deformity. Impaired range of motion after synovectomy is common, however, as are relapses of synovitis, making synovectomy subsequently more and more rarely performed.

Arthrodesis of the PIP joint

Since range of motion in the PIP joints is important for a functional hand grip, fusion is not an attractive alternative in these. Fusion is, however, widely used in spite of its obvious drawbacks, since results of arthroplasties are not consistent[71]. The surgical technique should imply rigid internal fixation in order to avoid prolonged splinting of the fingers, with subsequent loss of motion in neighbor joints.

Arthroplasty of the PIP joint

Replacement of the PIP joint is commonly performed with silicone implants of, for example, the Swanson-, Niebauer- or Sutter-type[72,73]. The pain-relieving effect is reasonably good, but range of motion and correction of deformities is unsatisfactory[74].

well[41]. A range of motion varying between 25° and 66° can be achieved. The fracture rate of the silicone can be up to 39%[38,59].

A new design of silicone implants has been introduced by Sutter, now Avanta. The implant surface against the resected bone ends is larger and prevents subsidence of the implant. Also the axis of motion is placed in a more volar position to improve the range of motion (Fig. 35.5). High fracture rates have, however, been reported with this implant[60]. No long-term studies are available.

Other polymeric materials such as polyurethane have been used in limited series as an alternative to silicone, but experience is limited[61].

Non-constrained implants

A non-constrained implant with a metal ball articulating in a plastic socket with implant stems fixed to surrounding bone with the help of bone cement has been described[62]. Extensive periarticular ectopic bone formation in 32%, and loosening of the distal stem in 17–18%, have contributed to a very limited use of this implant design.

There are also a few reports published on various kinds of non-cemented, non-constrained implants, for example with alumina–ceramic materials[63], polyester[64], pyrocarbon[65], or metal/polyethylene. The experiences from these methods are hitherto very limited.

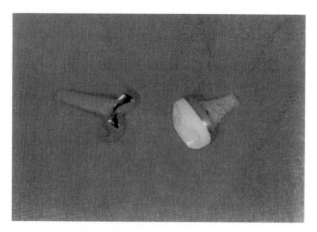

Fig. 35.7   Avanta® Anatomic Poly PIP implant.

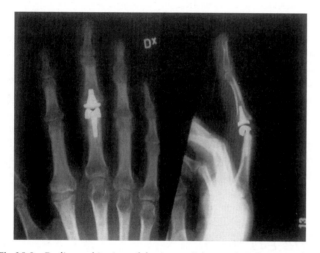

Fig.35.8   Radiographic view of the Avanta® Anatomic Poly PIP implant.

Non-constrained implants with cement fixation have been used without success[75,76]. A bicondylar non-constrained implant which can be used both with or without cement shows encouraging initial results[77]. Such an implant may be an attractive alternative to fusion in the future (Figs 35.7 and 35.8).

The DIP joint

Engagement of the DIP joints is not common in RA, but frequent in psoriatic arthritis. As range of motion in these joints is not important for hand function, fusion is the method of choice to achieve pain relief and to correct deformities. Bone resorption is often severe, necessitating the use of bone grafts when performing a DIP joint fusion.

The thumb

The main property of the thumb is to provide a stable pose against the fingers in grasping and pinching. Fusion is therefore

commonly used in the MCP and IP joints, even when both joints are operated simultaneously. The CMC joint is rarely fused in RA, but arthroplasty with or without endoprostheses is in most cases a reliable method to achieve pain relief and stability with preserved range of motion[78]. Soft-tissue stabilization of the MCP joint may be considered when the joint surfaces still allow motion.

Postoperative rehabilitation

Rigorous rules have to be followed in the postoperative phase in order to avoid complications. The rheumatoid patient is sensitive to prolonged. Bed rest, the use of wheelchairs, and prolonged splinting should be avoided. The surgical technique must include rigid internal fixation of fusions, fractures, and soft tissue stabilization procedures. Early mobilization, often controlled with splints, is commonly used after hand surgery. A specialized team, including nurses and physical and occupational therapists, is essential in the postoperative period.

Splints

Immobilization of the hand and wrist is often performed with the help of splints, which are lighter and easier to use than plaster. Splints are custom-made from various plastic materials by occupational therapists. Static splints are used for immobilization. Dynamic splints use rubber bands acting on fingers or finger joints in order to counteract muscle forces or to facilitate range of motion. After correction of ulnar drift, for example, a dynamic splint with rubber bands providing radial traction of the fingers is used for 6–8 weeks postoperatively. The use of dynamic splints has to be supervised by an occupational therapist.

Functional assessment

The indication for many hand surgical procedures is the need to improve hand function, which might be essential for a patient's occupation, independence, and ability to perform activities of daily living. Exercises to improve hand function are an important part of a treatment program in rheumatoid arthritis. Certain methods are available for measuring hand function, and for registering function before a surgical procedure and during the postoperative training period[79], but these have not been applied in controlled studies yet.

References

1. Larsen, A., Dale, K., and Eek, M. Radiographic evaluation of rheumatoid arthritis and related conditions by standard reference films. *Acta Radiol (Diagn)* 1977; **18**: 481–91.
2. SBU-TSCoTAiHC. (The Swedish Council Technology Assessment in Health Care). *Rheumatoid Arthritis: Surgical Treatment* [in Swedish]. SBU-rapport 1998; 136 (1 + 2).
3. Ferlic, D. Rheumatoid flexor tenosynovitis and rupture. *Hand Clin* 1996; **12**: 561–72.

4. Connor, J., and Nalebuff, E. A. Current recommendations for surgery of the rheumatoid hand and wrist. *Curr Opin Rheumatol* 1995; **7**: 120–4.

5. Leslie, B. M. Rheumatoid extensor tendon ruptures. *Hand Clin* 1989; **5**: 191–202.

6. Ertel, A. N. Flexor tendon ruptures in rheumatoid arthritis. *Hand Clin* 1989; **5**: 177–90.

7. Moore, J. R., Weiland, A. J., and Valdata, L. Tendon ruptures in the rheumatoid hand: analysis of treatment and functional results in 60 patients. *J Hand Surg (Am)* 1987; **12**: 9–14.

8. Chang, D. J., and Paget, S. A. Neurologic complications of rheumatoid arthritis. *Rheum Dis Clin of North Am* 1993; **19**: 955–73.

9. Schmidt, V. A. Nervenkompressionssyndrome in Bereich des Ellenbogengelenkes bei Patienten mit chronischer Polyarthritis. Eine Literaturübrsicht. *Handchir Mikrochir Plast Chir* 1993; **25**: 70–5.

10. Rask, M. R. Anterior interosseous nerve entrapment (Kiloh—Nevin syndrome): report of seven cases. *Clin Orthop Relat Res* 1979; **142**: 176–81.

11. Ishikawa, H., and Hirohata, K. Posterior interosseous nerve syndrome associated with rheumatoid synovial cysts of the elbow joint. *Clin Orthop* 1990; **254**: 134–9.

12. Vahvanen, V., and Patiala, H. Synovectomy of the wrist in rheumatoid arthritis and related diseases: a follow-up study of 97 consecutive cases. *Arch Orthop Trauma Surg* 1984; **102**: 230–7.

13. Allieu, Y., Lussiez, B., and Asencio, G. Long-term results of surgical synovectomies of the rheumatoid wrist: apropos 60 cases. *Rev Chir Orthop Reparatrice Appar Mot* 1989; **75**: 172–8.

14. Bohler, N., Lack, N., Schwagerl, W., Sollerman, C. T. J., Thabe, H., and Tillmann, K. Late results of synovectomy of wrist, MP, and PIP joints: multicenter study. *Clin Rheumatol* 1985; **4**: 23–5.

15. Evans, J. S., Blair, W. F., Andrews, J. G., and Crowninshield, R. D. The in vivo kinematics of the rheumatoid wrist. *J Orthop Res* 1986; **4**: 142–51.

16. Stanley, D., and Norris, S. H. The pathogenesis and treatment of rheumatoid wrist and hand deformities. *Br J Hosp Med* 1988; **39**: 156–60.

17. Backdahl, M. The caput ulnae syndrome in rheumatoid arthritis: a study of the morphology, abnormal anatomy and clinical picture. *Acta Rheumatol Scand* 1963; **5**: 1–75.

18. Nalebuff, E. A., Feldon, P. G., and Millender, L. H. (1988). Rheumatoid arthritis in hand and wrist. In *Operative Hand Surgery*, Vol. 3, 2nd edn (Green DP, ed.), pp. 1655–766. New York: Churchill Livingstone; 1988.

19. Simmen, B. R., and Huber, H. The rheumatoid wrist: a new classification related to the type of the natural course and its consequences for surgical therapy. *Rheumatology* 1992; **17**: 13–25.

20. Melone, C. P, Jr., and Taras, J. S. Distal ulna resection, extensor carpi ulnaris tenodesis, and dorsal synovectomy for the rheumatoid wrist. *Hand Clin* 1991; **7**: 335–43.

21. Taleisnik, J. The Sauvée-Kapandji procedure. *Clin Orthop Relat Res* 1992; **275**: 110–23.

22. Adolfsson, L., and Nylander, G. Arthroscopic synovectomy of the rheumatoid wrist. *J Hand Surg [Br]* 1993; **18**: 92–6.

23. Brown, F. E., and Brown, M. L. Long-term results after tenosynovectomy to treat the rheumatoid hand. *J Hand Surg [Am]* 1988; **13**: 704–8.

24. Culp, R. W., McGuigan, F. X., Turner, M. A., Lichtman, D. M., Osterman, A. L., and McCarrol, H. Proximal row carpectomy. *J Hand Surg [Am]* 1993; **18**: 19–25.

25. Mannerfelt, L., and Malmsten, M. Arthrodesis of the wrist in rheumatoid arthritis: a technique without external fixation. *Scand J Plast Reconstr Surg* 1971; **5**: 124–30.

26. Millender, L. H., and Nalebuff, E. A. Arthrodesis of the rheumatoid wrist: an evaluation of sixty patients and a description of a different surgical technique. *J Bone Joint Surg Am* 1973; **55**: 1026–34.

27. Rayan, G. M., Brentlinger, A., Purnell, D., and Garcia-Moral, C. A. Functional assessment of bilateral wrist arthrodeses. *J Hand Surg [Am]* 1987; **12**: 1020–4.

28. Vicar, A. J., and Burton, R. I. Surgical management of the rheumatoid wrist: fusion or arthroplasty. *J Hand Surg [Am]* 1986; **11**: 790–7.

29. Ishikawa, H., Hanyu, T., Saito, H., and Takahashi, H. Limited arthrodesis for the rheumatoid wrist. *J Hand Surg [Am]* 1992; **17**: 1103–9.

30. Della Santa, D., and Chamay, A. Radiological evolution of the rheumatoid wrist after radio-lunate arthrodesis. *J Hand Surg [Br]* 1995; **20**: 146–54.

31. Stanley, J. K., and Boot, D. A. Radio-lunate arthrodesis. *J Hand Surg [Br]* 1989; **14**: 283–7.

32. Palmer, A. K., Werner, F. W., and Eng, M. M. Functional wrist motion: a biomechanical study. *J Hand Surg [Am]* 1985; **19**: 39.

33. Cooney, W. P. I., Beckenbaugh, R. D., and Linscheid, R. L. Total wrist arthroplasty: problems with implant failures. *Clin Orthop* 1984; **187**: 121.

34. Jolly, S. L., Ferlic, D. E., Clayton, M. L., Dennis, D. A., and Stringer, E. A. Swanson silicone arthroplasty of the wrist in rheumatoid arthritis: a long-term follow-up. *J Hand Surg [Am]* 1992; **17**: 142–9.

35. Lundkvist, L., and Barfred, T. Total wrist arthroplasty: experience with Swanson Flexible Silicone Implants 1982–1988. *Scand J Plast Reconstr Hand Surg* 1992; **26**: 97–100.

36. Nylén, S., Sollerman, C., Haffajee, D., and Ekelund, L. Swanson implant arthroplasty of the wrist in rheumatoid arthritis. *J Hand Surg [Br]* 1984; **9**: 295–9.

37. Simmen, B. R., and Gschwend, N. Swanson silicone rubber interpositional arthroplasty of the wrist and of the metacarpophalangeal joints in rheumatoid arthritis. I. Wrist arthroplasty. *Acta Orthop Belg* 1988; **54**: 196–209.

38. Stanley, J. K., and Tolat, A. R. Long-term results of Swanson silastic arthroplasty in the rheumatoid wrist. *J Hand Surg [Br]* 1993; **18**: 381–8.

39. Swanson, A. B., De Groot Swanson, G., and Maupin, B. K. Flexible implant arthroplasty of the radiocarpal joint: surgical technique and long-term study. *Clin Orthop Rel Res* 1984; **187**: 94–106.

40. Smith, R. J., Atkinson, R. E., and Jupiter, J. B. Silicone synovitis of the wrist. *J Hand Surg [Am]* 1985; **10**: 47–60.

41. Peimer, C., Medige, J., Eckert, B., Wright, J., and Howard, C. Reactive synovitis after silicone arthroplasty. *J Hand Surg [Am]* 1986; **11**: 624–38.

42. Volz, R. G. Total wrist arthroplasty: a clinical review. *Clin Orthop* 1984; **187**: 112–20.

43. Meuli, H. C., and Fernandez, D. L. Uncemented total wrist arthroplasty. *J Hand Surg [Am]* 1995; **20**: 115–22.

44. Menon, J. Total wrist replacement using the modified Volz prosthesis. *J Bone Joint Surg [Am]* 1987; **69**: 998–1006.

45. Beckenbaugh, R. Preliminary experience with a noncemented nonconstrained total joint arthroplasty for the metacarpophalangeal joints. *Orthopedics* 1983; **6**: 962–5.

46. Divelbiss, B. J., *et al.* Early results of the Universal total wrist arthoplasty in rheumatoid arthritis. *J Hard Surg* 2002; **27**: 195–204.

47. Wilson, R. L., and Carlblom, E. R. The rheumatoid metacarpophalangeal joint. *Hand Clin* 1989; **5**: 223–37.

48. Fearnley, G. R. Ulnar deviation of fingers. *Ann Rheumat Dis* 1951; **10**: 126–36.

49. Wood, V. E., Ichtertz, D. R., and Yahiku, H. Soft tissue metacarpophalangeal reconstruction for treatment of rheumatoid hand deformity. *J Hand Surg [Am]* 1989; **14**: 163–74.

50. Straub, L. R. Surgical rehabilitation of the hand and upper extremity in rheumatoid arthritis. *Bull Rheumat Dis* 1962; **12**: 265–8.

51. Vainio, K. Vainio arthroplasty of the metacarpophalangeal joints in rheumatoid arthritis. *J Hand Surg [Am]* 1989; **14**: 367–8.

52. Tupper, J., W. The metacarpophalangeal volar plate arthroplasty. *J Hand Surg [Am]* 1989; **54**: 2: 371–5.

53. Beevers, D. J., and Seedhom, B. B. Metacarpophalangeal joint prostheses. *J Hand Surg [Am]* 1995; **20**: 125–36.

54. Gschwend, N., and Zimmerman. Analyse von 200 MCP-Artroplastiken. *Handchirurgie* 1974; **6**: 7–14.

55. Kirschenbaum, D., Schneider, L. H., Adams, D. C., and Cody, R. A. Arthroplasty of the metacarpophalangeal joints with use of silicone rubber implants in patients who have rheumatoid arthritis. *J Bone Joint Surg Am* 1993; **75**: 3–12.

56. Maurer, R., Ranawat, C., and McCormack, R., Inglis ALRS. Long-term follow-up of the Swanson MP arthroplasty for rheumatoid arthritis. *J Hand Surg [Am]* 1990; **15**: 810–11.

57. Swanson, A. B. Flexible implant arthroplasty for arthritic finger joints: rationale, technique and results of treatment. *J Bone Joint Surg Am* 1972; **54**: 435–55.

58. Hagert, C., Eiken, O., Ohlsson, N., Aschan, W., and Movin, A. Metacarpophalangeal joint implants. I. Roentgenographic study of the silastic finger joint implant, Swanson design. *Scand J Plast Reconstr Surg* 1975; **9**: 147–57.

59. Wilson, Y. G., Sykes, P. J., and Niranjan, N. S. Long-term follow-up of Swanson's silastic arthroplasty of the metacarpophalangeal joints in rheumatoid arthritis. *J Hand Surg [Br]* 1993; **18**: 81–91.

60. Bass, R. L., Stern, P. J., and Nairus, J. G. High implant fracture incidence with Sutter silicone metacarpophalangeal joint arthroplasty. *J Hand Surg [Am]* 1996; **21**: 813–18.

61. Sollerman, C. J., and Geijer, M. Polyurethane versus silicone for endoprosthetic replacement of the metacarpophalangeal joints in rheumatoid arthritis. *Scand J Plast Reconstr Hand Surg* 1996; **30**: 145–50.

62. Steffee, A., Beckenbaugh, R., and Lindsheid, R. H. D. The development, technique and early results of total joint replacement for the metacarpophalangeal joint of the fingers. *Orthopedics* 1981; **4**: 175–80.

63. Minami, M., Yamasaki, J., Kato, S., and Ischii, S. Alumina ceramic prosthesis arthroplasty of the metacarpophalangeal joint in the rheumatoid hand: a 2–4 year follow-up study. *J Arthroplasty* 1988; **3**: 157–66.

64. Vermeiren, J. A. M., Dapper, M. M., Schoonhoven, L. A., and Merx, P. W. J. Isoelastic arthroplasty of the metacarpophalangeal joints in rheumatoid arthritis: a preliminary report. *J Hand Surg [Am]* 1994; **19**: 319–24.

65. Beckenbaugh, B. D. Arthroplasty of the metacarpophalangeal joint using pyrocarbonate implants. *Orthopade* 2003; **9**: 794–7.

66. Brånemark, P. I., Breine, U., Lindström, J., Adell, R., Hansson, B. O., and Ohlsson, Å. Intraosseus anchorage of dental prosthesis. I. Experimental studies. *Scand J Plast Reconstr Surg* 1969; **3**: 81–100.

67. Lundborg, G., Brånemark, P-I., and Carlsson, I. Metacarpophalangeal joint arthroplasty based on the osseointegration concept. *J Hand Surg [Br]* 1993; **18**: 693–703.

68. Möller, K., Sollerman, C., Geijer, M., and Brånemark, P. I. Osseointegrated silicone implants: 57 MCP-joints followed for two years. *Acta Orthop Scand* 1999 **70**; **2**: 109–15.

69. Möller, K., Sollerman. C., and Lundborg, G. Radiographic evaluation of osseointegration and loosening of titanium implants in the MCP and PIP joints. *J Hand Surg [Am]* 2004; **29**: 1; 32–8.

70. Hagert, C-G., Brånemark, P-I., Albrektsson, T., Strid, K-G., and Irstam, L. Metacarpophalangeal joint replacement with osseointegrated endoprostheses. *Scand J Plast Reconstr Hand Surg* 1986; **20**: 207–18.

71. Osterman, A. H. J. Synovectomy, arthroplasty, and arthrodesis in the reconstruction of the rheumatoid wrist and hand. *Curr Opin Rheumatol* 1991; **3**: 102–8.

72. Pellegrini, V. D., and Burton, R. I. Osteoarthritis of the proximal interphalangeal joint of the hand: arthroplasty or fusion? *J Hand Surg [Am]* 1990; **15**: 194–209.

73. Swanson, A. B., and de Groot Swanson, G. Flexible implant arthroplasty of the proximal interphalangeal joint. *Hand Clin* 1994; **10**: 261–6.

74. Adamson, G. J., Gellman, H., Brumfield, R. H., Kuschner, S. H., and Lawler, J. W. Flexible implant resection arthroplasty of the proximal interphalangeal joint in patients with systemic inflammatory arthritis. *J Hand Surg [Am]* 1994; **19**: 378–84.

75. Beckenbaugh, R. D. New concepts in arthroplasty of the hand and wrist. *Arch Surg* 1977; **112**: 1094–8.

76. Linscheid, R. I., Dobyns, J. H., Beckenbaugh, R. D., and Cooney, W. P. Proximal interphalangeal joint arthroplasty with a total joint design. *Mayo Clin Proc* 1979; **54**: 227–40.

77. Linscheid, R. L., Murray, P. M., Vidal, M. A., and Beckenbaugh, R. D. Development of a surface replacement arthroplasty for proximal interphalangeal joints. *J Hand Surg [Am]* 1997; **22**: 286–98.

78. Amadio, P., Millender, L., and Smith, R. Silicone spacer or tendon spacer for trapezium resection arthoplasty: comparison of results. *J Hand Surg [Am]* 1982; **7**: 237–44.

79. Sollerman, C., and Ejeskär, A. Sollerman hand function test: a standardised method and its use in tetraplegic patients. *Scand J Plast Reconstr Hand Surg* 1995; **29**: 167–76.

36 | The cervical spine

A. T. H. Casey and H. A. Crockard

Introduction

Cervical spine involvement characteristically involves the atlantoaxial complex, the most mobile part of the spine, with the radiological abnormalities being classified into those of atlantoaxial subluxation (AAS), which may be horizontal or vertical in direction. Significant subaxial disease is less common and usually coexists with the above deformities (Fig. 36.1).

In many cases these radiological abnormalities remain asymptomatic for years, but these patients nonetheless are at continued risk from a range of neurological complications and even sudden death from medullary compression. Despite the predilection that rheumatoid arthritis has for the cervical spine and the severe consequences that may ensue, there has been surprisingly little work in determining the factors that influence which patients will become myelopathic, and if and when they do, what role has surgery to play.

The purpose of this chapter is to review the available surgical knowledge from the medical literature examining the clinical features, the size of the problem, and also the current surgical approaches and possible instrumentation solutions. It is notable that over the last five years there has been an apparent decrease in surgical patients. It is difficult to know the reasons behind this phenomenon. It is possible to speculate that use of disease-modifying anti-rheumatic drugs (DMARDs), with concomitant decreased use of steroids, is the major factor involved. Alternatively it may just be that more surgeons are prepared to operate on these challenging patients now that the ground rules are clearly established and instrumentation has come so far. Finally we will audit the results of surgery, comparing the surgical results with the natural history of the condition.

Radiographic patterns of disease

Common radiographic patterns of disease are illustrated below. Although some authors have tried to implicate cranial nerve findings with vertical translocation (also known as cranial settling or basilar invagination or impression) the symptoms of dysphagia and dysarthria are no more common in uncomplicated horizontal atlantoaxial subluxation than in vertical translocation[1]. There are different definitions of vertical translocation[2-8], Many of these are historical (McRae, McGregor's method). We prefer the Redlund-Johnell method, which measures from the base of C2 to the McGregor's palato-occipital line. If this measurement is less than a certain length (<34 mm for males, <29 mm for females),

it implies that there has been collapse of the lateral masses of C1 and C2 and vertical translocation (VT) is present[3].

Epidemiology

There are few epidemiological studies concentrating purely on rheumatoid manifestations in the cervical spine and many have serious methodological problems, with bias introduced by selecting only hospital-based patients or those who have a cervical spine X-ray for various reasons. There is one good quality study from Finland with a captive, geographically isolated population[9]. Their results are summarized in Table 36.1, with extrapolated figures for the UK and USA given in the adjacent columns. One problem with this study and most of the others is that it only provides a snapshot in time of the incidence (point incidence) and this depends very much on the disease duration and age distribution of the selected patient population. What is lacking from the literature is a prospective community-based study that gives information about the prevalence of AAS, VT, or other important manifestations of rheumatoid involvement of the cervical spine at predefined time intervals, that is, 2 years, 5 years, 10 years, 15 years, etc. Also, more importantly, what percentage of patients with these radiographic abnormalities develops neurological symptoms or signs?

A literature meta-analysis is provided in Tables 36.2 and 36.3, but problems with retrospective data, biased population groups and the lack of any agreement on what constitutes a neurological problem allow only broad conclusions to be drawn. AAS has been recorded in a range of 5.5–73% (mean 32%)! The average incidence of neurological problems is 17%. These epidemiology studies do not bring out the fact that is so obvious, from the surgical papers, that neurological complications are a late manifestation of the disease process (see below).

Natural history

The findings of the major non-surgical series have already been summarized in Table 36.3[10-14]. There is an overall fall-out rate of 33%, with many patients lost to follow-up.

One prospective study, which originated from the Middlesex Hospital, found subluxation to be an early complication of the rheumatoid process[15]. In this series, 12% of patients developed AAS, a further 20% developed subaxial subluxation, and 3% developed vertical translocation. Over 80% of these patients

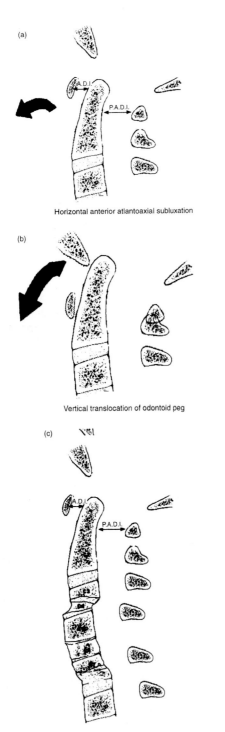

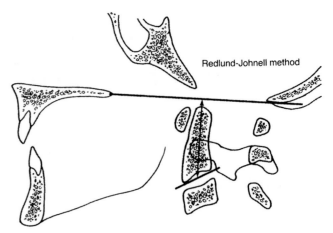

Fig. 36.2 Method of measuring vertical translocation by Redlund-Johnell. The disease from the base of C2 (axis) to McGregor's palato-occipital line is measured. As vertical translocation (aka cranial setting) progresses this distance gets smaller.

Fig. 36.1 (a) Horizontal atlantoaxial subluxation as the ADI (atlantodens interval) increases the space available for the cord (posterior atlantodens interval—PADI) decreases. (b) Vertical translocation—the odontoid peg has transgressed the foramen magnum. (c) Subaxial diseases—staircase deformity.

showed the first evidence of subluxation within two years of the disease presentation, and all their cases were apparent within five years[15]. Their message that atlantoaxial subluxation was not a late development of the disease contradicted the perceived wisdom of that time, and in many ways was an unexpected finding. A dilemma is therefore created: Why are these individuals neurologically normal, despite the fact that they have an obvious radiographic abnormality? And why do patients present with myelopathy, at average of 19 years after the disease onset, when subluxation has been present since 'year 2' in many individual cases? *We hypothesize that the damage is due to multiple repetitive microtrauma over many years. Our neuropathological analyses bears this out*[1,16].

The Swedish post mortem study by Mikulowski of 104 patients with RA is an important contribution. This revealed 11 patients with unexpected AAS and cord compression. Sudden death was experienced by 7 of the 11; medullary compression by a translocated peg was clearly demonstrable in all these individuals[17]. The findings of this study raise serious doubts about the benign nature of the disease as suggested by the natural history studies detailed in Table 36.3.

Once cervical myelopathy is established, mortality appears to be common. A report on 31 patients with RA and cervical myelopathy revealed that 19 died, with 15 of the deaths occurring within six months of presentation. All those who were untreated died, and half of those treated by collar alone died[18]. In another study, nine patients with myelopathy treated non-operatively all died within 12 months, with four deaths directly attributable to cord compression according to their death certificates[19]. However, the latter are unreliable in a multisystems disease and may seriously underestimate the incidence of cervical myelopathy as a cause of death[17,20]. Evidence from our own series of patients selected for surgery who refused decompression and fixation also suggests a very poor outcome once myelopathy is established, with all seven patients dead within five years[21]. These findings are echoed by 21 rheumatoid arthritis patients with myelopathy resulting from atlantoaxial dislocation who were studied by Sunahara *et al.* from Kagoshima University, Japan[22]. All of these patients were recommended for surgery, but they refused. Patients were reviewed by direct examination yearly. Radiographic changes and clinical course, including the survival rate, were observed. All patients became bedridden within three years of the onset of myelopathy. Of the 21 patients, 7 died suddenly for unknown reasons, 3 died of pneumonia, and 1 died of

Table 36.1 The incidence and prevalence of cervical rheumatoid arthritis and calculated estimates of the potential surgical workloads in the United Kingdom and United States of America (data extrapolated from Refs 9, 40, and 41)

Demographics	UK	USA	Comment
1. Population	57 M	248 M	Census data
2. Prevalence of RA	1.1%	0.9%	Based on Lawrence and Cathcart population studies
3. Number with RA	627 000	2.2 M	Calculated from the above
4. Incidence of RA	25 per 100 000	29 per 100 000	Based on large population studies in Norfolk, UK and Rochester, USA
5. Per cent with AAS at 3 years	15%	N/A	Personal communication A. Young on behalf of the ERAS group (prospective study of 650 patients)
6. Annual incidence at 3 years	2325(*)	10 788(*)	* calculated from 1. and 5.
7. Prevalence a) AAS (33%) b) VS (27 %)	206 910 169 000	726 000 594 000	Based on point prevalence population study in Finland % shown in brackets.
8. Potential surgical candidates fulfilling radiological criteria for surgery—10%.	62 700	220 000	AAS of >9 mm was found in 4% and a combination of AAS of 6–9 mm and vertical translocation in 6%. Subaxial subluxation >4mm was present in 1%.

Table 36.2 Incidence of atlantoaxial subluxation in rheumatoid arthritis reported in non-surgical series

Author	Total no. of patients	Number with AAS	% with AAS	Vertical translocation (VT)	% with VT	Neurologically affected	% with neurological symptoms or signs	Source of patients
Serre 1964[42]		60	23	38	n/a	n/a	n/a	n/a admissions
Cabot 1978[43]	53	19	36	4/53	7.5	6/19	32	Hospital admissions
Conlon 1966[45]	333	84	25	n/a	n/a	11/84	13	Hospital admissions
Marrtel 1961[44]	34	24	73	n/a	n/a	n/a	n/a	n/a
Halla 1990[46]	650	36	5.5	8/650	1.2	3/61	4.9	Outpatient study admissions
Mathews 1969[47]	76	19	25	6/76	18	5/76	6.6	Hospital admissions
Meikle 1971[48]	118	44	37.3	n/a	n/a	n/a	n/a	Outpatients with neck pain
Ornilla 1972[49]	100	14	14	n/a	n/a	n/a	n/a	Arthroplasty patients
Pellici 1981[12]	163	40	25	4/163	2.5	11/74	15	Outpatients with radiographs
Rasker 1978[50]	62	26	42	20/62	32	n/a	n/a	Inpatients (age 55–64)
Stevens 1971[10]	100	36	36	n/a	n/a	24/36	67	Outpatient clinic
Meta-analysis	1749	365	32	42/1004	4.2	60/350	17	Mixture

Table 36.3 Natural history studies on atlantoaxial subluxation in the rheumatoid cervical spine

Author	Length of follow-up (years)	Total number in series	%follow-up achieved	Source of patients	Neurological problems	% with neurological problems	Number with AAS	% with AAS	Radiological progression	
									Horizontal	Vertical
Isdale 1971[51]	6	171	62	Hospital admissions	'no change in 49 pts. by 3 years'	n/a	79	46	14/171 (8%)	n/a
Mathews 1974[11]	5	54	71	Outpatient clinic	12/54	22	6	11	9/54 (17%)	18/54 (33%)
Pellici 1981[12]	5	106	65	Outpatient clinic	33/106	31	41	39 (27%)	28/106	10/106 (9.4%)
Rana 1989[13]	10	41	100	Clinic and hospital patients with AAS	6/41	15	41	n/a	11/41 (27%)	4/41 (9.8%)
Smith 1972[14]	7.8	84	65	Cervical luxation cohort	10/130	7.7	55	65	19/55 (35%)	n/a
Winfield 1981[15]	7.2	100	100	Prospective study Patients within 1 year of diagnosis	0	0	12	12	12/100	3/100 (3%) (12%)
Meta-analysis	6.8 (mean)	556 (toal) (mean)	77	Mixed	61/431	15	234	35 (mean)	21% (mean)	14% (mean)

Several discrepancies appear to exist in the baseline number of patients (denominator). This is due to the fact that not all patients were followed up for both radiological and clinical examination. The abbreviation n/a is used when the authors of the original paper did not analyze their data for the relevant reading or value.

multiple organ failure. The three sudden-death cases showed progressive upward migration of the odontoid process at post mortem examination.

The overall impact of cervical spine involvement is highlighted in Corbett's prospective study of 102 patients[23], which is a follow-up to her original paper of 1981[15]. In this she has demonstrated for the first time that cervical subluxation appearing within the first two years of disease onset is a predictor of eventual poor functional outcome.

All these studies therefore seem to provide conflicting evidence. On the one hand there are reports of only modest radiographic progression over time, with only 15% of patients developing neurological problems. On the other hand we are presented with fairly compelling evidence that the incidence of myelopathy is probably underestimated and that once it develops the outlook is grim.

These apparent contradictions arise from the difficulty in diagnosing cervical myelopathy in the presence of a painful deforming arthritis with an oft-associated peripheral neuropathy and myopathy. Also it is important to bear in mind that the radiographic abnormalities described in many of these studies are plain X-rays. Many deal solely with horizontal atlantoaxial subluxation and fail to take into account the less common manifestations of rheumatoid involvement of the cervical spine, that is, vertical translocation, lateral and rotatory atlantoaxial subluxation, and subaxial disease. Plain radiographs cannot visualize compression by soft tissue, notably pannus. These facts in part explain the poor correlation of radiographic abnormalities and the development of cervical myelopathy described in the literature.

One of the issues that we have tried to address in this work is the more accurate characterization of the radiographic abnormalities associated with cervical myelopathy, taking into account findings from computerized tomography (CT) myelography which can visualize the neuraxis and soft tissue compression. Many of these radiographic parameters can be measured directly or via computerized morphometric analysis. We have also tried to quantify the level of disability secondary to rheumatoid cervical myelopathy[24].

Surgical indications

There is a consensus view that surgery should be offered to those individuals with neurological symptoms or signs. Patients with atlantoaxial instability and severe unremitting pain unresponsive to conservative measures are also usually offered surgery.

There is a significant gray area. This is whether prophylactic surgery should be offered to patients with severe radiographic abnormalities, for example a large atlantodens interval (>6–10 mm) who are at risk of imminent neurological catastrophe[25,26]. There is no compelling evidence to support prophylactic surgery. Circumstantial evidence in its favor comes from several sources. Agarwal's group has demonstrated that patients who undergo surgery at an early stage of disease (atlantoaxial fixation) fare better in the long run than patients who have surgery at a later stage of their disease (occipitocervical fixation). Our group has highlighted the very poor prognosis for the end-stage patient

(Ranawat class IIIB)[2]. The incidence of surgical complications is double that of Ranawat class IIIA patients. Finally the post-mortem studies of Mikulowski and Wollheim reveal that sudden death is a not infrequent complication[17].

Boden has suggested the PADI (space available for the cord) as an alternate radiographic indicator based on an analysis of 73 patients over a 20-year period[27]. he problem with relying on the atlantodens interval (ADI or PADI) is that it takes no account of soft tissue inflammation (pannus) or that the ADI actually decreases with advanced disease as vertical translocation occurs[1,28]. The presence of vertical translocation is an ominous sign and in our analysis of 116 patients with this condition they were more severely disabled than those patients with simple horizontal atlantoaxial subluxation, and ultimately had a poorer long-term survival as assessed by Kaplan–Meier survival curves[1,29,30]. Dvorak has suggested that a spinal cord diameter of less than 6 mm in flexion[31] as assessed by magnetic resonance imaging (MRI) should be an indication for surgery. Our own analysis of spinal cord morphometry has shown that once the spinal cord area is below 45 mm^2, the chances of a neurological recovery are very poor indeed[28]. Finally, some interesting work from Zygmunt *et al.*, based on a careful analysis of pre- and postoperative MRI studies, has shown that the periodontoid pannus diminishes in size after spinal fixation.

Surgical techniques

A full description of all the surgical approaches and methods of fixation is beyond the scope or remit of this chapter. A transoral decompression of the dens is illustrated below, along with a posterior occipitocervical fixation (Figs 36.3 and 36.4).

From careful inspection of the preoperative radiological studies the surgeon has to decide where the major area of compression anterior *or posterior* is, and at what level(s) is it occurring, that is, *cervicomedullary, atlantoaxial, subaxial, or a combination of these*. The next problem is to decide whether there is instability present preoperatively, or will it be created following surgical decompression? The influence of resection of the dens has been formally studied by Dickman *et al.* but the answer to these questions almost by definition is yes as the rheumatoid inflammatory process will destroy both ligaments and bone alike. For the atlantoaxial region this will involve the transverse ligament with atlantoaxial subluxation occurring, and this would have been the indication for surgery originally.

Anterior approaches include the transoral approach for resection of the dens or associated pannus, and the standard Cloward anterolateral approach to the anterior subaxial spine[32,33].

The **posterior approach** to either the posterior craniocervical junction or cervical spine is through the standard midline approach, with subperiosteal dissection of the muscles from the spinous processes, lamina, and occipital bone.

Healing in the rheumatoid patient may be compromised due to a combination of steroids, cytotoxic agents, osteopenia, and general debility. Therefore careful attention has to be paid to stabilization. In the opinion of the authors too much attention has been given to achieving bony fusion. This is important but an

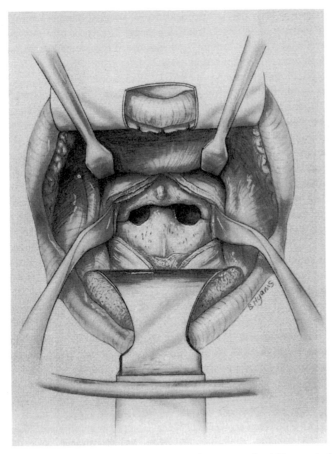

Fig. 36.3 Schematic drawing of transoral exposure. A midline vertical incision in the pharynx exposes the arch of C1 and anterior bony of C2.

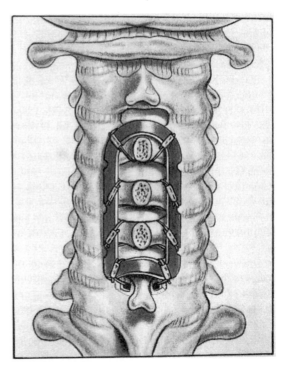

Fig. 36.4 A titanium loop (Ti-Frame) fixed to the subaxial cervical spine with titanium multistranded cables (Sof'wire). This can be attached to the occiput to effect an occipitocervical fixation.

instrumented fixation will rarely fail in the elderly rheumatoid patient, who will place few demands on the spinal instrumentation. Harvesting a bone graft is not without complications and will cause significant pain. For occipitocervical fixations we rely purely on instrumentation and do not supplement this with a bone graft in order to decrease operative morbidity. In our prospective follow-up of 256 patients there have been very few instances of instrumentation failure (only 3% of patients had broken wires; there were no instances of failure of Ransford loop—unpublished data). We currently use a posterior transarticular screw fixation method to stabilize the atlantoaxial joint. This technique is inappropriate in 20% of patients due to variations of the vertebral artery groove[34], and also in patients with significant vertical translocation[35]. Nonetheless this provides true three-point fixation and is superior to the previously used methods of Brooks and Gallie[36].

Surgical results

There are many ways of assessing outcome following spinal fixation. These would include the fusion rates, and standard operative morbidity and mortality figures, which are summarized in Tables 36.4 and 36.5. But surely patients are interested in more than this? They would be interested to know whether their pain

will improve, whether their neurological deficit will get better, and if so, by how much? A summary of the findings in the literature is presented in Table 36.6.

The use of neurological outcome scales, such as the Ranawat class or Steinbrocker's grades used by previous investigators, has the advantage of standardization but really only provides a thumbnail sketch of outcome (Table 36.7).

A useful way of describing outcome is by the use of functional questionnaires. A popular questionnaire which has been well validated is the Stanford Health Assessment Questionnaire (HAQ) devised by Fries *et al.*[37]. Wollheim's group used this to characterize functional recovery following occipitocervical fixation in 20 patients[38], and found there was little functional improvement. We have also used the Stanford HAQ and reported the change in function following surgery for 134 Ranawat class IIIA–B patients[21]. We then attempted to reduce the extraneous noise or redundant questions from the original instrument by statistical manoeuvres, including Principal Components Analysis. The resulting questionnaire, which we have called the Myelopathy Disability Index (Table 36.8), has good psychometric properties including reliability, validity, and responsiveness. Eigen analysis shows that it is measuring mainly one dimension of disability. There are statistical associations with the Myelopathy Disability Index and spinal cord area, response to surgery, and indeed long-term survival (Kaplan–Meier Analysis)[24]. Occipitocervical pain is best assessed by means of a visual analogue scale and the results of surgery are very good indeed in this respect. Unfortunately there is no literature on the success of C2 nerve blocks with local anesthetic and steroid, which these two authors have found to be successful for both surgical and non-surgical patients alike.

Table 36.4 Fusion rates reported in the literature from 'pure rheumatoid' series

Author	Successful osseous fusion	Fusion rate %
Boden[27]	32/35	91
Clark[52]	36/41	88
Conaty and Mongan[53]	25/31	81
Fehring[54]	12/16	75
Ferlic[55]	6/12	50
Heywood[25]	21/30	70
Milbrink[56]	11/12	92
Papadopoulos[26]	13/17	76
Peppelman[57]	67/77	87
Ranawat[2]	20/25	80
Santavirta[58]	16/18	89
Thompson[59]	10/11	91
Zoma[60]	18/30	60
Overall	287/355	83

Table 36.5 Documented mortality rates for cervical spine surgery on patients with rheumatoid arthritis

Authors	Series	Mortality (%)
Boden[27]	7/42	18
Clark[52]	0/41	0
Conaty and Mongan[53]	3/38	8
Crellin[61]	2/11	18
Fehring[54]	1/17	6
Ferlic[55]	2/15	13
Heywood[25]	2/26	8
Papadopoulos[26]	1/17	6
Peppelman[57]	4/110	4
Ranawat[2]	3/33	9
Santavirta[62]	0/34	0
Stanley[63]	2/25	8
Stirrat[64]	0/28	0
Thompson[59]	1/12	8
Zina[60]	3/32	10
Overall	31/481	6.4

New frontiers

The management of the rheumatoid spine is an exciting area with many still unresolved issues. Surgical technique is fairly well established, indications and complication management are not[68–70]. Future developments are likely in the field of surgical instrumentation but will essentially be refinements rather than any radical change of direction. It should be emphasized that surgery to the rheumatoid spine is not commonly performed and should stay concentrated in centers of excellence as there is little margin for error in these frail, debilitated patients. The concentration of surgical experience will hopefully continue to produce dividends. Other areas of interest are in the commercial availability of human bone morphogenic protein. In animal experiments this evokes very prompt bony fusion[39]. Phase 1 clinical trials are currently underway. It might be that it is the rheumatologist who fuses these patients in the fusion with a C2 nerve block and then percutaneous

Table 37.7 Ranawat neurological disability classification and the American Rheumatism Association grading system (ARA) for functional disability[2, 67]

STEINBROCKER or ARA grading system for functional disability
  I—Complete ability to carry out al the usual duties without handicaps.
  II—Adequate for normal activities despite handicap of discomfort or limited motion of one of the joints.
  III—Limited to little or none of the duties of usual occupation or self-care.
  IV—Incapacitated largely or wholly bed-ridden or confined to a wheelchair with little or no self-care.

RANAWAT'S neurological classification
  I—No neurological deficit (normal neurological condition)
  II—Subjective weakness with hyperreflexia and dyesthesias
  III A—Objective weakness and long-tract signs but able to walk
  III B—Quadraparetic and non-ambulatory

Table 36.6 Outcome in several recent surgical series

Author	No. with neurological improvement	% with neurological improvement	No. with significantly reduced pain	% with pain reduction	No. with overall non-specified improvement
Boden[27]	25/42	60	–		–
Clark[52]	11/41	27	21/23	91	27/41 'clinical'
Conaty[53]	12/22	55	31/35	89	22/35 'satisfactory'
Fehring[54]	8/11	73	7/11	63	10/14
Heywood[65]	7/8	88	12/12	100	
Milbrink[56]	8/9	75	–	–	5/12 by 1ARA grade
Milbrink[56]	10/12	83	16/19	84	–
Peppelman[57]	78/90	87	–	–	–
Ranawat[2]	8/17	47	–	–	18/33
Santavira[62]	8/14	57	12/15	80	–
Santavirta[66]	6/8	75	12/15	80	–
Thompson[59]	3/6	50	–	–	84% 'satisfactory'
Zoma[60]	19/29	66	23/32	72	23/40 'overall success'
Total	203/309	66%	160/199	80%	N/A

Table 37.8   The Myelopathy Disability Index[24] derived from the Stanford HAQ[37]

Please tick the response which best describe your usual abilities over the past week.	Without ANY diffculty	With SOME difficulty	With MUCH difficulty	Unable to do
Score (office use only)	0	1	2	3
STANDING Are you able to:				
• Get in and out of bed?		√		
• Stand up from an armless chair?	√			
EATING Are you able to:				
• Cut your meat?		√		
• Lift a full cup or glass to your mouth?	√			
WALKING Are you able to:				
• Walking outdoors on flat ground?	√			
• Climb up five steps?	√			
HYGIENE Are you able to:				
• Wash and dry your entire body?	√			
• Get on and off the toilet?		√		
• GRIP Are you able to:				
• Open jars which have previously opened?	√	√		
ACTIVITIES Are you able to:				
• Get in and out of car?	√			
DRESSING Are you able to:				
• Dress yourself, –including tying shoelaces, and doing buttons on a shirt or blouse?			√	
• TOTAL (office use only)	0	4	2	0

administration of BMP! Neuroprotective agents are being developed for use following spinal cord injury, with much of the research background to the development of these new agents being common to traumatic brain injury.

References

1. Casey, A. T., Crockard, H. A., Geddes, J. F., and Stevens, J. Vertical translocation: the enigma of the disappearing atlantodens interval in patients with myelopathy and rheumatoid arthritis. Part I. Clinical, radiological, and neuropathological features. *J Neurosurg* 1997; **87**: 856–62.
2. Ranawat, C. S., O'Leary, P., Pellicci, P., Tsairis, P., Marchisello, P., and Dorr, L. Cervical spine fusion in rheumatoid arthritis. *J Bone Joint Surg Am* 1979; **61**: 1003–10.
3. Redlund-Johnell, I., and Pettersson, H. Radiographic measurements of the cranio-vertebral region: designed for evaluation of abnormalities in rheumatoid arthritis. *Acta Radiol Diagn (Stockh)* 1984; **25**: 23–8.
4. Teigland, J., Ostensen, H., and Gudmundsen, T. E. Radiographic measurements of occipito-atlanto-axial dislocation in rheumatoid arthritis. *Scand J Rheumatol* 1990; **19**: 105–14.
5. McRae, D. L. The significance of abnormalities of the cervical spine. *Am J Roentgenol* 1960; **84**: 3–25.

6. McRae, D. L., and Barnum, A. S. Occipitalization of the atlas. *Am J Roentgenol* 1953; **70**: 23–46.

7. McGregor, M. The significance of certain measurements of the skull in the diagnosis of basilar impression. *Brit J Radiol* 1948; **21**: 171–81.

8. Clark, C. R. Cervical spine involvement in rheumatoid arthritis. *Iowa Med* 1984; **74**: 57–62.

9. Kauppi, M., and Hakala, M. Prevalence of cervical spine subluxations and dislocations in a community-based rheumatoid arthritis population. *Scand J Rheumatol* 1994; **23**: 133–6.

10. Stevens, J. C., Cartlidge, N. E., Saunders, M., Appleby, A., Hall, M., and Shaw, D. A. Atlanto-axial subluxation and cervical myelopathy in rheumatoid arthritis. *Q J Med* 1971; **40**: 391–408.

11. Mathews, J. A. Atlanto-axial subluxation in rheumatoid arthritis: a 5-year follow-up study. *Ann Rheum Dis* 1974; **33**: 526–31.

12. Pellicci, P. M., Ranawat, C. S., Tsairis, P., and Bryan, W. J. A prospective study of the progression of rheumatoid arthritis of the cervical spine. *J Bone Joint Surg Am* 1981; **63**: 342–50.

13. Rana, N. A. Natural history of atlanto-axial subluxation in rheumatoid arthritis. *Spine* 1989; **14**: 1054–6.

14. Smith, P. H., Sharp, J., and Kellgren, J. H. Natural history of rheumatoid cervical subluxations. *Ann Rheum Dis* 1972; **31**: 222–3.

15. Winfield, J., Cooke, D., Brook, A. S., and Corbett, M. A prospective study of the radiological changes in the cervical spine in early rheumatoid disease. *Ann Rheum Dis* 1981; **40**: 109–14.

16. Henderson, F. C., Geddes, J. F., and Crockard, H. A. Neuropathology of the brainstem and spinal cord in end-stage rheumatoid arthritis: implications for treatment. *Ann Rheum Dis* 1993; **1993**: 629–37.

17. Mikulowski, P., Wollheim, F. A., Rotmil, P., and Olsen, I. Sudden death in rheumatoid arthritis with atlanto-axial dislocation. *Acta Med Scand* 1975; **198**: 445–51.

18. Marks, J. S., and Sharp, J. Rheumatoid cervical myelopathy. *Q J Med* 1981; **50**: 307–19.

19. Meijers, K. A., van Beusekom, G. T., Luyendijk, W., and Duijfjes, F. Dislocation of the cervical spine with cord compression in rheumatoid arthritis. *J Bone Joint Surg Br* 1974; **56B**: 668–80.

20. Allebeck, P., Ahlbom, A., and Allander, E. Increased mortality among persons with rheumatoid arthritis, but where RA does not appear on the death certificate. *Scand J Rheumatol* 1981; **10**: 301–6.

21. Casey, A. T., Crockard. H. A., Bland, J. M., Stevens, J., Moskovich, R., and Ransford, A. O. Surgery on the rheumatoid cervical spine for the non-ambulant myelopathic patient: too much, too late? *Lancet* 1996; **347**: 1004–7.

22. Sunahara, N., Matsunaga, S., Mori, T., Ijiri, K., and Sakou, T. Clinical course of conservatively managed rheumatoid arthritis patients with myelopathy. *Spine* 1997; **22**: 2603–7.

23. Corbett, M., Dalton, S., Young, A., Silman, A., and Shipley, M. Factors predicting death, survival and functional outcome in a prospective study of early rheumatoid disease over fifteen years. *Br J Rheumatol* 1993; **32**: 717–23.

24. Casey, A. T., Bland, J. M., and Crockard, H. A. Development of a functional scoring system for rheumatoid arthritis patients with cervical myelopathy. *Ann Rheum Dis* 1996; **55**: 901–6.

25. Heywood, A.W., Learmonth, I. D., and Thomas, M. Cervical spine instability in rheumatoid arthritis. *J Bone Joint Surg Br* 1988; **70**: 702–7.

26. Papadopoulos, S. M., Dickman, C. A., and Sonntag, V. K. Atlantoaxial stabilization in rheumatoid arthritis. *J Neurosurg* 1991; **74**: 1–7.

27. Boden, S. D., Dodge, L. D., Bohlman, H. H., and Rechtine, G. R. Rheumatoid arthritis of the cervical spine: a long-term analysis with predictors of paralysis and recovery. *J Bone Joint Surg Am* 1993; **75**: 1282–97.

28. Casey, A. T., Crockard, H. A., Bland, J. M., Stevens, J., Moskovich, R., and Ransford, A. Predictors of outcome in the quadriparetic nonambulatory myelopathic patient with rheumatoid arthritis: a prospective study of 55 surgically treated Ranawat class IIIb patients. *J Neurosurg* 1996; **85**: 574–81.

29. Casey, A. T., and Crockard, A. In the rheumatoid patient: surgery to the cervical spine. *Br J Rheumatol* 1995; **34**: 1079–86.

30. Casey, A. T., Crockard, H. A., and Stevens, J. Vertical translocation. Part II. Outcomes after surgical treatment of rheumatoid cervical myelopathy. *J Neurosurg* 1997; **87**: 863–9.

31. Dvorak, J., Grob, D., Baumgartner, H., Gschwend, N., Grauer, W., and Larsson, S. Functional evaluation of the spinal cord by magnetic resonance imaging in patients with rheumatoid arthritis and instability of upper cervical spine. *Spine* 1989; **14**: 1057–64.

32. Crockard, H. A., Essigman, W. K., Stevens, J. M., Pozo, J. L., Ransford, A. O., and Kendall, B. E. Surgical treatment of cervical cord compression in rheumatoid arthritis. *Ann Rheum Dis* 1985; **44**: 809–16.

33. Crockard, H. A., Pozo, J. L., Ransford, A. O., Stevens, J. M., Kendall, B. E., and Essigman, W. K. Transoral decompression and posterior fusion for rheumatoid atlanto-axial subluxation. *J Bone Joint Surg Br* 1986; **68**: 350–6.

34. Madawi, A. A., Casey, A. T., Solanki, G. A., Tuite, G., Veres, R., and Crockard, H. A. Radiological and anatomical evaluation of the atlantoaxial transarticular screw fixation technique. *J Neurosurg* 1997; **86**: 961–8.

35. Casey, A. T. H., Madawi, A. A., Veres, R., and Crockard, H. A. Is the technique of posterior transarticular screw fixation suitable for rheumatoid atlantoaxial subluxation. *Br J Neurosurg* 1997; **11**: 508–19.

36. Montesano, P. X. Biomechanics of cervical spine internal fixation. *Spine* 1991; **16** (Suppl.): S10–S16.

37. Fries, J. F., Spitz, P. W., and Young, D. Y. The dimensions of health outcomes: the health assessment questionnaire, disability and pain scales. *J Rheumatol* 1982; **9**: 789–93.

38. Hultquist, R., Zygmunt, S., Saveland, H., Birch, I. M., and Wollheim, F. A. Characterization and functional assessment of patients subjected to occipito-cervical fusion for rheumatoid atlanto-axial dislocation. *Scand J Rheumatol* 1993; **22**: 20–4.

39. Urist, M., and Hudak, R. Radioimmunoassay of bone morphogenetic protein in serum: a tissue-specific parameter of bone metabolism. *Proc Soc Exp Biol Med* 1984; **4**: 472–5.

40. Lawrence, J. S. Radiological cervical arthritis in populations. *Ann Rheum Dis* 1976; **35**: 365–71.

41. Symmons, D. P. M., Barrett, E. M., Bankhead, C. R., Scott, D. G. I., and Silman, A. J. The incidence of rheumatoid arthritis in the United Kingdom: results from the Norfolk Arthritis Register. *Br J Rheumatol* 1994; **33**: 735–9.

42. Serre, H., and Simon, L. Atlanto-axial dislocation in rheumatoid arthritis. *Rheumatism* 1966; **22**: 53–8.

43. Cabot, A., and Becker, A. The cervical spine in rheumatoid arthritis. *Clin Orthop Relat Res* 1978; **131**: 130–40.

44. Martel, W. The occipito-atlanto-axial joints in rheumatoid arthritis and ankylosing spondylitis. *Am J Roentgenol Radium Ther Nucl Med* 1961; **86**: 230–40.

45. Conlon, P. W., Isdale, I. C., and Rose, B. S. Rheumatoid arthritis of the cervical spine: an analysis of 333 cases. *Ann Rheum Dis* 1966; **25**: 120–6.

46. Halla, J. T., and Hardin, J. J. The spectrum of atlantoaxial facet joint involvement in rheumatoid arthritis [see comments]. *Arthritis Rheum* 1990; **33**: 325–9.

47. Mathews, J. A. Atlanto-axial subluxation in rheumatoid arthritis. *Ann Rheum Dis* 1969; **28**: 260–6.

48. Meikle, J. A., and Wilkinson M. Rheumatoid involvement of the cervical spine: radiological assessment. *Ann Rheum Dis* 1971; **30**: 154–61.

49. Ornilla, E., Ansell, B. M., and Swannell, A. J. Cervical spine involvement in patients with chronic arthritis undergoing orthopaedic surgery. *Ann Rheum Dis* 1972; **31**: 364–8.

50. Rasker, J. J., and Cosh, J. A. Radiological study of cervical spine and hand in patients with rheumatoid arthritis of 15 years' duration: an assessment of the effects of corticosteroid treatment. *Ann Rheum Dis* 1978; **37**: 529–35.

51. Isdale, I. C., and Conlon, P. W. Atlanto-axial subluxation: a six-year follow-up report. *Ann Rheum Dis* 1971; **30**: 387–9.

52. Clark, C. R., Goetz, D. D., and Menezes, A. H. Arthrodesis of the cervical spine in rheumatoid arthritis. *J Bone Joint Surg Am* 1989; **71**: 381–92.

53. Conaty, J. P., and Mongan, E. S. Cervical fusion in rheumatoid arthritis. *J Bone Joint Surg Am* 1981; **63**: 1218–27.

54. Fehring, T. K., and Brooks, A. L. Upper cervical instability in rheumatoid arthritis. *Clin Orthop Relat Res* 1987; **221**: 137–48.

55. Ferlic, D. C., Clayton, M. L., Leidholt, J. D., and Gamble, W. E. Surgical treatment of the symptomatic unstable cervical spine in rheumatoid arthritis. *J Bone Joint Surg Am* 1975; **57**: 349–54.

56. Milbrink, J., and Nyman, R. Posterior stabilization of the cervical spine in rheumatoid arthritis: clinical results and magnetic resonance imaging correlation. *J Spinal Disord* 1990; **3**: 308–15.

57. Peppelman, W. C., Kraus, D. R., and Donaldson, W. F., 3rd, and Agarwal, A. Cervical spine surgery in rheumatoid arthritis: improvement of neurologic deficit after cervical spine fusion. *Spine* 1993; **18**: 2375–9.

58. Santavirta, S., Slatis, P., Kankaanpaa, U., Sandelin, J., and Laasonen, E. Treatment of the cervical spine in rheumatoid arthritis. *J Bone Joint Surg Am* 1988; **70**: 658–67.

59. Thompson, R. J., and Meyer, T. J. Posterior surgical stabilization for atlantoaxial subluxation in rheumatoid arthritis. *Spine* 1985; **10**: 597–601.

60. Zoma, A., Sturrock, R. D., Fisher, W. D., Freeman, P. A., and Hamblen, D. L. Surgical stabilisation of the rheumatoid cervical spine: a review of indications and results. *J Bone Joint Surg Br* 1987; **69**: 8–12.

61. Crellin, R. Q., MacCabe, J. J., and Hamilton, E. B. Surgical management of severe subluxations of the rheumatoid cervical spine. *Ann Rheum Dis* 1970; **29**: 565.

62. Santavirta, S., Konttinen, Y. T., Laasonen, E., Honkanen, V., Antti, P. I., and Kauppi, M. Ten-year results of operations for rheumatoid cervical spine disorders. *J Bone Joint Surg Br* 1991; **73**: 116–20.

63. Stanley, D., Laing, R. J., Forster, D. M., and Getty, C. J. Posterior decompression and fusion in rheumatoid disease of the cervical spine: redressing the balance. *J Spinal Disord* 1994; **7**: 439–43.

64. Stirrat, A. N., and Fyfe, I. S. Surgery of the rheumatoid cervical spine: correlation of the pathology and prognosis. *Clin Orthop Relat Res* 1993; **293**: 135–43.

65. Heywood, A. W., and Meyers, O. L. Rheumatoid arthritis of the thoracic and lumbar spine. *J Bone Joint Surg Br* 1986; **68**: 362–8.

66. Santavirta, S., Konttinen, Y. T., Sandelin, J., and Slatis, P. Operations for the unstable cervical spine in rheumatoid arthritis: sixteen cases of subaxial subluxation. *Acta Orthop Scand* 1990; **61**: 106–10.

67. Steinbrocker, O., Traeger, C. H., and Batterman, R. C. Therapeutic criteria in rheumatoid arthritis. *JAMA* 1949; **140**: 659–62.

68. Casey, A. T., Crockard, H. A., Pringle, J., O'Brien, M. F., and Stevens, J. M. Rheumatoid arthritis of the cervical spine: current techniques for management. *Orthop Clin North Am* 2002; **33**: 291–309.

69. Nguyen, H. V., Ludwig, S. C., Silber, J., Gelb, D. E., Anderson, P. A., Frank, L., and Vaccaro, A. R. Rheumatoid arthritis of the cervical spine. *Spine J* 2004; **4**: 329–34.

70. Grob, D. Surgical aspects of the cervical spine in rheumatoid arthritis [in German]. *Orthopade* 2004; **33**: 1201–14.

SECTION
7 | *Frontiers of therapy*

37 | Design of trials involving clinical end-points

Louise Pollard, Gabrielle Kingsley, and David L. Scott

Introduction

The primary aim of this chapter is to discuss the design of clinical trials, which use, to assess outcome, clinical end-points such as pain or disease activity. Though the chapter focuses primarily on trials of therapeutic agents in rheumatoid arthritis (RA), the basic principles apply to all types of clinical trials in a variety of rheumatic and other diseases.

Strategies for drug development

In recent years, many new drugs and biological treatments have become available for RA. The ongoing stream of new research means that many novel therapies are being developed which need evaluating in well-designed trials.

Traditionally, the first stage of drug development involved assessing a series of chemicals using *in vitro* systems and animal models chosen for their relevance to the target disease. For RA, studies usually involved *in vitro* models of inflammation and animal models of arthritis or relevant processes such as pain. More recently, as our understanding of RA pathogenesis has developed, molecules have been selected as potential targets based on their known function. For example, human clinical studies of interleukin (IL)-10 were conducted because the molecule had been shown to be inhibitory in model systems; conversely, tumor necrosis factor-α (TNF-α) antagonists were investigated in humans because TNF-α appeared to be pro-inflammatory and TNF-α antagonists inhibitory in such systems. Once a promising candidate has been identified, the next stage is to examine toxicity in animal studies. If the agent is not shown to have unacceptable toxicity in animals, it passes to human studies. Four human study phases (I–IV) are usually required before regulatory approval can be granted.

Phase I studies are usually conducted in healthy volunteers. They focus on human toxicity and pharmacokinetics and do not generally involve conventional clinical trials. Phases II and III, the most crucial phases in testing new drugs, do involve clinical trials. Conventionally Phase II trials evaluate short-term efficacy and safety. If successful, the product will move into Phase III studies, which are usually large, multicenter, and multinational. For drugs, like those in RA, which are going to be used long term, Phase III studies also last for prolonged periods; in RA they may

last up to one year. Because such Phase III studies are large, multicenter, and prolonged, they require careful monitoring, which is usually beyond the resources of agencies other than pharmaceutical companies. Traditionally two large Phase III trials with positive results are needed before a drug is approved. Finally, post-marketing, Phase IV studies are conducted to assess cost–benefit, examine rare side-effects, refine dosing regimes, and to extend indications. These use a variety of methods, which may include further clinical trials but will also use other methods such as post-marketing surveillance, pharmacokinetic studies, and health economic analyses.

Designing clinical trials

General aspects of trial design

Clinical trials are research studies in human volunteers to answer specific health questions. They are the quickest and safest way to identify what works and find ways to improve health. Interventional trials—the subject of this chapter—determine whether experimental treatments or new ways of using known therapies are safe and effective in controlled settings.

All trials need a purpose, which generally means they have to test a specific hypothesis. The process of developing a trial includes deciding whether a trial is needed, including a comprehensive literature review, defining the optimal design and methodology to be used, and predetermining the outcome measures, including agreeing which is primary and which are secondary. A predefined single primary outcome measure is needed to avoid investigators picking the outcome at the end of the study on the basis of what gives a positive result.

It is also essential to predetermine trial size and analytical techniques to be used with the help of an experienced statistician, which will include a realistic assessment of recruitment rates. Many studies fail to enrol enough patients as a consequence of unrealistic ideas about recruitment.

Non-randomized trial design

Observational trials address health issues in large groups of people or populations in natural settings. They are useful in establishing important questions but they cannot provide any definitive answers because they do not test a specific question about treatment.

Randomized controlled trial design

There are essentially two approaches for testing two or more treatments or treatment strategies in a clinical trial in a group of patients. The first approach is for patients to have one or other of the treatments—a parallel design. The second is for patients to have both treatments—a crossover design. In both designs the treatments should be given on the basis of random choice and ideally patients and observers should be blinded to which patients received what treatment. Trials have to show that two treatments are genuinely different from each other. To do so requires showing that any difference between treatments was unlikely to have occurred by chance. The natural assumption is that both treatments are the same and so trials must reject this so-called 'null hypothesis'. Conventionally they need to reject the null hypothesis with 95% confidence; in other words they must be 95% certain that a difference was genuine, leaving only a 5% likelihood that it occurred by chance.

Parallel group design

The most common design of trial is the parallel group[1]. In the simplest design patients are randomized to receive one of two treatments or interventions and outcome measurements are made at one time point at the end of the treatment period. A recent example of a parallel group design trial is a study comparing 10 mg and 20 mg leflunomide in active RA[2]. This multinational, randomized, double blind, parallel group study evaluated 402 RA patients over 24 weeks. It was designed to show non-inferiority of 10 mg compared with 20 mg leflunomide. It rejected the null hypothesis because patients given 20 mg had better responses and fewer adverse events.

Standard parallel group designs can be adapted in several ways. For example they can have three or more treatment groups, such as different doses of the same drug or comparing different drugs. Another example is comparing an experimental intervention with both a standard intervention and placebo. Trials may have outcome measures assessed at several time points rather than just at the end of the trial. Parallel group design is preferable when there may be carryover effects of an intervention or treatment, or if the natural history of a disease makes progression likely. Their major limitation is within-patient variability. Large sample sizes often balance out variability.

Crossover design

In a crossover trial, patients are randomized to a series of treatments or interventions. In the simplest design there are only two treatments[3]. An example of this design is a crossover trial of custom-made and commercially available wrist splints[4]. The study compared the effects of three wrist splints on wrist pain, hand function, and upper extremity function. The trial randomly assigned 45 patients to treatment order in a three-phase crossover trial. Each splint was worn for four weeks, separated by one-week washouts. Two splints performed well and one was less effective.

One of the main advantages of crossover trials is that there is no variation between treatment and control groups. This also means that in practice, for the same number of patients, a crossover design will be statistically more powerful than parallel group design trials, so a smaller number of patients can be recruited. There are several drawbacks. There may be a prolonged effect of the first treatment, which can in part be avoided by a 'washout period'. However, the extra period of time before each patient starts the next treatment can result in high dropout rates. In addition the patients' conditions may change over time.

Other designs

The single patient (*n*-of-1) trial design, which uses a randomized, controlled, multi-crossover study design, is an interesting alternative[5]. Such *n*-of-1 studies have similar limitations to center-based crossover trials. In such trials, the patient undergoes pairs of treatment periods organized so that one period involves the use of experimental treatment and the other involves the use of an alternate or placebo therapy. The patient and physician are blinded, if possible, and outcomes are monitored. Treatment periods are replicated until the clinician and patient are convinced that the treatments are definitely different or definitely not different.

Clinical outcome measures

Background

Chronic diseases like diabetes mellitus have a key abnormality such as elevated blood sugar levels that presents a single, simple treatment target. In RA there are a variety of clinical, laboratory, functional, and X-ray assessments that are all surrogate markers for activity or progression. They represent different areas or domains of the disease; for example swollen joint and disability are both characteristic of RA, but are different aspects of the disease, and can therefore be described as different domains. Some markers are inter-related (joint counts and acute phase response); others overlap domains (for example functional assessments reflect activity and progression)[6]. Optimal measures for trials have been agreed[7] as the core data set. Outcome markers need to be cheap, limited in number, reproducible, and easy to use.

Single measures

Joint counts

A large number of different methods for assessing joint counts have been developed over the years. The main ones in current use involve counting 66 joints or 28 joints. For simplicity, the 28-joint index is often considered preferable[8] (Fig. 37.1). The rationale for assessing 66 joints is that it includes the feet, therefore giving a more comprehensive evaluation, and that by measuring more joints it has greater sensitivity to change. These benefits are offset by it taking longer and being less accurate.

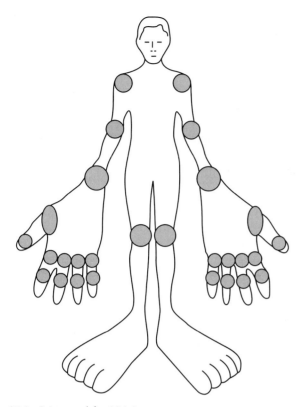

Fig. 37.1 Joints used for 28-joint counts.

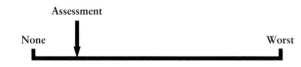

Fig. 37.2 Generic Visual Analogue Scale.

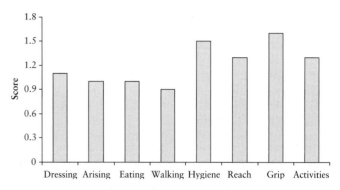

Fig. 37.3 Scores in different domains of the HAQ in 130 RA patients at one center.

Pain scores

Pain is often considered 'subjective' as it is based on data obtained from the patient, contrasting with 'objective' data from physical examination and laboratory tests. However, quantitative estimations of levels of pain can only be obtained from patients and a number of self-report questionnaires have been developed. The visual analogue scale (VAS) is the simplest approach and can be applied in both research and clinical settings[9]. The standard VAS is a 10-cm scale bordered on each side. At the '0' mark, it says 'No pain at all', and at the '10' mark, 'Pain as bad as it could be' (Fig. 37.2). The VAS is also often used to assess overall health status and disease activity.

Global assessments

Patient and assessor (or physician) global assessments of disease are measured using similar visual analogue scales.

The Health Assessment Questionnaire and other health status measures

Health status spans impairment, disability, and handicap. Impairment means loss of psychological or anatomical structure or function. Disability implies a restriction or lack of ability to perform an activity in the manner considered normal, as a consequence of impairment. Handicap, which is specific for an individual, indicates limitations in fulfilling normal roles for that individual due to impairment or disability.

Historically assessments of health status in RA concentrated on measures of function. More recently they have extended to include measures of quality of life. Although function can be measured using 'objective' measures of observed performance, self-completed or interviewer administered questionnaires of the patient's perception of function are generally preferred.

The Health Assessment Questionnaire (HAQ)[10] is the self-completed questionnaire most widely used to assess disability (Fig. 37.3). It was developed 25 years ago at Stanford University as a comprehensive measure of outcome in patients with a variety of rheumatic diseases. It focuses on self-reported, patient-oriented outcome measures. HAQ scores usually focus on the physical disability scale. This assesses upper and lower limb function related to the degree of difficulty encountered in performing a range of specified daily living tasks. HAQ scores range from 0 (without any difficulty) to 3 (unable to do). Scores for each section are transformed to give an overall disability score of 0–3, with 0 representing no disability and 3 very severe disability.

There are many other functional assessments that have been used in RA, including the Arthritis Impact Score[11] and the Lee functional index[12]. None of these have achieved the wide usage of HAQ scores. RA patients can also be assessed using generic health status measures such as the Short Form-36 Health Survey (SF-36)[13], the Nottingham Health Profile (NHP)[14], and the EuroQol[15]. These latter measures are rarely used in clinical practice.

Laboratory assessments

Though not strictly speaking clinical outcomes, quantitative laboratory markers like the erythrocyte sedimentation rate (ESR) are useful for monitoring because they are a consequence of systemic disease[16]. In contrast, qualitative markers like rheumatoid factor indicate prognosis and may have pathogenic relevance[17], but are not useful for monitoring.

The acute phase response can be measured indirectly using the ESR or directly using C-reactive protein (CRP) or serum amyloid A. ESR and CRP levels usually correlate with clinical measures of disease activity. However, in over-one third of patients both ESR and CRP are normal at presentation. In early RA they correlate most with joint swelling. A persistently elevated acute phase response is associated with high rates of progressive joint damage; the aim of treatment is to return these elevated acute phase proteins towards normal. The changes in individual measures can be summated over time and expressed as an 'area under the curve'. This approach may be particularly important for linking together measures of inflammation such as the 'under the curve for CRP' with joint damage and functional outcomes.

Using multiple measures to assess disease

Core data set

In RA no single measure is universally appropriate. Rather than achieving a cure, treatment benefits are derived by reducing symptoms or slowing disease progression. Until recently there was no agreement on which, if any, measure was best in either clinical trials or routine practice. In the last few years a limited 'core' set of preferred outcome measures has been defined by international consensus (Table 37.1). These should be included in every clinical trial in RA and are suitable for routine practice[18].

Using composite measures to assess disease and treatment response

Composite disease activity indices

A number of these are available (summarized in Table 37.2). The leading European index is the Disease Activity Score (DAS)[19]. The

Table 37.1   Core data set for RA

Number of swollen joints
Number of tender joints
Pain assessed by the patient
Patient's global assessments of disease activity
Assessor's global assessments of disease activity
Laboratory evaluation (ESR, CRP, or equivalent)
Self-administered functional assessment (e.g. HAQ)
X-ray assessment for joint damage

DAS, which has been modified for use with 28-joint counts for tenderness and swelling, is simple to use and as equally valid as more comprehensive articular indices, which can be time consuming in routine practice.

American College of Rheumatology (ACR) response criteria

These were developed in 1995 to simplify the assessment of response in clinical trials[29]. They use components of the core data set and involve improvements in both swollen and tender joint counts and three out of: patient global assessment, physician global assessment, pain, ESR, and a functional measure such as HAQ. Improvements can be at 20%, 50% or 70% levels (termed ACR-20 to ACR-70 responses).

Adverse events

Evidence of efficacy must be offset against potential toxicity. The nature and frequency of adverse events varies between different types of drug. In general, the less specific the assessment of adverse events the better it is. However, this is offset by many complex factors, including what effects are considered likely.

It is better to assess adverse events over a prolonged period in large numbers of patients. With some drugs, particularly new classes of non-steroidal anti-inflammatory drugs (NSAIDs), where the aim is to show reduction of toxicity, especially gastrointestinal effects, the studies have become increasingly large and of longer duration.

Outcome measures for different treatments

Analgesics

Analgesics like paracetamol, tramadol, and opioids control pain[30], though little clinical trial data supports their use[31], and patients often prefer NSAIDs[32]. There is slender evidence that adding paracetamol to NSAIDs improves symptoms[33]. Analgesics are effective within hours; efficacy studies need only last a few weeks. Adverse effects, like headaches, nausea, and constipation, are also identifiable in short-term trials.

Table 37.2   Composite disease activity scores

Year	Authors	Main features
1958	Lansbury[20]	EMS, fatigue, aspirin consumption, grip strength, ESR, hemoglobin
1956	Lansbury and Haut[21]	As above plus area-weighted articular index
1981	Mallya and Mace[22]	An index of disease activity
1990	Davis *et al.*[23]	Stoke index
1990	Van der Heijde *et al.*[24]	DAS
1990	Stewart *et al.*[25]	The index of disease activity
1993	Jones *et al.*[26]	Modified Stoke index
1995	Symmons *et al.*[27]	Overall status in RA (OSRA)—activity and damage score
1995	Prevoo *et al.*[28]	Modified DAS (for 28-joint counts)

EMS, early morning stiffness.

Table 37.3 Criteria for active RA—aimed at RCTs of DMARDs and biologics

Area	Change	Criteria
Current		3 out of 4 of EMS ≥ 45; ESR ≥ 28; SJ ≥ 6; TJ ≥ 6;
EMS	Remove	All of ESR ≥ 28; SJ ≥ 6; TJ ≥ 6
ESR	Reduce to ≥20 mm/h	3 out of 4 of EMS ≥ 45; ESR ≥ 20; SJ ≥ 6; TJ ≥ 6
Swollen joint count (SJ)	Reduce to ≥3;	3 out of 4 of EMS ≥ 45; ESR ≥ 28; SJ ≥ 3; TJ ≥ 6;
Tender joint count (TJ)	Reduce to ≥3	3 out of 4 of EMS ≥ 45; ESR ≥ 28; SJ ≥ 6; TJ ≥ 3
DAS	Single criterion	DAS ≥ 5.2

NSAIDs

The benefits of this diverse and frequently used group of drugs must be set against significant risks from gastrointestinal and renal toxicity[34]. Their main effects are ascribed to inhibiting cyclooxygenase (COX), which exists in two isoforms: COX-1, which is important for gastric mucosal integrity and vascular hemostasis, and COX-2, which is up-regulated at sites of inflammation. Conventional NSAIDs like diclofenac and ibuprofen and newer COX-2s like celecoxib have rapid effects on pain and joint tenderness. Trials of NSAIDs that focus on showing efficacy need only last 3–6 months, and can be of shorter duration, perhaps only 2–4 weeks, in exceptional circumstances. Studies that evaluate toxicity need to continue for 12 months or longer.

Disease-modifying anti-rheumatic drugs (DMARDs) and biologics

These diverse agents improve symptoms and modify the course of the disease by slowing radiological progression and reducing disability[35]. Although ideally they should also cause remission, there is little evidence that they often do so. Commonly used DMARDs include methotrexate and leflunomide, and commonly used biologics are the TNF inhibitors such as infliximab and etanercept.

The effect of DMARDs and biologics in reducing the signs and symptoms of RA involves improvements over six months. A proportion of patients will achieve a major clinical response, in which there is a marked reduction in evidence of joint inflammation that lasts up to 12 months. A small minority of patients will enter a period of sustained remission with these drugs. It is likely that very effective drugs, which result in remission in a substantial number of cases, will also stop erosive damage and improve function, even though until now these have remained elusive.

Trial entry criteria

Trials cannot enter all patients with RA, only those likely to benefit from a particular therapy and, with new drugs, less likely to have serious adverse effects. It is also important to facilitate recruitment and maximise generalizability by avoiding inappropriate restrictions, especially age restrictions.

Disease activity

The level of disease activity required may also constitute a barrier, yet therapeutic responses cannot be shown in inactive patients. A common definition of patients who are 'trial active' is that they should meet three out of four of the following: ≥6 tender joints, ≥6 swollen joints, ESR ≥ 28 mm/h and ≥ 45 min EMS. This is sometimes based on 66 swollen joints rather than the 28 joints used to construct the DAS. The main trial entry criteria are shown in Table 37.3.

In contrast to the detailed evaluation of outcome measures such as the DAS and the ACR response criteria, relatively little attention has been paid to the choice of these empirical disease entry criteria. Somewhat illogically, therefore, patients are recruited to randomized clinical trials (RCTs) using measures not used to assess their response. Pincus[36–38] has specifically criticized the disease activity aspect of current trial recruitment criteria and showed that many routine clinic patients had insufficiently active disease to be eligible for RCTs of new DMARDs and biologics.

There is a strong case to rationalize the definition of 'trial active' RA. Studies currently use varying numbers of tender or swollen joints[39], levels of ESR[40], and duration of EMS[41], and may combine domains differently[42]. There is something to be said for abandoning EMS in the definition of 'trial active' RA, especially as it is not included within current outcome assessment in RCTs. Individual measures could be replaced with DAS, which is a widely used composite outcome measure. Using a single summary assessment, like patient or physician global assessment, is superficially attractive, but when McConkey used this approach previously there was marked variation between assessors at different centers.

There is continual debate on the optimal outcome measures for RCTs of DMARDs and a similar debate is needed about trial entry criteria. Although current criteria provide answers about the efficacy of new drugs, they may be less relevant in defining how best to further improve moderately active disease. It may be rational to start with patients who have DAS scores of 4.2 or more. An alternative would be two out of the following: three or more swollen joints, three or more tender joints, and an ESR of 20 mm/h or more.

Other inclusion and exclusion criteria

Theoretically all RA patients should be eligible to participate in an RCT. However, many variables besides the therapies may affect outcomes, and randomization cannot be expected to adjust adequately for all variables. Therefore, almost all clinical trials have explicit exclusion criteria, such as extensive comorbidities, so that the randomization groups may be similar. However, many RA patients are old and have substantial comorbidities, and excluding such patients limits the generalizability of the findings. This issue is discussed in more detail in the section dealing with effectiveness trials.

Organization of trials

Randomization

Randomization in clinical trials plays an important role in balancing variability amongst patients so that results are more meaningful. Patients are randomly assigned into each arm of the trial, usually by a computer-generated program (e.g. by simple random numbers, permuted blocks, or minimization) so there is no chance of bias. However, if the investigator (or patient) is able to identify the treatment allocation, bias may be introduced. One way in which to minimize this is to ensure that patients are randomized according to when they present.

In trials with recruitment from GP practices, patients may be subject to cluster randomization. That is, that patients within each practice will receive the same treatment. However, there are flaws within this system as patients from the same practice may have similar characteristics and may be very different to other practices. The effect of cluster randomization is to increase the size of standard error and widen confidence intervals, and the study loses power[43].

Patients commonly misunderstand the randomization process, so careful explanation is needed[44]. They are often unaware that treatment allocation is random and they frequently believe that the doctor will ensure that they receive the best treatment offered or the most appropriate drug depending on their condition.

Blinding

Another source of bias in clinical trials is in blinding of investigators and patients. This is not possible in all trials depending on the intervention. There are various types of blinding techniques. In single-blinded trials either the patient or the investigator (usually the patient) is unaware of which treatment had been allocated. Double-blinded trials try to remove any bias by blinding both to the allocated treatment and are desirable for most studies. When the organization monitoring safety of a treatment or assessing outcomes is also blinded this is termed triple blind. Open-label studies of a drug are often continued after a double-blind trial, where both patient and investigator are aware of the treatment being received. An open-label trial is often required for some surgical procedures where it is impossible to blind the investigator or patient.

Patients often assume the new treatment is superior to standard treatments and if not blinded this can influence their reporting and responses. This equally can influence the reporting or management by the investigator.

Analysis by intention to treat and alternative approaches

Analysis by intention to treat (ITT) is a strategy that compares the study groups in terms of the treatment to which they were randomly allocated. Regardless of protocol deviations and participant compliance or withdrawal, analysis is performed according to the assigned treatment group[45].

Random allocation aims to ensure that trial participants' risk factors that may affect the outcome under investigation are balanced between the allocated treatments. This is to ensure that any differences in outcomes observed between groups are actually a result of the trial interventions. Importantly, there can be no guarantee that participants from each group who do not comply with the allocated treatment have the same risk-factor profile. Any analysis other than an ITT analysis (e.g. one that excludes non-compliant participants) will potentially compromise the balance of these factors and introduce bias into the treatment comparisons.

Thus, the ITT strategy generally gives a conservative estimate of the treatment effect compared with what would be expected if there were full compliance. By accepting that non-compliance and protocol deviations are likely to occur in actual clinical practice, ITT essentially tests a treatment policy or strategy, and avoids overoptimistic estimates of the efficacy of an intervention resulting from the removal of non-compliers.

The reality of conducting clinical trials means that the ITT principle is not usually fully met, especially when outcome data are missing for some participants. However, clinical trial researchers should consider this principle an ideal, and steps to achieve it should be considered in both the design and conduct of a trial.

Eligibility errors can be avoided by careful scrutiny before random allocation. All efforts should be pursued to ensure minimal dropouts from treatment, crossover of participants between groups, and losses to follow-up. An active run-in phase may identify patients who are likely to drop out. A thorough consent process should minimize the number of dropouts. Adequate warning of the potential side-effects of treatment, together with ongoing clinical support and reassurance, should be available to all participants. When a proportion of participants are expected to receive a treatment different from the assigned one, a dilution effect generally results. The subsequent potential loss of study power can be accounted for by increasing the planned sample size.

There is a view that only patients who sufficiently complied with the trial's protocol should be considered in the analysis. Compliance covers exposure to treatment, availability of measurements, and absence of major protocol violations. Such an analysis is often referred to as a 'per-protocol' (PP) or 'on treatment' analysis. The main issue arising from this approach is that it might introduce bias related to excluding participants from analysis. Therefore, the ITT analysis should always be considered as the ideal primary analysis, possibly supplemented by a secondary analysis using the PP approach. However, if investigators decide differently, their choice must be justified and should be subject to strict rules.

Another approach is to analyze all participants according to the treatment they actually received, regardless of what treatment

Table 37.4 CONSORT key points from checklist to include in reporting an RCT

Section	Topic	Description
Introduction	Background	scientific background and rationale
Methods	participants	Eligibility criteria and *settings and locations of data collection*
	Interventions	Details of interventions and how and when they were administered
	Objectives	Specific objectives and hypotheses
	Outcomes	Clearly defined primary and secondary outcome measures
	sample size	How sample size was determined and explanation of any interim analyses
	Randomization	Methods used to generate, conceal, and implement the random allocation sequence
	Blinding	Whether participants and those administering interventions and assessing outcomes were blinded
	Statistics	Methods used to compare groups for primary outcome and any subgroup analyses
Results	Participant flow	Flow of participants through each stage
	Recruitment	Dates of recruitment and follow-up
	Baseline data	Baseline demographic and clinical characteristics
	Numbers	Number of participants in each group in each analysis and whether the analysis was by ITT
	Outcomes	For each primary and secondary outcome, a summary of results for each group, estimated effect size, and its precision
	Ancillary analyses	Other analyses, indicating pre-specified and exploratory
	Adverse events	Important adverse events in each group
Discussion	Interpretation	Interpretation of results, taking into account study hypotheses, sources of bias, and dangers associated with multiplicity of analyses and outcomes

they were originally allocated. While this may have some initial appeal, once again the effect of random allocation is compromised, making the interpretation of the results difficult.

Assessing the quality of clinical trials

CONSORT (consolidated standards of reporting trials) guidelines

The CONSORT statement is a key tool that takes an evidence-based approach to improve the quality of reporting RCTs[46]. It is accepted by all the leading medical journals. Its value to researchers, healthcare providers, and health policy makers is the guarantee of integrity in the reported results of research.

It involves a checklist (Table 37.4) and flow diagram to improve and standardize the quality of reporting. The aim is to make the experimental process clear, so that users of the data can fully evaluate its validity.

Jadad scores

There is often a need to review the quality of published RCTs and a classical instrument developed for this purpose is the Jadad Score[47]. This was devised by a multidisciplinary panel of judges and it involves three key items of quality: randomization, being

Table 37.5 Summary of Jadad scores

Items	Score 1 point for 'yes' or 0 points for each 'no'
1.	Was the study randomized?
2.	Was the study double blind?
3.	Was there a description of withdrawals and dropouts?

Refinements	
Give 1 additional point if:	For question 1, the method to generate the sequence of randomization was described *and* was appropriate
And/or:	For question 2 the method of double blinding was described and was appropriate
Deduct 1 point if:	For question 1, the method used to generate the sequence of randomization was inappropriate
And/or:	For question 2, the study was described as double blind but the method of blinding was inappropriate

double-blind, and if there was a description of withdrawals and dropouts. There are some subsequent refinements to the score (Table 37.5). The end result is a five-point score. Trials that do not score maximally will not be highly regarded.

Ethical issues

There are several benefits for patients who enter trials. They may get access to new drugs before they are generally available and these new drugs may be superior to those routinely available. Patients taking part in trials often have better medical care as they are closely monitored. There are also drawbacks. In placebo-controlled trials patients may not receive active treatment. With new drugs patients may suffer unanticipated adverse reactions. The guidelines on ethical standards are within 'The Declaration of Helsinki', drafted after the Nuremberg trials and since updated[48]. These guidelines are that the well-being of the individual patient is the most important consideration and that she/he should be assured of the best treatment when enrolled in a clinical trial.

In RA it is no longer common practice to design a simple placebo-controlled trial. There is good evidence that RA does not follow a slow benign course, but if untreated leads to functional decline, disability, and increased mortality. There are effective DMARDs and withholding these drugs during a prolonged trial where the patient may receive placebo may be unethical. It is now commonplace that if a placebo-controlled trial is undertaken some DMARD (e.g. methotrexate) is taken by all patients in addition to the new therapy.

There are often criteria for withdrawal from a trial in the event of a serious adverse event. In order to protect patients from further functional decline and disability, there should also be criteria for withdrawal for those who do not respond to treatment satisfactorily.

There is always a worry of undue influence on patients to take part in a trial if their physician has a financial interest. Ways in which this can be minimized include advertising ongoing trials on posters or flyers, asking patients who are interested to speak to their physician. Occasionally patients are paid to take part in trials; in these circumstances patients should be paid a total sum rather than per visit. This prevents the patient being penalized if they withdraw and stops incentives to keep patients in long-term trials without evidence of efficacy.

Efficacy versus effectiveness

Efficacy trials differ from effectiveness trials[49,50]. The key difference is their aims. Efficacy trials seek to show if a treatment works in the best possible circumstances to meet regulatory approval. Fixed drug doses are used to maximize the efficacy/toxicity ratio. Effectiveness trials seek to test how a treatment works in routine practice to convince formularies and payers of usefulness in practice. Flexible drug regimens are used and patients may be allowed to switch to alternate drugs. The management protocol is the subject of the investigation, not the individual treatment.

Efficacy trials recruit a homogeneous population to maximize response to treatment while effectiveness trials reflect the patients seen in clinical practice and enrol atypical patients and those with comorbidities. Outcome measures also differ. Efficacy trials use outcomes related to the biological basis of the treatment. In RA these are usually effects on synovitis and systemic inflammation. Effectiveness trials use outcomes to reflect the range of benefits expected from the treatment relevant to patients and payers. In RA these include improvements in function and quality of life.

References

1. Lavori, P. W., Louis, T. A., Bailar, J. C. 3rd, and Polansky, M. Designs for experiments: parallel comparisons of treatment. *N Engl J Med* 1983; **309**: 1291–9.
2. Poor, G., and Strand, V. Leflunomide Multinational Study Group. Efficacy and safety of leflunomide 10 mg versus 20 mg once daily in patients with active rheumatoid arthritis: multinational double-blind, randomized trial. *Rheumatology* 2004; **43**: 744–9.
3. Carriere, K. C. Crossover designs for clinical trials. *Stat Med* 1994; **13**: 1063–9.
4. Haskett, S., Backman, C., Porter, B. *et al.* A crossover trial of custom-made and commercially available wrist splints in adults with inflammatory arthritis. *Arthritis Rheum* 2004; **51**: 792–9.
5. Backman, C. L., and Harris, S. R. Case studies, single-subject research, and N of 1 randomized trials: comparisons and contrasts. *Am J Phys Med Rehabil* 1999; **78**: 170–6.
6. Wolfe, F. A. reappraisal of HAQ disability in rheumatoid arthritis. *Arthritis Rheum* 2000; **43**: 2751–61.
7. Brooks, P., and Hochberg, M. ILAR; OMERACT. Outcome measures and classification criteria for the rheumatic diseases: a compilation of data from OMERACT (Outcome Measures for Arthritis Clinical Trials), ILAR (International League of Associations for Rheumatology), regional leagues and other groups. *Rheumatology* 2001; **40**: 896–906.
8. van Gestel, A. M., Haagsma, C. J., and van Riel, P. L. Validation of rheumatoid arthritis improvement criteria that include simplified joint counts. *Arthritis Rheum* 1998; **41**: 1845–50.
9. McCormack, H. M., Horne, D. J., and Sheather, S. Clinical applications of visual analogue scales: a critical review. *Psychol Med* 1988; **18**: 1007–19.
10. Bruce, B., and Fries, J. F. The Stanford Health Assessment Questionnaire: dimensions and practical applications. *Health Qual Life Outcomes* 2003; **1**: 20.
11. Meenan, R. F., Mason, J. H., Anderson, J. J., Guccione, A. A., and Kazis, L. E. The content and properties of a revised and expanded arthritis impact measurement scales health status questionnaire. *Arthritis Rheum* 1992; **35**: 1–10.
12. Lee, P., Jasani, M. K., Dick, W. C., and Buchanan, W. W. Evaluation of a functional index in rheumatoid arthritis. *Scand J Rheumatol* 1973; **2**: 71–7.
13. Ware, J. E., and Sherbourne, C. D. The MOS 36-Item Short-Form Health Survey (SF-36). Conceptual framework and item selection. *Med Care* 1992; **30**: 473–83.
14. Houssien, D. A., McKenna, P., and Scott, D. L. The Nottingham Health Profile as a measure of disease activity and outcome in rheumatoid arthritis. *Br J Rheumatol* 1997; **36**: 69–73.
15. Wolfe, F., and Hawley, D. J. Measurement of the quality of life in rheumatic disorders using the EuroQol. *Br J Rheumatol* 1997; **36**: 786–93.
16. Bull, B. S., Westengard, J. C., Farr, M., Bacon, P. A., Meyer, P. J., and Stuart, J. Efficacy of tests used to monitor rheumatoid arthritis. *Lancet* 1989; **2**: 965–7.
17. Dorner, T., Egerer, K., Feist, E., and Burmester, G. R. Rheumatoid factor revisited. *Curr Opin Rheumatol* 2004; **16**: 246–53.
18. Pincus, T., and Sokka, T. Quantitative measures for assessing rheumatoid arthritis in clinical trials and clinical care. *Best Pract Res Clin Rheumatol* 2003; **17**: 753–81.
19. van der Heijde, D. M., van't Hof, M., van Riel, P. L., and van de Putte L. B. Development of a disease activity score based on

judgment in clinical practice by rheumatologists. *J Rheumatol* 1993; **20**: 579–81.

20. Lansbury, J. Numerical method of evaluating the status of rheumatoid arthritis. *Ann Rheum Dis* 1958; **17**: 101–7.

21. Lansbury, J., and Haut, D. D. Quantitation of the manifestations of rheumatoid arthritis. 4. Area of joint surfaces as an index to total joint inflammation and deformity. *Am J Med Sci* 1956; **232**: 150–5.

22. Mallya, R. K., and Mace, B. E. The assessment of disease activity in rheumatoid arthritis using a multivariate analysis. *Rheumatol Rehabil* 1981; **20**: 14–17.

23. Davis, M. J., Dawes, P. T., Fowler, P. D., Sheeran, T. P., Shadforth, M. F., Ziade, F., Collins, M., and Jones, P. Comparison and evaluation of a disease activity index for use in patients with rheumatoid arthritis. *Br J Rheumatol* 1990; **29**: 111–15.

24. van der Heijde, D. M., van't Hof, M. A., van Riel, P. L., Theunisse, L. A., Lubberts, E. W., van Leeuwen, M. A. *et al*. Judging disease activity in clinical practice in rheumatoid arthritis: first step in the development of a disease activity score. *Ann Rheum Dis* 1990; **49**: 916–20.

25. Stewart, M. W., Palmer, D. G., and Knight, R. G. A self-report articular index measure of arthritic activity: investigations of reliability, validity and sensitivity. *J Rheumatol* 1990; **17**: 1011–15.

26. Jones, P. W., Ziade, M. F., Davis, M. J., and Dawes, P. T. An index of disease activity in rheumatoid arthritis. *Stat Med* 1993; **12**: 1171–81.

27. Symmons, D. P., Hassell, A. B., Gunatillaka, K. A., Jones, P. J., Schollum, J., and Dawes, P. T. Development and preliminary assessment of a simple measure of overall status in rheumatoid arthritis (OSRA) for routine clinical use. *QJM* 1995; **88**: 429–37.

28. Prevoo, M. L., van't Hof, M. A., Kuper, H. H., van Leeuwen, M. A., van de Putte, L. B., and van Riel, P. L. Modified disease activity scores that include twenty-eight-joint counts: development and validation in a prospective longitudinal study of patients with rheumatoid arthritis. *Arthritis Rheum* 1995; **38**: 44–8.

29. Felson, D. T., Anderson, J. J., Boers, M., Bombardier, C., Furst, D., Goldsmith, C., Katz, L. M., Lightfoot, R. Jr., Paulus, H., Strand, V. *et al*. American College of Rheumatology: preliminary definition of improvement in rheumatoid arthritis. *Arthritis Rheum* 1995; **38**: 727–35.

30. Management of Early Rheumatoid Arthritis SIGN. Publication No. 48. ISBN 1899893 37 7. Published December 2000.

31. Wienecke, T., and Gotzsche, P. C. Paracetamol versus nonsteroidal anti-inflammatory drugs for rheumatoid arthritis. *Cochrane Database Syst Rev* 2004; (1): CD003789.

32. Wolfe, F., Zhao, S., and Lane, N. Preference for nonsteroidal antiinflammatory drugs over acetaminophen by rheumatic disease patients: a survey of 1,799 patients with osteoarthritis, rheumatoid arthritis, and fibromyalgia. *Arthritis Rheum* 2000; **43**: 378–85.

33. Seideman, P. Additive effect of combined naproxen and paracetamol in rheumatoid arthritis. *Br J Rheumatol* 1993; **32**: 1077–82.

34. Fries, J. F., Williams, C. A., Bloch, D. A., and Michel, B. A. Nonsteroidal anti-inflammatory drug-associated gastropathy: incidence and risk factor models. *Am J Med* 1991; **91**: 213–22.

35. Kremer, J. M. Rational use of new and existing disease-modifying agents in rheumatoid arthritis. *Ann Intern Med* 2001; **134**: 695–706.

36. Pincus, T., and Stein, C. M. Why randomized controlled clinical trials do not depict accurately long-term outcomes in rheumatoid arthritis: some explanations and suggestions for future studies. *Clin Exp Rheumatol* 1997; **15** (Suppl. 17): S27–S38.

37. Sokka, T., and Pincus, T. Eligibility of patients in routine care for major clinical trials of anti-tumor necrosis factor alpha agents in rheumatoid arthritis. *Arthritis Rheum* 2003; **48**: 313–18.

38. Sokka, T., and Pincus, T. Most patients receiving routine care for rheumatoid arthritis in 2001 did not meet inclusion criteria for most recent clinical trials or American College Of Rheumatology criteria for remission. *J Rheumatol* 2003; **30**: 1138–46.

39. Bathon, J. M., Martin, R. W., Fleischmann, R. M. *et al*. A comparison of etanercept and methotrexate in patients with early rheumatoid arthritis. *N Engl J Med* 2000; **343**: 1586–93.

40. Ahern, M. J., Harrison, W., Hollingsworth, P., Bradley, J., Laing, B., and Bayliss, C. A randomized double-blind trial of cyclosporin and azathioprine in refractory rheumatoid arthritis. *Aust NZ J Med* 1991; **21**: 844–9.

41. Furst, D., Felson, D., Thoren, G., and Gendreau, R. M. Immunoadsorption for the treatment of rheumatoid arthritis: final results of a randomized trial. *Ther Apher* 2000; **4**: 363–73.

42. Tugwell, P., Bombardier, C., Gent, M. *et al*. Low-dose cyclosporin versus placebo in patients with rheumatoid arthritis. *Lancet* 1990; **335**: 1051–5.

43. Bland, J. M., and Kerry, S. M. Statistic notes: trials randomised in clusters. *BMJ* 1997; **315**: 600.

44. Kerr, C., Robinson, E., Stevens, A. *et al*. Randomisation in trials: do potential trial participants understand it and find it acceptable? *J Med Ethics* 2004; **30**: 80–4.

45. Fisher, L., Dixon, D., Jerson, J. *et al*. Intention to treat in clinical trials. In *Statistical Issues in Drug Research and Development* (Peace K, ed.), pp. 331–50. New York: Marcel Dekker; 1990.

46. Moher, D., Schulz, K. F., and Altman, D. The CONSORT statement: revised recommendations for improving the quality of reports of parallel-group randomized trials. *JAMA* 2001; **285**: 1987–91.

47. Jadad, A. R., Moore, R. A., Carroll, D., Jenkinson, C., Reynolds, D. J., Gavaghan, D. J., and McQuay, H. J. Assessing the quality of reports of randomized clinical trials: is blinding necessary? *Control Clin Trials* 1996; **17**: 1–12.

48. World Medical Association declaration of Helsinki. Recommendations guiding physicians in biomedical research involving human subjects. *JAMA* 1997; **277**: 925–6.

49. Schwartz, D., and Lellouch, J. Explanatory and pragmatic attitudes in clinical trials. *J Chron Dis* 1967; **20**: 637–48.

50. Feinstein, A. R. An additional basic science for clinical medicine. II. The limitations of randomized trials. *Ann Intern Med* 1983; **99**: 544–50.

38 | Clinical trials with imaging and biomarker end-points

Jane Freeston and Paul Emery

Principles of outcome measurement in clinical trials

A major goal in the treatment of rheumatoid arthritis (RA) is the prevention of erosive joint disease and therefore the prevention of irreversible functional disability[1]. To achieve this goal in clinical practice, combinations of disease-modifying anti-rheumatic drugs (DMARDs) and, more recently, biologic agents such as those blocking TNF (tumor necrosis factor)-α are used. To fully evaluate the benefit of such drugs, the randomized clinical trial (RCT) is used, which produces the highest level of evidence for or against a certain treatment. The evidence confirms the efficacy of such disease-modifying medication in preventing damage, which has made it unethical to do placebo-controlled trials, and consequently studies have now to be designed to actively compare treatments.

Randomized controlled trials in rheumatoid arthritis have examined the therapeutic effects of DMARDs using a variety of outcome measures. In this chapter we will examine these outcome measures in more detail, looking at their validity and highlighting those which have been particularly useful in trials to date. We will also discuss outcome measures that are likely to be of use in the future.

A major ambition in rheumatology is to identify inflammatory disease at the earliest time point when disease activity is reversible. Intervening at this time point allows prevention of subsequent irreversible damage and functional disability. We therefore need to be able to distinguish disease activity from damage. Methods to measure disease activity have been developed in the areas of biological markers and radiographic, ultrasound, and computerized imaging techniques, and utilized as outcome measures in clinical trials.

Traditionally many trials have looked at established biomarkers such as rheumatoid factor and their effect on radiological progression. However, over the last 20 years both the number of biomarkers being investigated and the imaging modalities available for assessing structural damage have increased. First of all, biomarkers and their relative value both in diagnosis and prognostication in RA will be discussed.

Biomarkers as outcome measures

A biomarker refers to a specific biochemical substance present in the body which has a particular molecular feature that makes it useful for measuring the progress of disease or the effects of treatment. Ideally it needs to be present at the onset of disease and it is additionally useful if it is independent of disease activity.

Acute phase reactants

Acute phase reactants or acute phase proteins refer to proteins produced in higher quantities by the liver as part of the acute phase response to an inflammatory stimulus, examples of which are C-reactive protein (CRP) and serum amyloid A. The erythrocyte sedimentation rate (ESR) is also commonly used as a measure of the acute phase response, providing an indirect measure of the amount of fibrinogen in the blood, the production of which is increased as part of the acute phase. A raised acute phase response, especially when analyzed as the 'area under the curve', has been shown by many groups to correlate with bone damage[2], loss of bone mineral density (BMD)[3], and functional impairment[4]. Acute phase reactants have been shown to correlate with subsequent bony erosions in multiple studies[5-7]. However, when CRP is analyzed on a population basis it does not predict RA[8] and indeed CRP may be normal at presentation in up to 60% of new RA patients[9]. Baseline CRP may not be a predictor of persistence or disease severity in very early disease, as suggested both by Green[10] and van der Heijde[11]. Indeed in patients with less than 12 weeks symptoms it is suggested that outcome measures other than CRP should be used. Thus whilst in established disease the level of CRP reflects the cytokine and overall inflammatory load (and therefore is a useful surrogate marker), in early disease it may not be helpful diagnostically in distinguishing different forms of arthritis.

Antibodies

IgM and IgA rheumatoid factor

Rheumatoid factor (RF) refers to autoantibodies produced against the Fc portion of the immunoglobulin G (IgG) molecule. These autoantibodies can be of the immunoglobulin M, A, or G variety, M being the most abundant.

Work on RF has examined both IgA and IgM types. Kaltenhauser et al.[12] looked at a cohort with disease duration of less than two years, scoring hand and feet X-rays as an outcome measure by the Larsen method. They found that the rate of joint destruction in RA was influenced by the disease-associated, shared epitope positive human leukocyte antigen (HLA)-DR4 alleles, IgA RF level, sex, and presence of erosive disease at presentation. These prognostic markers were independent of the inflammatory disease activity. However, seropositivity for IgA RF frequently developed rather late in the disease course, unlike IgM where almost all the seropositive patients were positive for IgM at initial presentation, making IgM actually more useful in early disease.

In an early RA cohort, van Zeben[13] showed that RF acts as a prognostic marker for later joint damage in early RA regardless of the test used to measure RF. Gough[14] similarly showed that RF positivity had a strong correlation with development of erosions in an early arthritis cohort, independent of shared epitope, emphasizing its predictive role in early patients. Paimela[15] showed that initial RF levels correlated with radiologically determined joint damage (using hand and feet X-rays) up to three years but there was no correlation with other initially determined conventional variables of disease activity such as ESR, CRP, and swollen joint count. Houssien[16] and Van Zeben[13] both confirmed in their studies that IgA RF correlates better with disease activity than IgM RF, Houssien also showing that IgA RF is associated with more erosive disease. Finally, the EIRA study group[17] have shown that smokers have an increased risk of developing seropositive (but not seronegative) RA.

Anti-filaggrin and anti-cyclic citrullinated peptide antibodies

Anti-perinuclear factor (APF) and anti-keratin antibodies (AKAs) are molecules which been found to recognize human epidermal filaggrin and are often referred to as 'antifilaggrin antibodies' (AFAs). AFAs have been shown to bind to sites involving the amino acid citrulline and as a result enzyme-linked immunosorbent assays (ELISAs) were developed using human filaggrin or citrullinated filaggrin-derived synthetic peptides. These ELISAs were shown to have sensitivities and specificities at least comparable to those of indirect immunofluorescence assays and the ELISA that used a modified peptide variant known as cyclic citrullinated peptide (CCP) was found to have a higher sensitivity, and thus the anti-CCP test was developed[18].

Anti-CCP antibodies are RA-specific IgG antibodies against cyclic citrullinated peptides. These antibodies have been shown both to be specific to RA and in many patients to precede the onset of symptoms, as shown by Nielen *et al.* using a cohort who had enrolled as blood donors before the onset of symptoms[19]. Such antibodies are especially useful for prognosis in patients who are RF negative. Kroot[20] looked at a cohort with less than one year of disease symptoms and showed that anti-CCP antibodies were present in almost 70% of early RA patients, and that these developed significantly more severe radiological damage than those who were anti-CCP negative ($p < 0.03$ after six years of follow-up). However, in multiple regression analysis the additional predictive value was rather moderate, that is, anti-CCP antibodies have only a moderate predictive value on radiological damage in patients with recent onset RA. Schellekens[21] similarly showed that anti-CCP antibodies were very specific for RA, being present in a significant percentage of the patients they studied.

Berglin *et al.*[22] looked at 96 patients with early RA who had donated blood when asymptomatic and analyzed various biomarkers, including anti-CCP antibodies. Patients with predating anti-CCP antibodies had significantly higher Larsen scores at disease onset and after 24 months of disease, confirming that anti-CCP antibodies can predict more erosive disease. Van Gaalen[23] and team in Leiden looked at a prospective cohort to assess the predictive value of anti-CCP antibodies in patients with undifferentiated arthritis. They found that RA developed in 25% of those with a negative anti-CCP test and in 93% with a positive anti-CCP test (odds ratio (OR): 37.8, 95% confidence interval (CI): 13.8–111.9). Multivariate analysis identified anti-CCP antibodies, amongst other factors, as a significant predictor of RA. Jansen *et al.*[24] looked specifically at the role of anti-CCP positivity in those who were IgM–RF negative in his analysis, and found that the prognostic value of anti-CCP was accentuated in this group. Thus the major value of this autoantibody is likely to be in the early phase of arthritis when the diagnosis is unclear.

Anti-neutrophil cytoplasmic antibody

Anti-neutrophil cytoplasmic antibodies (ANCAs) can be divided into those which produce perinuclear (pANCA) staining and are directed against myeloperoxidase and those which produce cytoplasmic (cANCA) staining directed against proteinase 3. Mustila[25] and Braun[26] have looked at pANCA and produced similar findings, showing that pANCA is significantly associated with parameters indicating active RA, such as RF positivity, APF/AKA, laboratory markers of active inflammation, and clinical scoring, such as a higher Disease Activity Score (DAS). In addition, Braun found that vasculitic involvement was more frequent ($p < 0.05$) in his pANCA-positive group. Cambridge[27] found that rheumatoid nodules were more common in those who were pANCA positive but did not find a similar relationship between pANCA and the presence of cutaneous vasculitis. Overall this suggests a distinct and severe disease course in ANCA-positive patients. However, RF still remains more useful than pANCA as a biomarker because of its better sensitivity.

MHC associated markers: HLA class II alleles/the shared epitope

Many studies have looked at the association of major histocompatibility complex (MHC) genes such as the HLA alleles and their predisposition to RA. In particular, the so-called 'shared epitope' conserved amino acids of the HLA-DR4/DR1 cluster, which constitutes one of the peptide binding sites of certain HLA-DR molecules associated with RA, has been shown to be a significant risk factor for RA.

Gough[14] showed that when compound heterozygotes or homozygotes for the shared epitope were studied, there was a significant relationship with persistence (relative risk (RR): 3.25, sensitivity 23%, specificity 91%) in early disease. The same group also showed that possession of the shared epitope or rheumatoid factor produced a RR of 13.49 for erosions (sensitivity 95%, specificity 39%). Huang *et al.*[28] have shown that possession of the shared epitope correlates with synovitis score, as measured by the rate of gadolinium enhancement using magnetic resonance imaging (MRI).

Possessing the shared epitope may also predict response to therapy. O'Dell *et al.*[29] showed that epitope positive patients were significantly more likely to achieve an ACR50 response if treated with triple therapy rather than methotrexate alone ($p < 0.0001$). In contrast, patients negative for the shared epitope responded equally well regardless of treatment.

Kaltenhauser[12] showed shared epitope positive DR4 alleles were a prognostic marker for the pace of joint destruction in RA. Weyand *et al.*[30], along the same lines, showed that there was a higher frequency of joint replacements in those patients in their cohort who were homozygous for the shared epitope.

Markers of bone and cartilage turnover

Markers of subchondral bone and articular cartilage turnover have been studied as surrogate markers of erosive bone destruction, such as that which occurs with synovitis in RA. The majority of collagen in cartilage is type II and in bone predominantly type I. Collagen in cartilage forms a network of fibrils which form the basis of a matrix and, when combined with proteoglycans, provide considerable tensile strength. In addition, other proteins such as cartilage oligomeric protein (COMP) may help to stabilize the structure.

Looking for appropriate markers requires candidate molecules that should ideally reflect the total cartilage and bone damage within an individual, and thus both urine and serum assays offer this potential. The corollary to this is that for each molecule it must be known whether it is metabolized prior to detection or whether it is subject to interference from other non-relevant sources of the same molecule.

Examples of markers studied include cartilage markers such as type II collagen, procollagen peptides, and hydroxyproline, as well as bone markers such as osteocalcin and procollagen extension peptides (formation) and hydroxyproline (resorption).

Type II collagen, serum YKL-40 levels, and COMP

Fraser *et al.*[31] looked at turnover of articular cartilage type II collagen and the proteoglycan aggrecan in synovial fluid and membrane obtained at arthroscopy, and compared these to synovial fluid levels of molecules such as TNF-α and matrix metalloproteinase 1 (MMP-1). They demonstrated a reduction in type II collagen synthesis and a direct correlation between the increases in TNF-α and MMP-1 production and collagen degradation, hypothesizing that the cleavage of cartilage collagen is related to the activities of TNF-α and MMP-1.

YKL-40 (also known as human cartilage glycoprotein 39) has been shown by many studies to be secreted by chondrocytes, macrophages, neutrophils, and cells within the synovium[32], and in addition it is a possible candidate auto-antigen in RA[33]. Matsumoto[34] showed a positive correlation between YKL-40 level in an RA cohort and interleukin (IL)-6, CRP, and radiological score but Harvey *et al.*[35] found that the baseline YKL-40 was a poor predictor of radiographic progression. It may be that tissue-derived markers such as YKL-40 may better reflect large joint rather than small joint damage (the latter seen predominantly in

RA). Saxne[36], however, looked at the ability of a positive serum COMP at baseline (defined as a value over the 95th percentile) to predict joint damage and impaired physical function after two years of RA and found statistically significant values for these outcome variables ($p = 0.036$, $p = 0.001$, respectively).

Urinary markers of collagen degradation

Landewe *et al.*[37] used data from the COBRA cohort to compare patients' urinary C-terminal cross-linking telopeptide of type I collagen (CTX-1) and type II collagen (CTX-II) levels with radiographic progression on plain film scored by the modified Sharp system. They showed that the individual CTX-II response measured after three months of therapy in patients with active RA who had increased CTX-II levels at baseline independently predicted long-term radiographic progression, concluding that urinary CTX-II levels could be used as early markers of treatment efficacy in patients with RA.

IL-6 and other cytokines

A variety of macrophage derived, pro-inflammatory cytokines such as IL-1, IL-6, and IL-8, and TNF-α have been studied with a view to defining them as potential biomarkers, as their production is closely related to that of the acute phase reactants CRP and indirectly to ESR. IL-6 in particular is known to induce the production of CRP by the liver. It is therefore not surprising that studies have shown a close correlation between IL-6 and CRP levels in RA patients[38]. For example, Straub[39] showed a decrease in IL-6 serum levels during the first year of therapy (gold or methotrexate) which correlated significantly with the decrease (after 36 months) in the number of inflamed joints ($p < 0.005$), Lansbury index ($p < 0.005$), and early morning stiffness ($p < 0.005$). IL-6 reduction was independent of the drug used.

Whilst an extensive review of this subject is not within the scope of this chapter, to date results from the literature do not support the value of measuring cytokines as biomarkers except in mode of action studies.

Use of biomarker combinations

Combinations of biomarkers have also been studied in an effort to produce an improved diagnostic effect. Combe[40] performed a prospective study of 191 patients with RA and disease duration of less than one year where hand, feet, and wrist radiological progression were used as outcome measures. Logistic regression analysis showed that the only baseline values that were predictive of the three-year radiological scores were IgM RF positivity, DRB1*04 genes, pain score, and total radiological score. Progression of joint damage was predicted by the ESR, IgM RF positivity, DRB1*04 genes, and erosion score at baseline. They therefore proposed a combination of radiographic score, IgM RF, DRB1*04 RA-associated genes, and ESR or pain score, modulated by coefficients based on the importance of each variable. Similarly, Emery[9] produced a prognostic severity score PISA (persistent inflammatory symmetrical arthritis) for patients with arthritis of >12 weeks, using five known prognostic factors for poor functional outcome and radiographic damage. These were RF, HLA-DR4 shared epitope, Health Assessment Questionnaire (HAQ) score, CRP, and female sex. The contribution from HAQ to the final score was doubled if the individual HAQ score was more than 1.5. Patients with a total PISA score of ≥3 have been shown to have a poor outcome.

Van Zeben[41] has proposed combining IgM RF positivity, erosions, and disease activity/functional capacity/ESR/CRP/presence of DR4 (accuracy 70–80%). Van der Heijde[42] recommended an association of high disease activity at baseline (ESR/CRP/DAS) with DR4 or DR2 (which was protective in their study) and RF positivity (83% accuracy). Evidence has also been published for the combination of RF and anti-CCP antibodies in early arthritis patients, as shown by Raza *et al.*[43] in patients with synovitis of three months duration, providing high specificity and positive predictive value for the development of persistent RA.

Imaging modalities as outcome measures in clinical trials

Imaging, in the form of plain film radiography, has historically been used in RA clinical trials as an outcome measure because of its ability to detect structural damage such as erosions and joint space narrowing. More recently, imaging has allowed dissection of the pathological inter-relationship between synovitis and bone damage[44], as newer imaging modalities, such as ultrasound and MRI, allow simultaneous detection of both synovitis and structural damage. In addition, the increased sensitivity of these newer modalities increases the statistical power of studies. Consequently these modalities are becoming increasingly utilized in studies and are even being used to identify features for entry criteria for clinical trials. However, plain film radiography remains the gold standard for assessing damage and will be discussed first.

Plain film radiography

As radiographs are both cheap to perform and widely available, in the majority of RA clinical trials hand and feet radiographs are the marker for structural damage. The hands and feet are chosen because they are amenable to quantitation, and joint destruction in these anatomical areas is known to occur early in the disease course[45]. Radiographs are able to detect many pathological changes such as erosions, joint space narrowing, periarticular osteoporosis, and subluxation. The first two are the most important as they occur in the early stages of RA. Radiographs, however, cannot detect soft tissue changes or cartilage deterioration, although joint space narrowing implies loss of cartilage. Consecutive plain films act as a permanent record representing cumulative damage. Radiographic changes have been shown to correlate with functional capacity, a correlation which increases with time[46]. The images can now also be digitally recorded and retrieved, allowing electronic transmission and standardized reading.

As reproducibility is the key, scoring systems with various modifications have been developed to allow the same standardized method to be applied in different centers involved in clinical trials. The two most well known and used (and consequently the most validated) methods are the Sharp and Larsen scores, with the van der Heijde and Scott modifications, respectively.

The original Sharp score[47] involved scoring 27 areas in the hands (including wrists) for erosions and joint space narrowing, although this was subsequently reduced[48] based on the frequency with which certain joints were affected. Erosions in each joint were assigned a maximal score of 5, and joint space narrowing 4. Van der Heijde's subsequent modification mainly involved the incorporation of the feet into the scoring system (as changes in the feet have been shown to occur early in RA). A further simplification called the Simple Erosion Narrowing Score (SENS) was developed for clinical use as the full, modified score was difficult to use in clinical practice.

The original paper written by Larsen[49] described a radiographic scoring system to assess RA progression, in which a variety of joints were graded on a scale of 0–5 against an atlas of standard radiographs for each joint. The final score was obtained by adding the individual joint scores, after weighting the wrist and subtalar joints. The Larsen method was less useful when used to assess early and mild disease so the subsequent Scott modification[50] involved relevant alterations. The modifications improved inter-observer correlation (assessed by Spearman's method).

Molenaar *et al.*[51] looked at the ability to train readers in the Sharp and Larsen methods, examining the variability in the scores generated for a fixed set of radiographs. This showed that the Sharp method produced greater variance in the scores compared to the Larsen method, implying that the latter was easier to learn and apply. Other studies, however, have shown that the modified Sharp method is more sensitive[52]. This clearly has implications for the design of clinical trials with radiographic end-points.

An important problem is the 'ceiling effect'; that is, when the maximum score is reached for that joint, it is not possible to score any further pathological progression. This effect has been shown by Kuper *et al.*[53] (with the modified Sharp scoring system) to influence the scoring results within six years of disease onset. The authors did show, however, that the modified Sharp score was especially valid when used in early RA.

The OMERACT (Outcomes Measures in Rheumatology) subgroup looking at plain radiography made preliminary recommendations in 2001, advising that a minimum of two trained observers should be used where possible, a scoring system with documented quality, such as the Larsen or Sharp methods, should be used, and their modifications (though not necessarily limited to these) and intra- and inter-observer agreement should be reported by intraclass correlation coefficients[54]. In addition, the smallest detectable difference in each study should be reported.

MRI: high and low field

MRI is the most sensitive imaging modality[55–57] and, because of its tomographic quality, gives a much greater field of view, visualizing the field of interest in three orthogonal planes. It produces a highly detailed view of both the bony aspect of the joint and the surrounding soft tissues without any ionizing radiation exposure for the patient. This is clearly a considerable advance compared to plain film radiography, although with disadvantages that include cost and lack of availability.

MRI is now available in several field strengths: the conventional high field 1.5 Tesla (T) magnet machines, the higher field 2 T machines, and the new low field 0.2 T dedicated extremity MRI machines. Sequences used in routine high field MRI imaging of musculoskeletal structures include T1-weighted images which provide good anatomical detail, T2-weighted, where fluid/edema and fat produce a high signal, T2-weighted, fat-suppressed images where bone edema is highlighted, short tau inversion recovery (STIR) images, and T1 images post-intravenous injection of the contrast agent gadolinium (Gd-DTPA). The gadolinium is preferentially taken up at sites of inflammation such as synovitis. Sequences available on low field machines are essentially restricted to T1 and STIR, although images post-contrast injection are possible though time consuming.

MRI, as shown by Ostergaard et al.[56], can identify most new bone erosions at least one year earlier than conventional radiography. Their study found a significantly increased risk of progression of radiographic erosions in bones with baseline MRI erosions, showing that MRI has a prognostic value in terms of long-term radiographic outcome. In addition, MRI can identify pre-erosive features such as synovitis and bone edema.

The use of a contrast agent such as gadolinium allows further delineation between fluid collection and synovitis, and produces greater sensitivity in terms of erosion detection. It has been shown that the synovitis and bone edema changes identified by MRI act as predictors of erosion formation[58]. In addition, MRI allows the identification of progressive erosive disease when clinical activity is suppressed[59].

MRI is a rapidly developing field, where techniques such as contrast-enhancement, dynamic views, and quantification of synovitis and erosion volume, for example, are becoming more and more widespread. Quantification of synovitis can be done by several methods: by manual or semi-automated volume measures of single/multiple sections, or as a dynamic estimation where the rate of Gd-DTPA enhancement and/or the maximum Gd-DTPA enhancement is measured.

Studies attempting to demonstrate a significant association between conventional measures of inflammation such as CRP and the synovial volumes or grading scores generated by imaging such as MRI have raised concerns about the accuracy of conventional measures in reflecting the pathological processes in the joint and surrounding bone[54,55]. One possible explanation may be that the MRI process is extremely focal in the area of interest, whereas inflammatory markers such as ESR reflect a systemic overview. This area clearly requires further work.

Inter-observer variability has been studied extensively, an example of such a study being that by Ostergaard et al.[60], which used a simple scoring system for RA changes on MRI. Their preliminary results showed that basic interpretation of MRI changes was relatively consistent among readers from different countries and medical backgrounds but that further training, calibration, and standardization of imaging protocols were required to produce acceptable inter-group reproducibility. The OMERACT MRI collaborative subgroup has been set up to address such

issues and it has produced acceptable definitions and a valid scoring system for MRI findings in RA[60,61].

The issue of validation in MRI has been extensively addressed by using arthroscopy and synovial biopsy, and by comparing these with MRI synovial volume estimates[62–65]. This has been performed mainly in knees as well as by mini-arthroscopy, macroscopic evaluation, and histology in the metacarpophalangeal (MCP) joints. The study by Ostendorf et al.[63] found that synovial enhancement post-gadolinium on MRI correlated with macroscopic signs of synovitis, and that joint space narrowing on MRI was significantly correlated with bony changes on arthroscopy. Further work, though, still needs to be done before we can conclude that MRI is an accurate representation of erosive change, synovitis, and bone edema, that is, the changes of inflammatory arthritis.

The future in MRI is likely to involve movement from scoring to measuring, the aim being to show that MRI measures are predictive of functional outcome. MRI synovitis measures could become the main outcome measure in clinical trials as better treatments are likely to reduce progressive structural joint damage to a minimum[66]. Histological correlation with imaging findings will also be emphasized. It may be that the use of MRI as an outcome measure will be combined with, for example, the American College of Rheumatology (ACR) classification tree criteria for the diagnosis of RA to improve our diagnostic capability in early RA (as done by Sugimoto et al.[55]). In contrast to ultrasound, MRI is more validated as a technique, but currently available data suggest that findings on ultrasonography are equivalent to those on MRI when looking at peripheral joints in RA patients[67].

Low field MRI

Dedicated extremity MRI using a significantly smaller 0.2 T magnet has many obvious advantages over its high field counterpart[68]. Cost is significantly reduced and the machine can be situated conveniently in a suitable clinic room rather than requiring a purpose-built home as for conventional MRI. The machine consists essentially of a 'cradle' in which the peripheral joints of interest are placed, such as the MCP joints of the dominant hand. There are no issues, therefore, of claustrophobia and the positioning of arthritic limbs which present so many problems with conventional MRI. Disadvantages include smaller fields of view with longer imaging times and, due to the reduction in the magnet strength, there is clearly some reduction in image quality. Studies have looked at whether this impacts significantly on the ability to detect synovitis and erosions.

Taouli et al.[69], for example, compared conventional high field strength 1.5 T MRI with 0.2 T low field dedicated extremity MRI and radiography, looking at the ability to detect and grade bone erosions, joint space narrowing, and synovitis in the hands and wrist of patients with RA, showing similar results. The inter-observer agreement for MRI scores was good to excellent, with intra-class correlation coefficients of 0.83–0.94. Hottya et al.[70] provide similar evidence. The only complication was that of motion artefact limiting the value of a few of the low field studies. Low field has been compared with clinical examination by

Lindegaard[71], who showed that low field MRI was significantly better, being able to identify synovial hypertrophy in joints in patients without clinical signs of joint inflammation, that is, swelling and/or tenderness. In addition, Olech[72] has shown superiority of low field MRI over radiography.

Ultrasound

Musculoskeletal ultrasound is extremely versatile, allowing the ultrasonographer to image many joints at the same, sitting in a safe environment with no X-ray exposure. Ultrasound is less expensive than computerized tomography (CT) or MRI. Machines can be situated in rheumatology outpatient clinics, allowing immediate access as clinically indicated. Ultrasound has been shown to be more sensitive than conventional radiography in the detection of erosions[73], and in the same study sonographic erosions not visible on radiography corresponded by site to MRI bone abnormalities. Backhaus et al.[74] compared ultrasound with clinical examination, conventional radiography, three-phase bone scintigraphy, and contrast-enhanced MRI in a variety of inflammatory arthritis patients and found that, not surprisingly, all techniques were significantly more sensitive than radiography for detecting inflammatory soft tissue lesions, as well as structural damage in those with effectively normal radiographs (grade 0–1 Larsen score). They also found ultrasound to be even more sensitive than MRI in the detection of synovitis, a finding not replicated by others.

Hau et al.[75] have shown that ultrasound is better than clinical examination alone and Wakefield et al.[73] demonstrated its superiority to plain radiography. Kraan et al.[76] showed that ultrasound and MRI are both able to detect subclinical synovitis with corroborative macro- and microscopic data from arthroscopy in clinically normal knees of RA patients. Karim et al.[77] compared ultrasound of the knee against the gold standard of arthroscopy as well as clinical examination in order to validate ultrasonic images in terms of accurate representation of the pathology present in the joint. They concluded that ultrasound was valid and reproducible, as well as superior to clinical examination for detecting knee synovitis.

The development of power Doppler techniques to look at blood flow in the vascular synovium (indicating inflammatory activity) has also enhanced the diagnostic power of ultrasound[78,79]. Terslev et al.[80] found that both Doppler ultrasound and post-contrast MRI produced comparable results in terms of estimation of synovial inflammatory activity; that is, there was a highly significant association between ultrasound indices of inflammation and post-contrast MRI scores. However, no association between the MRI or ultrasound estimates of inflammation and values obtained for the VAS (visual activity score), HAQ, duration of early morning stiffness, ESR, or CRP were found. Similar results were found by Szkudlarek et al.[81].

Early work has been done on the use of echo-contrast agents such as Levovist[82] that, following injection, produce a qualitative increase in power Doppler signal from synovial vessels (which is the first sign of synovial changes in inflammatory disease), although use of such contrast medium in clinical practice is not currently routine.

Disadvantages of ultrasound include issues of standardization and reliability, inter- and intra-observer variability being of particular concern. Szkudlarek et al.[83] looked at inter-observer agreement and showed that an experienced musculoskeletal radiologist and a rheumatologist with limited ultrasound training achieved high inter-observer agreement rates for identification of synovitis and bone erosions using a semiquantitative scoring system. Further work, however, is currently underway on the validation of ultrasound as an outcome measure.

Dual energy X-ray absorptiometry (DXA)

DXA has an accepted mainstream clinical role in the assessment of BMD in a wide range of patients. Loss of bone mineral density has been the subject of a significant amount of research in RA and it is likely that it will become part of the imaging assessment in patients with early arthritis, both in diagnosis and monitoring of disease.

The maximum rate of bone loss has been shown to occur in early disease stages when inflammation and potential for reversibility are greatest. Gough et al.[3] showed that femoral and spinal BMD correlated with systemic inflammation (measured by the CRP level). The bone loss stabilized when patients responded to treatment with normalization of CRP. Devlin et al.[84] found that loss of hand BMD occurred even prior to the onset of systemic disease and before lumbar BMD loss in 202 early patients. Early loss of hand BMD has been shown to be predictive of long-term BMD and outcome in terms of function by Deodhar et al.[85]. Deodhar showed that loss of more than 3% of hand bone mineral content within the first six months correlated with a significantly worse functional outcome at five years.

Following on from this research data, a trial looking at the role of zoledronic acid (ZA) in protecting patients from erosions and local and systemic bone loss associated with active inflammatory arthritis has been undertaken, with encouraging results[86]. The use of the bisphosphonate drug zoledronic acid is based on the knowledge that increased osteoclast activity is a key factor in bone loss in RA and zoledronic acid is known to be one of the most potent agents for blocking osteoclast function. Human TNF-transgenic mice with severe destructive arthritis and osteoporosis were used. Bone erosion was shown to be retarded by a single dose of ZA (-60%) and was almost completely blocked by repeated administration of ZA (-95%). Synovial osteoclast counts were significantly reduced with ZA treatment. Systemic bone mass dramatically increased after administration of ZA, which was attributed to an increase in trabecular number and connectivity. In addition, bone resorption parameters were significantly lowered after administration of ZA.

The future

So what does the future hold for diagnosis and prognosis in the early arthritis clinic? It is clear from the biomarkers discussed that those with sufficient specificity and sensitivity to merit use in clinical trials include RF, the shared epitope, anti-CCP antibodies, and CRP/ESR. Combining the measurement of such biomarkers with imaging can improve population homogeneity and the earlier classification of such patients can therefore improve outcome.

The use of imaging as an outcome measure will move away from the concept of scoring to that of measuring, and consistent with this there will be a move from plain radiography to MRI, possibly with a significant role for low field imaging. The role of musculoskeletal ultrasound will be as an alternative to MRI in those centers with easier access to the former or as an adjunct, as suggested by Ostergaard et al.[67]. The case can be made for MRI as the gold standard in RA assessment, with ultrasound used as a 'bedside tool' for improved joint evaluation (compared to clinical examination alone) and for better targeting of joint injections. Other imaging techniques likely to become more available in the future include positron emission tomography (PET) and quantitative CT[87].

References

1. Emery, P. The optimal management of early rheumatoid disease: the key to preventing disability. *Br J Rheumatol* 1994; 33: 765–8.
2. van Leeuwen, M. A., van Rijswijk, M. H., Sluiter, W. J. *et al.* Individual relationship between progression of radiological damage and the acute phase response in early rheumatoid arthritis: towards development of a decision support system. *J Rheumatol* 1997; 24: 20–7.
3. Gough, A. K., Lilley, J., Eyre, S., Holder, R. L., and Emery, P. Generalised bone loss in patients with early rheumatoid arthritis. *Lancet* 1994; 344: 23–7.
4. Devlin, J., Gough, A., Huisoon, A. *et al.* The acute phase and function in early rheumatoid arthritis: C-reactive protein levels correlate with functional outcome. *J Rheumatol* 1997; 24: 9–13.
5. Wollheim, F. A., Pettersson, H., Saxne, T., and Sjoblom, K. G. Radiographic assessment in relation to clinical and biochemical variables in rheumatoid arthritis. *Scand J Rheumatol* 1988; 17: 445–53.
6. Caruso, I., Santandrea, S., Sarzi Puttini, P. *et al.* Clinical, laboratory and radiographic features in early rheumatoid arthritis. *J Rheumatol* 1990; 17: 1263–7.
7. Otterness, I. G. The value of C-reactive protein measurement in rheumatoid arthritis. *Semin Arthritis Rheum* 1994; 24: 91–104.
8. Aho, K., Palosuo, T., Knekt, P., Alha, P., Aromaa, A., and Heliovaara, M. Serum C-reactive protein does not predict rheumatoid arthritis. *J Rheumatol* 2000; 27: 1136–8.
9. Emery, P. The Dunlop-Dottridge Lecture. Prognosis in inflammatory arthritis: the value of HLA genotyping and the oncological analogy. *J Rheumatol* 1997; 24: 1436–42.
10. Green, M., Marzo-Ortega, H., McGonagle, D. *et al.* Persistence of mild, early inflammatory arthritis: the importance of disease duration, rheumatoid factor, and the shared epitope. *Arthritis Rheum* 1999; 42: 2184–8.
11. van der Heijde, D. M., van Riel, P. L., van Rijswijk, M. H., and van de Puttem, L. B. Influence of prognostic features on the final outcome in rheumatoid arthritis: a review of the literature. *Semin Arthritis Rheum* 1988; 17: 284–92.
12. Kaltenhauser, S., Wagner, U., Schuster, E. *et al.* Immunogenetic markers and seropositivity predict radiological progression in early rheumatoid arthritis independent of disease activity. *J Rheumatol* 2001; 28: 735–44.
13. Van Zeben, D., Hazes, J. M., Zwinderman, A. H., Cats, A., van der Voort, E. A., and Breedveld, F. C. Clinical significance of rheumatoid factors in early rheumatoid arthritis: results of a follow up study. *Ann Rheum Dis* 1992; 51: 1029–35.
14. Gough, A., Faint, J., Salmon, M. *et al.* Genetic typing of patients with inflammatory arthritis at presentation can be used to predict outcome. *Arthritis Rheum* 1994; 37: 1166–70.
15. Paimela, L., Palosuo, T., Leirisalo-Repo, M., Helve, T., and Aho, K. Prognostic value of quantitative measurement of rheumatoid factor in early rheumatoid arthritis. *Br J Rheumatol* 1995; 34: 1146–50.
16. Houssien, D. A., Jonsson, T., Davies, E., and Scott, D. L. Rheumatoid factor isotypes, disease activity and the outcome of rheumatoid arthritis: comparative effects of different antigens. *Scand J Rheumatol* 1998; 271: 46–53.
17. Stolt, P., Bengtsson, C., Nordmark, B., Lindblad, S., Lundberg, I., Klareskog, L., and Alfredsson, L. Quantification of the influence of cigarette smoking on rheumatoid arthritis: results from a population based case-control study, using incident cases. *Ann Rheum Dis* 2003; 62: 835–41.
18. Vittecoq, O., Incaurgarat, B., Jouen-Beades, F., Legoedec, J., Letourneur, O., Rolland, D. *et al.* Autoantibodies recognising citrullinated rat filaggrin in an ELISA using citrullinated and non-citrullinated recombinant proteins as antigens are highly diagnostic for rheumatoid arthritis. *Clin Exp Immunol* 2004; 135: 173–80.
19. Nielen, M. M., van Schaardenburg, D., Reesink, H. W. *et al.* Specific autoantibodies precede the symptoms of rheumatoid arthritis: a study of serial measurements in blood donors. *Arthritis Rheum* 2004; 50: 380–6.
20. Kroot, E. J., de Jong, B. A., van Leeuwen, M. A. *et al.* The prognostic value of anti-cyclic citrullinated peptide antibody in patients with recent-onset rheumatoid arthritis. *Arthritis Rheum* 2000; 43: 1831–5.
21. Schellekens G. A., Visser. H., de Jong, B. A. *et al.* The diagnostic properties of rheumatoid arthritis antibodies recognizing a cyclic citrullinated peptide. *Arthritis Rheum* 2000; 43: 155–63.
22. Berglin, E., Sundin, U., Wadell, G., Hallmans, G., and Dahlqvist, S. R. Antibodies against cyclic citrullinated peptide before disease onset predict radiological outcome of rheumatoid arthritis. *Arthritis Rheum* 2004; 50 (Suppl.): S161.
23. van Gaalen, F. A., Linn-Rasker, S. P., van Venrooij, W. J. *et al.* Autoantibodies to cyclic citrullinated peptides predict progression to rheumatoid arthritis in patients with undifferentiated arthritis: a prospective cohort study. *Arthritis Rheum* 2004; 50: 709–15.
24. Jansen, L. M., van Schaardenburg, D., van der Horst-Bruinsma, I., van der Stadt, R. J., de Koning, M. H., and Dijkmans, B. A. The predictive value of anti-cyclic citrullinated peptide antibodies in early arthritis. *J Rheumatol* 2003; 30: 1691–5.
25. Mustila, A., Paimela, L., Leirisalo-Repo, M., Huhtala, H., and Miettinen, A. Antineutrophil cytoplasmic antibodies in patients with early rheumatoid arthritis: an early marker of progressive erosive disease. *Arthritis Rheum* 2000; 43: 1371–7.
26. Braun, M. G., Csernok, E., Schmitt, W. H., and Gross, W. L. Incidence, target antigens, and clinical implications of antineutrophil cytoplasmic antibodies in rheumatoid arthritis. *J Rheumatol* 1996; 23: 826–30.
27. Cambridge, G., Williams, M., Leaker, B., Corbett, M., and Smith, C. R. Anti-myeloperoxidase antibodies in patients with rheumatoid arthritis: prevalence, clinical correlates, and IgG subclass. *Ann Rheum Dis* 1994; 53: 24–9.
28. Huang, J., Stewart, N., Crabbe, J. *et al.* A 1-year follow-up study of dynamic magnetic resonance imaging in early rheumatoid arthritis reveals synovitis to be increased in shared epitope-positive patients and predictive of erosions at 1 year. *Rheumatol* 2000; 39: 407–16.
29. O'Dell, J. R., Nepom, B. S., Haire, C. *et al.* HLA-DRB1 typing in rheumatoid arthritis: predicting response to specific treatments. *Ann Rheum Dis* 1998; 57: 209–13.
30. Weyand, C. M., Hicok, K. C., Conn, D.L., and Goronzy, J. J. The influence of HLA-DRB1 genes on disease severity in rheumatoid arthritis. *Ann Intern Med* 1992; 117: 801–6.
31. Fraser, A., Fearon, U., Billinghurst, R. C. *et al.* Turnover of type II collagen and aggrecan in cartilage matrix at the onset of inflammatory arthritis in humans: relationship to mediators of systemic and local inflammation. *Arthritis Rheum* 2003; 48: 3085–95.
32. Johansen, J. S., Jensen, H. S., and Price, P. A. A new biochemical marker for joint injury: analysis of YKL-40 in serum and synovial fluid. *Br J Rheumatol* 1993; 32: 949–55.

33. Verheijden, G. F., Rijnders, A. W., Bos, E., Coenen-de Roo, C. J., van Staveren, C. J., Miltenburg, A. M. *et al*. Human cartilage glycoprotein-39 as a candidate autoantigen in rheumatoid arthritis. *Arthritis Rheum* 1997; **40**: 1115–25.

34. Matsumoto, T., Tsurumoto, T., and Serum, Y. K. L-40 levels in rheumatoid arthritis: correlations between clinical and laboratory parameters. *Clin Exp Rheumatol* 2001; **19**: 655–60.

35. Harvey, S., Whaley, J., and Eberhardt, K. The relationship between serum levels of YKL-40 and disease progression in patients with early rheumatoid arthritis. *Scand J Rheumatol* 2000; **29**: 391–3.

36. Saxne, T., and Svensson, B. Serum cartilage oligomeric matrix protein (COMP): a predictor of joint damage and physical function in early rheumatoid arthritis. *Arthritis Rheum* 2004; **50** (Suppl.): S158.

37. Landewe, R., Geusens, P., Boers, M. *et al*. Markers for type II collagen breakdown predict the effect of disease-modifying treatment on long-term radiographic progression in patients with rheumatoid arthritis. *Arthritis Rheum* 2004; **50**: 1390–9.

38. Boss, B., and Neeck, G. Correlation of IL-6 with the classical humoral disease activity parameters ESR and CRP and with serum cortisol, reflecting the activity of the HPA axis in active rheumatoid arthritis. *Z Rheumatol* 2000; **59** (Suppl. 2): II/62–4.

39. Straub, R. H., Muller-Ladner, U., Lichtinger, T., Scholmerich, J., Menninger, H., and Lang, B. Decrease of interleukin 6 during the first 12 months is a prognostic marker for clinical outcome during 36 months treatment with disease-modifying anti-rheumatic drugs. *Br J Rheumatol* 1997; **36**: 1298–303.

40. Combe, B., Dougados, M., Goupille, P. *et al*. Prognostic factors for radiographic damage in early rheumatoid arthritis: a multiparameter prospective study. *Arthritis Rheum* 2001; **44**: 1736–43.

41. van Zeben, D., Hazes, J. M., Zwinderman, A. H., Vandenbroucke, J. P., and Breedveld, F. C. Factors predicting outcome of rheumatoid arthritis: results of a followup study. *J Rheumatol* 1993; **20**: 1288–96.

42. van der Heijde, D. M., van Riel, P. L., van Leeuwen, M. A., van't Hof, M. A., van Rijswijk, M. H., and van de Putte, L. B. Prognostic factors for radiographic damage and physical disability in early rheumatoid arthritis: a prospective follow-up study of 147 patients. *Br J Rheumatol* 1992; **31**: 519–25.

43. Raza, K., Breese, M., Nightingale, P. *et al*. Predictive value of antibodies to cyclic citrullinated peptide in patients with very early inflammatory arthritis. *J Rheumatol* 2005; **32**: 231–8.

44. Conaghan, P. G., O'Connor, P., McGonagle, D. *et al*. Elucidation of the relationship between synovitis and bone damage: a randomized magnetic resonance imaging study of individual joints in patients with early rheumatoid arthritis. *Arthritis Rheum* 2003; **48**: 64–71.

45. Brook, A., and Corbett, M. Radiographic changes in early rheumatoid disease. *Ann Rheum Dis* 1977; **36**: 71–3.

46. van Leeuwen, M. A., van der Heijde, D. M. F. M., van Rijswijk, M. H. *et al*. Interrelationship of outcome measures and process variables in early rheumatoid arthritis: a comparison of radiologic damage, physical disability, joint counts, and acute phase reactants. *J Rheumatol* 1994; **21**: 425–9.

47. Sharp, J. T., Lidsky, M. D., Collins, L. C., and Moreland, J. Methods of scoring the progression of radiologic changes in rheumatoid arthritis: correlation of radiologic, clinical and laboratory abnormalities. *Arthritis Rheum* 1971; **14**: 706–20.

48. Sharp, J. T., Young, D. Y., Bluhm, G. B. *et al*. How many joints in the hands and wrists should be included in a score of radiologic abnormalities used to assess rheumatoid arthritis? *Arthritis Rheum* 1985; **28**: 1326–35.

49. Larsen, A., Dale, K., and Eek, M. Radiographic evaluation of rheumatoid arthritis and related conditions by standard reference films. *Acta Radiol Diagn (Stockh)* 1977; **18**: 481–91.

50. Scott, D. L., Houssien, D. A., and Laasonen, L. Proposed modification to Larsen's scoring method for hand and wrist radiographs. *Br J Rheumatol* 1995; **34**: 56.

51. Molenaar, E. T. H., Edmonds, J., Boers, M., van der Heijde, D. M., and Lassere, M. A practical exercise in reading RA radiographs by the Larsen and Sharp methods. *J Rheumatol* 1999; **26**: 746–8.

52. Bruynesteyn, K., van der Heijde, D., Boers, M., van der Linden, S., Lassere, M., and van der Vleuten, C. The Sharp/van der Heijde method out-performed the Larsen/Scott method on the individual patient level in assessing radiographs in early rheumatoid arthritis. *J Clin Epidemiol* 2004; **57**: 502–12.

53. Kuper, I. H., van Leeuwen, M. A., van Riel, P. L. C. M. *et al*. Influence of a ceiling effect on the assessment of radiographic progression in rheumatoid arthritis during the first 6 years of disease. *J Rheumatol* 1999; **26**: 268–76.

54. Klarlund, M., Ostergaard, M., Rostrup, E., Skjodt, H., and Lorenzen, I. Dynamic magnetic resonance imaging of the metacarpophalangeal joints in rheumatoid arthritis, early unclassified polyarthritis, and healthy controls. *Scand J Rheumatol* 2000; **29**: 108–15.

55. Sugimoto, H., Takeda, A., Masuyama, J., and Furuse, M. Early-stage rheumatoid arthritis: diagnostic accuracy of MR imaging. *Radiology* 1996; **198**: 185–92.

56. Ostergaard, M., Hansen, M., Stoltenberg, M. *et al*. New radiographic bone erosions in the wrists of patients with rheumatoid arthritis are detectable with magnetic resonance imaging a median of two years earlier. *Arthritis Rheum* 2003; **48**: 2128–31.

57. Klarlund, M., Ostergaard, M., Jensen, K. E., Madsen, J. L., Skjodt, H., and Lorenzen, I. Magnetic resonance imaging, radiography, and scintigraphy of the finger joints: one year follow up of patients with early arthritis. The TIRA group. *Ann Rheum Dis* 2000; **59**: 521–8.

58. McGonagle, D., Conaghan, P. G., O'Connor, P. *et al*. The relationship between synovitis and bone changes in early untreated rheumatoid arthritis: a controlled magnetic resonance imaging study. *Arthritis Rheum* 1999; **42**: 1706–11.

59. McQueen, F. M., Stewart, N., Crabbe, J. *et al*. Magnetic resonance imaging of the wrist in early rheumatoid arthritis reveals progression of erosions despite clinical improvement. *Ann Rheum Dis* 1999; **58**: 156–63.

60. Ostergaard, M., Klarlund, M., Lassere, M. *et al*. Interreader agreement in the assessment of magnetic resonance imaging of rheumatoid arthritis wrist and finger joints: an international multicenter study. *J Rheumatol* 2001; **28**: 1143–50.

61. Ostergaard, M., Peterfy, C., Conaghan, P. *et al*. OMERACT Rheumatoid Arthritis Magnetic Resonance Imaging Studies: core set of MRI acquisitions, joint pathology definitions, and the OMERACT RA-MRI scoring system. *J Rheumatol* 2003; **30**: 1385–6.

62. Ostergaard, M., Stoltenberg, M., Løvgreen-Nielsen, P., Volck, B., Jensen, C.H., and Lorenzen, I. Magnetic resonance imaging-determined synovial membrane and joint effusion volumes in rheumatoid arthritis and osteoarthritis: comparison with the macroscopic and microscopic appearance of the synovium. *Arthritis Rheum* 1997; **40**: 1856–67.

63. Ostendorf, B., Peters, R., Dann, P. *et al*. Magnetic resonance imaging and mini-arthroscopy of metacarpophalangeal joints: sensitive detection of morphologic changes in rheumatoid arthritis. *Arthritis Rheum* 2001; **44**: 2492–502.

64. Gaffney, K., Cookson, J., Blake, D., Coumbe, A., and Blades, S. Quantification of rheumatoid synovitis by magnetic resonance imaging. *Arthritis Rheum* 1995; **38**: 1610–17.

65. Tamai, K., Yamato, M., Yamaguchi, T., and Ohno, W. Dynamic magnetic resonance imaging for the evaluation of synovitis in patients with rheumatoid arthritis. *Arthritis Rheum* 1994; **37**: 1151–7.

66. Østergaard, M., Duer, A., Møller, U., and Ejbjerg, B. Magnetic resonance imaging of peripheral joints in rheumatic diseases. *Best Prac Res Clin Rheumatol* 2004; **18**: 861–79.

67. Ostergaard, M., and Szkudlarek, M. Imaging in rheumatoid arthritis: why MRI and ultrasonography can no longer be ignored. *Scand J Rheumatol* 2003; **32**: 63–73.

68. Peterfy, C. G., Roberts, T., and Genant, H. K. Dedicated extremity MR imaging: an emerging technology. *Magn Reson Imaging Clin N Am* 1998; **6**: 849–70.

69. Taouli, B., Zaim, S., Peterfy, C. *et al*. Rheumatoid arthritis of the hand and wrist: comparison of three imaging techniques. *Am J Roentgenol* 2004; **182**: 937–43.

70. Hottya, G. A., Peterfy, C. G., Uffmann, M. *et al.* Dedicated extremity MR imaging of the foot and ankle. *Eur Radiol* 2000; **10**: 467–75.

71. Lindegaard, H., Vallo, J., Horslev-Petersen, K., Junker, P., and Ostergaard, M. Low field dedicated magnetic resonance imaging in untreated rheumatoid arthritis of recent onset. *Ann Rheum Dis* 2001; **60**: 770–6.

72. Olech, E., and Yocum, D. Use of portable in-office magnetic resonance imaging in assessing hand and feet erosions in patients with early rheumatoid arthritis. *Arthritis Rheum* 2004; **50** (Suppl.): S170.

73. Wakefield, R. J., Gibbon, W. W., and Conaghan, P. G. *et al.* The value of sonography in the detection of bone erosions in patients with rheumatoid arthritis: a comparison with conventional radiography. *Arthritis Rheum* 2000; **43**: 2762–70.

74. Backhaus, M., Kamradt, T., Sandrock, D. *et al.* Arthritis of the finger joints: a comprehensive approach comparing conventional radiography, scintigraphy, ultrasound, and contrast-enhanced magnetic resonance imaging. *Arthritis Rheum* 1999; **42**: 1232–45.

75. Hau, M., Schultz, H., Tony, H. P. *et al.* Evaluation of pannus and vascularization of the metacarpophalangeal and proximal interphalangeal joints in rheumatoid arthritis by high-resolution ultrasound (multidimensional linear array). *Arthritis Rheum* 1999; **42**: 2303–8.

76. Kraan, M. C., Versendaal, H., Jonker, M. *et al.* Asymptomatic synovitis precedes clinically manifest arthritis. *Arthritis Rheum* 1998; **41**: 1481–8.

77. Karim, Z., Wakefield, R. J., Quinn, M. *et al.* Validation and reproducibility of ultrasonography in the detection of synovitis in the knee: a comparison with arthroscopy and clinical examination. *Arthritis Rheum* 2004; **50**: 387–94.

78. Wakefield, R. J., Brown, A. K., O'Connor, P. J., and Emery, P. Power Doppler sonography: improving disease activity assessment in inflammatory musculoskeletal disease. *Arthritis Rheum* 2003; **48**: 285–8.

79. Wakefield, R. J., Brown, A. K., O'Connor, P. J., Karim, Z., Grainger, A., and Emery, P. Musculoskeletal ultrasonography: what is it and should training be compulsory for rheumatologists? *Rheumatology* 2004; **43**: 821–2.

80. Terslev, L., Torp-Pedersen, S., Savnik, A. *et al.* Doppler ultrasound and magnetic resonance imaging of synovial inflammation of the hand in rheumatoid arthritis: a comparative study. *Arthritis Rheum* 2003; **48**: 2434–41.

81. Szkudlarek, M., Court-Payen, M., Strandberg, C., Klarlund, M., Klausen, T., and Ostergaard, M. Power Doppler ultrasonography for assessment of synovitis in the metacarpophalangeal joints of patients with rheumatoid arthritis: a comparison with dynamic magnetic resonance imaging. *Arthritis Rheum* 2001; **44**: 2018–23.

82. Magarelli, N., Guglielmi, G., Di Matteo, L., Tartaro, A., Mattei, P. A., and Bonomo, L. Diagnostic utility of an echo-contrast agent in patients with synovitis using power Doppler ultrasound: a preliminary study with comparison to contrast-enhanced MRI. *Eur Radiol* 2001; **11**: 1039–46.

83. Szkudlarek, M., Court-Payen, M., Jacobsen, S., Klarlund, M., Thomsen, H. S., and Ostergaard, M. Interobserver agreement in ultrasonography of the finger and toe joints in rheumatoid arthritis. *Arthritis Rheum* 2003; **48**: 955–62.

84. Devlin, J., Lilley, J., Gough, A. *et al.* Clinical associations of dual-energy X-ray absorptiometry measurement of hand bone mass in rheumatoid arthritis. *Br J Rheumatol* 1996; **35**: 1256–62.

85. Deodhar, A. A., Brabyn, J., Pande, I., Stanley, E., and Woolf, A. D. A five years longitudinal study of hand bone densitometry in early rheumatoid arthritis. *Arthritis Rheum* 1998; **41** (Suppl.): S52.

86. Herrak, P., Görtz, B., Hayer, S. *et al.* Zoledronic acid protects against local and systemic bone loss in tumor necrosis factor-mediated arthritis. *Arthritis Rheum* 2004; **50**: 2327–37.

87. Wakefield, R. J., Conaghan, P. G., Jarrett, S., and Emery, P. Noninvasive techniques for assessing skeletal changes in inflammatory arthritis: imaging technique. *Curr Opin Rheumatol* 2004; **16**: 435–42.

39 | *New biologics: cytokines*
Jeffrey R. Curtis and Larry W. Moreland

Introduction

Few milestones have advanced our understanding of disease etiopathogenesis and expanded our therapeutic options as dramatically as the introduction of biologic response modifiers (specifically tumor necrosis factor alpha antagonists) for use in rheumatoid arthritis (RA). Engineered to antagonize specific components of the inflammatory process, biologic response modifiers ('biologics') have been described as 'targeted' therapies to distinguish their mechanism of action from the more non-specific immunosuppression common to small molecules (i.e. disease-modifying anti-rheumatic drugs, DMARDs). Despite continuing uncertainties regarding the triggering event leading to incident RA, blocking even a single component of the downstream inflammatory cascade has proved highly effective in a large percentage of patients to reduce signs and symptoms and to reduce long-term radiographic damage. Although many RA patients derive a significant benefit from use of these agents, not all respond, and for some individuals the durability of response is less than optimal. The state of the art at this time likely represents only the initial foray into an ever-expanding array of strategies that may be useful to achieve control of RA and other inflammatory diseases.

This chapter will briefly review cytokines believed to be pathogenic in the inflammatory process in RA and will discuss various approaches to targeting these mediators. Approved therapies that target tumor necrosis factor alpha (TNF-α) and interleukin-1 (IL-1) have been discussed in Chapter 27, but strategies to block these two cytokines that differ from those currently in use will be discussed. Biologics that inhibit other inflammatory cytokines will be reviewed in the context of their initial results in animal and human clinical trials.

TNF-α blockade

TNF-α as a pro-inflammatory cytokine

TNF-α, a member of the TNF superfamily of receptors and ligands that includes CD-40/CD40 ligand, Fas/Fas-ligand, and lymphotoxin-a and -b[1], is a transmembrane protein produced principally by macrophages and fibroblasts. TNF-α, unlike some members of the TNF superfamily, has been found within the RA synovium, where it is produced by synovial macrophages and typically is present in high concentrations in active disease states. Initially synthesized intracellularly and incorporated into the cell membrane, TNF-α is cleaved by a membrane metalloproteinase

called TNF-α-converting enzyme (TACE) and is released in a soluble form. Among its effects relevant to RA, TNF-α has been shown to up-regulate RANK (receptor activator of NF-κB)-ligand expression, leading to bone resorption, and to induce adhesion molecules, metalloproteinases, collagenases, chemokines, prostaglandins, and other pro-inflammatory molecules[2–6]. It also activates numerous cell types, including B and T cells, and participates in a number of other physiologic functions.

TNF-α induces the production of two forms of soluble receptors, p55 (TNFR-I) and p75 (TNFR-II), which can be found in human serum and on most mammalian cell surfaces[3]. Some evidence suggests that the concentrations of these receptors increase in certain inflammatory diseases, including RA, and may be used to differentiate RA from other forms of arthritis such as gout and osteoarthritis[7]. TNF receptors can also be solubilized by TACE and can be found in a free form (sTNFR), where they may act as natural antagonists of soluble TNF-α as the host attempts to down-regulate the inflammatory response[8]. Serum concentrations of TNF receptors have also been shown to decrease in RA patients, following treatment with TNF-α antagonists[9,10].

Animal studies in the 1980s and early 1990s demonstrated the importance of TNF-α in models of collagen-induced arthritis and suggested benefit with TNF-α blockade[11,12]. TNF transgenic mice were observed to have an exuberant and erosive synovitis, which was reduced with TNF inhibition. Success with animal models led to the development of several strategies to block TNF-α in humans. A discussion of the efficacy, durability of response, and safety of the currently approved anti-TNF-α therapies for RA in humans (i.e. infliximab, etanercept, adalimumab) are discussed in Chapter 27.

New ways to antagonize TNF-α

Other biologics that target TNF-α are currently being studied, with the goal of increasing the circulating half-life of the agent and decreasing the frequency of administration. Pharmaceutical companies are attempting to minimize the immunogenicity of these compounds, which may decrease the incidence of anti-drug antibodies and prolong efficacy. Other strategies besides biologics, which will not be discussed further in this chapter, involve more durable mechanisms of cytokine inhibition using gene therapy. Strategies using this technology have delivered TNF-α receptors using an adenoviral vector injected into either the systemic circulation or the joint itself[13,14]. The potential for TNF gene therapy to impact on the course of chronic inflammatory diseases such as RA remains of interest[15], but has received limited attention in humans. Novel biologic strategies to block TNF-α that are under investigation in clinical trials will now be reviewed.

CDP 870 and other monoclonal antibodies against TNF-α

CDP 870 is a humanized Fab' antibody fragment linked to two polyethylene glycol molecules (PEGylation) that increases the half-life to ~14 days. An eight-week, dose-ranging study in 36 RA patients who failed DMARD therapy demonstrated a 50% ACR50 response with a reasonable safety profile[16]. A somewhat larger study of 92 Crohn's patients also reported good efficacy and safety in a 12-week, single-dose study. Results from phase III trials using CDP 870 for RA both as monotherapy and in combination with methotrexate (MTX) are pending. Another monoclonal antibody currently under investigation for RA is CNTO148. Phase I studies have found that it was well-tolerated in both intravenous and subcutaneous forms[17]. The half-life of the subcutaneous preparation ranged from 12 to 26 days, and no immunogenicity was observed even among individuals with repeated administration. Ongoing trials with CNTO148 are being conducted.

Soluble TNF-α receptors

Pegsunercept is a truncated form of the p55 TNF-α receptor that is PEGylated at the amino terminus. Phase II trials have shown a beneficial effect on signs and symptoms of RA at 12 weeks[18], although full efficacy results have not yet been published. Another p55 soluble receptor linked to an IgG1 (lenercept) was studied in 247 RA patients. Despite adequate safety, no benefit over MTX monotherapy was observed, and the drug was withdrawn from further RA clinical trials. Onercept, another p55 receptor construct linked to IgG1, has been shown to decrease disease activity in a small pilot study of 12 patients with active Crohn's disease[19], and this drug may be useful in RA as well.

TACE inhibitors

TNF-α activation requires cleavage from its membrane-bound form to a soluble form by TACE[20]. Inhibition of this enzyme might therefore reduce the biologically active concentration of TNF-α and retard its pro-inflammatory effect. However, TACE inhibition also increases levels of membrane-bound TNF-α, although the net effect of this result is unclear. Several oral agents which inhibit TACE in conjunction with inhibition of matrix metalloproteinases (which cause joint damage through degradation of the extracellular matrix) are in development (e.g. GW3333, TMI-0005, Ro32–7315). These dual inhibitors have shown benefit in animal models of adjuvant arthritis[21] and are currently under study in clinical trials.

IL-1 antagonism

Biologic rationale for IL-1 blockade

IL-1 appears to be an important mediator in the inflammatory process of RA. Produced by macrophages, synoviocytes, chondrocytes, and osteoclasts, IL-1 has numerous functions, similar to TNF-α[22,23]. IL-1 recruits neutrophils, stimulates lymphocyte growth and differentiation, promotes neoangiogenesis (associated with synovitis), and activates a number of cells, including macrophages. It also induces a variety of cytokines, chemokines, matrix metalloproteinases, and other enzymes that effect cartilage damage and bone resorption. IL-1α exists as a membrane bound molecule, and IL-1β requires activation from a precursor form into a soluble active form by a separate enzyme, IL-1 converting enzyme (ICE), also known as caspace-1. Both forms of IL-1 bind to a common receptor (IL-1R1) and subsequently recruit an accessory protein necessary for signal transduction (IL-1RAcP).

The role of IL-1 in RA was demonstrated by murine models that showed that IL-1 accelerated collagen-induced arthritis[24] and rabbit studies that demonstrated that IL-1 delivered intra-articularly into knee joints induced an arthritis similar to RA[25]. IL-1 has a natural receptor antagonist (IL-1Ra) that is able to inhibit IL-1 from binding to its receptor and prevent signaling. Mice deficient in IL-1Ra have been shown to spontaneously develop an inflammatory arthritis, which was reversible by re-administration of IL-1Ra.

IL-1 was subsequently shown to be present in excess in inflamed RA joints and its serum concentrations correlate with disease activity[26]. IL-1Ra is also present in RA synovium, but in RA, the ratio of IL-1Ra to IL-1 appears to be too low to adequately block the destructive effects of IL-1[27]. This observation led to interest in increasing the concentration of IL-1Ra with a recombinant human IL-1Ra. The first IL-1Ra, anakinra, was developed as a non-glycosylated form of endogenous IL-1Ra and is identical to native human IL-1Ra except for a single amino acid substitution at the N terminus. Anakinra demonstrated efficacy in reducing inflammation and bone resorption when studied in animal models of arthritis, especially when high serum levels could be sustained[28]. However, the efficacy in humans has been somewhat disappointing (further details are discussed in Chapter 27), but new strategies to block IL-1 are being developed.

New strategies to block IL-1

IL-1 Trap

A 'trap' is a cytokine inhibitor that uses different high-affinity receptor components to bind the target ligand. A molecule targeting IL-1 ('IL-1 Trap') consists of the extracellular domains of both IL-1 receptor components (Type I receptor and receptor accessory protein) linked to the Fc portion of a human IgG1. This recombinant molecule binds to IL-1α and IL-1β and prohibits interaction with the IL-1 receptor. A recent 12-week trial of IL-1 Trap in 201 RA patients who had failed at least one DMARD and who had moderate to severe disease activity showed that even at the highest dose of IL-1 Trap (100 mg/week) no significant differences between IL-1 Trap and placebo could be demonstrated[29]. Of treated patients, 46% achieved the primary end-point of an ACR20 response, compared to 31% of placebo patients ($p = 0.11$). IL-1 Trap was well tolerated, and DAS28 scores and acute phase reactants (i.e. C-reactive protein (CRP), erythrocyte sedimentation rate (ESR), and IL-6) did show statistically significant dose-dependent decreases with IL-1 Trap. Further evaluation with higher doses may be warranted.

ICE inhibition

Because IL-1β requires conversion from a precursor into an active form similar to TNF-α, blocking the necessary converting enzyme (ICE) is a rational approach to reducing IL-1-induced inflammation. ICE inhibition might also achieve the secondary goal of IL-18 blockade (discussed later), which may have an independent benefit. An orally available ICE inhibitor, pralnacasan, has been developed, which showed efficacy in animal models of osteoarthritis[30]. However, in a 12-week trial of 285 RA patients on standard DMARD therapy, pralnacasan showed no significant benefit in ACR20 response rates (44%) compared to placebo (33%). Dose-dependent decreases in acute phase reactants were observed in treated patients, and the drug was well tolerated. In 2003, the phase IIb study was suspended due to hepatotoxicity observed in animal studies treated with high dose pralnacasan for nine months. Pralnacasan is still under investigation for other inflammatory conditions such as colitis where it may prove beneficial[31].

Beyond TNF-α and IL-1: new cytokine targets in active development

Despite the advances in RA therapy represented by the available or investigational biologics targeting TNF-α and IL-1 summarized in Table 39.1, many patients exhibit only partial response or no response. The success of single cytokine blockade despite the synergy of the inflammatory milieu in the RA synovium suggests that certain cytokines may be key mediators of the propagation of inflammation. Antagonism of these cytokines may achieve dramatic disease control without systemic immunosuppression. Among the most promising cytokine targets are IL-6, IL-15, IL-18, IL-17, and macrophage migration inhibitory factor.

IL-6

Role of IL-6 in RA

Like TNF-α, IL-6 is a pleiotropic cytokine with a variety of biologic effects. In fact, prior to its identification on chromosome 7, IL-6 was referenced by a variety of names, including cytotoxic T cell differentiation factor, B cell stimulating/differentiating factor, hepatocyte stimulating factor, interferon β2, and monocyte granulocyte inducing factor type 2. These names aptly describe its diverse functions. IL-6 is a 184-amino acid glycoprotein produced by a wide range of cells, including lymphocytes, monocytes, neutrophils, eosinophils, B cells, fibroblasts, mast cells, synoviocytes, and endothelial cells. IL-6 shares structural homology with a number of other cytokines, including IL-11, leukemia inhibitory factor, cardiotrophin-1, oncostatin M, and ciliary neurotrophic factor, together forming the IL-6 superfamily. These cytokines also produce biologic effects through similar receptor interactions and signaling pathways.

IL-6 binds to the human IL-6 receptor (IL-6R) with low affinity. IL-6R is an 80 kDa, transmembrane glycoprotein which does not have an intracellular signal transduction domain[32]. Consequently IL-6/IL-6R engagement alone does not lead to cellular activation, and cell surface expression of IL-6R does not mean the cell is responsive to IL-6 stimulation. Proteolytic cleavage leads to the release of soluble forms of IL-6R, which can also bind to circulating IL-6. IL-6 binds to either cell bound IL-6R or sIL-6R, and the heterodimeric complex then associates with a cell surface glycoprotein called gp130. The resulting tripartite heterocomplex binds to another IL-6/IL-6R/gp130 and signal transduction ensues[33]. Hence both cell bound and soluble IL-6Rs contribute to cellular activation. Cells expressing gp130 but no IL-6R can be stimulated by IL-6 through sIL-6R, and the biological effects of IL-6 can be blocked by inhibiting IL-6, IL-6R, or gp130. However, blocking IL-6 or sIL-6R will inhibit the biological effect of IL-6 alone, but inhibition of gp130 will impede the function of all the cytokines in the IL-6 superfamily.

Table 39.1 TNF-α and IL-1 antagonism using currently approved biologics and compounds in development

Name	Date approved	Structure	Route of administration
Currently approved			
Etanercept (TNF-α)	1998	p75 TNF receptor fused to Fc portion of IgG1	Subcutaneous
Infliximab (TNF-α)	1999	Human/murine chimeric monoclonal antibody	Intravenous
Adalimumab (TNF-α)	2002	Human monoclonal antibody	Subcutaneous
Anakinra (IL-1)	2001	Recombinant human IL-1 receptor antagonist	Subcutaneous
In development			
CDP870 (TNF-α)	Phase III	Fab' antibody linked to two PEG molecules	Subcutaneous
CNTO 148 (TNF-α)	Phase I	Monoclonal antibody	Intravenous/ Subcutaneous
sTNFR-I (e.g. pegsunercept) (TNF-α)	Phase II	p55 TNF-α receptor PEGylated at N terminus	Subcutaneous
TACE inhibitor (e.g. TMI-0005, GW3333, TMI-1) (TNF α)	Phase II or earlier	Small molecule (i.e. non-peptide)	Oral
IL-1 Trap (IL-1)	Phase II	Recombinant IL-1 receptor + IL-1 receptor accessory protein linked to human IgG1	Subcutaneous

Relevant to RA, IL-6 stimulates B cells to proliferate, produce immunoglobulins, and differentiate into plasma cells[34]. It also encourages the proliferation and differentiation of T cells into cytotoxic T cells. Through its effects on hepatocytes, it promotes the systemic inflammatory response, including pyrexia, and it induces acute phase reactants such as C-reactive protein. IL-6 may have a role in juxta-articular osteoporosis and joint damage through differentiation of osteoclasts and potentiation of aggre-canase activity and increased proteoglycan breakdown[35]. High levels of IL-6 have been found in the serum and synovium of patients with active RA[36], as has IL-6 receptor, although whether IL-6 mediates or regulates inflammation remains unclear. Cells in the rheumatoid joint that produce IL-6 include lymphocytes, monocytes, fibroblasts, synoviocytes, and endothelial cells. IL-6 levels were correlated with RA disease activity and joint damage[37] and have been observed to decrease following effective treatment with DMARDs.

Compelling evidence for the important role of IL-6 in RA disease pathogenesis was evidenced by the resistance of IL-6-deficient transgenic mice to antigen-induced arthritis despite normal concentrations of TNF-α and IL-1[38]. Injecting these animals with subcutaneous IL-6 made them susceptible to antigen-induced arthritis.

IL-6 blockade in inflammatory arthritis

In animal models of collagen-induced arthritis, IL-6 blockade with a monoclonal antibody was shown to abrogate disease if given early (≤3 days) after immunization, suggesting that IL-6 is present as an early mediator of the inflammatory response[39]. The therapeutic potency of a humanized anti-IL-6R monoclonal antibody, MRA, was tested in a primate model of RA where Cynomolgus monkeys were immunized with bovine type II collagen[40]. MRA was given as an intravenous infusion weekly for 13 weeks. At 10 mg/kg, MRA led to significant disease improvement. Acute phase reactants, including ESR and CRP, were suppressed and joint damage was reduced.

Phase I/II trials conducted in the UK from 1998 to 2000 used a single dose of a recombinant human IgG1 fused to a humanized IL-6 receptor monoclonal antibody (MRA) in 45 RA patients randomized to active drug or placebo[41]. All patients had failed at least one DMARD, and MRA doses of 0.1, 1, 5, or 10 mg/kg were given. At two weeks, 56% of the patients in the 5 mg/kg group and no placebo patients achieved an ACR20 response (the primary end-point), although efficacy was not seen in the other MRA cohorts. A statistically significant improvement in ACR20 was also noted between the 10 mg/kg MRA group and placebo at weeks 6 and 8. ESR and CRP were normalized two weeks after treatment in the 5 and 10 mg/kg cohort. Diarrhea was the commonest adverse event, occurring in 18% of patients.

A Phase I/II Japanese study administered a single intravenous infusion every two weeks for six months to 15 RA patients[42]. At 24 weeks, 40% achieved an ACR50 response, and 90% achieved an ACR20 response. No serious adverse reactions were reported, although two-thirds of the cohort had an increase in serum cholesterol levels. A larger phase II study randomized 164 RA patients with refractory disease to placebo or 4 mg/kg or 8 mg/kg MRA given intravenously every four weeks for three months[43].

In the 8 mg/kg group 40% achieved an ACR50 response, compared to 2% in the placebo group ($p < 0.001$). Similar to previous studies, a significant proportion of treated patients (44%) had an increase in serum cholesterol. Several other side-effects including elevated liver function tests were observed although they were mild and transient.

In the largest study reported to date, MRA was evaluated in a phase II dose-ranging randomized, controlled trial of 359 RA patients partially responsive or non-responsive to MTX[44]. In the three active therapy subgroups (2, 4, 8 mg/kg), MRA was administered monthly for three months as monotherapy or in combination with MTX. A dose-dependent improvement in signs and symptoms as measured by the EULAR (European League Against Rheumatism) response was reported (73% moderate-to-good response on monotherapy; 85% in the combination group). At the highest dose, the DAS28 improved 2.9 units with monotherapy and 3.6 units with combination therapy, compared with an improvement of 1.7 units for MTX alone ($p < 0.001$). Significant reductions in ESR and CRP levels were noted, as expected with an IL-6 inhibitor; CRP normalized in 61% of patients treated with the 8 mg/kg dose compared to 4% in the methotrexate-alone group. Anaphylaxis was reported in 5 of 107 patients with lower-dose monotherapy. Sepsis, osteomyelitis, and other serious adverse effects were reported in five patients. Continuing studies of the safety and efficacy of IL-6 antagonism are in progress, and MRA is now in Phase III trials.

IL-15

IL-15, a cytokine found in 4-α helix conformation that shares structural homology with IL-2[45], was first described as a T cell activator but has subsequently been shown to manifest a variety of effector functions. Both IL-15 mRNA and the more tightly controlled and parsimoniously expressed IL-15 protein have been found in the serum of RA patients and appear to increase with RA disease duration[46]. Located both bound to the cell surface and in a soluble form, IL-15 has been found in inflamed RA synovium and the granulomatous histology of RA nodules[47]. It functions to activate neutrophils, T cells, natural killer (NK) cells, and B cells; to induce T cell-dependent cytokine release, including TNF-α; and to sustain T cell interactions with macrophages[48-51]. IL-15 also has been shown to increase expression of CD40L and the chemokine receptor CCR5 on RA T cells[52]. Synovial fibroblasts appear to require direct contact with T cells to produce IL-15, and this cellular contact has been shown to be blocked by methotrexate[53].

In vivo, murine models of collagen-induced arthritis were effectively treated by antagonizing IL-15 or its receptor[54,55]. One study used a recombinant fusion protein (CRB-15) consisting of the constant region of IgG2a and a point-mutated IL-15 that bound the IL-15 receptor with high affinity but did not trigger IL-15-mediated signaling. CRB-15 was shown to be able to block both incident and established disease. Moreover, in contrast to the results of earlier studies that antagonized IL-15 directly, blockade of the IL-15 receptor appeared to provide a sustained benefit that persisted weeks beyond the two-week treatment window.

A fully human IgG1/K antibody, HuMax-IL15, has been developed that can bind both membrane-bound and soluble IL-15 and blocks IL-15-induced signaling. Pooled data using all six dosing regimens from a phase I/II trial in 30 RA patients demonstrated that 39% of treated participants reached an ACR50, and 61% reached an ACR20[56]. A larger trial studied 110 biologic-naïve RA patients on background MTX administered a human monoclonal IgG1k antibody (AMG-714) twice monthly[57]. The highest dose group demonstrated a 62% ACR20 response compared to 26% in the placebo arm ($p = 0.01$). A 20% or greater reduction in CRP was observed in 63% of the treated group and 39% of the placebo group at 14 weeks. The drug was well-tolerated and had an adverse effect profile similar to placebo. Further results from phase II trials should be forthcoming to better clarify the potentially promising role for IL-15 blockade in RA.

IL-18

IL-18 is produced as an inactive precursor and requires ICE to generate the biologically active cytokine. Its receptor is expressed on neutrophils, macrophages, NK cells, CD4+ T cells, and endothelial cells and can be up-regulated by IL-12. Induced by TNF-α and acting synergistically with IL-12 and IL-15, IL-18 promotes further release of TNF-α and interferon gamma (IFN-γ), through direct effects on macrophages and T cells[58–60]. IL-18 also up-regulates the expression of vascular cell adhesion molecule (VCAM)-1 and intercellular adhesion molecule (ICAM)-1 on monocytes, which mediate the enhancing effects of IL-18 on T cell–monocyte contact. It also appears to regulate expression of Toll-like receptor-2 and -4 in RA synovial tissue. IL-18 bioactivity has been shown to correlate with RA disease activity[61].

A variety of approaches have been suggested to target IL-18, including monoclonal antibodies to IL-18, recombinant IL-18 receptor binding protein (IL-18BP)[62], or inhibition of IL-18 release or processing. A collagen-induced arthritis model found that administration of an anti-IL-18 monoclonal antibody decreased disease activity and levels of TNF-α, IFN-γ, and IL-6[63]. These results have been confirmed in other animal studies of collagen-induced arthritis[64] and have also been observed in an experimental model of group B streptococcal arthritis, resulting in a decrease in mortality and in the incidence and severity of the arthritis[65]. A murine IL-18 binding protein fused to the Fc portion of an IgG1 showed efficacy in a murine model of collagen-induced arthritis with a 50% reduction in disease activity score and histologic score of joint damage with either of two doses of IL-18BP[66]. ICE inhibition, which concomitantly blocks IL-1 and IL-18, has been previously discussed. Because IL-18 appears to be synergistic with many other cytokines in a Th1 inflammatory response, further data are needed to understand whether blockade of IL-18 alone will be effective in reducing RA disease activity.

IL-12

IL-12 is a potent pro-inflammatory cytokine produced by activated inflammatory cells, including neutrophils, macrophages, and dendritic cells[67]. IL-12 promotes differentiation of naïve T cells into Th1 cells and stimulates IFN-γ production from T cells, NK cells, dendritic cells, and macrophages[68–70]. IL-12 is a heterodimeric molecule comprised of two proteins linked by disulfide bonds encoded by two separate genes, p35 and p40, located on chromosomes 3 and 5, respectively. The IL-12 receptor is expressed on activated T and NK cells and is composed of two subunits that belong to the gp130 subgroup of the cytokine receptor superfamily[71]. IL-12 appears to play a pivotal role in the host response to early infection as it transitions from an innate to an adaptive immune response[67].

In RA patients, IL-12 is expressed by macrophages and synovial lining cells[72]. Some data suggest that IL-12 production in RA is regulated by two different pathways. One is T cell dependent, predominantly mediated through a CD40–CD154 interaction; the other is T cell independent, mediated through TNF-α[73]. Inhibition of IL-12 has also been posited as a potential mechanism by which gold compounds have efficacy in rheumatic diseases[74]. Mice with established collagen-induced arthritis were treated with an anti-IL-12 antibody and/or anti-TNF-α therapy for 10 days from the onset of disease[75]. Anti-IL-12 had limited efficacy alone but appeared to show synergism with TNF-α in reducing inflammation, and results were better with the combination than anti-TNF-α alone. Other studies have found that IL-12 antibodies were not able to decrease the incidence of arthritis but significantly lowered the severity of the disease[76].

More recent data suggest that the apparent blockade of IL-12 may in fact exert benefit through concomitant blockade of a recently discovered and structurally related cytokine, IL-23[77,78]. The p40 subunit of IL-12 is a shared component of IL-23 (which has a separate subunit, p19), and the IL-12 and IL-23 receptors also have overlapping homology[79]. IL-23 appears to be an essential factor in the expansion of a CD4+ T cell population capable of driving autoimmune inflammation and inducing a variety of pro-inflammatory cytokines, including TNF-α and IL-17[80]. In contrast to IL-12, IL-23 appears to be an effector cytokine and to act directly on macrophages[77]. An even more recently discovered member of the IL-12 cytokine family, IL-27, may also be important in autoimmunity[79]. Antibodies that block IL-12 will need to be carefully examined to understand the relevant biology to make sure that the observed effects are not, in fact, due to concurrent blockade of a more pathogenic cytokine also found in IL-12 family.

IL-17

IL-17, first described in 1995, is an attractive target in RA although it has been less studied than many of the previously described cytokines. It has pro-inflammatory activity both *in vitro* and *in vivo* and has been shown to induce a variety of inflammatory mediators, including TNF, IL-6, and IL-1[81]. Predominantly produced by CD4+ T cells, IL-17 appears to be involved in early stages of inflammation[82]. Detectable in the serum and synovial fluids of RA patients but not in osteoarthritis patients or controls[83], IL-17 may have direct catabolic properties in cartilage through up-regulation of nitric oxide production from chondrocytes. It also appears to effect osteoclastic bone resorption through RANK ligand[84–86]. It appears to act synergistically with IL-1 and TNF-α to increase cytokine production by synoviocytes[87], and may also regulate the expression and/or stability of cyclooxygenase-2 mRNA and matrix metalloproteinases through its effects on p38 mitogen-activated protein (MAP) cascade[88,89]. In RA synovium, IL-17 appears to be dependent on upstream NF-κB and phosphoinositide 3-kinase signaling[90].

In models of murine collagen-induced arthritis, IL-17 promotes bone erosions[86], and its deficiency or blockade is protective, perhaps through inhibition of collagen-specific T cell activation and IgG2a production[91–94]. Moreover, IL-1 blockade was not able to abrogate IL-17-induced inflammation, suggesting an independent pathway[95]. Studies in humans will provide further information on whether IL-17 inhibition will be as protective as the animal data have suggested.

Macrophage migration inhibitory factor (MMIF)

MMIF, a pro-inflammatory cytokine first described in the 1960s, was initially studied in the systemic inflammatory response of shock. Subsequent work suggested that it has an important role in both innate and adaptive immunity. MMIF has been localized to fibroblast-like synoviocytes, macrophages, and endothelial cells and is overexpressed in both the serum and synovial fluid of RA patients[96,97]. MMIF induces macrophages to release a plethora of cytokines, including IL-1, TNF-α, and IL-8, and it also up-regulates matrix metalloproteinases (e.g. MMP-1 and MMP-3), cyclooxygenase 2, and prostacyclin E2[98–100]. It may also recruit inflammatory cells into RA synovium via IL-8 induction[101]. Independent of NF-κB signaling and at least partially dependent on extracellular signal-regulated kinase (ERK)-MAP kinase signaling[100], MMIF also appears to inactivate endogenous p53, which in turn leads to synoviocyte proliferation and impaired apoptosis, invasion into cartilage, and neoangiogenesis[102,103]. MMIF correlates with RA disease activity and inflammatory markers like CRP[104]. Polymorphisms in the MMIF gene have been associated with the presence of juvenile idiopathic arthritis (JIA)[105] and the severity of adult RA[106].

A variety of animal models reflect the potential importance of MMIF in experimental arthritis. Pre-treatment with an anti-MMIF antibody leads to lower incidence and reduced severity of disease in models of collagen-induced arthritis and adjuvant-induced arthritis[107,108]. Although small molecules that antagonize the effects of MMIF have been described[109], the potential role for biologic agents to inhibit MMIF remains an attractive possibility as well.

Less promising cytokine targets for RA

A number of other cytokines have been found in inflamed RA synovium. However, early studies of antagonism of several of these have demonstrated only modest clinical benefit. The biologic rationale for their inhibition and the available clinical data will be presented, although the benefit of targeting these cytokines in RA appears to be limited.

IL-10

IL-10 is produced by macrophages, CD5+ B cells, CD4+ T cells, and monocytes. It is able to inhibit expression of a variety of cytokines, including IL-1, IL-6, IL-8, TNF-α, and a variety of metalloproteinases. It blocks T cell responses to specific antigens and inhibits the costimulatory action of macrophages. Its anti-inflammatory effects may be tempered by the fact that it promotes B cell proliferation and differentiation and enhances class II major histocompatibility complex (MHC) expression. Inflammatory disease states such as rheumatoid arthritis and psoriasis have been postulated to represent an IL-10-deficient state.

Adenoviral transfer of the IL-10 gene suppressed collagen-induced arthritis in rabbits[110,111] and provided impetus to study IL-10 in humans. However, small clinical studies in RA patients showed little efficacy. Although the reasons for this lack of response are unclear, up-regulation of Fcγ R expression in RA with IL-10 treatment has been hypothesized to counteract the otherwise anti-inflammatory effects of IL-10[112]. A better understanding of the anti-inflammatory signaling pathways used by IL-10 may help identify more efficacious targets for therapy.

IL-4

Similar to IL-10, IL-4 is a Th2 cytokine that is able to inhibit T cell production of Th1 cytokines, including IL-1, IL-6, TNF-α, IL-2, and IFN-γ. It does have proliferative and activating effects on B cells and induces IgE production. RA patients appear to have a deficiency of IL-4, leading to interest in using this cytokine therapeutically. A phase I trial of IL-4 for RA was conducted but was halted due to lack of efficacy[113]. The bone-protective effects of IL-4 on osteoclast formation, osteoprotegerin, and RANK ligand expression have been shown to be similar to the effects of several traditional DMARDs in RA patients[114]. These data suggest that downstream pathways from IL-4 may be more effectively targeted than IL-4 itself.

IFN-γ

IFN-γ is produced by activated T cells and minimally expressed in RA synovium, suggesting the potential for a deficiency state. Trials from the 1980s and 1990s studied recombinant human IFN-γ with disappointing results. A trial randomized 105 RA patients to recombinant human IFN-γ or placebo. At 12 weeks, the treated group failed to show at least 50% improvement in any single outcome measure compared to placebo-treated patients[115], and further investigation of this strategy has been largely curtailed.

IL-2

In light of the growing interest in the role for T cells in the pathogenesis of RA, T cell-derived cytokines would seem to be a relevant target for therapy. IL-2 functions as a T cell growth factor and affects the activation, proliferation, and differentiation of T cells, NK cells, and B cells. T cell inhibitors such as cyclosporine or tacrolimus block these effects and inhibit pro-inflammatory cells such as neutrophils, and the antigen presentation function of dendritic cells[116].

Early studies of a recombinant fusion protein of monoclonal antibody to IL-2 and diphtheria toxin (DAB486IL-2) in refractory

RA showed limited efficacy for this approach[117]. Only 4 of 22 patients in the treated group compared to none in the placebo group demonstrated a clinical response, and only about one-third of the patients in the open-label phase responded. Moreover, adverse effects were relatively common, including elevated liver enzymes[55], nausea/vomiting (50%), and transient fever/chills (45%). Further evaluation of this compound was halted. A truncated version (DAB389IL-2) also failed to show efficacy in a phase II trial in RA patients[118] but is approved for use in cutaneous T cell lymphoma.

More recently, a humanized monoclonal antibody directed against the IL-2 receptor (daclizumab) was shown to significantly reduce joint inflammation and erosions in a rhesus monkey model of collagen-induced arthritis[119]. Although daclizumab may be beneficial for some inflammatory diseases such as psoriasis, no data on the efficacy of daclizumab for RA patients are yet available. Despite continued enthusiasm for targeting T cells for the treatment of RA, IL-2 antagonism may have only a limited role.

IFN-β

Therapeutic administration of IFN-β would seem reasonable in light of its observed role in inhibiting IL-1β, TNF-α, and metalloproteinases[120–122]. IFN-β also has anti-inflammatory properties by induction of IL-10 and through promotion of IL-1Ra from monocytes, chondrocytes, and synovial fibroblasts. Success in animal models of collagen-induced arthritis also supported its potential benefit in reducing inflammation and inhibiting bone erosions[123,124]. A small study of 12 RA patients demonstrated gradual improvement in tender and swollen joint count and patient and physician global assessment of pain[124]; 4 of the 10 patients completing the study fulfilled ACR20 response criteria, although none achieved an ACR50 response.

A subsequent phase II, randomized, double-blind, placebo-controlled trial examined the safety and efficacy of weekly intramuscular IFN-β at 24 weeks in 22 RA patients[125]. Despite the safety of the drug (the primary outcome), IFN-β failed to demonstrate any significant improvement in the treated group compared to placebo, and fewer than 20% of patients achieved an ACR20 response (a secondary outcome). Two-thirds of the patients in each group withdrew early from the study, most due to perceived lack of efficacy. Similarly, a larger phase II trial of 209 RA patients on background MTX randomized to IFN-β thrice-weekly for 24 weeks failed to show any benefit in ACR20 or radiographic end-points[126]. Levels of urinary collagen cross-links and histologic specimens from a subset of patients also failed to demonstrate any efficacy of this therapy. Based on these results, targeting IFN-β appears to provide minimal benefit for RA patients.

Antagonism of neovascularization

Neoangiogenesis is an important process in RA, since hyperplastic synovial tissue requires adequate tissue oxygenation[127,128]. A number of signals are required for this process, among them vascular endothelial growth factor (VEGF). Serum levels of VEGF have been shown to correlate with RA disease activity, levels of acute phase reactants, and radiographic progression at one year[129,130]. VEGF gene polymorphisms have also been shown to be associated with RA susceptibility[131]. Synergistic with TNF-α and IL-1, IL-6 has been observed to induce VEGF from synovial cells, and the benefits of IL-6 blockade may be partially mediated through decreased VEGF levels[132].

Success with a monoclonal antibody against VEGF demonstrated its ability to reduce both the incidence and severity of collagen-induced arthritis[133] and suggested that it may have a therapeutic role in RA. A slightly different approach targeting soluble VEGF receptors used a chimeric protein against soluble VEGF receptor 1 fused to the Fc portion of human IgG1 and showed dose-dependent efficacy in inhibiting angiogenesis in human rheumatoid synovium[134]. Another potential mechanism to block VEGF is using VEGF-Trap, which consists of an IgG1 fused to the first three domains of the VEGF receptor. VEGF-Trap has shown promise in anti-tumor studies and may be useful in RA as well[135]. Finally, inhibition of VEGF tyrosine kinase receptors, which mediate signaling[136], may also be useful to block VEGF.

Blockade of angiogenesis may also be achieved via recombinant forms of one of several endogenous inhibitors. One of them, thrombospondin 1 (TSP-1) inhibits both angiogenesis and tumor growth. Direct administration of adenoviral vector encoding TSP-1 has been shown to significantly improve the severity of collagen-induced arthritis, with a resulting decrease in synovial hypertrophy and vasculature[137]. Certain endothelial precursor cells that may give rise to the neovasculature necessary for synovial hypertrophy may also be useful targets. Several studies have identified CD34+ cells in both the marrow and synovium of RA patients[138,139]. Depletion of these cells may have a therapeutic benefit in RA and is currently being explored.

Chemokine blockade

Chemokines and their receptors appear to be important in the cellular trafficking of the inflammatory response. A number of specific chemokines appear to promote or reduce movement of Th1 cells into rheumatoid synovium, including CCL5[140]. One study examined 155 RA patients compared to an equal number of controls and found that CD4+ T cells in the RA synovium had significantly higher CCR5 expression compared to controls and that this expression was up-regulated by IL-15[52]. Success in CCR5 blockade with small molecules in collagen-induced arthritis models[141] suggests that there may be a role for CCR5 antagonism with biologic therapies[142].

Ectopic lymphoid structures appear to form in the synovial tissues of RA patients, and another chemokine, CXCL13, localizes with follicular dendritic cells at these sites[143]. Mice receiving a neutralizing antibody to CXCL13 showed significant improvement in a collagen-induced arthritis model, demonstrating a potential target that may be useful in RA patients[144]. Levels of IL-10 with CXCL13 blockade were significantly increased, suggesting that CXCL13 may at least partially mediate its effects through this anti-inflammatory cytokine. Moreover, CXCL13 neutralization appeared to suppress the formation of ectopic

Table 39.2   Chemokines and chemokine receptor targets potentially therapeutic in RA[140,145–150]

Ligand	Receptor	Cells expressing receptor	Function
CCL5	CCR1, CCR3, CCR5	Monocytes, T cells, DCs (CCR1 & 5 only), NK cells (CCR5 only), neutrophils (CCR1 only)	
CCL2	CCR2	Monocytes, T cells, NK cells, endothelial cells, fibroblasts, DCs	Recruitment of cells to the synovium
CCL3	CCR1, CCR5	Monocytes, T cells, DCs, NK cells (CCR5 only), neutrophils (CCR1 only)	
CCL21	CCR7	B cells, T cells	Ectopic lymphoid structure (germinal center) formation
CXCL13	CXCR5	B cells	
CX3CL1	CX3CR1	Th1 cells, NK cells, DCs, macrophages	
CXCL1, CXCL5, CXCL6, CXCL8	CXCR1 (CXCL5, 6, 8 only)	Neutrophils, endothelial cells, monocytes	
	CXCR2 (CXCL1, 5, 8 only)	B cells, T cells, DCs, monocytes, neutrophils	Recruitment of cells to the synovium and Angiogenesis
CXCL12	CXCR4		

DC, dendritic cell.

lymphoid follicles in the joints, which may be another mechanism by which CXCL13 neutralization may be beneficial.

A variety of other chemokines and chemokine receptors have been studied in models of experimental arthritis (Table 39.2). Their role in recruiting and retaining inflammatory cells within the synovium and involvement in ectopic germinal center formation within the inflamed RA pannus suggest that chemokines and chemokine receptor blockade may be therapeutic and perhaps even synergistic with other biologic agents.

Conclusions

The last several years have witnessed tremendous excitement over the use of biologic agents in the treatment of RA, although the nascent field of biologic agents has been largely limited to antagonizing TNF-α and IL-1. A more complete understanding of other cytokines and chemokines pathogenic in RA will continue to expand the therapeutic arsenal of agents available for treatment. Combinations of these drugs may also provide synergistic benefit compared to blockade of any of them in isolation, although the safety of this approach will need to be carefully studied. Moreover, the role of various cytokines in the evolution of the inflammatory response suggests that the approach to RA treatment may be significantly dependent on disease duration. Finally, prognostic markers that identify those with severe disease likely to benefit from blockade of particular cytokines are needed to help guide clinicians in their selection of the most rational therapies for individual patients.

References

1. Beutler, B., Greenwald, D., Hulmes, J., *et al.* Identity of tumour necrosis factor and the macrophage secreted factor cachectin. *Nature* 1985; **316**: 552–4.

2. Dayer, J., Beutler, B., and Cerami, A. Cachectin/tumor necrosis factor stimulates collagenase and prostaglandin E2 production by human synovial cells and dermal fibroblasts. *J Exp Med* 1985; **162**: 2163.

3. Bazzoni, F., and Beutler, B. The tumor necrosis factor ligand and receptor families. *N Engl J Med* 1996; **334**: 1717–25.

4. Fox, D. Cytokine blockade as a new strategy to treat rheumatoid arthritis. *Arch Intern Med* 2000; **160**: 437–44.

5. Koch, A., Kunkel, S., and Strieter, R. Cytokines in rheumatoid arthritis. *J Invest Med* 1995; **43**: 28.

6. Beutler, B., and Cerami, A. The biology of cachectin/TNF: a primary mediator of the host response. *Annu Rev Immunol* 1989; **7**: 625–55.

7. Lee, C. S., Chen, K. H., and Wang, P. C. Soluble tumor necrosis factor receptor in serum of patients with arthritis. *J Formos Med Assoc* 1997; **96**: 573–8.

8. Wildbaum, G., Nahir, M., and Karin, N. Beneficial autoimmunity to proinflammatory mediators restrains the consequences of self destructive immunity. *Immunity* 2003; **19**: 679–88.

9. Charles, P., Elliott, M., Davis, D. *et al.* Regulation of cytokines, cytokine inhibitors, and acute phase proteins following anti-TNF-a therapy in rheumatoid arthritis. *J Immunol* 1999; **163**: 1521–8.

10. Ohshima, S., Saeki, Y., Mima, T. *et al.* Long term follow up of the changes in circulating cytokines, soluble cytokine receptors, and white blood cell subset counts in patients with rheumatoid arthritis (RA) after monoclonal anti-TNF alpha antibody therapy. *J Clin Immunol* 1999; **19**: 305–13.

11. Williams, R., Mason, L., Feldmann, M., and Maini, R. Synergy between anti-CD4 and anti-tumor necrosis factor in the amelioration of established collagen induced arthritis. *Proc Natl Acad Sci U S A* 1994; **91**: 2762.

12. Williams, R., Feldmann, M., and Maini, R. Anti-tumor necrosis factor ameliorates joint disease in murine collagen-induced arthritis. *Proc Natl Acad Sci U S A* 1992; **89**: 9785.

13. Le, C., Nicolson, A., Morales, A., and Sewell, K. Suppression of collagen induced arthritis through adenovirus mediated transfer of a modified tumor necrosis factor alpha receptor gene. *Arthritis Rheum* 1997; **40**: 1662–9.

14. Quattrocchi, E., Walmsley, M., Browne, K. *et al.* Paradoxical effects of adenovirus mediated blockage of TNF activity in murine collagen induced arthritis. *J Immunol* 1999; **163**: 1000–9.

15. Robbins, P., Evans, C., and Chaernajovsky, Y. Gene therapy for rheumatoid arthritis. *Springer Semin Immunopathol* 1998; **20**: 197–209.

16. Choy, E., Hazleman. B., and Smith, M. Efficacy of a novel PEGylated humanized anti-TNF fragment (CDP870) in patients with rheumatoid arthritis: a phase II double blinded, randomized dose-escalating trial. *Rheumatology* 2002; **41**: 1133–7.

17. Fleischmann, R., Cohen, S., Caldwell, J. R. *et al*. Phase I studies evaluating the safety, pharmacokinetics, and pharmacodynamics of intravenous and subcutaneous administration of a fully human monoclonal antibody to human TNF-α (CNTO 148) in rheumatoid arthritis patients. *Arthritis Rheum* 2004; **48**: S178.

18. Davis, M. W., Feige, U., Bendele, A. M., Martin, S. W., and Edwards. C. K., 3rd. Treatment of rheumatoid arthritis with PEGylated recombinant human soluble tumour necrosis factor receptor type I: a clinical update. *Ann Rheum Dis* 2000; **59** (Suppl. 1): i41–i43.

19. Rutgeerts, P., Lemmens, L., Van Assche, G., Noman, M., Borghini-Fuhrer, I., and Goedkoop, R. Treatment of active Crohn's disease with onercept (recombinant human soluble p55 tumour necrosis factor receptor): results of a randomized, open-label, pilot study. *Aliment Pharmacol Ther* 2003; **17**: 185–92.

20. Newton, R. C, Solomon K. A., Covington, M. B., Decicco, C. P., Haley, P. J., Friedman, S. M., and Vaddi, K. Biology of TACE inhibition. *Ann Rheum Dis* 2001; **60** (Suppl. 3): iii25–iii32.

21. Conway, J., Andrews, R., Beaudet, B. *et al*. Inhibition of tumor necrosis factor-alpha (TNF-alpha) production and arthritis in the rat by GW3333, a dual inhibitor of TNF-alpha-converting enzyme and matrix metalloproteinases. *J Pharmacol Exp Ther* 2001; **298**: 900–8.

22. Dinarello, C. A. Interleukin-1 beta, interleukin-18, and the interleukin-1 beta converting enzyme. *Ann N Y Acad Sci* 1998; **856**: 1–11.

23. Dinarello, C. A. Interleukin-1, interleukin-1 receptors and interleukin-1 receptor antagonist. *Int Rev Immunol* 1998; **16**: 457–99.

24. Hom, J. T., Bendele, A. M., and Carlson, D. G. In vivo administration with IL-1 accelerates the development of collagen-induced arthritis in mice. *J Immunol* 1988; **141**: 834–41.

25. Feige, U., Karbowski, A., Rordorf-Adam, C., and Pataki, A. Arthritis induced by continuous infusion of hr-interleukin-1 alpha into the rabbit knee-joint. *Int J Tissue React* 1989; **11**: 225–38.

26. Eastgate, J. A., Symons, J. A., Wood, N. C., Grinlinton, F. M., di Giovine, F. S., and Duff, G. W. Correlation of plasma interleukin 1 levels with disease activity in rheumatoid arthritis. *Lancet* 1988; **2**: 706–9.

27. Firestein, G. S., Boyle, D. L., Yu, C. *et al*. Synovial interleukin-1 receptor antagonist and interleukin-1 balance in rheumatoid arthritis. *Arthritis Rheum* 1994; **37**: 644–52.

28. Bendele, A., McAbee, T., Sennello, G., Frazier, J., Chlipala, E., and McCabe, D. Efficacy of sustained blood levels of interleukin-1 receptor antagonist in animal models of arthritis: comparison of efficacy in animal models with human clinical data. *Arthritis Rheum* 1999; **42**: 498–506.

29. Bingham, C., Genovese, M., Moreland, L., Grimes, I., and Parsey, M. Results of a Phase II study of IL1-Trap in moderate to severe rheumatoid arthritis. *Arthritis Rheum* 2004; **48**: S237.

30. Rudolphi, K., Gerwin, N., Verzijl, N., van der Kraan, P., and van den Berg, W. Pralnacasan, an inhibitor of interleukin-1beta converting enzyme, reduces joint damage in two murine models of osteoarthritis. *Osteoarthritis Cartilage* 2003; **11**: 738–46.

31. Loher, F., Bauer, C., Landauer, N. *et al*. The interleukin-1 beta-converting enzyme inhibitor pralnacasan reduces dextran sulfate sodium-induced murine colitis and T helper 1 T-cell activation. *J Pharmacol Exp Ther* 2004; **308**: 583–90.

32. Kishimoto, T., Tanaka, T., Yoshida, K., Akira, S., and Taga, T. Cytokine signal transduction through a homo- or heterodimer of gp130. *Ann N Y Acad Sci* 1995; **766**: 224–34.

33. Bravo, J., and Heath, J. K. Receptor recognition by gp130 cytokines. *EMBO J* 2000; **19**: 2399–411.

34. Akira, S., Isshiki, H., Nakajima, T. *et al*. Regulation of expression of the interleukin 6 gene: structure and function of the transcription factor NF-IL6. *Ciba Found Symp* 1992; **167**: 47–62; discussion 62–7.

35. Flannery, C. R., Little, C. B., Hughes, C. E., Curtis, C. L., Caterson, B., and Jones, S. A. IL-6 and its soluble receptor augment aggrecanase-mediated proteoglycan catabolism in articular cartilage. *Matrix Biol* 2000; **19**: 549–53.

36. Brozik, M., Rosztoczy, I., Meretey, K. *et al*. Interleukin 6 levels in synovial fluids of patients with different arthritides: correlation with local IgM rheumatoid factor and systemic acute phase protein production. *J Rheumatol* 1992; **19**: 63–8.

37. Dasgupta, B., Corkill, M., Kirkham, B., Gibson, T., and Panayi, G. Serial estimation of interleukin 6 as a measure of systemic disease in rheumatoid arthritis. *J Rheumatol* 1992; **19**: 22–5.

38. Boe, A., Baiocchi, M., Carbonatto, M., Papoian, R., and Serlupi-Crescenzi, O. Interleukin 6 knock-out mice are resistant to antigen-induced experimental arthritis. *Cytokine* 1999; **11**: 1057–64.

39. Takagi, N., Mihara, M., Moriya, Y. *et al*. Blockage of interleukin-6 receptor ameliorates joint disease in murine collagen-induced arthritis. *Arthritis Rheum* 1998; **41**: 2117–21.

40. Mihara, M., Kotoh, M., Nishimoto, N. *et al*. Humanized antibody to human interleukin-6 receptor inhibits the development of collagen arthritis in cynomolgus monkeys. *Clin Immunol* 2001; **98**: 319–26.

41. Choy, E. H., Isenberg, D. A., Garrood, T. *et al*. Therapeutic benefit of blocking interleukin-6 activity with an anti-interleukin-6 receptor monoclonal antibody in rheumatoid arthritis: a randomized, double-blind, placebo-controlled, dose-escalation trial. *Arthritis Rheum* 2002; **46**: 3143–50.

42. Nishimoto, N., Yoshizaki, K., Maeda, K. *et al*. Toxicity, pharmacokinetics, and dose-finding study of repetitive treatment with the humanized anti-interleukin 6 receptor antibody MRA in rheumatoid arthritis: phase I/II clinical study. *J Rheumatol* 2003; **30**: 1426–35.

43. Nishimoto, N., Yoshizaki, K., Miyasaka, N. *et al*. Treatment of rheumatoid arthritis with humanized anti-interleukin-6 receptor antibody: a multicenter, double-blind, placebo-controlled trial. *Arthritis Rheum* 2004; **50**: 1761–9.

44. Maini, R., Taylor, P., and Pavelka, K. Efficacy of IL-6 receptor antagonist MRA in rheumatoid arthritis patients with an incomplete response to methotrexate (CHARISMA). *Arthritis Rheum* 2003; **46**: S652.

45. Grabstein, K. H., Eisenman, J., Shanebeck, K. *et al*. Cloning of a T cell growth factor that interacts with the beta chain of the interleukin-2 receptor. *Science* 1994; **264**: 965–8.

46. Gonzalez-Alvaro, I., Ortiz, A. M., Garcia-Vicuna, R., Balsa, A., Pascual-Salcedo, D., and Laffon, A. Increased serum levels of interleukin-15 in rheumatoid arthritis with long-term disease. *Clin Exp Rheumatol* 2003; **21**: 639–42.

47. Hessian, P. A., Highton, J., Kean, A., Sun, C. K., and Chin, M. Cytokine profile of the rheumatoid nodule suggests that it is a Th1 granuloma. *Arthritis Rheum* 2003; **48**: 334–8.

48. McInnes, I. B., Leung, B. P., Sturrock, R. D., Field, M., and Liew, F. Y. Interleukin-15 mediates T cell-dependent regulation of tumor necrosis factor-alpha production in rheumatoid arthritis. *Nat Med* 1997; **3**: 189–95.

49. Liew, F. Y., and McInnes, I. B. Role of interleukin 15 and interleukin 18 in inflammatory response. *Ann Rheum Dis* 2002; **61** (Suppl. 2): ii100–2.

50. McInnes, I. B., al-Mughales, J., Field, M. *et al*. The role of interleukin-15 in T-cell migration and activation in rheumatoid arthritis. *Nat Med* 1996; **2**: 175–82.

51. McInnes, I. B., Leung, B. P., and Liew, F. Y. Cell-cell interactions in synovitis: interactions between T lymphocytes and synovial cells. *Arthritis Res* 2000; **2**: 374–8.

52. Wang, C. R., and Liu, M. F. Regulation of CCR5 expression and MIP-1alpha production in CD4+ T cells from patients with rheumatoid arthritis. *Clin Exp Immunol* 2003; **132**: 371–8.

53. Miranda-Carus, M. E., Balsa, A., Benito-Miguel, M., Perez de Ayala, C., and Martin-Mola, E. IL-15 and the initiation of cell contact-dependent synovial fibroblast-T lymphocyte cross-talk in rheumatoid arthritis: effect of methotrexate. *J Immunol* 2004; **173**: 1463–76.

54. Ruchatz, H., Leung, B. P., Wei, X. Q., McInnes, I. B., and Liew, F. Y. Soluble IL-15 receptor alpha-chain administration prevents murine collagen-induced arthritis: a role for IL-15 in development of antigen-induced immunopathology. *J Immunol* 1998; **160**: 5654–60.

55. Ferrari-Lacraz, S., Zanelli, E., Neuberg, M. *et al*. Targeting IL-15 receptor-bearing cells with an antagonist mutant IL-15/Fc protein prevents disease development and progression in murine collagen-induced arthritis. *J Immunol* 2004; **173**: 5818–26.

56. Baslund, B., Tvede, N., Danneskiold-Samsoe, B. *et al*. A novel human monoclonal antibody against IL-15 (HuMax-IL15) in patients with

57. McInnes, I. B., Martin, R, W., Zimmerman, I. *et al.* Safety and efficacy of a human monoclonal antibody to IL-15 (AMG 714) in patients with rheumatoid arthritis (RA): results from a multicenter, randomized, double-blind, placebo-controlled trial. *Arthritis Rheum* 2004; **48**: S241.

58. Gracie, J. A., Robertson, S. E., and McInnes, I. B. Interleukin-18. *J Leukoc Biol* 2003; **73**: 213–24.

59. Gobel, T. W., Schneider, K., Schaerer, B. *et al.* IL-18 stimulates the proliferation and IFN-gamma release of CD4+ T cells in the chicken: conservation of a Th1-like system in a nonmammalian species. *J Immunol* 2003; **171**: 1809–15.

60. Dai, S. M., Matsuno, H., Nakamura, H., Nishioka, K., and Yudoh, K. Interleukin-18 enhances monocyte tumor necrosis factor alpha and interleukin-1beta production induced by direct contact with T lymphocytes: implications in rheumatoid arthritis. *Arthritis Rheum* 2004; **50**: 432–43.

61. Yamamura, M., Kawashima, M., Taniai, M. *et al.* Interferon-gamma-inducing activity of interleukin-18 in the joint with rheumatoid arthritis. *Arthritis Rheum* 2001; **44**: 275–85.

62. Novick, D., Kim, S. H., Fantuzzi, G., Reznikov, L. L., Dinarello, C. A., and Rubinstein, M. Interleukin-18 binding protein: a novel modulator of the Th1 cytokine response. *Immunity* 1999; **10**: 127–36.

63. Plater-Zyberk, C., Joosten, L. A., Helsen, M. M. *et al.* Therapeutic effect of neutralizing endogenous IL-18 activity in the collagen-induced model of arthritis. *J Clin Invest* 2001; **108**: 1825–32.

64. Ye, X. J., Tang, B., Ma, Z., Kang, A. H., Myers, L. K., and Cremer, M. A. The roles of interleukin-18 in collagen-induced arthritis in the BB rat. *Clin Exp Immunol* 2004; **136**: 440–7.

65. Tissi, L., McRae, B., Ghayur, T. *et al.* Role of interleukin-18 in experimental group B streptococcal arthritis. *Arthritis Rheum* 2004; **50**: 2005–13.

66. Banda, N. K., Vondracek, A., Kraus, D. *et al.* Mechanisms of inhibition of collagen-induced arthritis by murine IL-18 binding protein. *J Immunol* 2003; **170**: 2100–5.

67. Trinchieri, G. Interleukin-12 and the regulation of innate resistance and adaptive immunity. *Nat Rev Immunol* 2003; **3**: 133–46.

68. Trinchieri, G. Interleukin-12 and interferon-gamma: do they always go together? *Am J Pathol* 1995; **147**: 1534–8.

69. Trinchieri, G. Interleukin-12: a proinflammatory cytokine with immunoregulatory functions that bridge innate resistance and antigen-specific adaptive immunity. *Annu Rev Immunol* 1995; **13**: 251–76.

70. Trinchieri, G., and Scott, P. Interleukin-12: a proinflammatory cytokine with immunoregulatory functions. *Res Immunol* 1995; **146**: 423–31.

71. Desai, B. B., Quinn, P. M., Wolitzky, A. G., Mongini, P. K., Chizzonite, R., and Gately, M. K. IL-12 receptor. II. Distribution and regulation of receptor expression. *J Immunol* 1992; **148**: 3125–32.

72. Sakkas, L. I., Johanson, N. A., Scanzello, C. R., and Platsoucas, C. D. Interleukin-12 is expressed by infiltrating macrophages and synovial lining cells in rheumatoid arthritis and osteoarthritis. *Cell Immunol* 1998; **188**: 105–10.

73. Kitagawa, M., Mitsui, H., Nakamura, H. *et al.* Differential regulation of rheumatoid synovial cell interleukin-12 production by tumor necrosis factor alpha and CD40 signals. *Arthritis Rheum* 1999; **42**: 1917–26.

74. Kim, T. S., Kang, B. Y., Lee, M. H., Choe, Y. K., and Hwang, S. Y. Inhibition of interleukin-12 production by auranofin, an antirheumatic gold compound, deviates CD4(+) T cells from the Th1 to the Th2 pathway. *Br J Pharmacol* 2001; **134**: 571–8.

75. Butler, D. M., Malfait, A. M., Maini, R. N., Brennan, F. M., and Feldmann, M. Anti-IL-12 and anti-TNF antibodies synergistically suppress the progression of murine collagen-induced arthritis. *Eur J Immunol* 1999; **29**: 2205–12.

76. Malfait, A. M., Butler, D. M., Presky, D. H., Maini, R. N., Brennan, F. M., and Feldmann, M. Blockade of IL-12 during the induction of collagen-induced arthritis (CIA) markedly attenuates the severity of the arthritis. *Clin Exp Immunol* 1998; **111**: 377–83.

77. Cua, D. J., Sherlock, J., Chen, Y. *et al.* Interleukin-23 rather than interleukin-12 is the critical cytokine for autoimmune inflammation of the brain. *Nature* 2003; **421**: 744–8.

78. Vandenbroeck, K., Alloza, I., Gadina, M., and Matthys, P. Inhibiting cytokines of the interleukin-12 family: recent advances and novel challenges. *J Pharm Pharmacol* 2004; **56**: 145–60.

79. Watford, W. T., and O'Shea, J. J. Autoimmunity: a case of mistaken identity. *Nature* 2003; **421**: 706–8.

80. Langrish, C. L., Chen, Y., Blumenschein, W. M. *et al.* IL-23 drives a pathogenic T cell population that induces autoimmune inflammation. *J Exp Med* 2005; **201**: 233–40.

81. Fossiez, F., Djossou, O., Chomarat, P. *et al.* T cell interleukin-17 induces stromal cells to produce proinflammatory and hematopoietic cytokines. *J Exp Med* 1996; **183**: 2593–603.

82. Bush, K. A., Walker, J. S., Lee, C. S., and Kirkham, B. W. Cytokine expression and synovial pathology in the initiation and spontaneous resolution phases of adjuvant arthritis: interleukin-17 expression is upregulated in early disease. *Clin Exp Immunol* 2001; **123**: 487–95.

83. Ziolkowska, M., Koc, A., Luszczykiewicz, G. *et al.* High levels of IL-17 in rheumatoid arthritis patients: IL-15 triggers in vitro IL-17 production via cyclosporin A-sensitive mechanism. *J Immunol* 2000; **164**: 2832–8.

84. Kotake, S., Udagawa, N., Takahashi, N. *et al.* IL-17 in synovial fluids from patients with rheumatoid arthritis is a potent stimulator of osteoclastogenesis. *J Clin Invest* 1999; **103**: 1345–52.

85. Attur, M. G., Patel, R. N., Abramson, S. B., and Amin, A. R. Interleukin-17 up-regulation of nitric oxide production in human osteoarthritis cartilage. *Arthritis Rheum* 1997; **40**: 1050–3.

86. Lubberts, E., van den Bersselaar, L., Oppers-Walgreen, B. *et al.* IL-17 promotes bone erosion in murine collagen-induced arthritis through loss of the receptor activator of NF-kappa B ligand/osteoprotegerin balance. *J Immunol* 2003; **170**: 2655–62.

87. Miossec, P. Interleukin-17 in rheumatoid arthritis: if T cells were to contribute to inflammation and destruction through synergy. *Arthritis Rheum* 2003; **48**: 594–601.

88. Rifas, L., and Arackal, S. T cells regulate the expression of matrix metalloproteinase in human osteoblasts via a dual mitogen-activated protein kinase mechanism. *Arthritis Rheum* 2003; **48**: 993–1001.

89. Faour, W. H., Mancini, A., He, Q. W., and Di Battista, J. A. T-cell-derived interleukin-17 regulates the level and stability of cyclooxygenase-2 (COX-2) mRNA through restricted activation of the p38 mitogen-activated protein kinase cascade: role of distal sequences in the 3′-untranslated region of COX-2 mRNA. *J Biol Chem* 2003; **278**: 26897–907.

90. Kim, K., Cho, M., Park, M. *et al.* Increased interleukin-17 production via a phosphoinositide 3-kinase/Akt and nuclear factor kappaB-dependent pathway in patients with rheumatoid arthritis. *Arthritis Res Ther* 2005; 7: R139–48.

91. Nakae, S., Nambu, A., Sudo, K., and Iwakura, Y. Suppression of immune induction of collagen-induced arthritis in IL-17-deficient mice. *J Immunol* 2003; **171**: 6173–7.

92. Burchill, M. A., Nardelli, D. T., England, D. M. *et al.* Inhibition of interleukin-17 prevents the development of arthritis in vaccinated mice challenged with Borrelia burgdorferi. *Infect Immun* 2003; **71**: 3437–42.

93. Nakae, S., Saijo, S., Horai, R., Sudo, K., Mori, S., and Iwakura, Y. IL-17 production from activated T cells is required for the spontaneous development of destructive arthritis in mice deficient in IL-1 receptor antagonist. *Proc Natl Acad Sci U S A* 2003; **100**: 5986–90.

94. Lubberts, E., Koenders, M. I., Oppers-Walgreen, B. *et al.* Treatment with a neutralizing anti-murine interleukin-17 antibody after the onset of collagen-induced arthritis reduces joint inflammation, cartilage destruction, and bone erosion. *Arthritis Rheum* 2004; **50**: 650–9.

95. Lubberts, E., Joosten, L. A., Oppers, B. *et al.* IL-1-independent role of IL-17 in synovial inflammation and joint destruction during collagen-induced arthritis. *J Immunol* 2001; **167**: 1004–13.

96. Morand, E. F., Bucala, R., and Leech, M. Macrophage migration inhibitory factor: an emerging therapeutic target in rheumatoid arthritis. *Arthritis Rheum* 2003; **48**: 291–9.

The top of the first column also shows the end of reference 56:

active rheumatoid arthritis (RA): results of a double-blind, placebo-controlled phase I/II trial. *Arthritis Rheum* 2003; **46**: S652.

97. Leech, M., Metz, C., Hall, P. *et al*. Macrophage migration inhibitory factor in rheumatoid arthritis: evidence of proinflammatory function and regulation by glucocorticoids. *Arthritis Rheum* 1999; **42**: 1601–8.

98. Calandra, T., Bernhagen, J., Metz, C. N. *et al*. MIF as a glucocorticoid-induced modulator of cytokine production. *Nature* 1995; **377**: 68–71.

99. Onodera, S., Nishihira, J., Iwabuchi, K. *et al*. Macrophage migration inhibitory factor up-regulates matrix metalloproteinase-9 and -13 in rat osteoblasts: relevance to intracellular signaling pathways. *J Biol Chem* 2002; **277**: 7865–74.

100. Santos, L. L., Lacey, D., Yang, Y., Leech, M., and Morand, E. F. Activation of synovial cell p38 MAP kinase by macrophage migration inhibitory factor. *J Rheumatol* 2004; **31**: 1038–43.

101. Onodera, S., Nishihira, J., Yamazaki, M., Ishibashi, T., and Minami, A. Increased expression of macrophage migration inhibitory factor during fracture healing in rats. *Histochem Cell Biol* 2004; **121**: 209–17.

102. Mitchell, R. A., Liao, H., Chesney, J. *et al*. Macrophage migration inhibitory factor (MIF) sustains macrophage proinflammatory function by inhibiting p53: regulatory role in the innate immune response. *Proc Natl Acad Sci U S A* 2002; **99**: 345–50.

103. Firestein, G. S., Nguyen, K., Aupperle, K. R., Yeo, M., Boyle, D. L., and Zvaifler N. J. Apoptosis in rheumatoid arthritis: p53 over-expression in rheumatoid arthritis synovium. *Am J Pathol* 1996; **149**: 2143–51.

104. Morand, E. F., Leech, M., Weedon, H., Metz, C., Bucala, R., and Smith, M. D. Macrophage migration inhibitory factor in rheumatoid arthritis: clinical correlations. *Rheumatology (Oxford)* 2002; **41**: 558–62.

105. Donn, R. P., Shelley, E., Ollier, W. E., and Thomson, W. A. novel 5′-flanking region polymorphism of macrophage migration inhibitory factor is associated with systemic-onset juvenile idiopathic arthritis. *Arthritis Rheum* 2001; **44**: 1782–5.

106. Baugh, J. A., Chitnis, S., Donnelly, S. C. *et al*. A functional promoter polymorphism in the macrophage migration inhibitory factor (MIF) gene associated with disease severity in rheumatoid arthritis. *Genes Immun* 2002; **3**: 170–6.

107. Leech, M., Metz, C., Santos, L. *et al*. Involvement of macrophage migration inhibitory factor in the evolution of rat adjuvant arthritis. *Arthritis Rheum* 1998; **41**: 910–17.

108. Mikulowska, A., Metz, C. N., Bucala, R., and Holmdahl, R. Macrophage migration inhibitory factor is involved in the pathogenesis of collagen type II-induced arthritis in mice. *J Immunol* 1997; **158**: 5514–17.

109. Senter, P. D., Al-Abed, Y., Metz, C. N. *et al*. Inhibition of macrophage migration inhibitory factor (MIF) tautomerase and biological activities by acetaminophen metabolites. *Proc Natl Acad Sci U S A* 2002; **99**: 144–9.

110. Whalen, J. D., Lechman, E. L., Carlos, C. A. *et al*. Adenoviral transfer of the viral IL-10 gene periarticularly to mouse paws suppresses development of collagen-induced arthritis in both injected and uninjected paws. *J Immunol* 1999; **162**: 3625–32.

111. Lechman, E. R., Jaffurs, D., Ghivizzani, S. C. *et al*. Direct adenoviral gene transfer of viral IL-10 to rabbit knees with experimental arthritis ameliorates disease in both injected and contralateral control knees. *J Immunol* 1999; **163**: 2202–8.

112. van Roon, J., Wijngaarden, S., Lafeber, F. P., Damen, C., van de Winkel, J., and Bijlsma, J. W. Interleukin 10 treatment of patients with rheumatoid arthritis enhances Fc gamma receptor expression on monocytes and responsiveness to immune complex stimulation. *J Rheumatol* 2003; **30**: 648–51.

113. Van den Bosch, F., Russell, A., and Keystone, E. rhuIL-4 in subjects with active rheumatoid arthritis (RA): a phase I dose escalating safety study. *Arthritis Rheum* 1998; **41**: S56.

114. Lee, C. K., Lee, E. Y., Chung, S. M., Mun, S. H., Yoo, B., and Moon, H. B. Effects of disease-modifying antirheumatic drugs and antiinflammatory cytokines on human osteoclastogenesis through interaction with receptor activator of nuclear factor kappaB, osteoprotegerin, and receptor activator of nuclear factor kappaB ligand. *Arthritis Rheum* 2004; **50**: 3831–43.

115. Cannon, G. W., Pincus, S. H., Emkey, R. D. *et al*. Double-blind trial of recombinant gamma-interferon versus placebo in the treatment of rheumatoid arthritis. *Arthritis Rheum* 1989; **32**: 964–73.

116. Chen, T., Guo, J., Yang, M. *et al*. Cyclosporin A impairs dendritic cell migration by regulating chemokine receptor expression and inhibiting cyclooxygenase-2 expression. *Blood* 2004; **103**: 413–21.

117. Moreland, L. W., Sewell, K. L., Trentham, D. E. *et al*. Interleukin-2 diphtheria fusion protein (DAB486IL-2) in refractory rheumatoid arthritis: a double-blind, placebo-controlled trial with open-label extension. *Arthritis Rheum* 1995; **38**: 1177–86.

118. Sewell, K., Moreland, L., Cush, J., Furst, D., Woodworth, T., and Mechan, R. Phase I/II double-blind dose-response trial of a second fusion toxin DAB389-IL-2 in rheumatoid arthritis. *Arthritis Rheum* 1993; **36**: S130.

119. Brok, H. P., Tekoppele, J. M., Hakimi, J. *et al*. Prophylactic and therapeutic effects of a humanized monoclonal antibody against the IL-2 receptor (DACLIZUMAB) on collagen-induced arthritis (CIA) in rhesus monkeys. *Clin Exp Immunol* 2001; **124**: 134–41.

120. Smeets, T. J., Dayer, J. M., Kraan, M. C. *et al*. The effects of interferon-beta treatment of synovial inflammation and expression of metalloproteinases in patients with rheumatoid arthritis. *Arthritis Rheum* 2000; **43**: 270–4.

121. Palmer, G., Mezin, F., Juge-Aubry, C. E., Plater-Zyberk, C., Gabay, C., and Guerne, P. A. Interferon beta stimulates interleukin 1 receptor antagonist production in human articular chondrocytes and synovial fibroblasts. *Ann Rheum Dis* 2004; **63**: 43–9.

122. Coclet-Ninin, J., Dayer, J. M., and Burger, D. Interferon-beta not only inhibits interleukin-1beta and tumor necrosis factor-alpha but stimulates interleukin-1 receptor antagonist production in human peripheral blood mononuclear cells. *Eur Cytokine Netw* 1997; **8**: 345–9.

123. van Holten, J., Reedquist, K., Sattonet-Roche, P. *et al*. Treatment with recombinant interferon-beta reduces inflammation and slows cartilage destruction in the collagen-induced arthritis model of rheumatoid arthritis. *Arthritis Res Ther* 2004; **6**: R239–R249.

124. Tak, P. P., Hart, B. A., Kraan, M. C., Jonker, M., Smeets, T. J., and Breedveld, F. C. The effects of interferon beta treatment on arthritis. *Rheumatology (Oxford)* 1999; **38**: 362–9.

125. Genovese, M. C., Chakravarty, E. F., Krishnan, E., and Moreland, L. W. A. randomized, controlled trial of interferon-beta-1a (Avonex(R)) in patients with rheumatoid arthritis: a pilot study [ISRCTN03626626]. *Arthritis Res Ther* 2004; **6**: R73–R77.

126. van Holten, J., Pavelka, K., Vencovsky, J. *et al*. A multicentre, randomised, double blind, placebo controlled phase II study of subcutaneous interferon beta-1a in the treatment of patients with active rheumatoid arthritis. *Ann Rheum Dis* 2005; **64**: 64–9.

127. Folkman, J. Angiogenesis in cancer, vascular, rheumatoid and other disease. *Nat Med* 1995; **1**: 27–31.

128. Koch, A. E. Angiogenesis as a target in rheumatoid arthritis. *Ann Rheum Dis* 2003; **62** (Suppl. 2): ii60–ii67.

129. Sone, H., Sakauchi, M., Takahashi, A. *et al*. Elevated levels of vascular endothelial growth factor in the sera of patients with rheumatoid arthritis correlation with disease activity. *Life Sci* 2001; **69**: 1861–9.

130. Taylor, P. C. Serum vascular markers and vascular imaging in assessment of rheumatoid arthritis disease activity and response to therapy. *Rheumatology (Oxford)* 2005; **44**: 721–8.

131. Han, S. W., Kim, G. W., Seo, J. S. *et al*. VEGF gene polymorphisms and susceptibility to rheumatoid arthritis. *Rheumatology (Oxford)* 2004; **43**: 1173–7.

132. Nakahara, H., Song, J., Sugimoto, M. *et al*. Anti-interleukin-6 receptor antibody therapy reduces vascular endothelial growth factor production in rheumatoid arthritis. *Arthritis Rheum* 2003; **48**: 1521–9.

133. Sone, H., Kawakami, Y., Sakauchi, M. *et al*. Neutralization of vascular endothelial growth factor prevents collagen-induced arthritis and ameliorates established disease in mice. *Biochem Biophys Res Commun* 2001; **281**: 562–8.

134. Sekimoto, T., Hamada, K., Oike, Y. *et al*. Effect of direct angiogenesis inhibition in rheumatoid arthritis using a soluble vascular

endothelial growth factor receptor 1 chimeric protein. *J Rheumatol* 2002; **29**: 240–5.

135. Holash, J., Davis, S., Papadopoulos, N. *et al.* VEGF-Trap: a VEGF blocker with potent antitumor effects. *Proc Natl Acad Sci U S A* 2002; **99**: 11393–8.

136. Grosios, K., Wood, J., Esser, R., Raychaudhuri, A., and Dawson, J. Angiogenesis inhibition by the novel VEGF receptor tyrosine kinase inhibitor, PTK787/ZK222584, causes significant anti-arthritic effects in models of rheumatoid arthritis. *Inflamm Res* 2004; **53**: 133–42.

137. Jou, I. M., Shiau, A. L., Chen, S. Y. *et al.* Thrombospondin 1 as an effective gene therapeutic strategy in collagen-induced arthritis. *Arthritis Rheum* 2005; **52**: 339–44.

138. Ruger, B., Giurea, A., Wanivenhaus, A. H. *et al.* Endothelial precursor cells in the synovial tissue of patients with rheumatoid arthritis and osteoarthritis. *Arthritis Rheum* 2004; **50**: 2157–66.

139. Hirohata, S., Yanagida, T., Nampei, A. *et al.* Enhanced generation of endothelial cells from CD34+ cells of the bone marrow in rheumatoid arthritis: possible role in synovial neovascularization. *Arthritis Rheum* 2004; **50**: 3888–96.

140. Shadidi, K. R., Aarvak, T., Henriksen, J. E., Natvig, J. B., and Thompson, K. M. The chemokines CCL5, CCL2 and CXCL12 play significant roles in the migration of Th1 cells into rheumatoid synovial tissue. *Scand J Immunol* 2003; **57**: 192–8.

141. Vierboom, M. P., Zavodny, P. J., Chou, C. C. *et al.* Inhibition of the development of collagen-induced arthritis in rhesus monkeys by a small molecular weight antagonist of CCR5. *Arthritis Rheum* 2005; **52**: 627–36.

142. Bruhl, H., Cihak, J., Stangassinger, M., Schlondorff, D., and Mack, M. Depletion of CCR5-expressing cells with bispecific antibodies and chemokine toxins: a new strategy in the treatment of chronic inflammatory diseases and HIV. *J Immunol* 2001; **166**: 2420–6.

143. Shi, K., Hayashida, K., Kaneko, M. *et al.* Lymphoid chemokine B cell-attracting chemokine-1 (CXCL13) is expressed in germinal center of ectopic lymphoid follicles within the synovium of chronic arthritis patients. *J Immunol* 2001; **166**: 650–5.

144. Zheng, B., Ozen, Z., Zhang, X. *et al.* CXCL13 neutralization reduces the severity of collagen-induced arthritis. *Arthritis Rheum* 2005; **52**: 620–6.

145. Takemura, S., Braun, A., Crowson, C. *et al.* Lymphoid neogenesis in rheumatoid synovitis. *J Immunol* 2001; **167**: 1072–80.

146. Katschke, K. J., Jr, Rottman, J. B., Ruth, J. H. *et al.* Differential expression of chemokine receptors on peripheral blood, synovial fluid, and synovial tissue monocytes/macrophages in rheumatoid arthritis. *Arthritis Rheum* 2001; **44**: 1022–32.

147. Hjelmstrom, P. Lymphoid neogenesis: de novo formation of lymphoid tissue in chronic inflammation through expression of homing chemokines. *J Leukoc Biol* 2001; **69**: 331–9.

148. Weyand, C. M., and Goronzy, J. J. Ectopic germinal center formation in rheumatoid synovitis. *Ann N Y Acad Sci* 2003; **987**: 140–9.

149. Keane, M. P., and Strieter, R. M. The role of CXC chemokines in the regulation of angiogenesis. *Chem Immunol* 1999; **72**: 86–101.

150. Nanki, T., Imai, T., Nagasaka, K. *et al.* Migration of CX3CR1-positive T cells producing type 1 cytokines and cytotoxic molecules into the synovium of patients with rheumatoid arthritis. *Arthritis Rheum* 2002; **46**: 2878–83.

New biologics: T and B modulators

Ernest Choy

Introduction

Untreated, rheumatoid arthritis (RA) is a disease with high mortality and morbidity[1]. Disease severity[2] and response to treatment[3] are important predictors of prognosis. Mortality of patients with persistent synovitis despite treatment by disease modifying antirheumatic drugs (DMARDs) is comparable to triple vessel coronary artery disease and Hodgkin's lymphoma[4]. Although DMARDs reduce inflammation, they rarely abort disease completely. Continued synovial inflammation leads to progressive destruction of the synovial joints. Consequently, disability is common[5]. More effective treatment is therefore needed to improve the prognosis of RA.

Over the last decade, greater understanding of the pathogenesis of RA and advances in biotechnology have made targeted therapy a reality. This is epitomized by the success of cytokine inhibition in RA especially tumor necrosis factor alpha (TNF-α) antagonists. In patients with active RA, cytokines are found in abundance not only in synovial joints but also in the blood. Some cytokines such as interleukin (IL)-1 and TNF-α are pro-inflammatory while others like tissue growth factor beta (TGF-β) are anti-inflammatory. Both pro-inflammatory and anti-inflammatory cytokines are present at the site of the inflammation. The balance between pro-inflammatory and anti-inflammatory cytokines determines whether the tissue becomes inflamed. Inhibiting inflammatory cytokines, thereby tilting the balance towards anti-inflammatory cytokines, is a treatment strategy that has proved successful in RA, as exemplified by the benefit of TNF-α inhibitors.

Despite the success of TNF-α antagonists, some patients are ineligible because of contraindications such as chronic infection and severe cardiac failure. Moreover, the number of treatment failures due to either lack of response or side-effects is increasing. There is a growing need for alternative treatments in these patients.

Pathogenesis of rheumatoid arthritis

Although the precise pathogenesis of RA remains unknown, there is considerable evidence implicating T and B cells. The rheumatoid synovial membrane is heavily infiltrated by T cells in a perivascular and diffuse distribution[6]. Monocytes and macrophages infiltrate the subsynovium as well as the synovial lining layer[7]. In some patients, T and B cells may organize into aggregates akin to germinal centers in lymphoid organs. They synthesize and secrete immunoglobulins, of which a variable proportion is rheumatoid factor (RF). These B lymphocytes, macrophages, and dendritic cells express human leukocyte antigen (HLA) molecules and are all capable of presenting antigenic peptides to T cells.

Interactions between T and B cells have several potential consequences in RA. First, B cells express HLA class II molecules and therefore can present antigens and provide costimulatory signals for T cell activation and proliferation. Second, B cells can produce cytokines such as TNF-α. Third, B cell activation, along with help from T cells, results in the production of antibodies, especially auto-antibodies such as RF and antibodies against cyclic citrullinated peptide[8]. These antibodies may form immune complexes and activate complement complexes, which perpetuate synovial inflammation and joint damage. Edwards *et al.* suggested that immune complexes formed by IgG RF may have an important role in the pathogenesis of RA[9]. By virtue of its small size, it may readily gain access to the extra-vascular space and activate tissue macrophages which express Fcγ receptors. Furthermore, IgG RF may also promote the survival of B cells in lymphoid aggregates in the rheumatoid synovia. This could lead to a self-perpetuation of the immune response by B cells and IgG RF immune complexes.

T cells in the synovium are activated and express HLA-DR, CD69[10], and CCR5[11], the latter being selectively expressed by Th1 cells. Studies using sensitive immunohistological techniques and semi-quantitative polymerase chain reaction have demonstrated the presence of the Th1 lymphokines IL-2 and interferon gamma (IFN-γ). Therefore, these activated T cells are capable of sustaining synovitis through the release of lymphokines and direct contact with mesenchymal cells. Activated CD4 T cells stimulate monocytes/macrophages and synovial fibroblasts to produce cytokines such as IL-1, IL-6, and TNF-α through the release of IFN-γ and direct cell surface contact via CD69 and leukocyte function antigen-1 (LFA-1) molecules, respectively. IL-1 and TNF-α stimulate the release of the matrix metalloproteinases (MMPs) such as collagenase and stromelysin, which degrade connective tissue and cause joint damage[12]. They also up-regulate the expression of adhesion molecules, such as intercellular adhesion molecule-1 (ICAM-1) and vascular cellular adhesion molecule-1 (VCAM-1), on endothelial cells. These molecules bind to LFA-1 and very late adhesion molecule-4 (VLA-4) on the surface of leukocytes, leading to migration of inflammatory cells into the synovial joints and perpetuation of inflammation.

The ideal treatment of RA is one that is safe, disease specific, and produces sustained disease remission after a brief course of treatment. While the TNF-α antagonists are powerful anti-inflammatory and disease-modifying agents, repeated treatments are necessary to sustain clinical improvement. This is probably due to unabated lymphocyte activation that continues to perpetuate inflammation[13]. Therefore, there is an increasing interest in targeting lymphocytes in order to achieve disease remission.

Anti-T cell therapy

Rationale of targeting T cells

The immunogenetic basis of RA is one of the strongest pieces of evidence for the importance of T cells in disease pathogenesis. RA is strongly linked to HLA-DRB10404[14] and -DRB10401[15]. The HLA-DR molecule consists of an invariant α and a polymorphic β chain. They form a groove in which an antigenic peptide is presented to the T cell receptor (TCR) of a CD4+ T cell. This is the only known function of HLA molecules. The third hypervariable region of the β chain is thought to be especially important since it binds to the antigenic peptide. Molecular analysis of this region in HLA-DRB10404 and DRB10401 molecules shows that they are identical apart from a conserved substitution. This leads to the proposal of the shared epitope hypothesis[16] in which HLA-DR molecules sharing similar third hypervariable regions are capable of binding an arthritogenic peptide, thus rendering individuals susceptible to RA. The arthritogenic peptide in RA remains unknown, but recently a human chondrocyte antigen, HC-gp39, has been identified as a possible candidate autoantigen[17], as well as the endoplasmic reticulum chaperone BiP. For a full discussion of the genetics of RA see Chapter 1.

Further compelling evidence for the involvement of T cells in the pathogenesis of destructive inflammatory arthritis comes from animal models. There are three commonly used animal models of RA: adjuvant arthritis in rats, collagen arthritis in mice and rats, and streptococcal cell wall arthritis in rats. In all three models Th1 T cells are central to the pathogenesis. Arthritis cannot be induced in T cell-deficient animals; it is linked to a particular mouse or rat MHC, and disease can be transferred from one animal to another by extracting T cells from the arthritic animal and administering them to a healthy one.

History of anti-T cell therapy

In T cell-based treatment strategies in RA, the ideal target is the arthritogenic T cell itself. Clearly, such specific therapy will be less toxic than a general anti-T cell therapy. However, it is a more elusive goal, especially in established disease, since the arthritogenic peptide and disease specific T cells in RA remain unknown. Therapies against T cells can be broadly divided into those that deplete T cells and those that modulate their function.

T cell depletion

The initial strategy in anti-T cell therapy was to deplete all or a subset of T cells. Overall, the clinical effects of these depleting monoclonal antibodies have been disappointing. Three major factors probably contributed to the lack of efficacy. First, the majority of the T cells targeted are not the pathogenic T cells in RA. Second, severe and prolonged lymphopenia after treatment increases the risk of long-term immunosuppression and precludes the use of high doses of monoclonal antibodies. Third, depleting antibodies are more efficient in eliminating naïve, circulating T cells than the activated, pathogenic T cells present in the joint. Fourth, depleting treatments may preferentially deplete regulatory T cells. see Waldmann infectious tolerance.

The first point is illustrated by the experience of murine and chimeric anti-CD7 monoclonal antibodies, which produced no significant clinical improvement yet circulating CD7+ T cells were depleted[18,19]. Lazarovits et al. later showed that in the RA synovial joint, lymphocytes are predominantly CD7— when compared with peripheral blood[20]. Therefore, CD7+ lymphocytes are unlikely to have a major pathogenic role in RA

The second point is borne out by the experience with CD5-PLUS, which is an immunotoxin composed of the murine anti-CD5 monoclonal antibody conjugated to the A chain of the toxin, ricin. CD5 is expressed by all mature T cells and a subset of mature B cells. The initial open study[21] led to a 50% reduction in disease activity, and a further study in early RA to a 70% clinical improvement. Both studies showed a marked reduction in the number of circulating CD3+CD5+ T cells. In common with other murine monoclonal antibodies, all but one patient developed a human anti-murine antibody response. Unfortunately, a double-blind, placebo-controlled trial of CD5-PLUS failed to show any significant clinical improvement despite inducing significant lymphopenia[22]. However, this study suffered from one major problem. In the open studies, CD5-PLUS was given daily for five days, while in the placebo-controlled trial patients were treated only for two days. Indeed, the degree of lymphopenia was less than that obtained in the open studies, raising doubts regarding the biological equivalence of the open and controlled studies. The placebo-controlled trial was further compounded by an uncommonly high placebo response of ~40%.

The fact that depleting antibodies are more efficient in eliminating naïve circulating T cells than the activated, memory pathogenic T cells resident in the joint was illustrated by experience with both Campath-1H and cM-T412 antibodies. Campath-1H is a humanized anti-CDw52 monoclonal antibody. The CDw52 molecule is present on the surface of T cells, monocytes, and B cells. Campath-1H is extremely potent in inducing complement-mediated lysis. In open studies, tender and swollen joint scores reduced by 50% without significant changes in erythrocyte sedimentation rate (ESR) or C-reactive protein (CRP)[23,24]. Campath-1H induced a profound and protracted lymphopenia after treatment. In the high dose groups there was a prolonged absence of circulating lymphocytes. Nevertheless, disease improvement did not correlate with lymphopenia such that disease relapse occurred in the presence of severe lymphopenia. Synovial biopsies in lymphopenic patients who relapsed showed that there were diffuse mononuclear infiltrates with CD4+ and CD8+ lymphocytes still present[25], so that the changes in peripheral blood were not reflected in the synovium.

The experience with the chimeric depleting anti-CD4 monoclonal antibody, cM-T412 (Centocor Inc.), further highlights this problem. cM-T412 produced a dose-dependent reduction in the number of circulating CD4+ lymphocytes which was protracted when high doses were given, especially with concomitant methotrexate[26,27]. Clinical improvement was variable and correlated with synovial fluid but not peripheral blood changes. After a single 50 mg dose of cM-T412, there was a severe CD4 lymphopenia and over 90% of the peripheral blood CD4+ lymphocytes were coated with cM-T412. In contrast, there was no change in synovial fluid CD4+ lymphocyte number and only 11% of synovial CD4+ cells were coated with cM-T412. After five daily treatments with cM-T412, there was a statistically significant reduction in the number of synovial fluid CD4+ lymphocytes. Interestingly, the percentage of synovial fluid lymphocytes coated with cM-T412 varied greatly among patients; crucially, the percentage of cM-T412-coated synovial lymphocytes correlated with the percentage of clinical improvement[27].

These results suggested that, when cM-T412 is given intravenously, it binds to peripheral blood CD4+ T cells. Most of these cells do not contribute significantly to synovitis. One may construe that the dose and treatment regimen of cM-T412 is critical in producing a clinical response because these determine the amount of cM-T412 entering the joint. Among the synovial CD4+ lymphocytes, most are recruited non-specifically to the joint and only a small proportion are the disease-driving arthritogenic lymphocytes. Therefore, if one aims to improve arthritis by depleting synovial CD4+ lymphocytes, sufficiently high doses must be given to achieve significant concentration in the joint. However, at these doses of depleting monoclonal antibodies, there may be severe depletion of peripheral CD4+ lymphocytes for a prolonged period, resulting in an unacceptable level of immunosuppression, although this has not been reported in the cM-T412-treated patients even after several years of lymphopenia. This principle is likely to apply to all depleting anti-T cell monoclonal antibodies. Therefore, the T cell depletion strategy has been abandoned in favor of a strategy aiming to modulate T cells.

Semi-specific T cell immunomodulation

Non-depleting anti-CD4 monoclonal antibodies

The rationale for using non-depleting anti-CD4 monoclonal antibody in RA was developed initially in animal models of disease[28]. In streptococcal cell wall arthritis, a single course of a non-depleting anti-CD4 monoclonal antibody, given at the time of disease induction, prevented the development of arthritis. Moreover, the treated animals acquired a resistance to further attempts at disease induction. This phenomenon is known as 'immunological tolerance'. In non-obese diabetic mice, an animal model of Type I diabetes, anti-CD4 monoclonal antibody can induce tolerance even in established disease[29]. Interestingly, CD4 lymphocyte depletion was not necessary to produce tolerance[30]. On the contrary, established anti-CD4 monoclonal antibody-mediated tolerance could be broken by lymphocyte depletion, suggesting tolerance is an active lymphocyte-mediated process[31]. If anti-CD4 monoclonal antibodies could induce tolerance in established human autoimmune diseases, such as RA, it is hypothesized that this could result in 're-programing' of the immune response and, hence, long-term disease improvement[32].

Four non-depleting anti-CD4 monoclonal antibodies have been tested in RA:

IDEC-CE9.1/SB-210396 (Smith Kline and Beecham) IDEC-CE9.1/SB-210396 is a primatized, non-depleting anti-CD4 monoclonal antibody. It is known as a primatized monoclonal antibody because it was raised initially in macaques. In a randomized, placebo-controlled trial[33], patients with refractory RA were treated either with placebo or three different doses (40, 80, and 140 mg) of IDEC-CE9.1/SB-210396 twice weekly for four weeks. In the two high dose groups, there were statistically significant clinical improvements although some patients in the 140 mg group developed leukocytoclastic vasculitis that necessitated termination of treatment.

4162W94 (Glaxo Wellcome) 4162W94 is a humanized, non-depleting anti-CD4 monoclonal antibody. In an open-labelled dose-escalating study, 24 RA patients in four cohorts were treated with five daily doses of 10, 30, 100, or 300 mg monoclonal antibody, respectively. Clinical improvement with reduction in ESR and CRP was seen in patients treated with either 100 or 300 mg doses[34]. Interestingly, there were reductions in synovial fluid IL-6 and TNF-α levels. Treatments were well tolerated but half the patients developed a cytokine release syndrome. The concentration of synovial fluid 4162W94 was ~30% of the corresponding plasma level[34]. In a subsequent placebo-controlled trial 48 patients with RA were dosed with one (cohort 1), two (cohort 2) or three (cohort 3) cycles of 5×300 mg 4162W94 or placebo (12 and 4 patients, respectively, per cohort) at monthly intervals[35]. Sixteen patients were dosed in each of the first two cohorts; however, the dose was reduced in cohort 3 after five patients received ≥ 2 dose cycles due to accumulating evidence of a high frequency of rash. These patients were analyzed according to the number of cycles received. A further eight patients received 5×100 mg for 1–3 cycles prior to stopping the study for administrative reasons. An American College of Rheumatology (ACR)20 response was observed in 4/13 ($p = 0.119$ vs. placebo) and 7/13 ($p = 0.015$ vs. placebo) in cohorts 1 and 2, respectively. No 5×100 mg/day or placebo patients achieved ACR20. Four patients were still responding at the end of the three month follow-up period. CD4 lymphocyte suppression ($<0.2 \times 10^9$/L on ≥ 2 successive occasions) occurred in 11/34 patients who received 4162W94 compared to none on placebo. Rash occurred in 21/34 monoclonal antibody-treated patients, including one case of biopsy-confirmed cutaneous vasculitis, and 1/11 placebo patients. 4162W94 demonstrated significant clinical efficacy in this study. However, because of unacceptable CD4 lymphopenia and rash, the original hypothesis of prolonged CD4 'blockade' to give lasting clinical benefit could not be tested.

Humax-CD4/HM6G (Genmab) Humax-CD4/HM6G is a fully human anti-CD4 IgG1 monoclonal antibody. A single dose of Humax-CD4 of 0.005, 0.05, 0.15, 0.5, or 1.0 mg/kg was given by subcutaneous injection to cohorts of five patients, with four patients randomized to active treatment and one patient to placebo[36]. Between days 1 and 7, CD4+ lymphocyte counts transiently decreased after treatment but recovered by day 7. Improvements in the disease during the follow-up period were reported in the highest dose groups. For most patients the maximal improvement occurred 28 days after treatment. Further trials will be required to confirm its clinical efficacy.

OKT4-cdr4a (Johnson & Johnson) The results of a placebo-controlled trial using the humanized, non-depleting anti-CD4 monoclonal antibody OKT4-cdr4a have not been published in full, but a preliminary communication suggested that it might be efficacious[37].

Development of IDEC-CE9.1/SB-210396 and 4162W94 have been stopped because of lymphocyte depletion and side-effects. Although short-term clinical trials suggest that non-depleting anti-CD4 monoclonal antibodies suppress inflammation, long-term studies are necessary to assess whether they could achieve the holy grail of immunotherapy, the induction of prolonged disease remission without the need for ongoing long-term treatment.

Non-depleting anti-IL-2 receptor α chain (CD25) monoclonal antibody

A chimeric, non-depleting anti-CD25 monoclonal antibody (Novartis Pharmaceuticals) has recently been tested in six RA patients who had a partial response to methotrexate[38]. Intravenous bolus injections were administered on day 0 (0.02 mg), day 4 (0.2 mg), day 8 (2.0 mg), and day 12 (20 mg). Treatment led to significant CD25 saturation 2 h post-injection without evidence of depletion. Moreover, phytohemagglutinin-stimulated mononuclear cell proliferation, which is IL-2 dependent, was significantly reduced after treatment. Randomized controlled trials will be required to assess its efficacy in RA.

T cell vaccination

In animal models, it is fairly easy to identify the arthritogenic clones, which induce disease since they can be transferred from one animal to another. This has led to the development of the technique of T cell vaccination[39], analogous to bacterial vaccination, in which animals are immunized with pathogenic T cells, attenuated by chemicals or irradiation such that they can no longer induce disease. The animals develop an anti-vaccine immune response, which also inhibits the non-attenuated but otherwise immunologically identical pathogenic T cells responsible for the disease. T cell vaccination in animal models is able both to prevent and to treat established disease. Attempts have been made to apply this technique to humans, using synovial T cells, which are postulated to contain a higher proportion of pathogenic T cells than those in the blood; studies have been small and no firm conclusions can be drawn. No further studies are currently planned in RA, though more success has been reported in multiple sclerosis where a better potential candidate exists for the disease-causing antigen, myelin basic protein, enabling identification of possible disease-inducing T cells.

T cell receptor vaccination

An alternative approach to the identification of pathogenic T cells examined whether T cells with particular T cell receptor Vα or Vβ chains were expanded in lesional sites, such as the synovium, compared to blood. It was proposed that such expansions would be pathogenetically relevant. It was further suggested, by analogy with experiments in animals, that vaccination with unique peptides, derived from the sequence of the T cell receptors found on the surface of the pathogenic T cells, would inhibit disease[39]. Sadly, T cell populations expressing many different Vα and Vβ chains were reported as expanded by various groups of investigators. However,

one group looked at Vβ usage by recently activated T cells, defined as T cells expressing the IL-2 receptor; they felt these recently activated cells were more relevant to disease pathogenesis. On the basis of results showing an increase of Vβ17+ usage by IL-2 receptor positive (IL-2R+) T cells in the synovium, these investigators embarked on a clinical trial of a Vβ17-derived peptide in RA. This was an uncontrolled, open dose-finding study so evidence of clinical and biological efficacy must be treated cautiously. However, the investigators noted that patients' joint scores decreased at all follow-up visits, as did the frequency of Vβ17+ IL-2R+ T cells in the blood. Indeed, ~40% of patients developed a T cell response to the vaccinated peptide. No toxicity was observed. Subsequently, these investigators have used a combination of three TCR peptides (Vβ3, Vβ14, Vβ17) in incomplete Freund's adjuvant as a vaccine (IR501, Immune Response Corp.) in a placebo-controlled trial of 99 RA patients[40]. The vaccine (90 or 300 mg) or placebo was administered as intramuscular injections at weeks 0, 4, 8, and 20. In the 90 mg group there was a statistically significant improvement when compared with placebo, although only a third of the patients showed a response to the vaccine. A subsequent randomized, placebo-controlled trial assessed the effect of IR501 and IR703 in 340 RA patients[41]. IR703 consists of three, 40 amino acid peptides, which encompass the IR501 peptides. Patients were randomized into five groups and received IR501 (30 mg, 90 mg), IR703 (30 mg, 90 mg), or placebo. Four intramuscular injections were given at weeks 0, 4, 8, and 20. Of the patients in the IR501 30 mg group, 34% showed a statistically significant ACR20 improvement compared with 18% in the placebo group. The IR501 90 mg and IR703 90 mg groups also showed improvement but these did not reach statistical significance. Patients not receiving concomitant steroids and those with disease of less than three years showed greater clinical improvement.

MHC and MHC-peptide vaccines

Since RA is linked with the HLA-DRB1*0404 and DRB1*0401 in Northern Europeans and North Americans, vaccination using the disease-associated MHC or MHC-peptide may be efficacious. This approach is effective in experimental allergic encephalomyelitis, an animal model of multiple sclerosis. In RA, three doses (1.3, 4, and 13 mg) of HLA-DRB1*0404/B1*04041-peptide (Anergen) were administered to 52 RA patients who were heterozygous for the shared epitope as an adjunct to methotrexate[42]. Treatment was well tolerated and no significant immunosuppression was seen. However, only 33% and 31% of the patients developed antibody response to the vaccine.

A further study investigated the use of HLA-DRB1*0404/B1*04041 conjugated with the putative cartilage-derived RA autoantigen HC gp-39 as a vaccine. AG4263 is HLA-DRB1*0404/CDP263 (13mer peptide from HC gp-39). It was given to 31 HLA-DRB1*0404-positive RA patients in a randomized, placebo-controlled trial as an adjunct to methotrexate[43]. Seven intravenous doses of either placebo or (0.5–150 mg/kg) AG4263 were infused weekly. Eighty-nine percent of all AG4263-treated patients, compared with 57% of placebo patients, achieved Paulus 20 improvement criteria at any time point. Response was greatest among patients receiving the highest doses of AG4263, with 85.7%, 28.6%, and 0% in the 150 mg, 60 mg, and placebo patients responding, respectively, at day 28.

Interestingly, T cell response to tetanus toxoid and tuberculin protein product derivative was unaffected by treatment.

Oral tolerance with bovine collagen

The gut-associated lymphoid tissue (GALT) consists of the Peyer's patches, villi with epithelial cells, intraepithelial and lamina propria lymphocytes. These lymphocytes are highly specialized to protect the host from ingested pathogens and prevent the host from reacting to ingested foreign proteins. This local 'tolerance' to ingested foreign antigen can be spread systemically. In 1911, Wells first demonstrated that guinea pigs, fed with hen egg protein, were less likely to develop anaphylaxis when challenged systemically with hen egg protein[44].

Oral tolerance has been investigated as a possible therapy in many animal models of autoimmune diseases, including collagen-induced arthritis, experimental allergic encephalomyelitis, non-obese diabetes, and uveitis. Thompson and Staines first demonstrated that feeding with type II collagen prevented collagen-induced arthritis in disease susceptible rats[45]. WA/KIR rats were fed with 2.5 or 25 mg/g of type II collagen by gavage before immunization with type II collagen in incomplete Freund's adjuvant. The onset of inflammatory arthritis was delayed and the severity was reduced at both dosages. Similar suppression was seen in DBA/I mice using 300 mg/g of type II collagen[46]. Interestingly, collagen peptides are also capable of inducing arthritis and similarly they could be used to induce oral tolerance.

Bystander suppression describes the phenomenon where a fed antigen suppresses the immune responses stimulated by different antigens as long as the fed antigen is present in the anatomic vicinity. It solves a major conceptual problem in the therapeutic use of oral tolerance in inflammatory autoimmune diseases in which the autoantigens remain unknown, such as RA.

Bystander tolerance was first demonstrated *in vitro* when cells from myelin basic protein-fed animals could suppress proliferation of an ovalbumin cell line across a transwell[47]. Suppression was triggered only by the fed antigen. Subsequently, bystander suppression was demonstrated *in vivo* when feeding with ovalbumin suppressed experimental allergic encephalomyelitis[48]. Similarly, in animal models of RA, feeding with type II collagen suppressed adjuvant arthritis, antigen-induced arthritis, pristane-induced arthritis, silicone-induced arthritis, and streptococcal cell wall arthritis[49–52].

The mechanisms that lead to oral tolerance are complex and, in animal models, depend on the dose of the antigen fed. When animals are fed with a high dose of antigen, the major mechanism appears to be clonal deletion or anergy of antigen-specific T cells. In contrast, when animals are fed with a low dose of antigen, the mode of action is active immunosuppression mediated by a subset of T cells. These immunoregulatory T cells are generated initially in the GALT, which then migrate to the systemic immune system. Such regulatory T cells produce the Th2 cytokines IL-4, IL-10, and TGF-β[53,54]. These anti-inflammatory cytokines suppress the production of IL-1, IL-6, and TNF-α. In collagen-induced arthritis, there is evidence of switching from Th1 to Th2 response as anti-collagen antibodies shift from IgG2b to IgG1 isotype. Furthermore, in treated animals, TNF-α and IL-6 levels are decreased in the joints, and cells lines producing IL-4 and IL-10 could be established. Interestingly, anti-IL4

monoclonal antibodies can reverse the immunosuppressive effect of oral collagen in collage-induced arthritis[55].

Native type II collagen has been used to induce mucosal tolerance in RA. The initial study[56] showed a clinical improvement in patients treated with chicken-derived type II collagen compared to placebo; there was also an increase in the number of patients who went into remission. Disappointingly, a study from a different group, using bovine type II collagen[57], failed to demonstrate any significant effect. Both studies were underpowered and the former had serious trial design faults. In a large, randomized, placebo-controlled trial, 274 patients were treated with either placebo, or 20, 100, 500, or 2500 mg/day of chicken type II collagen for 24 weeks[58]. Three response criteria were used: Paulus, ACR, and 30% reduction in both tender and swollen joint counts. Statistically significant improvement was only detected in the 20 mg/day group when compared with placebo (39% vs. 19%) using Paulus criteria. Interestingly, presence of serum antibody to type II collagen was associated with clinical improvement.

Another randomized, placebo-controlled trial examined the effect of bovine type II collagen tablets with a lactose base in patients with RA59. The trial studied 55 patients with established RA for more than two years who had failed at least one DMARD. They were randomly assigned to receive placebo, 0.05 mg, 0.5 mg, or 5 mg daily of bovine type II collagen or placebo tablets for three months. All DMARDs were stopped at least four weeks before starting treatment but prednisolone was permitted at doses of less than 10 mg/day. There was no significant difference in disease activity between the placebo, 0.05 mg, and 5 mg groups. However, in the 0.5 mg group, disease activity reduced by ~15% from weeks 8 to 24, which is statistically significant when compared with the placebo-treated group. This unusual dose response could be explained by different modes of action at high and low dose. A high dose of antigen led to deletion or anergy of antigen specific T cells, while a low dose of antigen suppressed disease through release of cytokines such as IL-4, IL-10, and TGF-b. Since chicken and bovine type II collagen are not the autoantigens in all RA patients, depletion of collagen specific T cells is not the treatment objective. The main therapeutic aim of type II collagen in RA is the induction of bystander suppression. Therefore, the therapeutic dose range should be low and narrow. There were no side-effects associated with type II collagen treatment.

Current evidence suggests that oral tolerance may be efficacious, although the clinical effect is small. New strategies to enhance the immunomodulatory effect of mucosal tolerance may lead to more effective therapies.

Costimulation blockade

Proliferation and full activation of an effective antigen-specific T cell response require a specific TCR-mediated signal and at least one additional costimulatory signal provided by an antigen-presenting cell[60]. Triggering of the antigen-specific T cell receptor in the absence of a costimulatory signal can inhibit T cell responses or leads to programed cell death, and in some cases results in immunological tolerance. A number of costimulatory molecules have been identified but one of the major pathway involves interactions between the CD28 and CTLA4 molecules on T cells and their ligands CD80 (B7-1) and CD86 (B7-2) molecules on the surface of antigen-presenting cells. CD28 is constitutively expressed by all CD4 and some CD8 T cells while CTLA4 is expressed only on activated T cells[61]. Monocytes and dendritic cells express CD86 constitutively but other antigen-presenting cells only express CD86 when activated. CD80 is expressed primarily on activation. Binding of CD28 to CD80 or CD86 stimulates T cell growth. Conversely, binding of CTLA4 to CD80 or CD86 suppresses T cell activation. CD86 is expressed by macrophages, monocytes, dendritic cells, and some T cells in the rheumatoid synovium. The expression of CD86 and CD80 has been linked to disease status and treatment by DMARDs. Proliferation of synovial T cells can be inhibited by CTLA4-Ig fusion protein or anti-B7 or anti-CTLA4 monoclonal antibodies[62].

Animal models of blockade of costimulatory molecules

Ijima *et al.* constructed an adenovirus vector carrying a gene encoding a soluble form CTLA4-Ig fusion protein[63]. They tested its efficacy in collagen-induced arthritis. The vector was administered by intra-articular injections to mice prior to immunization with type II collagen. A single intra-articular injection was able to inhibit or delay the development of arthritis both clinically and histologically.

Abatacept (Bristol Meyer Squibb) in RA

Abatacept is a fusion protein formed by conjugating the external domain of human CTLA4 to the heavy-chain constant region of human IgG1 genetically. It binds both CD80 and CD86 on antigen-presenting cells, thereby preventing these molecules from engaging CD28 on T cells. Abatacept has high avidity for both CD80 and CD86, binding ~500–2500 times as avidly to these ligands as does CD28.

A preliminary study of Abatacept in RA showed that it was well tolerated as well as demonstrating efficacy, although the number of patients was small[64]. A double-blind, placebo-controlled trial randomized 214 adults with active RA, who had treated unsuccessfully with at least one DMARD, to either Abatacept (0.5, 2, or 10 mg/kg), LEA29Y (a second-generation T cell inhibitor now discontinued for further development), or placebo on days 1, 15, 29, and 57. DMARD was discontinued for at least 28 days prior to treatment[65]. ACR20 responses on day 85, the primary end-point of the trial, was met by 23%, 44%, and 53% of patients in the 0.5, 2, and 10 mg/kg groups, respectively, versus 31% in the placebo group.

Abatacept is also effective when given in combination with methotrexate. A large phase II, double-blind, randomized, placebo-controlled trial enrolled a total of 339 patients with RA taking concurrent methotrexate[66]. Patients were randomized to receive placebo, or 2 mg/kg or 10 mg/kg of Abatacept. Treatment was administered by intravenous infusions initially on days 1, 15, and 30, then monthly for six months. All patients continued with methotrexate. The primary end-point of the study was ACR20 response at six months. 259 patients completed the study. The study was completed by 259 patients, with more in the placebo group discontinuing therapy than in either of the Abatacept groups, the most common reason being lack of efficacy. The proportion of patients with an ACR20 response was significantly higher in the 10 mg group than placebo (60% vs. 35%). The rates of ACR50 and ACR70 response at six months were also significantly higher in both Abatacept groups than in the placebo group.

ACR50 was 37%, 23%, and 12%, while ACR70 was 17%, 11%, and 2% for 10 mg, 2 mg, and placebo, respectively. Quality of life scores measured by the Short Form-36 Health Survey (SF-36) also showed significant improvement from baseline in the 10 mg/kg group, compared to placebo. Abatacept was well tolerated; upper respiratory tract infection, nausea and vomiting, cough, diarrhea, and pharyngitis were more frequently reported in the 10 mg/kg group but statistically these were not significant.

Another double-blind, placebo-controlled, phase II trial randomized 121 patients with active RA who were partial responders to etanercept[67]. They were randomized to either 2 mg/kg Abatacept (85 patients) or placebo (36 patients) in addition to etanercept. There was an ACR20 response of 20% versus 28%, an ACR50 response of 26% versus 19%, and an ACR70 response of 11% versus 0%, in the Abatacept versus placebo groups, respectively. These data do not support major synergy between etanercept and abatacept.

A recently reported phase III trial of Abatacept in 547 RA patients with inadequate response to methotrexate or TNF-α was presented at the ACR annual scientific meeting of 2004. Of patients on Abatacept, 73.1% achieved an ACR20 response compared to 39.7% on placebo. ACR50 and ACR70 responses in the abatacept group were 48.3% and 28.8%, respectively, compared with 18.2% and 6.1% in the placebo group. There was also a statistically significant reduction in joint damage assessed by X-ray.

T cell immunomodulation using costimulatory signal inhibitor: Abatacept is efficacious in RA. It is likely that it will soon be available for use in routine clinical practice.

Anti-B cell therapy

B cell depletion

Rationale for deleting B cells in RA

The B cell had not been a main target for the treatment of RA until 1999 when Edwards *et al.* suggested that IgG RF immune complex might have a specific pathogenic role in RA[9]. They also argued that IgG RF is generated by chance mutation in the lymphoid aggregates of the synovium. Depleting B cells that produce IgG RF would be therapeutically beneficial. However, as there is no specific antibody that targets IgG RF B cells, the effect of nonspecific B cell depletion was examined.

Rituximab

Rituximab (Roche) is a genetically engineered, chimeric, anti-CD20 monoclonal antibody that depletes CD20+ B cells. CD20 is a 33–35kD antigen present on B cells but it is not expressed by stem cells, early pre-B cells, dendritic cells, or plasma cells. Rituximab is licensed for the treatment of non-Hodgkin's lymphoma.

Clinical trials of rituximab in RA

Edwards and Cambridge first published the beneficial effect of B cell depletion in RA[68]. In this open-label study, five patients were given rituximab. They also received concomitant high dose steroids and cyclophosphamide, a therapeutic regime used in non-Hodgkin's lymphoma, so the exact effect of rituximab was unclear. After a single course of treatment, CD20+ B cells became undetectable in the blood. All the patients met the ACR50 response criteria at 26 weeks, with three patients also achieving ACR70. Three patients received further treatments after disease relapsed. The encouraging result of this study led to the first randomized, double-blind, placebo-controlled trial of rituximab in RA[69]. This multi-center trial included 161 patients with active RA. The patients were assigned to one of four groups: methotrexate alone, rituximab, rituximab plus cyclophosphamide (750 mg on days 3 and 17), or rituximab plus methotrexate. Patients were given 1000 mg of rituximab or placebo intravenously on days 1 and 15 and followed up for 48 weeks. In addition to the above treatment all patients, including the methotrexate group, were given a 17-day course of corticosteroids, including intravenous methylprednisolone and high dose oral steroids. ACR20 and -50 responses were significantly higher in all the rituximab groups compared with the control group. Only the rituximab plus methotrexate group had significantly higher ACR70 responses (23% compared with 5% in the control group). There were a number of serious adverse events in the rituximab groups (highest in the rituximab plus cyclophosphamide group) and one patient in the rituximab alone group died from bronchopneumonia. Therefore, close monitoring for infection is needed in patients receiving rituximab.

These results suggest that rituximab may have a place in the treatment RA. In view of the increased infections in the cyclophosphamide group and the favorable results from the rituximab and methotrexate group, this would seem a more logical combination. The issue of the high dose steroids needs further clarification.

Conclusion

B and T cells are important mediators of rheumatoid synovitis. Therapies that target B and T cells such as rituximab and Abatacept showed promising results in randomized control trials in RA. Although they improve symptoms and signs, the best treatment regime for achieving long-term remission remains unknown. Nevertheless, elucidating the biological effect of these agents could lead to the design of better such treatment regimes in the future.

References

1. Pincus, T., Callahan, L.F., Sale, W. G., Brooks, A. L., Payne, L. E., and Vaughn, W. K. Severe functional declines, work disability, and increased mortality in seventy-five rheumatoid arthritis patients studied over nine years. *Arthritis Rheum* 1984; **27**: 864–72.
2. Pincus, T., and Callahan, L. F. Rheumatology function tests: grip strength, walking time, button test and questionnaires document and predict longterm morbidity and mortality in rheumatoid arthritis. *J Rheumatol* 1992; **19**: 1051–7.
3. Choi, H. K., Hernan, M. A., Seeger, J. D., Robins, J. M., and Wolfe, F. Methotrexate and mortality in patients with rheumatoid arthritis: a prospective study. *Lancet* 2002; **359**: 1173–7.
4. Pincus, T. Long-term outcome in rheumatoid arthritis. *Br J Rheumatol* 1995; **34** (Suppl. 2): 59–73.
5. Scott, D. L., Symmons, D. P., Coulton, B. L., and Popert, A. J. Long-term outcome of treating rheumatoid arthritis: results after 20 years. *Lancet* 1987; **1**: 1108–11.
6. Duke, O., Panayi, G. S., Janossy, G., and Poulter, L. W. An immunohistological analysis of lymphocyte subpopulations and their micro-environment in the synovial membranes of patients with RA using monoclonal antibodies. *Clin Exp Immunol* 1982; **49**: 23–30.
7. Duke, O., and Panayi, G. S. The pathogenesis of rheumatoid arthritis. *In vivo* 1988; **2**: 95–104.
8. Reparon-Schuijt, C. C., van Esch, W. J., van Kooten, C., Schellekens, G. A., de Jong, B. A., van Venrooij, W. J. *et al.* Secretion of anti-citrulline-containing peptide antibody by B lymphocytes in rheumatoid arthritis. *Arthritis Rheum* 2001; **44**: 41–7.
9. Edwards, J. C., Cambridge, G., and Abrahams, V. M. Do self-perpetuating B lymphocytes drive human autoimmune disease? *Immunology* 1999; **97**: 188–96.
10. Galeazzi, M., Afeltra, A., Porzio, F., and Bonomo, L. The activation markers on synovial T cells of rheumatoid arthritis. *Clin Rheumatol* 1990; **9**.
11. Loetscher, P., Uguccioni, M., Bordoli, L., Baggiolini, M., Moser, B., and Chizzolini. *et al.* CCR5 is characteristic of Th1 lymphocytes. *Nature* 1998; **391**: 344–5.
12. Brennan, F. M., and Feldmann M. Cytokines in autoimmunity. *Curr Opin Immunol* 1992; **4**: 754–9.
13. Choy, E. H. S, Rankin, E. C. C., Kassimos, D., Vetterlein, O., Sopwith, M., Eastell, R. *et al.* Engineered human anti-tumour necrosis factor alpha (TNF) antibody (Ab) reduces serum interleukin-6 (IL-6) and urine bone markers but has no effect on soluble CD4 (sCD4) and soluble interleukin-2 receptor (sIL2R) in rheumatoid arthritis (RA). *Br J Rheumatol* 1996; **35** (Suppl.), 172.
14. Lanchbury, J. S., Sakkas, L. I., and Panayi, G. S. Genetic factors in rheumatoid arthritis. In *Rheumatoid Arthritis: Recent Research Advances* (Smolen, J. R., Kalden, J. R., Maini, R. N., eds), pp. 17–28. Berlin: Springer-Verlag; 1992.
15. Boki, K. A., Panayi, G. S., Vaughan, R. W., Drosos, A. A., Moutsopoulos, H. M., and Lanchbury, J. S. HLA class II sequence polymorphisms and susceptibility to rheumatoid arthritis in Greeks: the HLA-DR beta shared-epitope hypothesis accounts for the disease in only a minority of Greek patients. *Arthritis Rheum* 1992; **35**: 749–55.
16. Gregersen, P. K., Silver, J., and Winchester, R. J. The shared epitope hypothesis: an approach to understanding the molecular genetics of susceptibility to rheumatoid arthritis. *Arthritis Rheum* 1987; **30**: 1205–13.
17. Verheijden, G. F., Rijnders, A. W., Bos, E., Coenen-de Roo, C. J., van Staveren, C. J. *et al.* Human cartilage glycoprotein-39 as a candidate autoantigen in rheumatoid arthritis. *Arthritis Rheum* 1997; **40**: 1115–25.
18. Kirkham, B. W., Pitzalis, C., Kingsley, G. H., Chikanza, I. C., Sabharwal, S., Barbatis, C. *et al.* Monoclonal antibody treatment in rheumatoid arthritis: clinical and immunological effects of a CD7 monoclonal antibody. *Br J Rheumatol* 1991; **30**: 459–63.
19. Kirkham, B. W., Thien. F., Pelton, B. K., Pitzalis, C., Amlot, P., Denman, A. M. *et al.* Chimeric CD7 monoclonal antibody therapy in rheumatoid arthritis. *J Rheumatol* 1992; **19**: 1348–52.
20. Lazarovits, A. I., White, M.J., and Karsh, J. CD7- T cells in rheumatoid arthritis. *Arthritis Rheum* 1992; **35**: 615–24.
21. Strand, V., Lipsky, P. E., Cannon, G. W., Calabrese, L. H., Wiesenhutter, C., Cohen, S. B. *et al.* Effects of administration of an anti-CD5 plus immunoconjugate in rheumatoid arthritis: results of two phase II studies. The CD5 Plus Rheumatoid Arthritis Investigators Group. *Arthritis Rheum* 1993; **36**: 620–30.
22. Olsen, N. J., Brooks, R. H., Cush, J. J., Lipsky, P. E., St Clair, E. W., Matteson, E. L. *et al.* A double-blind, placebo-controlled study of anti-CD5 immunoconjugate in patients with rheumatoid arthritis. *Arthritis Rheum* 1996; **39**: 1102–8.
23. Isaacs, J. D., Watts, R. A., Hazelman, B. L., Hale, G., Keogan, M. T., Cobbold, S. P. *et al.* Humanised monoclonal antibody therapy for rheumatoid arthritis. *Lancet* 1992; **340**: 748–52.

24. Isaacs, J. D., Manna, V. K., Rapson, N., Bulpitt, K. J., Hazleman, B. L., Matteson, E. L. *et al*. Campath-1H in rheumatoid arthritis: an intravenous dose-ranging study. *Br J Rheumatol* 1996; **35**: 231–40.

25. Ruderman, E. M., Weinblatt, M. E., Thurmond, L. M., Pinkus, G. S., and Gravallese, E. M. Synovial tissue response to treatment with Campath-1H. *Arthritis Rheum* 1995; **38**: 254–8.

26. Choy, E. H. S., Chikanza, I. C., Kingsley, G. H., Corrigall, V., and Panayi, G. S. Treatment of rheumatoid arthritis with single dose or weekly pulses of chimaeric anti-CD4 monoclonal antibody. *Scand J Immunol* 1992; **36**: 291–8.

27. Choy, E. H., Pitzalis, C., Cauli, A., Bijl, J. A., Schantz, A., Woody, J. *et al*. Percentage of anti-CD4 monoclonal antibody-coated lymphocytes in the rheumatoid joint is associated with clinical improvement: implications for the development of immunotherapeutic dosing regimens. *Arthritis Rheum* 1996; **39**: 52–6.

28. Van den Broek, M. F., Van de Langerijt, L. G., Van Bruggen, M. C., Billingham, M. E., and Van den Berg, W. B. Treatment of rats with monoclonal anti-CD4 induces long-term resistance to streptococcal cell wall-induced arthritis. *Eur J Immunol* 1992; **22**: 57–61.

29. Hutchings, P., O'Reilly, L., Parish, N. M., Waldmann, H., and Cooke, A. The use of a non-depleting anti-CD4 monoclonal antibody to re-establish tolerance to beta cells in NOD mice. *Eur J Immunol* 1992; **22**: 1913–18.

30. Carteron, N. L., Wofsy, D., and Seaman, W. E. Induction of immune tolerance during administration of monoclonal antibody to L3T4 does not depend on depletion of L3T4+ cells. *J Immunol* 1988; **140**: 713–16.

31. Parish, N. M., Hutchings, P. R., Waldmann, H., and Cooke, A. Tolerance to IDDM induced by CD4 antibodies in nonobese diabetic mice is reversed by cyclophosphamide. *Diabetes* 1993; **42**: 1601–5.

32. Cobbold, S. P., Qin, S. X., and Waldmann, H. Reprogramming the immune system for tolerance with monoclonal antibodies. *Semin Immunol* 1990; **2**: 377–87.

33. Levy, R., Weisman, M., Wiesenhutter, C., Yocum, D., Schnitzer, T., Goldman, A. *et al*. Results of a placebo-controlled, multicenter trial using a primatized, non-depleting, anti-CD4 monoclonal antibody in the treatment of rheumatoid arthritis. *Arthritis Rheum* 1996; **39** (Suppl.): S122.

34. Choy, E. H., Connolly, D. J. A., Rapson, N., Jeal, S., Brown, J. C., Kingsley, G. H. *et al*. Pharmacokinetic, pharmacodynamic and clinical effects of a humanised IgG1 anti-CD4 monoclonal antibody in the peripheral blood and synovial fluid of rheumatoid arthritis patients. *Rheumatology* 2000; **39**: 1139–46.

35. Panayi, G. S., Choy, E. H. S., Emery, P., Madden, S., Breedveld, F. C., Kraan, M. C. *et al*. Repeat-cycle study of high-dose intravenous (iv) 4162w94 anti-CD4 monoclonal antibody (mAb) in rheumatoid arthritis (RA). *Arthritis Rheum* 1998; **41**: S56.

36. Baslund, J., Skjoedt, H., Klausen, T., Moreland, L. M., Svedberg, A., Moeller, C., and Petersen, J. A phase I, double-blind, randomized, placebo-controlled study of a non-depleting fully human anti-CD4 monoclonal antibody (HUMAX-CD4/HM6G) in patients with active rheumatoid arthritis. *Arthritis Rheum* 2000; **43** (Suppl.): S289.

37. Schulze-Koops, H., Davis, L. S., Haverty, P., Wacholtz, M. C., and Lipsky, P. Reduction of Th1 cell activity in patients with rheumatoid arthritis after treatment with a non-depleting monoclonal antibody to CD4. *Arthritis Rheum* 1997; **40** (Suppl.): S191.

38. Hammaker, D. R., McGowan, P. F., and Yocum, D. E. Chimeric anti IL-2 receptor α chain (CD25) antibody in rheumatoid arthritis (RA) patients receiving concomitant methotrexate (MTX): immunopharmacological effects. *Arthritis Rheum* 1999; **42** (Suppl.): S238.

39. Choy, E. H. S., Kingsley, G. H., and Panayi, G. S. (1995). T-cell regulation. In *Innovative treatment approaches for rheumatoid arthritis* (Brooks PM, Furst DE, eds), pp. 653–71. London, Baillière Tindall.

40. Moreland, L. W., Heck, Jr., L. W., Koopman, W. J., Saway, P.A., Adamson, T. C., Fronek, Z. *et al*. Vβ17 T cell receptor peptide vaccination in rheumatoid arthritis: results of phase I dose escalation study. *J Rheumatol* 1996; **23**: 1353–62.

41. Moreland, L., Koopman, W. J., Adamson, T., Calabrese, L., Cash, J., Markenson, J. *et al*. Results of phase II rheumatoid arthritis clinical trial using T cell receptor peptides. *Arthritis Rheum* 1997; **40**: S223.

42. St Clair, E. W., Cohen, S. B., Fleischmann, R. M., Lee, S., Moreland, L., Olsen, N. J. *et al*. Vaccination of rheumatoid arthritis patients with DR4/1-peptide. *Arthritis Rheum* 1997; **40**: S96.

43. Kivitz, A. J., Paulus, H. E., Olsen, N. J., Weisman, M. H., Matteson, E. L., Furst, D. E. *et al*. Allele- and antigen-specific treatment of rheumatoid arthritis: final results from a double blind placebo controlled phase I trial. *Arthritis Rheum* 2000; **43** (Suppl.): S392.

44. Wells, H. Studies on the chemistry of anaphylaxis. III. Experiments with isolated proteins, especially those of hen's egg. *J Infect Dis* 1911; **9**: 147–51.

45. Thompson, H. S., and Staines, N. A. Gastric administration of type II collagen delays the onset and severity of collagen-induced arthritis in rats. *Clin Exp Immunol* 1986; **64**: 581–6.

46. Nagler-Anderson, C., Bober, L. A., Robinson, M. E., Siskind, G. W., and Thorbecke, G. J. Suppression of type II collagen-induced arthritis by intragastric administration of soluble type II collagen. *Proc Natl Acad Sci U S A* 1986; **83**: 7443–6.

47. Miller, A., Lider, O., and Weiner, H. L. Antigen-driven bystander suppression after oral administration of antigens. *J Exp Med* 1991; **174**: 791–8.

48. Miller, A., Lider, O., Roberts, A. B., Sporn, M. B., and Weiner, H. L. Suppressor T cells generated by oral tolerization to myelin basic protein suppress both in vitro and in vivo immune responses by the release of transforming growth factor beta after antigen- specific triggering. *Proc Natl Acad Sci U S A* 1992; **89**: 421–5.

49. Yoshino, S., Quattrocchi, E., and Weiner, H. L. Suppression of antigen-induced arthritis in Lewis rats by oral administration of type II collagen. *Arthritis Rheum* 1995; **38**: 1092–6.

50. Thompson, S. J., Thompson, H. S., Harper, N., Day, M. J., Coad, A. J. *et al*. Prevention of pristane-induced arthritis by the oral administration of type II collagen. *Immunology* 1993; **79**: 152–7.

51. Yoshino, S. Downregulation of silicone-induced chronic arthritis by gastric administration of type II collagen. *Immunopharmacology* 1995; **31**: 103–8.

52. Zhang, Z. J., Lee, C. S. Y., Lider, O., and Weiner, H. L. Suppression of adjuvant arthritis in Lewis rats by oral administration of type II collagen. *J Immunol* 1990; **145**: 2489–93.

53. Khoury, S. J., Hancock, W. W., and Weiner, H. L. Oral tolerance to myelin basic protein and natural recovery from experimental autoimmune encephalomyelitis are associated with downregulation of inflammatory cytokines and differential upregulation of transforming growth factor beta, interleukin 4, and prostaglandin E expression in the brain. *J Exp Med* 1992; **176**: 1355–64.

54. Chen, Y., Kuchroo, V. K., Inobe, J., Hafler, D. A., and Weiner, H. L. Regulatory T cell clones induced by oral tolerance: suppression of autoimmune encephalomyelitis. *Science* 1994; **265**: 1237–40.

55. Yoshino, S. Treatment with an anti-IL-4 monoclonal antibody blocks suppression of collagen-induced arthritis in mice by oral administration of type II collagen. *J Immunol* 1998; **160**: 3067–71.

56. Trentham, D. E., Dynesius-Trentham, R. A., Orav, E. J., Combitchi, D., Lorenzo, C., Hafler, D. A. *et al*. Effects of oral administration of type II collagen on rheumatoid arthritis. *Science* 1993; **261**: 1727–30.

57. Sieper, J., Kary, S., Sorensen, H., Alten, R., Eggens, U., Huge, W. *et al*. Oral type II collagen treatment in early rheumatoid arthritis: a double-blind, placebo-controlled, randomized trial. *Arthritis Rheum* 1996; **39**: 41–51.

58. Barnett, M. L., Kremer, J. M., St Clair, E. W., Clegg, D. O., Furst, D., Weisman, M. *et al*. Treatment of rheumatoid arthritis with oral type II collagen: results of a multicenter, double-blind, placebo-controlled trial. *Arthritis Rheum* 1998; **41**: 290–7.

59. Choy, E. H. S., Scott, D. L., Kingsley, G. H., Thomas, S., Murphy, T., Staines, N., and Panayi, G. S. Control of rheumatoid arthritis (RA) by oral tolerance with bovine type II collagen (CII). *Ann Rheum Dis* 1999; **58** (Suppl.): 5 (OP10).

60. Davis, S. J., Ikemizu, S., Evans, E. J., Fugger, L., Bakker, T. R., and van der Merwe, P. A. The nature of molecular recognition by T cells. *Nat Immunol* 2003; **4**: 217–24.

61. Coyle, A. J., and Gutierrez-Ramos, J. C. The expanding B7 superfamily: increasing complexity in costimulatory signals regulating T cell function. *Nat Immunol* 2001; **2**: 203–9.

62. Verwilghen, J., Lovis, R., de Boer, M., Linsley, P. S., Haines, G. K., Koch, A. E. *et al.* Expression of functional B7 and CTLA4 on rheumatoid synovial T cells. *J Immunol* 1994; **153**: 1378–85.

63. Ijima, K., Murakami, M., Okamoto, H., Inobe, M., Chikuma, S., Saito, I. *et al.* Successful gene therapy via intraarticular injection of adenovirus vector containing CTLA4IgG in a murine model of type II collagen-induced arthritis. *Hum Gene Ther* 2001; **12**: 1063–77.

64. Russell, A., Shergy, W., Sany, J., Nuamah, I., Aranda, R., and Becker, J. Abatacept (CTLA4Ig; BMS 188667) treatment demonstrates rapid, persistent and sustained increases in ACR response rates over 1 year in patients with active rheumatoid arthritis. *[JOURNAL NAME]* 2004; **63**: 284.

65. Moreland, L. W., Alten, R., Van den, B. F., Appelboom, T., Leon, M., Emery, P. *et al.* Costimulatory blockade in patients with rheumatoid arthritis: a pilot, dose-finding, double-blind, placebo-controlled clinical trial evaluating CTLA-4Ig and LEA29Y eighty-five days after the first infusion. *Arthritis Rheum* 2002; **46**: 1470–9.

66. Kremer, J. M., Westhovens, R., Leon, M., Di Giorgio, E., Alten, R., Steinfeld, S. *et al.* Treatment of rheumatoid arthritis by selective inhibition of T-cell activation with fusion protein CTLA4Ig. *N Engl J Med* 2003; **349**: 1907–15.

67. Schiff, M., Genovese, M., Nuamah, I., Becker, J., and Weinblatt, M. CTLA4Ig (BMS-188667) in a phase IIb, multi-center, randomised, double-blind, placebo controlled study in rheumatoid arthritis patients receiving etanercept: association between clinical response and key biomarkers. *Ann Rheum Dis* 2003; **62** (Suppl. 1): 178.

68. Edwards, J. C., and Cambridge, G. Sustained improvement in rheumatoid arthritis following a protocol designed to deplete B lymphocytes. *Rheumatology (Oxford)* 2001; **40**: 205–11.

69. Edwards, J. C., Szczepanski, L., Szechinski, J., Filipowicz-Sosnowska, A., Emery, P., Close, D. R. *et al.* Efficacy of B-cell-targeted therapy with rituximab in patients with rheumatoid arthritis. *N Engl J Med* 2004; **350**: 2572–81.

41 | *Inhibition of proteolytic activity involved in cartilage breakdown*

Tim E. Cawston and David A. Young

Introduction

In severe cases of arthritis both cartilage and the underlying bone are destroyed and this prevents joints from functioning normally. Cartilage tissue consists of a single cell type, chondrocytes[1], which are embedded within an extracellular matrix (ECM) of aggrecan, type II collagen, and other minor components. The rod-shaped collagen molecules aggregate in a staggered array to form cross-linked fibers giving connective tissues strength and rigidity. Trapped between these collagen fibers are the aggrecan molecules[2] that, in the presence of hyaluronic acid, form highly charged aggregates that attract water into the tissue and allow cartilage to resist compression. Chondrocytes in normal adult cartilage maintain a steady state where the rate of matrix synthesis equals the rate of degradation. Any change in this steady state will affect the functional integrity of the cartilage. During growth and development synthesis of matrix components exceeds the rate of degradation; a reduction in the rate of matrix synthesis and an increase in the rate of degradation occurs during matrix resorption[3].

The primary cause of cartilage and bone destruction in joint pathology involves the elevated levels of active proteinases, secreted from a variety of cells, which degrade the ECM. These proteinases are regulated by different cytokines and growth factors acting on cells found within the joint. In osteoarthritis (OA) the proteinases produced by chondrocytes play a major role[4]. In contrast, in a highly inflamed rheumatoid joint the proteinases produced by chondrocytes, synovial cells, and inflammatory cells all contribute to the loss of tissue matrix[5]. This review will describe the different proteolytic enzymes that are produced by cells and implicated in the destruction of cartilage and bone tissue, and consider inhibition of the matrix metalloproteinases (MMPs) as a therapeutic target.

Articular cartilage and its destruction: the role of proteolytic enzymes

The five main classes of proteinases are classified according to the chemical group which participates in the hydrolysis of peptide bonds[6]. Cysteine, aspartate, and threonine proteinases are predominantly active at acid pH and act intracellularly; the serine and metalloproteinases are active at neutral pH, and act extracellularly (Fig. 41.1). Some proteinases are membrane-bound rather than secreted from the cell and such enzymes are associated with cytokine processing, receptor shedding, and the removal of proteins that are associated with cell-cell or cell-matrix interactions[7]. Some enzymes such as elastase are released when neutrophils are stimulated, whilst others may not participate in the cleavage of matrix proteins but activate proenzymes that degrade the matrix. All classes of proteinase play a part in the turnover of connective tissues and one proteinase pathway may precede another. For example, in bone the removal of the osteoid layer by metalloproteinases precedes the attachment of the osteoclast and subsequent breakdown of the ECM by cysteine proteinases[8]. A close apposition of intra- and extracellular pathways will be found in many conditions where there is connective tissue turnover.

Extracellular proteolysis: neutral proteinases

The metzincin superfamily

These metalloproteinases are distinguished by a highly conserved motif containing three histidines that bind zinc at the catalytic site and a conserved methionine turn that lies beneath the active-site zinc[9]. Metalloproteinases are further divided into four multigene families: the serralysins, the astacins, ADAMs (a disintegrin and metalloproteinase)/adamalysins, and MMPs[10]. These families are classified according to the sequence around the three conserved histidines that bind zinc. A fifth group, the pappalysins, has been proposed[11] that cleaves insulin-like growth factor binding protein (IGFBP)-4 and -5[12].

MMPs

The MMPs constitute a multigene family of over 23 secreted and cell surface zinc-dependent endopeptidases that process or degrade numerous substrates at neutral pH[13]. All MMPs contain common domains (Fig. 41.2), zinc is present at the catalytic center, and all are produced in a proenzyme form. Latency of the proMMP is maintained by the interaction of a conserved cysteine

Proteinases

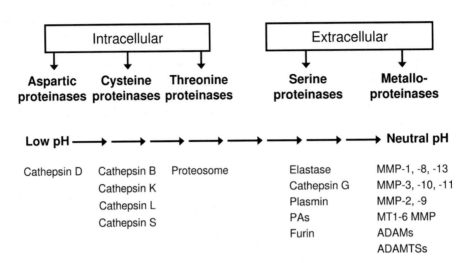

Fig. 41.1 The five classes of proteinase, three of which act predominantly intracellularly (aspartate, cysteine, and threonine) and two predominantly extracellularly (metallo- and serine). Examples are shown of enzymes from each class. ADAMTS, a disintegrin and metalloproteinase with thrombospondin motif.

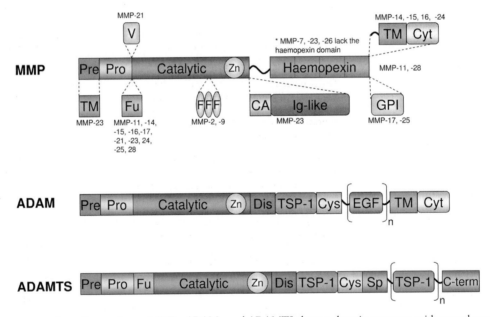

Fig. 41.2 Domain structures of metalloproteinases. MMPs, ADAMs, and ADAMTSs have a domain structure, with several common domains across the family. All have a zinc binding domain and propeptide that preserves latency. Other domains influence the behavior of the protein; the transmembrane (TM) domain anchors the proteinase onto the membrane surface whilst other domains bind to different components of the extracellular matrix. The MMPs were originally classified according to their substrate specificity but are now more commonly grouped according to their domain structure. All MMPs have a catalytic domain containing the active site zinc (Zn). Some MMPs contain a furin recognition motif (Fu) that allows intracellular activation by furin-like proteinases. Apart from MMP -7, -26, and -23, all MMPs contain a hemopexin domain that often determines substrate specificity. Other domains found within the MMPs are the fibronectin-like domains (F) in MMP-2 and -9 and the vitronectin-like domain (v) in MMP-21. Some MMPs are anchored to the cell surface via a TM with a cytoplasmic tail (Cyt) or via a GPI anchor. MMP-23 is structurally unique amongst the MMPs and contains an N-terminal TM (actually an N-terminal signal anchor), a cysteine array (CA), and an immunoglobulin-like domain (Ig-like) (adapted from Ref. 10). The ADAMs and ADAMTSs contain a disintegrin and a metalloprotease domain. The metalloprotease domains of ADAMs can induce ectodomain shedding and cleave ECM proteins. The ADAMs disintegrin (Dis) and cysteine-rich (Cys) domains have adhesive activities. All ADAMs contain a TM and their activities may be controlled in part via phosphorylation of their cytoplasmic tails (Cyt). The ADAMTSs uniquely contain a thrombospondin type-1 (TSP-1) repeat, then a Cys domain and one or more additional TSP-1 repeats (except ADAMTS-4). This is frequently followed by a C-terminal domain often containing a recently described protease and lacunin motif[34]. See also colour plate section.

residue in the prodomain with the catalytic zinc in the active site[14,15]. The MMP family are best known for their ability to cleave components of the ECM, but also cleave other proteinases, proteinase inhibitors, latent growth factors, chemotactic molecules, growth factor binding proteins, cell surface receptors, and cell-cell adhesion molecules (Table 41.1)[16].

Traditionally MMPs were divided into different groups, according to their substrates, called the stromelysins, collagenases, and gelatinases[13]. MMP-3 and MMP-10 (stromelysin-1

and -2, respectively) have a broad and similar substrate specificity[17] but the expression pattern of these enzymes is often distinct. Their natural substrates are probably proteoglycans, fibronectin, and laminin. Both enzymes are able to activate latent collagenases[18-20] and are present in articular cartilage and synovium from patients with either rheumatoid arthritis (RA) or OA[21-23].

There are three mammalian collagenases: MMP-1, MMP-8, and MMP-13 (collagenase-1, -2, and -3, respectively). These enzymes cleave fibrillar collagens, producing three-quarter- and

Table 41.1   MMP substrates

Enzyme		ECM substrates	Non-ECM substrates
MMP-1	Collagenase 1	Aggrecan, collagens I, II, III, VII, VIII, X, XI, entactin, fibronectin, gelatin, laminin, link protein, myelin basic, perlecan, tenascin, versican, vitronectin	α_1AC, α_2M, α_1PI, IL-1β, proMMP-2, proTNF-α
MMP-2	Gelatinase A	Aggrecan, collagen I, III, IV, V, VII, X, XI, decorin, elastin, entactin, fibrillin, fibronectin, fibulins, gelatin, laminin, link protein, myelin basic, osteonectin, tenascin, versican, vitronectin	α_1AC, α_1PI, FGF-R1, MCP-3, proIL-1β, proMMP-1,-13, proTGF-β, proTNF-α, plasminogen
MMP-3	Stromelysin 1	Aggrecan, collagen III, IV, V, VII, IX, X, XI, decorin, elastin, entactin, fibrillin, fibronectin, gelatin, laminin, link protein, myelin basic, osteonectin, osteopontin, tenascin, versican	α_1AC, α_2M α_1PI, E-cadherin, MCP-3, proIL-1β, proMMP-1,-7,-8,-9,-13, proTGF-β, proTNF-α, plasminogen
MMP-7	Matrilysin	Aggrecan, collagen I, IV, decorin, elastin, entactin, fibronectin, fibulins, gelatin I, laminin, link protein, myelin basic, osteonectin, osteopontin, tenascin, vitronectin	β4 integrin, cell surface-bound Fas-L, pro-α-defensin, proMMP-2, α_1PI, proTNF-α, plasminogen, E-cadherin
MMP-8	Collagenase 2	Aggrecan, collagen I, II, III	α_2M, α_1PI
MMP-9	Gelatinase B	Aggrecan, collagen IV, V, XI, XIV, decorin, elastin, fibrillin, gelatin, laminin, link protein, myelin basic, osteonectin, versican, vitronectin	α_2M, α_1PI, proIL-1β, proTGF-β2, proTNF-α, plasminogen
MMP-10	Stromelysin 2	Aggrecan, collagen III, IV, V, elastin, fibronectin, gelatin, link protein	ProMMP-1,-8
MMP-11	Stromelysin 3	Aggrecan, fibronectin, laminin	α_2M, α_1PI,
MMP-12	Macrophage metalloelastase	Aggrecan, bone sialoprotein, collagen I, IV, elastin, entactin, fibrillin, fibronectin, gelatin I, laminin, myelin basic, osteopontin, vitronectin	α_2M, α_1PI, factor XII, proTNF-α, plasminogen, uPAR
MMP-13	Collagenase 3	Aggrecan, collagen I, II, III, VI, IX, X, XIV, fibrillin, fibronectin, gelatin I, osteonectin	α_1AC, α_2M factor XII, proMMP-9
MMP-14	MT1-MMP	Aggrecan, collagen I, II, III, entactin, fibrillin, fibronectin, gelatin I, laminin, vitronectin	α_2M, α_1PI, cell-bound CD44, factor XII, proMMP-2,-13, proTNF-α
MMP-15	MT2-MMP	Aggrecan, elastin, fibronectin, gelatin, laminin, vitronectin,	
MMP-16	MT3-MMP	Collagen III, fibronectin	ProMMP-2
MMP-17	MT4-MMP		ProMMP-2, proTNF-α
MMP-18	*Xenopus* collagenase	Collagen I, gelatin	
MMP-19		Collagen I, IV, fibronectin, gelatin, laminin, tenascin	
MMP-20	Enamelysin	Amelogenin	
MMP-21	*Xenopus* MMP		
MMP-22	Chicken MMP	Gelatin	
MMP-23			
MMP-24	MT5-MMP	Gelatin	ProMMP-2, -9
MMP-25	MT6-MMP	Collagen IV, gelatin, fibronectin, fibrin	ProMMP-2
MMP-26	Endometase	Collagen IV, fibrinogen, fibronectin, gelatin, vitronectin	α_1PI, proMMP-9
MMP-27			
MMP-28	Epilysin		

α_2M, α2macroglobulin; α_1PI, α1proteinase inhibitor; α_1AC, α1antichymotrypsin; FGF, fibroblast growth factor; IL, interleukin; MCP, monocyte chemotactic protein; MT, membrane-type; TGF, transforming growth factor; TNF, tumor necrosis factor; uPAR: urokinase plasminogen activator receptor.
Adapted from Refs 16, 34, and 151.

one-quarter-sized fragments; MMP-2 and MMP-14 (membrane-type matrix metalloproteinases, MT1-MMP) can also cleave at this site[24,25]. The enzymes differ in their specificity for different collagens; MMP-13 prefers to cleave type II collagen[26] whilst MMP-1 and MMP-8 prefer types III and I, respectively. Both MMP-1 and MMP-13 are synthesized by macrophages, fibroblasts, and chondrocytes when these cells are stimulated with inflammatory mediators. MMP-8 is predominantly released from neutrophils upon stimulation of the cell but is also produced by chondrocytes. All three collagenases are present in diseased cartilage[27], although their control can be different; for example, retinoic acid, which down-regulates MMP-1, is known to up-regulate MMP-13 in some cells[28].

The two gelatinases cleave denatured collagens, type IV and V collagen, and elastin[24,29]. MMP-2 (gelatinase A) is the most widespread of all the MMPs and can activate proMMP-13[20]. MMP-9 (gelatinase B) is expressed in a wide variety of transformed and tumor-derived cells[30]. MMP-2 and MMP-9 protein levels are elevated in RA synovial fluids and tissues[31–33].

With the increasing numbers, complexity, and range of substrates MMPs are now often grouped according to their domain structure[34] (Fig. 41.2). Most MMPs resemble MMP-1; MMP-2 and MMP-9 have fibronectin-like inserts, whilst MMP-21 has a vitronectin-like domain insert. MMP-17 and MMP-25 both have a cytoplasmic glycosylphosphatidyl inositol (GPI) anchor, MMP-23 has a C-terminal immunoglobulin-like domain, and neither MMP-7 (matrilysin) nor MMP-26 has a hemopexin domain[10].

There is an increase in levels of different MMPs in rheumatoid synovial fluid, in conditioned culture media from rheumatoid synovial tissues and cells, synovial tissue at the cartilage–pannus junction from rheumatoid joints, osteoarthritic cartilage, and in animal models of arthritis[27,30,35,36]. In OA, both the rate of matrix synthesis and breakdown are increased, leading to the formation of excess matrix in some regions (such as osteophytes) with focal loss of matrix in other areas.

Control of MMPs

MMPs regulate many biological processes and consequently are precisely controlled at a number of critical steps that include: synthesis and secretion, activation of the proenzymes, inhibition of the active enzymes, and localization and clearance of MMPs (Fig. 41.3).

Synthesis and secretion

Cytokines such as IL-1, TNF-α, and IL-17 stimulate numerous cell types to produce MMPs[37,38]. Within the arthritic joint different cell types produce specific cytokines and growth factors which can be found in synovial fluids from RA patients. These cytokines often differ in their action on individual cell types and many cytokines can synergize to increase the production of MMPs by cells.

Activation of the proenzymes

The control of activation of the proenzyme form of MMPs is important in connective tissue breakdown[39,40]. The proteolytic removal of the propeptide is likely to be achieved in a tightly controlled environment close to the cell surface. Plasmin and other serine proteinases can activate some proMMPs[20,41–43] and are involved in the activation cascades of the pro-collagenases[40]. Active MMP-3 can activate pro-collagenases and other proMMPs[18,19,26,44]. Some MMPs (Fig. 41.2) have a furin recognition sequence between the propeptide and the catalytic domain and these enzymes are often activated within the golgi. Recent data show that cartilage explant

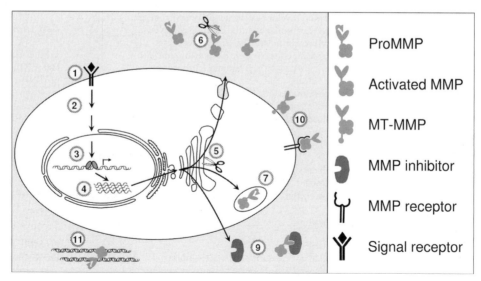

Fig. 41.3 Control of MMP activity. Cytokines and growth factors can up-regulate or down-regulate MMP expression (1). Different intracellular signalling pathways combine (2) to activate or suppress transcription (3). RNA can be unstable and rapidly processed (4). ProMMPs can be activated intracellularly by furin (5) or after they have left the cell (6). Some MMPs are stored in granules within the cell (7) prior to secretion. All active MMPs can be inhibited by TIMPs (9). Secreted MMPs can be expressed on the cell surface, bound to cell surface receptor proteins or sequestered by ECM proteins (10). Other control mechanisms include secretion to specific regions of the plasma membrane, proteolytic processing and inactivation of MMPs, and endocytosis and lysosomal breakdown. See also colour plate section.

cultures, treated with cytokines and an inhibitor of furin, have reduced levels of active collagenases and low collagen release[45]. Several members of the MT-MMP family (MMP-14, -16, -24, and -25) can activate proMMP-2[46–50], and MMP-14 can also activate proMMP-13[20].

Inhibition of the active enzymes

All active MMPs are inhibited by tissue inhibitors of metalloproteinases (TIMPs)[35,51], which bind tightly to active MMPs in a 1:1 ratio (Fig. 41.3) and so can control connective tissue breakdown. If TIMP levels exceed those of active enzyme then connective tissue turnover is prevented. TIMP-2 is known to be associated with the activation of proMMP-2. TIMP-3 is bound by the ECM after secretion and inhibits some members of the ADAM family, whilst TIMP-4 is predominantly localized in the heart but can be produced by joint tissues[52]. TIMP-1 and -3 are up-regulated by growth factors such as TGFβ, IGF-1, and oncostatin M (OSM), and these agents also induce matrix synthesis[53]. All active MMPs bind to α2-macroglobulin and these complexes are rapidly cleared via endocytosis and degradation within the lysosomal system.

Localization and clearance

Proteolysis often occurs in the immediate vicinity of the cell in pericellular pockets close to the cell membrane where MMPs can be secreted to specific areas at the cell surface (Fig. 41.3)[54]. This allows a high degree of control and these localization mechanisms can enhance MMP activity, prevent access of MMP inhibitors, concentrate MMPs to their precise target substrate, and limit the extent of proteolysis to a discrete region. Although the MMPs with transmembrane domains are the most important cell surface enzymes, some MMPs bind to cell surface receptors, to cell surface activating enzymes, or to pericellular matrix proteins. Cell surface heparan sulfate can bind MMPs such as MMP-7[55], and also TIMP-3, whilst MMP-1 can bind to the cell surface protein EMMPRIN[56].

ADAM family of proteinases

To date, over 25 ADAM genes and 19 ADAMTS (A Disintegrin And Metalloproteinase with ThromboSpondin motifs) genes have been described. ADAMs are usually membrane-anchored proteinases with diverse functions conferred by the addition of different protein domains[7,57] (see Fig. 41.2). The disintegrin domain can bind to integrins and prevent cell–cell interactions; cysteine-rich, epidermal growth factor-like, transmembrane and cytoplasmic tail domains are also found (see Fig. 41.2). ADAM-17 is known for its ability to release TNF-α from the cell surface[58]. In addition to ADAM-17, ADAM-10, -12 and -15 have also been described in cartilage[59]. The ADAMTS family members are distinguished from the ADAMs in that they lack these latter three domains but have additional thrombospondin-1 (TSP-1) domains predominantly at the C-terminus which are thought to mediate interactions with the ECM[60].

The major aggrecan fragments from resorbing cartilage are cleaved at a specific Glu(373)–Ala(374) bond[61]. ADAMTS-1, -4, -5, -8, and -15 are all able to cleave proteoglycan at this bond[3,60,62–67], but recent compelling data from mouse knockout

(KO) studies indicate that ADAMTS-5 is the pathophysiological mediator of aggrecan catabolism[68,69]. Purified chondrocyte membranes also cleave at this site but it is not known if this activity is associated with a known aggrecanase or a different enzyme[62]. Recently, ADAMTS-9 was also identified as an aggrecanase, but cleaved aggrecan at the Glu(1771)–Ala(1772) bond[70].

Proteoglycan release from cartilage occurs following stimulation with a variety of mediators such as IL-1, TNF-α, IL-17, retinoic acid, and fibronectin fragments[71–73]. Levels of ADAMTS-4 are up-regulated in cartilage in response to IL-1 and TNF-α, and in synovial fibroblasts in response to TGF-β[67,74], whilst ADAMTS-5 appears to be unaffected. In an immortalized chondrocyte line, ADAMTS-1, -4, -5, and -9 were all regulated by a mixture of IL-1 and OSM, although the speed of induction differed between these enzymes[75,76]. Aggrecanase activity can be blocked by specific synthetic inhibitors[77] and by TIMP-3[78]. A role for neprilysin-induced aggrecanase activity via the generation of regulatory peptides has also been proposed[79].

Serine proteinases

Many *in vitro* experiments with tissue or cells point to a role for the plasminogen-plasmin system in the activation of proMMPs[13,80]. IL-1 and TNF-α-induced proteoglycan release can be blocked with an inactivator of urokinase-type plasminogen activator[81]. Inclusion of α1 proteinase inhibitor to resorbing cartilage effectively blocks the release of collagen, implicating serine proteinase(s) in the activation cascades of pro-inflammatory cytokine-induced proMMPs[40]. Both tissue- and urokinase-type plasminogen activators (tPAs and uPAs) are found in cartilage and cleave plasminogen to plasmin.

Other serine proteinase activities have been implicated in arthritis. Granzyme B can initiate proteoglycan degradation (but not collagen); granzyme B-positive cells can be detected in synovium and at the invasive front in RA[82]. Many enzymes have furin recognition motifs in their prodomains and studies have shown that blocking furin can prevent the release of collagen from resorbing cartilage[45].

Intracellular pathways: acid proteinases

Cysteine proteinases

Cysteine proteinase inhibitors prevent the resorption of bone explants[83,84], suggesting an involvement of lysosomal cysteine proteinases[85] in matrix resorption; they can degrade type I collagen at acidic pH[86,87]. Cathepsin B is raised in OA tissue and raised levels of cathepsins B, L, and H are found in antigen-induced rat arthritis models and within the rheumatoid joint. Incubation of resorbing cartilage with specific cathepsin B inhibitors blocked the release of proteoglycan fragments[88], suggesting an involvement in cartilage proteoglycan breakdown. Everts[89] showed that substantial amounts of fibrillar collagen accumulate intracellularly in the presence of cysteine proteinase inhibitors[90]. Cathepsin K plays a key role in collagen turnover and subsequent bone resorption[91,92]. It cleaves type I collagen at the N-terminal end of the triple helix at pH values as high as 6.5[93], and is produced by synovial fibroblasts, contributing to synovium-initiated bone destruction in the rheumatoid joint[94]. Both cathepsins K and S are expressed in RA and OA synovia[95] and there is evidence that cathepsin K is localized to sites of cartilage erosion[96]. Cathepsin K has potent aggrecan-degrading activity and the resulting degradation products potentiate the collagenolytic activity of cathepsin K toward types I and II collagen[97]. Inhibitors of cathepsin K are under development; however, their use in pathological conditions such as RA is currently problematic as delivery of the inhibitor to specific sites of action is required to prevent the inhibition of the normal physiological function of the enzyme[98].

Calpain (calcium-dependent neutral cysteine proteinase) can cleave proteoglycan[99] and its presence correlates with arthritis and tissue destruction[100]. However, the significance of calpain in arthritic disease is currently unclear[101].

Threonine proteinases

Threonine proteinases represent a relatively new class of proteinases[102]. The proteasome is a ubiquitously expressed, essential intracellular protease complex belonging to this new proteinase class. It performs many intracellular roles, including the degradation of phosphorylated and ubiquitinated inhibitor of kappa B (IκB).

Inhibition of MMPs

Relevance of knockout studies to discovering novel therapeutic drug targets

Mouse KO studies are a powerful approach for defining protein function but these data need to be interpreted carefully in humans and then used to develop novel targets for therapeutic intervention. Overall, mouse and human MMP orthologues appear to retain 65–80% identity at the amino acid levels[103]. However, there are significant differences; for example, the expression of the mouse orthologues of human MMP-1 is restricted exclusively to the uterus and testis[104]. Other limitations may include gene redundancy or compensation and whether the loss of a gene throughout development gives reliable information of the role of that gene in the adult. Humans and mice differ with respect to the distribution of load across the joints, which may be particular relevant when investigating arthritic diseases[105]. KO studies have highlighted many novel functions of MMPs[106,107]. The relevance of a KO phenotype to developing a small-molecule drug is high. A study of the KO phenotypes for the targets of the 100 best-selling drugs indicates that these phenotypes correlate well with known drug efficacy[108]. These studies demonstrate that highly specific MMP inhibitors could show great potential for the effective treatment of arthritis.

Mouse studies have shown that MMP activity is not always associated with pathology. For example, MMP-14 deficiency gives rise to severe connective tissue defects and the development

of arthritis[109,110], demonstrating that MMP-14 is necessary for maintaining healthy joints. A defect in the formation of osteocyte processes is found in these animals, indicating that the pathology could be caused by a disruption of bone development and function[111]. Thus the arthritic changes in MMP-14 KO mice could develop as a consequence of inappropriate remodeling of the ECM during growth or as a result of a disruption of the nutrient supply to the joint tissues during growth.

In antibody-induced arthritis (AbIA) MMP-2 KO mice show significantly exacerbated arthritis compared to wild-type mice[112], whilst MMP-9 KO mice show reduced signs of arthritis, indicating that whilst MMP-2 protects, MMP-9 enhances arthritis in this model[112]. Disruption of the MMP-3 gene has been investigated in three models of arthritis: antigen-induced arthritis (AIA)[113], collagen-induced arthritis (CIA)[114], and the induction of OA by surgical procedures[115]. All studies show no significant differences in either inflammation or proteoglycan depletion between the MMP-3 KO and controls. The major MMP cleavage site in aggrecan is at the Asn341–Phe342 bond, generating the carboxy-terminal neoepitope VDIPEN[116]. In the AIA model VDIPEN staining in cartilage was eliminated in MMP-3 KO mice; however, in CIA and surgical model mice VDIPEN staining were the same as in the wild-type mice. Collagen cleavage was eliminated in MMP-3 KO mice compared to wild-type controls in the AIA model and appears to have an important role in the mechanisms leading to cleavage of type II collagen[113]. This contrasts with the surgical model MMP-3 KO mice, which exhibited accelerated formation of OA lesions compared with wild-type mice. Clements *et al.* postulate that MMP-3 may play an important role in homeostasis in healthy cartilage, balancing anabolism and catabolism of the cartilage matrix[115].

Mice homozygous for the deletion of the catalytic domain of both ADAMTS-4 and ADAMTS-5 show no apparent developmental dysfunction and appear normal at birth and as adults. The ADAMTS-4 KO mice and wild-type littermates showed no differences in OA progression or severity after surgical induction of joint instability by transection of the meniscotibial ligament[68,117]. These data indicate that ADAMTS-4 is not the aggrecanase responsible for aggrecan degradation, at least in murine OA[68,117]. In the same OA model and in an AIA model the ADAMTS-5 KO mice were protected against aggrecan loss and cartilage erosion[68,69]. These two reports suggest ADAMTS-5 is the major aggrecanase in murine arthritic cartilage, although further studies are required to confirm the importance of the gene in human disease[68,69].

Synthetic MMP inhibitors

The important early advances involved in the design of MMP inhibitors were to discover potent inhibitors that avoid modification within the gut and to avoid any musculoskeletal side-effects. The early inhibitors were broad range inhibitors produced using conventional pharmaceutical screening processes. As the crystal structures of the catalytic domains of many MMPs became available, they explained in part the variation in substrate specificity amongst MMPs and have allowed the design of more specific synthetic inhibitors[118].

The challenges for MMP inhibition in the arthritides is to decide whether broad spectrum or targeted inhibition is best and if proteoglycan or collagen release should be the focus. Other considerations would involve the inclusion or avoidance of sheddase inhibition and to ensure that compounds avoid inhibition of MMPs that have essential and beneficial effects on tissue integrity.

MMP inhibitors and arthritis: animal and clinical trials

Relatively few synthetic MMP inhibitors have been studied in terms of their ability to prevent joint destruction in patients with arthritis but many have been shown to be effective in animal models of arthritis. Trocade (Ro 32-3555), a selective collagenase inhibitor, has a low nanomolar inhibition constant (Ki) against MMP-1, -8 and -13, with ~10–100-fold lower potency against MMP-2, -3, and -9. It blocks IL-1α-induced collagen release from cartilage explants and, *in vivo*, prevented cartilage degradation in a rat granuloma model, a *P. acnes*-induced rat arthritis model and OA model using the SRT mouse[119]. Over 1000 RA patients were treated with Trocade in a large-scale trial which was terminated after one year because of a lack of efficacy, although this drug was reported to be well tolerated in patients with RA[120].

Novartis have described an orally active hydroxamate MMP inhibitor, CGS 27023A. This broad spectrum inhibitor with nanomolar Ki against MMP-1, -2, -3, -9, -12, and -13 was chondroprotective in both the rabbit meniscectomy model of OA and the guinea pig model of spontaneous OA[121,122]. However, phase I clinical trials with this compound were halted due to concerns of toxicity, with musculoskeletal side-effects being reported.

Tanomastat (BAY 12-9566), a synthetic MMP inhibitor that targets MMP-3, -2, -8, -9, and -13, with low activity against MMP-1, is effective in guinea pig and canine models of OA[123]. Tanomastat was given to 300 OA patients for three months and no musculoskeletal side-effects were reported. The drug could be detected in human cartilage of treated patients undergoing joint replacement[124]. However, this compound was withdrawn from an 1800-patient phase III trial in OA following negative results in a separate trial of the same drug in cancer patients[125] (see later section on safety).

It is reported that Pfizer is developing an MMP-13 inhibitor, CP-544439, which is currently in phase II clinical trials. CPA-926, developed by Kureha and Sanyo for the potential treatment of OA, is also in phase II clinical trials, while the ONO-developed, broad-spectrum MMP inhibitor, ONO-4817, is in phase I clinical trials for OA. Furthermore, Pharmacia, Wyeth and Proctor & Gamble have all reported on the preclinical evaluation of MMP inhibitors for the treatment of arthritis[34].

Several recent reports have demonstrated efficacy of other MMP inhibitors in animal models of arthritis. Sabatini *et al.* have shown that S-34291, a wide-spectrum MMP inhibitor with a preferential effect on MMP-13 as compared with MMP-1, prevented the loss of cartilage *ex vivo* and in a guinea pig model of OA[126]. Two recent papers from Ishikawa *et al.* (Fujisawa Pharmaceuticals) established that the broad-spectrum metalloproteinase inhibitors FR217840 and FR255031 suppressed joint destruction in adjuvant and collagen-induced arthritis rat models, respectively, and have suggested these inhibitors may be novel anti-rheumatic drugs[127,128].

The antibiotic doxycycline is known to inhibit MMPs. Some recent derivatives can be shown to inhibit MMPs but have no antibiotic activity and have been proposed as a treatment to prevent cartilage damage in the arthritides[129]. These compounds are effective in animal models[130], but their effectiveness in RA patients is currently unclear[131,132]. A trial of 430 OA patients randomly assigned to receive either doxycycline or placebo was recently completed[133]. X-rays of the two groups were compared at 30 months: the initial results suggest that protection of the affected joint was seen in the treated patients. Interestingly, Periostat (CollaGenex Pharmaceuticals, Inc.), a subantimicrobial dose of doxycycline, is currently the only US Food and Drugs Administration-approved MMP inhibitor and is licensed for the treatment of periodontal disease.

A variety of explanations have been offered to explain why the metalloproteinase inhibitors have been unsuccessful in clinical trials in patients with joint diseases. There is no doubt that MMPs are present and active in joint diseases but if compounds are unable to penetrate the cartilage/bone/synovial interface they would be ineffective. Early inhibitors were originally screened against a limited set of available MMPs and so may not inhibit some MMPs that have subsequently been discovered. Further, data from MMP knockout mouse experiments clearly show that while certain MMPs are involved in cartilage destruction (e.g. MMP-9), others (e.g. MMP-2) may play a chondroprotective role[112].

Further studies are required to demonstrate the effectiveness of MMP inhibitors in the prevention of joint destruction, although the clinical evaluation of these drugs is difficult and expensive. Radiographs are still the most reliable measure of joint damage but any change in joint damage is impossible to detect over short periods of time. Whilst some progress has been made with the use of magnetic resonance imaging (MRI) to image joints, this technology is still to be proven and routine centers do not have access to validated methods for quantitation.

Safety of MMP inhibitors

MMPs are involved in many physiological processes so their inhibition could affect the rate of wound healing, growth, and fetal development. Metalloproteinases are involved in the activation and/or release of cytokines and growth factors from the ECM (Table 41.1)[16]. These released factors have a myriad of effects on cellular proliferation and behavior. Inhibition of these enzymes could lead to fibrosis, although dose-ranging studies should avoid such complications. The most advanced safety data available concern the musculoskeletal pain and tendonitis identified as a side-effect in treated patients[134]. These effects commence in the small joints of the hand and upper limbs, and the symptoms are time and dose dependent and reversible. These symptoms were seen with a Roche compound, Ro 31-9790, and this led to its development as an arthritis treatment being stopped. All new compounds can be very effectively screened in rodent models for these musculoskeletal events and compounds that cause these side-effects discarded. BAY 12–9566 was withdrawn as it was associated with increased tumor growth and poor survival times in small cell lung cancer, but no other cases of these effects have been reported. It is not necessarily logical to assume that an effect seen with one member of this class of compounds will automatically be seen with all and there are significant differences in chemical structure and metabolism of individual inhibitors. Finally, deleterious side-effects preventing the appropriate therapeutic dose from being administered may explain the lack of efficacy of MMP inhibitors such as Trocade in clinical trials[135].

Future prospects for the inhibition of MMP activity and expression

Signalling pathway inhibitors and MMP expression

The efficacy of anti-cytokine biotherapies in the treatment of RA patients provides supporting evidence that the inhibition of a signal-transduction pathway could be a potential therapeutic target. Cytokine-mediated transcriptional regulation has been shown to be a key mechanism in controlling the expression of many MMPs. The four main pathways involved in the inflammatory response are believed to be those acting through nuclear factor kappa B (NF-κB), mitogen-activated protein kinase (MAPK), phosphatidylinositol-3 protein (PI3) kinase, and janus kinase-signal transducer and activator of transcription (Jak-STAT). Both synthetic and natural inhibitors, along with biologics, of these pathways have been developed and tested both *in vitro* and *in vivo* with varying degrees of success[136]. For example, SP600125, a pharmacological inhibitor of the MAPK JNK (c-Jun N-terminal kinase) pathway decreases joint destruction in an adjuvant arthritis model, in part by diminishing the production of MMP-1[137]. IL-1α and OSM signal via the NF-κB and Jak-STAT pathways, respectively, a cytokine combination that *in vivo* causes a RA-like phenotype and rapid joint destruction concomitantly with an up-regulation of specific MMPs[138]. Gene therapies using inhibitors of both these pathways appear efficacious in arthritis animal models[139,140] and represent excellent potential methodologies to prevent the induction of the degradative MMPs.

Acetylation is a key post-translational protein modification that controls signal transduction and gene transcription events[141]. Substrates for acetylation include NF-kB and STATs, transcription factors that represent the end-points of IL-1 and OSM signalling, respectively. Deacetylation is mediated by a family of 11 enzymes, the histone deacetylases (HDAC). Many structurally divergent HDAC inhibitors (HDACi) have been developed as cancer therapies as they cause cancer cells specifically to undergo growth arrest, differentiation, or apoptosis *in vivo* and *in vitro*[142]. Several recent reports demonstrate that HDACi modulate gene expression in synovial cells *in vivo*[143–145]. Four structurally different HDACi (phenylbutyrate and the bacterial/fungal metabolites trichostatin A, FK228, and FR235222 (Fujisawa Pharmaceuticals)) blocked the proliferation of synovial fibroblasts, all probably by a similar mechanism involving the up-regulation of cell cycle inhibitors (p16[INK4] and p21[Cip1]). *In vivo*, this was mirrored with inhibition of TNF-α expression, leading to an abrogation of cartilage destruction[143,145]. These and other authors suggest that HDACi may represent a new class of compounds for treatment of inflammatory diseases[143,146].

The HDACi trichostatin A and sodium butyrate potently inhibit cartilage degradation in an explant assay. These compounds decreased the level of collagenolytic enzymes in explant-conditioned culture media and blocked the cytokine (IL-1α and OSM) induction of key MMPs (e.g. MMP-1, -3, -8, and -13) and aggrecanases (e.g. ADAMTS-4, ADAMTS-5, and ADAMTS-9) at the mRNA level[76]. These data indicate that HDACi function as potent repressors of metalloproteinase expression in chondrocytes and may therefore not only be a new treatment for RA but also potentially for any of the destructive arthritides mediated by metalloproteinases.

MMP—substrate interactions

As more detailed information about the interaction of MMPs with their substrates becomes available it may be possible to design inhibitors that target areas of the enzyme other than the active site. For example, the C-terminal hemopexin-like domain of collagenases has long been known to be required for collagenolysis, presumably because of interactions with substrate. The activation of the proenzyme is also a valid target, again requiring a detailed knowledge of the underlying biology[147].

Modification of TIMP function or expression

One further possibility for inhibiting metalloproteinase activity is to induce the expression of their natural inhibitors the TIMPs or exogenously deliver modified TIMPs that are specifically targeted to inhibit specific enzymes[147–149]. Both TIMP-1 and TIMP-2 are capable of preventing cartilage destruction *ex vivo*, while the N-terminal domain of TIMP-3 in a similar system can prevent aggrecan release. Adenoviral delivery of TIMP-1 and -3 prevented cartilage degradation and invasion by rheumatoid synovial fibroblasts *in vitro*[150]; however, their efficacy in arthritis animal model studies requires further confirmation.

Finally, like many metalloproteinases, TIMP-1, -3, and -4 are regulated at the transcriptional level and can be induced by a number of growth factors and cytokines. Modulation of these cytokine pathways may re-address the local balance of metalloproteinase and TIMP activities believed to be pivotal in determining the extent of ECM turnover in disease.

Conclusions

Inhibition of cartilage collagen destruction still remains an important and viable target to prevent joint damage in arthritic disease.

Although the trials of MMP inhibitors in patients have been disappointing, new agents are still under development and these may overcome some of the problems of both delivery and side-effects. A key to future success is to identify the specific MMPs that are responsible for destruction within arthritic joints in different diseases. This will allow highly specific inhibitors that target individual enzymes and potentially reduce side-effects.

It is likely that blocking MMPs will be more effective if combined with treatments that target earlier steps in inflammation. Furthermore, as noted above, MMPs are not alone in being implicated in joint disease. Serine proteinases are believed to be involved in MMP activation and cysteine proteinases have been shown to degrade collagen, particularly in the resorption of bone. It may be necessary to combine proteinase inhibitors, either in sequence or with other agents that hit other specific steps in the pathogenesis, before the chronic cycle of joint destruction found in these diseases can be broken.

Acknowledgements

We thank the arthritis research campaign, the Wellcome Trust, FARNE, Dunhill Medical Trust, JGW Pattinson Trust, and the Nuffield Foundation (Oliver Bird Fund) for financial support.

References

1. Goldring, M. B. The role of the chondrocyte in osteoarthritis. *Arthritis Rheum* 2000; **43**: 1916–26.
2. Iozzo, R. V. Matrix proteoglycans: from molecular design to cellular function. *Annu Rev Biochem* 1998; **67**: 609–52.
3. Mort, J. S., and Billington C. J. Articular cartilage and changes in arthritis: matrix degradation. *Arthritis Res* 2001; **3**: 337–41.
4. van den Berg, W. B. Pathophysiology of osteoarthritis. *Joint Bone Spine* 2000; **67**: 555–6.
5. Firestein, G. S. Evolving concepts of rheumatoid arthritis. *Nature* 2003; **423**: 356–61.
6. Barrett, A. J., Rawlings, N. D., and Woessner, J. F., Jr. *Handbook of Proteolytic Enzymes*. San Diego: Academic Press; 1998.
7. Becherer, J. D., and Blobel, C. P. Biochemical properties and functions of membrane-anchored metalloprotease-disintegrin proteins (ADAMs). *Curr Top Dev Biol* 2003; **54**: 101–23.
8. Everts, V., Delaisse, J. M., Korper, W., Niehof, A., Vaes, G., and Beertsen, W. Degradation of collagen in the bone-resorbing compartment underlying the osteoclast involves both cysteine-proteinases and matrix metalloproteinases. *J Cell Physiol* 1992; **150**: 221–31.
9. Stocker, W., Grams, F., Baumann, U., Reinemer, P., Gomis-Ruth, F. X., McKay, D. B. *et al.* The metzincins: topological and sequential relations between the astacins, adamalysins, serralysins, and matrixins (collagenases) define a superfamily of zinc-peptidases. *Protein Sci* 1995; **4**: 823–40.
10. Egeblad, M., and Werb, Z. New functions for the matrix metalloproteinases in cancer progression. *Nat Rev Cancer* 2002; **2**: 161–74.
11. Boldt, H. B., Overgaard, M. T., Laursen, L. S., Weyer, K., Sottrup-Jensen, L., and Oxvig, C. Mutational analysis of the proteolytic domain of pregnancy-associated plasma protein-A (PAPP-A): classification as a metzincin. *Biochem J* 2001; **358** (Pt 2): 359–67.
12. Overgaard, M. T., Boldt, H. B., Laursen, L. S., Sottrup-Jensen, L., Conover, C. A., and Oxvig, C. Pregnancy-associated plasma protein-A2 (PAPP-A2), a novel insulin-like growth factor-binding protein-5 proteinase. *J Biol Chem* 2001; **276**: 21849–53.
13. Nagase, H., and Woessner, J. F., Jr. Matrix metalloproteinases. *J Biol Chem* 1999; **274**: 21491–4.
14. Springman, E. B., Angleton, E. L., Birkedal-Hansen, H., and Van Wart, H. E. Multiple modes of activation of latent human fibroblast collagenase: evidence for the role of a Cys^{73} active- site zinc complex in latency and a 'cysteine switch' mechanism for activation. *Proc Natl Acad Sci U S A* 1990; **87**: 364–8.
15. Van Wart, H. E., and Birkedal-Hansen, H. The cysteine switch: a principle of regulation of metalloproteinase activity with potential applicability to the entire matrix metalloproteinase gene family. *Proc Natl Acad Sci U S A* 1990; **87**: 5578–82.
16. Sternlicht, M. D., and Werb, Z. How matrix metalloproteinases regulate cell behavior. *Annu Rev Cell Dev Biol* 2001; **17**: 463–516.
17. Nagase, H. Stromelysins 1 and 2. *Methods Enzymol* 1995; **248**: 449–70.
18. Murphy, G., Cockett, M. I., Stephens, P. E., Smith, B., and Docherty, A. J. P. Stromelysin is an activator of procollagenase. *J Biochem* 1987; **248**: 265–8.
19. Knäuper, V., Wilhelm, S. M., Seperack, P. K., DeClerck, Y. A., Langley, K. E., Osthues, A. *et al.* Direct activation of human neutrophil procollagenase by recombinant stromelysin. *Biochem J* 1993; **295**: 581–6.
20. Knäuper, V., Will, H., López-Otin, C., Smith, B., Atkinson, S. J., Stanton, H. *et al.* Cellular mechanisms for human procollagenase-3 (MMP-13) activation. *J Biol Chem* 1996; **271**: 17124–31.
21. Hembry, R. M., Bagga, M. R., Reynolds, J. J., and Hamblen, D. L. Immunolocalisation studies on six matrix metalloproteinases and their inhibitors, TIMP-1 and TIMP-2, in synovia from patients with osteo- and rheumatoid arthritis. *Ann Rheum Dis* 1995; **54**: 25–32.
22. Okada, Y., Shinmei, M., Tanaka, O., Naka, K., Kimura, A., Nakanishi, I. *et al.* Localization of matrix metalloproteinase 3 (stromelysin) in osteoarthritic cartilage and synovium. *Lab Invest* 1992; **66**: 680–90.
23. Wolfe, G. C., MacNaul, K. L., Buechel, F. F., McDonnell, J., Hoerrner, L. A., Lark, M. W. *et al.* Differential in vivo expression of collagenase messenger RNA in synovium and cartilage: quantitative comparison with stromelysin messenger RNA levels in human rheumatoid arthritis and osteoarthritis patients and in two animal models of acute inflammatory arthritis. *Arthritis Rheum* 1993; **36**: 1540–7.
24. Aimes, R. T., and Quigley, J. P. Matrix metalloproteinase-2 is an interstitial collagenase: inhibitor-free enzyme catalyzes the cleavage of collagen fibrils and soluble native type I collagen generating the specific 3/4 and 1/4-length fragments. *J Biol Chem* 1995; **270**: 5872–6.
25. Ohuchi, E., Imai, K., Fujii, Y., Satio, H., Seiki, M., and Okada, Y. Membrane type 1 matrix metalloproteinase digests interstitial collagenase and other extracellular macromolecules. *J Biol Chem* 1997; **272**: 2446–51.
26. Knäuper, V., López-Otin, C., Smith, B., Knight, G., and Murphy, G. Biochemical characterization of human collagenase-3. *J Biol Chem* 1996; **271**: 1544–50.
27. Tetlow, L. C., Adlam, D. J., and Woolley, D. E. Matrix metalloproteinase and proinflammatory cytokine production by chondrocytes of human osteoarthritic cartilage. *Arthritis Rheum* 2001; **44**: 585–94.
28. Shingleton, W. D., Ellis, A. J., Rowan, A. D., and Cawston, T. E. Retinoic acid combines with interleukin-1 to promote the degradation of collagen from bovine nasal cartilage: matrix metalloproteinases-1 and -13 are involved in cartilage collagen breakdown. *J Cell Biochem* 2000; **79**: 519–31.
29. Fosang, A. J., Neame, P. J., Last, K., Hardingham, T. E., Murphy, G., and Hamilton, J. A. The interglobular domain of cartilage aggrecan is cleaved by PUMP, gelatinases, and cathepsin B. *J Biol Chem* 1992; **267**: 19470–4.
30. Murphy, G., and Crabbe, T. Gelatinases A and B. *Methods Enzymol* 1995; **248**: 470–84.
31. Ahrens, D., Koch, A. E., Pope, R. M., Stein-Picarella, M., and Niedbala, M. J. Expression of matrix metalloproteinase 9 (96-kd gelatinase B) in human rheumatoid arthritis. *Arthritis Rheum* 1996; **39**: 1576–87.
32. Gruber, B. L., Sorbi, D., French, D. L., Marchese, M. J., Nuovo, G. J., Kew, R. R. *et al.* Markedly elevated serum MMP-9 (gelatinase B)

levels in rheumatoid arthritis: a potential useful laboratory marker. *Clinical Immunol Immunopathol* 1996; **78**: 161–171.

33. Yoshihara, Y., Nakamura, H., Obata, K., Yamada, H., Hayakawa, T., Fujikawa, K. *et al.* Matrix metalloproteinases and tissue inhibitors of metalloproteinases in synovial fluids from patients with rheumatoid arthritis or osteoarthritis. *Ann Rheum Dis* 2000; **59**: 455–61.

34. Clark, I. M., Parker, A. E. Metalloproteinases: their role in arthritis and potential as therapeutic targets. *Expert Opin Ther Targets* 2003; **7**: 19–34.

35. Cawston, T. E. Metalloproteinases inhibitors and the prevention of connective tissue breakdown. *Pharmacol Ther* 1996; **70**: 163–82.

36. Konttinen, Y. T., Ainola, M., Valleala, H., Ma, J., Ida, H., Mandelin, J. *et al.* Analysis of 16 different matrix metalloproteinases (MMP-1 to MMP-20) in the synovial membrane: different profiles in trauma and rheumatoid arthritis. *Ann Rheum Dis* 1999; **58**: 691–7.

37. van den Berg, W. B. The role of cytokines and growth factors in cartilage destruction in osteoarthritis and rheumatoid arthritis. *Z Rheumatol* 1999; **58**: 136–41.

38. Koshy, P. J., Henderson, N., Logan, C., Life, P. F., Cawston, T. E., and Rowan, A. D. Interleukin 17 induces cartilage collagen breakdown: novel synergistic effects in combination with proinflammatory cytokines. *Ann Rheum Dis* 2002; **61**: 704–13.

39. Kleiner, D. E., Jr., and Stetler-Stevenson, W. G. Structural biochemistry and activation of matrix metalloproteases. *Curr Opin Cell Biol* 1993; **5**: 891–7.

40. Milner, J. M., Elliott, S. F., and Cawston, T. E. Activation of procollagenases is a key control point in cartilage collagen degradation: interaction of serine and metalloproteinase pathways. *Arthritis Rheum* 2001; **44**: 2084–96.

41. Eeckhout, Y., and Vaes, G. Further studies on the activation of procollagenase, the latent precursor of bone collagenase: effects of lysomal cathepsin B, plasmin and kallikrein and spontaneous activation. *Biochem J* 1977; **166**: 21–31.

42. He, C., Wilhelm, S. M., Pentland, A. P., Marmer, B. L., Grant, G. A., Eisen, A. Z. *et al.* Tissue cooperation in a proteolytic cascade activating human interstitial collagenase. *Proc Natl Acad Sci U S A* 1989; **86**: 2632–6.

43. Werb, Z., Mainardi, C. L., Vater, C. A., and Harris, E. D. Endogenous activation of latent collagenase by rheumatoid synovial cells: evidence for a role of plasminogen activator. *N Engl J Med* 1977; **296**: 1017–23.

44. Ogata, Y., Enghild, J. J., and Nagase, H. Matrix metalloproteinase 3 (stromelysin) activates the precursor for the human matrix metalloproteinase 9. *J Biol Chem* 1992; **267**: 3581–4.

45. Milner, J. M., Rowan, A. D., Elliott, S. F., and Cawston, T. E. Inhibition of furin-like enzymes blocks interleukin-1alpha/oncostatin M-stimulated cartilage degradation. *Arthritis Rheum* 2003; **48**: 1057–66.

46. Sato, H., Takino, T., Okada, Y., Cao, J., Shinagawa, A., Yamamoto, E. *et al.* A matrix metalloproteinase expressed on the surface of invasive tumour cells. *Nature* 1994; **370**: 61–5.

47. Takino, T., Sato, H., Shinagawa, A., and Seiki, M. Identification of the second membrane-type matrix metalloproteinase (MT-MMP-2) gene from a human placenta cDNA library: MT-MMPs form a unique membrane-type subclass in the MMP family. *J Biol Chem* 1995; **270**: 23013–20.

48. Butler, G. S., Will, H., Atkinson, S. J., and Murphy, G. Membrane-type-2 matrix metalloproteinase can initiate the processing of progelatinase A and is regulated by the tissue inhibitors of metalloproteinases. *Eur J Biochem* 1997; **244**: 653–7.

49. Pei, D. Identification and characterization of the fifth membrane-type matrix metalloproteinase MT5-MMP. *J Biol Chem* 1999; **274**: 8925–32.

50. Velasco, G., Cal, S., Merlos-Suárez, A., Ferrando, A. A., Alvarez, S., Nakano, A. *et al.* Human MT6-matrix metalloproteinase: identification, progelatinase A activation, and expression in brain tumors. *Cancer Res* 2000; **60**: 877–82.

51. Brew, K., Dinakarpandian, D., and Nagase, H. Tissue inhibitors of metalloproteinases: evolution, structure and function. *Biochim Biophys Acta* 2000; **1477**: 267–83.

52. Greene, J., Wang, M., Liu, Y. E., Raymond, L. A., Rosen, C., and Shi, Y. E. Molecular cloning and characterization of human tissue inhibitor of metalloproteinase 4. *J Biol Chem* 1996; **271**: 30375–80.

53. Varga, J., Rosenbloom, J., and Jimenez, S. A. Transforming growth factor beta (TGF beta) causes a persistent increase in steady-state amounts of type I and type III collagen and fibronectin mRNAs in normal human dermal fibroblasts. *Biochem J* 1987; **247**: 597–604.

54. Zucker, S., Pei, D., Cao, J., and Lopez-Otin, C. Membrane type-matrix metalloproteinases (MT-MMP). *Curr Top Dev Biol* 2003; **54**: 1–74.

55. Yu, W. H., and Woessner, J. F., Jr. Heparan sulfate proteoglycans as extracellular docking molecules for matrilysin (matrix metalloproteinase 7). *J Biol Chem* 2000; **275**: 4183–91.

56. Guo, H., Li, R., Zucker, S., and Toole, B. P. EMMPRIN (CD147), an inducer of matrix metalloproteinase synthesis, also binds interstitial collagenase to the tumor cell surface. *Cancer Res* 2000; **60**: 888–91.

57. Primakoff, P., and Myles, D. G. The ADAM gene family: surface proteins with adhesion and protease activity. *Trends Genet* 2000; **16**: 83–7.

58. Black, R. A., Rauch, C. T., Kozlosky, C. J., Peschon, J. J., Slack, J. L., Wolfson, M. F. *et al.* A metalloproteinase disintegrin that releases tumour-necrosis factor-α from cells. *Nature* 1997; **385**: 729–33.

59. McKie, N., Edwards, T., Dallas, D. J., Houghton, A., Stringer, B., Graham, R. *et al.* Expression of members of a novel membrane linked metalloproteinase family (ADAM) in human articular chondrocytes. *Biochem Biophys Res Comm* 1997; **230**: 335–9.

60. Porter, S., Clark, I. M., Kevorkian, L., and Edwards, D. R. The ADAMTS metalloproteinases. *Biochem J* 2005; **386** (Pt 1): 15–27.

61. Sandy, J. D., Flannery, C. R., Neame, P. J., and Lohmander, L. S. The structure of aggrecan fragments in human synovial fluid: evidence for the involvement in osteoarthritis of a novel proteinase which cleaves the Glu 373-Ala 374 bond. *J Clin Invest* 1992; **89**: 1512–16.

62. Tortorella, M. D., Liu, R. Q., Burn, T., Newton, R. C., and Arner, E. Characterization of human aggrecanase 2 (ADAM-TS5): substrate specificity studies and comparison with aggrecanase 1 (ADAM-TS4). *Matrix Biol* 2002; **21**: 499–511.

63. Rodriguez-Manzaneque, J. C., Westling, J., Thai, S. N., Luque, A., Knauper, V., Murphy, G. *et al.* ADAMTS1 cleaves aggrecan at multiple sites and is differentially inhibited by metalloproteinase inhibitors. *Biochem Biophys Res Commun* 2002; **293**: 501–8.

64. Collins-Racie, L. A., Flannery, C. R., Zeng, W., Corcoran, C., Annis-Freeman, B., Agostino, M. J. *et al.* ADAMTS-8 exhibits aggrecanase activity and is expressed in human articular cartilage. *Matrix Biol* 2004; **23**: 219–30.

65. Yamanouchi-Pharmaceutical-Co. Patent WO0134785. 2001.

66. Tortorella, M. D., Malfait, A. M., Deccico, C., and Arner, E. The role of ADAM-TS4 (aggrecanase-1) and ADAM-TS5 (aggrecanase-2) in a model of cartilage degradation. *Osteoarthritis Cartilage* 2001; **9**: 539–52.

67. Caterson, B., Flannery, C. R., Hughes, C. E., and Little, C. B. Mechanisms involved in cartilage proteoglycan catabolism. *Matrix Biology* 2000; **19**: 333–44.

68. Glasson, S. S., Askew, R., Sheppard, B., Carito, B., Blanchet, T., Ma, H. L. *et al.* Deletion of active ADAMTS5 prevents cartilage degradation in a murine model of osteoarthritis. *Nature* 2005; **434**: 644–8.

69. Stanton, H., Rogerson, F. M., East, C. J., Golub, S. B., Lawlor, K. E., Meeker, C.T. *et al.* ADAMTS5 is the major aggrecanase in mouse cartilage in vivo and in vitro. *Nature* 2005; **434**: 648–52.

70. Somerville, R. P., Longpre, J. M., Jungers, K. A., Engle, J. M., Ross, M., Evanko, S. *et al.* Characterization of ADAMTS-9 and ADAMTS-20 as a distinct ADAMTS subfamily related to Caenorhabditis elegans GON-1. *J Biol Chem* 2003; **278**: 9503–13.

71. Arner, E. C., Hughes, C. E., Decicco, C. P., Caterson, B., and Tortorella, M. D. Cytokine-induced cartilage proteoglycan degradation is mediated by aggrecanase. *Osteoarthritis Cartilage* 1998; **6**: 214–28.

72. Stanton, H., Ung, L., and Fosang, A. J. The 45 kDa collagen-binding fragment of fibronectin induces matrix metalloproteinase-13 synthesis by chondrocytes and aggrecan degradation by aggrecanases. *Biochem J* 2002; **364** (Pt 1): 181–90.

73. Dudler, J., Renggli-Zulliger, N., Busso, N., Lotz, M., and So, A. Effect of interleukin 17 on proteoglycan degradation in murine knee joints. *Ann Rheum Dis* 2000; **59**: 529–32.

74. Yamanishi, Y., Boyle, D. L., Clark, M., Maki, R. A., Tortorella, M. D., Arner, E. C. *et al.* Expression and regulation of aggrecanase in arthritis: the role of TGF-beta. *J Immunol* 2002; **168**: 1405–12.

75. Koshy, P. J., Lundy, C. J., Rowan, A. D., Porter, S., Edwards, D. R., Hogan, A. *et al.* The modulation of matrix metalloproteinase and ADAM gene expression in human chondrocytes by interleukin-1 and oncostatin M: a time-course study using real-time quantitative reverse transcription-polymerase chain reaction. *Arthritis Rheum.* 2002; **46**: 961–7.

76. Young, D. A., Lakey, R. L., Pennington, C. J., Kevorkian, L., Edwards, D. R., Cawston, T. E. *et al.* Histone deacetylase inhibitors modulate metalloproteinase gene expression in chondrocytes and block cartilage resorption. *Arthritis Res Ther* 2005; **7**: R503–12.

77. Ellis, A. J., Curry, V. A., Powell, E. K., and Cawston, T. E. The prevention of collagen breakdown in bovine nasal cartilage by TIMP-1, TIMP-2 and a low molecular weight synthetic inhibitor. Biochem Biophys *Res Commun* 1994; **201**: 94–101.

78. Kashiwagi, M., Tortorella, M., Nagase, H., and Brew, K. TIMP-3 is a potent inhibitor of aggrecanase 1 (ADAM-TS4) and aggrecanase 2 (ADAM-TS5). *J Biol Chem* 2001; **276**: 12501–4.

79. Chevrier, A., Mort, J. S., Crine, P., Hoemann, C. D., and Buschmann, M. D. Soluble recombinant neprilysin induces aggrecanase-mediated cleavage of aggrecan in cartilage explant cultures. *Arch Biochem Biophys* 2001; **396**: 178–86.

80. Campbell, I. K., Wojta, J., Novak, U., Hamilton, J. A. Cytokine modulation of plasminogen activator inhibitor-1 (PAI-1) production by human articular cartilage and chondrocytes. Down-regulation by tumor necrosis factor α and up-regulation by transforming growth factor-β and basic fibroblast growth factor. *Biochimica et Biophysica Acta* 1994; **1226**: 277–85.

81. Bryson, H., Bunning, R. A. D., Feltell, R., Kam, C. M., Kerrigan, J., Powers, J. C. *et al.* A serine proteinase inactivator inhibits chondrocyte-mediated cartilage proteoglycan breakdown occurring in response to proinflammatory cytokines. *Arch Biochem Biophys* 1998; **355**: 15–25.

82. Ronday, H. K., van der Laan, W. H., Tak, P. P., de Roos, J. A., Bank, R. A., TeKoppele, J. M. *et al.* Human granzyme B mediates cartilage proteoglycan degradation and is expressed at the invasive front of the synovium in rheumatoid arthritis. *Rheumatology (Oxford)* 2001; **40**: 55–61.

83. Delaisse, J. M., Eeckhout, Y., and Vaes, G. Inhibition of bone resorption in culture by inhibitors of thiol proteinases. *Biochem J* 1980; **192**: 365–8.

84. Delaisse, J. M., Eeckhout, Y., and Vaes, G. In vivo and in vitro evidence for the involvement of cysteine proteinases in bone resorption. *Biochem Biophys Res Commun* 1984; **125**: 441–7.

85. Turk, V., Turk, B., and Turk, D. Lysosomal cysteine proteases: facts and opportunities. *EMBO J* 2001; **20**: 4629–33.

86. Etherington, D. J. The nature of the collagenolytic cathepsin of rat liver and its distribution in other rat tissues. *Biochem J* 1972; **127**: 685–92.

87. Burleigh, M. C., Barrett, A. J., and Lazarus, G. S. Cathepsin B1: a lysosomal enzyme that degrades native collagen. *Biochem J* 1974; **137**: 387–98.

88. Buttle, D. J., Bramwell, H., and Hollander, A. P. Proteolytic mechanisms of cartilage breakdown: a target for arthritis therapy? *Clin Pathol Mol Pathol* 1995; **48**: M167–M177.

89. Everts, V., Van der Zee, E., Creemers, L., and Beertsen, W. Phagocytosis and intracellular digestion of collagen, its role in turnover and remodelling. *Histochem J* 1996; **28**: 229–45.

90. Everts, V., Beertsen, W., and Tigchelaar-Gutter, W. The digestion of phagocytosed collagen is inhibited by the proteinase inhibitors leupeptin and E-64. *Coll Relat Res* 1985; **5**: 315–36.

91. Inaoka, T., Bilbe, G., Ishibashi, O., Tezuka, K., Kumegawa, M., and Kokubo, T. Molecular cloning of human cDNA for cathepsin K: novel cysteine proteinase predominantly expressed in bone. *Biochem Biophys Res Commun* 1995; **206**: 89–96.

92. Bossard, M. J., Tomaszek, T. A., Thompson, S. K., Amegadzie, B. Y., Hanning, C. R., Jones, C. *et al.* Proteolytic activity of human osteoclast cathepsin K: expression, purification, activation, and substrate identification. *J Biol Chem* 1996; **271**: 12517–24.

93. Kafienah, W., Bromme, D., Buttle, D. J., Croucher, L. J., and Hollander, A. P. Human cathepsin K cleaves native type I and II collagens at the N-terminal end of the triple helix. *Biochem J* 1998; **331** (Pt 3): 727–32.

94. Hummel, K. M., Petrow, P. K., Franz, J. K., Muller-Ladner, U., Aicher, W. K., Gay, R. E *et al.* Cysteine proteinase cathepsin K mRNA is expressed in synovium of patients with rheumatoid arthritis and is detected at sites of synovial bone destruction. *J Rheumatol* 1998; **25**: 1887–94.

95. Hou, W. S., Li, W., Keyszer, G., Weber, E., Levy, R., Klein, M. J. *et al.* Comparison of cathepsins K and S expression within the rheumatoid and osteoarthritic synovium. *Arthritis Rheum* 2002; **46**: 663–74.

96. Li, Z., Hou, W. S., and Bromme, D. Collagenolytic activity of cathepsin K is specifically modulated by cartilage-resident chondroitin sulfates. *Biochemistry* 2000; **39**: 529–36.

97. Hou, W. S., Li, Z., Gordon, R. E., Chan, K., Klein, M. J., Levy, R. *et al.* Cathepsin K is a critical protease in synovial fibroblast-mediated collagen degradation. *Am J Pathol* 2001; **159**: 2167–77.

98. Wang, D., Li, W., Pechar, M., Kopeckova, P., Bromme, D., and Kopecek, J. Cathepsin K inhibitor-polymer conjugates: potential drugs for the treatment of osteoporosis and rheumatoid arthritis. *Int J Pharm* 2004; **277**: 73–9.

99. Suzuki, K., Shimizu, K., Hamamoto, T., Nakagawa, Y., Murachi, T., and Yamamoto, T. Characterization of proteoglycan degradation by calpain. *Biochem J* 1992; **285** (Pt 3): 857–62.

100. Szomor, Z., Shimizu, K., Fujimori, Y., Yamamoto, S., and Yamamuro, T. Appearance of calpain correlates with arthritis and cartilage destruction in collagen induced arthritic knee joints of mice. *Ann Rheum Dis* 1995; **54**: 477–83.

101. Ishikawa, H., Nakagawa, Y., Shimizu, K., Nishihara, H., Matsusue, Y., and Nakamura, T. Inflammatory cytokines induced down-regulation of m-calpain mRNA expression in fibroblastic synoviocytes from patients with osteoarthritis and rheumatoid arthritis. *Biochem Biophys Res Commun* 1999; **266**: 341–6.

102. Wlodawer, A. Proteasome: a complex protease with a new fold and a distinct mechanism. *Structure* 1995; **3**: 417–20.

103. Shapiro, S. D. Mighty mice: transgenic technology 'knocks out' questions of matrix metalloproteinase function. *Matrix Biol* 1997; **15**: 527–33.

104. Nuttall, R. K., Sampieri, C. L., Pennington, C. J., Gill, S. E., Schultz, G. A., Edwards, D. R. Expression analysis of the entire MMP and TIMP gene families during mouse tissue development. *FEBS Lett* 2004; **563**: 129–34.

105. Helminen, H. J., Saamanen, A. M., Salminen, H., and Hyttinen M. M. Transgenic mouse models for studying the role of cartilage macromolecules in osteoarthritis. *Rheumatology (Oxford)* 2002; **41**: 848–56.

106. Li, Q., Park, P. W., Wilson, C. L., and Parks, W. C. Matrilysin shedding of syndecan-1 regulates chemokine mobilization and transepithelial efflux of neutrophils in acute lung injury. *Cell* 2002; **111**: 635–46.

107. Churg, A., Wang, R. D., Tai, H., Wang, X., Xie, C., Dai, J. *et al.* Macrophage metalloelastase mediates acute cigarette smoke-induced inflammation via TNF-alpha release. *Am J Respir Crit Care Med* 2003; **167**: 1083–9.

108. Zambrowicz, B. P., and Sands, A. T. Knockouts model the 100 best-selling drugs: will they model the next 100? *Nat Rev Drug Discov* 2003; **2**: 38–51.

109. Holmbeck, K., Bianco, P., Caterina, J., Yamada, S., Kromer, M., Kuznetsov, S. A. *et al.* MT1-MMP-deficient mice develop dwarfism, osteopenia, arthritis and connective tissue disease due to inadequate collagen turnover. *Cell* 1999; **99**: 81–92.

110. Zhou, Z., Apte, S. S., Soininen, R., Cao, R., Baaklini, G. Y., Rauser, R. W. *et al.* Impaired endochondral ossification and angiogenesis in mice deficient in membrane-type matrix metalloproteinase I. *Proc Natl Acad Sci U S A* 2000; **97**: 4052–7.

111. Holmbeck, K., Bianco, P., Pidoux, I., Inoue, S., Billinghurst, R. C., Wu, W. *et al.* The metalloproteinase MT1-MMP is required for normal development and maintenance of osteocyte processes in bone. *J Cell Sci* 2005; **118** (Pt 1): 147–56.

112. Itoh, T., Matsuda, H., Tanioka, M., Kuwabara, K., Itohara, S., and Suzuki, R. The role of matrix metalloproteinase-2 and matrix metalloproteinase-9 in antibody-induced arthritis. *J Immunol* 2002; **169**: 2643–7.

113. Van Meurs, J., Van Lent, P., Stoop, R., Holthuysen, A., Singer, I., Bayne, E. *et al*. Cleavage of aggrecan at the Asn[341]-Phe[342] site coincides with the initiation of collagen damage in murine antigen-induced arthritis. *Arthritis Rheum* 1999; **42**: 2074–84.

114. Mudgett, J. S., Hutchinson, N. I., Chartrain, N. A., Forsyth, A. J., McDonnell, J., Singer, I. I. *et al*. Susceptibility of stromelysin 1-deficient mice to collagen-induced arthritis and cartilage destruction. *Arthritis Rheum* 1998; **41**: 110–21.

115. Clements, K. M., Price, J. S., Chambers, M. G., Visco, D. M., Poole, A. R., and Mason, R. M. Gene deletion of either interleukin-1beta, interleukin-1beta-converting enzyme, inducible nitric oxide synthase, or stromelysin 1 accelerates the development of knee osteoarthritis in mice after surgical transection of the medial collateral ligament and partial medial meniscectomy. *Arthritis Rheum* 2003; **48**: 3452–63.

116. Flannery, C. R., Lark, M. W., and Sandy, J. D. Identification of a stromelysin cleavage site within the interglobular domain of human aggrecan: evidence for proteolysis at this site in vivo in human articular cartilage. *J Biol Chem* 1992; **267**: 1008–14.

117. Glasson, S. S., Askew, R., Sheppard, B., Carito, B. A., Blanchet, T., Ma, H. L. *et al*. Characterization of and osteoarthritis susceptibility in ADAMTS-4-knockout mice. *Arthritis Rheum* 2004; **50**: 2547–58.

118. Borkakoti, N. Matrix metalloprotease inhibitors: design from structure. *Biochem Soc Trans* 2004; **32** (Pt 1): 17–20.

119. Lewis, E. J., Bishop, J., Bottomley, K. M., Bradshaw, D., Brewster M., Broadhurst, M. J. *et al*. Ro 32–3555, an orally active collagenase inhibitor, prevents cartilage breakdown in vitro and in vivo. *Br J Pharmacol* 1997; **121**: 540–6.

120. Hemmings, F. J., Farhan, M., Rowland, J., Banken, L., and Jain, R. Tolerability and pharmacokinetics of the collagenase-selective inhibitor Trocade in patients with rheumatoid arthritis. *Rheumatology (Oxford)* 2001; **40**: 537–43.

121. MacPherson, L. J., Bayburt, E. K., Capparelli, M. P., Carroll, B. J., Goldstein, R., Justice, M. R. *et al*. Discovery of CGS 27023A, a non-peptidic, potent, and orally active stromelysin inhibitor that blocks cartilage degradation in rabbits. *J Med Chem* 1997; **40**: 2525–32.

122. O'Byrne, E. M., Blancuzzi, V., Singh, H., MacPherson, L. J., Parker, D. T., and Roberts, E. D. Chondroprotective activity of a matrix metalloproteinase inhibitor, CGS 27023A in animal models of osteoarthritis. Tokyo: Springer-Verlag; 1999.

123. Chau, T., Jolly, G., Plym, M. J., McHugh, M., Bortolon, E., Wakefield, J. *et al*. Inhibition of articular cartilage degradation in dog and guinea-pig models of osteoarthritis by the stromelysin inhibitor, BAY-12–9566. *Arthritis Rheum* 1998; **41**: S300.

124. Leff, R. L., Elias, I., Ionescu, M., Reiner, A., and Poole, A. R. Molecular changes in human osteoarthritic cartilage after 3 weeks of oral administration of BAY 12–9566, a matrix metalloproteinase inhibitor. *J Rheumatol* 2003; **30**: 544–9.

125. Bayer drug casts shadow over MMP inhibitors in cancer. *Scrip* 1999; **2476**: 7.

126. Sabatini, M., Lesur, C., Thomas, M., Chomel, A., Anract, P., de Nanteuil, G. *et al*. Effect of inhibition of matrix metalloproteinases on cartilage loss in vitro and in a guinea pig model of osteoarthritis. *Arthritis Rheum* 2005; **52**: 171–80.

127. Ishikawa, T., Nishigaki, F., Miyata, S., Hirayama, Y., Minoura, K., Imanishi, J. *et al*. Prevention of progressive joint destruction in adjuvant induced arthritis in rats by a novel matrix metalloproteinase inhibitor, FR217840. *Eur J Pharmacol* 2005; **508**: 239–47.

128. Ishikawa, T., Nishigaki, F., Miyata, S., Hirayama, Y., Minoura, K., Imanishi, J. *et al*. Prevention of progressive joint destruction in collagen-induced arthritis in rats by a novel matrix metalloproteinase inhibitor, FR255031. *Br J Pharmacol* 2005; **144**: 133–43.

129. Ryan, M. E., Greenwald, R. A., and Golub, L. M. Potential of tetracyclines to modify cartilage breakdown in osteoarthritis. *Curr Opin Rheumatol* 1996; **8**: 238–47.

130. de Bri, E., Lei, W., Svensson, O., Chowdhury, M., Moak, S. A., and Greenwald, R. A. Effect of an inhibitor of matrix metalloproteinases on spontaneous osteoarthritis in guinea pigs. *Adv Dent Res* 1998; **12**: 82–5.

131. Stone, M., Fortin, P. R., Pacheco-Tena, C., and Inman, R. D. Should tetracycline treatment be used more extensively for rheumatoid arthritis? Metaanalysis demonstrates clinical benefit with reduction in disease activity. *J Rheumatol* 2003; **30**: 2112–22.

132. van der Laan, W., Molenaar, E., Ronday, K., Verheijen, J., Breedveld, F., Greenwald, R. *et al*. Lack of effect of doxycycline on disease activity and joint damage in patients with rheumatoid arthritis: a double blind, placebo controlled trial. *J Rheumatol* 2001; **28**: 1967–74.

133. Mazzuca, S. A., Brandt, K. D., Lane, K. A., and Katz, B. P. Subject retention and adherence to dosing regimen in a 30-month clinical trial of doxycycline (doxy) as a disease-modifying osteoarthritis drug (DMOARD). *Arthritis Rheum* 2003; **48** (S9): 294.

134. Nemunaitis, J., Poole, C., Primrose, J., Rosemurgy, A., Malfetano, J., Brown, P. *et al*. Combined analysis of studies of the effects of the matrix metalloproteinase inhibitor marimastat on serum tumor markers in advanced cancer: selection of a biologically active and tolerable dose for longer-term studies. *Clin Cancer Res* 1998; **4**: 1101–9.

135. Pavlaki, M., and Zucker, S. Matrix metalloproteinase inhibitors (MMPIs): the beginning of phase I or the termination of phase III clinical trials. *Cancer Metastasis Rev* 2003; **22**: 177–203.

136. Morgan, K., and Kalsheker, N. A. Regulation of the serine proteinase inhibitor (SERPIN) gene α_1-antitrypsin: a paradigm for other SERPINs. *Int J Biochem Cell Biol* 1997; **29**: 1501–11.

137. Han, Z., Boyle, D. L., Chang, L., Bennett, B., Karin, M., Yang, L. *et al*. c-Jun N-terminal kinase is required for metalloproteinase expression and joint destruction in inflammatory arthritis. *J Clin Invest* 2001; **108**: 73–81.

138. Rowan, A. D., Hui, W., Cawston, T. E., and Richards, C. D. Adenoviral gene transfer of interleukin-1 in combination with oncostatin M induces significant joint damage in a murine model. *Am J Pathol* 2003; **162**: 1975–84.

139. Tak, P. P., Gerlag, D. M., Aupperle, K. R., van de Geest, D. A., Overbeek, M., Bennett, B. L. *et al*. Inhibitor of nuclear factor kappaB kinase beta is a key regulator of synovial inflammation. *Arthritis Rheum* 2001; **44**: 1897–907.

140. Shouda, T., Yoshida, T., Hanada, T., Wakioka, T., Oishi, M., Miyoshi, K. *et al*. Induction of the cytokine signal regulator SOCS3/CIS3 as a therapeutic strategy for treating inflammatory arthritis. *J Clin Invest* 2001; **108**: 1781–8.

141. Kouzarides, T. Acetylation: a regulatory modification to rival phosphorylation? *EMBO J* 2000; **19**: 1176–9.

142. Johnstone, R. W. Histone-deacetylase inhibitors: novel drugs for the treatment of cancer. *Nat Rev Drug Discov* 2002; **1**: 287–99.

143. Chung, Y. L., Lee, M. Y., Wang, A. J., Yao, L. F. A therapeutic strategy uses histone deacetylase inhibitors to modulate the expression of genes involved in the pathogenesis of rheumatoid arthritis. *Mol Ther* 2003; **8**: 707–17.

144. Mori, H., Abe, F., Furukawa, S., Sakai, F., Hino, M., and Fujii, T. FR235222, a fungal metabolite, is a novel immunosuppressant that inhibits mammalian histone deacetylase (HDAC) II. Biological activities in animal models. *J Antibiot (Tokyo)* 2003; **56**: 80–6.

145. Nishida, K., Komiyama, T., Miyazawa, S., Shen, Z. N., Furumatsu, T., Doi, H. *et al*. Histone deacetylase inhibitor suppression of autoantibody-mediated arthritis in mice via regulation of p16INK4a and p21(WAF1/Cip1) expression. *Arthritis Rheum* 2004; **50**: 3365–76.

146. Blanchard, F., and Chipoy, C. Histone deacetylase inhibitors: new drugs for the treatment of inflammatory diseases? *Drug Discov Today* 2005; **10**: 197–204.

147. Nagase, H., and Brew, K. Designing TIMP (tissue inhibitor of metalloproteinases) variants that are selective metalloproteinase inhibitors. *Biochem Soc Symp* 2003: 201–12.

148. Lee, M. H., Rapti, M., Knauper, V., and Murphy, G. Threonine 98, the pivotal residue of tissue inhibitor of metalloproteinases (TIMP)-1 in metalloproteinase recognition. *J Biol Chem* 2004; **279**: 17562–9.

149. Lee, M. H., Rapti, M., and Murphy, G. Total conversion of tissue inhibitor of metalloproteinase (TIMP) for specific metalloproteinase targeting: fine-tuning TIMP-4 for optimal inhibition of TNF-a converting enzyme (TACE). *J Biol Chem* 2005; **280**: 15967–75.

150. van der Laan, W. H., Quax, P. H., Seemayer, C. A., Huisman, L. G., Pieterman, E. J., Grimbergen, J. M. *et al*. Cartilage degradation and invasion by rheumatoid synovial fibroblasts is inhibited by gene transfer of TIMP-1 and TIMP-3. *Gene Ther* 2003; **10**: 234–42.

151. McCawley, L. J., and Matrisian, L. M. Matrix metalloproteinases: they're not just for matrix anymore! *Curr Opin Cell Biol* 2001; **13**: 534–40.

42 | *Signal transduction in rheumatoid arthritis*

Di Chen and Edward M. Schwarz

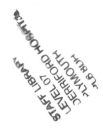

Introduction

Cellular activation, suppression, replication, differentiation, and apoptosis occur as a consequence of extracellular signals. The biochemical events utilized by cells to perceive and respond to these signals appropriately is known as signal transduction. Extensive research over the last twenty years has elucidated many of the critical signal transduction pathways that are operant in rheumatic diseases[1]. Moreover, this knowledge has been used to develop novel therapeutic interventions, both small molecules (i.e. cyclooxygenase (COX)-2 selective inhibitors) and biologics (i.e. tumor necrosis factor (TNF) antagonists), which have completely transformed rheumatology and our ability to effectively treat arthritis. In this chapter we will review the fundamental basis of signal transduction using the TNF, interleukin (IL), interferon (IFN), T-cell receptor (TCR), steroid, and transforming growth factor-beta (TGF-β) signaling pathways as examples of host inflammatory/immune responses. Since a new research focus to understand the pathways involved in healing and skeletal repair has emerged, we will also review bone morphogenetic protein (BMP) and Wnt signal transduction as examples.

The end product of signal transduction is a change in gene expression, which allows the cell to respond to the environmental signals. There are five fundamental components to every signal transduction pathway which cells use to modulate both immediate and long-term changes in gene expression. They are: (1) the ligand; (2) the receptor; (3) the cytoplasmic transduction molecule(s); (4) the transcription factor(s); and (5) the negative regulator(s). These proteins can be enzymes (i.e. kinases, phosphatases, ubiquitin ligases) or function solely by physical association to activate a transcription factor such that it will bind to its specific DNA recognition sequence in the promoter of the target gene and facilitate transcription by RNA polymerase II. In inflammatory responses, these target genes include the cytokines, adhesion molecules, oxygenases, and proteases that precipitate tissue destruction. An established paradigm to explain chronic autoimmune diseases like rheumatoid arthritis (RA) posits that the central etiologic mechanism is the inability to down-regulate pro-inflammatory signal transduction pathways. To emphasize this critical point, here we focus on these negative regulators and how they function to autoregulate signal transduction to inhibit constitutive activation and a chronic response.

The TNF signal transduction pathway

The clinical success of anti-TNF therapy over the last decade provides formal proof that the selective inhibition of a single signal transduction pathway can ameliorate autoimmuninty in some patients. However, it is noteworthy to mention that this pathway has long been recognized for its importance in inflammatory and immune responses[2]. The first indication of the importance of this pathway for innate immunity was highlighted by its extraordinary conservation during evolution, as homologues for all five components of the pathway are conserved from *Drosophila* to humans. Our current knowledge of the TNF signaling includes information on the three-dimensional structure and the *in vivo* function of most of the molecules in this pathway as defined by X-ray crystallography and targeted gene disruption (knockout) in mice.

Tumor necrosis factor was originally named to define its anticancer activity in the nineteenth century[3]. It is now known that there is a large family of TNF ligands, which are characterized by homologous C-terminal domains. TNF receptors are type I membrane proteins that are characterized by cysteine rich extracellular domains. Three unique features distinguish TNF receptor signaling from all other pathways. Signaling commences via ligand binding, which mediates activation by oligomerization of three identical receptors to form a homotrimer. Since TNF receptors are void of catalytic activity, the next step in the cascade involves the recruitment of adaptor proteins called TNF receptor-associated factors (TRAFs), which bind to sites in the TNF receptors created by homotrimerization[4]. TRAF binding allows for the recruitment and activation of mitogen-activated protein kinases (MAPKs), which trigger nuclear factor kappa B (NF-κB)- and activator protein-1 (AP-1)-mediated transcription[5]. The final unique property of TNF signaling is that it is the only receptor-mediated pathway known to directly trigger programed cell death, known as apoptosis. This feature of TNF signaling is arguably the most dominant, and has been demonstrated to be central in disease pathogenesis in many different organ systems.

Death receptor signaling through caspases

While it is known that all TNF receptors can influence apoptosis, only a subset, known as the death receptors (DRs), can activate this process directly[6]. This function is mediated by a unique amino acid motif in the cytoplasmic tail of the receptor call the death domain (DD). TNF receptors containing a DD trigger apoptosis by recruiting adapter proteins (TRADD and FADD), which associate with the receptor through mutual DD binding. Instead of recruiting MAPKs like the TRAFs, DD-adapter proteins recruit cysteine proteases called caspases. The binding of caspase-8 or -10 results in autoproteolytic processing and the release of the active enzyme, which mediates a cleavage cascade of family members, culminating in the processing of caspase-3. Once caspase-3 is processed apoptosis is irreversible, as this enzyme directly activates the DNases, lipases, and proteases that destroy the cell. Prior to caspase-3 cleavage, apoptosis can be prevented by the synthesis of inhibitor of apoptosis proteins (IAPs) via NF-κB-dependent signaling.

MAP kinase signal transduction

The most common mechanism by which cells respond to extracellular signals involves protein phosphorylation. The MAPK family is responsible for transducing the majority of inflammatory signals that ultimately lead to NF-κB-, AP-1-, and STAT-mediated transcription[1]. The phosphorylation cascade consist of a three- or four-tiered signaling module in which the MAPK is activated by a MAP kinase kinase (MAPKK), which in turn is activated by a MAP kinase kinase kinase (MAPKKK). The MAPKKK is itself activated by a small G protein such as Ras directly or by an intermediate kinase as a direct consequence of membrane receptor activation.

Currently, investigators are working to understand how identical MAPK signals in the same cell derived from different receptors can have opposing biological outcomes[7]. One example is the response of neuroendocrine cells to epidermal growth factor (EGF) and nerve growth factor (NGF)[7]. While both of these signals require Raf (the MAPKKK), MEK (the MAPKK), and extracellular signal-regulated kinases (ERK) (the MAPK), EGF signals for proliferation and NGF signals for differentiation. There are two theories to explain these phenomena. The first is the concept of 'cross-talk,' which posits that different signaling pathways (i.e. MAPK and cAMP) that are simultaneously active can interact with each other at some point to produce an effect that is different from either one alone. The other mechanism is the duration of the signal. MAPK activity is negatively regulated by protein phosphatases that dephosphorylate the kinases. Thus, the time interval from when the MAPKs become phosphorylated to the time they are dephosphorylated may control the strength of the signal and the ultimate biological response.

NF-κB signal transduction

NF-κB is a transcription factor that was first described to be a B cell-specific protein that bound to a short DNA sequence motif located in the immunoglobulin κ light chain enhancer[8]. Subsequently, it was discovered that NF-κB is expressed in virtually all cell types and is involved in the transcription of a wide array of genes[9]. NF-κB is comprised of a family of proteins (termed Rel), that share a Rel homology domain. This region mediates dimerization and DNA binding of the transcription factor. The most ubiquitous form of NF-κB is a heterodimer of Rel-A (p65) and NF-κB1 (p50), but almost all combinations of homo- and heterodimers are known to exist. It is believed that through these different combinations target gene specificity is derived. Among these are genes known to play a critical role in rheumatic diseases, including cytokines (TNF, IL-1β, IL-6), adhesion molecules (intercellular adhesion molecule (ICAM)-1, vascular cell adhesion molecule (VCAM)-1, E-selectin), oxygenases (iNOS, COX-2) and matrix metalloproteinases (MMPs). Furthermore, the efficacy of aspirin, gold compounds, sulfasalazine, and corticosteroids in the treatment of RA has been attributed to their inhibitory effects on NF-κB.

The central mechanism through which NF-κB is regulated involves post-translational modifications by phosphorylation and proteolysis. In resting cells, NF-κB is sequestered in the cytoplasm by proteins termed inhibitor of NF-κB (IκB). This protein family is characterized by common ankyrin-like repeat domains, which functions by binding to NF-κB in a manner that masks the nuclear translocation signal (NLS). Following the appropriate signal (i.e. TNF), activation of the transcription factor occurs through the signal-induced proteolytic degradation of IκB in the cytoplasm, which liberates NF-κB to translocate to the nucleus. The critical MAPKKKs in this pathway are the IκB kinases (IKK1,2), which directly phosphorylate IκB to trigger ubiquitination and degradation by the proteosome[10]. Although the true MAPKK that phosphorylates the IKKs in response to TNF has yet to be determined, several upstream kinases have been identified, including receptor-interacting protein (RIP), NF-κB-inducing kinase (NIK), and MEKK-1. Phosphorylation of NF-κB is also important in the regulation of this pathway. The transcriptional activity of NF-κB is stimulated upon phosphorylation of its p65 subunit by protein kinase A (PKA)[11]. This phosphorylation is required for efficient association with the transcriptional coactivator CBP/p300, and high transcriptional activity.

Negative autoregulation of NF-κB signaling occurs by the induction of three different NF-κB target genes, IκB, IAP, and A20. One of the first genes transcribed by NF-κB following nuclear translocation is IκBα[12]. This resynthesized IκB enters the nucleus, binds to NF-κB, and relocates it to the cytoplasm, thus extinguishing NF-κB activity[13]. As described above, NF-κB-mediated transcription of IAP genes is required to protect cells from TNF-induced apoptosis via caspase inhibition[14]. Similarly, NF-κB-mediated transcription of A20 is also required to down-regulate TNF responses, including apoptosis[15]. While the mechanism of A20 activity is unclear, there is evidence that it plays a role in the inactivation of the IKK complex. *In vivo* loss of these negative feedback pathways has severe consequences, as seen in the embryonic lethal phenotype of the RelA[16] and IKK-2 knockout mice[17], and the severe runting and postnatal wasting observed in the RIP[18] and A20[15] knockout mice. It has also been shown that the chronic inflammation found in RA synovium is associated with constitutive NF-κB activity[19].

AP-1 signal transduction

Even though AP-1 is a distinct signaling pathway from NF-κB, it is activated by many of the same signals and mediates a similar gene expression profile. Therefore, AP-1 is also a central regulator of the inflammatory responses that control rheumatic diseases. The AP-1 transcription factor is also composed of a family of proteins that are subdivided into two groups, Jun (c-Jun, Jun B, Jun D) and Fos (c-Fos, Fos B, Fra-1, Fra-2)[20]. Structurally, AP-1 proteins have two characteristic domains, a basic domain for transactivation, and a leucine-zipper domain for dimerization and DNA binding, which is referred to as bZIP. These motifs are also shared by activating transcription factor-2 (ATF-2), which can heterodimerize with Jun. While AP-1 complexes can bind to DNA as Jun homodimers, Jun–Jun heterodimers, and Jun–Fos heterodimers, the prototypic AP-1 is a c-Jun–c-Fos heterodimer. Three distinct MAPK pathways, the extracellular signal-regulated kinases (ERK), Jun N-terminal kinases (JNK), and the p38 kinases activate AP-1. The ERKs are activated by mitogens and growth factors via a Ras-dependent pathway, while the JNK and p38 kinases are activated in response to the pro-inflammatory cytokines and cellular stress (e.g. reactive oxygen metabolites, ultraviolet light, heat, and osmotic shock). Based on these stimuli, the JNKs and p38 kinases have been termed stress-activated protein kinases (SAPKs).

The MAPKs activate the AP-1 pathway by two distinct mechanisms. First, they directly phosphorylate c-Jun and ATF-2, which markedly increases their transcriptional activity by allowing for efficient association with CBP/p300 and the RNA polymerase II complex. They also signal for c-Fos de novo synthesis. This c-Fos binds with phosphorylated c-Jun to generate the AP-1 transcription factor that is responsible for the induction of the inflammatory response genes. Negative regulation of the AP-1 pathway is tripartite, which involves dephosphorylation of the MAPKs, proteolysis of c-Fos and de novo synthesis of Fos-related antigens (Fra-1 and -2). After their synthesis, Fra-1 and -2 bind to Jun to make a DNA binding AP-1 complex, but since they lack the potent transactivation domain of c-Fos they act as transcriptional inhibitors.

NF-AT signal transduction

The nuclear factor of activated T cell (NF-AT)-signaling pathway was elucidated as a result of an intense investigation to understand the molecular mechanism of cyclosporine/FK506 activity and the independent Ca^{++} and protein kinase C (PKC)-derived signals from the T cell receptor[21]. These studies revealed that PKC activation leads to c-Fos expression and inducible AP-1 activity. Ca^{++} mobilization activates the calmodulin-dependent phosphatase calcineurin, which functions to dephosphorylate NF-AT in the cytoplasm of resting cells. This cyclosporine/FK506 sensitive step allows the active transcription factor to translocate to the nucleus, where it binds to its cognate DNA binding site, which is usually adjacent to an AP-1 binding site. As a complex, NF-AT and AP-1 cooperate to mediate transcription of a large set of target genes that are critical for antigen and Fc receptor-mediated response. This activation is autoregulated by the proteolysis of c-Fos as described above, and the nuclear activity of JNK, which phosphorylates NF-AT, relocating it back to the cytoplasm[22].

More recent studies have found that NF-AT is a family of transcription factors that are encoded by at least four genes (NF-AT 1–4). While there are immune cell-specific isoforms, NF-AT is also ubiquitously expressed to activate a wide array of genes. Interestingly, NF-AT has been shown to be a repressor of cartilage cell growth and differentiation, and may be a critical regulator of the changes seen in osteoarthritis[23].

STAT signal transduction

Two critical cytokine families that are involved in immunity against pathogens and tumors are the interferons and the interleukins. While these factors bind to different kinds of receptors, they heavily rely on the signal transducer and activator of transcription (STAT) pathways to mediate their responses[24]. The STATs are a highly conserved family of proteins, for which seven mammalian homologues are known, and contain three functional domains. The C-terminus contains the transactivation domain, while the DNA binding domain is in the center of the molecule. The unique STAT feature is its Src-homology 2 (SH2) domain, which is a protein motif that specifically binds to phosphorylated tyrosine residues. The STAT SH2 domain functions by binding to the activated receptor after ligation to the cytokine. This activation occurs through phosphorylation by a novel family of cytoplasmic tyrosine kinases, termed Janus kinases (JAKs). JAKs bind specifically to intracellular domains of cytokine receptor signaling chains and catalyze ligand-induced phosphorylation of themselves and the receptor, generating STAT binding sites. Then, STAT phosphorylation on activating tyrosine residues leads to the formation of STAT homo- and heterodimers, which rapidly translocate to the nucleus to mediate transcription of the target genes.

The STAT pathway is negatively regulated by common mechanisms like receptor internalization and dephosphorylation. It is also down-regulated specifically by de novo synthesis of the pathway inhibitors: suppressors of cytokine signaling (SOCS) and protein inhibitors of activated STATs (PIAS). The SOCS family consists of eight proteins: SOCS1–SOCS7 and CIS, each of which contains a central SH2 domain and a C-terminal SOCS box[25]. SOCS are STAT target genes that function in a negative feedback loop by occupying the STAT binding site on the cytokine receptor and preventing further activation. SOCS proteins also function to direct a response to a particular cytokine when the cell is also in the presence of other cytokines. For example Th1 responses are mediated in part by IFN-γ induction of SOCS-1 through the STAT-1 pathway, which binds to the IL-4 receptor, inhibiting signaling through STAT-6 and preventing Th2 responses[26]. The PIAS function by associating with phosphorylated STAT dimers and preventing DNA binding[24].

Steroid receptor signal transduction

Steroid receptors are a family of transcription factors, which includes the sex hormone receptors (i.e. estrogen, androgen) and the glucocorticoid receptors (the targets of steroidal drug therapy), mediate a very simple signal transduction that is completely void of intermediate molecules. Since steroids are hydrophobic and can readily diffuse through membranes, receptor ligation can occur in the nucleus, triggering immediate DNA binding and transactivation. In the case of inflammatory diseases, the inhibitory functions of steroid receptors are perhaps more important than their transcriptional activity. This inhibition occurs through two mechanisms. First, after ligand binding, steroid receptors can inhibit other transcription factors (i.e. NF-κB) through direct interaction[27]. Second, they also inhibit transcription through a process known as 'squelching,' whereby the steroid receptors occupy a large proportion of the available co-activators CBP/p300 and RNA polII complexes, thereby creating a shortage for other transcription factors.

This signal transduction cascade is down-regulated primarily by proteolysis of the receptors and *de novo* synthesis of steroid receptors with limited transactivation potential. As an example, the effects of estrogens are manifested almost entirely by estrogen receptor-alpha (ERα). One of ERα's target genes is ERβ, which acts as an efficient dominant inhibitor of ERα transcriptional activity in cells in which both receptors are expressed[28]. Thus, this pathway is also tightly controlled in an autoregulatory loop.

Signal transduction by the TGF-β superfamily

Following the establishment of a concrete understanding of proinflammatory/catabolic signal transduction that has occurred over the last decade, a new trust of research has been focused toward understanding the signal transduction events that mediate tissue regeneration and repair. Based on the cytokines and signal transduction pathways involved, it has become clear that regeneration and repair processes are essentially a recapitulation of embryonic development at the tissue level. With respect to mesenchymal cells and the repair of skeletal tissue, the TGF-β/BMP superfamily has been defined as central to this process. Two of its members (BMP-2 and BMP-7) are already in clinical use to facilitate fracture healing and spinal fusion.

The first member of the superfamily, TGF-β1, was discovered ~20 years ago[29]. Currently there are more than 30 known vertebrate members; many of these have invertebrate homologues.

TGF-β signaling plays a critical role in development and homeostasis. TGF-β and BMP ligands signal by binding to a transmembrane heterodimer composed of a type I and type II receptor. Both receptor subunits are serine–threonine kinase receptors. Following ligand binding, the type II receptor phosphorylates the type I receptor. This activates its kinase domain and leads to the phosphorylation of bound transcription factors known as receptor-associated Sma- and Mad-related proteins (Smads) (Smads 2 and 3 for TGF-β, Smads 1, 5, and 8 for BMP). This signal allows the receptor associated Smads to dissociate and bind the common Smad (Smad4), which then triggers the heteromeric complex to translocate to the nucleus where it binds to its cognate DNA sequence. Like NF-AT, Smad-mediated transcription is virtually always mediated by cooperation with other transcription factors (i.e. AP-1, ATF-2). This can be accomplished by direct activation of the MAPKKK TGF-β receptor associated kinase (TAK), which leads to the activation of IKK, JNK, and p38.

Another elegant component of this pathway is the mechanism by which opposing signals in the cell are avoided by direct competition for Smad4. Thus, in mesenchymal stem cells, the TGF-β signal for proliferation prevents a subsequent BMP signal for differentiation by consuming the cytoplasmic Smad4 in TGF-β receptor-specific Smad complexes and vice versa. In this section, we will review some of recent progresses on BMP studies.

BMPs and bone and cartilage formation

Cumulative evidence demonstrates that BMPs play a critical role in the formation of cartilage and bone. Using a dominant-negative approach to probe the function of BMP receptor signaling in chondrocytes and in osteoblasts has demonstrated that BMP receptor signaling plays an essential role in chondrocyte maturation, osteoblast differentiation, and postnatal bone formation[30-32]. Studies of naturally occurring mutations have also demonstrated the importance of BMPs in several inherited diseases. In mice with short ear mutations BMP-5 gene is disrupted. This mutation in the BMP-5 gene is associated with a wide range of skeletal defects, including reductions in long bone width and the size of several vertebral processes, and an overall lower body mass[33,34]. Mutations in growth/differentiation factor-5 (Gdf5) gene result in brachypodism in mice[35] and chondrodysplasia in humans[36,37]. Gdf5 has been shown to bind BMPR-IB specifically[38] and null mutations in the Bmpr1b gene cause a skeletal phenotype similar to that observed in Gdf5 mutant mice[39].

Most of the animal models with null mutations in BMP ligands, receptors or Smads are embryonic lethal resulting in death before limb development. These animal models include BMP-2, BMP-4, Bmpr1a, Smad1, and Smad5 null mutant mice. Tissue-specific or inducible conditional knockout approaches should be employed to further investigate the function of these genes. Mice lacking Bmpr1b are viable and exhibit defects in the appendicular skeleton. In these mice, proliferation of prechondrogenic cells and differentiation of chondrocytes in the phalangeal region are markedly decreased. In adult mutant mice, the proximal interphalangeal joint is absent, and the phalanges are replaced by a single rudimentary element, while the distal phalanges are unaffected[39]. The appendicular defects in Bmpr1b mutant mice resemble those seen in mice homozygous for the Gdf5 null mutant mice. Since Gdf5 has been shown to play a critical role in cartilage formation and binds the type IB BMP receptors with high affinity[38], these findings suggest that BMPR-IB plays a non-redundant role in cartilage formation *in vivo*. Mutations in the amino acid residues in the GS domain of BMPR-IB cause brachydactyly (BD) type A2 in humans. BD type A2 is an autosomal dominant hand malformation characterized by shortening and lateral deviation of the index fingers and the first and second toes[40]. BMP ligands may utilize multiple type I BMP receptors to mediate their signaling during cartilage and bone formation. In Bmpr1b and BMP-7 double mutant mice, severe appendicular skeletal defects have been observed in the forelimbs and hindlimbs. The ulna and radius are severely affected (absent or shortened)[39]. Since BMP-7 binds efficiently to both BMPR-IB and ActR-IA (ALK2), it is conceivable that BMPR-IB and ActR-IA (ALK2) play important synergistic or overlapping roles in cartilage and bone formation *in vivo*.

The role of BMP signaling in joint formation and the development of arthritis has been examined in Bmpr1a conditional knockout mice in which the gene is inactivated in developing joints, including early joint interzones, adult articular cartilage, and the joint capsule. Mice with conditional deletion of the Bmpr1a gene form normally. However, articular cartilage within the joints gradually wears away in receptor-deficient mice after birth in a process resembling human osteoarthritis (OA)[41]. These findings provide evidence that BMP signaling plays a critical role in the development of OA.

Negative regulation of BMP signaling

BMP activity is controlled at different molecular levels. First, there are a series of BMP antagonists (i.e. noggin, chordin, gremlin), which bind BMP ligands and prevent receptor activation. Second, Smad6 acts as a dominant-negative protein that binds type I BMP receptors and prevents the binding and phosphorylation of Smads 1 and 5. And third, Smad ubiquitin regulatory factor 1 (Smurf1) acts as an E3 ubiquitin ligase (Table 42.1). It interacts with Smads 1 and 5, type I BMP receptor, and the bone-specific transcription factor Runx2, and it mediates the degradation of these proteins.

Mutations in the BMP antagonists have shown how important the activity is in a given system. For example, proximal symphalangism is an autosomal-dominant disorder with ankylosis of the proximal interphalangeal joints, carpal and tarsal bone fusion, and conductive deafness. These symptoms are shared by another disorder of joint morphogenesis, multiple synostoses syndrome. Recently, it was reported that both disorders were caused by heterozygous mutations of the human *noggin* gene. To date, seven mutations in *noggin* have been identified from unrelated families affected with joint morphogenesis[42,43]. Noggin is a secreted polypeptide that binds and inactivates BMPs 2, 4, and 7. Co-crystal structures of noggin and BMP-7 show that noggin inhibits BMP signaling by blocking the molecular interfaces of the binding epitopes for both type I and type II BMP receptors[44], thus preventing BMP-7 from binding to BMP receptors. A transgenic mouse model has recently been established using the osteocalcin promoter to drive the *noggin* transgene. The animals develop a severe osteoporosis. Significant reductions in bone mineral density, bone volume, and bone formation rates are observed[45,46].

Sclerostosis is a recessive inherited osteosclerotic disorder caused by mutations in the protein sclerostin. Recently it was found that sclerostin is related in sequence to the family of secreted BMP antagonists, which includes noggin, chordin, gremlin and dan. Sclerostin is expressed in osteoblasts and osteocytes and binds BMPs 5, 6, and 7 with high affinity. Expression of sclerostin in multipotent fibroblast C3H10T1/2 cells blocks osteoblast differentiation and overexpression of sclerostin in osteoblasts under the control of the osteocalcin promoter in transgenic mice causes osteoporosis[47]. In addition to its inhibitory effect of sclerostin on BMP ligands, a recent report demonstrates that sclerostin also blocks Wnt-3a-induced osteoblast differentiation[48], suggesting that Wnt-3a may regulate osteoblasts through increasing BMP expression and that there is a cross-talk between Wnt/β-catenin and BMP signaling pathways. Taken together, these findings provide evidence that activation of endogenous BMP signaling can enhance bone formation, and regulation of the BMP activity in postnatal stage is required for normal bone homeostasis.

Smad6 is another member of the Smad family, which plays a negative regulatory role in BMP signaling by stably binding to type I BMP receptors. Smad6 interrupts the phosphorylation of Smads 1 and 5 and the subsequent heterodimerization with Smad4[49]. Expression of Smad6 is regulated by BMPs. In the

Table 42.1 Ubiquitin–proteasome system and TGFβ/BMP signaling

Smads	Signaling	E3 ligase	PY motif	Modification	As an adaptor	Effect	References
Smad1	BMP	Smurf1	+	Ub	−	Inhibition	53, 62, 94
Smad2	TGF-β	Smurf1	+	Ub	+	Inhibition	95
Smad3	TGF-β	ROCK1−SCF^β-TrCP	+	Ub	−	Inhibition	96
Smad4	TGF-β/	Jab1	−	Ub	−	Inhibition	97
	BMP	Sumo1		Sumoylation	−	Stimulation	98
Smad5	BMP	Smurf1	+	Ub		Inhibition	53
Smad6	BMP	Smurf1/2	+	Ub	+	Inhibition	58, 59
Smad7	TGF-β	Smurf1/2	+	Ub	+	Inhibition	54, 57
		Arkadia	−	Ub	−	Stimulation	99
Smad8	BMP	?	−	?	?	?	

Smad6 promoter, four overlapping copies of the GCCGnCGC-like motif, which is the binding element for Smads 1 and 5, have been identified[50]. These findings establish a negative feedback regulation mechanism for BMP signaling.

Ubiquitin–proteasome regulation of BMP signaling

Another important regulatory mechanism by which the activity of BMP signaling proteins is modulated involves ubiquitin-mediated proteasomal degradation. The formation of ubiquitin-protein conjugates requires three enzymes that participate in a cascade of ubiquitin transfer reactions: ubiquitin-activating enzyme (E1), ubiquitin-conjugating enzyme (E2), and ubiquitin ligase (E3). The specificity of protein ubiquitination is determined by E3 ubiquitin ligases, which play a crucial role in defining substrate specificity and subsequent protein degradation by 26S proteasomes[52,52].

Smurf1 was identified in the yeast two-hybrid assay by its ability to interact with Smads 1 and 5[53], and later studies show that Smurf1 has much higher affinity to bind Smads 6 and 7[54]. Smurf1 is a member of the Hect domain family of E3 ubiquitin ligases. Smurf1 contains a conserved cysteine, located at the carboxyl terminal of the Hect domain, which is capable of forming a thioester bond with ubiquitin[55,56]. Mutation of this conserved cysteine residue to an alanine (C710A) abolished the ubiquitination and degradation activity of Smurf1[53]. Another motif often found in the Hect domain family of E3 ligase is the WW domain, which contains two highly conserved tryptophans and a conserved proline in an ~30-amino acid region[56,53]. The WW domains have a preference for binding to small proline-rich sequences, PPXY motifs, and different WW domains possess different substrate specificity. Mutations of the PY motif of Smads 1 and 5 prevent them interacting with Smurf1 and inhibit the degradation of these Smad proteins[53]. Smurf1 is located in the cytoplasm and the nucleus and it is exported with Smads 6 or 7, which are located in the nucleus, to the cell membrane or cytoplasm and induces the degradation of type I TGF-β and BMP receptors on cell membrane and Smads 1 and 5 in cytoplasm[54,57,58]. Several lines of evidence suggest that Smurf1 may have a synergistic effect with Smad6 to inhibit BMP signaling[58,59].

Since bone-specific transcription factor Runx2 interacts with Smad1 protein[60,61], whose degradation is mediated by Smurf1[53], the effect of Smurf1 on Runx2 degradation has been examined in osteoblast precursor cells. Smurf1 induces Runx2 degradation in a ubiquitin–proteasome-dependent manner[62]. Similar findings were also reported when Smurf1 is transfected into osteoblastic OB-6 cells[63]. Smurf1 may interact with Runx2 in a direct or indirect mechanism. The conserved PY motif has been identified in all Runx family members. It has been reported that Smurf1 mediates Runx3 degradation and Runx3 protein with a PY motif deletion is resistant to Smurf1-induced degradation in 293 cells[64].

The role of Smurf1 in bone formation *in vivo* was examined by generating Smurf1 transgenic mice in which expression of a Smurf1 transgene is targeted to osteoblasts using the type I collagen promoter (murine 2.3 kb Colla1). In Coll–Smurf1 transgenic mice, the bone mass as well as dynamic bone formation rates are decreased, and osteoblast function, including proliferation and differentiation, is inhibited[65]. Recent studies also demonstrate that bone formation is enhanced in Smurf1 null mutant mice[66]. These findings demonstrate that regulatory proteins of BMP signaling may also play an important physiological role in bone homeostasis *in vivo*.

Wnt/β-catenin signaling

The Wnt family consists of a number of small, cysteine-rich, secreted glycoproteins involved in regulation of a variety of cellular activities, and plays critical roles early during development, for instance controlling mesoderm induction, patterning, cell fate determination, and morphogenesis[67–69]. Wnt proteins trigger signaling pathways inside cells that proceed through several protein complexes. One protein in these pathways is β-catenin. The canonical Wnt signaling pathway affects cellular functions by regulating β-catenin expression and its subcellular localization. In the absence of Wnt signaling, β-catenin levels are kept at a steady-state. Any β-catenin molecules that are not bridging cadherins to the actin cytoskeleton or participating in other activities are ubiquitinated and degraded by the 26S proteasome[70]. A multiprotein complex containing kinases (glycogen synthase kinase (GSK) 3β and casein kinase (CK) 1) and scaffolding proteins (Axin, Axin2, adenomatous polyposis coli (APC) and disheveled (Dsh)) mediate the degradation of excess β-catenin by phosphorylating specific amino terminal residues and creating docking sites for F-box protein/E3 ligase complexes[69,71,72]. Therefore, inhibition of β-catenin phosphorylation prevents its degradation and increases its cytoplasmic level and nuclear translocation. Signaling from Wnt releases β-catenin from its binding proteins, allowing it to move to the nucleus, where it interacts with the T-cell factor (TCF)/lymphoid enhancer factor (LEF) transcription factors, to activate expression of target genes[68,69,73].

At the surface of cells, Wnts interact with two kinds of protein: Frizzled receptor and low-density-lipoprotein (LDL) receptor-related protein 5 or 6 (Lrp5/6). Wnt proteins can form a complex with the cysteine-rich domain (CRD) of Frizzled and with Lrp5/6, leading to the formation of a dual-receptor complex[74,75]. The intracellular parts of the receptors pass on this information, turning on the pathways that feed through β-catenin inside the cell. Lrp5 or 6 receptors have a second function. They bind to Dickkopf-1 (Dkk1), a molecule that counteracts Wnt and blocks Wnt function. Binding of Dkk1 to Lrp5/6 might alter the confirmation of Lrp5/6 so that it can no longer interact with Wnt and Frizzled, thus halting the intracellular signaling. Kremen-1 associates with Dkk1 and interacts with Lrp5 to induce Lrp5 endocytosis[76]. The intracellular tail of Lrp5/6 binds Axin and causes dissociation of β-catenin from its protein complex and activates β-catenin signaling (Fig. 42.1)[77].

The osteoporosis pseudoglioma (OPPG) syndrome and the high bone mass (HBM) syndrome are mapped to the human chromosome 11q12–13 locus[78,79]. OPPG is an autosomal recessive childhood disorder with both skeletal and eye abnormalities. OPPG patients have normal bone growth associated with severe osteopenia without abnormal collagen synthesis or hormonal

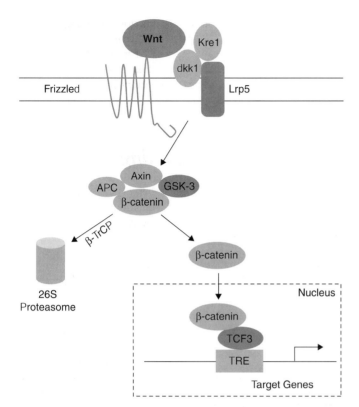

Fig. 42.1 Wnt/β-catenin signaling pathway. See also colour plate section.

defects. They also have congenital or juvenile-onset blindness due primarily to hyperplasia of the primary vitreous. In contrast, carriers of the autosomal dominant HBM trait have very high spinal bone mineral density compared to unaffected individuals[79]. OPPG patients harbor inactivating mutations in the Lrp5 gene[80] and heterozygous carriers of the mutations have reduced bone mass. An activating mutation (Gly171Val) in Lrp5 is responsible for the high bone mass syndrome[81–84]. The finding that Lrp5 deficiency does not cause developmental defects[80,85] suggests the importance of the Wnt pathway to the regulation of perinatal and postnatal functions. Several lines of evidence have suggested that Lrp5-mediated control of bone mass is through canonical β-catenin pathway[80] but the role of β-catenin in bone formation and osteoblast function remain to be defined.

It has been reported that Wnt4, Wnt14, and Wnt16 as well as β-catenin are expressed in an overlapping pattern in the developing synovial joints. Removal of β-catenin early in mesenchymal progenitor cells promotes chondrocyte differentiation and blocks the activity of Wnt14 in joint formation. Ectopic expression of an activated form of β-catenin or Wnt14 in early differentiating chondrocytes induces ectopic joint formation and genetic removal of β-catenin in chondrocytes leads to joint fusion [86,87]. These findings indicate that the Wnt/β-catenin signaling pathway is necessary for the induction of early steps of synovial joint formation. Expression of Wnt5a and frizzled5 is up-regulated in RA synovial tissues in comparison to normal adult tissues. Compared with normal synovial fibroblasts, cultured RA fibroblast-like synoviocytes express higher levels of IL-15. Transfection of Wnt5a into normal fibroblasts stimulates IL-15 secretion[88]. These

findings suggest that Wnt/frizzled signaling may contribute to the phenotypic changes in RA fibroblasts.

Therapeutic application

TNF-α plays an essential role in the pathophysiology of RA and other autoinflammatory diseases. Etanercept (Enbrel, Immunex Wyeth Research, Seattle, WA) is a soluble receptor TNF-α antagonist that competitively inhibits the interaction of TNF-α with cell-surface receptors, preventing TNF-α-mediated cellular responses and modulating the activity of other pro-inflammatory cytokines and processes that are regulated by TNF-α. The results from a multicenter, randomized, double-blind, placebo-controlled trial of etanercept (25 mg, twice a week or 50 mg, once a week) show that etanercept reduces signs and symptoms in patients with moderately to severely active RA and inhibits the progression of structural damage in patients with RA[89,90]. Patients treated with methotrexate for RA often improve but continue to have active disease. The combination therapy of etanercept with methotrexate provides a significantly greater clinical benefit than methotrexate alone[91].

Recent studies demonstrate that p38 MAPK regulates TNF-α production in RA synovium. Inhibition of p38 MAPK results in reduction of TNF-α mRNA in human macrophages. The kinase regulates TNF-α expression by a dual mechanism, in part by controlling TNF-α mRNA stability but also via the 5′-promoter region through NF-κB in macrophages[92]. These observations suggest that p38 MAPK could serve as a target for inhibitors of TNF-α expression and anti-inflammatory drugs.

A cell-permeable peptide inhibitor of the IκB–kinase complex, a crucial component of signal transduction pathways to NF-κB, has been developed. This peptide inhibits RANKL (receptor activator of NF-κB ligand)-stimulated NF-κB activation and osteoclast formation *in vitro* and *in vivo*. This peptide also significantly reduces the severity of collagen-induced arthritis in mice by reducing levels of TNF-α and IL-1β, abrogating joint swelling and reducing destruction of bone and cartilage[93]. These findings clearly demonstrate that selective inhibition of NF-κB activation provides effective therapeutic benefit for the treatment of RA and other inflammatory diseases.

Conclusions

As a result of elucidating the signal transduction pathways involved in inflammation and immunity we now have a firm biochemical basis for the etiology of rheumatic diseases. From this knowledge we now understand how over-activation and/or defective inhibition of selective receptors, kinases, and transcription factors can convert a normal phlogistic or immune response into a chronic disease state. More importantly, targets for intervention have been identified and the promise of rational drug design has come to fruition. As the gaps in our knowledge of signal transduction continue to be filled, and new advances in drug development are made, it is likely that our ability to treat patients will also markedly improve. From this approach we may also see the development of the first therapeutics designed for tissue repair and regeneration.

References

1. Firestein, G. S., and Manning, A. M. Signal transduction and transcription factors in rheumatic disease. *Arthritis Rheum* 1999; **42**: 609.

2. Smith, C. A., Farrah, T., and Goodwin, R. G. The TNF receptor superfamily of cellular and viral proteins: activation, costimulation, and death. *Cell* 1994; **76**: 959.

3. Locksley, R. M., Killeen, N., and Lenardo, M. J. The TNF and TNF receptor superfamilies: integrating mammalian biology. *Cell* 2001; **104**: 487.

4. Arch, R. H., Gedrich, R. W., and Thompson, C. B. Tumor necrosis factor receptor-associated factors (TRAFs): a family of adapter proteins that regulates life and death. *Genes Dev* 1998; **12**: 2821.

5. Chen, G. and Goeddel, D. V. TNF-R1 signaling: a beautiful pathway. *Science* 2002; **296**: 1634.

6. Wajant, H. The Fas signaling pathway: more than a paradigm. *Science* 2002; **296**: 1635.

7. Vaudry, D., Stork, P. J., Lazarovici, P., and Eiden, L. E. Signaling pathways for PC12 cell differentiation: making the right connections. *Science* 2002; **296**: 1648.

8. Sen, R., and Baltimore, D. Multiple nuclear factors interact with the immunoglobulin enhancer sequences. *Cell* 1986; **46**: 705.

9. Verma, I. M., Stevenson, J. K., Schwarz, E. M., Van Antwerp, D., and Miyamoto. S. Rel/NF-kappa B/I kappa B family: intimate tales of association and dissociation. *Genes Dev* 1995; **9**: 2723.

10. Verma, I. M. and Stevenson, J. IkappaB kinase: beginning, not the end. *Proc Natl Acad Sci U S A* 1997; **94**: 11758–60.

11. Zhong, H., Voll, R. E., and Ghosh, S. Phosphorylation of NF-kappa B p65 by PKA stimulates transcriptional activity by promoting a novel bivalent interaction with the coactivator CBP/p300. *Mol Cell* 1998; **1**: 661.

12. Chiao, P. J., Miyamoto, S., and Verma, I. M. Autoregulation of I kappa B alpha activity. *Proc Natl Acad Sci U S A* 1994; **91**: 28.

13. Arenzana-Seisdedos, F., Turpin, P., Rodriguez, M., Thomas, D., Hay, R. T., Virelizier, J. L., and Dargemont, C. Nuclear localization of I kappa B alpha promotes active transport of NF-kappa B from the nucleus to the cytoplasm. *J Cell Sci* 1997; **110**: 369.

14. Wang, C. Y., Mayo, M. W., Korneluk, R. G., Goeddel, D. V., and Baldwin, Jr. A. S. NF-kappaB antiapoptosis: induction of TRAF1 and TRAF2 and c-IAP1 and c-IAP2 to suppress caspase-8 activation. *Science* 1998; **281**: 1680.

15. Lee, E. G., Boone, D. L., Chai, S., Libby, S. L., Chien, M., Lodolce, J. P., and Ma, A. Failure to regulate TNF-induced NF-kappaB and cell death responses in A20-deficient mice. *Science* 2000; **289**: 2350.

16. Beg, A. A., Sha, W. C., Bronson, R. T., Ghosh, S., and Baltimore, D. Embryonic lethality and liver degeneration in mice lacking the RelA component of NF-kappa B. *Nature* 1995; **376**: 167.

17. Li, Q., Van Antwerp, D., Mercurio, F., Lee, K. F., and Verma, I. M. Severe liver degeneration in mice lacking the IkappaB kinase 2 gene. *Science* 1999; **284**: 321.

18. Kelliher, M. A., Grimm, S., Ishida, Y., Kuo, F., Stanger, B. Z., and Leder, P. The death domain kinase RIP mediates the TNF-induced NF-kappaB signal. *Immunity* 1998; **8**: 297.

19. Marok, R., Winyard, P. G., Coumbe, A., Kus, M. L., Gaffney, K., Blades S. *et al.* Activation of the transcription factor nuclear factor-kappaB in human inflamed synovial tissue. *Arthritis Rheum* 1996; **39**: 583.

20. Ransone, L. J., and Verma, I. M. Nuclear proto-oncogenes fos and jun. *Annu Rev Cell Biol* 1990; **6**: 539.

21. Rao, A., Luo, C., and Hogan, P. G. Transcription factors of the NFAT family: regulation and function. *Annu Rev Immunol* 1997; **15**: 707.

22. Chow, C. W., Rincon, M., Cavanagh, J., Dickens, M., and Davis, R. J. Nuclear accumulation of NFAT4 opposed by the JNK signal transduction pathway. *Science* 1997; **278**: 1638.

23. Ranger, A. M., Gerstenfeld, L. C., Wang, J., Kon, T., Bae, H., Gravallese E. M. *et al.* The nuclear factor of activated T cells (NFAT) transcription factor NFATp (NFATc2) is a repressor of chondrogenesis. *J Exp Med* 2000; **191**: 9.

24. Aaronson, D. S., and Horvath, C. M. A road map for those who know JAK-STAT. *Science* 2002; **296**: 1653.

25. Krebs, D. L., and Hilton, D. J. SOCS: physiological suppressors of cytokine signaling. *J Cell Sci* 2000; **113**: 2813.

26. Dickensheets, H. L., Venkataraman, C., Schindler, U., and Donnelly, R. P. Interferons inhibit activation of STAT6 by interleukin 4 in human monocytes by inducing SOCS-1 gene expression. *Proc Natl Acad Sci U S A* 1999; **96**: 10800.

27. Doucas, V., Shi, Y., Miyamoto, S., West, A., Verma, I., and Evans, R. M. Cytoplasmic catalytic subunit of protein kinase A mediates cross- repression by NF-kappa B and the glucocorticoid receptor. *Proc Natl Acad Sci U S A* 2000; **97**: 11893.

28. McDonnell, D. P., and Norris, J. D. Connections and regulation of the human estrogen receptor. *Science* 2002; **296**: 1642.

29. Attisano, L., and Wrana, J. L. Signal transduction by the TGF-beta superfamily. *Science* 2002; **296**: 1646.

30. Enomoto-Iwamoto, M., Iwamoto, M., Mukudai, Y., Kawakami, Y., Nohno, T., Higuchi, Y. *et al.* Bone morphogenetic protein signaling is required for maintenance of differentiated phenotype, control of proliferation, and hypertrophy in chondrocytes. J Cell Biol 1998; **140**: 409–18.

31. Chen, D., Ji, X., Harris, M. A., Feng, J. Q., Karsenty, G., Celeste A. J. *et al.* Differential roles for BMP receptor type IB and IA in differentiation and specification of mesenchymal precursor cells to osteoblast and adipocyte lineages. *J Cell Biol* 1998; **142**: 295–305.

32. Zhao, M., Harris, S. E., Horn, D., Geng, Z., Nishimura, R., Mundy, G. R., and Chen, D. Bone morphogenetic protein receptor signaling is necessary for normal murine postnatal bone formation. *J Cell Biol* 2002; **157**: 1049–60.

33. Kingsley, D. M., Bland, A. E., Grubber, J. M., Marker, P. C., Russell, L.B., Copeland N.C., and Jenkins N.A. The mouse short ear skeletal morphogenesis is associated with defects in a bone morphogenetic member of the TGFβ superfamily. *Cell* 1992; **71**: 399–410.

34. Mikic, B., van der Meulen, M. C., Kingsley, D. M., Carter, D.R., Long bone geometry and strength in adult BMP-5 deficient mice. *Bone* 1995; **16**: 445–54.

35. Storm, E. E., Huynh, T. V., Copeland, N. G., Jenkins, N. A., Kingsley, D. M., and Lee, S. J. Limb alterations in *brachypodism* mice due to mutations in a new member of the TGFβ? superfamily. *Nature* 1994; **368**: 639–43.

36. Thomas, J. T., Lin, K., Nandedkar, M., Camargo, M., Cervenka, J., and Luyten, F. P. A human chondrodysplasia due to a mutation in a TGFβ superfamily member. *Nat Genet* 1996; **12**: 315–17.

37. Thomas, J. T., Kilpatrick, M. W., Lin, K., Erlacher, L., Lembessis, P., Costa, T. *et al.* Disruption of human limb morphogenesis by a dominant negative mutation in CDMP1. *Nat Genet* 1997; **17**: 58–64.

38. Nishitoh, H., Ichijo, H., Kimura, M., Matsumoto, T., Makishima, F., Yamaguchi, A. *et al.* Identification of type I and type II serine/threonine kinase receptors for growth/differentiation factor-5. *J Biol Chem* 1996; **271**: 21345–52.

39. Yi, S. E., Daluiski, A., Pederson, A. R., Rosen, V., and Lyons, K. M. The type I BMP receptor BMPRIB is required for chondrogenesis in the mouse limb. *Development* 2000; **127**: 621–30.

40. Lehmann, K., Seemann, P., Stricker, S., Sammar, M., Meyer, B., Suring, K. *et al.* Mutations in bone morphogenetic protein receptor 1B cause brachydactyly type A2. *Proc Natl Acad Sci U S A* 2003; **100**: 12277–82.

41. Rountree, R. B., Schoor, M., Chen, H., Marks, M. E., Harley, V., Mishina, Y., and Kingsley, D. M. BMP receptor signaling is required for postnatal maintenance of articular cartilage. *PLoS Biol* 2004; **2**: 1815–27.

42. Gong, Y., Krakow, D., Marcelino, J., Wilkin, D., Chitayat, D., Babul-Hirji, R. *et al.* Heterozygous mutations in the gene encoding noggin affect human joint morphogenesis. *Nat Genet* 1999; **21**: 302–4.

43. Takahashi, T., Takahashi, I., Komatsu, I., Sawaishi, Y., Higashi, K., Nishimura, G. *et al.* Mutations of the NOG gene in individuals with

proximal symphalangism and multiple synostosis syndrome. *Clin Genet* 2001; **60**: 447–51.

44. Groppe, J., Greenwald, J. E., Wiater, J., Rodrizuez-Leon, A. N., Economides, W., Kwiatkowshi, *et al*. Structural basis of BMP signaling inhibition by the cystine knot protein Noggin. *Nature* 2002; **420**: 636–42.

45. Devlin, R. D., Du, Z., Pereira, R. C., Kimble, R. B., Economides, N., Jorgetti, V., and Canalis, E. Skeletal over-expression of noggin results in osteopenia and reduced bone formation. *Endocrinology* 2003; **144**: 1972–8.

46. Wu, X. B., Li, Y., Schneider, A., Yu, W., Rajendren, G., Iqbal, J. *et al*. Impaired osteoblastic differentiation, reduced bone formation, and severe osteoporosis in noggin-overexpressing mice. *J Clin Invest* 2003; **112**: 924–34.

47. Winkler, D. G., Sutherland, M. K., Geoghegan, J. C., Yu, C., Hayes, T., Skonier, J. E. *et al*. Osteocyte control of bone formation via sclerostin, a novel BMP antagonist. *EMBO J* 2003; **22**: 6267–76.

48. Winkler, D. G., Sutherland, M. S., Ojala, E., Turcott, E., Geoghegan, J. C., Shpektor, D. *et al*. Sclerostin inhibition of Wnt-3a-induced C3H10T1/2 cell differentiation is indirect and mediated by bone morphogenetic proteins. *J Biol Chem* 2005; **280**: 2498–502.

49. Imamura, T., Takase, M., Nishihara, A., Oeda, E., Hanai, J., Kawabata, M., and Miyazono K. Smad6 inhibits signalling by the TGF-beta superfamily. *Nature* 1997; **389**: 622–6.

50. Ishida, W., Hamamoto, T., Kusanagi, K., Yagi, K., Kawabata, M., Takehara, K. *et al*. Smad6 is a Smad1/5-induced smad inhibitor: characterization of bone morphogenetic protein-responsive element in the mouse Smad6 promoter. *J Biol Chem* 2000; **275**: 6075–9.

51. Hershko, A. Ubiquitin: roles in protein modification and breakdown. *Cell* 1983; **34**: 11–12.

52. Ciechanover, A., Orian, A., and Schwartz, A. L. The ubiquitin-mediated proteolytic pathway: mode of action and clinical implications. *J Cell Biochem* 2000; **77**: 40–51.

53. Zhu, H., Kavsak, P., Abdollah, S., Wrana, J., and Thomsen, G. H. A SMAD ubiquitin ligase targets the BMP pathway and affects embryonic pattern formation. *Nature* 1999; **400**: 687–93.

54. Ebisawa, T., Fukuchi, M., Murakami, G., Chiba, T., Tanaka, K., Imamura, T., and Miyazono, K. Smurf1 interacts with transforming growth factor-beta type I receptor through Smad7 and induces receptor degradation. *J Biol Chem* 2001; **276**: 12477–80.

55. Hochetrasser, M. Ubiquitin-dependent protein degradation. *Annu Rev Genet* 1996; **30**: 405–39.

56. Rotin, D. WW (WWP) domains: from structure to function. *Curr Top Microbiol Immunol* 1998; **228**: 115–33. [Review.]

57. Suzuki, C., Murakami, G., Fukuchi, M., Shimanuki, T., Shikauchi, Y., Imamura, T., and Miyazono, K. Smurf1 regulates the inhibitory activity of Smad7 by targeting Smad7 to the plasma membrane. *J Biol Chem* 2002; **277**: 39919–25.

58. Murakami, G., Watabe, T., Takaoka, K., Miyazono, K., and Imamura, T Cooperative inhibition of bone morphogenetic protein signaling by Smurf1 and inhibitory Smads. *Mol Biol Cell* 2003; **14**: 2809–17.

59. Horiki, M., Imamura, T., Okamoto, M., Hayashi, M., Murai, J., Myoui, A. *et al*. Smad6/Smurf1 overexpression in cartilage delays chondrocyte hypertrophy and causes dwarfism with osteopenia. *J Cell Biol* 2004; **165**: 433–45.

60. Hanai, J. I., Chen, L. F., Kanno, T., Ohtani-Fujita, N., Kim, W. Y., Guo, W. H. *et al*. Interaction and functional cooperation of PEBP2/CBF with Smads: synergistic induction of the immunoglobulin germline Calpha promoter. *J Biol Chem* 1999; **274**: 31577–82.

61. Lee, K. S., Kim, H. J., Li, Q. L., Chi, X. Z., Ueta, C., Komori, T. *et al*. Runx2 is a common target of transforming growth factor-beta1 and bone morphogenetic protein 2, and cooperation between Runx2 and Smad5 induces osteoblast-specific gene expression in the pluripotent mesenchymal precursor cell line C2C12. *Mol Cell Biol* 2000; **20**: 8783–92.

62. Zhao, M., Qiao, M., Oyajobi, B., Mundy, G. R., and Chen, D. E3 ubiquitin ligase Smurf1 mediates core-binding factor α1/Runx2 degradation and plays a specific role in osteoblast differentiation. *J Biol Chem* 2003; **278**: 27939–44.

63. Bellido, T., Ali, A. A., Plotkin, L. I., Fu, Q., Gubrij, I., Roberson, P. K. *et al*. Proteasomal degradation of Runx2 shortens parathyroid hormone-induced anti-apoptotic signaling in osteoblasts: a putative explanation for why intermittent administration is needed for bone anabolism. *J Biol Chem* 2003; **278**: 50259–72.

64. Jin, Y. H., Jeon, E. J., Li, Q. L., Lee, Y. H., Choi, J. K., Kim, W. J. *et al*. Transforming growth factor-beta stimulates p300-dependent RUNX3 acetylation, which inhibits ubiquitination-mediated degradation. *J Biol Chem* 2004; **279**: 29409–17.

65. Zhao, M., Qiao, M., Harris, S. E., Oyajobi, B., Mundy, G. R., and Chen, D. Smurf1 inhibits osteoblast differentiation and bone formation in vitro and in vivo. *J Biol Chem* 2004; **279**: 12854–9.

66. Yamashita, M., Ying, S., Zhang, G., Li, C., Deng, C. and Zhang, Y. Ubiquitin ligase smurf1 controls osteblast activity and bone homeostasis by targeting MEKK2 for degradation. *Cell* 2005; **121**: 101–13.

67. Huelsken, J., and Birchmeier, W. New aspects of Wnt signaling pathways in higher vertebrates. *Curr Opin Genet Dev* 2001; **11**: 547–53.

68. Moon, R. T., Bowerman, B., Boutros, M., and Perrimon, N. The promise and perils of Wnt signaling through beta-catenin. *Science* 2002; **296**: 1644–6. [Review.]

69. Westendorf, J. J., Kahler, R. A., and Schroeder, T. M. Wnt signaling in osteoblasts and bone diseases. *Gene* 2004; **341**: 19–39. [Review.]

70. Aberle, H., Bauer, A., Stappert, J., Kispert ,A., and Kemler, R. beta-catenin is a target for the ubiquitin-proteasome pathway. *EMBO J* 1997; **16**: 3797–804.

71. Behrens, J., Jerchow, B. A., Wurtele, M., Grimm, J., Asbrand, C., Wirtz, R. *et al*. Functional interaction of an axin homolog, conductin, with beta-catenin, APC, and GSK3beta. *Science* 1998; **280**: 596–9.

72. Jiang, J., and Struhl, G. Regulation of the Hedgehog and Wingless signalling pathways by the F-box/WD40-repeat protein Slimb. *Nature* 1998; **391**: 493–6.

73. Staal, F. J., and Clevers, H. Tcf/Lef transcription factors during T-cell development: unique and overlapping functions. *Hematol J* 2000; **1**: 3–6.

74. Bejsovec, A. Wnt signaling: an embarrassment of receptors. *Curr Biol* 2000; **10**: R919–R922.

75. Huelsken, J., and Birchmeier, W. New aspects of Wnt signaling pathways in higher vertebrates. *Curr Opin Genet Dev* 2001; **11**: 547–53.

76. Mao, B., Wu, W., Davidson, G., Marhold, J., Li, M., Mechler, B. M *et al*. Kremen proteins are Dickkopf receptors that regulate Wnt/beta-catenin signalling. *Nature* 2002; **417**: 664–7.

77. Mao, J., Wang, J., Liu, B., Pan, W., Farr, G. H., 3rd, Flynn, C. *et al*. Low-density lipoprotein receptor-related protein-5 binds to Axin and regulates the canonical Wnt signaling pathway. *Mol Cell* 2001; **7**: 801–9.

78. Gong, Y., Vikkula, M., Boon, L. *et al*. Osteoporosis-pseudoglioma syndrome, a disorder affecting skeletal strength and vision, is assigned to chromosome region 11q12–13. *Am J Hum Genet* 1996; **59**: 146–51.

79. Johnson, M. L., Gong, G., Kimberling, W., Recker, S. M., Kimmel, D. B., and Recker, R. B. Linkage of a gene causing high bone mass to human chromosome 11 (11q12–13) *Am J Hum Genet* 1997; **60**: 1326–32.

80. Gong, Y., Slee, R. B., Fukai, N., Rawadi, G., Roman-Roman, S., Reginato, A. M. *et al*. LDL receptor-related protein 5 (LRP5) affects bone accrual and eye development. *Cell* 2001; **107**: 513–23.

81. Little, R. D., Carulli, J. P., Del Mastro, R. G., *et al*. A mutation in the LDL receptor-related protein 5 gene results in the autosomal dominant high-bone-mass trait. *Am J Hum Genet* 2002; **70**: 11–19.

82. Boyden, L. M., Mao, J., Belsky, J., Mitzner, L., Farhi, A., Mitnick, M. A *et al*. High bone density due to a mutation in LDL-receptor-related protein 5. *N Engl J Med* 2002; **346**: 1513–21.

83. Babij, P., Zhao, W., Small, C., Kharode, Y., Yaworsky, P. J., Bouxsein, M. L. *et al*. High bone mass in mice expressing a mutant LRP5 gene. *J Bone Miner Res* 2003; **18**: 960–74.

84. Zhang, Y., Wang, Y., Li, X., Zhang, J., Mao, J., Li, Z. *et al*. The LRP5 high-bone-mass G171V mutation disrupts LRP5 interaction with Mesd. *Mol Cell Biol* 2004; **24**: 4677–84.

85. Kato, M., Patel, M. S., Levasseur, R., Lobov, I., Chang, B. H., Glass, D. A., 2nd *et al.* Cbfa1-independent decrease in osteoblast proliferation, osteopenia, and persistent embryonic eye vascularization in mice deficient in Lrp5, a Wnt coreceptor. *J Cell Biol* 2002; **157**: 303–14.

86. Hartmann, C., and Tabin, C. J. Wnt-14 plays a pivotal role in inducing synovial joint formation in the developing appendicular skeleton. *Cell* 2001; **104**: 341–51.

87. Guo, X., Day, T. F., Jiang, X., Garrett-Beal, L., Topol, L., and Yang, Y. Wnt/beta-catenin signaling is sufficient and necessary for synovial joint formation. *Genes Dev* 2004; **18**: 2404–17.

88. Sen, M., Lauterbach, K., El-Gabalawy, H., Firestein, G. S., Corr, M., and Carson, D. A. Expression and function of wingless and frizzled homologs in rheumatoid arthritis. *Proc Natl Acad Sci U S A* 2000; **97**: 2791–6.

89. Bathon, J. M., Martin, R. W., Fleischmann, R. M., Tesser, J. R., Schiff, M. H., Keystone, E. C. *et al.* A comparison of etanercept and methotrexate in patients with early rheumatoid arthritis. *N Engl J Med* 2000; **343**: 1586–93.

90. Keystone, E. C., Schiff, M. H., Kremer, J. M., Kafka, S., Lovy, M., DeVries, T., and Burge, D. J. Once-weekly administration of 50 mg etanercept in patients with active rheumatoid arthritis: results of a multicenter, randomized, double-blind, placebo-controlled trial. *Arthritis Rheum* 2004; **50**: 353–63.

91. Weinblatt, M. E., Kremer, J. M., Bankhurst, A. D., Bulpitt, K. J., Fleischmann, R. M., Fox, R. I. *et al.* A trial of etanercept, a recombinant tumor necrosis factor receptor: Fc fusion protein, in patients with rheumatoid arthritis receiving methotrexate. *N Engl J Med* 1999; **340**: 253–9.

92. Campbell, J., Ciesielski, C. J., Hunt, A. E., Horwood, N. J., Beech, J. T., Hayes, L. A *et al.* A novel mechanism for TNF-alpha regulation by p38 MAPK: involvement of NF-kappa B with implications for therapy in rheumatoid arthritis. *J Immunol* 2004; **173**: 6928–37.

93. Jimi, E., Aoki, K., Saito, H., D'Acquisto, F., May, M. J., Nakamura, I. *et al.* Selective inhibition of NF-kappa B blocks osteoclastogenesis and prevents inflammatory bone destruction in vivo. *Nat Med* 2004; **10**: 617–24.

94. Zhang, Y., Chang, C., Gehling, D. J., Hemmati-Brivanlou, A., and Derynck, R. Regulation of Smad degradation and activity by Smurf2, an E3 ubiquitin ligase. *Proc Natl Acad Sci U S A* 2000; **98**: 974–9.

95. Lin, X., Liang, M., and Feng, X. H. Smurf2 is an ubiquitin E3 ligase mediating proteasome-dependent degradation of Smad2 in transforming growth factor-beta signaling. *J Biol Chem* 2000; **275**: 36818–22.

96. Fukuchi, M., Imamura, T., Chiba, T., Ebisawa, T., Kawabata, M., Tanaka, K., and Miyazono, K. Ligand-dependent degradation of Smad3 by a ubiquitin ligase complex of ROC1 and associated proteins. *Mol Biol Cell* 2001; **12**: 1431–43.

97. Wan, M., Cao, X., Wu, Y., Bai, S., Wu, L., Shi, X. *et al.* Jab1 antagonizes TGF-beta signaling by inducing Smad4 degradation. *EMBO Rep* 2002; **3**: 171–6.

98. Lin, X., Liang, M., Liang, Y. Y., Brunicardi, F. C., Feng, X. H. SUMO-1/Ubc9 promotes nuclear accumulation and metabolic stability of tumor suppressor Smad4. *J Biol Chem* 2003; **278**: 31043–8.

99. Koinuma, D., Shinozaki, M., Komuro, A., Goto, K., Saitoh, M., Hanyu, A. *et al.* Arkadia amplifies TGF-beta superfamily signalling through degradation of Smad7. *EMBO J* 2003; **22**: 6458–70.

43 | Mesenchymal stem cells in arthritis

Frank P. Luyten

Introduction

Recent advances in our understanding of the biology of stem cells have attracted the attention of the biomedical community[1-4]. Basic scientists and clinicians are moving in concert, trying to bridge the gap from 'bench to bedside', and to unravel the biology of stem cell populations in development, growth, homeostasis, and disease. Adult stem cells are found in most adult tissues. Adult stem cells, hematopoietic and non-hematopoietic, are more restricted than embryonic stem cells, although recent findings have revealed the existence, at least *in vitro*, of adult marrow-derived, pluripotent stem cells (MAPCs) with a differentiation potential close to embryonic stem cells[5]. However, more critical studies directed toward hematopoietic stem cells have disputed the concept of stem cell plasticity, suggesting that experimental artifact or somatic cell fusion may account for some reported observations of plasticity. Animal and human models with appropriate cell tracking and *in vivo* imaging technologies to explore the biology and therapeutic potential of human stem cells will be vital to advance the field over the coming years[6]. Regardless, cumulative data suggest that precursor cells, residing in 'niches' or recruited from circulating stem cells, can participate in tissue homeostasis and repair, but also potentially contribute to disease processes.

In this chapter, an overview is presented on the existing knowledge regarding the characterization of mesenchymal stem cells (MSCs), a distinct population of non-hematopoietic stem cells, and their potential role in arthritic diseases. MSCs are pluripotent cells, capable of self-renewal and considered the progenitors of connective tissue cell lineages, including chondrocytes, osteoblasts, muscle cells, and adipocytes, and also of other joint-associated tissues such as meniscus, ligaments, and tendons (for review see Ref. 7). This makes MSCs relevant to joint biology and pathology. Much has been done on the characterization and biology of MSCs, because of their potential for cell-based therapeutic strategies in clinical applications such as osteogenesis imperfecta[8], bone engineering[9,10], cardiac muscle repair[11,12], and several applications in the field of hematology/oncology, mostly related to facilitating the engraftment process of allogeneic bone marrow and donor-specific tolerance (for review see Ref. 13).

Besides bone marrow, it appears now that most musculoskeletal tissues, including joint tissues such as articular cartilage[14-17], retropatellar fat[18], and synovium[19], contain a cell population that upon culture on plastic/polystyrene substrates will attach, proliferate, and display pluripotentiality, both *in vitro* and *in vivo*. However, there is little data about the presence, biology, and role of MSCs *in vivo* before any *in vitro* selection. Looking into the joint and the synovio-enthesial complex, it is anticipated that the MSC pool belongs for the most part to the so-called synovial fibroblast-like cells; some call them progenitor cells, some mesenchymal fibroblasts. There is increasing evidence that this MSC pool is diverse and may play very distinct roles in the joint environment. They may be considered as 'reparative' cell populations[20], but their role may go far beyond that; it may include a pro- or anti-inflammatory effect, they may interfere with cell trafficking or the functioning of immune cells, they may play a critical role in epithelial–mesenchymal interactions, guide and influence neo-angiogenesis, and by doing so contribute to a microenvironment that is unique for the normal or diseased joint. The MSC pool can ultimately contribute to the formation of new 'signaling centers', a term used in developmental biology and referring to a group of cells that coordinates a complex biological process in a precise spatio-temporal cascade at a specific developmental stage, thereby orchestrating the arthritic disease process.

In the first part of this chapter, we will examine in more detail the data and their possible interpretations with respect to the role of MSCs in arthritic disease. It may not escape the attention of the reader that in this chapter no clear distinction is always made between the different clinical classifications of arthritis, such as rheumatoid arthritis (RA), osteoarthritis (OA), spondyloarthropathies (SAs), or other forms of arthritis. This has merely to do with the fact that it is my intention to look at MSCs and arthritis from a mechanistic point of view, and that the existing classification of arthritis made by clinicians may not necessarily be of much value to the disease processes when investigating MSC populations and their relevant molecular pathways[21].

The second part of this chapter will briefly touch upon and refer to a variety of potential therapeutic implications when manipulating the MSC pool, and applications by delivering, systemically or locally, selected or engineered MSC populations. Finally, some conclusions and future challenges will be presented.

The characterization and biology of the MSCs in chronic arthritis

Characterization of MSCs in chronic arthritis

Considerable progress has been made towards the characterization of culture-expanded MSCs, and using fluorescence-activated cell sorting (FACS) a cell surface antigen marker profile has evolved for MSCs, apparently regardless of their tissue of origin[22,23]. MSCs typically express a number of adhesion molecules (integrins/CD49, vascular cell adhesion molecule (VCAM)-1/CD106), and other markers such as Thy1/CD90 and endoglin/CD105; they lack the hematopoietic markers such as CD34 and CD45, and are generally regarded as negative for the major histocompatibility II complex (MHCII, human leukocyte antigen (HLA)-DR). However, this marker profile has not been rigorously validated and these characteristics have been established on a cell population selected by its inherent ability to adhere to plastic and proliferate in the presence of serum or specific growth factors, and there are few data correlating this population to the *in vivo* 'real life' MSCs. For instance, it has been recently reported that the synovium of end-stage osteoarthritic joints contains sub-populations (3–10 %) of adherent cells expressing triplicate combinations of cell surface markers associated with the MSC phenotype such as CD9, CD44, CD54, CD90, and CD166[24]. Upon cultivation and expansion, the relative percentages of these sub-populations markedly increased to values of up to 50%, or by a factor of 3 to 7.

There are some indications that, at least for bone marrow-derived stromal cells, some cell surface receptors detected on cultured MSCs are relevant to human MSCs found *in vivo*, but this was only shown for a few markers and in a limited number of samples[22]. Therefore, and due to the lack of a highly sensitive and specific marker, it is of importance to realize that there are only limited data establishing the presence, distribution, and characteristics of MSCs *in vivo*[25]. This is obviously even more so when investigating the MSC pool in normal and diseased joints.

It has long been known that the synovial membrane and synovial fluid contain fibroblast-like cells that can proliferate. These so-called synovial fibroblasts appear to undergo in arthritic disease a number of changes, also referred to as 'activation' or 'transformation', but not all synovial fibroblasts have these altered phenotypes, leading to the concept that sub-populations of fibroblasts are present in the arthritic joint (for review see Refs 26, 27). More recent studies have revealed the presence of fibroblast-like cells with mesenchymal stem cell characteristics both in normal[19,28] and arthritic synovium[29,30], as well as in synovial fluid of arthritic individuals[31]. Very recent data have provided additional evidence for the heterogeneity of the fibroblast-like cells in the synovium using complementary DNA microarrays and hierarchical cluster analysis[32]. Interestingly, they report a striking increased conversion to an earlier developmental 'myofibroblast' phenotype in highly inflamed RA synovia.

It is unclear at this point what the origins are of the MSCs in the synovial joint. However, several sources are possible, including the subchondral bone marrow, the articular cartilage, the synovium, the periosteum, the blood vessels, or even circulating MSCs in the blood[33,34]. Synovium-derived culture-expanded MSCs may originate from the synovial lining and appear to be highly similar to type B synoviocytes[35]. The MSCs may come from the vascular pericytes associated with the vascular networks in the synovio-enthesial complex[36–38]. In models of inflammation the origin of MSCs may be even more complex, as demonstrated in experimentally induced renal inflammation and fibrosis, where local fibroblast proliferation, transdifferentiation, and recruitment from the bone marrow contribute to the local accumulation of fibroblast-like cells, some of which may have MSC characteristics[39]. Synovial MSCs, defined by morphological appearance and characterized by the expression of bone morphogenetic protein receptor Ia (BMPR/Alk3), have been demonstrated in RA synovium but not synovium obtained from patients with OA[40]. The same authors detected similar cells in the initial stages of collagen-induced arthritis, a well characterized mouse model[40]. Remarkably, in the pre-arthritic phase of this model, BMPR-positive cells were present in increased numbers in the subchondral bone marrow and within enlarged bone canals connecting the bone marrow with the synovium. Although these vascular connections have not been described in human arthritis, these findings have led to the intriguing hypothesis that in human arthritis also, these BMP receptor positive cells may be derived from bone marrow or the circulation[41]. Importantly, these data suggested MSCs as potential critical players also in the early phase of arthritic disease, as they appear even before neutrophils and lymphocytes. This phenomenon may not only play a role in RA, but even more so in other chronic arthritides involving extensive subchondral bone remodelling such as the spondyloarthropathies.

The existing data suggest that more MSC-like cells, as judged by the presence of BMPRs, are found in RA synovial tissues as compared to OA synovium[33]. However, it is unclear and not very likely that they represent the total pool of MSCs. The number of presumed MSCs could be further evaluated by *in vitro* approaches with a number of limitations, including the attachment, growth, and proliferation being affected by drug treatment[42]. By carefully enumerating MSCs in synovial fluid, the number of MSCs characterized by *in vitro* multilineage potential is larger in OA than in RA synovial fluid[31]. The higher number of clonogenic multipotential cells was apparently not related to the influx of inflammatory cells into the joint. These data suggest that the appearance and accumulation of MSCs in synovial fluid may be uncoupled from inflammation and rather be the result of tissue damage.

These findings are certainly provocative and provide a strong impetus to further investigate the role of MSCs in arthritis. We are only beginning to address the question of whether there is indeed in arthritis an altered stem cell compartment, and if so, whether this is associated with the initiation and progression of the disease. The characterization of the stem cell compartment will not be easy, and requires a systematic and careful analysis of the stem cell pools involved. This includes the study of the presence of cell surface markers on freshly obtained MSC populations, and the distribution of these cells and associated markers in the discrete niches or tissue compartments. The lack of markers to clearly identify MSCs, and associate these markers with a functional behavior and pluripotentiality, continues to hamper the field. Currently available cell surface markers may not be sufficient to discriminate between physiology and disease. Recent findings suggest that cadherins, in particular cadherin-11, may play a role in the adhesion and synovial tissue organization in both normal and RA patients[43]. These data add to the increasing evidence that molecular players involved in tissue formation and organization are also key signals in postnatal tissue response to injury, regardless of the nature of the injury. The expression of specific intracellular genes, such as transcriptional regulators, and post-translational modifications such as phosphorylation of proteins, may be more informative.

Functional analysis of MSCs in chronic arthritis

Very little has been reported on the *in vivo* biology of MSCs in diseased tissues such as the joints in chronic arthritis and the role of the microenvironment on their *in vivo* biological behavior. There is little doubt that the functional analysis of MSCs, derived from the different tissue sources of the joint and studied in a relevant environment mimicking early or advanced disease, will be of great importance. These tissue-derived MSCs may be of local origin, but some cells of the tissue MSC pool may have been recruited from a distance, and they may have very different functions linked to the severity of the disease state and its progression. Manipulating the stem cell compartment and thereby modulating and possibly slowing down disease progression may then be the proof of principle to convince the scientific community that mesenchymal stem cells are a therapeutic target in arthritic disease.

The rapid advances in our understanding of the biology of mesenchymal stem cells have revealed an increasing number of potential functions[7]. MSCs, by local activation or recruitment from a distance, may be involved in the restoration of tissue homeostasis. Examples are the low frequency replacement of hepatocytes by bone marrow-derived stem cells even in the absence of liver injury[44]. There is sufficient proof of principle of the contribution of stem cells to local tissue repair, as seen in models of wound healing[45], skeletal muscle repair[46,47], cardiac muscle repair[48-51], and pulmonary fibrosis[52]. These regulatory and repair functions may be mediated by an autocrine mechanism, that is, the direct contribution to the differentiated functional cell pool. However, a paracrine mechanism such as releasing specific regulatory instructions to the microenvironment, or even an endocrine mechanism, may play a role. MSCs may enhance the angiogenesis and cardiac function of ischemic hearts by increasing the local expression of vascular endothelial growth factor (VEGF)[53]. The release of specific chemokines from injured liver can recruit distinct stem cell populations to the site of injury[54]. It is well known that MSCs can secrete a whole range of cytokines with many potential effects on the environment, locally and at a distance. They include a number of well-studied hematopoietic cytokines such as macrophage colony stimulating factor, interleukin (IL)-6, IL-7, IL-8, IL-12, IL-14, and IL-15[55]. Recent reports have brought to attention that embryonic signaling molecules, such as Wnts and bone morphogenetic proteins (BMPs), are also secreted by synovial-derived MSCs, and that these peptides are clearly integrated in the cytokine signaling networks, responding to inflammatory cytokines and in turn affecting downstream signaling pathways involved in inflammation and tissue remodeling[56-58].

The potential functional roles of MSCs may be affected and altered by age and disease. There has been accumulating evidence that the proliferative activity and osteogenic potential of bone marrow-derived MSCs (BM-MSCs) diminish with age[59-61]. Regardless of an age-associated decline in stem cell function, the concept that MSCs may be deficient or behave differently in chronic diseases has been further supported by the findings that MSCs from osteoporotic patients have significantly reduced osteogenic activity[62]. In contrast, cultures of BM-MSCs from OA patients did not show altered *in vitro* behavior when compared with normal individuals[63]. Recently, a more comprehensive study reported a significant reduction in the proliferation rate of OA-derived BM-MSCs, and in their chondrogenic and adipogenic differentiation *in vitro*[64]. Interestingly, there was no difference in osteogenic activity. These findings were independent of the site of harvest and appeared to be disease- and not age-related. It is important to keep in mind that these data suggest a possible association, but do not indicate a causal relationship.

Most interestingly, and of direct relevance to arthritic disease, is the potential immunoregulatory role of MSCs both *in vitro* and *in vivo* (for review see Ref. 22). MSCs appear to be quite resistant to rejection and they suppress proliferation of allogenic T cells in an MHC-independent manner[65-68]. Interestingly, some of the observed effects are clearly dose dependent, with high numbers of MSCs suppressing alloreactive T cells, whereas low numbers stimulate lymphocyte proliferation[65]. The ability of MSCs to regulate the immune response has been exploited to reduce graft versus host disease (GVHD), and to induce immune tolerance. Administration of bone marrow-derived MSCs can prolong donor skin-graft survival in mice and non-human primates[68]. Using a preclinical model of human hematopoietic engraftment in NOD-SCID mice, it was shown that unrelated human bone marrow-derived culture-expanded MSCs may improve the outcome of allogeneic transplantation[69]. Early findings in clinical trials of allogeneic bone marrow transplantation indicated that patients who received allogeneic MSCs along with a bone marrow transplant had a low incidence of GVHD[70]. Most recently, encouraging results have been reported in another clinical study for the treatment of severe GVHD with third party haploidentical MSCs[71]. It is noteworthy that, although mesenchymal stem cells are transplantable across allogeneic barriers, transplant rejection can occur in a xenogenic model[72,73].

This surprising immunomodulatory role may be mediated by a number of mechanisms[74]. These include an interaction with, and altering of the secretion profile of several immune cell populations such as dendritic cells, naïve and effector T cells, and natural killer cells to induce a more tolerant and anti-inflammatory phenotype[75]. The observed inhibition of the secretion of TNF α by dendritic cells may lead to immunological tolerance. Interestingly, in this study the human bone marrow-derived MSCs produced constitutively prostaglandin E2 (PGE2) in culture, and inhibitors of PGE2 production affected the MSC-mediated immune modulation. Some of the effects, such as the suppression of T cell proliferation, have been associated with the release of specific signaling molecules, including TGF-β and hepatocyte growth factor by the MSC cell population, and points again towards the potential critical paracrine functions of stem cell populations *in vivo*[40,66,76,77].

It is important to remember that the *in vivo* usefulness of MSCs in humans is still open, and some of the observed effects may be *in vitro* artefacts. The mechanism of action of MSC-mediated immunomodulation is still not well understood. Furthermore, most of the data have been established using bone marrow-derived MSCs and there is no guarantee that MSCs present in the normal or arthritic joints, most probably derived from different sources (see discussion above), have similar immunomodulatory functions. Regardless, the observations so far imply that MSCs are present in an inflammatory environment, also in arthritis, and there is sufficient proof of principle that they can affect local immune responses by interacting with dendritic cell and T cell subsets, thereby potentially interfering with the initiation, progression, and outcome of arthritic and autoimmune diseases.

Therapeutic use of MSCs

Targeting the MSC compartment

Based on the above-described functional characteristics of MSCs, several therapeutic opportunities for manipulating the adult mesenchymal stem cell pool can be recognized. Most importantly, more studies are required to provide insights into the role of the stem cell pool *in vivo* in specific and well-defined diseases, before interfering with MSC biology, involving enhanced and appropriate stem cell activation, stem cell recruitment, stem cell homing, and *in situ* stem cell differentiation. A better understanding of the stem cell pool may lead to therapeutic targets. There have been recent reports indicating that targeting adult stem cell populations may be valuable. The mobilization of endothelial precursor cells by granulocyte-macrophage colony stimulating factor accelerates re-endothelialization and reduces vascular inflammation in a model of intravascular radiation in rabbits[78]. At this point, a further understanding of the processes involved and the relationship to inflammation is essential to assess the risk–benefit of these interventions[79].

The stem cell pool, as a cell phenotype with developmental characteristics, most likely responds to embryonic signaling. Therefore, it is expected that modulating these embryonic signaling pathways will selectively affect the stem cell pool. A striking example is seen in models of kidney injury, an excellent model system in which to study stem cell plasticity and epithelial–mesenchymal transitions. There is overwhelming evidence that modulating BMP signaling by administration of exogenous BMP-7/osteogenic protein-1, enhances recovery of kidney function in animal models of both acute and chronic renal injury[80,81]. Collectively, the therapeutic effect appears to be the result of a direct influence on tubular epithelial cells and interstitial fibroblasts[82]. Mechanistically, the experimental findings suggest that renal 'fibroblasts' retain parts of their original epithelial imprint and plasticity, which can be re-activated by modulating BMP signaling, resulting in epithelial cell formation mediating repair of tubular injury in an inflamed and fibrotic kidney[82].

Although similar processes may take place in the inflamed synovium, very little is known about the mechanisms of action of the stem cell pool in arthritic diseases. As described above, recent data have indicated the recruitment of BMPRs expressing stem cells in the early phase of inflammatory destructive joint disease such as rheumatoid arthritis[33,40]. Further *in vivo* experimental approaches are needed to identify the role of these MSC populations in the arthritic disease models.

MSCs and joint tissue repair

Treatments with cell-based products are reaching the clinical arena, and with some success. A number of these applications have been described in more detail in recent reviews[7,20,25,83]. Understanding the role of the stem cell pool may lead to the isolation and expansion of well-defined multipotent MSCs *ex vivo*, with functional characteristics appropriate for the envisioned therapeutic intervention. In the field of joint surface repair, autologous chondrocyte implantation (ACI) as a promising treatment for deep symptomatic cartilage defects is based on mostly retrospective studies[84–86]. Very recent prospective studies confirm the good clinical outcome of ACI, but positioning this treatment versus other standard treatments such as microfracture is still unclear[87,88]. Nonetheless, retrospective data indicate a potential for long-term tissue repair using these cell-based approaches in the joint environment[85,86]. Careful prospective long-term follow-up is required to confirm and extend these findings. Although the implanted cell populations appear to directly contribute to the articular cartilage repair[89], there is still an important lack of understanding of the mechanisms of repair in this application. Dedifferentiation of the articular cartilage-derived cells due to the expansion process is regarded as a major limitation, and results in an inconsistent cellular product[90]. More careful analysis and characterization of expanded cell populations convincingly demonstrated the presence of substantial numbers of cells with MSC characteristics in these expanded cell populations, and their relative amount depended on the culture conditions[14,15,91].

The use of 'pure' MSCs for cartilage and bone repair has been reported both in animal models and in pilot clinical studies (for review see Ref. 83). They can be isolated from multiple sources, including bone marrow, fat, and also synovium. Indeed, the routine use of needle arthroscopy in rheumatology clinics allows the harvesting of synovial biopsies from which various cell types can be obtained, including synovial-derived mesenchymal stem cells (SM-MSCs). SM-MSCs are multipotent both *in vitro* and *in vivo*[19,46,92,93] Interestingly, the *in vitro* behavior may not necessarily reflect their *in vivo* biology, as was demonstrated using SM-MSCs[92]. The choice of the source of MSCs and the use of properly characterized and selected MSCs is not trivial. As has been shown for kidney repair (see under the section Targeting the MSC compartment), it makes sense to use cell populations that have retained the original tissue imprint and plasticity, suggesting the preferred use of 'niche' MSCs or at least MSCs with the proper imprints, regardless of the tissue source. Therefore, the use of SM-MSCs or MSCs with characteristics of the joint interzone, the region of the prospective joint consisting of a few cell layers of MSCs, expressing *Gdf5* and present postnatally in the synovium, may be a good choice, as they contain the precursors of articular cartilage and joint-associated tissues[94].

It is important to indicate that ACI is performed for cartilage defects in an otherwise healthy joint. Therefore, it is unclear at this point what the potential role and success of cell-based repair is in an arthritic joint. Loss of joint homeostasis and arthritic disease are creating a very different microenvironment, and thus will influence cell engraftment and tissue differentiation. Regardless of this, remarkable results with MSCs were recently reported in a large animal model of osteoarthritis[95]. OA-like disease was induced by medial meniscectomy and resection of the anterior cruciate ligament in the knee joints of goats. Local delivery of labelled adult MSCs, isolated from bone marrow, to injured joints resulted in engraftment in meniscus, fat pad, and synovium, and some, although very limited, in the articular surface. Regeneration of a neo-menisceal-like tissue and retardation of joint destruction, particularly of the articular surface, were the most striking results. These data indicate that, since OA is often a local disease, restricted to one or a few large weight-bearing joints, there are opportunities for these local MSC-based treatments.

A platform for gene delivery

MSCs can be used to locally deliver specific signals, thereby contributing by a paracrine mechanism to more successful tissue repair[96] or any other envisioned therapeutic effect, such as immunomodulation in autoimmune diseases[97]. It is not the purpose of this chapter to discuss the gene delivery modalities in detail, and the reader is referred to recent reviews[98,25].

The tissue homing capacities of MSCs may become of particular importance for this purpose, provided we understand better what determines their homing. So far, it appears that bone marrow-derived MSCs predominantly go to the bone marrow when injected systemically[99]. However, data indicate that MSCs will also preferentially seek engraftment in damaged tissues, regardless of the tissue source[46]. Taken together, it is evident that proper tissue homing coupled with a contribution to local tissue repair and secreting locally a therapeutic agent, makes MSCs very attractive candidates for the treatment of arthritic disease. Proof of principle experiments have been published for cytokine delivery such as IL-3[100], soluble TNF receptor[101], and other therapeutic genes relevant to hematopoietic diseases such as haemophilia[102]. Some authors have advocated the use of MSCs as a platform of overexpressing growth factors such as BMP-2 for the repair of local cartilage defects[103]. Indeed, MSCs appear mostly not to be successful in the repair of cartilage defects unless they are stimulated and supported by the proper chondrogenic factor[104].

Toxicity and potential unforeseen events

As for all therapeutic interventions, there is always a possible downside. Cell fusion has been described using bone marrow-derived MSCs, but this is a rare event, and it is not well understood what the biological implications of this phenomenon are[105]. Although apparently fairly successful in repairing cartilage lesions, the associated effects of MSCs engineered to secrete growth factors such as BMPs may result in side-effects or 'unforeseen events' such as osteophyte formation[103]. More worrisome are the findings in a murine melanoma tumor model, where it was shown that the subcutaneous injection of B16 melanoma cells led to tumor growth in allogeneic recipients only when MSCs were co-injected[106]. This raises the concern of favoring tumor growth in patients receiving MSCs for therapeutic purposes such as tissue repair. This effect is probably related to their immunomodulatory and immunosuppressive effects on regulatory T cells. Tumor formation, however, is possible due to a different mechanism. Data in a recent publication indicated that chronic infection in a mouse model with *Helicobacter*, a known carcinogen, induced repopulation of the stomach with bone marrow-derived MSCs. Subsequently, these cells progressed through metaplasia and dysplasia to intra-epithelial cancer[107]. Although the existing clinical experience does not identify this as a major concern, it is clear that a careful prospective follow-up will be needed to evaluate these potentially serious adverse events. Potential toxicity associated with gene therapy is outside the scope of this chapter.

Conclusions and future challenges

The presence of MSCs in arthritis, both in the synovium and synovial fluid, is reasonably well established. The potential involvement and roles of MSC populations in arthritic diseases are far from clear. The expression and reactivation of embryonic signaling pathways associated with stem cells in the context of arthritis, previously suggested and not sufficiently recognized, may have a profound impact on pathogenetic mechanisms of arthritic disease[41,108]. Tissue damage and inflammation elicit a tissue response and repair mechanisms that happen routinely in our body. However, at some point this process may go wrong and lead to the accumulation of fetal or 'developmental' fibroblasts with MSC characteristics, generated locally by proliferation or trans-differentiation, or recruited from a distance. This may result in new 'signaling centers', as defined by developmental biologists, eventually leading to a shift in the local 'stromal code' as conceptualized by immunologists[109,110], and is likely involved in the switch of normal physiological inflammation and restoration of tissue homeostasis to chronic inflammation and loss of homeostasis (see Fig. 43.1). The mechanisms responsible for an irreversible shift into new populations of stromal cells with developmental characteristics and an autonomous behavior are still unknown, but may involve local dedifferentiation with epigenetic alterations, DNA mutations, and chromosomal rearrangements, or recruitment of distant stem cell populations with an inappropriate phenotype for the local environment. It may be overstated, due to lack of sufficient convincing data, that rheumatoid arthritis may be regarded as premature osteoarthritis with fetal-like healing[111], but this concept should be investigated further. The study of the role of embryonic signaling pathways, guiding and modulating the stem cell pool, is part of a strategy to try to 'deconstruct' arthritis[21].

This new field of research requires more comprehensive technological approaches including genetic models allowing stem cell tracking, *in situ* identification of the stem cell populations and microdissection technology, and cell and molecular imaging.

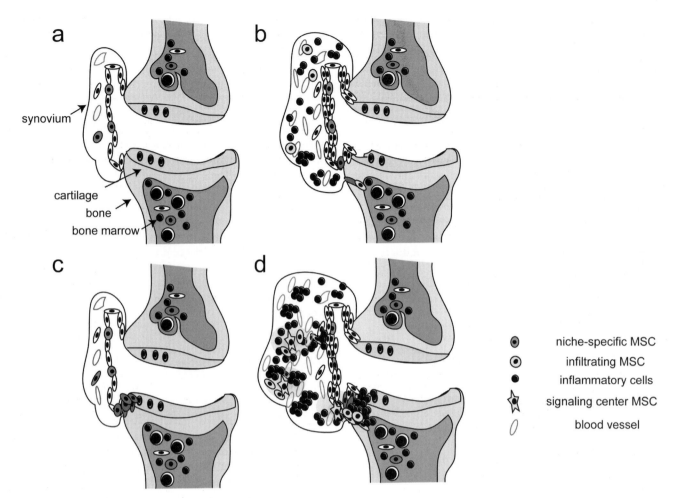

Fig. 43.1 Schematic drawing of stem cell biology and pathology in synovium. (a) In the normal joint, a limited number of 'niche' MSCs are present in the synovial lining, the interstitium, and other joint-associated tissues, as well as the subchondral bone marrow. They contribute to the maintenance of joint homeostasis. (b) Upon joint 'injury', regardless of the type of injury, MSC recruitment (infiltrating MSCs) and proliferation (niche or infiltrating MSCs) takes place, and cell differentiation. This tissue response is considered an attempt to repair. (c) A 'successful' tissue response results in proper tissue repair and the restoration of joint homeostasis. (d) However, this process may go wrong and lead to the accumulation of 'developmental' fibroblasts with MSC characteristics, generated locally by proliferation or recruited from a distance, some of them undergoing a process of dedifferentiation or transdifferentiation. This may induce the formation of new 'signaling centers', creating gradients of signals (e.g. chemokines) attracting inflammatory cells and enhanced angiogenesis. At some point, this becomes an irreversible alteration of the stromal environment, and leads to chronic disease. See also colour plate section.

Local activation and recruitment of stem cell populations are opportunities in the search for new therapeutic approaches contributing to the restoration of joint homeostasis and repair for arthritic diseases[20,108]. Understanding the mechanisms of action of these stem cell-based approaches is critical in their development towards clinical applications. Using the stem cells as a platform for local gene delivery may also be a promising treatment approach for the future.

Acknowledgement

The author expresses his gratitude to Rik Lories, who provided excellent support for the figure.

References

1. Weissman, I. L. Translating stem and progenitor cell biology to the clinic: barriers and opportunities. *Science* 2000; **287**: 1442–6.
2. Korbling, M., and Estrov, Z. Adult stem cells for tissue repair: a new therapeutic concept? *New Engl J Med* 2003; **349**: 570–82.
3. Hochedlinger, K., and Jaenisch, R. Mechanisms of disease: nuclear transplantation, embryonic stem cells, and the potential for cell therapy. *New Engl J Med* 2003; **349**: 275–86.
4. Rosenthal, N. Medical progress: Prometheus's vulture and the stem-cell promise. *New Engl J Med* 2003; **349**: 267–74.
5. Jiang, Y., Jahagirdar, B. N., Reinhardt, R. L. *et al*. Pluripotency of mesenchymal stem cells derived from adult marrow. *Nature* 2002; **418**: 41–9.
6. Horwitz, E. M. Stem cell plasticity: the growing potential of cellular therapy. *Arch Med Res* 2003; **34**: 600–6.

7. Barry, F. P., and Murphy, J. M. Mesenchymal stem cells: clinical applications and biological characterization. *Int J Biochem Cell Biol* 2004; **36**: 568–84.

8. Horwitz, E. M., Gordon, P. L., Koo, W. K. K. *et al.* Isolated allogeneic bone marrow-derived mesenchymal cells engraft and stimulate growth in children with osteogenesis imperfecta: implications for cell therapy of bone. *Proc Natl Acad Sci U S A* 2002; **99**: 8932–7.

9. Petite, H., Viateau, V., Bensaid, W. *et al.* Tissue-engineered bone regeneration. *Nat Biotechnol* 2000; **18**: 959–63.

10. Quarto, R., Mastrogiacomo, M., Cancedda, R. *et al.* Repair of large bone defects with the use of autologous bone marrow stromal cells. *New Engl J Med* 2001; **344**: 385–6.

11. Stamm, C., Westphal, B., Kleine, H. D. *et al.* Autologous bone-marrow stem-cell transplantation for myocardial regeneration. *Lancet* 2003; **361**: 45–6.

12. Stamm, C., Kleine, H. D., Westphal, B. *et al.* CABG and bone marrow stem cell transplantation after myocardial infarction. *Thorac Cardiovasc Surg* 2004; **52**: 152–8.

13. Tabbara, I. A., Zimmerman, K., Morgan, C., and Nahleh, Z. Allogeneic hematopoietic stem cell transplantation: complications and results. *Arch Int Med* 2002; **162**: 1558–66.

14. Dell'Accio, F., De Bari, C., and Luyten, F. P. Microenvironment and phenotypic stability specify tissue formation by human articular cartilage-derived cells in vivo. *Exp Cell Res* 2003; **287**: 16–27.

15. Barbero, A., Ploegert, S., Heberer, M., and Martin, I. Plasticity of clonal populations of dedifferentiated adult human articular chondrocytes. *Arthritis Rheum* 2003; **48**: 1315–25.

16. Tallheden, T., Dennis, J. E., Lennon, D. P., Sjogren-Jansson, E., Caplan, A. I., and Lindahl, A. Phenotypic plasticity of human articular chondrocytes. *J Bone Joint Surg Am* 2003; **85A**: 93–100.

17. Dowthwaite, G. P., Bishop, J. C., Redman, S. N. *et al.* The surface of articular cartilage contains a progenitor cell population. *J Cell Sci* 2004; **117**: 889–97.

18. Wickham, M. Q., Erickson, G. R., Gimble, J. M., Vail, T.P., and Guilak, F. Multipotent stromal cells derived from the infrapatellar fat pad of the knee. *Clin Orthop Relat Res* 2003; **412**: 196–212.

19. De Bari, C., Dell'Accio, F., Tylzanowski, P., and Luyten, F. P. Multipotent mesenchymal stem cells from adult human synovial membrane. *Arthritis Rheum* 2001; **44**: 1928–42.

20. Luyten, F. P. Mesenchymal stem cells in osteoarthritis. *Curr Opin Rheumatol* 2004; **16**: 599–603.

21. Lories, R. J. U., and Luyten, F. P. Bone Morphogenetic Protein signaling in joint homeostasis and disease. *Cytokine Growth Factor Rev* 2005; **16**: 287–98.

22. Majumdar, M. K., Keane-Moore, M., Buyaner, D. *et al.* Characterization and functionality of cell surface molecules on human mesenchymal stem cells. *J Biomed Sci* 2003; **10**: 228–41.

23. De La Fuente, R., Abad, J. L., Garcia-Castro, J. *et al.* Dedifferentiated adult articular chondrocytes: a population of human multipotent primitive cells. *Exp Cell Res* 2004; **297**: 313–28.

24. Fickert, S., Fiedler, J., and Brenner, R. E. Identification, quantification and isolation of mesenchymal progenitor cells from osteoarthritic synovium by fluorescence automated cell sorting. *Osteoarthritis and Cartilage* 2003; **11**: 790–800.

25. Baksh, D., Song, L., and Tuan, R. S. Adult mesenchymal stem cells: characterization, differentiation, and application in cell and gene therapy. *J Cell Mol Med* 2004; **8**: 301–16.

26. Firestein, G. S. Invasive fibroblast-like synoviocytes in rheumatoid arthritis: passive responders or transformed aggressors? *Arthritis Rheum* 1996; **39**: 1781–90.

27. Neumann, E., Gay, R. E., Gay, S., and Muller-Ladner, U. Functional genomics of fibroblasts. *Curr Opin Rheumatol* 2004; **16**: 238–45.

28. Nishimura, K., Solchaga, L.A., Caplan, A.I., Yoo, J.U., Goldberg, V. M., and Johnstone, B. B. Chrondroprogenitor cells of synovial tissue. *Arthritis Rheum* 1999; **42**: 2631–7.

29. Zvaifler, N. J., Tsai, V., Alsalameh, S., vonKempis, J., Firestein, G.S., and Lotz, M. Pannocytes: distinctive cells found in rheumatoid arthritis articular cartilage erosions. *Am J Pathol* 1997; **150**: 1125–38.

30. Imamura, F., Aono, H., and Hasunuma, T. *et al.* Monoclonal expansion of synoviocytes in rheumatoid arthritis. *Arthritis Rheum* 1998; **41**: 1979–86.

31. Jones, E. A., English, A., Henshaw, K. *et al.* Enumeration and phenotypic characterization of synovial fluid multipotential mesenchymal progenitor cells in inflammatory and degenerative arthritis. *Arthritis Rheum* 2004; **50**: 817–27.

32. Kasperkovitz, P. V., Timmer, T. C., Smeets, T. J. *et al.* Fibroblast-like synoviocytes derived from patients with rheumatoid arthritis show the imprint of synovial tissue heterogeneity: evidence a link between an increased myofibroblast-like phenotype and high-inflammation synovitis. *Arthritis Rheum* 2005; **52**: 430–41.

33. Marinova-Mutafchieva, L., Taylor, P., Funa, K., Maini, R. N., and Zvaifler, N. J. Mesenchymal cells expressing bone morphogenetic protein receptors are present in the rheumatoid arthritis joint. *Arthritis Rheum* 2000; **43**: 2046–55.

34. Kuznetsov, S. A., Mankani, M. H., Gronthos, S., Satomura, K., Bianco, P., and Robey, P. G. Circulating skeletal stem cells. *J Cell Biol* 2001; **153**: 1133–9.

35. Vandenabeele, F., De Bari, C., Moreels, M. *et al.* Morphological and immunocytochemical characterization of cultured fibroblast-like cells derived from adult human synovial membrane. *Arch Histol Cytol* 2003; **66**: 145–53.

36. Doherty, M. J., Ashton, B. A., Walsh, S., Beresford, J. N., Grant, M. E., and Canfield, A. E. Vascular pericytes express osteogenic potential in vitro and in vivo. *J Bone Miner Res* 1998; **13**: 828–38.

37. Bou-Gharios, G., Ponticos, M., Rajkumar, V., and Abraham, D. Extra-cellular matrix in vascular networks. *Cell Prolif* 2004; **37**: 207–20.

38. Ruger, B., Giurea, A., Wanivenhaus, A. H. *et al.* Endothelial precursor cells in the synovial tissue of patients with rheumatoid arthritis and osteoarthritis. *Arthritis Rheum* 2004; **50**: 2157–66.

39. Iwano, M., Plieth, D., Danoff, T. M., Xue, C., Okada, H., and Neilson, E. G. Evidence that fibroblasts derive from epithelium during tissue fibrosis. *J Clin Invest* 2002; **110**: 341–50.

40. Marinova-Mutafchieva, L., Williams, R. O., Funa, K., Maini, R. N., and Zvaifler, N. J. Inflammation is preceded by tumor necrosis factor-dependent infiltration of mesenchymal cells in experimental arthritis. *Arthritis Rheum* 2002; **46**: 507–13.

41. Corr, M., and Zvaifler, N. J. Mesenchymal precursor cells. *Ann Rheum Dis* 2002; **61**: 3–5.

42. Lories, R. J. U., Derese, I., De Bari, C., and Luyten, F. P. In vitro growth rate of fibroblast-like synovial cells is reduced by methotrexate treatment. *Ann Rheum Dis* 2003; **62**: 568–71.

43. Valencia, X., He, L. S., Illei, G., and Lipsky, P. E. CD4+CD25+T regulatory cells in autoimmune diseases. *FASEB J* 2004; **18**: A832.

44. Theise, N. D., Badve, S., Saxena, R. *et al.* Derivation of hepatocytes from bone marrow cells in mice after radiation-induced myeloablation. *Hepatology* 2000; **31**: 235–40.

45. MacKenzie, T. C., and Flake, A. W. Human mesenchymal stem cells persist, demonstrate site-specific multipotential differentiation, and are present in sites of wound healing and tissue regeneration after transplantation into fetal sheep. *Blood Cell Mol Dis* 2001; **27**: 601–4.

46. De Bari, C., Dell'Accio, F., Vandenabeele, F., Vermeesch, J. R., Raymackers, J. M., and Luyten, F. P. Skeletal muscle repair by adult human mesenchymal stem cells from synovial membrane. *J Cell Biol* 2003; **160**: 909–18.

47. Gussoni, E., Soneoka, Y., Strickland, C. D. *et al.* Dystrophin expression in the mdx mouse restored by stem cell transplantation. *Nature* 1999; **401**: 390–4.

48. Orlic, D., Kajstura, J., Chimenti, S. *et al.* Bone marrow cells regenerate infarcted myocardium. *Nature* 2001; **410**: 701–5.

49. Jackson, K. A., Majka, S. M., Wang, H. Y. *et al.* Regeneration of ischemic cardiac muscle and vascular endothelium by adult hematopoietic stem cells. *Circulation* 2001; **104**: 289.

50. Bittira, B., Shum-Tim, D., Al Khaldi, A., and Chiu, R. C. J. Mobilization and homing of bone marrow stromal cells in myocardial infarction. *Eur J Cardiothorac Surg* 2003; **24**: 393–8.

51. Wu, G. D., Nolta, J. A., Jin, Y. S. *et al.* Migration of mesenchymal stem cells to heart allografts during chronic rejection. *Transplantation* 2003; **75**: 679–85.

52. Ortiz, L. A., Gambelli, F., McBride, C. *et al.* Mesenchymal stem cell engraftment in lung is enhanced in response to bleomycin exposure and ameliorates its fibrotic effects. *Proc Natl Acad Sci U S A* 2003; **100**: 8407–11.

53. Tang, Y. L., Zhao, Q., Zhang, Y. C. *et al.* Autologous mesenchymal stem cell transplantation induce VEGF and neovascularization in ischemic myocardium. *Regul Pept* 2004; **117**: 3–10.

54. Hatch, H. M., Zheng, D., Jorgensen, M. L., and Petersen, B. E. SDF-1alpha/CXCR4: a mechanism for hepatic oval cell activation and bone marrow stem cell recruitment to the injured liver of rats. *Cloning Stem Cells* 2002; **4**: 339–51.

55. Deans, R. J., and Moseley, A. B. Mesenchymal stem cells: biology and potential clinical uses. *Expl Hematol* 2000; **28**: 875–84.

56. Sen, M., Lauterbach, K., El Gabalawy, H., Firestein, G. S., Corr, M., and Carson, D. A. Expression and function of wingless and frizzled homologs in rheumatoid arthritis. *Proc Natl Acad Sci U S A* 2000; **97**: 2791–6.

57. Sen, M., Chamorro, M., Reifert, J., Corr, M., and Carson, D. A. Blockade of Wnt-5A/Frizzled 5 signaling inhibits rheumatoid synoviocyte activation. *Arthritis Rheum* 2001; **44**: 772–81.

58. Lories, R. J. U., Derese, I., Ceuppens, J. L., and Luyten, F. P. Bone morphogenetic proteins 2 and 6, expressed in arthritic synovium, are regulated by proinflammatory cytokines and differentially modulate fibroblast-like synoviocyte apoptosis. *Arthritis Rheum* 2003; **48**: 2807–18.

59. Oreffo, R. O., Bord, S., and Triffitt, J. T. Skeletal progenitor cells and ageing human populations. *Clin Sci (Lond)* 1998; **94**: 549–55.

60. Majors, A. K., Boehm, C. A., Nitto, H., Midura, R. J., and Muschler, G. F. Characterization of human bone marrow stromal cells with respect to osteoblastic differentiation. *J Orthop Res* 1997; **15**: 546–57.

61. Quarto, R., Thomas, D., and Liang, C. T. Bone progenitor cell deficits and the age-associated decline in bone repair capacity. *Calcif Tissue Int* 1995; **56**: 123–9.

62. Rodriguez, J. P., Garat, S., Gajardo, H., Pino, A. M., and Seitz, G. Abnormal osteogenesis in osteoporotic patients is reflected by altered mesenchymal stem cells dynamics. *J Cell Biochem* 1999; **75**: 414–23.

63. Oreffo, R. O. C., Bennett, A., Carr, A. J., and Triffitt, J. T. Patients with primary osteoarthritis show no change with ageing in the number of osteogenic precursors. *Scand J Rheumatol* 1998; **27**: 415–24.

64. Murphy, J. M., Dixon, K., Beck, S., Fabian, D., Feldman, A., and Barry, F. Reduced chondrogenic and adipogenic activity of mesenchymal stem cells from patients with advanced osteoarthritis. *Arthritis Rheum* 2002; **46**: 704–13.

65. Le Blanc, K., Tammik, L., Sundberg, B., Haynesworth, S. E., and Ringden, O. Mesenchymal stem cells inhibit and stimulate mixed lymphocyte cultures and mitogenic responses independently of the major histocompatibility complex. *Scand J Immunol* 2003; **57**: 11–20.

66. Di Nicola, M., Carlo-Stella, C., Magni, M. *et al.* Human bone marrow stromal cells suppress T-lymphocyte proliferation induced by cellular or nonspecific mitogenic stimuli. *Blood* 2002; **99**, 3838–43.

67. Potian, J. A., Aviv, H., Ponzio, N. M., Harrison, J. S., and Rameshwar, P. Veto-like activity of mesenchymal stem cells: functional discrimination between cellular responses to alloantigens and recall antigens. *J Immunol* 2003; **171**: 3426–34.

68. Bartholomew, A., Sturgeon, C., Siatskas, M. *et al.* Mesenchymal stem cells suppress lymphocyte proliferation in vitro and prolong skin graft survival in vivo. *Exp Hematol* 2002; **30**: 42–8.

69. Maitra, B., Szekely, E., Gjini, K. *et al.* Human mesenchymal stem cells support unrelated donor hematopoietic stem cells and suppress T-cell activation. *Bone Marrow Transplant* 2004; **33**: 597–604.

70. Lazarus, H., Curtin, P., and Devine, S. Role of mesenchymal stem cells in allogeneic transplantation: early phase 1 clinical results. [Abstract.] *Blood* 2000; **96**: 392.

71. Le Blanc, K., Rasmusson, I., Sundberg, B. *et al.* Treatment of severe acute graft-versus-host disease with third party haploidentical mesenchymal stem cells. *Lancet* 2004; **363**: 1439–41.

72. Grinnemo, K. H., Mansson, A., Dellgren, G. *et al.* Xenoreactivity and engraftment of human mesenchymal stem cells transplanted into infarcted rat myocardium. *J Thorac Cardiovasc Surg* 2004; **127**: 1293–300.

73. Xia, Z., Ye, H., Choong, C. *et al.* Macrophagic response to human mesenchymal stem cell and poly(E-caprolactone) implantation in nonobese diabetic/severe combined immunodeficient mice. *J Biomed Mat Res* 2004; **71A**: 538–48.

74. Zhao, R. C., Chen, L., Ge, W. *et al.* Mesenchymal stem cells inhibit T-lymphocyte proliferation through secreting TGFbeta. *Exp Hematol* 2004; **32**: 72.

75. Aggarwal, S., and Pittenger, M. F. Human mesenchymal stem cells modulate allogeneic immune cell responses. *Blood* 2005; **105**: 1815–22.

76. Kuroiwa, T., Kakishita, E., Hamano, T. *et al.* Hepatocyte growth factor ameliorates acute graft-versus-host disease and promotes hematopoietic function. *J Clin Invest* 2001; **107**: 1365–73.

77. Krampera, M., Glennie, S., Dyson, J. *et al.* Bone marrow mesenchymal stem cells inhibit the response of naive and memory antigen-specific T cells to their cognate peptide. *Blood* 2003; **101**: 3722–9.

78. Cho, H. J., Kim, H. S., Lee, M. M. *et al.* Mobilized endothelial progenitor cells by granulocyte-macrophage colony-stimulating factor accelerate reendothelialization and reduce vascular inflammation after intravascular radiation. *Circulation* 2003; **108**: 2918–25.

79. Rabelink, T. J., de Boer, H. C., de Koning, E. J. P., and van Zonneveld, A. J. Endothelial progenitor cells: more than an inflammatory response? *Arterioscler Thromb Vasc Biol* 2004; **24**: 834–8.

80. Vukicevic, S., Basic, V., Rogic, D. *et al.* Osteogenic protein-1 (Bone morphogenetic protein-7) reduces severity of injury after ischemic acute renal failure in rat. *J Clin Invest* 1998; **102**: 202–14.

81. Zeisberg, M., Hanai, J., Sugimoto, H. *et al.* BMP-7 counteracts TGF-beta 1-induced epithelial-to-mesenchymal transition and reverses chronic renal injury. *Nat Med* 2003; **9**: 964–8.

82. Zeisberg, M., and Kalluri, R. The role of epithelial-to-mesenchymal transition in renal fibrosis. *J Mol Med* 2004; **82**: 175–81.

83. Jorgensen, C., Gordeladze, J., and Noel, D. Tissue engineering through autologous mesenchymal stem cells. *Curr Opin Biotechnol* 2004; **15**: 406–10.

84. Brittberg, M., Lindahl, A., Nilsson, A., Ohlsson, C., Isaksson, O., and Peterson, L. Treatment of deep cartilage defects in the knee with autologous chondrocyte transplantation. *N Engl J Med* 1994; **331**: 889–95.

85. Peterson, L., Minas, T., Brittberg, M., Nilsson, A., Sjogren-Jansson, E., and Lindahl, A. Two-to 9-year outcome after autologous chondrocyte transplantation of the knee. *Clin Orthop Relat Res* 2000; **374**: 212–34.

86. Brittberg, M., Tallheden, T., Sjogren-Jansson, E., Lindahl, A., and Peterson, L. Autologous chondrocytes used for articular cartilage repair: an update. *Clin Orthop Relat Res* 2001; **391** (Suppl.): S337–S348.

87. Bentley, G., Biant, L. C., Carrington, R. W. J. *et al.* A prospective, randomised comparison of autologous chondrocyte implantation versus mosaicplasty for osteochondral defects in the knee. *J Bone Joint Surg Br* 2003; **85B**: 223–30.

88. Knutsen, G., Engebretsen, L., Ludvigsen, T. C. *et al.* Autologous chondrocyte implantation compared with microfracture in the knee: a randomized trial. *J Bone Joint Surg Am* 2004; **86A**: 455–64.

89. Dell'Accio, F., Vanlauwe, J., Bellemans, J., Neys, J., De Bari, C., and Luyten, F. P. Expanded phenotypically stable chondrocytes persist in the repair tissue and contribute to cartilage matrix formation and structural integration in a goat model of autologous chondrocyte implantation. *J Orthop Res* 2003; **21**: 123–31. [Erratum in *J Orthop Res* **21**, 572.]

90. De Bari, C., Dell'Accio, F., and Luyten, F. P. Human periosteum-derived cells maintain phenotypic stability and chondrogenic potential throughout expansion regardless of donor age. *Arthritis Rheum* 2001; **44**: 85–95.

91. Diaz-Romero, J., Gaillard, J. P., Grogan, S. P., Nesic, D., Trub, T., and Mainil-Varlet, P. Immunophenotypic analysis of human articular chondrocytes: changes in surface markers associated

with cell expansion in monolayer culture. *J Cell Physiol* **202**: 731–42.

92. De Bari, C., Dell'Accio, F., and Luyten, F. P. Failure of in vitro-differentiated mesenchymal stem cells from the synovial membrane to form ectopic stable cartilage in vivo. *Arthritis Rheum* 2004; **50**: 142–50.

93. Seto, H., Kamekura, S., Miura, T. *et al.* Distinct roles of Smad pathways and p38 pathways in cartilage-specific gene expression in synovial fibroblasts. *J Clin Invest* 2004; **113**: 718–26.

94. Rountree, R. B., Schoor, M., Chen, H. *et al.* BMP receptor signaling is required for postnatal maintenance of articular cartilage. *PLoS Biol* 2004; **2**: 1815–27.

95. Murphy, J. M., Fink, D. J., Hunziker, E. B., and Barry, F. P. Stem cell therapy in a caprine model of osteoarthritis. *Arthritis Rheum* 2003; **48**: 3464–74.

96. Evans, C. H., Ghivizzani, S. C., Smith, P., Shuler, F. D., Mi, Z., and Robbins, P. D. Using gene therapy to protect and restore cartilage. *Clin Orthop Rel Res* 2000; **379** (Suppl.): S214–S219.

97. Jorgensen, C., Djouad, F., Apparailly, F., and Noel, D. Engineering mesenchymal stem cells for immunotherapy. *Gene Therapy* 2003; **10**: 928–31.

98. Gafni, Y., Turgeman, G., Liebergal, M., Pelled, G., Gazit, Z., and Gazit, D. Stem cells as vehicles for orthopedic gene therapy. *Gene Therapy* 2004; **11**: 417–26.

99. Devine, S. M., Bartholomew, A. M., Mahmud, N. *et al.* Mesenchymal stem cells are capable of homing to the bone marrow of non-human primates following systemic infusion. *Exp Hematol* 2001; **29**: 244–55.

100. Allay, J. A., Dennis, J. E., Haynesworth, S. E. *et al.* LacZ and interleukin-3 expression in vivo after retroviral transduction of marrow-derived human osteogenic mesenchymal progenitors. *Hum Gene Ther* 1997; **8**: 1417–27.

101. Liu, W., Avent, N. D., Jones, J.W., Scott, M. L., and Voak, D. Molecular configuration of Rh D epitopes as defined by site-directed mutagenesis and expression of mutant Rh constructs in K562 erythroleukemia cells. *Blood* 1999; **94**: 3986–96.

102. Van Damme, A., Chuah, M. K. L., Dell'Accio, F. *et al.* Bone marrow mesenchymal cells for haemophilia A gene therapy using retroviral vectors with modified long-terminal repeats. *Haemophilia* 2003; **9**: 94–103.

103. Gelse, K., von der Mark, K., Aigner, T., Park, J., and Schneider, H. Articular cartilage repair by gene therapy using growth factor-producing mesenchymal cells. *Arthritis Rheum* 2003; **48**: 430–41.

104. Grande, D. A., Mason, J., Light, E., and Dines, D. Stem cells as platforms for delivery of genes to enhance cartilage repair. *J Bone Joint Surg Am* 2003; **85A**: 111–6.

105. Spees, J. L., Olson, S. D., Ylostalo, J. *et al.* Differentiation, cell fusion, and nuclear fusion during ex vivo repair of epithelium by human adult stem cells from bone marrow stroma. *Proc Natl Acad Sci U S A* 2003; **100**: 2397–402.

106. Djouad, F., Plence, P., Bony, C. *et al.* Immunosuppressive effect of mesenchymal stem cells favors tumor growth in allogeneic animals. *Blood* 2003; **102**: 3837–44.

107. Houghton, J., Stoicov, C., Nomura, S. *et al.* Gastric cancer originating from bone marrow-derived cells. *Science* 2004; **306**: 1568–71.

108. Luyten, F. P. A scientific basis for the biologic regeneration of synovial joints. *Oral Surg Oral Med Oral Pathol Oral Radiol Endod* 1997; **83**: 167–9.

109. Buckley, C. D., Pilling, D., Lord, J. M., Akbar, A. N., Scheel-Toellner, D., and Salmon, M. Fibroblasts regulate the switch from acute resolving to chronic persistent inflammation. *Trends Immunol* 2001; **22**: 199–204.

110. Parsonage, G., Filer, A. D., Haworth, O. *et al.* A stromal address code defined by fibroblasts. *Trends Immunol* 2005; **26**: 150–6.

111. Reines, B.P. Is rheumatoid arthritis premature osteoarthritis with fetal-like healing? *Autoimmunity Rev* 2004; **3**: 305–11.

Index

Note: Page numbers in *italic* refer to figures and/or tables.